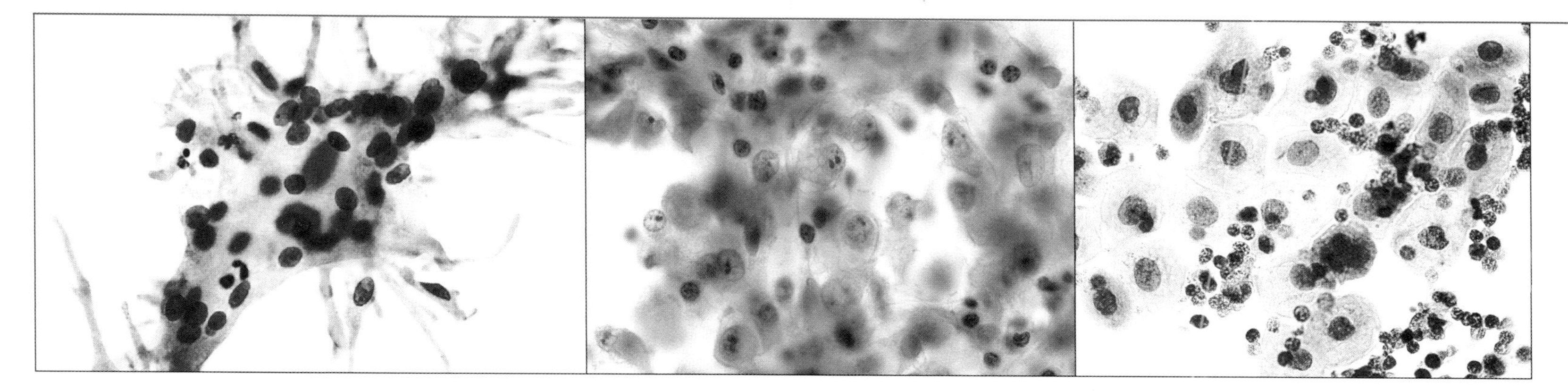

Diagnostic Atlas of Genitourinary Pathology

EDITED BY

Myron Tannenbaum MD PhD
Pathology and Laboratory Medicine Services (113)
Bay Pines VA Medical Center
Bay Pines, FL
Professor of Pathology and Surgery (Urology)
University of South Florida School of Medicine Tampa, FL
USA

John F. Madden MD PhD
Associate Professor
Department of Pathology
Duke University Medical Center
Durham, NC
USA

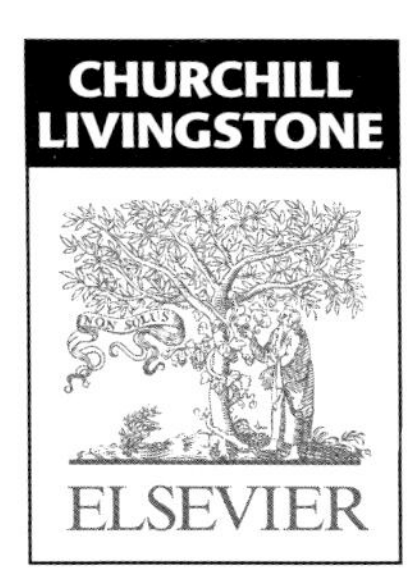
CHURCHILL LIVINGSTONE
ELSEVIER

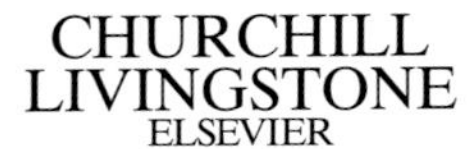

First published 2006

EAN: 9780443071300
ISBN: 0443071306

British Library Cataloguing in Publication Data
A catalogue record for this book is available from the British Library

Library of Congress Cataloging in Publication Data
A catalog record for this book is available from the Library of Congress

Notice
Medical knowledge is constantly changing. Standard safety precautions must be followed, but as new research and clinical experience broaden our knowledge, changes in treatment and drug therapy may become necessary or appropriate. Readers are advised to check the most current product information provided by the manufacturer of each drug to be administered to verify the recommended dose, the method and duration of administration, and contraindications. It is the responsibility of the practitioner, relying on experience and knowledge of the patient, to determine dosages and the best treatment for each individual patient. Neither the Publisher nor the author assume any liability for any injury and/or damage to persons or property arising from this publication.
The Publisher

Printed in China
Last digit is the print number: 9 8 7 6 5 4 3 2 1

Contents

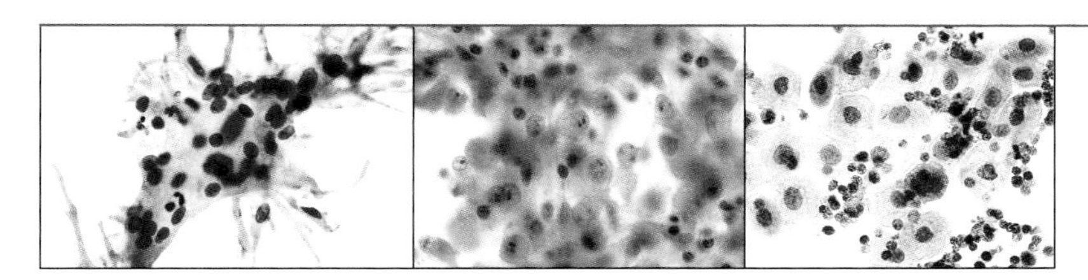

Diagnostic Atlas of

Genitourinary Pathology

Commissioning Editor: Michael Houston
Project Development Manager: Tim Kimber
Project Manager: Jess Thompson
Illustration Manager: Mick Ruddy
Design Manager: Erik Bigland
Marketing Manager(s): Ethel Cathers, Sarah Rogers

List of Contributors

Mahul B. Amin MD
Director of Surgical Pathology
Department of Pathology
Emory University Hospital
Atlanta, GA
USA

Ricardo H. Bardales MD
Director Cytology Laboratory
Hennepin County Medical Center
Associate Professor of Pathology
University of Minnesota School of Medicine
Minneapolis, MN
USA

James L. Burchette HT(ASCP) QIHC
Department of Pathology
Duke University Medical Center
Durham, NC
USA

April Chiu MD
Assistant Professor
Department of Pathology and Lab Medicine
Weill Medical College of Cornell University
New York, NY
USA

Antonio L. Cubilla MD
Professor of Pathology
Facultat de Ciencias Medicas
Instituto de Pathología e Investigación
Asunción
Paraguay

Scott Ely MD MPH
Associate Professor of Pathology
Department of Pathology
Weill Medical College of Cornell University
New York, NY
USA

Iqbal Kapadia MD
Pathologist
Pathology Department
Mercy Medical Center – Des Moines
Des Moines, IA
USA

Ruth L. Katz MD
Department of Cytopathology
MD Anderson Cancer Center
Houston, TX
USA

John F. Madden MD
Associate Professor
Department of Pathology
Duke University Medical Center
Durham, NC
USA

John Maksem MD
Department of Pathology
Mercy Hospital
Des Moines, IA
USA

Peter L. McEvoy MD
Chief
Division of Infectious and Tropical Disease Pathology
Environmental and Infectious Disease Sciences Department
Armed Forces Institute of Pathology
Washington, DC
USA

Michael B. Morgan MD
Professor of Pathology
Department Laboratory Service
James A Haley Veterans Memorial Hospital
Tampa, FL
USA

Klaus Schreiber MD
Department of Pathology
Montefiore Hospital
Bronx, NY
USA

M. Angelica Selim MD
Department of Pathology
Duke University Medical Center
Durham, NC
USA

Christopher R. Shea MD
Professor of Medicine
University of Chicago
Department of Medicine, Section of Dermatology
Chicago, IL
USA

Maria M. Shevchuk MD
Associate Professor of Pathology
Department of Pathology
Lenox Hill Hospital
New York, NY
USA

Aleksander Talerman MD FRCPath
Peter A. Herbut Professor of Pathology
Department of Pathology
Thomas Jefferson University
Philadelphia, PA
USA

Myron Tannenbaum MD PHD
Pathology and Laboratory Medicine Services (113)
Bay Pines VA Medical Center
Bay Pines, FL
Professor of Pathology and Surgery (Urology)
University of South Florida School of Medicine
Tampa, FL
USA

Satish Tickoo MD
Department of Pathology
Weill Medical School of Cornell University
New York, NY
USA

Elsa F. Velázquez MD
Assistant Professor
Departments of Pathology and Dermatology
NYU Medical Center
New York, NY
USA

Bruce M. Wenig MD
Professor of Pathology
Department of Pathology
Beth Israel Medical Center
New York, NY
USA

Preface

We would like to quote portions of letters that we routinely receive from our colleagues, "A lot of times, or at least it seems to me that way, when we have seen borderline lesions in the prostate, and urinary bladder, we usually pass the slides around to all of our pathologists before we come up with an answer that reassures us all. I don't know whether it is the lack of fine morphology or just the inexperience of picking up early lesions, but I certainly personally do not feel as confident about making a diagnosis in urologic pathology, especially with prostate and urinary bladder, as I would about cervical, endometrial, or breast lesions." Not only has this felling been expressed by many other pathologists throughout the country but we have especially encountered it during our years of teaching.

A diagnostic atlas in Urologic Pathology was conceived with the expectation of bridging the communication gap that exists between the general practitioner of urology and the surgical pathologist. Perusal of the table of contents demonstrates that the authors, all of whom are experts in their respective fields, have addressed themselves to numerous themes that are pertinent to genitourinary diseases. Special emphasis has been placed on issues that are of utmost importance to the clinician in order that the disease problems relating to tumor and infection may be better understood. Although this approach may inevitably be accompanied by some overlapping, the chapters were chosen because they would be of practical help to the pathologist and urologist whether he or she is in the operating room or reviewing the slides together with other pathologists and urologists. Consequently, this text not only provides information regarding the history and epidemiology of genitourinary disease but also presents information that will show the pathologist in what manner the urologist approaches the surgery of these organs. It is also hoped that those in various disciplines such as biochemistry, radiology, and other basic sciences interested in diseases of the genitourinary system, especially the prostate and urinary bladder will find some illuminating and rewarding pictorial illustrations and information in at least one of the chapters on the various organs that comprise the genitourinary system.

Our interpretation of the problems of genitourinary disease, and the editing of this reference work, is based on a cumulative personal experience and the cumulative teaching from our mentors in surgical pathology. They include the late Dr. Arthur Purdy Stout, Dr. Raffaele Lattes, and Dr. Meyer M. Melicow.

This atlas and text represents the cooperative efforts of numerous other people. They not only have contributed to what is known, but will bring new understanding and insight to the readers. We also want to thank our many other colleagues, which include Drs Stanley Robboy, Roger Zitman, Rahana Nawab, Ted Strickland, T-Y Wang, and John Mason.

In addition, our gratitude is great to those people who have supported the contributing authors. This includes Martino Friedman from Adorama and John Williams at Bay Pines VAMC for digital camera equipment. Dr. Thomas J. Madden for his practical love of pathology. Likewise we wish to express our appreciation to our wives, Sheila and Heidi, to whom we are greatly indebted, not only for their practical help with the chapters, but also for their deep understanding which has sustained us during the writing and editing of this book. To our publishers at Elsevier, we wish to impart our gratefulness for their encouragement, cooperation, and persistence in guiding us through this effort. This includes Michael Houston, Tim Kimber and Jess Thompson.

Myron Tannenbaum MD PhD
John Madden MD PhD

Dedication

To my wife Sheila Carol Tannenbaum
To my wife Heidi Madden and L, D, and L

EPITHELIAL TUMORS OF THE PENIS

Elsa F. Velazquez and Antonio L. Cubilla

NORMAL ANATOMY

The whole penis is divided into three anatomic parts:[1]

- the distal part (head);
- the mid part (body or shaft);
- the proximal part (root).

Most primary epithelial tumors occur in the distal part.

GROSS ANATOMY

(Figs 1.1–1.5)

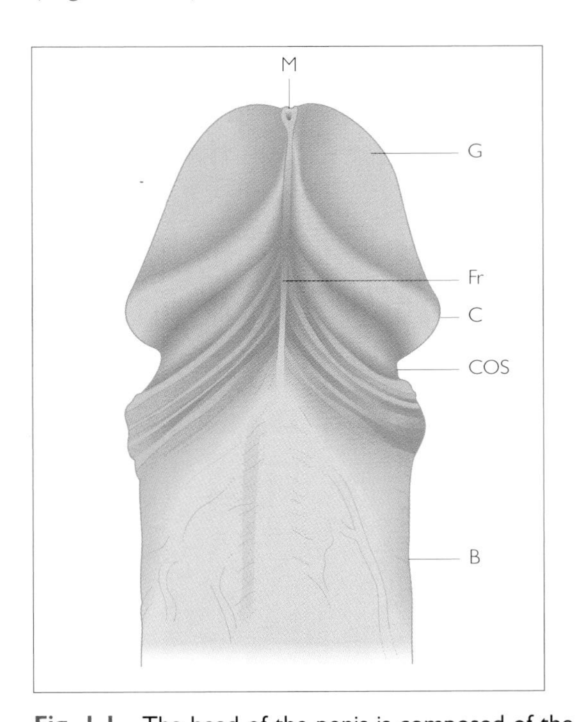

Fig. 1.1 The head of the penis is composed of the glans (G) and the coronal sulcus (COS). Both are encased by the foreskin, the inner surface of which is lined by a smooth membrane. The glans is composed of the meatus (M), frenulum (Fr), and corona (C). The frenulum arises at the ventral meatus and inserts at the attachment of the glans to the foreskin. The glans corona is a circumferential rim at the base of the glans, the widest part of penis. The foreskin covers the external surface of the penis and distally reflects over the preputial orifice.[2] The coronal sulcus (balano-preputial sulcus) is a cul-de-sac located between the glans corona and foreskin. Preputial length is variable. Long foreskins, entirely covering the glans, are associated with phimosis and an increased risk of penile cancer.[3] B, body.

MICROSCOPIC ANATOMY

(Figs 1.6–1.14)

EPITHELIAL ABNORMALITIES AND PRECANCEROUS LESIONS

Of the many epithelial lesions affecting the penile epithelium (see Chapter 2), several are statistically associated with squamous cell carcinoma, and a few are undoubtedly precancerous lesions.[7]

SQUAMOUS HYPERPLASIA

Squamous hyperplasia is acanthotic thickening of the epithelium, equally affecting the glans, coronal sulcus, and

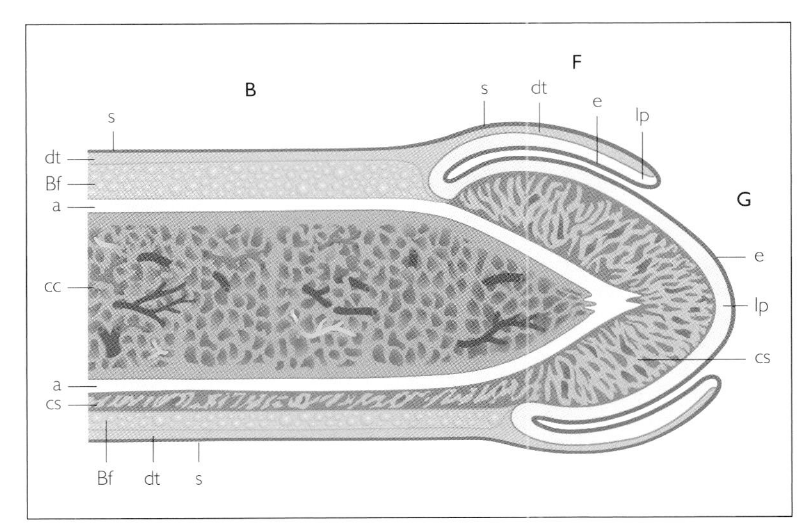

Fig. 1.2 In longitudinal section, the layers of the glans (G) are the squamous epithelium (e), lamina propria (lp), corpus spongiosum (cs), tunica albuginea (a), and corpora cavernosa (cc). The foreskin (F) consists of skin (s), dartos (dt), lamina propria (lp), and squamous epithelium (e). The body (B) consists of skin (s), penile dartos (dt), Buck's fascia (Bf), tunica albuginea (a), and corpora cavernosa (cc).

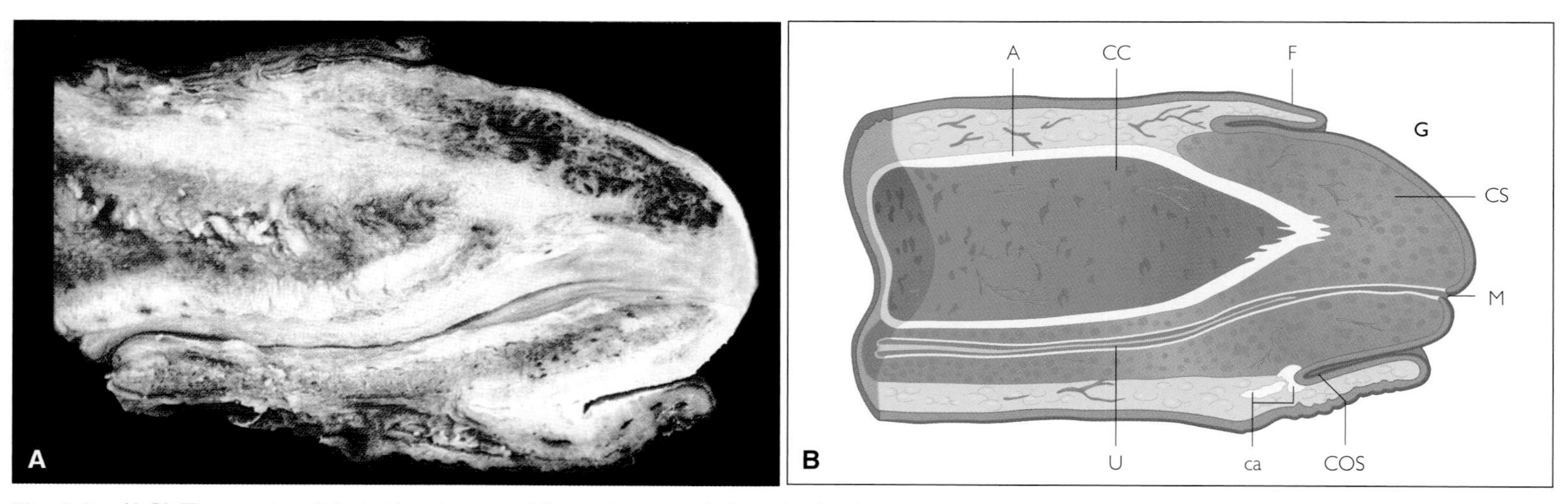

Fig. 1.3 (A,B) The urethra (U) divides the dorsal from the ventral glans. In this image, a small squamous cell carcinoma (ca) is present at the coronal sulcus (COS). A, tunica albuginea; CC, corpus cavernosum; F, foreskin; G, glans; CS, corpus spongiosum; M, meatus.

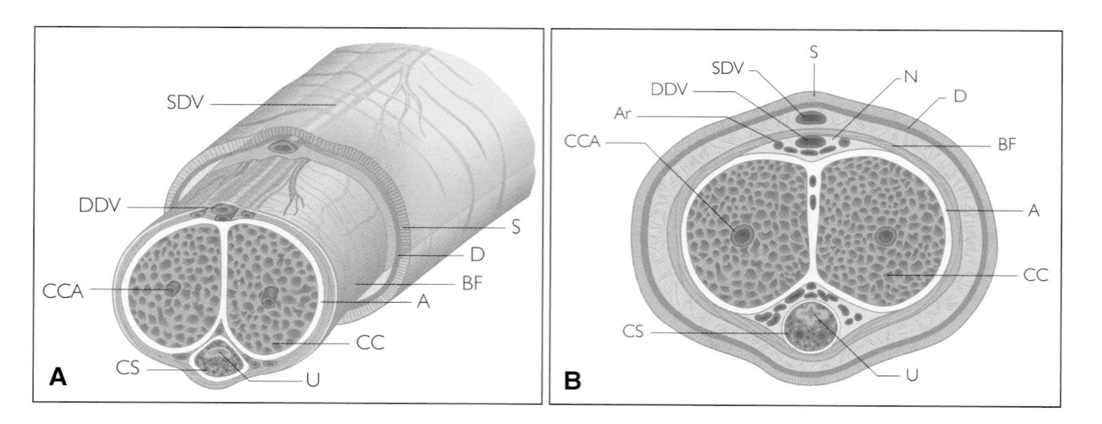

Fig. 1.4 (A,B) The penile urethra is located ventrally and is surrounded by corpus spongiosum. Primary urethral tumors may be confused with penile neoplasms.[4] SDV, superficial dorsal vein; DDV, deep dorsal vein; CCA, cavernous arteries; CS, corpus spongiosum; U, urethra, CC, corpus cavernosum; A, albuginea; BF, Buck's fascia; D, dartos; S, skin; N, nerves; Ar, arteries.

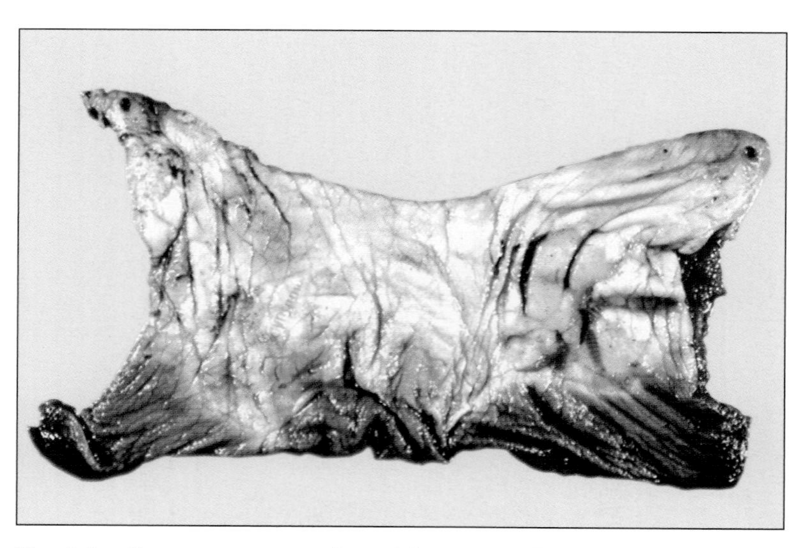

Fig. 1.5 Gross appearance of an adult prepuce. The mucosa is pale beige and slightly irregular. The cutaneous surface (bottom) is darker and more wrinkled.

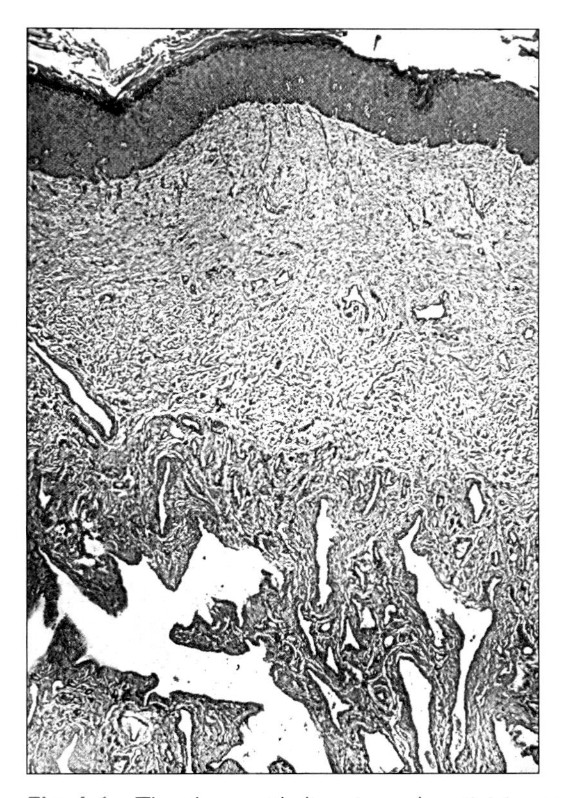

Fig. 1.6 The glans epithelium is nonkeratinizing squamous type, six to ten cell layers thick in uncircumcised patients. The lamina propria is 2–3 mm thick, composed of loose connective tissue with small blood and lymphatic vessels and nerves. Its boundary with the corpus spongiosum is not always sharp.

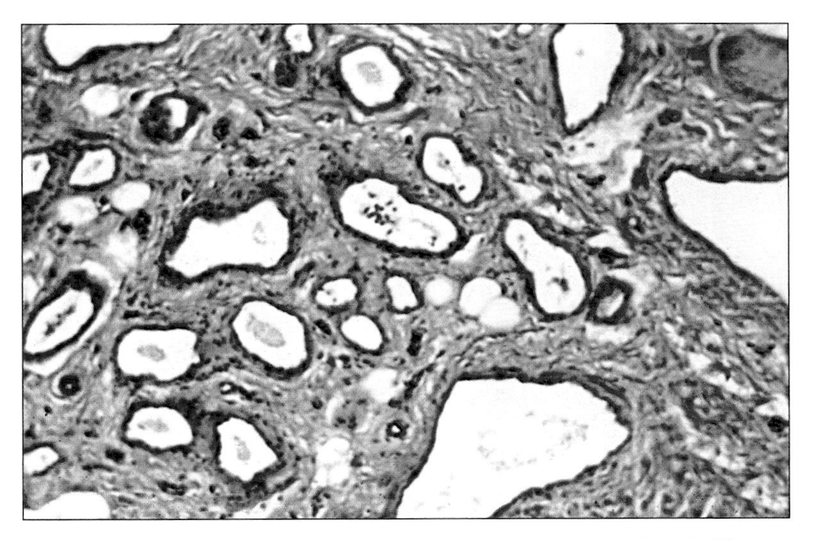

Fig. 1.7 Corpus spongiosum makes up most of the glans. It is 6–13 mm thick and consists of erectile tissue, with characteristic anastomosing venous sinuses. The walls of the corpus spongiosum are composed of thick bundles of smooth muscle. The vascular channels of the corpus spongiosum are thinner, less complex, and are separated by more abundant fibrous tissue than those of the corpora cavernosa.

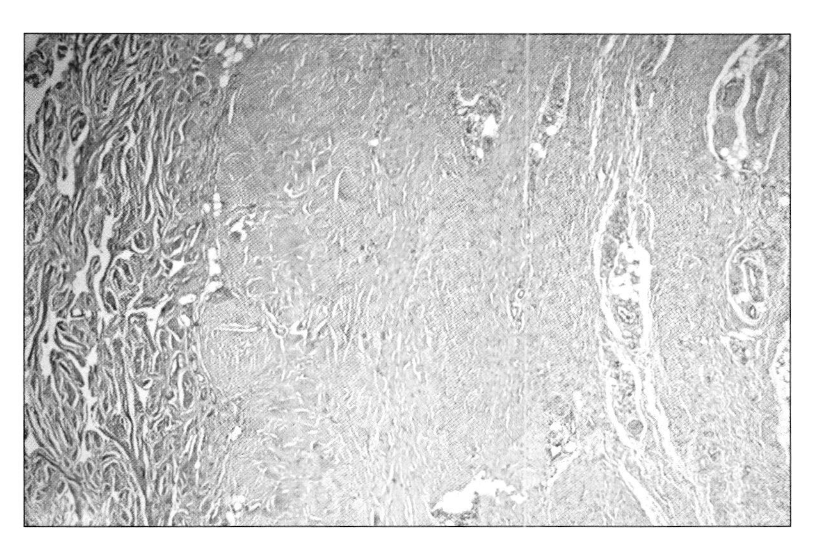

Fig. 1.8 The tunica albuginea (right) is a 2-mm hyaline fibrous band separating the corpus spongiosum (left) from the corpora cavernosa. It is composed of dense, highly collagenized connective tissue. Small nutrient vessels perforate the tunica into the corpora cavernosa, facilitating occasional tumor invasion of the latter. Also, adipose tissue may focally interrupt the tunica, explaining the occasional presence of fat in the corpora cavernosa.

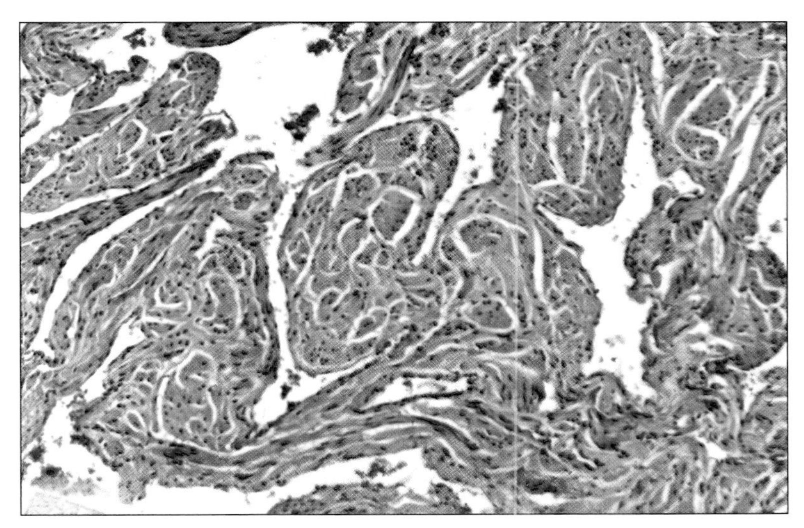

Fig. 1.9 Corpus cavernosum tissue is the main constituent of the shaft, but extends into the glans in more than two-thirds of the specimens.[5] Corpus cavernosum is composed of thick-walled, anastomosing vascular structures with scant fibrous matrix.

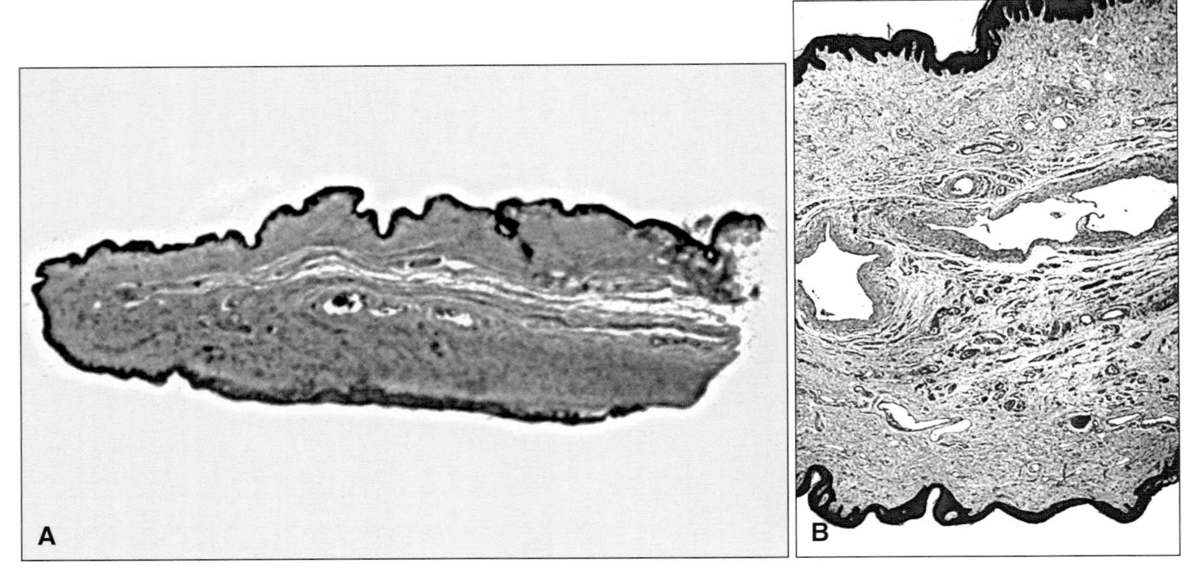

Fig. 1.10 (A,B) The foreskin shows five histologic layers: epidermis, dermis, dartos, lamina propria, and squamous mucosa (from top to bottom in these images).

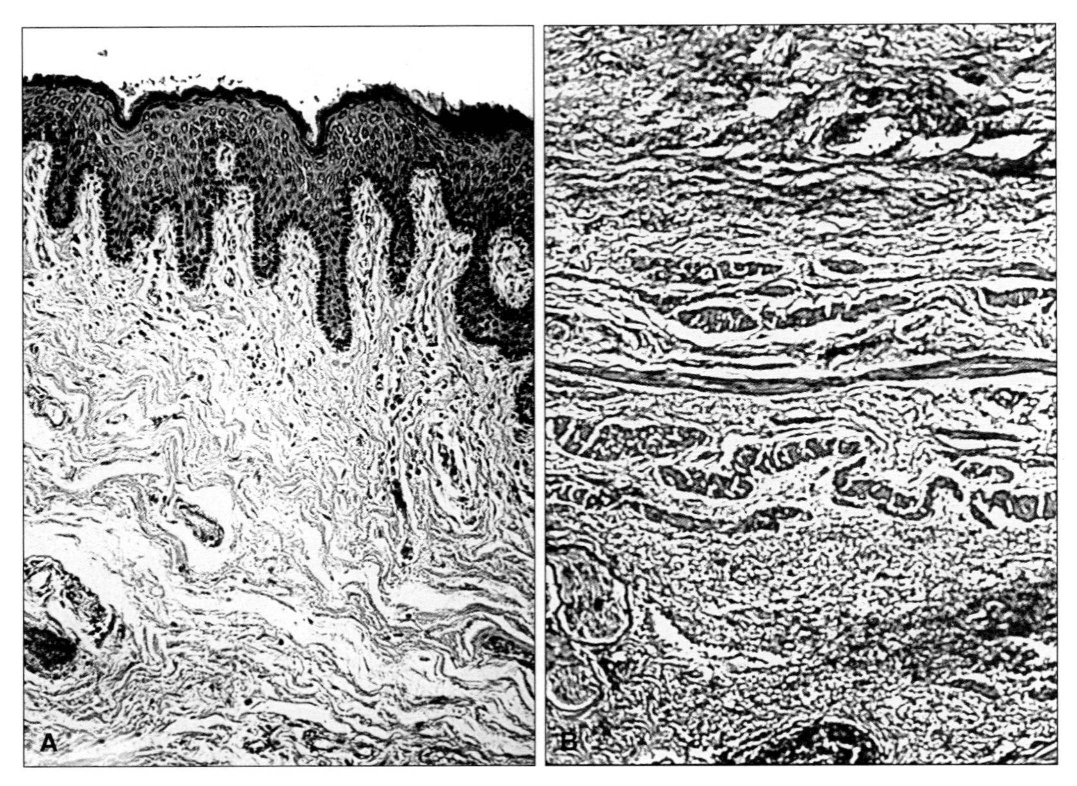

Fig. 1.11 The skin has a wrinkled epidermis and rare adnexal structures. The dartos is a discontinuous layer of smooth muscle, variably arranged in transverse and longitudinal fascicles embedded in a matrix of loose connective tissue with vessels and nerves. The dartos is thicker near the coronal sulcus, as is demonstrated in Fig. 1.2.

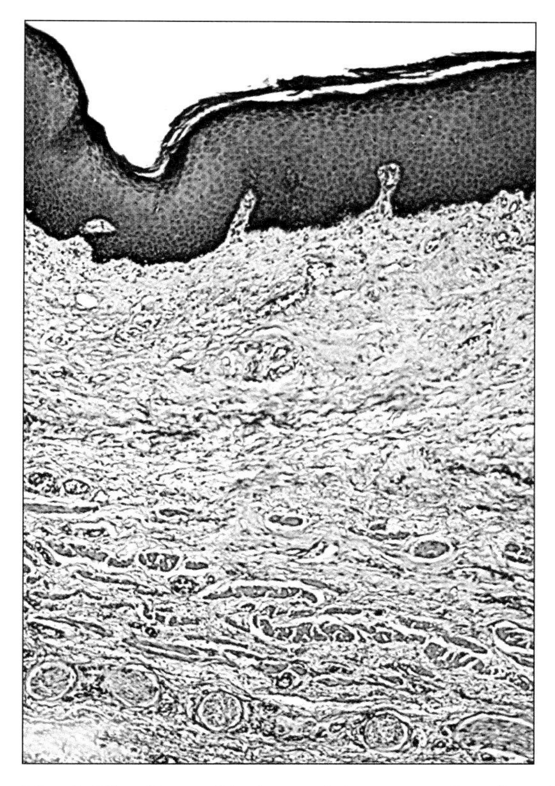

Fig. 1.12 The epithelium of the mucosal surface is normally nonkeratinized. The basal layer is flat and hypopigmented. No skin adnexa are present. The lamina propria is thin. The epithelium may show epithelial hyperplasia and/or hyperkeratosis. Rarely, mucinous metaplastic cells occur with chronic inflammation.[6] The epithelium of the coronal sulcus is similar to that of the glans and foreskin.

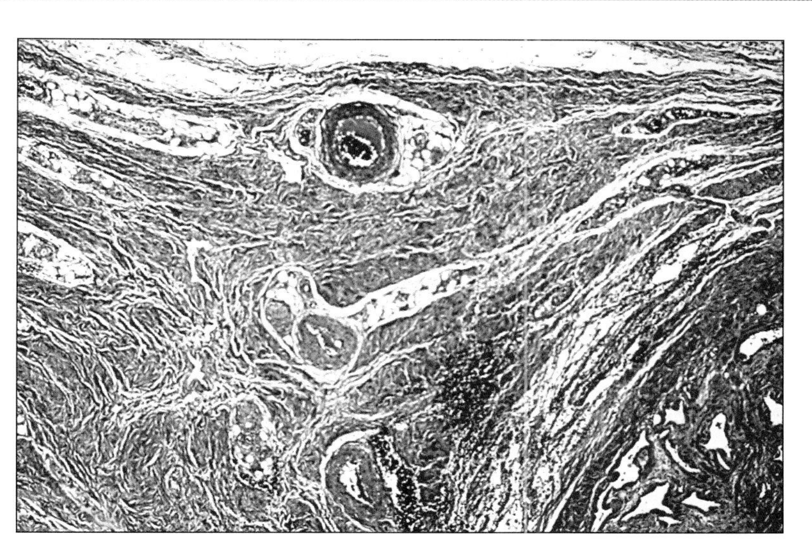

Fig. 1.13 Buck's fascia is located between dartos and albuginea and is a fibroelastic layer containing numerous blood vessels and nerves embedded in a loose connective tissue. It is important because it is a frequent pathway of tumor extension from the glans to the shaft to the resection margin, and from the shaft to the corpus cavernosum through slit-like spaces created by nutritional vessels and fat entering the corpus cavernosum through the albuginea.

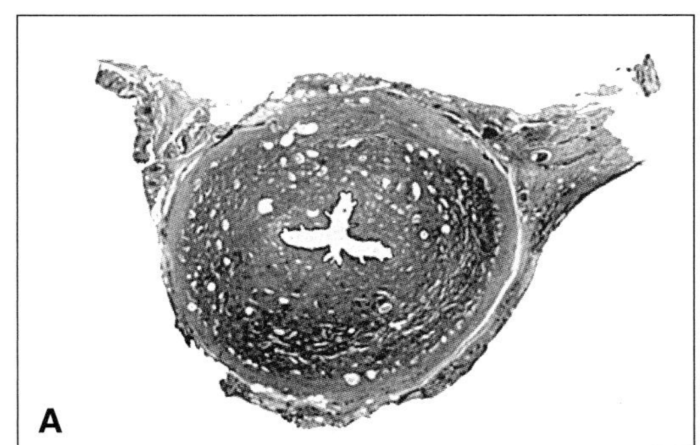

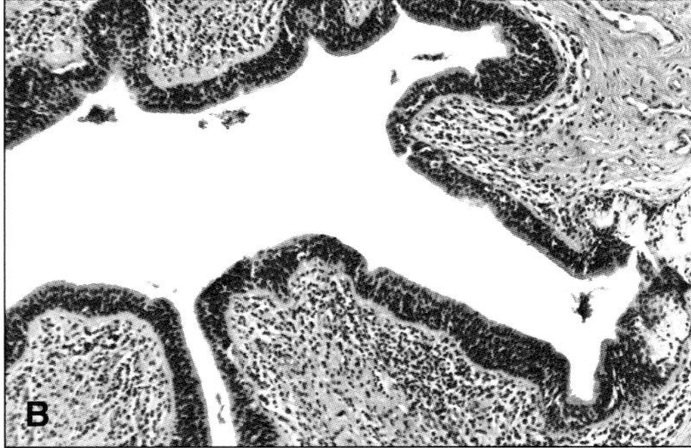

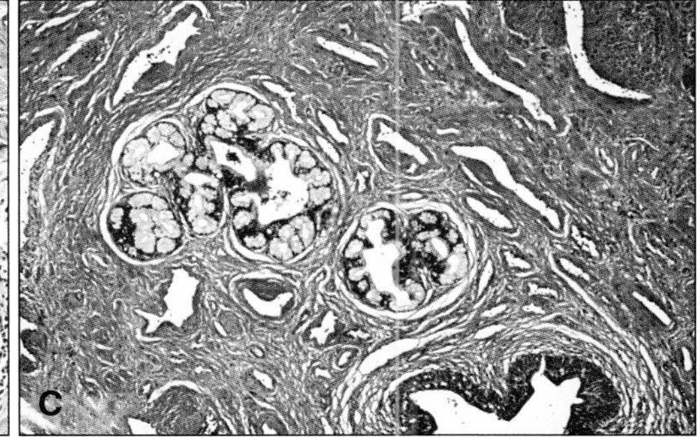

Fig. 1.14 (A) The penile urethra is surrounded by the corpus spongiosum, which forms a cylindrical sheath around it. Note the stellate shape of the lumen in this cross-section. (B) The penile urethra is lined by urothelial mucosa composed variably of transitional, intermediate, columnar, or squamous epithelium. (C) Morgagni´s lacunae are intraepithelial mucinous cells or glands related to adjacent periurethral (Littré) glands.

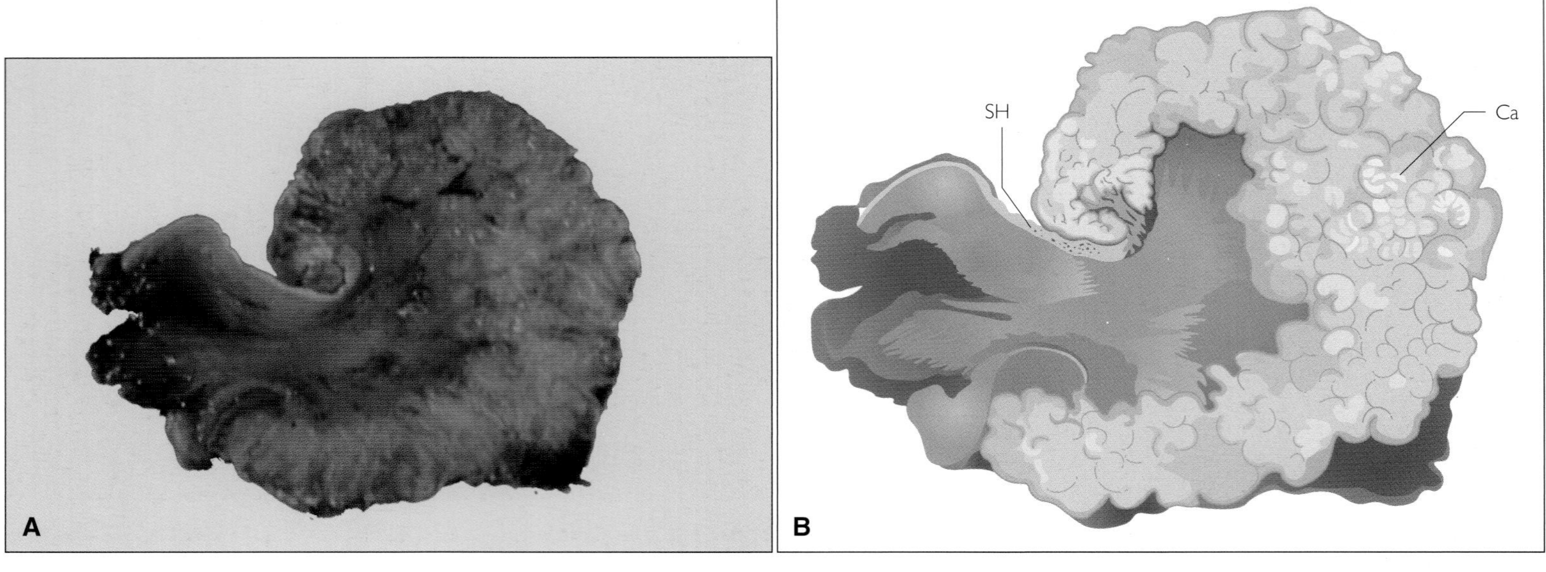

Fig. 1.15 (A) Grossly, squamous hyperplasia appears as a pearly white smooth plaque. (B) In this image, squamous hyperplasia (SH, gray) is present next to an invasive squamous cell carcinoma (Ca).

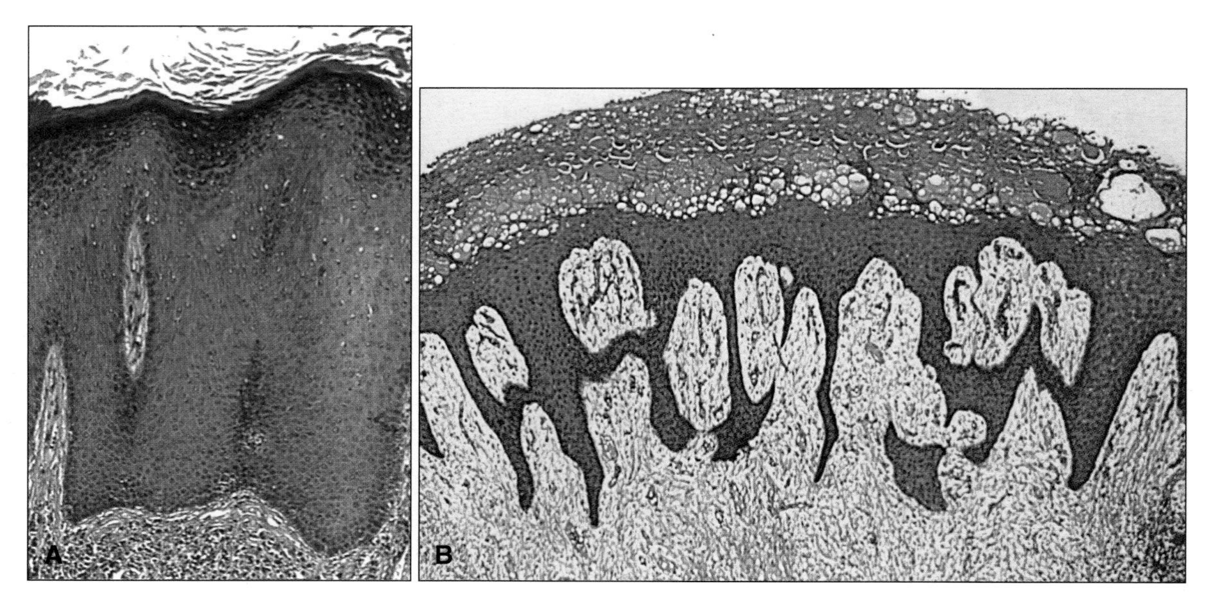

Fig. 1.16 (A) Microscopically, squamous hyperplasia usually presents as a flat-surfaced lesion. Hyper-orthokeratosis is present. Mild elongation of rete ridges (acanthosis) is typical. Cytologic atypia is absent. Squamous hyperplasia variants include pseudoepitheliomatous, verrucous, and papillary types. (B) Pseudoepitheliomatous squamous hyperplasia appears as a flat or slightly elevated lesion with hyperkeratosis. There is exaggerated, irregular acanthosis with sharply pointed, jagged, and irregular rete ridges. The differential diagnosis is well-differentiated squamous carcinoma, but nuclear enlargement, hyperchromasia, and single cell keratinization are minimal or absent.

foreskin mucosa. It is present next to invasive carcinoma in more than two-thirds of cases, and is especially common with verrucous and papillary carcinomas.[8] Coexistent lichen sclerosus is noted in nearly half of the cases. (Figs 1.15 & 1.16)

SQUAMOUS INTRAEPITHELIAL LESION

Squamous intraepithelial lesion (SIL) is plausibly a precursor of invasive carcinoma, with which it is commonly associated. Like carcinoma, SIL is most often seen in the glans,

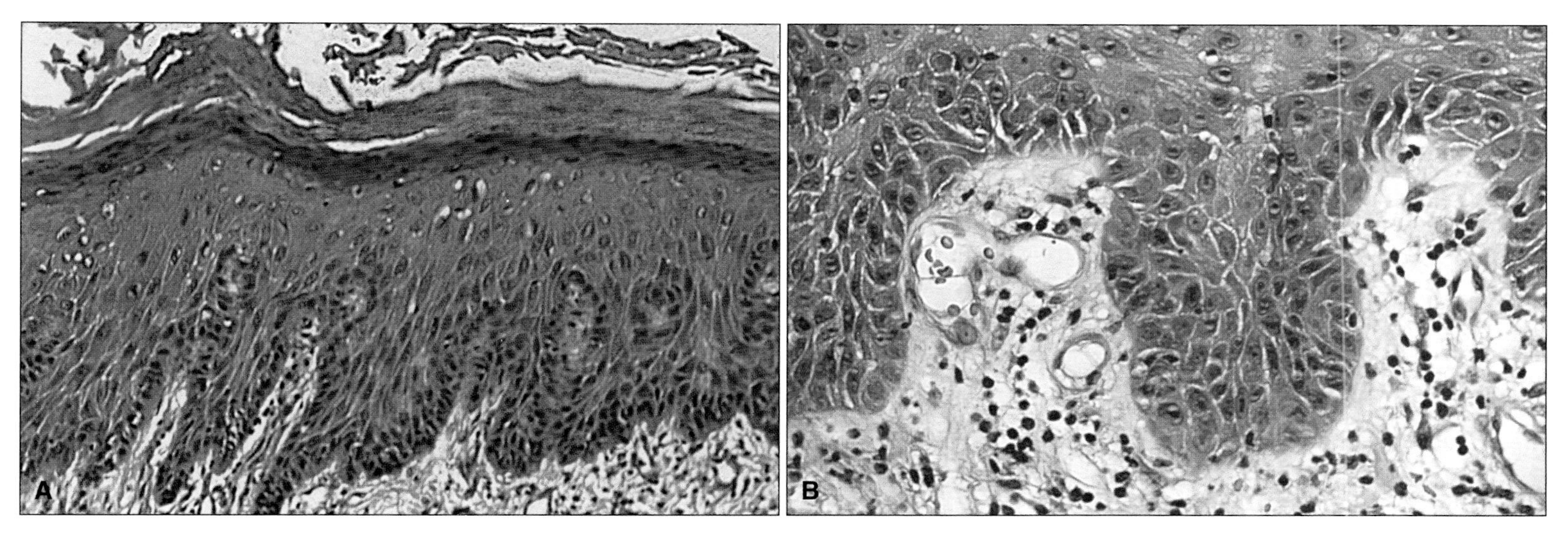

Fig. 1.17 (A,B) Microscopically, a low-grade squamous intraepithelial lesion shows atypical cells restricted to the lower third of epithelium. There is accompanying acanthosis and hyperkeratosis.

coronal sulcus, or foreskin mucosa, and is rare on the outer foreskin or shaft. On the other hand, human papillomavirus (HPV) has been demonstrated more often in SIL than in invasive carcinoma.[9-13] Many synonyms for SIL are in common use: erythroplasia of Queyrat, Bowen's disease, carcinoma in situ, penile intraepithelial neoplasia, and dysplasia.[10,14-22] We prefer the term squamous intraepithelial lesion, and differentiate between low-grade and high-grade lesions. Grossly, SIL appears as a flat or slightly raised plaque, macule, or papule. Typically, the lesion is white, but may be pink, red, dark, or variegated. SIL may present as single or multiple lesions. (Figs 1.17 & 1.18)

BOWENOID PAPULOSIS

Bowenoid papulosis is an unusual and poorly understood HPV-related intraepithelial proliferation affecting the anogenital region of both sexes.[23,24] In the penis, it commonly presents as multicentric papules on the skin of the shaft or the mucous membrane of the head. Bowenoid papulosis affects young patients, the course is indolent, and lesions sometimes spontaneously regress.[25] (Fig. 1.19)

LICHEN SCLEROSUS

Also called lichen sclerosus et atrophicus or balanitis xerotica obliterans, this penile lesion appears similar to its vulvar counterpart.[26-28] The condition affects the glans and foreskin, sometimes producing severe phimosis. It coexists with about 30% of cancers of the glans[29] and about 50–75% of preputial cancers.[30] The association is strongest with verrucous and papillary carcinomas, and weakest with warty or basaloid tumors. These findings suggest that lichen sclerosus may be a precursor condition to at least a subset of penile carcinomas that are unrelated to HPV. Other inflammatory conditions such as lichen planus have also been linked to penile cancer but a causal relationship to cancer is conjectural.[29,31-33] (Fig. 1.20)

GIANT CONDYLOMA

This HPV-related benign tumor occurs at a slightly older age than common condylomas, but at a younger age than carcinoma.[34] (The term 'Buschke–Löwenstein tumor' has been inconsistently applied to several similar lesions, and should not be used.[35,36]) Typically, the lesions have been present for many years at diagnosis. Longstanding giant condylomas may harbor foci of in situ or invasive squamous carcinoma, especially warty or basaloid types.[37] In giant condylomas, atypical cells are restricted to koilocytes in the superficial layers. Clinically, giant condyloma may be difficult to distinguish from warty carcinoma; however, microscopically, giant condyloma lacks high-grade atypia or frank invasion. Differentiation from verrucous carcinoma is straightforward, since the latter lacks koilocytosis and arborescent fronds. (Figs 1.21 & 1.22)

PENILE CARCINOMA

Most penile primary tumors are squamous cell carcinomas and originate in the glans or foreskin, less commonly in the coronal sulcus, and only rarely on the shaft. Carcinomas involving the foreskin are typically well differentiated, less deeply invasive, and associated with a better prognosis.[30] Basal cell or sweat gland carcinomas of the penis are

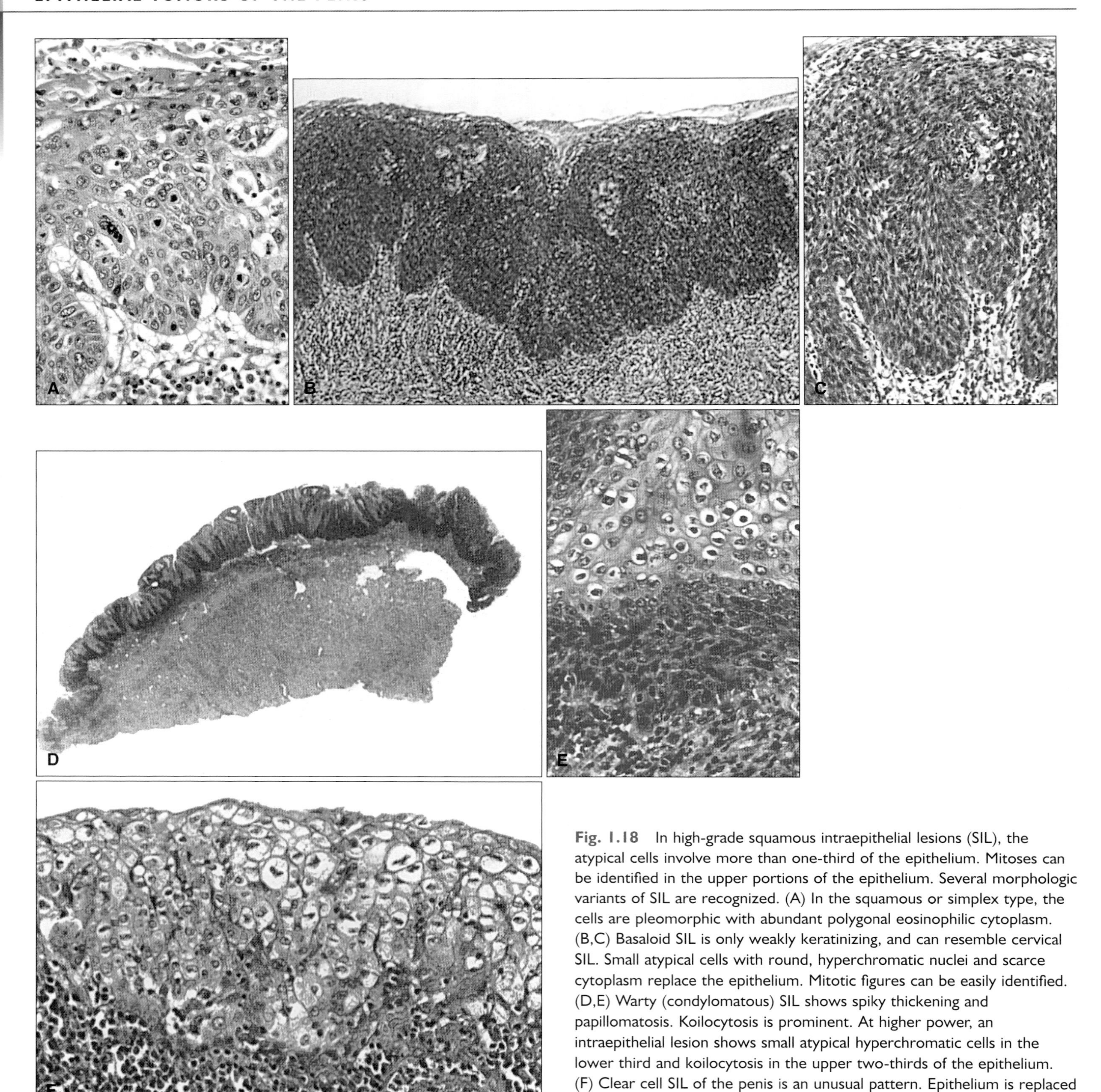

Fig. 1.18 In high-grade squamous intraepithelial lesions (SIL), the atypical cells involve more than one-third of the epithelium. Mitoses can be identified in the upper portions of the epithelium. Several morphologic variants of SIL are recognized. (A) In the squamous or simplex type, the cells are pleomorphic with abundant polygonal eosinophilic cytoplasm. (B,C) Basaloid SIL is only weakly keratinizing, and can resemble cervical SIL. Small atypical cells with round, hyperchromatic nuclei and scarce cytoplasm replace the epithelium. Mitotic figures can be easily identified. (D,E) Warty (condylomatous) SIL shows spiky thickening and papillomatosis. Koilocytosis is prominent. At higher power, an intraepithelial lesion shows small atypical hyperchromatic cells in the lower third and koilocytosis in the upper two-thirds of the epithelium. (F) Clear cell SIL of the penis is an unusual pattern. Epithelium is replaced by atypical squamous cells with clear cytoplasm.

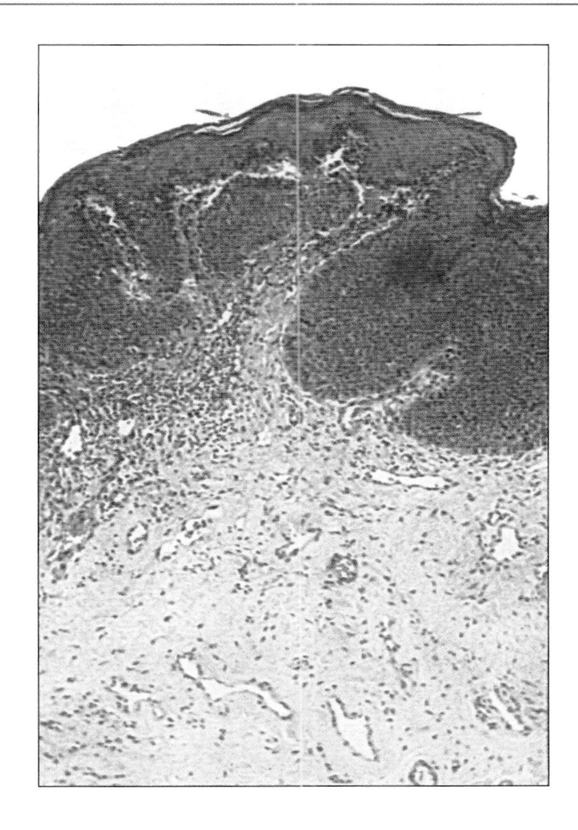

Fig. 1.19 Bowenoid papulosis is characterized by acanthosis and hyperkeratosis, with scattered atypical cells and some HPV-related changes. The microscopic appearance overlaps with that of squamous intraepithelial lesion. Diagnosis requires correlation with the clinical presentation as a multicentric papular eruption.

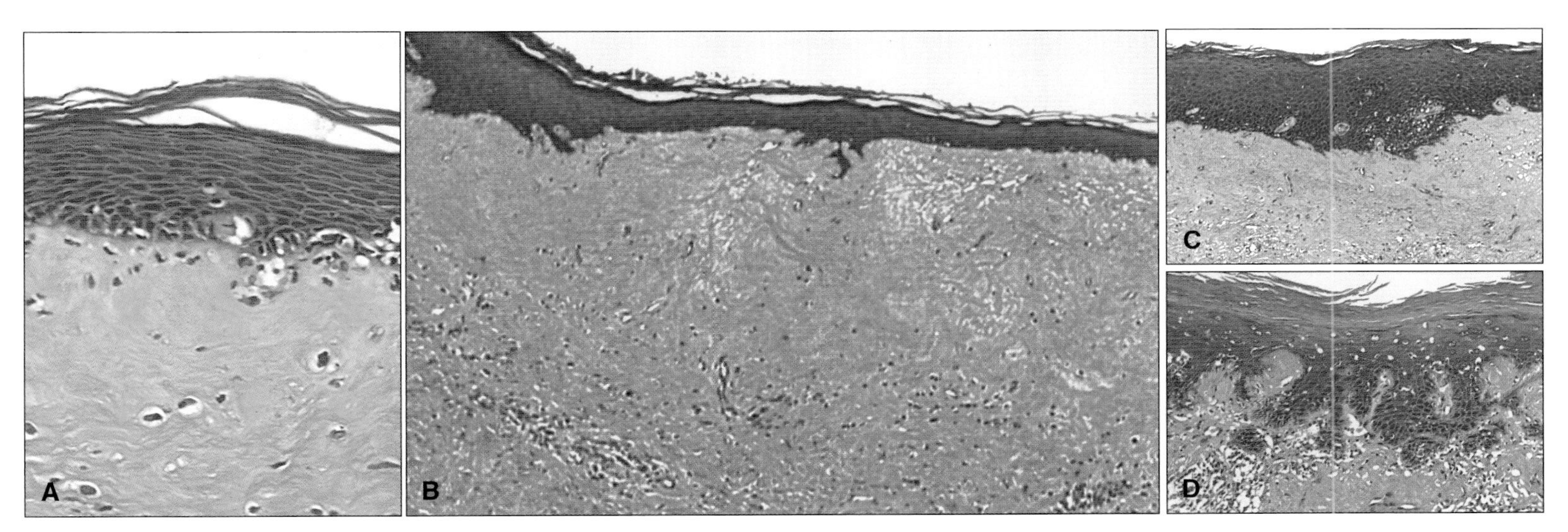

Fig. 1.20 Lichen sclerosus. (A–C) Microscopically, there is hyper-orthokeratosis, mild epithelial atrophy with hydropic degeneration of basal cells and homogenization of the collagen in the upper lamina propria. Lichen sclerosus is occasionally associated with acanthotic, hyperplastic squamous epithelium. There is no cytologic atypia. Hyperplastic lesions are often associated with carcinoma. (D) Lichen sclerosus can be associated with a low-grade squamous intraepithelial lesion.

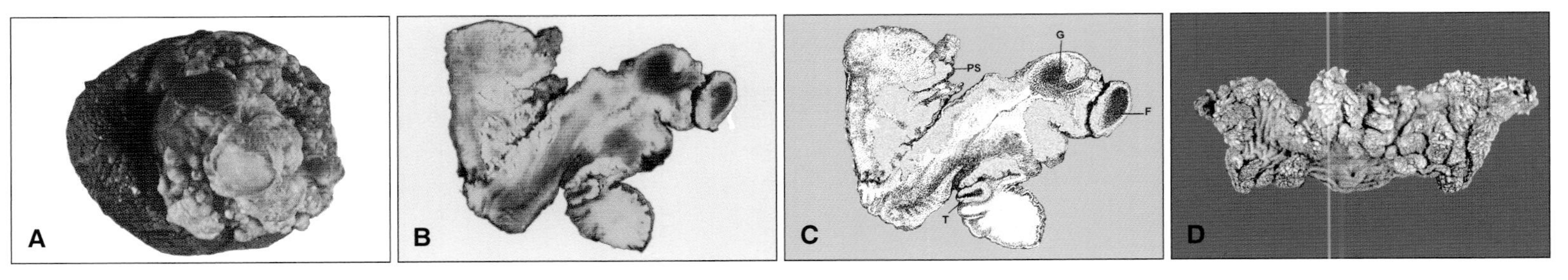

Fig. 1.21 (A) Giant condyloma is a large (5–10 cm), cauliflower-like neoplasm involving the coronal sulcus or foreskin, often with extension to the glans. This lobulated exophytic mass replaces most of the penis except for a part of the glans, which appears intact in the mid part of the specimen. (B,C) Cut surface of the same specimen discloses that the lesion (yellow) is superficial, but extends widely along the penile surface and pubic skin (PS). G, glans; F, foreskin; T, tunnelization phenomenon. (D) By contrast, this circumcision specimen shows extensive but non-destructive multifocal benign condylomata acuminata.

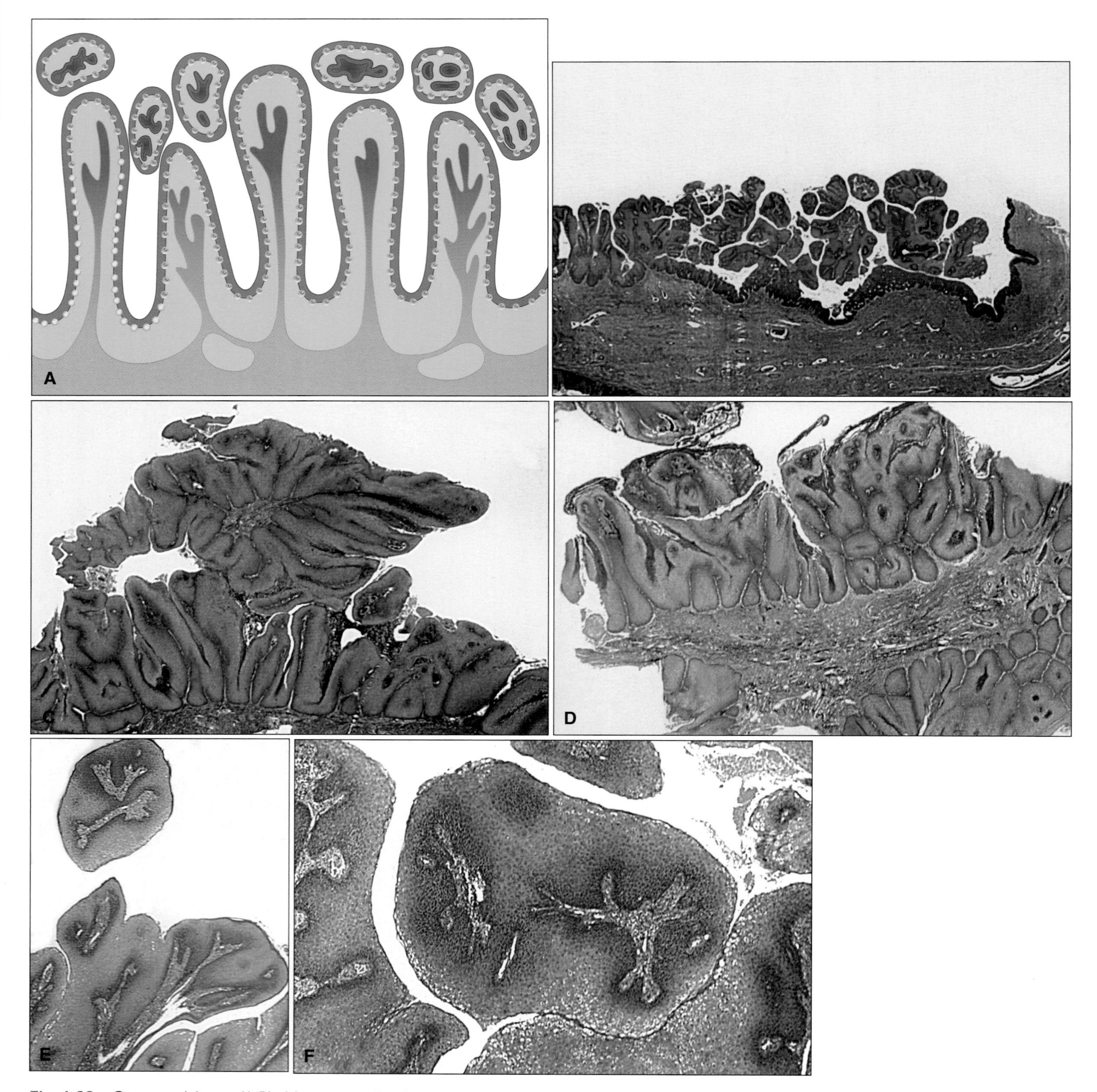

Fig. 1.22 Giant condyloma. (A,B) Microscopically, the tumor shows regular, condylomatous papillae with central fibrovascular cores and surface koilocytosis. The border between tumor and stroma is sharply delineated. The microscopic appearance is similar to that of common condyloma, despite the large size, unicentricity, older age, and destructive growth. (C–F) High-power findings are those of common condyloma. There is papillomatosis acanthosis and hyperkeratosis. The border between tumor and stroma is flat and broad.

unusual.[38-40] Benign epithelial tumors are restricted to condyloma acuminatum and the rare giant condyloma.

Penile cancer is a rare disease. Incidence varies widely by location, from 0.3 to 1 per 100 000. Rates are higher in Asia, Africa, and Latin America than in the USA and Europe.[41] Reported risk factors include lack of circumcision, phimosis, poor hygiene, tobacco use, inmunosuppression, irradiation, PUVA (psoralen plus ultraviolet A), and lichen sclerosus.[42-45] Basaloid and warty (condylomatous) carcinomas are highly associated with HPV infection; the association is less consistent for verrucous, papillary, sarcomatoid, and ordinary squamous cell carcinomas.[46,47]

Primary prognostic factors include stage, grade, and vascular invasion.[48-50] In addition, the tumor growth pattern independently predicts outcome.[51,52] Among histologic subtypes, verruciform tumors have the best prognosis, whereas poorly differentiated squamous cell, basaloid, and sarcomatoid carcinomas have the worst.[53]

GROWTH PATTERNS

(Figs 1.23–1.29)

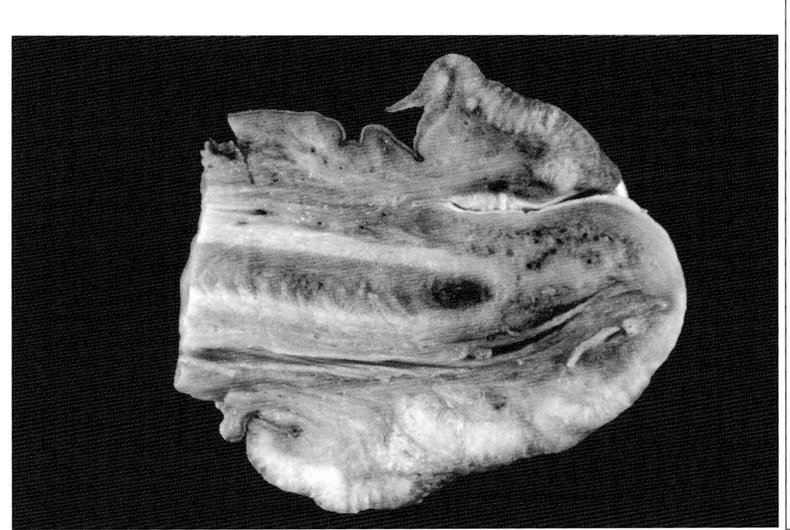

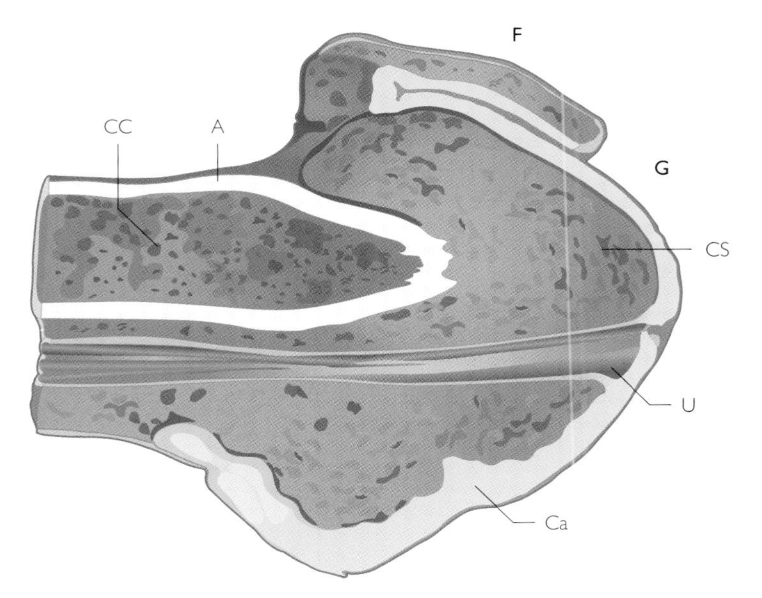

Fig. 1.23 Superficially spreading tumors grow slowly, invade superficially, and enlarge horizontally along the epithelium. This pattern accounts for about half of penile neoplasms. Inguinal node metastasis is rare. In the later stages, a vertical growth phase may develop, which worsens prognosis. CC, corpus cavernosum; A, albuginea; F, foreskin; G, glans; CS, corpus spongiosum; U, urethra; Ca, carcinoma.

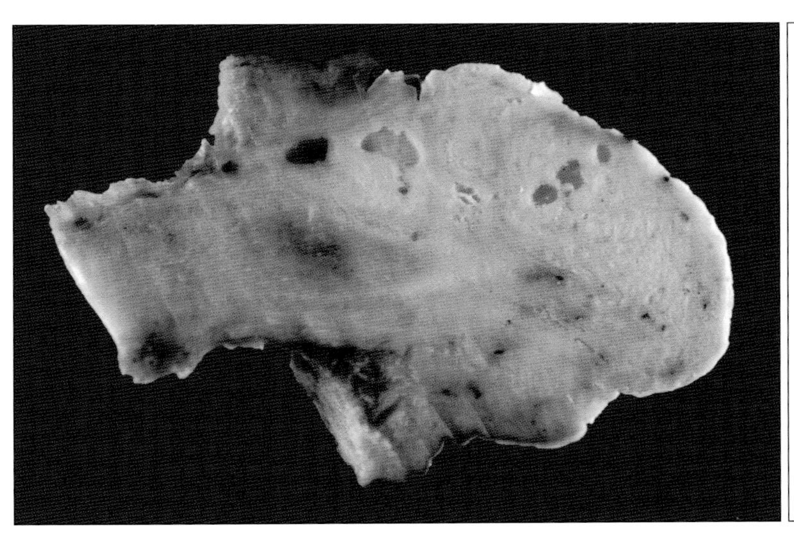

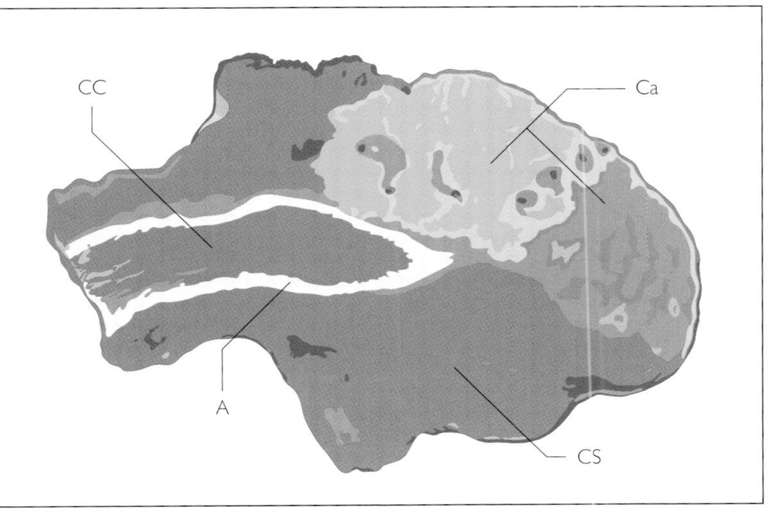

Fig. 1.24 Vertical-growth tumors typically penetrate rapidly into deep corpus spongiosum or cavernosum. Such tumors are typically high grade. About 20% of penile tumors show this pattern of growth. Nodal metastasis is common. CC, corpus cavernosum; Ca, carcinoma; CS, corpus spongiosum; A, tunica albuginea.

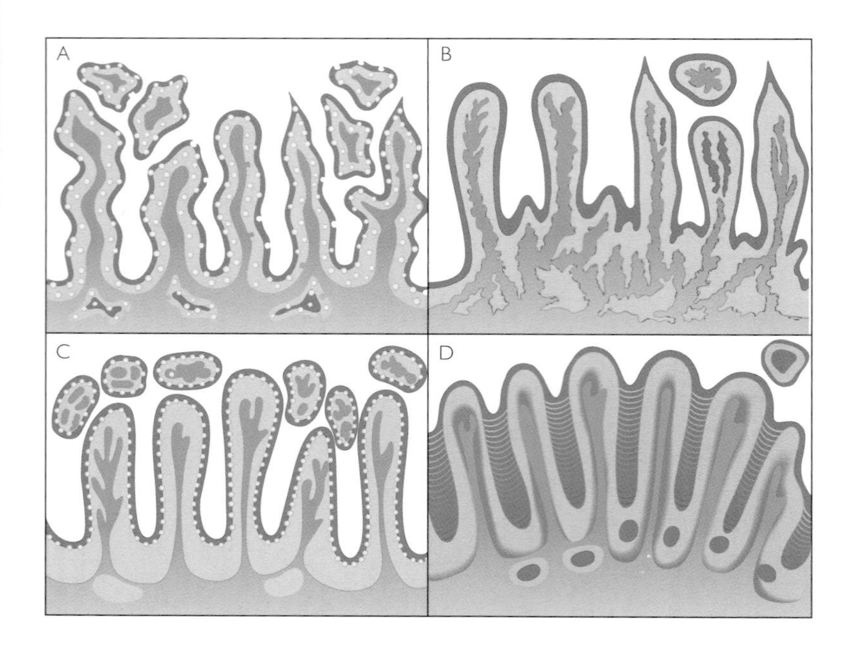

Fig. 1.25 Verruciform (or exophytic) tumors show limited invasion of superficial anatomic layers. These account for about 20% of penile cancers. Three variants of malignant verruciform tumors exist: warty or condylomatous (A), papillary (B), and verrucous (D). Giant condyloma (C), a benign penile exophytic tumor, must be differentiated. In these diagrams, epithelium is yellow, keratin orange, stroma pink. Dots show koilocytosis.

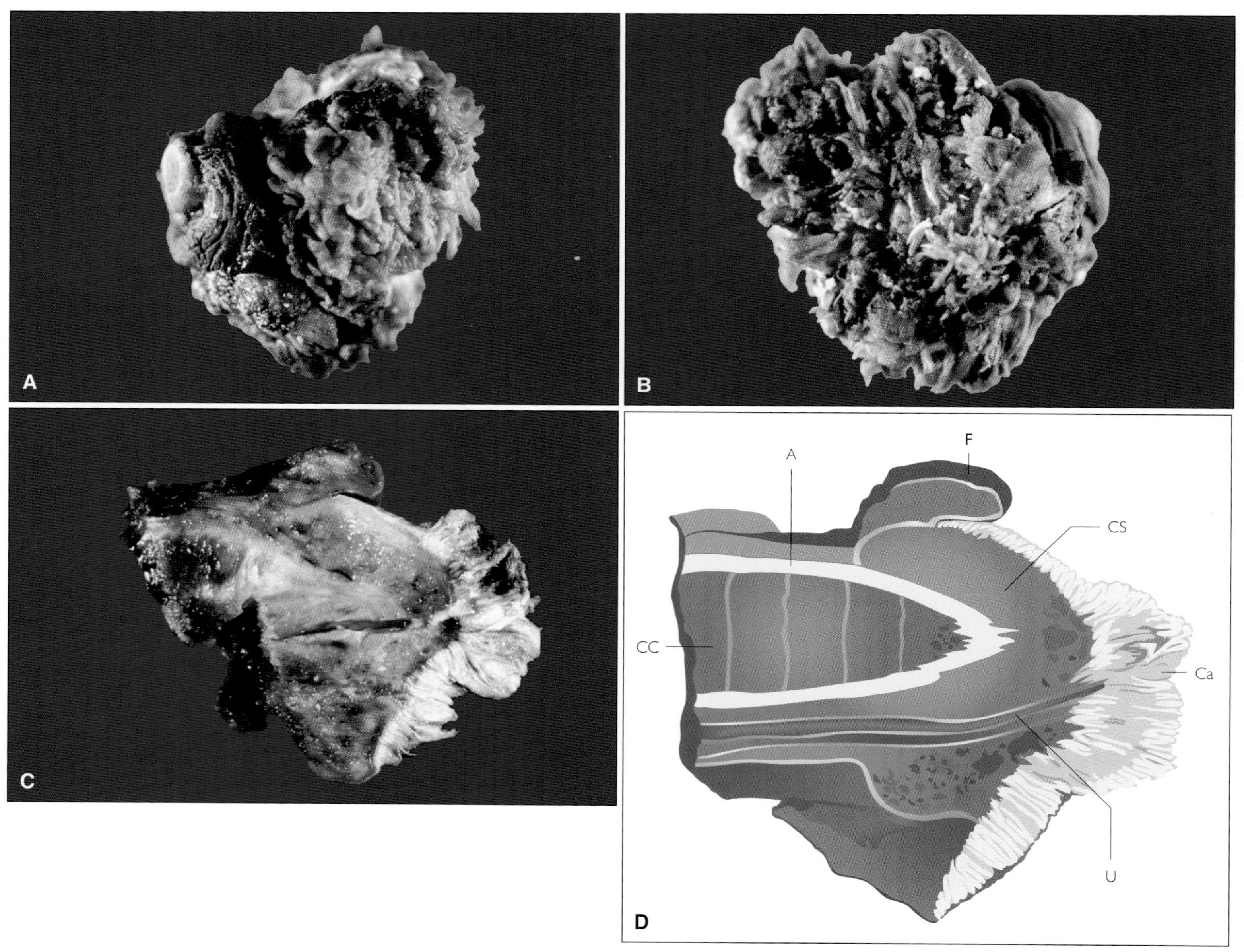

Fig. 1.26 (A–D) This example of the verrucous variant has a white–tan, filiform appearance. The cut surface shows spiky, papillomatous tumor superficially involving the glans. CC, corpus cavernosum; A, tunica albuginea; F, foreskin; CS, corpus spongiosum; Ca, carcinoma; U, urethra.

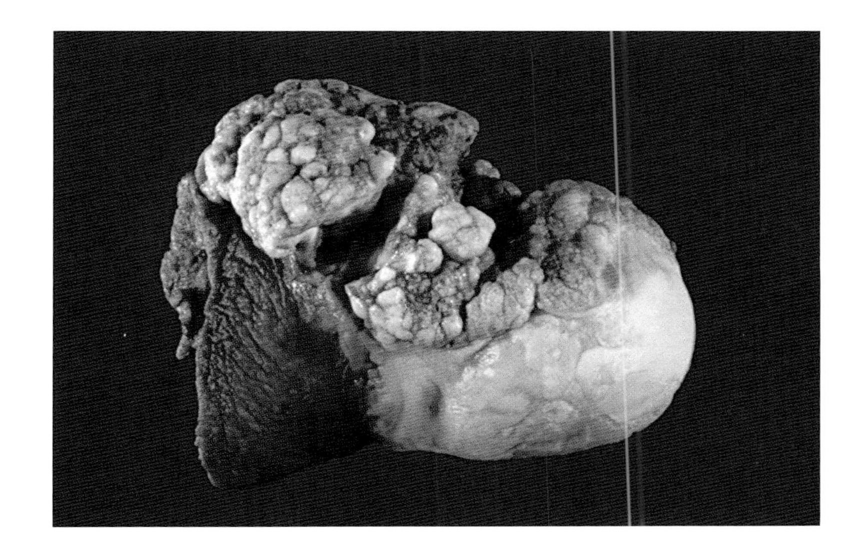

Fig. 1.27 This example of the warty (condylomatous) variant is seen in this specimen as a beige, exophytic mass involving the glans and coronal sulcus. The surface of the tumor has a cobblestone appearance.

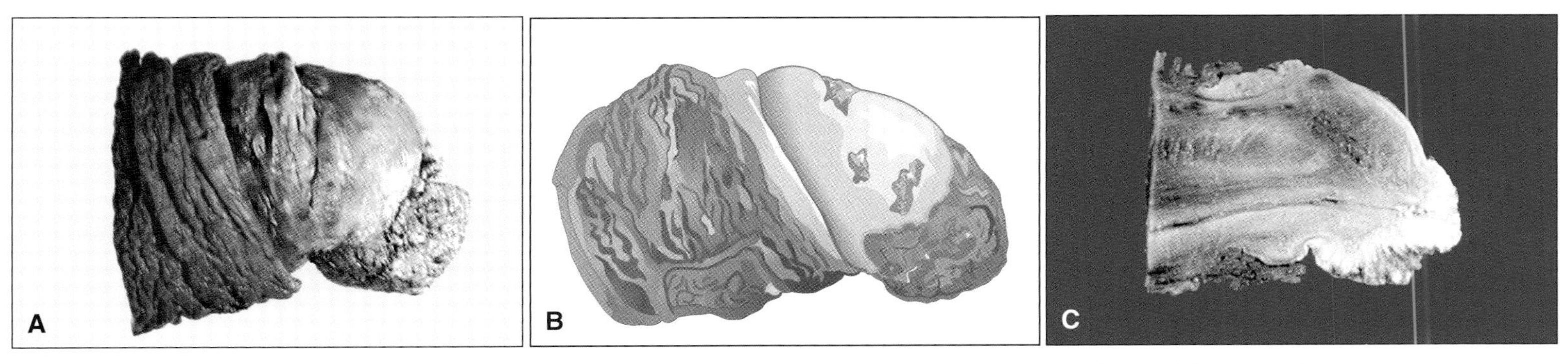

Fig. 1.28 (A–C) Multicentric carcinomas show two or more independent foci separated by normal epithelium. This unusual pattern is most common in the foreskin. Here, four separate, independent foci of carcinoma were found. The main tumor was at the apex of the glans; the other tumors were microscopic findings.

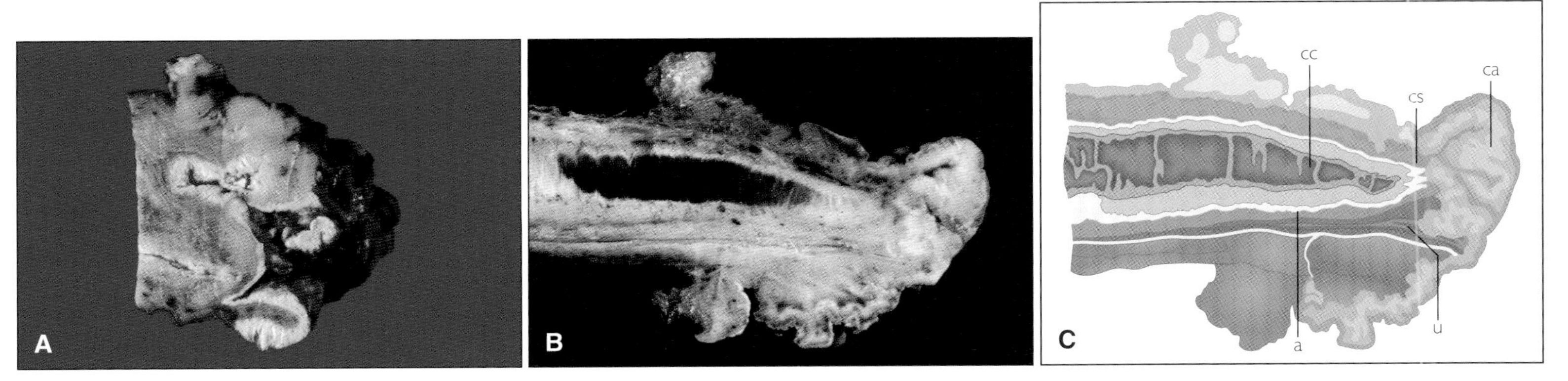

Fig. 1.29 Mixed growth patterns may be seen in clinically advanced tumors. (A) Mixed superficially spreading, verruciform (SS-VM). This superficial and extensive tumor (SS) covers all epithelial compartments. Ventrally, there is a papillomatous verruciform tumor (VM) growing along the preputial surface, including the cutaneous aspect. (B,C) Mixed superficially spreading, vertical growth. Specimen and diagram. Ventrally, there is a flat, superficially spreading pattern in the glans. Dorsally and above the urethra (u), the tumor (ca) shows a vertical growth pattern with deep invasion of the corpus spongiosum (cs). The corpus cavernosum (cc) and albuginea (a) are not involved.

HISTOLOGIC TYPES

Squamous cell carcinoma, usual type

Ordinary squamous cell carcinoma represents over half of all penile malignancies.[54] Mean age at presentation is 60 years. Overall, less than half of patients develop metastases, but some patients, after years of neglect, present with a massive primary tumor and inguinal nodal and skin metastasis. Overexpression of p53 correlates with metastatic risk.[55] Overall 5-year survival rate following surgery is 36%.[53] (Figs 1.30–1.34)

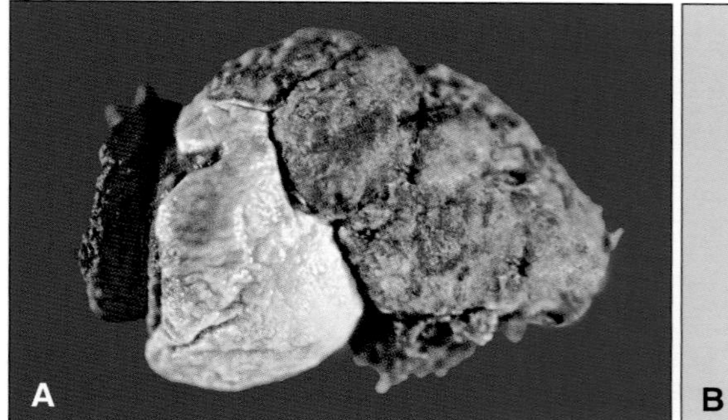

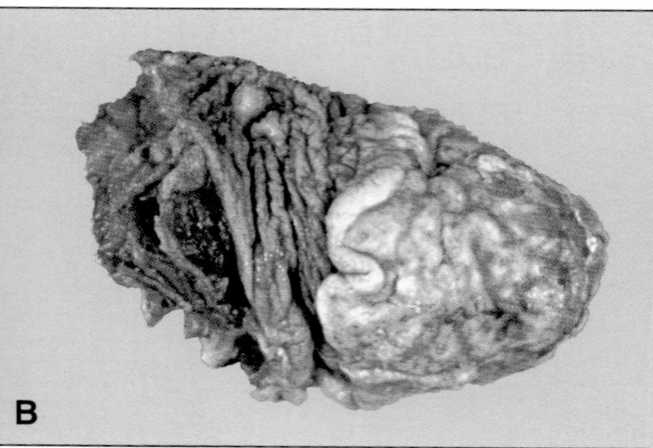

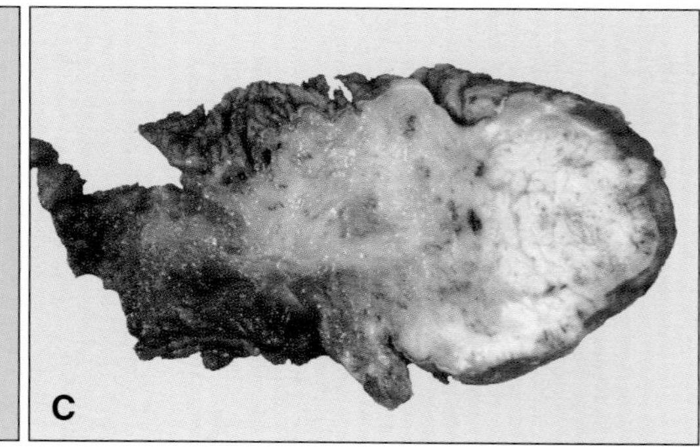

Fig. 1.30 Squamous cell carcinoma, usual type. Grossly, squamous cell carcinoma presents as an exophytic, gray–tan, firm, ulcerated mass involving (and often replacing) the head of the penis. The most common site is the glans, followed by the foreskin and coronal sulcus. Often, all anatomic compartments are involved. Pathologists should specifically inspect the specimen for evidence of tumor penetration into the corpus spongiosum or cavernosum, which is an important staging criterion. (A) Partial penectomy showing a large, exophytic, pink–tan, firm mass involving the distal portion of the glans. (B) Large, gray–tan, fungating and extensively ulcerated tumor replacing the glans. (C) Cut surface of the neoplasm seen in (B) shows a solid, white–gray, firm, deeply invasive tumor effacing normal anatomic landmarks.

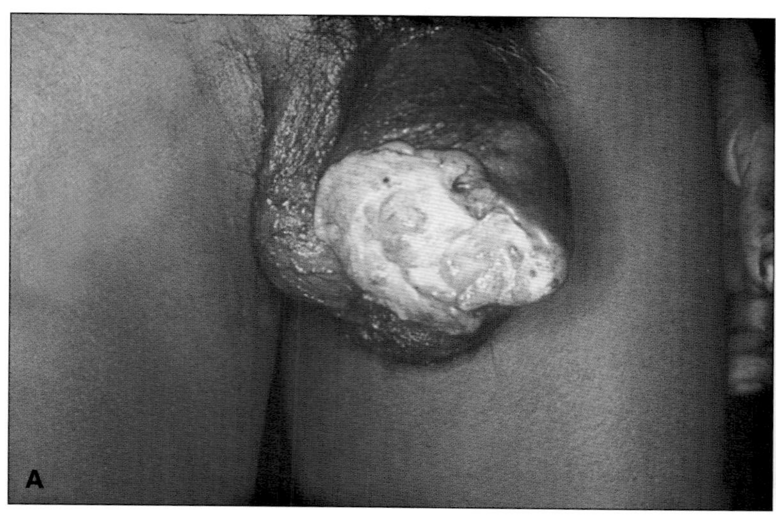

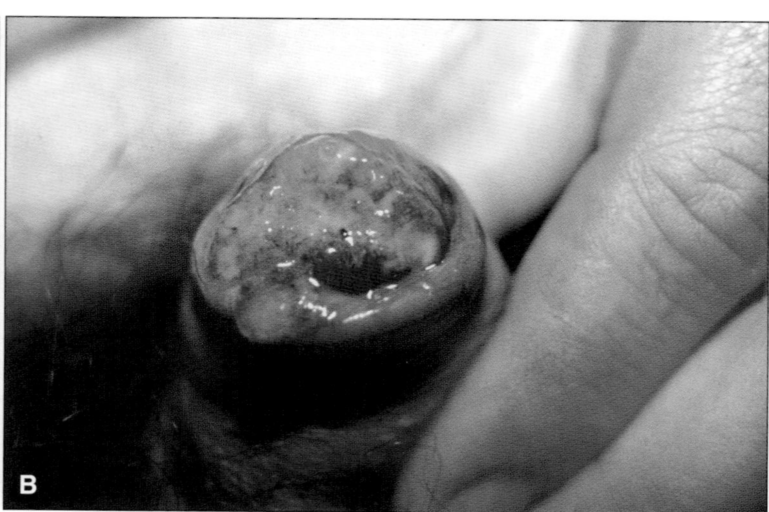

Fig. 1.31 Squamous cell carcinoma, usual type. Grossly, the tumor may show predominantly exophytic or endophytic growth. (A) Exophytic, fungating, destructive masses involving the distal penis; glans, coronal sulcus, and foreskin. (B) Flat, erythematous lesion replacing the glans. This tumor was deeply invasive on cut section. Invasion of the urethra or prostate can upstage the tumor, and must be documented.

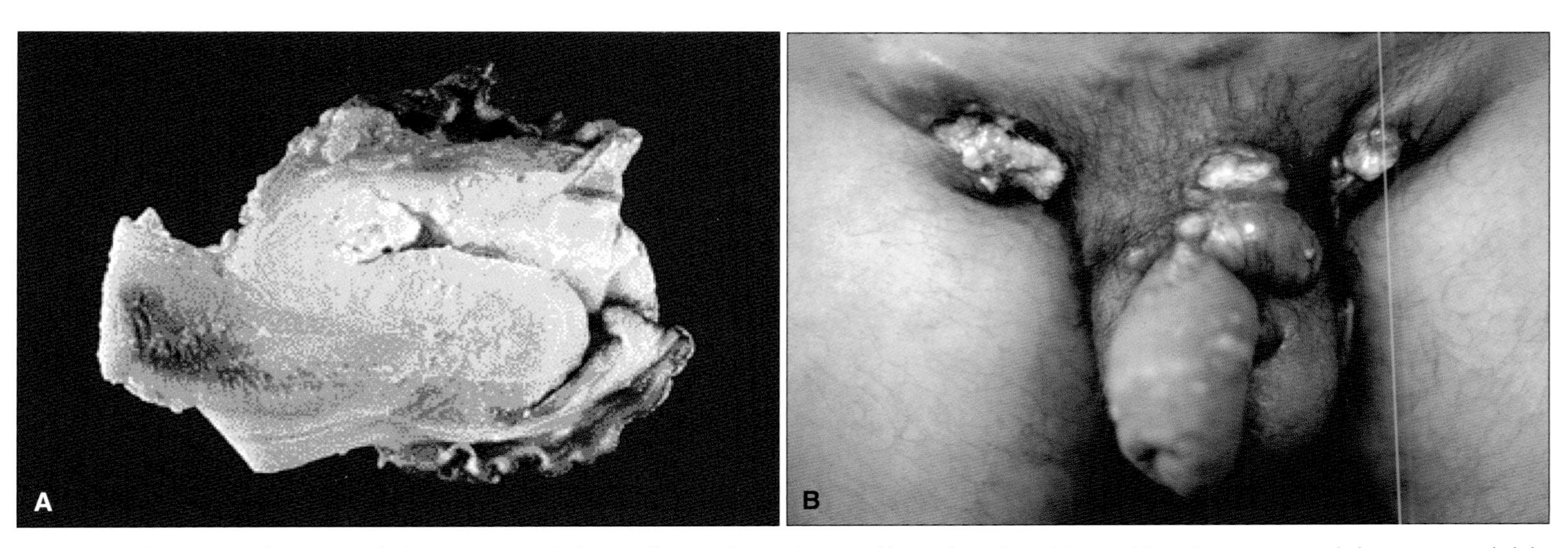

Fig. 1.32 Phimosis and poor penile hygiene are risk factors for penile carcinoma. Also, a long foreskin or phimosis may conceal the tumor and delay diagnosis. (A) Phimotic penis with a large, white, firm tumor growing into an enlarged preputial sac. (B) Patient with a long phimotic foreskin presented with an occult primary tumor in the glans and multiple inguinal nodal metastases.

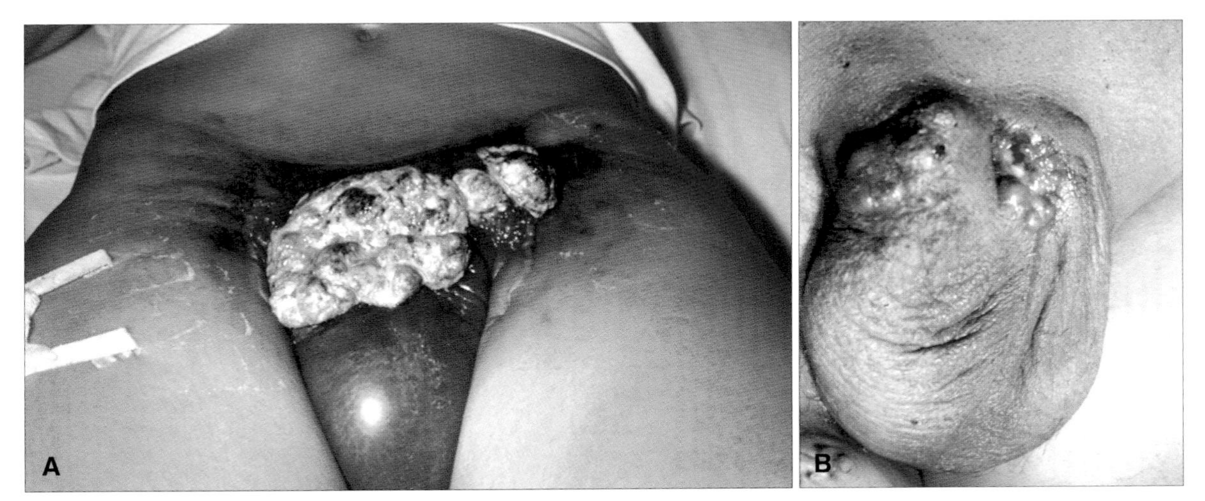

Fig. 1.33 (A,B) Advanced cases of squamous cell carcinoma may show continuous local extension into the scrotal and inguinal regions, as in the recurrent carcinoma seen in (B). Alternatively, satellite tumors are frequent in advanced cases, secondary to local vascular dissemination.

Basaloid squamous cell carcinoma

This HPV-related variant of squamous cell carcinoma occurs in slightly younger patients (median age, 52 years). The most common site is the glans, and tumors are usually deeply invasive at diagnosis. Regional metastasis is present in 60–70% of patients, but reported 5-year survival rates range from 20% to 60%.[56,57] (Figs 1.35–1.38)

Warty (condylomatous) carcinoma

This exophytic tumor is associated with HPV infection and coexisting condyloma.[35,37,58] It has been confused with verrucous carcinoma and giant condyloma. These are slow-growing tumors affecting patients younger than those with typical squamous cell carcinoma (median age, 50 years). Most penile tumors diagnosed

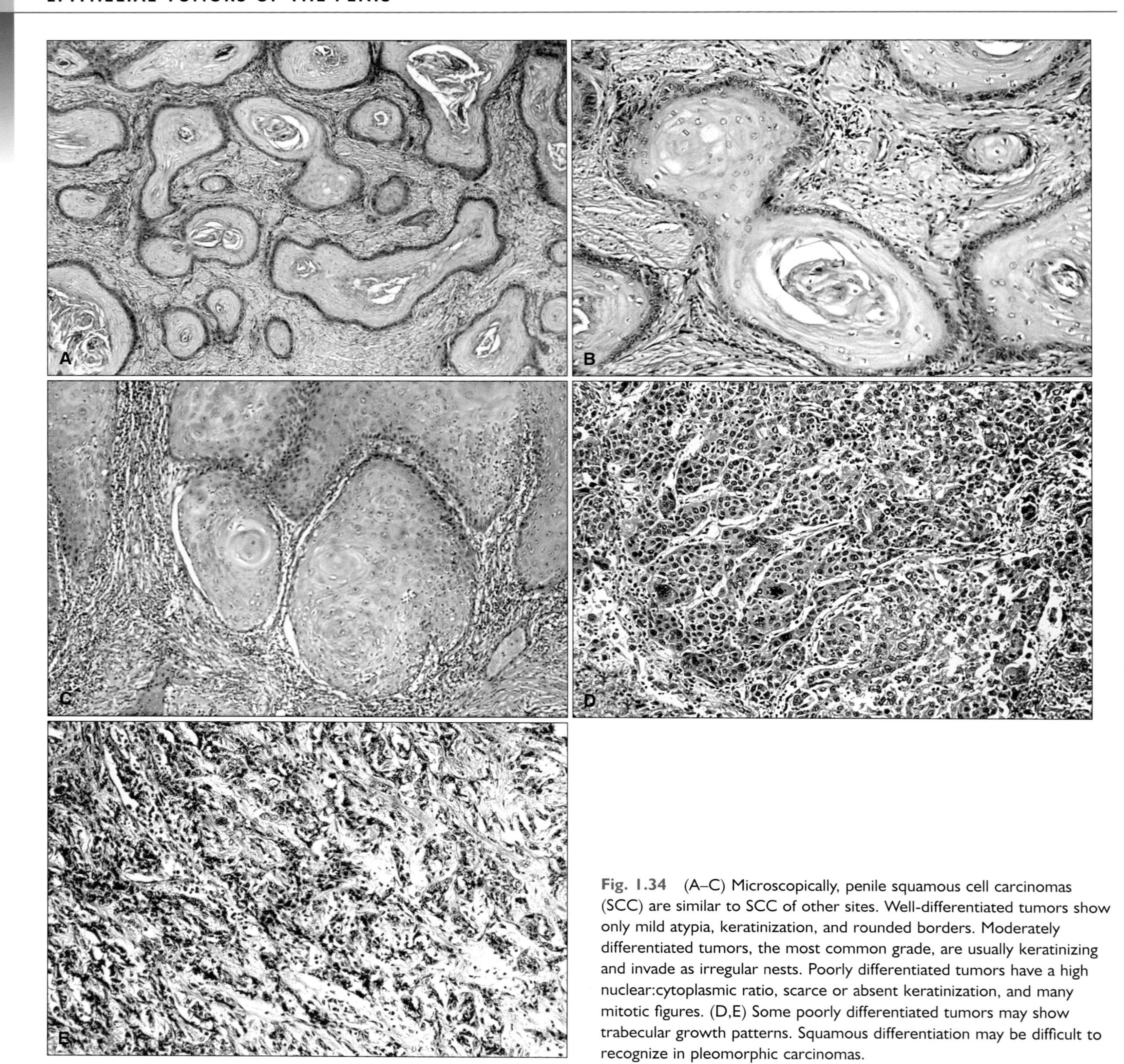

Fig. 1.34 (A–C) Microscopically, penile squamous cell carcinomas (SCC) are similar to SCC of other sites. Well-differentiated tumors show only mild atypia, keratinization, and rounded borders. Moderately differentiated tumors, the most common grade, are usually keratinizing and invade as irregular nests. Poorly differentiated tumors have a high nuclear:cytoplasmic ratio, scarce or absent keratinization, and many mitotic figures. (D,E) Some poorly differentiated tumors may show trabecular growth patterns. Squamous differentiation may be difficult to recognize in pleomorphic carcinomas.

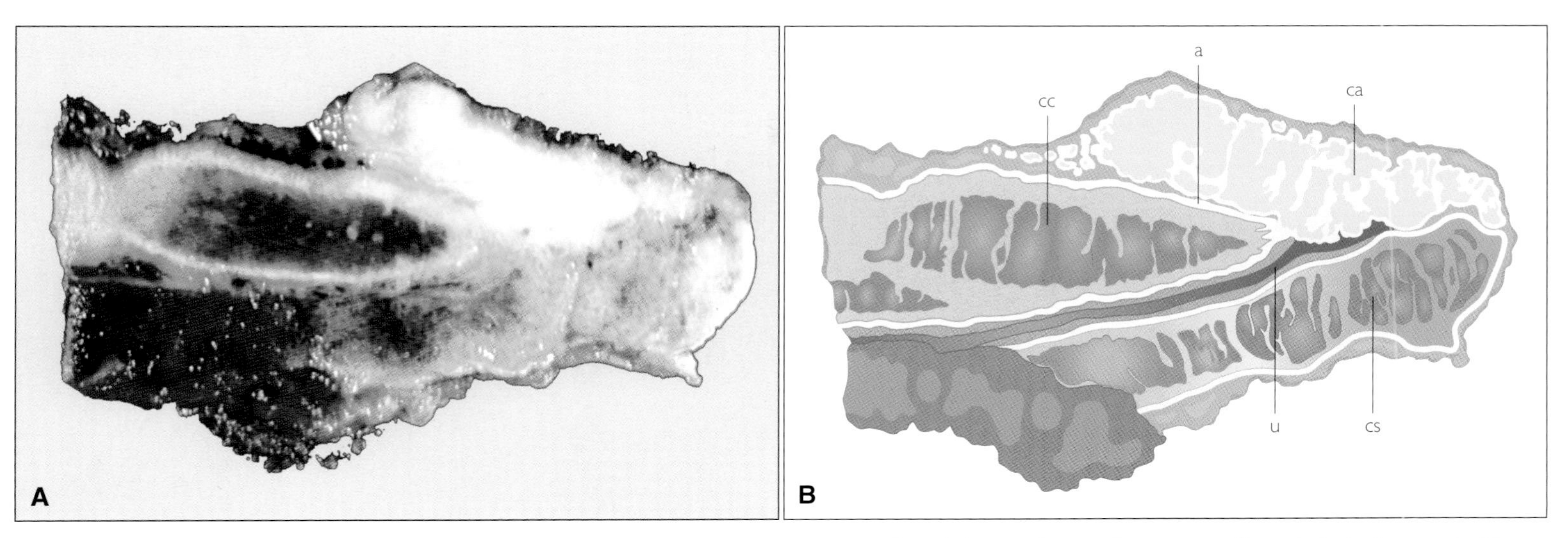

Fig. 1.35 (A,B) Basaloid squamous cell carcinoma. The cut surface is characteristically solid tan, often with minute yellowish foci of necrosis. Tumor margins are well circumscribed. Here, tumor (ca) deeply infiltrates the corpus spongiosum (cs) but does not penetrate the albuginea (a). cc, corpus cavernosum; u, urethra.

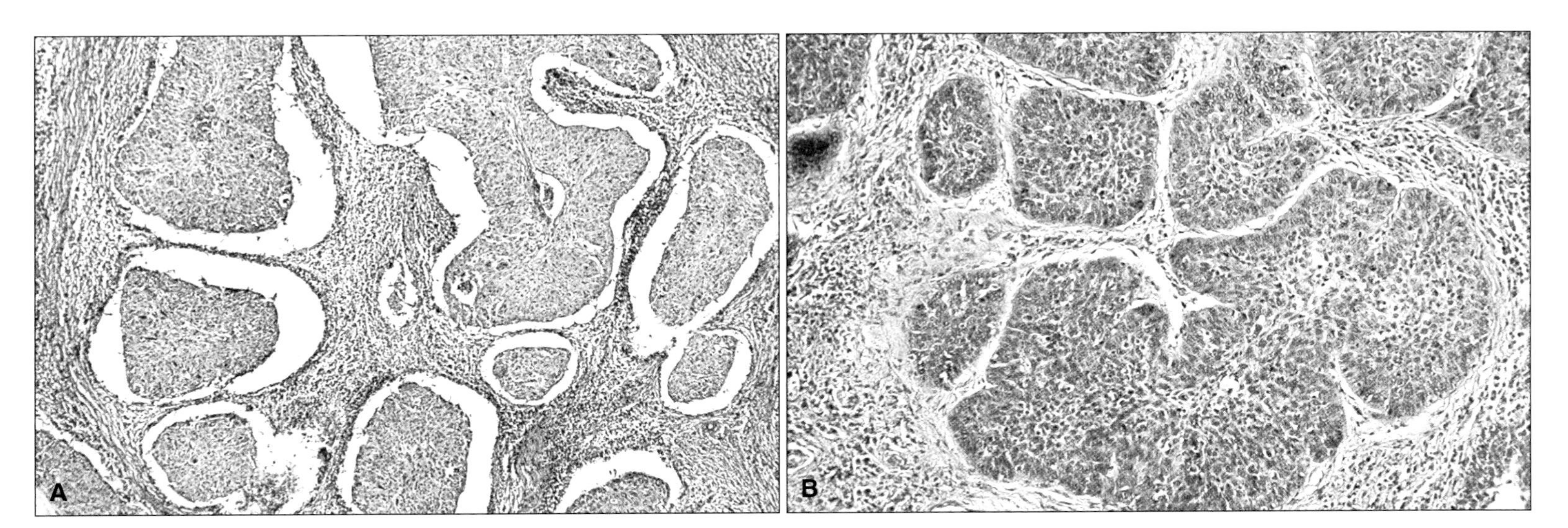

Fig. 1.36 (A,B) Basaloid squamous cell carcinoma. Microscopically, tumor shows a downward proliferation of solid or centrally necrotic nests of uniform small cells. Peripheral palisading with artifactual surrounding clefts and central keratinization may be noted. Mitotic figures are numerous. Invasion of lymphatic vascular spaces in lamina propria is common.

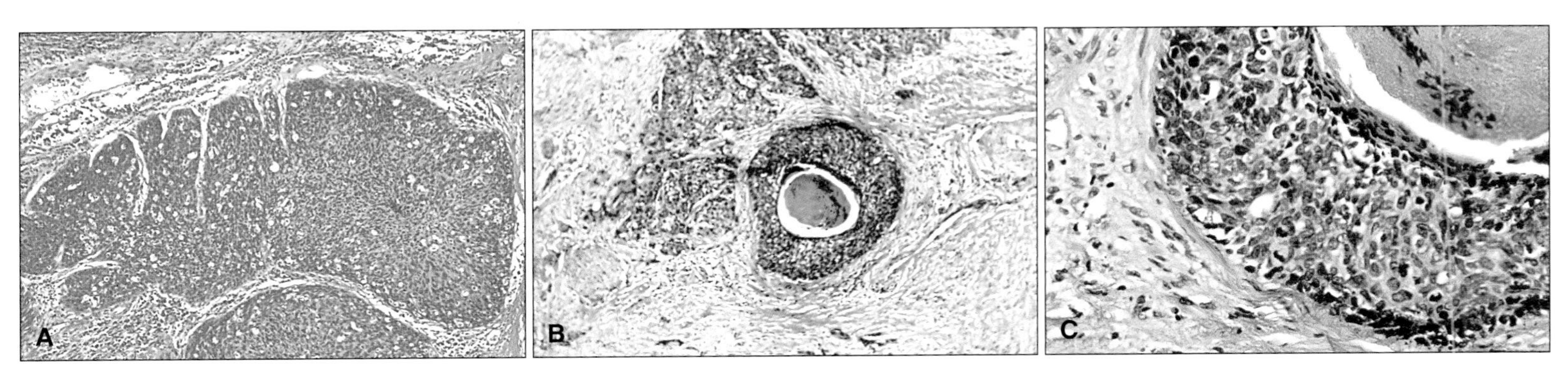

Fig. 1.37 (A–C) Basaloid squamous cell carcinoma. Individual cell necrosis ('starry-sky pattern') is common. Mitotic figures are numerous.

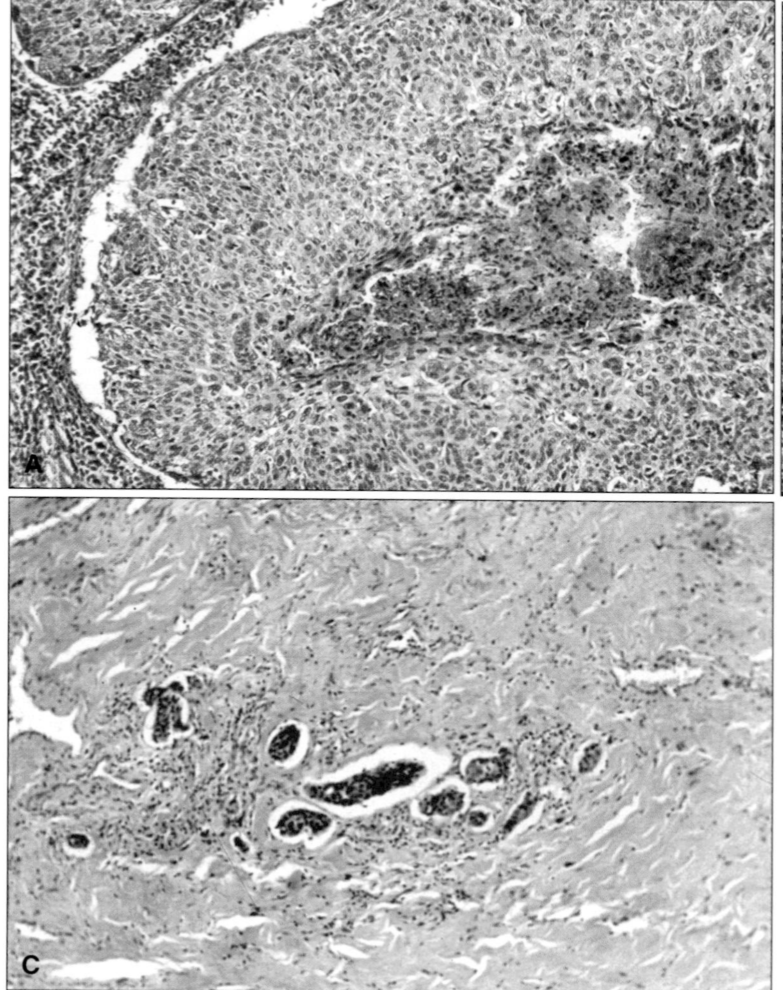

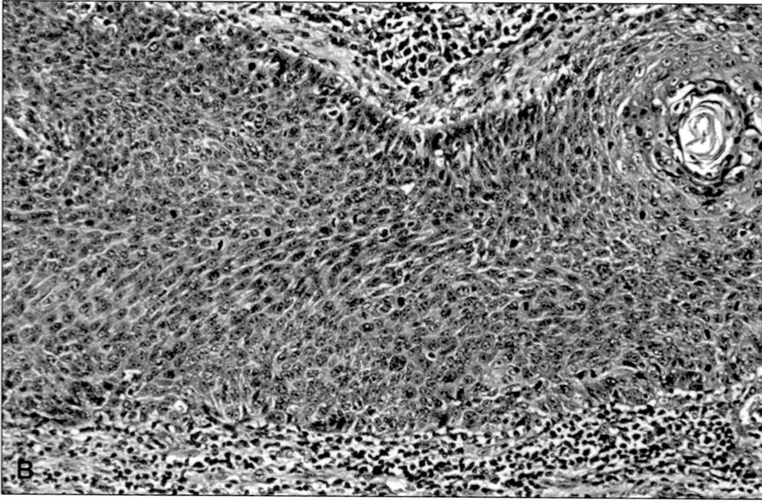

Fig. 1.38 (A–C) Basaloid carcinoma is typically highly invasive, and lymphatic vascular invasion is common. Irregular, invasive foci of carcinoma and desmoplasia are seen budding from a central nest with comedonecrosis. Minute tumor nests are seen perforating albuginea, with tumor emboli present in the corpus cavernosum.

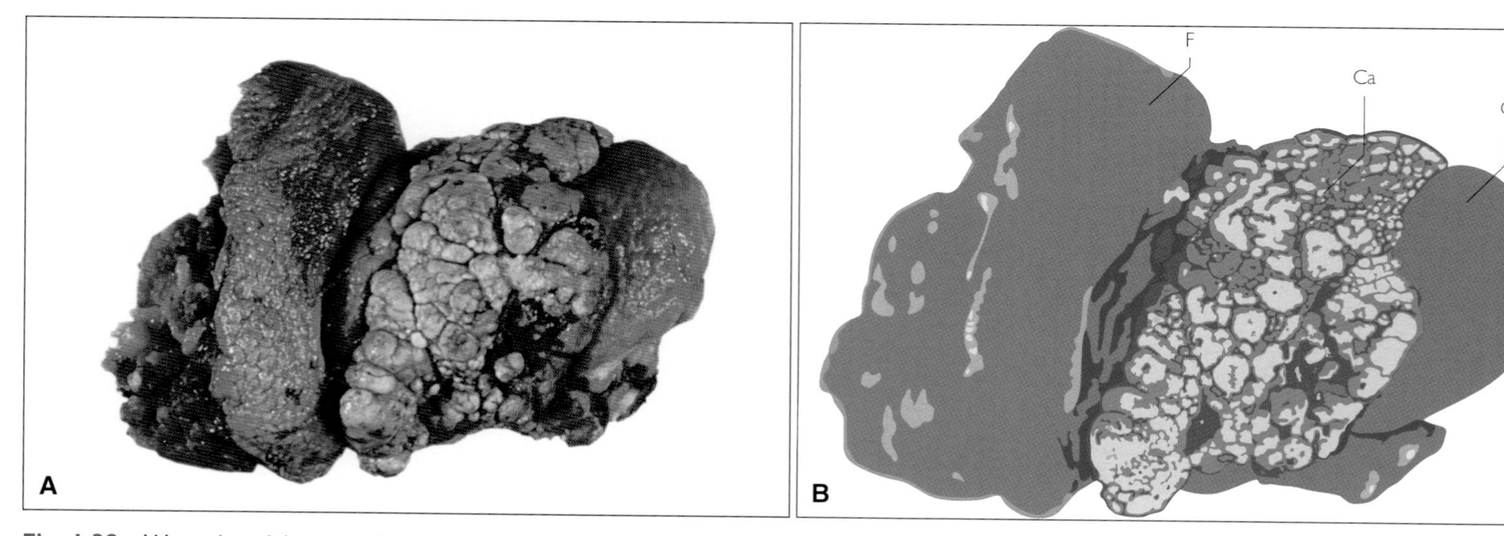

Fig. 1.39 Warty (condylomatous) carcinoma equally affects the foreskin and glans. This penectomy specimen (A) and diagram (B) show a white–gray tumor (Ca, blue in diagram) involving the coronal sulcus, foreskin (F), and glans (G). Grossly, warty carcinomas show a cauliflower-like appearance and average 5 cm in diameter. The neoplasm surface has a cobblestone appearance.

in patients with HIV are of this variety.[59,60] Regional metastasis is present in about 20% of cases. There are no literature reports of deaths due to this variant, but we know of one unpublished fatal case. (Figs 1.39–1.48)

Verrucous carcinoma

These slow-growing, well-differentiated squamous neoplasms are characterized by exophytic growth and a broad, 'pushing' tumor border.[61–63] Median age at diagnosis is 60

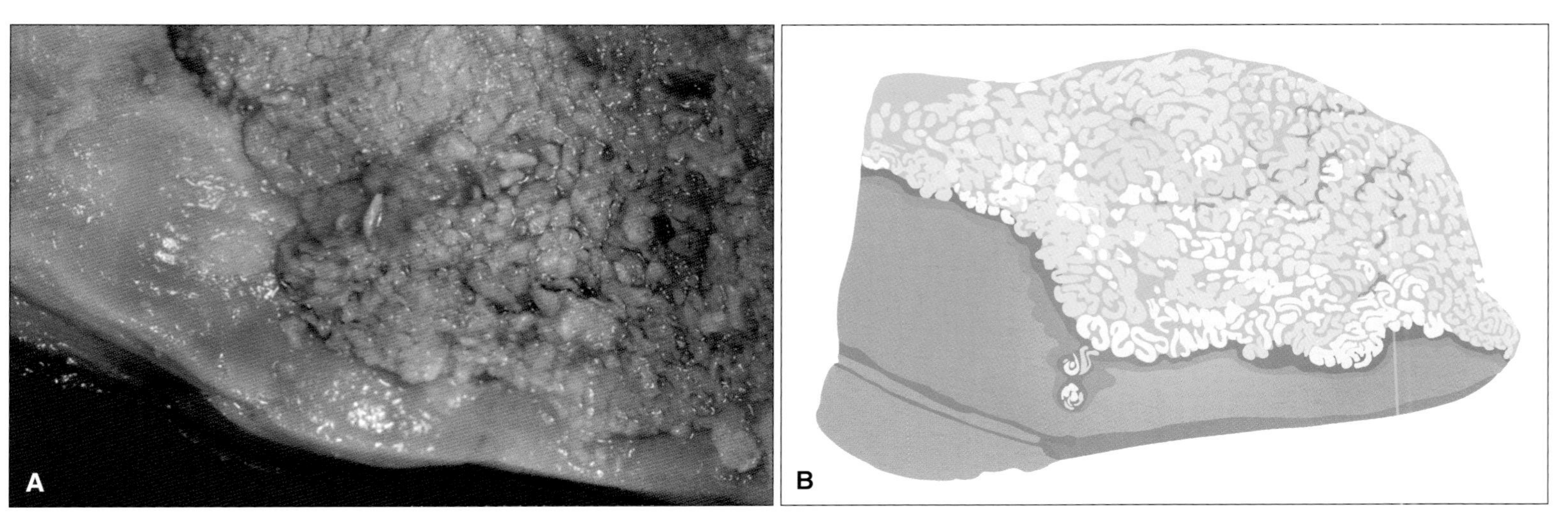

Fig. 1.40 (A,B) Warty (condylomatous) carcinoma. Here, the preputial mucosa is covered by a granular lesion. The surface of the tumor (yellow, diagram) shows a uniform cerebriform pattern.

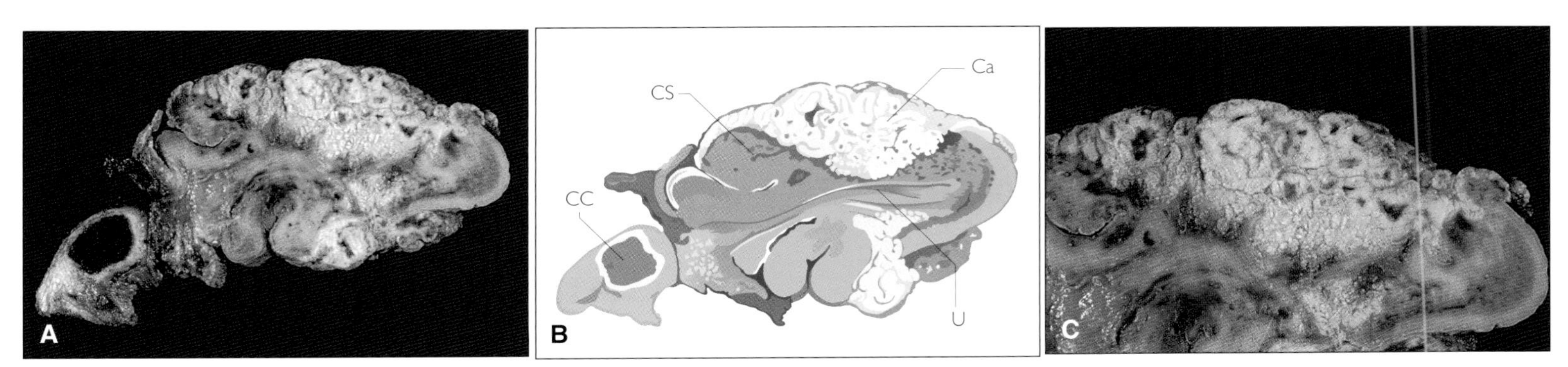

Fig. 1.41 (A–C) The cut surface of this partial penectomy specimen with warty carcinoma (Ca) involving the foreskin, coronal sulcus, and glans shows a complex, arborizing, and papillomatous tumor. Neoplastic epithelium is seen as gray–yellow lobules surrounding darker, tan, central fibrovascular cores. The neoplasm involves the whole thickness of the prepuce and invades the corpus spongiosum (CS) and cavernosum (CC); the urethra (U) is free of tumor.

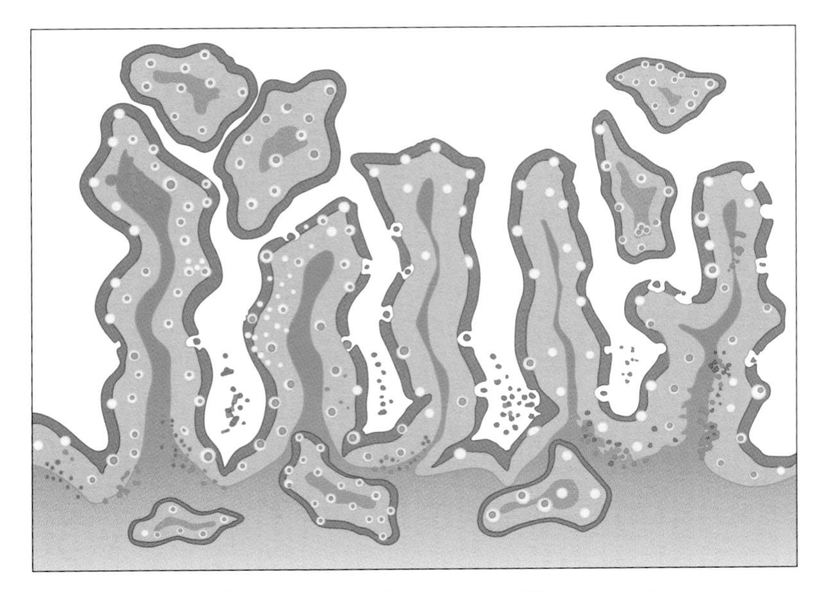

Fig. 1.42 Warty (condylomatous) carcinoma. Diagrammatic representation shows: long, condylomatous, and undulating papillae; jagged deep borders; HPV-related changes throughout the neoplasm. See Fig. 1.25 for color coding.

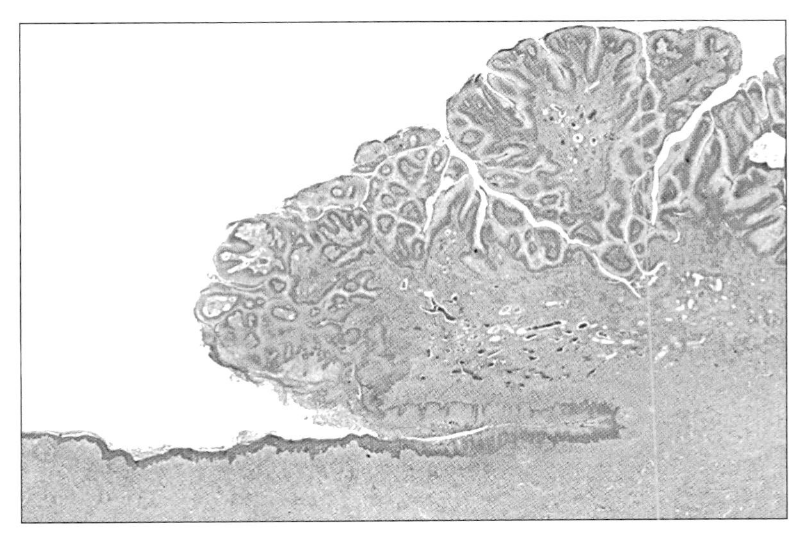

Fig. 1.43 Warty (condylomatous) carcinoma. Microscopically, an acanthotic, papillomatous appearance is present. Papillae are variably long and typically spiky, but sometimes undulating or round. The interface between tumor and stroma may be broad and flat, or, in deeply invasive tumors, irregular and jagged. Prominent central fibrovascular cores are seen.

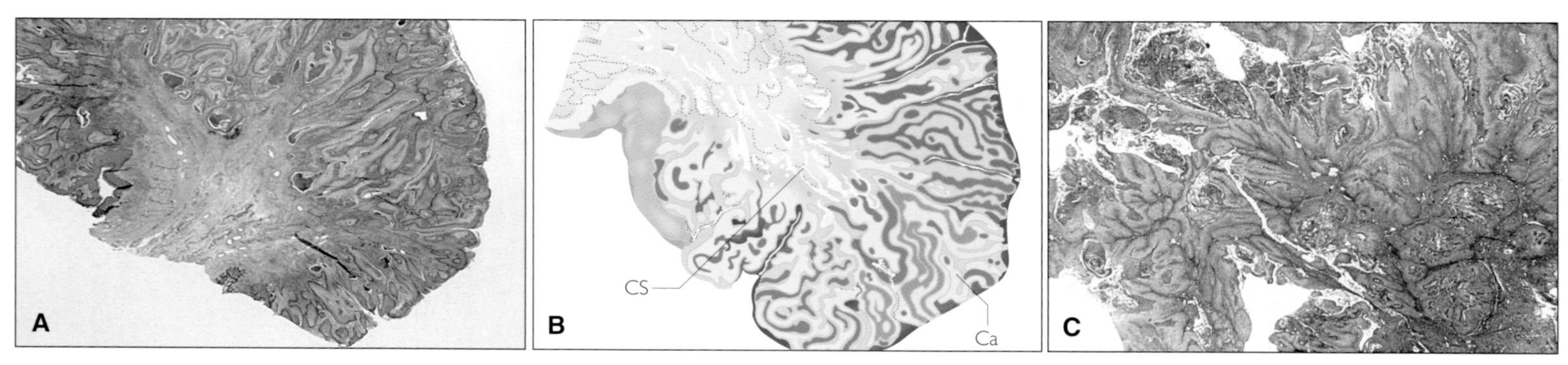

Fig. 1.44 (A–C) Warty (condylomatous) carcinoma. Low-power view shows an arborescent neoplasm with round, thick papillae. These cases show variations of papillary architecture: in some cases, long and undulating; in others, thin and complex. Note microabscesses at the base of papillae (A). Keratin cysts may be present (C). CS, corpus spongiosum; Ca, carcinoma.

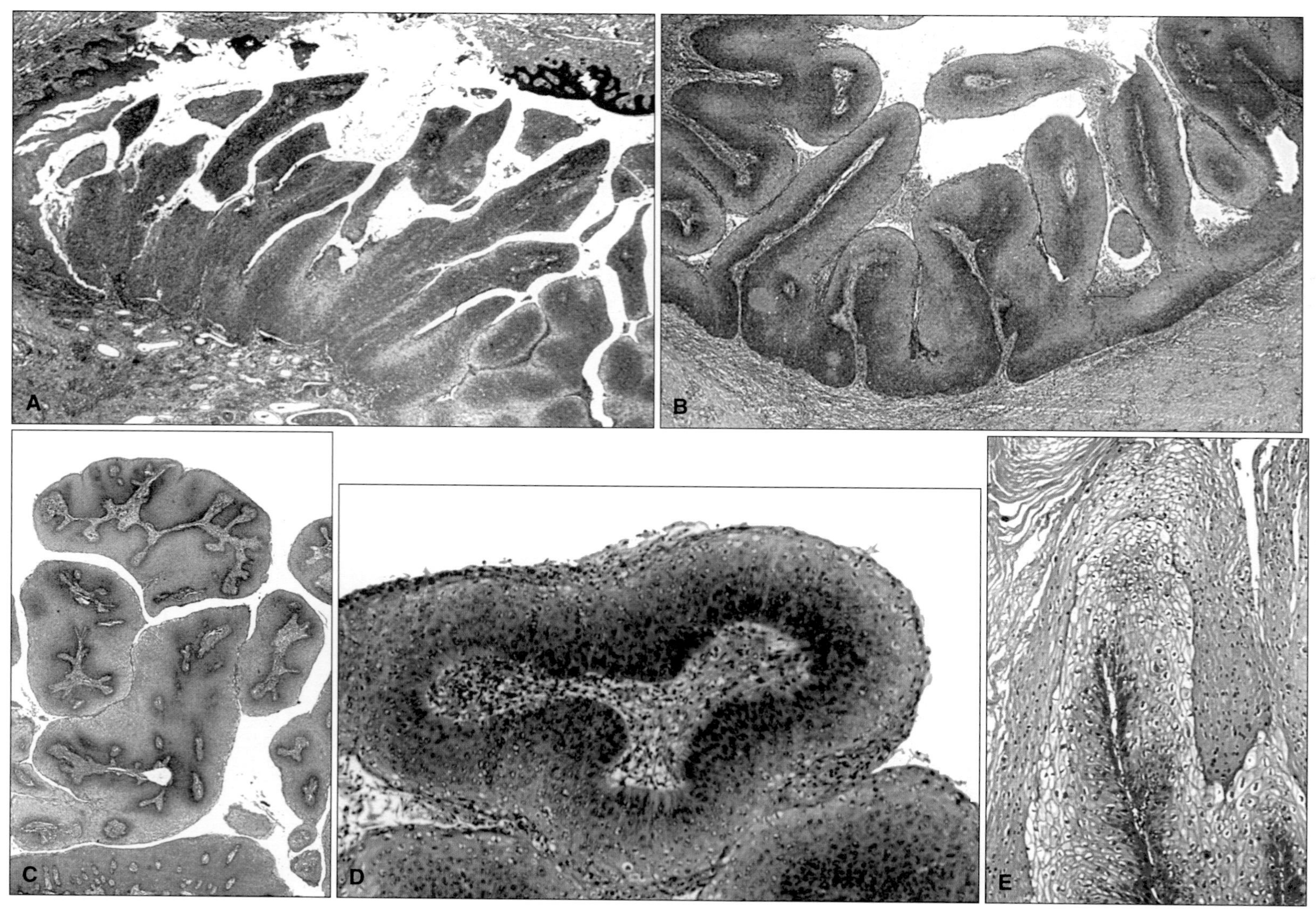

Fig. 1.45 (A–E) Warty (condylomatous) carcinoma. Clearing of cell cytoplasm and koilocytosis are noted throughout the tumor epithelium, including deep layers. Often a biphasic clear and dark cell pattern is present. Note the lymphatic vascular invasion in the lamina propria (A).

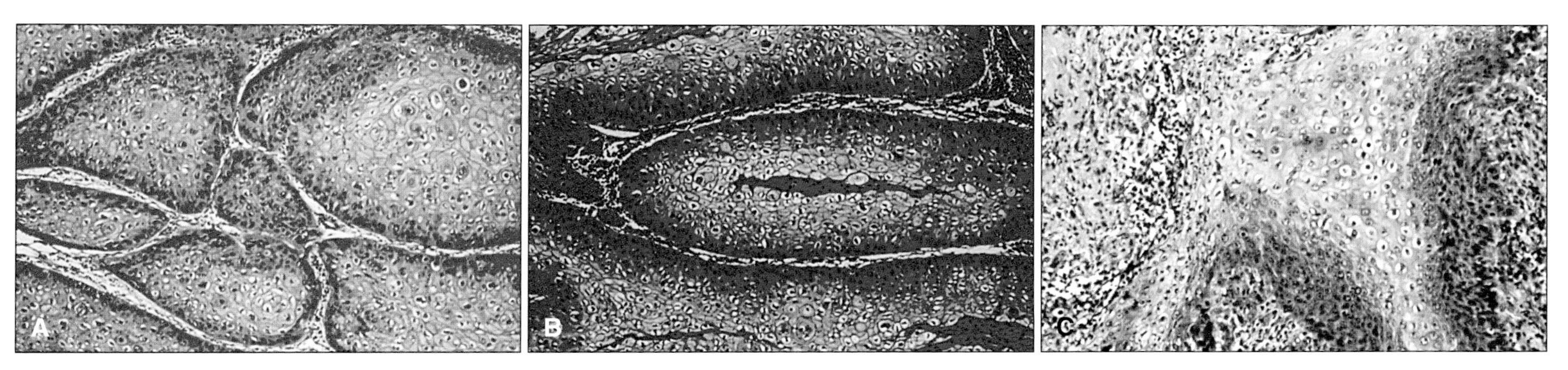

Fig. 1.46 (A–C) Warty carcinoma is usually cytologically low grade with prominent koilocytotic changes throughout. Though well differentiated, the cells are clearly malignant. Mitotic figures are identified.

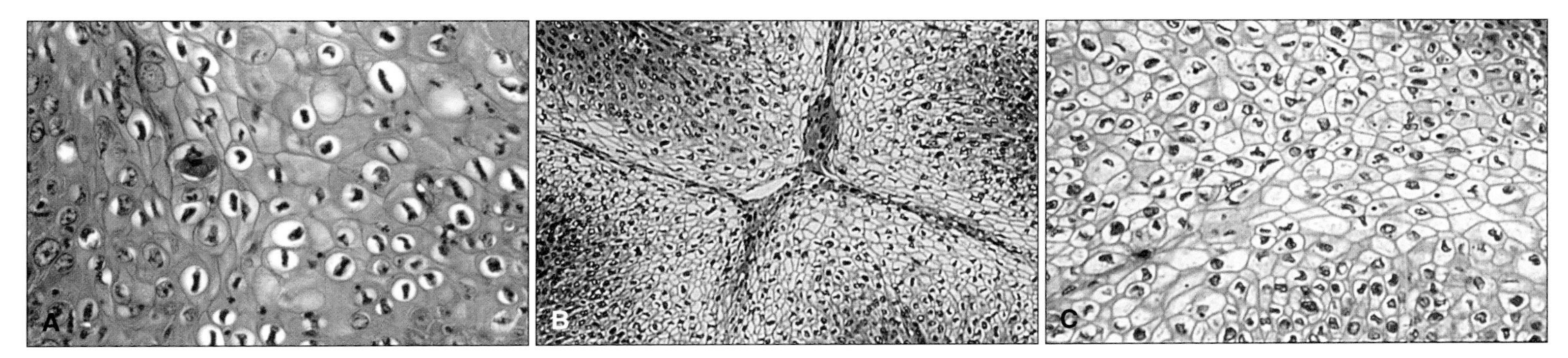

Fig. 1.47 (A–C) Warty (condylomatous) carcinoma. In these high- and medium-power views, atypical koilocytes show enlarged hyperchromatic nuclei with irregular contours, a prominent perinuclear halo, bi- and multinucleated cells, and dyskeratotic or apoptotic cells. Warty carcinomas occasionally show a prominent perinuclear halo simulating a clear cell carcinoma.

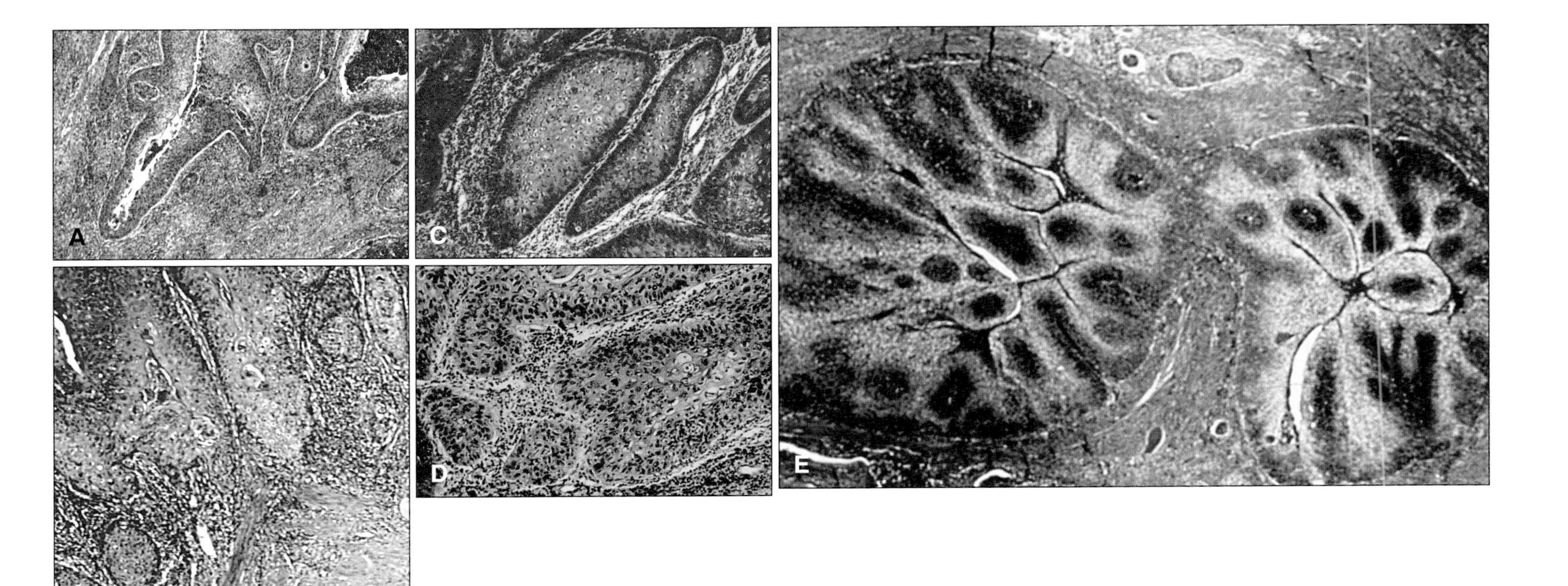

Fig. 1.48 (A–E) Warty (condylomatous) carcinoma. The interface between tumor and stroma is irregular and jagged. Koilocytotic changes are present throughout the neoplasm, including deeply invasive nests. Pseudo-invasion due to the 'tunnelization' phenomenon (tangential sectioning of deep portions of complex papillae) may simulate deep invasion (E).

years. Most occur on the glans or foreskin. Multicentricity is common, especially in the foreskin. The well-differentiated cytology makes interpretation of biopsy specimens difficult, and a large specimen may be needed to prove the malignant nature of the tumor. Pure verrucous carcinomas are not known to metastasize, but they commonly recur following incomplete resection. (Figs 1.49–1.56)

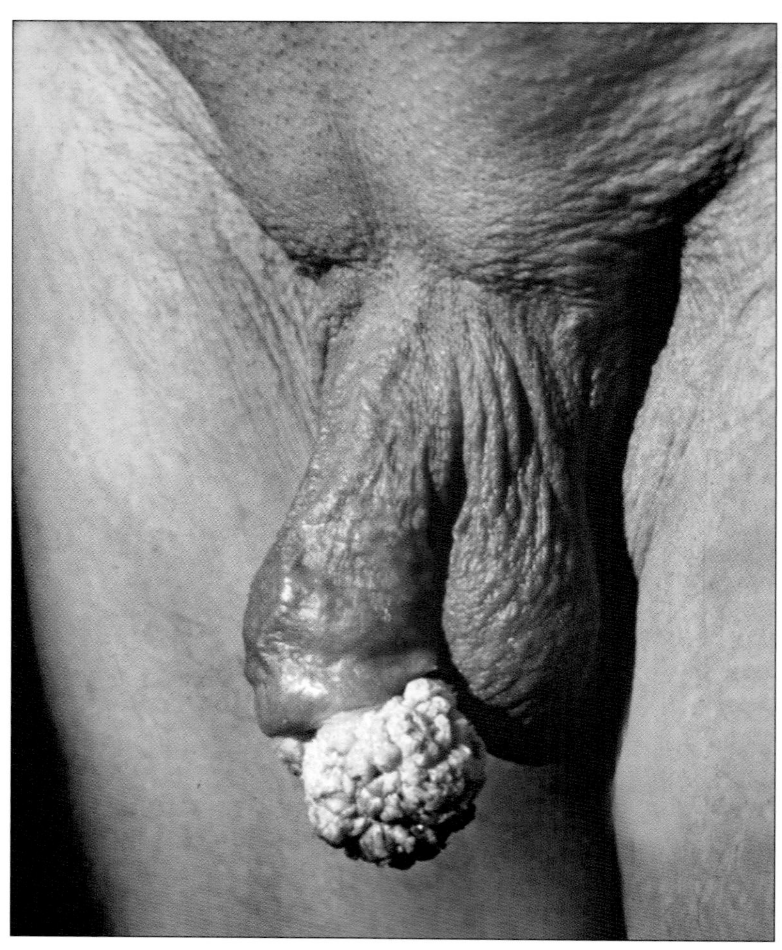

Fig. 1.49 Verrucous carcinoma is an exophytic, papillary, lobulated, gray–white tumor, typically 3–4 cm at diagnosis.

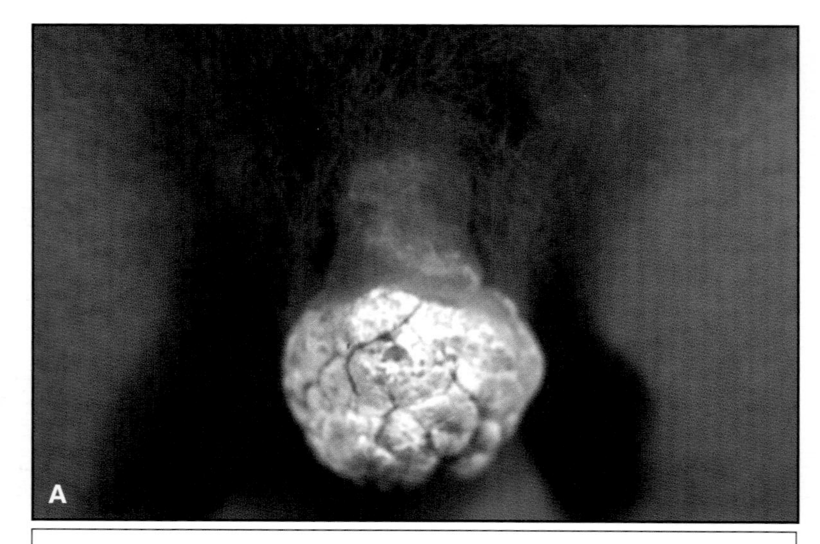

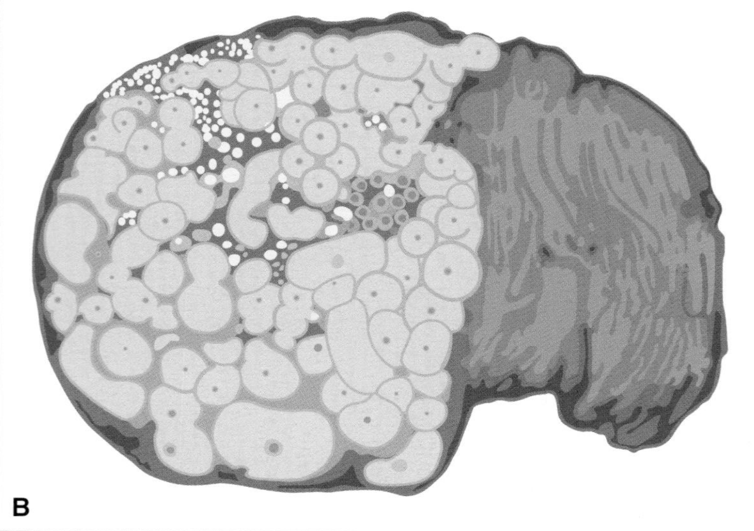

Fig. 1.50 This tumor primarily affects the head of the penis (A). The surface may be smooth and flat with fronds separated by irregular clefts. The diagram (B) stresses the broad lobulated papillae, characteristic of verrucous carcinomas.

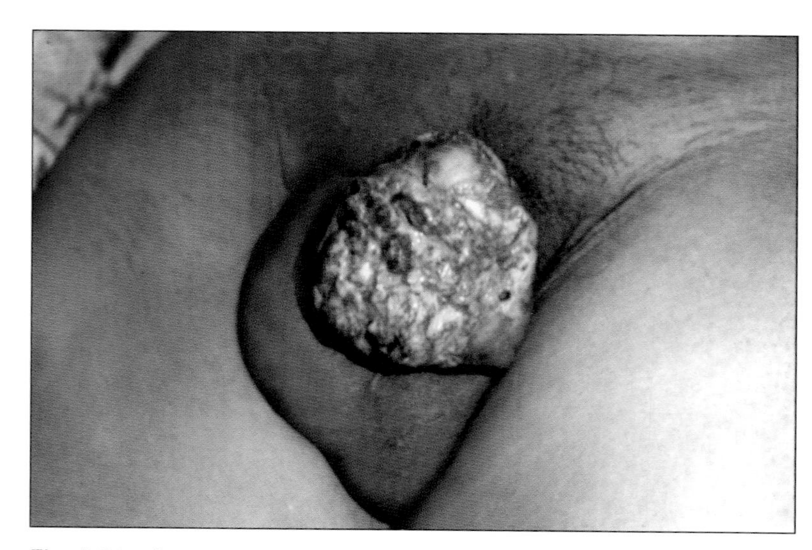

Fig. 1.51 Recurrent verrucous carcinoma.

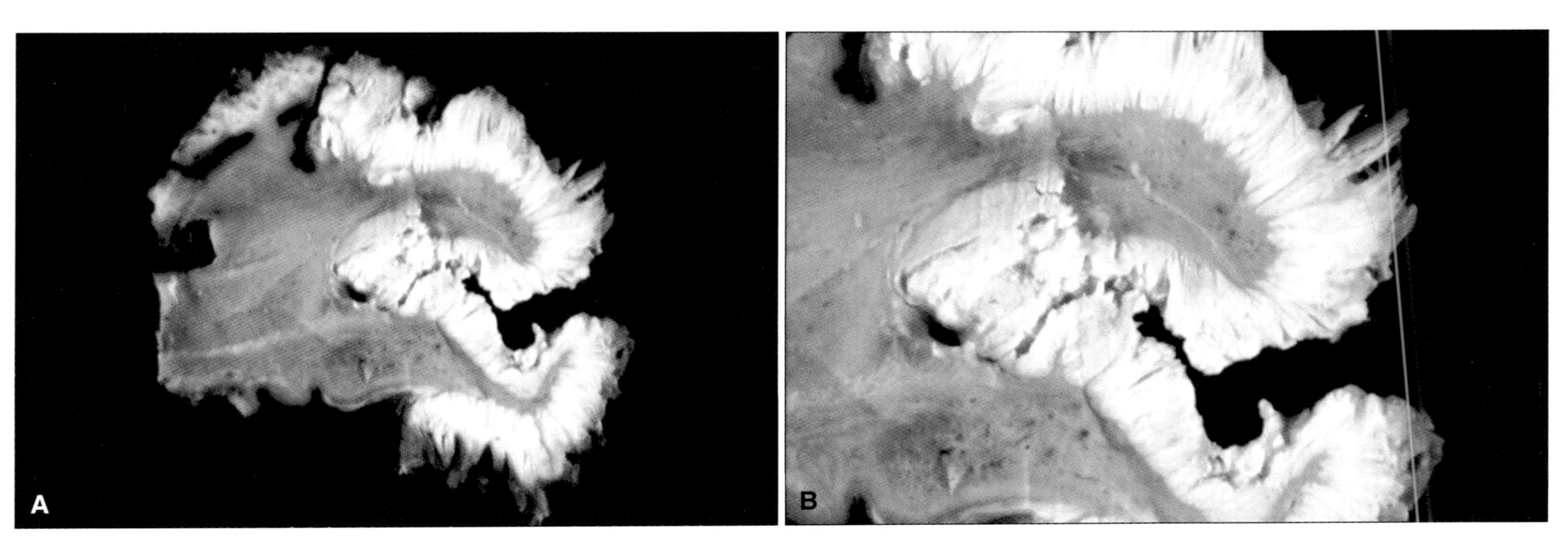

Fig. 1.52 (A,B) This verrucous carcinoma covers the entire penis. The cut surface shows a spiky appearance and a sharp boundary between tumor and stroma. There is deep invasion through the tunica albuginea into the corpus cavernosum, yet the advancing tumor border is broad and 'pushing'.

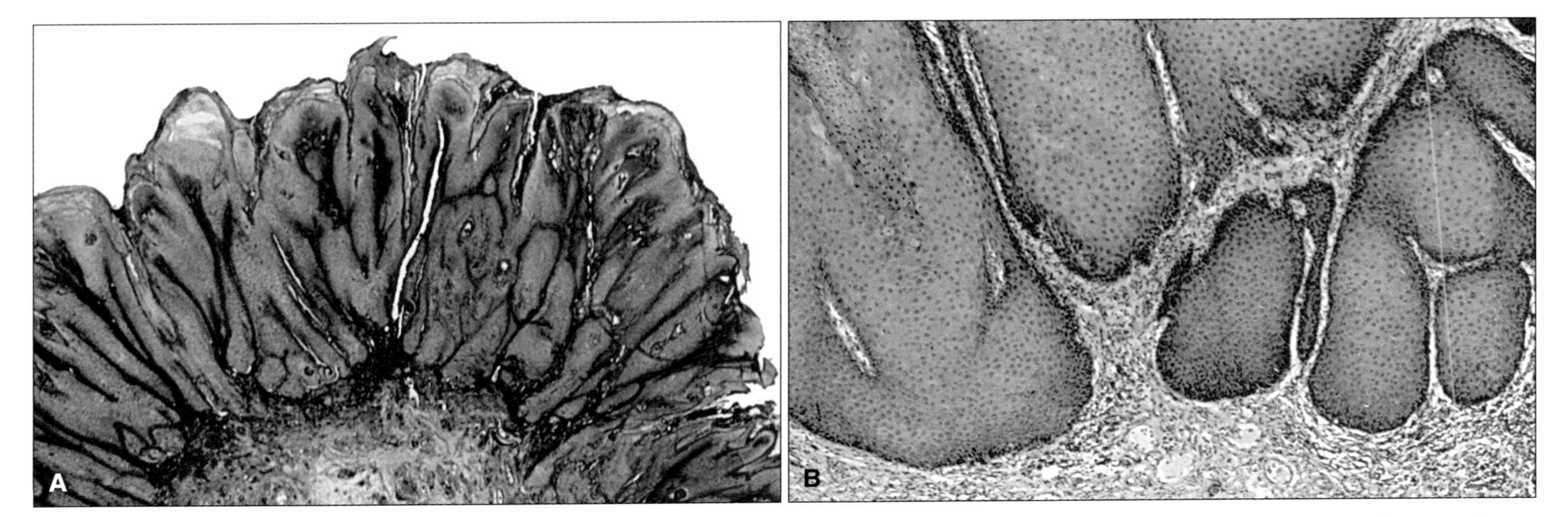

Fig. 1.53 (A,B) Microscopically, verrucous carcinoma shows hyper-orthokeratosis, papillomatosis, and acanthosis. Papillae have thin fibrovascular cores. Intraepithelial keratin plugs are usual. The interface between tumor and stroma is sharp, but a dense chronic inflammatory infiltrate may efface the border.

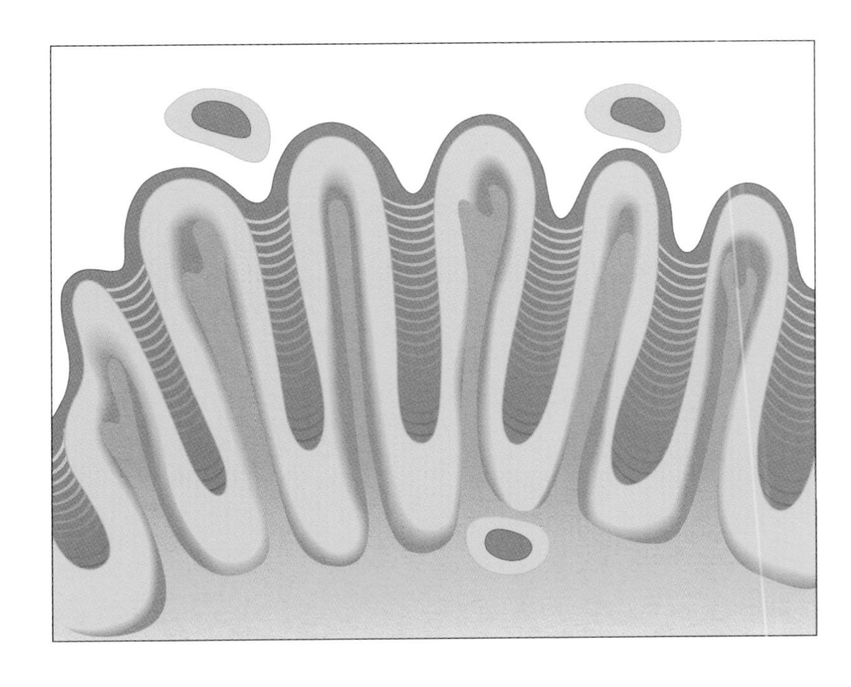

Fig. 1.54 Verrucous carcinoma. Diagrammatic representation showing regular papillae with scant fibrovascular cores, deep bulbous borders, and absent koilocytosis.

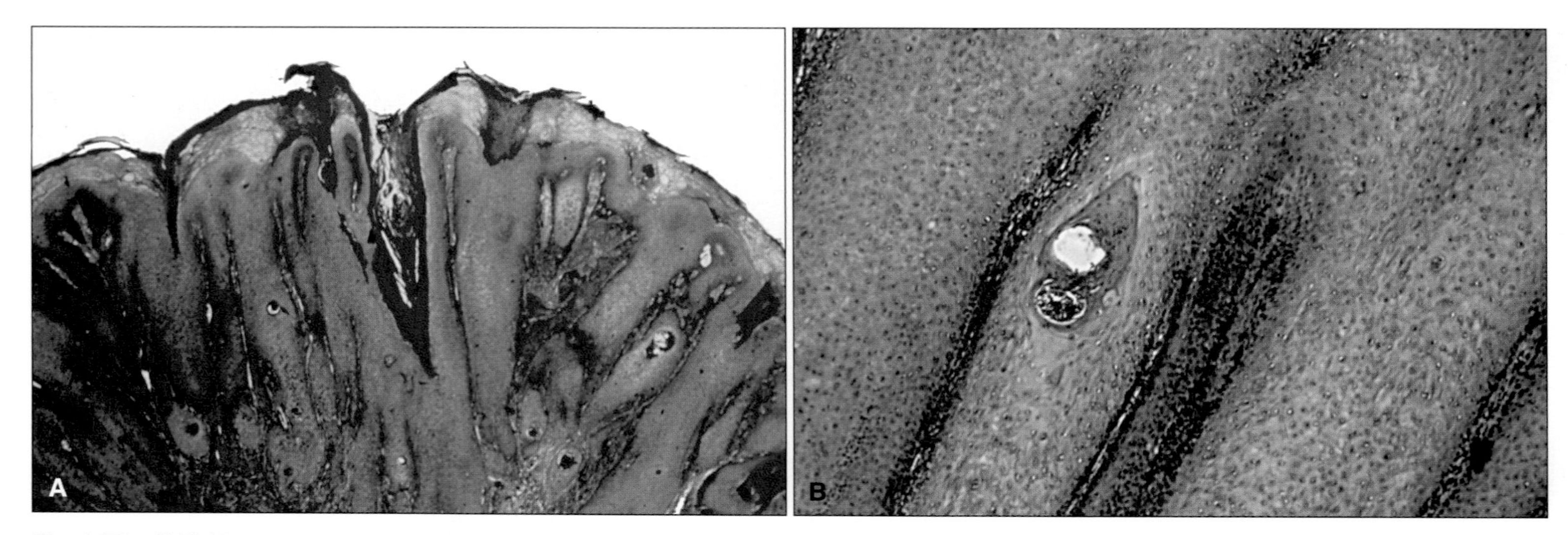

Fig. 1.55 (A,B) Verrucous carcinoma. A characteristic finding is keratin filling spaces between the papillae. In tangential sections, these keratin accumulations are seen as keratin cysts surrounded by epithelium, or may give the impression of papillae with a keratin core.

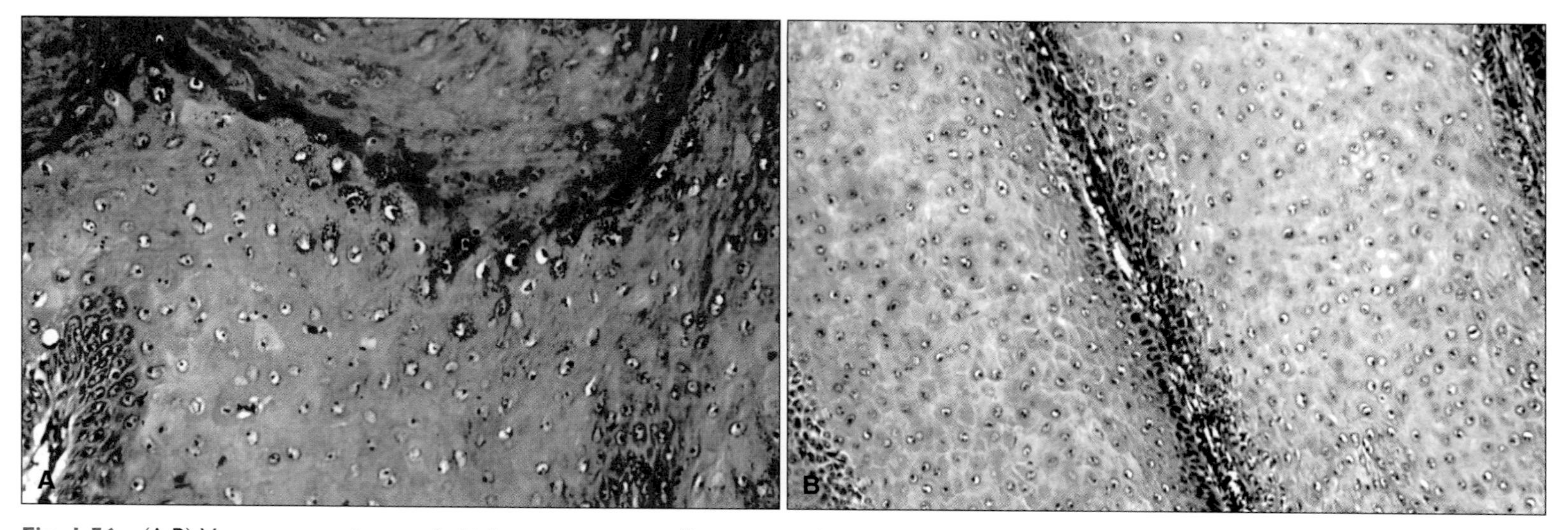

Fig. 1.56 (A,B) Verrucous carcinoma. At high power, tumor cells appear well differentiated, with little basal cell atypia. Mitoses are rare. Despite the name of this lesion, HPV-related changes are not identified.

Papillary carcinoma, not otherwise specified

This is an exophytic, low-grade, invasive penile neoplasm not classifiable as either warty or verrucous carcinoma. No metastasis occurred in a follow-up of nine patients with this neoplasm.[53] (Figs 1.57–1.60)

Sarcomatoid carcinoma

This unusual penile tumor (approximately 4% of penile malignancies) consists of spindle cells resembling fibrosarcoma or leiomyosarcoma. Median age at diagnosis is 60 years. The tumor is usually deeply invasive at diagnosis, and satellite nodules are often noted in the corpus cavernosum.[64] Heterologous differentiation (usually osteoid or cartilage) may be observed in the sarcomatoid component; osteosarcoma has even been reported in the penis.[65] Consequently, synonyms for this tumor include metaplastic carcinoma and carcinosarcoma.[66] Recurrence and metastasis to regional nodes are frequent, and mortality is high.[53,64] (Figs 1.61 & 1.62)

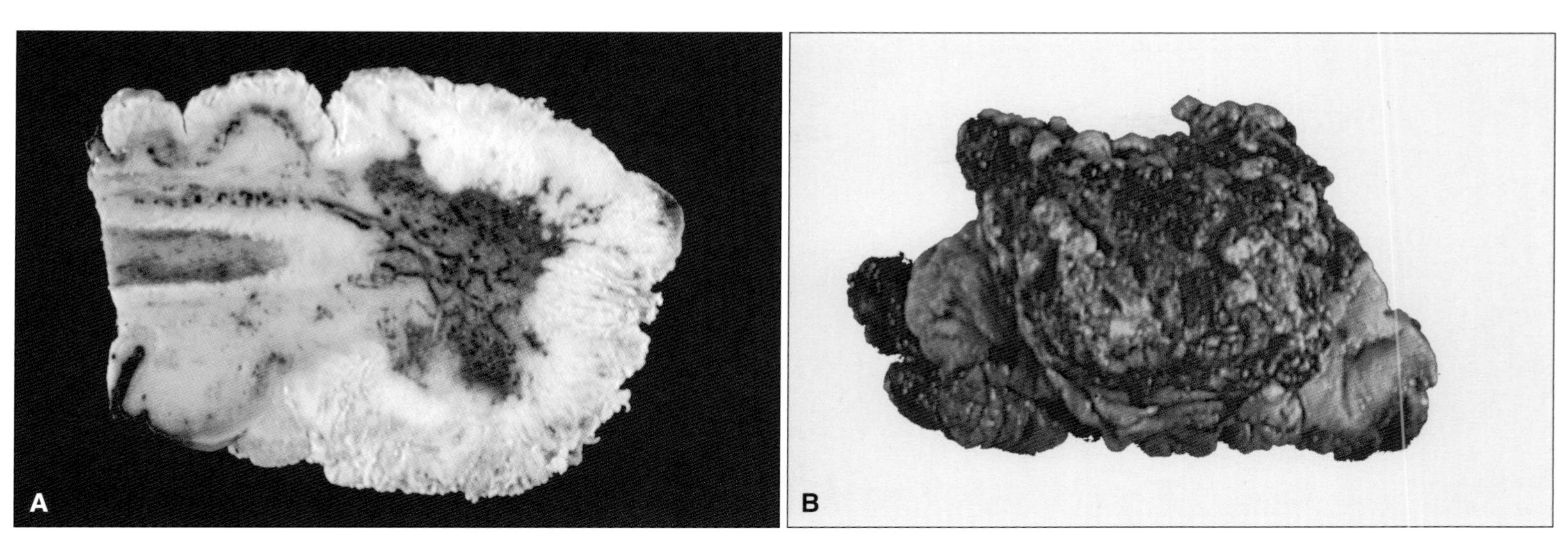

Fig. 1.57 (A,B) Papillary carcinomas are bulky, lobulated, verruciform tumors. At diagnosis, size is typically from 5 to 15 cm. The border between tumor and underlying stroma is characteristically irregular, similar to that seen in warty carcinoma, but distinct from the 'pushing' border of verrucous carcinoma.

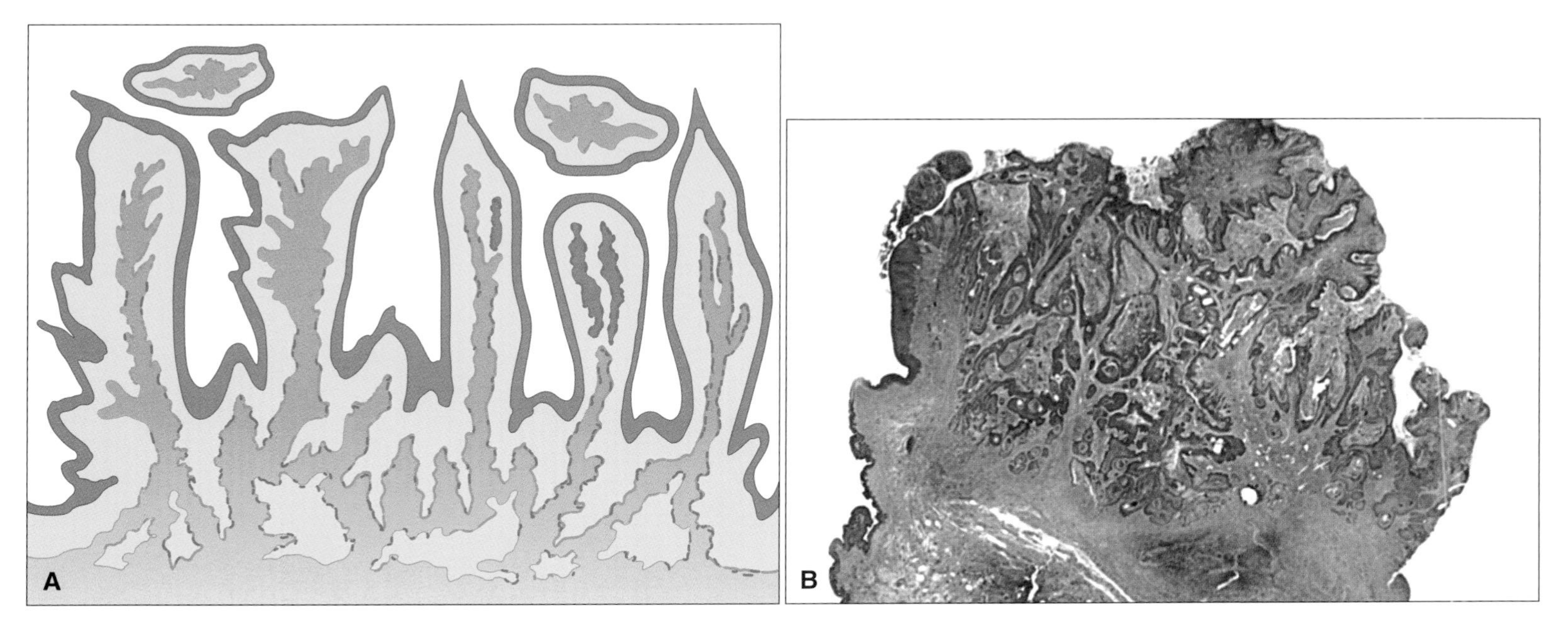

Fig. 1.58 (A,B) Microscopically, papillary carcinomas consist of long, irregular, and hyperkeratotic papillae with prominent fibrovascular cores. The absence of koilocytosis distinguishes this neoplasm from warty carcinoma. The infiltrative, irregular, and jagged invasive border distinguishes it from verrucous carcinoma.

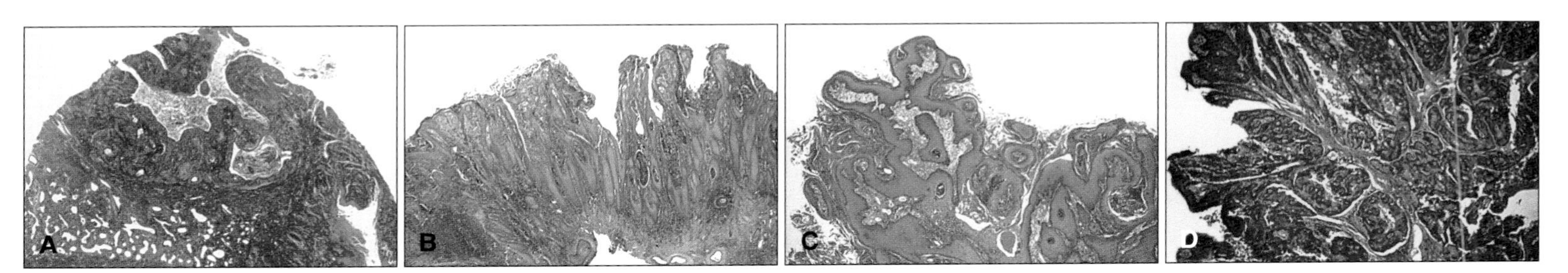

Fig. 1.59 (A–D) Papillary carcinoma. Papillae are variably long and wide, arborizing with prominent fibrovascular cores. Intermediate-power view showing the well-differentiated neoplastic cells with no koilocytotic changes. The absence of koilocytosis helps to differentiate papillary carcinoma from verrucous carcinoma.

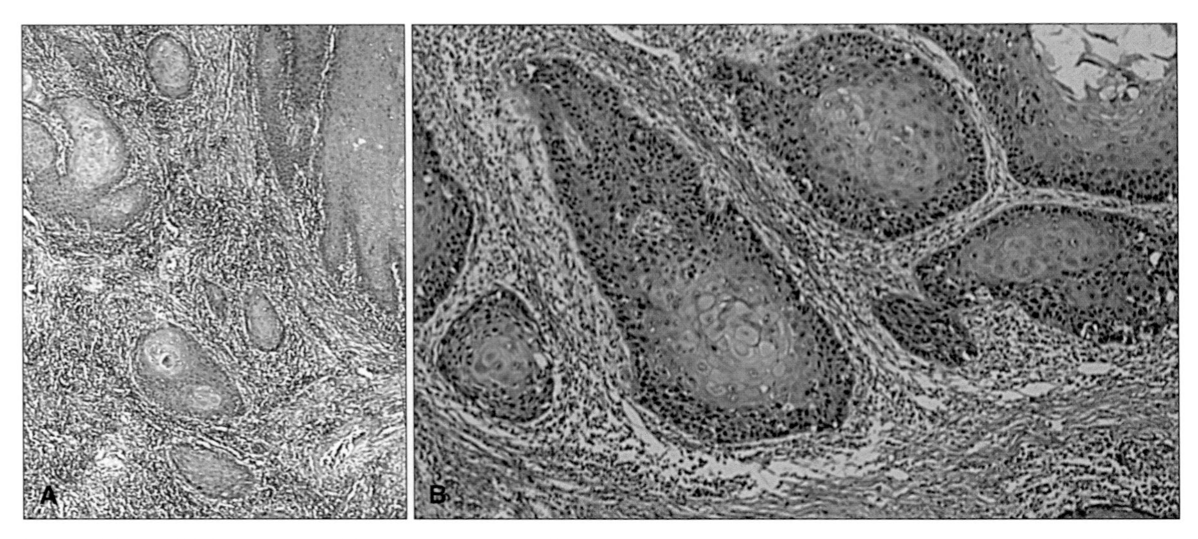

Fig. 1.60 (A,B) Although papillary carcinoma is a low-grade squamous cell carcinoma, it is never as well differentiated as verrucous carcinoma. The infiltrative, irregular, and jagged deep borders also distinguish papillary carcinoma from verrucous carcinoma, in which the border is broad and pushing.

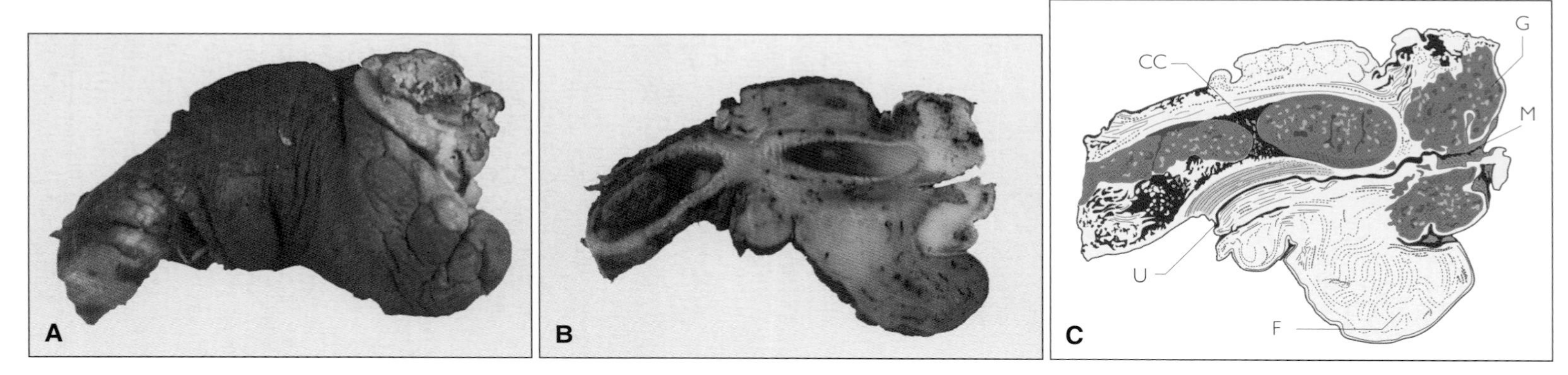

Fig. 1.61 Grossly, sarcomatoid carcinomas are gray–white, irregular masses. The distal glans of this subtotal penectomy (A) shows a granular, ulcerated mass. The cut surface (B) shows deep infiltration of the corpus spongiosum of the glans, and extension to the coronal sulcus and foreskin. Satellite nodules are present in the corpus cavernosum, a frequent finding in this highly aggressive neoplasm. In (C), the carcinoma is shown in red. CC, corpus cavernosum; G, glans; M, meatus; F, foreskin; U, urethra.

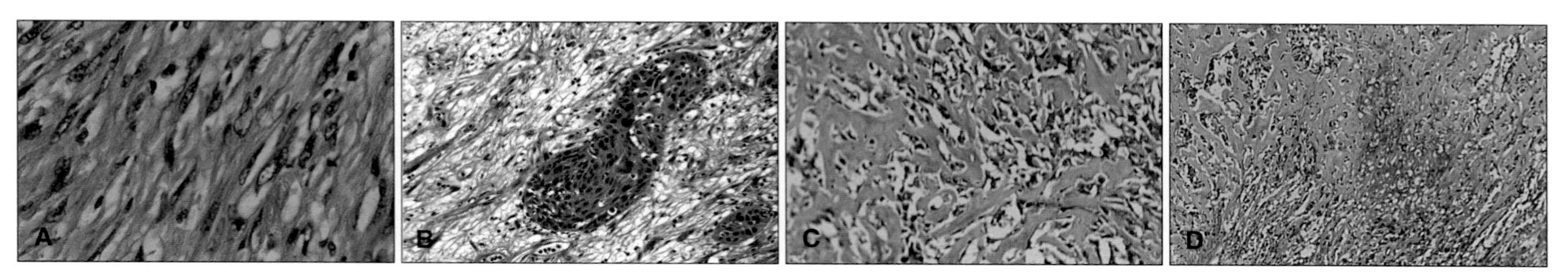

Fig. 1.62 Sarcomatoid carcinoma. (A) Fascicles of atypical spindle cells simulate sarcoma, yet, this component stained for cytokeratin and elsewhere was associated with obvious carcinoma. (B) Usually, sarcoma-like areas blend with foci of obvious squamous cell carcinoma. High-power view showing sarcomatoid areas intermixed with nests of squamous cell carcinoma. Sarcomatoid carcinoma may contain a mixture of neoplastic giant cells with bizarre, hyperchromatic nuclei, resembling a malignant fibrous histiocytoma. The tumor stroma may be myxoid, simulating myxoid fibrous histiocytoma. (C,D) Rarely, sarcomatoid carcinoma may show areas of osteoid and chondroid formation.

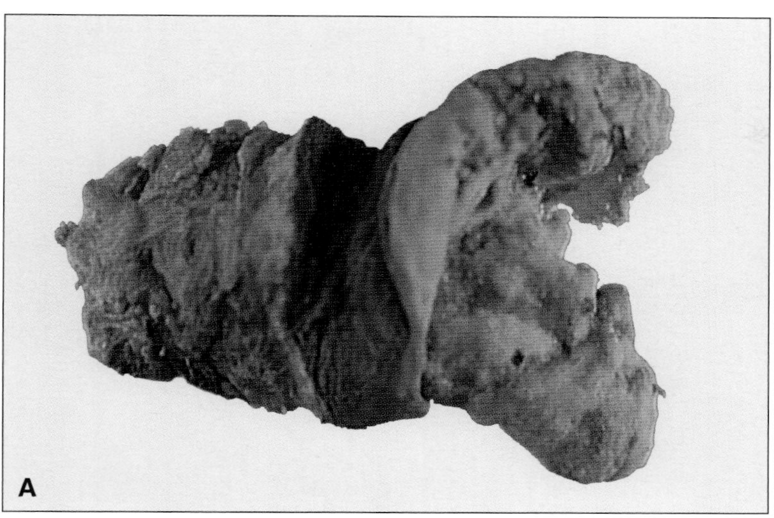
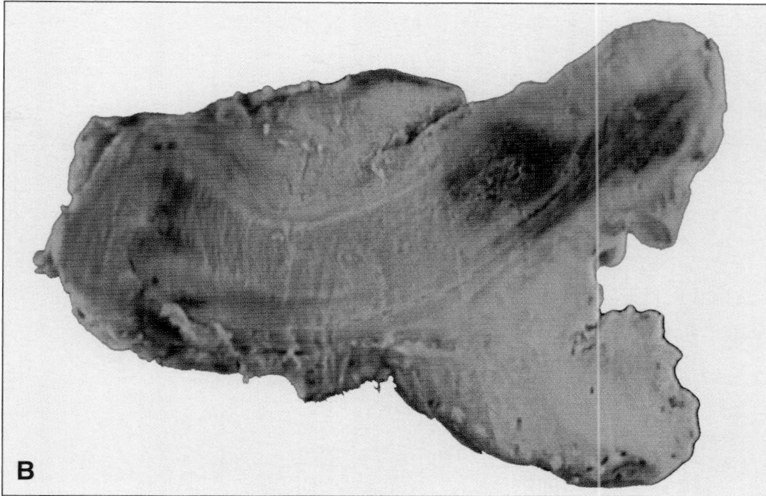

Fig. 1.63 Anaplastic carcinomas are large, destructive tumors affecting the coronal sulcus and foreskin, extending focally to the glans (A). (B) The cut surface shows a solid tan tumor growing from the foreskin to cover the glans surface.

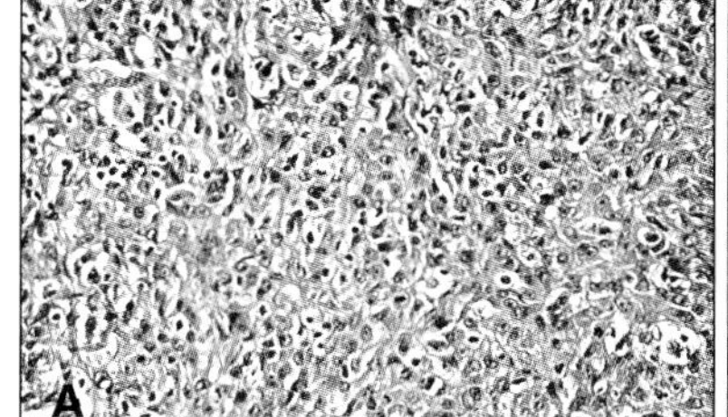
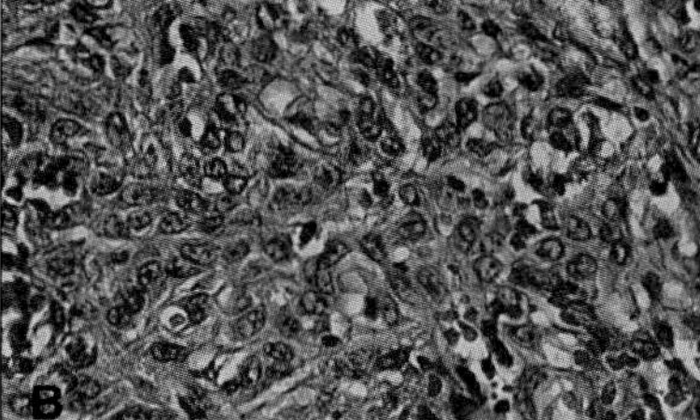
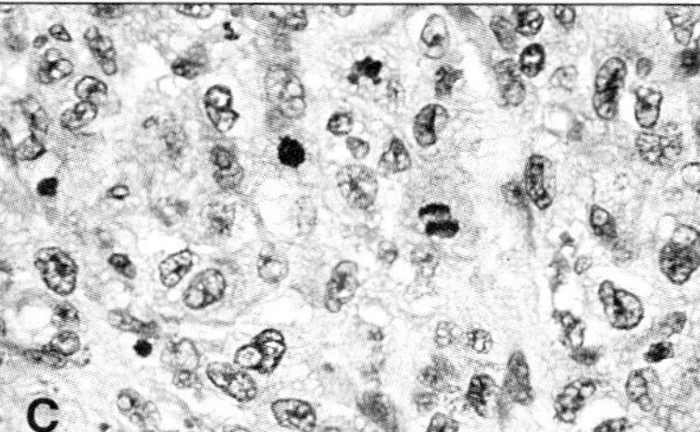
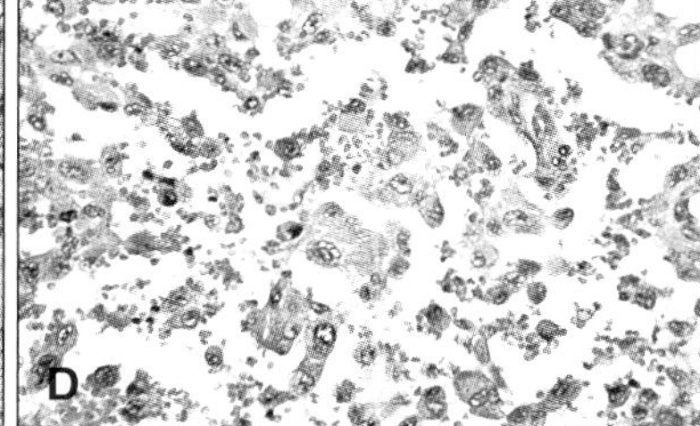

Fig. 1.64 (A,B) Anaplastic carcinoma is usually nonkeratinizing, and intercellular bridges are not identified. Neoplastic cells are round to ovoid with vesicular nuclei and prominent nucleoli. Foci of necrosis are often present. (C,D) High magnification shows many mitotic figures, and pleomorphic, undifferentiated, round to polygonal malignant cells. Loss of cohesion results in pseudovascular spaces containing erythrocytes, simulating epithelioid angiosarcoma.

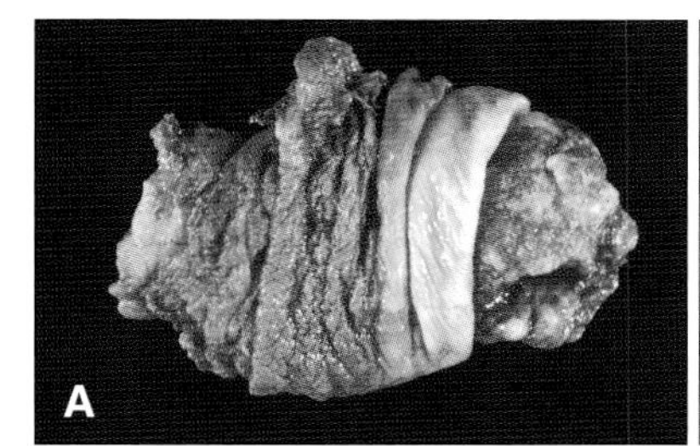
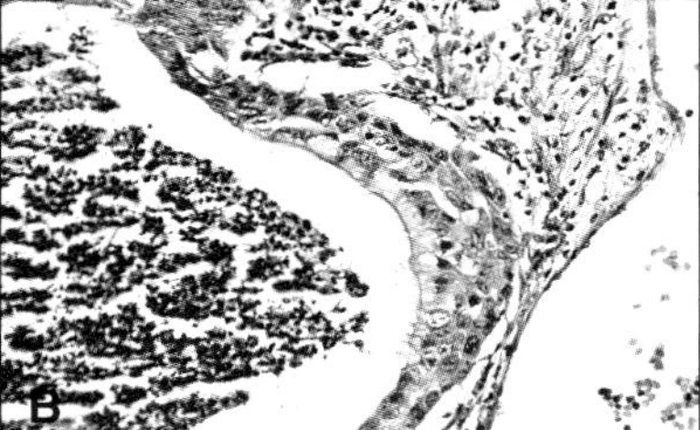
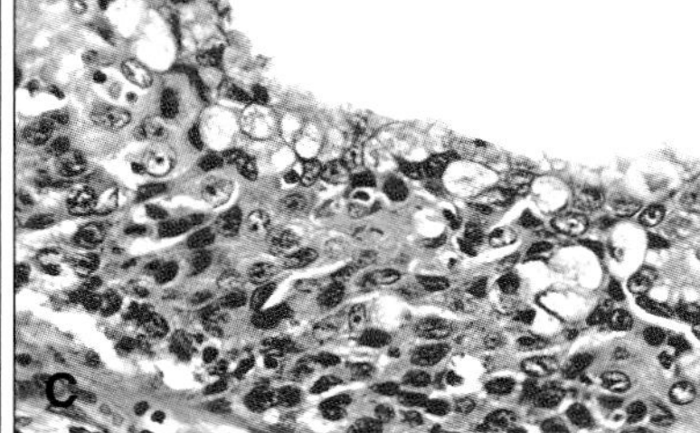
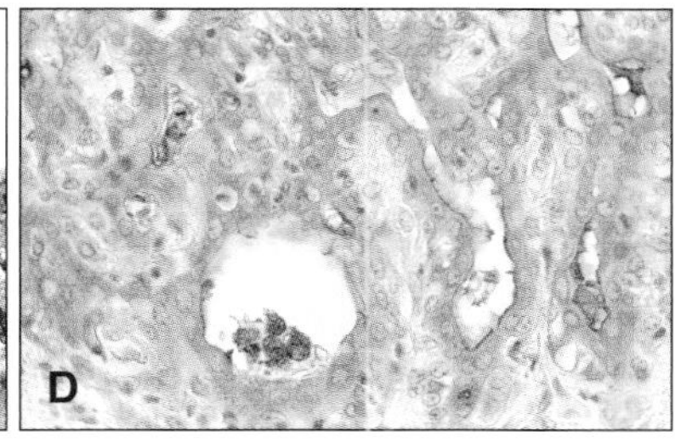

Fig. 1.65 (A) Grossly, adenosquamous carcinoma appears similar to ordinary squamous cell carcinoma. In this penectomy specimen, a granular pink–tan irregular tumor involves the distal glans. (B–D) Microscopically, nests of squamous cells contain admixed clear mucin-secreting cells or glandular structures. Glandular spaces may contain necrotic luminal debris. Carcinoembryonic antigen immunostaining (D) highlights the glandular component.

Anaplastic carcinoma

This unusual variant of penile carcinoma has a presentation similar to that of typical squamous cell carcinoma, but lacks histologic evidence of squamous differentiation. It is an aggressive neoplasm, with regional metastasis typical at diagnosis. (Figs 1.63 & 1.64)

Adenosquamous carcinoma

These composite tumors show both keratinizing squamous and mucinous glandular features.[67,68] The squamous cells predominate over the glandular component. When the mucinous features are focal, the tumor has been called mucoepidermoid carcinoma.[69,70] It must be distinguished from adenocarcinoma arising in periurethral (Littré) glands and from urothelial carcinoma with glandular metaplasia, neither of which show concomitant surface dysplasia. There is little information regarding the behavior of this rare neoplasm. (Fig. 1.65)

Mixed tumors

About a third of penile neoplasms contain a mixture of tumor subtypes. The so-called hybrid verrucous carcinoma,

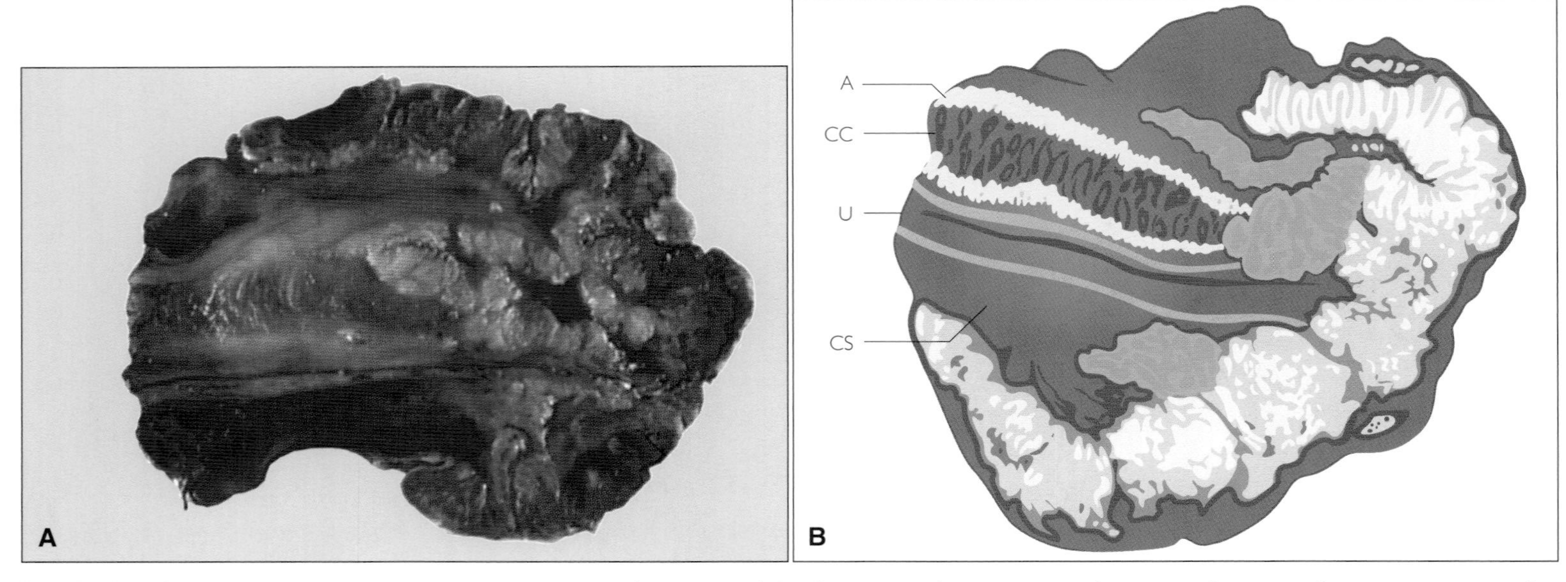

Fig. 1.66 (A) Mixed verrucous–squamous cell carcinoma (verrucous 'hybrid' carcinoma) presents as a large, exophytic, papillomatous tumor replacing the distal penis. (B) The cut surface shows an endophytic component (blue) of typical moderately differentiated squamous cell carcinoma deeply invading through the albuginea (A) into the corpora (CS, CC), but not involving the urethra (U). This tumor has gross features of a carcinoma cuniculatum.

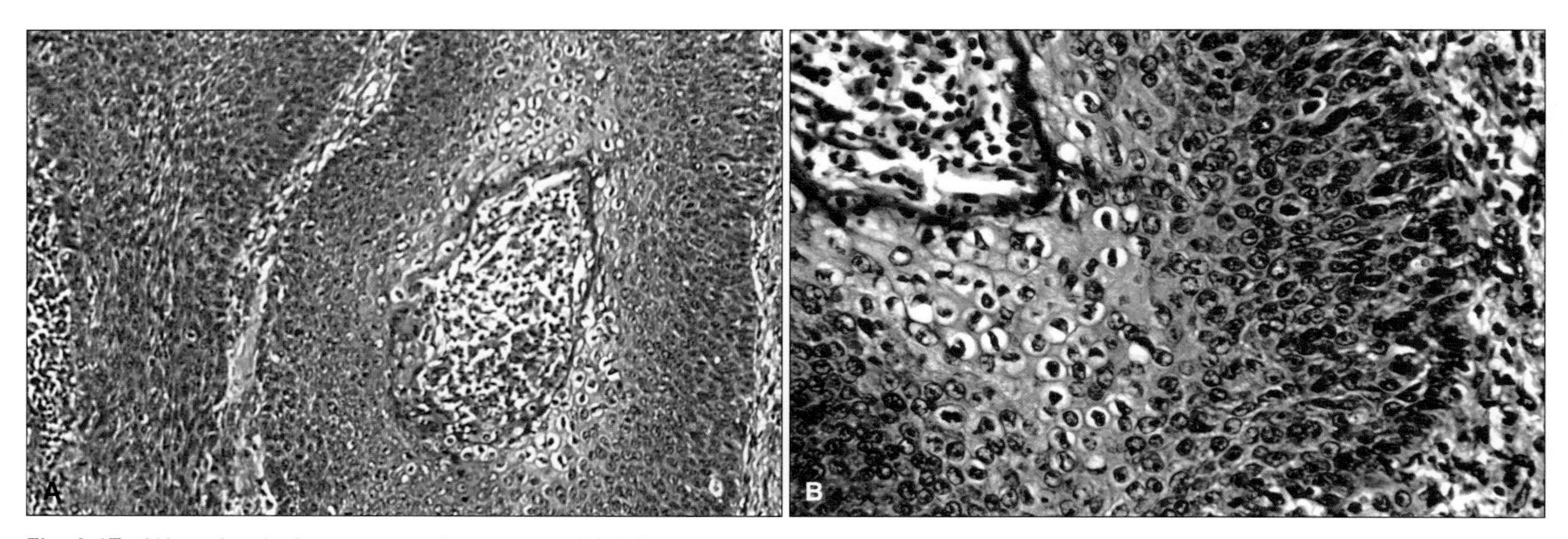

Fig. 1.67 Warty–basaloid squamous cell carcinoma. (A) Infiltrative neoplastic nests, with central necrosis, a mixed clear and dark cell pattern and the characteristic palisading of basaloid carcinoma. (B) Higher-power view reveals a mixed tumor composed of basaloid, undifferentiated cells at the periphery of the nests. In more superficial areas and at the center of the neoplastic nests, the cells are larger and exhibit koilocytotic changes similar to those seen in warty carcinoma.

a composite of typical squamous cell carcinoma and verrucous carcinoma, is the most common.[61] Recognition of these lesions is important because the metastatic potential is that of the more aggressive component.[71] Verrucous carcinomas may also occur mixed with sarcomatoid carcinoma.[72] Another interesting mixed tumor is the warty–basaloid carcinoma, an unusual combination of two tumors both related to HPV infection.[73] Another recently described, usually mixed variant of verrucous carcinoma is the so-called 'carcinoma cuniculatum' of the penis.[74] This tumor affects older patients and is characterized by labyrinthine endophytic growth simulating rabbit burrows. Similar neoplasms have been described in the skin and other sites. The term cuniculatum is attributed to Ayrd, who in 1954 described a group of plantar neoplasms with analogous morphologic characteristics. Initially the tumor resembles a plantar wart but it slowly progresses to an exophytic tumor, which eventually becomes ulcerated, developing numerous sinuses from which a foul-smelling keratinous material can be expressed.[74] Most carcinomata cuniculata represent mixed variants of verrucous and usual squamous cell carcinomas. Despite the deep invasion, they are usually not associated with regional or systemic dissemination at time of diagnosis. (Figs 1.66–1.68)

Rare tumors[75,76]

(Figs 1.69–1.73)

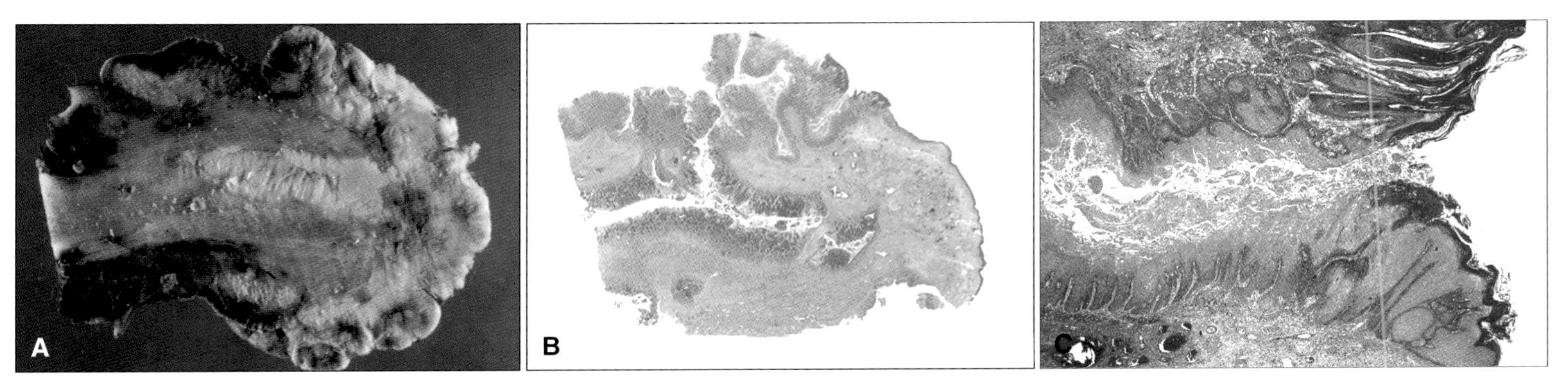

Fig. 1.68 Carcinoma cuniculatum. (A) Cut surface reveals the hallmark of this lesion: a deep labyrinthine endophytic growth simulating rabbit burrows. (B) Low-power view shows a verruciform, hyperkeratotic lesion with deep tumoral sinuses. (C) Hyperkeratotic opening of the deep sinuses into the surface.

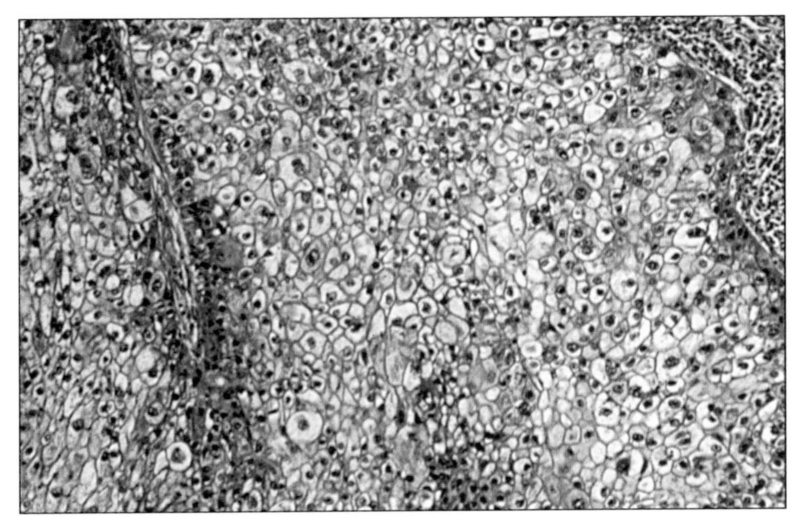

Fig. 1.69 Clear cell carcinoma is a solid nonkeratinizing variant of squamous cell carcinoma, with a heavily glycogenated cytoplasm. Polygonal cells with well-defined borders, clear cytoplasm, pleomorphic nuclei, and prominent nucleoli comprise the tumor. Clear cell change is a frequent focal finding in otherwise typical carcinoma; this category is reserved for rare tumors in which almost all the cells display this cytology.

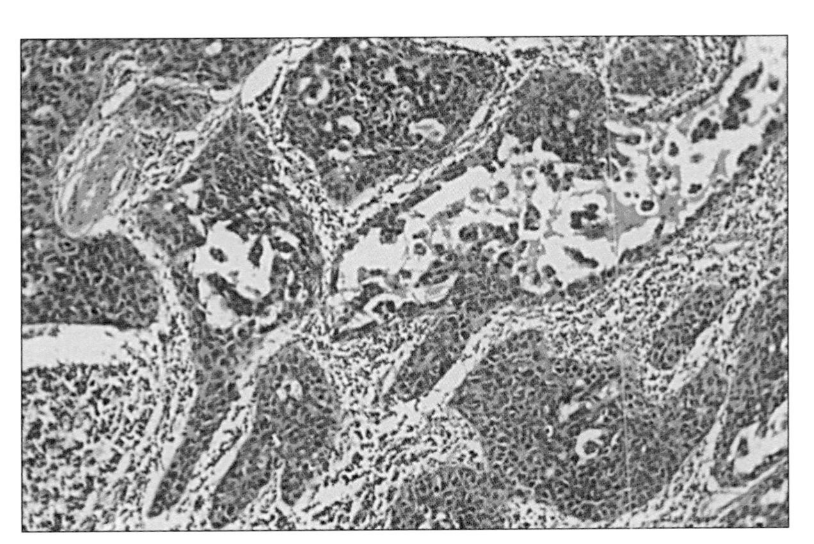

Fig. 1.70 Acantholytic (adenoid) carcinoma shows pseudoglandular features secondary to acantholysis of neoplastic cells. Acantholytic cells are numerous and easily identified in the center of the neoplastic nests. This variant of squamous cell carcinoma should not be confused with true adenosquamous carcinoma.

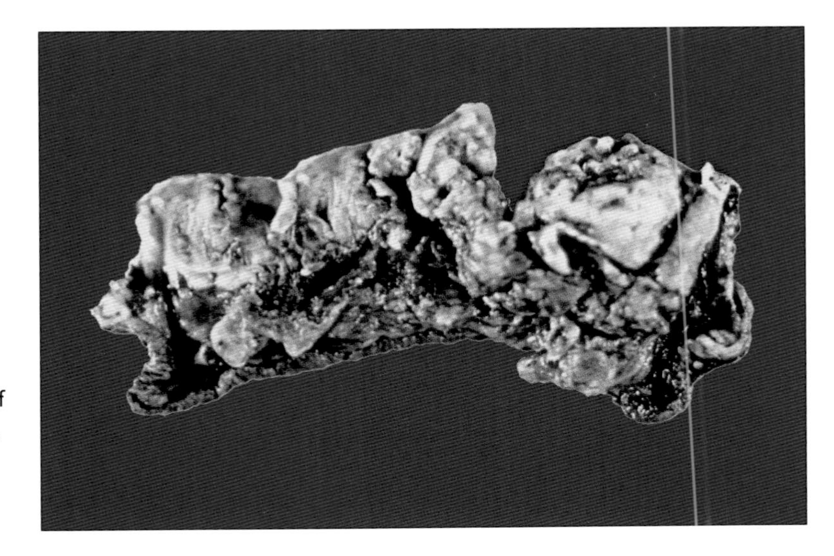

Fig. 1.71 An extremely well-differentiated 'pseudohyperplastic' variant of squamous cell carcinoma was recently described.[77] This unusual low-grade, verruciform neoplasm affects the prepuce of older patients and is often associated with lichen sclerosus. Grossly, the tumor appears as irregular nodules on the mucosal surface.

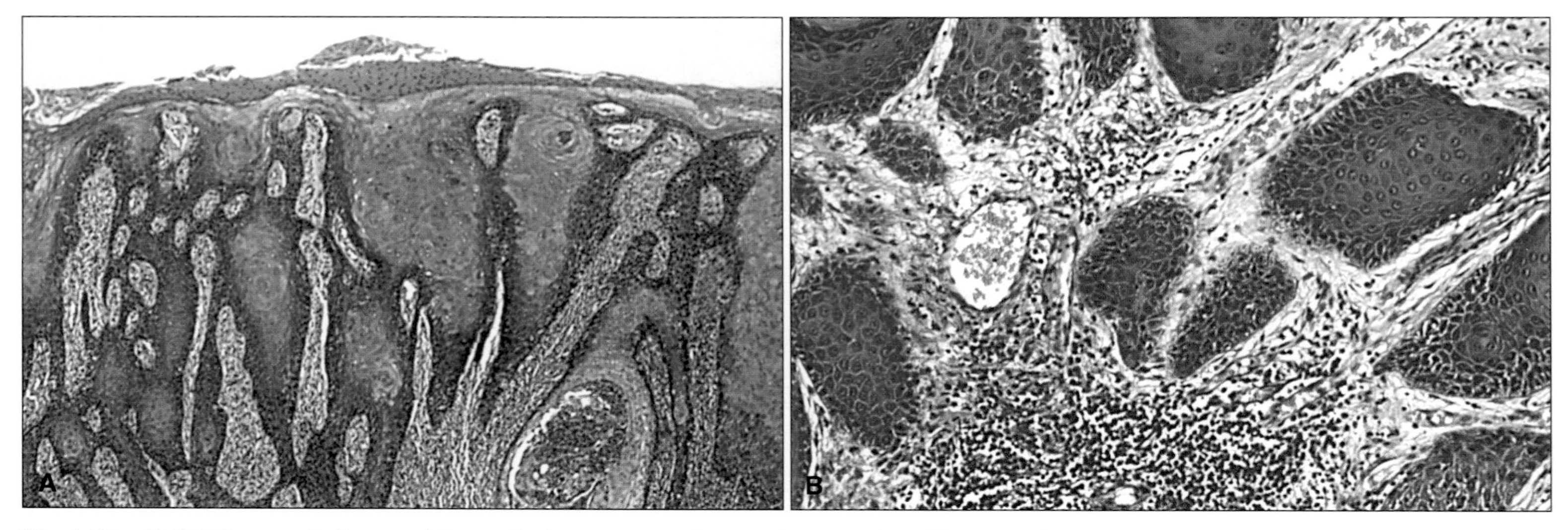

Fig. 1.72 (A,B) Microscopically, pseudohyperplastic carcinoma shows a downward proliferation of cytologically benign-appearing squamous cells. However, the border between tumor and stroma is irregular, signifying invasiveness.

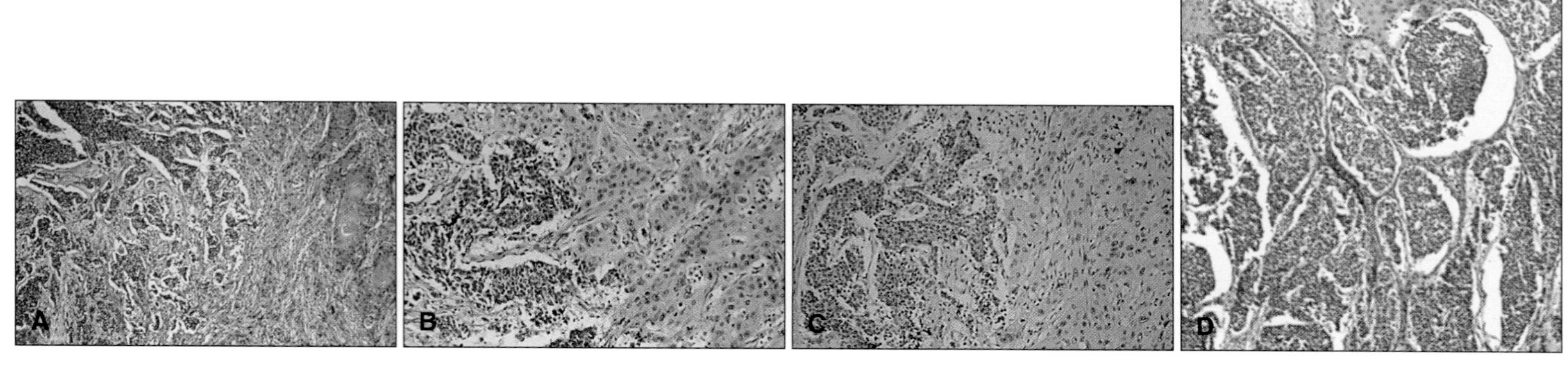

Fig. 1.73 (A–D) An unusual composite squamous–neuroendocrine carcinoma shows the small cell, neuroendocrine component to the left and the usual squamous cell carcinoma to the right. Chromogranin stain is diffusely positive in the small cell carcinoma. Nests of small, hyperchromatic, and undifferentiated cells invade the hyperplastic epidermis.

REFERENCES

1. Velazquez EF, Cold C, Barreto J, et al. Penis. In: Mills SE, ed. Sternberg's histology for pathologists. 3rd edn. Philadelphia: Lippincott Williams & Wilkins; 2005 (in press).
2. Cold CJ, Taylor JR. The prepuce. BJU Int 1999;83(Suppl 1):34–44.
3. Velazquez EF, Bock A, Soskin A, et al. Preputial variability and preferential association of long phimotic foreskins with penile cancer: an anatomic comparative study of types of foreskin in a general population and cancer patients. Am J Surg Pathol 2003;27:994–998.
4. Kageyama S, Ueda T, Kushima R, Sakamoto T. Primary adenosquamous cell carcinoma of the male distal urethra: magnetic resonance imaging using a circular surface coil. J Urol 1997;158:1913–1914.
5. Cubilla AL, Piris A, Pfannl R, Rodriguez I, Aguero F, Young RH. Anatomic levels: important landmarks in penectomy specimens: a detailed anatomic and histologic study based on examination of 44 cases. Am J Surg Pathol 2001;25:1091–1094.
6. Fang AW, Whittaker MA, Theaker JM. Mucinous metaplasia of the penis. Histopathology 2002;40:177–179.
7. Ayala TM, Piris A, Cubilla AL. Epithelial lesions associated with invasive squamous cell carcinoma of the penis: a study of 152 resected specimens. Lab Invest 1999;79:88A.
8. Cubilla AL, Meijer CJ, Young RH. Morphological features of epithelial abnormalities and precancerous lesions of the penis. Scand J Urol Nephrol Suppl 2000;(205):215–219.
9. Higgins GD, Uzelin DM, Phillips GE, Villa LL, Burrell CJ. Differing prevalence of human papillomavirus RNA in penile dysplasias and carcinomas may reflect differing etiologies. Am J Clin Pathol 1992;97:272–278.
10. Aynaud O, Ionesco M, Barrasso R. Penile intraepithelial neoplasia. Specific clinical features correlate with histologic and virologic findings. Cancer 1994;74:1762–1767.
11. Malek RS, Goellner JR, Smith TF, Espy MJ, Cupp MR. Human papillomavirus infection and intraepithelial, in situ, and invasive carcinoma of penis. Urology 1993;42:159–170.
12. von Krogh G, Horenblas S. Diagnosis and clinical presentation of premalignant lesions of the penis. Scand J Urol Nephrol Suppl 2000;(205): 201–214.
13. Horenblas S, von Krogh G, Cubilla AL, Dillner J, Meijer CJ, Hedlund PO. Squamous cell carcinoma of the penis: premalignant lesions. Scand J Urol Nephrol Suppl 2000;(205):187–188.

14. Gerber GS. Carcinoma in situ of the penis. J Urol 1994;151:829–833.
15. Lucia MS, Miller GJ. Histopathology of malignant lesions of the penis. Urol Clin North Am 1992;19:227–246.
16. Graham JH, Helwig EB. Erythroplasia of Queyrat. A clinicopathologic and histochemical study. Cancer 1973;32:1396–1414.
17. Kaye V, Zhang G, Dehner LP, Fraley EE. Carcinoma in situ of penis. Is distinction between erythroplasia of Queyrat and Bowen's disease relevant? Urology 1990;36:479–482.
18. Jaeger AB, Gramkow A, Hjalgrim H, Melbye M, Frisch M. Bowen disease and risk of subsequent malignant neoplasms: a population-based cohort study of 1147 patients. Arch Dermatol 1999;135:790–793.
19. Nuovo GJ, Hochman HA, Eliezri YD, Lastarria D, Comite SL, Silvers DN. Detection of human papillomavirus DNA in penile lesions histologically negative for condylomata. Analysis by in situ hybridization and the polymerase chain reaction. Am J Surg Pathol 1990;14:829–836.
20. Demeter LM, Stoler MH, Bonnez W, et al. Penile intraepithelial neoplasia: clinical presentation and an analysis of the physical state of human papillomavirus DNA. J Infect Dis 1993;168:38–46.
21. Ikenberg H, Gissmann L, Gross G, Grussendorf-Conen EI, zur Hausen H. Human papillomavirus type-16-related DNA in genital Bowen's disease and in Bowenoid papulosis. Int J Cancer 1983;32:563–565.
22. Barrasso R, De Brux J, Croissant O, Orth G. High prevalence of papillomavirus-associated penile intraepithelial neoplasia in sexual partners of women with cervical intraepithelial neoplasia. N Engl J Med 1987;317: 916–923.
23. Wade TR, Kopf AW, Ackerman AB. Bowenoid papulosis of the penis. Cancer 1978;42:1890–1903.
24. Wade TR, Kopf AW, Ackerman AB. Bowenoid papulosis of the genitalia. Arch Dermatol 1979;115:306–308.
25. Eisen RF, Bhawan J, Cahn TH. Spontaneous regression of bowenoid papulosis of the penis. Cutis 1983;32:269–272.
26. Hewitt J. Histologic criteria for lichen sclerosus of the vulva. J Reprod Med 1986;31:781–787.
27. Carlson JA, Ambros R, Malfetano J, et al. Vulvar lichen sclerosus and squamous cell carcinoma: a cohort, case control, and investigational study with historical perspective; implications for chronic inflammation and sclerosis in the development of neoplasia. Hum Pathol 1998;29: 932–948.
28. Powell JJ, Wojnarowska F. Lichen sclerosus. Lancet 1999;353: 1777–1783.
29. Velazquez EF, Cubilla AL. Lichen sclerosus in 68 patients with squamous cell carcinoma of the penis: frequent atypias and correlation with special carcinoma variants suggests a precancerous role. Am J Surg Pathol 2003; 27:1448–1453.
30. Oertell J, Duarte S, Ayala J, et al. Squamous cell carcinoma exclusive of the foreskin: distinctive association with low-grade variants, multicentricity and lichen sclerosus. Mod Pathol 2002;15:175A.
31. Nasca MR, Innocenzi D, Micali G. Penile cancer among patients with genital lichen sclerosus. J Am Acad Dermatol 1999;41:911–914.
32. Bain L, Geronemus R. The association of lichen planus of the penis with squamous cell carcinoma in situ and with verrucous squamous carcinoma. J Dermatol Surg Oncol 1989;15:413–417.
33. Powell J, Robson A, Cranston D, Wojnarowska F, Turner R. High incidence of lichen sclerosus in patients with squamous cell carcinoma of the penis. Br J Dermatol 2001;145:85–89.
34. Young RH, Srigley JR, Amin MB, Ulbright TM, Cubilla AL. Tumors of the prostate gland, seminal vesicles, male urethra, and penis. Atlas of tumor pathology. Third Series; no. 28. Rosai J, Sobin LH, series editors. Washington, DC: Armed Forces Institute of Pathology; 2000.
35. Cubilla AL, Velazquez EF, Reuter VE, Oliva E, Mihm MC Jr, Young RH. Warty (condylomatous) squamous cell carcinoma of the penis: a report of 11 cases and proposed classification of 'verruciform' penile tumors. Am J Surg Pathol 2000;24:505–512.
36. Niederauer HH, Weindorf N, Schultz-Ehrenburg U. [A case of giant condyloma acuminatum. On differential diagnosis of giant condylomas from Buschke-Lowenstein tumors and verrucous carcinoma.] Hautarzt 1993;44:795–799.
37. Velazquez EF, Barreto JE, Rodríguez I. Coexisting benign condylomas and squamous cell carcinoma of the penis: preferential association with the warty and basaloid variants. Mod Pathol 2001;14:127A.
38. Kim ED, Kroft S, Dalton DP. Basal cell carcinoma of the penis: case report and review of the literature. J Urol 1994;152(5 Pt 1):1557–1559.
39. Mitsudo S, Nakanishi I, Koss LG. Paget's disease of the penis and adjacent skin: its association with fatal sweat gland carcinoma. Arch Pathol Lab Med 1981;105:518–520.
40. Park S, Grossfeld GD, McAninch JW, Santucci R. Extramammary Paget's disease of the penis and scrotum: excision, reconstruction and evaluation of occult malignancy. J Urol 2001;166:2112–2116; discussion 2117.
41. Parkin DM, Muir CS, Whelan SL, Gao YT, Ferlay J, Powell J. Cancer incidence in five continents. Volume VI. IARC Scientific Publications; no. 120. Lyon, France: IARC Press; 1992.
42. Brinton LA, Li JY, Rong SD, et al. Risk factors for penile cancer: results from a case-control study in China. Int J Cancer 1991;47:504–509.
43. Maden C, Sherman KJ, Beckmann AM, et al. History of circumcision, medical conditions, and sexual activity and risk of penile cancer. J Natl Cancer Inst 1993;85:19–24.
44. Dillner J, Meijer CJ, von Krogh G, Horenblas S. Epidemiology of human papillomavirus infection. Scand J Urol Nephrol Suppl 2000;(205):194–200.
45. Tsen HF, Morgenstern H, Mack T, Peters RK. Risk factors for penile cancer: results of a population-based case-control study in Los Angeles County (United States). Cancer Causes Control 2001;12:267–277.
46. Rubin MA, Kleter B, Zhou M, et al. Detection and typing of human papillomavirus DNA in penile carcinoma: evidence for multiple independent pathways of penile carcinogenesis. Am J Pathol 2001;159: 1211–1218.
47. Gregoire L, Cubilla AL, Reuter VE, Haas GP, Lancaster WD. Preferential association of human papillomavirus with high-grade histologic variants of penile-invasive squamous cell carcinoma. J Natl Cancer Inst 1995;87:1705–1709.
48. Emerson RE, Ulbright TM, Eble JN, Geary WA, Eckert GJ, Cheng L. Predicting cancer progression in patients with penile squamous cell carcinoma: the importance of depth of invasion and vascular invasion. Mod Pathol 2001;14:963–968.
49. Slaton JW, Morgenstern N, Levy DA, et al. Tumor stage, vascular invasion and the percentage of poorly differentiated cancer: independent prognosticators for inguinal lymph node metastasis in penile squamous cancer. J Urol 2001;165:1138–1142.
50. Solsona E, Iborra I, Rubio J, Casanova JL, Ricos JV, Calabuig C. Prospective validation of the association of local tumor stage and grade as a predictive factor for occult lymph node micrometastasis in patients with penile carcinoma and clinically negative inguinal lymph nodes. J Urol 2001;165: 1506–1509.
51. Cubilla AL, Barreto J, Caballero C, Ayala G, Riveros M. Pathologic features of epidermoid carcinoma of the penis. A prospective study of 66 cases. Am J Surg Pathol 1993;17:753–763.
52. Villavicencio H, Rubio-Briones J, Regalado R, Chechile G, Algaba F, Palou J. Grade, local stage and growth pattern as prognostic factors in carcinoma of the penis. Eur Urol 1997;32:442–447.
53. Cubilla AL, Reuter V, Velazquez E, Piris A, Saito S, Young RH. Histologic classification of penile carcinoma and its relation to outcome in 61 patients with primary resection. Int J Surg Pathol 2001;9:111–120.
54. Cubilla AL, Tamboli P, Amin MB, et al. Geographical comparison of subtypes of penile squamous cell carcinoma from regions of high and low incidence. Lab Invest 2000;80:97A.
55. Lopes A, Bezerra AL, Pinto CA, Serrano SV, de Mell OC, Villa LL. p53 as a new prognostic factor for lymph node metastasis in penile carcinoma: analysis of 82 patients treated with amputation and bilateral lymphadenectomy. J Urol 2002;168:81–86.
56. Cubilla AL, Reuter VE, Gregoire L, et al. Basaloid squamous cell carcinoma: a distinctive human papilloma virus-related penile neoplasm: a report of 20 cases. Am J Surg Pathol 1998;22:755–761.
57. Tran TA, Tamboli P, Ayala G, et al. Basaloid squamous cell carcinoma of the penis: a clinicopathologic study of 11 cases. Lab Invest 2000;80:117A.
58. Bezerra AL, Lopes A, Landman G, Alencar GN, Torloni H, Villa LL. Clinicopathologic features and human papillomavirus DNA prevalence of warty and squamous cell carcinoma of the penis. Am J Surg Pathol 2001; 25:673–678.
59. Poblet E, Alfaro L, Fernander-Segoviano P, Jimenez-Reyes J, Salido EC. Human papillomavirus-associated penile squamous cell carcinoma in HIV-positive patients. Am J Surg Pathol 1999;23:1119–1123.
60. Aboulafia DM, Gibbons R. Penile cancer and human papilloma virus (HPV) in a human immunodeficiency virus (HIV)-infected patient. Cancer Invest 2001;19:266–272.
61. Johnson DE, Lo RK, Srigley J, Ayala AG. Verrucous carcinoma of the penis. J Urol 1985;133:216–218.
62. Masih AS, Stoler MH, Farrow GM, et al. Penile verrucous carcinoma: pathologic human papillomavirus typing and flow cytometric analysis. Mod Pathol 1992;5:48–55.
63. McKee PH, Lowe D, Haigh RJ. Penile verrucous carcinoma. Histopathology 1983;7:897–906.

64. Velazquez EF, Melamed J, Barreto JE, et al. Sarcomatoid carcinoma of the penis. A clinico-pathological study of 15 cases. Am J Surg Pathol 2005 (in press).
65. Fraser G, Harnett AN, Reid R. Extraosseous osteosarcoma of the penis. Clin Oncol (R Coll Radiol) 2000;12:238–239.
66. Somogyi L, Kalman E. Metaplastic carcinoma of the penis. J Urol 1998; 160(6 Pt 1):2152–2153.
67. Cubilla AL, Ayala MT, Barreto JE, Bellasai JG, Noel JC. Surface adenosquamous carcinoma of the penis. A report of three cases. Am J Surg Pathol 1996;20:156–160.
68. Masera A, Ovcak Z, Volavsek M, Bracko M. Adenosquamous carcinoma of the penis. J Urol 1997;157:2261.
69. Froehner M, Schobl R, Wirth MP. Mucoepidermoid penile carcinoma: clinical, histologic, and immunohistochemical characterization of an uncommon neoplasm. Urology 2000;56:154.
70. Layfield LJ, Liu K. Mucoepidermoid carcinoma arising in the glans penis. Arch Pathol Lab Med 2000;124:148–151.
71. Kato N, Onozuka T, Yasukawa K, Kimura K, Sasaki K. Penile hybrid verrucous-squamous carcinoma associated with a superficial inguinal lymph node metastasis. Am J Dermatopathol 2000;22:339–343.
72. Fukunaga M, Yokoi K, Miyazawa Y, Harada T, Ushigome S. Penile verrucous carcinoma with anaplastic transformation following radiotherapy. A case report with human papillomavirus typing and flow cytometric DNA studies. Am J Surg Pathol 1994;18:501–505.
73. Tamboli P, Tran TA, Ro JY, et al. Mixed basaloid-condylomatous (warty) squamous cell carcinoma of the penis: a report of 17 cases. Lab Invest 2000; 80:115A.
74. Barreto JE, Velazquez EF, Ayala E, et al. Carcinoma cuniculatum of the penis. Mod Pathol 2004;17:583A.
75. Tomic S, Warner TF, Messing E, Wilding G. Penile Merkel cell carcinoma. Urology 1995;45:1062–1065.
76. Eichhorn JH, Young RH. Neuroendocrine tumors of the genital tract. Am J Clin Pathol 2001;115(Suppl):S94–S112.
77. Cubilla AL, Velazquez EF, Young RH. Pseudohyperplastic squamous cell carcinoma of the penis associated with lichen sclerosus: an extremely well differentiated neoplasm that preferentially affects the foreskin and is frequently misdiagnosed. Report of 10 cases of a distinctive clinico-pathologic entity. Am J Surg Pathol 2004;28:895–900.

2

GENITAL SKIN

M. Angelica Selim, John F. Madden, Peter L. McEvoy, and Christopher R. Shea

INFECTIONS

The external genital skin, located at the confluence of the cutaneous, urinary, and genital tracts, poses complex problems for dermatologic diagnosis and management. Disorders of these systems may present with genital cutaneous manifestations. The local environment of warmth, humidity, irritation, and exposure to body fluids predisposes the external genital skin to many primary cutaneous lesions, especially infections.

FUNGAL INFECTIONS

Superficial dermatophytosis

Dermatophytosis (tinea) is a superficial fungal infection by *Trichophyton*, *Epidermophyton*, and *Microsporum* species, affecting keratinized tissues. It is the presenting complaint responsible for 3–4% of all dermatologic visits. Clinically, tinea is an erythematous well-demarcated plaque, often with scalloped borders and central clearing. These features and focal scaling differentiate dermatophytosis from erythrasma. *Tricrophyton rubrum*[1] and *T. mentagropytes*[2] are the most frequent agents. Dermatophytosis commonly affects the inguinal area (so-called tinea cruris). However, it may extend to the shaft of the penis and scrotum.[3] Patients with dermatophytosis of the feet (tinea pedis) can transfer the microorganism to the genital area by hand.[3,4] Predisposing factors for tinea cruris include the use of tight-fitting garments,[5] atopic dermatitis, immunosuppresion, and diabetes. (Fig. 2.1)

Pityriasis versicolor (tinea versicolor)

This superficial fungal infection is uncommon on the external genitalia, but can cause a hypo- or hyperpigmented macular eruption of the penile shaft.[6,7] The etiologic agent, lipophilic yeast of the *Malassezia* family, was recently reclassified as *M. globosa*. (Fig. 2.2)

Candidiasis (candidosis, moniliasis)

Candida albicans is part of the normal flora of the intertriginous skin, prepuce, and perineal area. Candidal balanoposthitis is the most common fungal infection of the penis.[8]

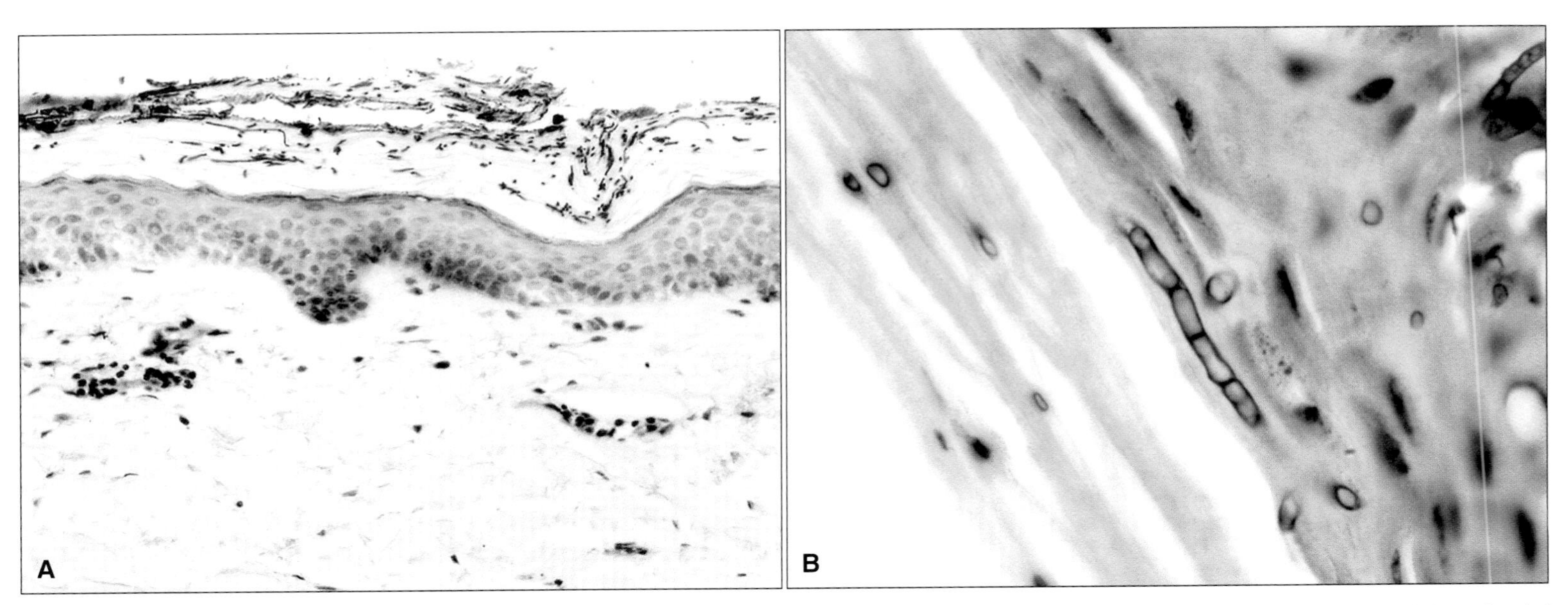

Fig. 2.1 Superficial dermatophytosis. (A,B) Dermatophytes appear on biopsy as basophilic nonpigmented septate hyphae, often with globose hyphal segments and chains of arthroconidia, characteristically located in the stratum corneum. Fungal stains highlight the organisms (periodic acid–Schiff or Grocott). The underlying dermis can show a scant lymphohistiocytic infiltrate.

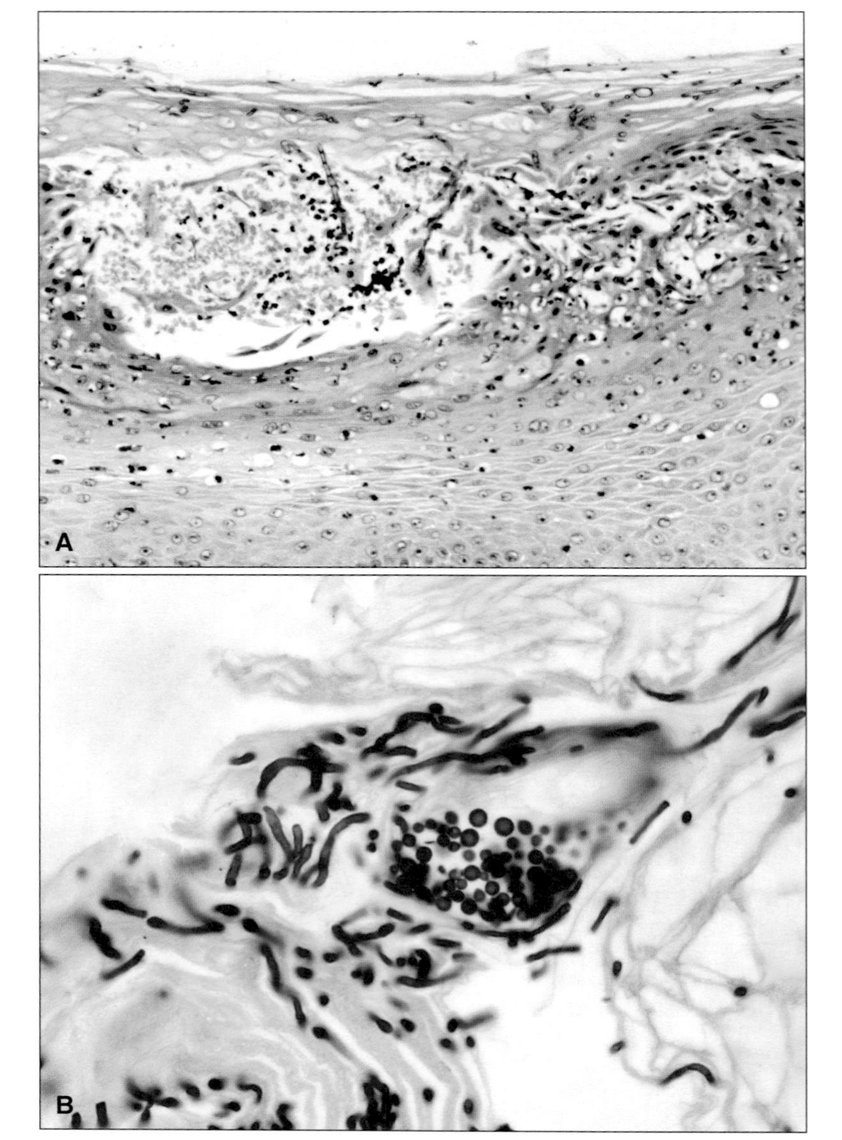

Fig. 2.2 Pityriasis versicolor. (A) The biopsy shows yeast and hyphae in the stratum corneum of a slightly acanthotic epidermis with an associated superficial perivascular lymphohistocytic infiltrate. (B) The combination of round budding yeasts (blastoconidia) and short septate hyphae (pseudomycelium) creates the characteristic 'spaghetti and meatballs' appearance.

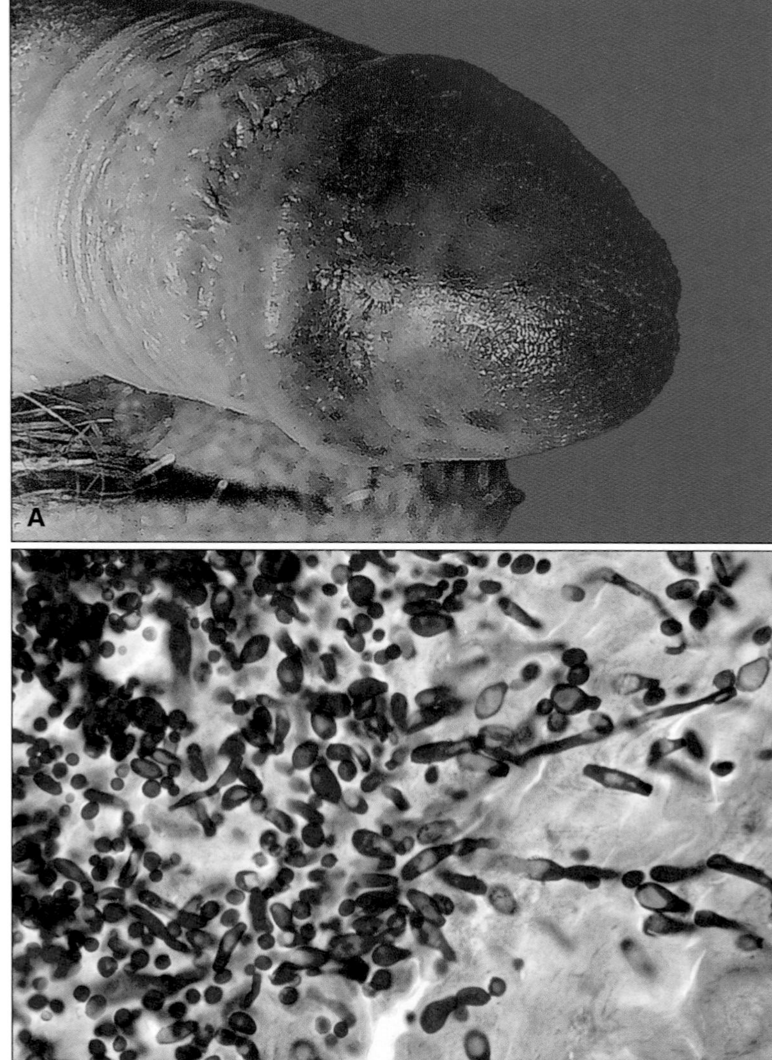

Fig. 2.3 Candidiasis. (A) The primary lesions are papules and pustules that expand rapidly to merge into erosive plaques surrounded by satellite pustules. Increased pain and exudate may herald superimposed bacterial infection.[10] (B) Budding yeast and pseudohyphae can be shown by KOH preparation.

There is usually a predisposing factor such as uncontrolled diabetes mellitus, impaired immunity, or severely debilitating illness. A sexual partner may be the source of infection;[9] over three-fourths of women experience at least one symptomatic episode of vulvovaginal candidiasis. (Fig. 2.3)

Deep mycotic infections

The differential diagnosis for deep fungal infection includes blastomycosis,[11] histoplasmosis,[12,13] coccidioidomycosis, and paracoccidioidomycosis. Cryptococcosis can involve the penis through hematogenous spread from the lungs or genitourinary tract.[14,15] (Fig. 2.4)

BACTERIAL INFECTIONS

Gram-positive bacteria

Several common Gram-positive bacterial infections affect the genital skin and may present to dermatologists, but are rarely biopsied.

Erythrasma is a chronic bacterial infection that affects humid cutaneous recesses like the inguinal folds and the vulva. It is common in warm weather. It presents as a sharply demarcated, brown to red, scaly plaque that fluoresces coral red under Wood's lamp due to the presence of porphyrins of bacterial origin. The diagnosis is made by ruling out a fungal infection by KOH. The etiologic factor is *Corynebacterium minutissimum*.[16]

Trichomycosis pubis[17] is an often-asymptomatic colonization of the hair by various corynebacteria (especially *C. tenuis*). It may cause an offensive odor and produce a yellow, red, or black coating around pubic hairs.

Cellulitis of the scrotum and the penis due to β-hemolytic streptococci can occur following an epidermal break, i.e. after circumcision. The genital skin is red, hot, and tender. The dermis shows marked edema with perivascular and interstitial acute inflammation. The clinical diagnosis is confirmed by culture.

Staphylococcus aureus produces primary lesions in the genital tract including folliculitis (Fig. 2.5), impetigo, bullous impetigo, and furuncles. It can also cause secondary infection in psoriatic plaques, lichen simplex chronicus, atopic dermatitis, or lesions primarily due to other infections such as candidiasis, genital herpes, or syphilitic chancre. Group A or B β-hemolytic streptococci can cause superficial erosive intertrigo.

Fournier's gangrene

Fournier's gangrene is a necrotizing infection of the genital and anorectal regions.[18] Risk factors include contaminated genitourinary trauma, lower urinary tract instrumentation,[19] periurethritis, septic injection into the penile vein,[20] diabetes, immunosuppression,[21] and poor nutritional status. Rarely, it can complicate *trans*-retinoic acid treatment of acute promyelocytic leukemia. A mixture of aerobic and anaerobic enteric organisms causes the infection. Rapidly developing cellulitis, fasciitis, and myositis accompany severe systemic toxicity, often out of proportion to the external findings. The physiologic basis is a localized vasculitis due to the Schwartzmann phenomenon. Mortality ranges from 10% to 30%. Early, aggressive debridement and broad-spectrum antibiotics can improve outcome. (Fig. 2.6)

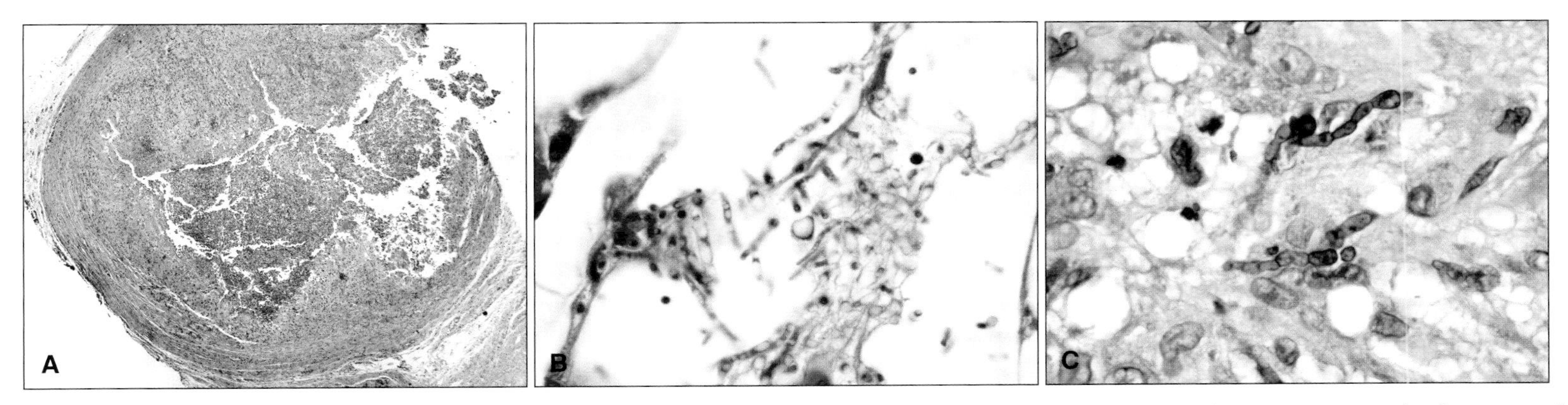

Fig. 2.4 Deep mycotic infection. (A–C) Pigmented fungal infections can affect the genital skin in immunosuppressed patients as part of a disseminated infection, but they occur only rarely in immunologically intact individuals.

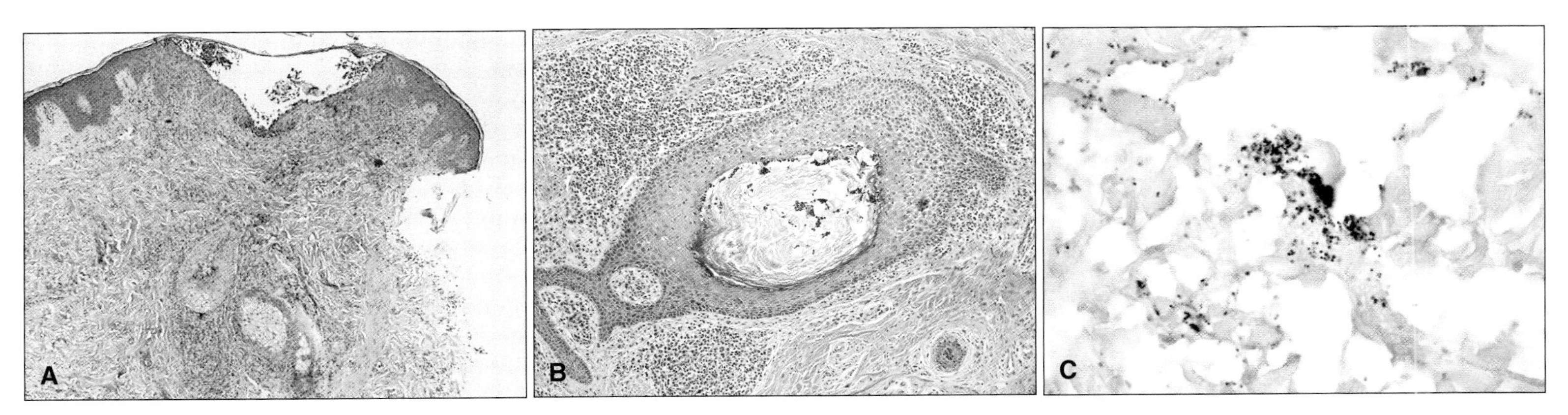

Fig. 2.5 Bacterial folliculitis. (A,B) This case of folliculitis shows a distended follicle filled with keratin, and acute inflammation. (C) The Brown–Brenn stain highlights Gram-positive cocci in the hair follicle.

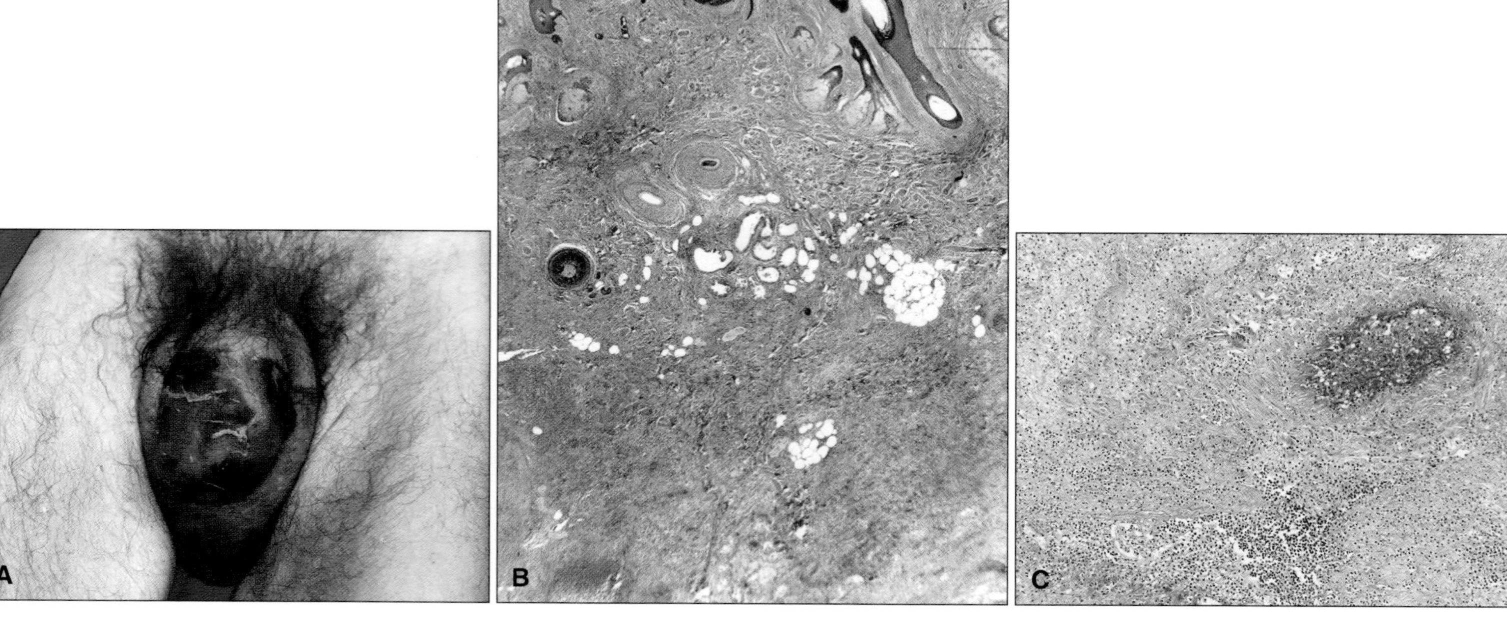

Fig. 2.6 Fournier's gangrene. (A) Clinically, Fournier's gangrene presents with edema, erythema, necrosis, crepitus, and bulla formation. The process involves the epidermis up to the subcutaneous tissue and spreads along fascial planes. (B,C) A mixed inflammatory cell infiltrate surrounds areas of necrosis with vasculitis. Basically, this disease is a gangrene of the subcutis followed by necrosis of the skin.

Pseudomonal cellulitis (ecthyma gangrenosum)

This complication of pseudomonal sepsis presents as an erythematous or purpuric cutaneous macule that rapidly develops into a bulla with subsequent ulceration. The disease is bacterial vasculitis leading to cutaneous infarction. Penile ecthyma gangrenosum has been reported in neutropenic patients[22,23] and drug abusers.[24] (Fig. 2.7)

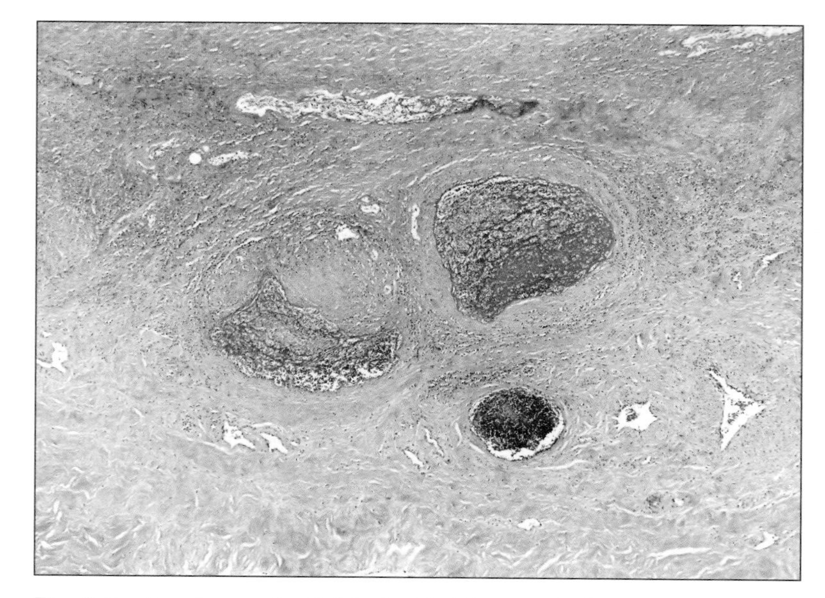

Fig. 2.7 Pseudomonal cellulitis. In this infection the lesions appear 'gun-metal gray', with a surrounding halo of erythema. The biopsy shows epidermal and upper dermal necrosis with hemorrhage. Necrotizing vasculitis with thrombosis occurs at the periphery of the necrosis. Gram-negative bacteria are present in the dermis and surrounding vessels.

Mycobacterial disease

Tuberculosis of the penis can result from a sexual contact with a partner with active genital or oral tuberculosis. *Mycobacterium tuberculosis* is the most frequent species, with a few reported cases caused by *Mycobacterium celatum*.[25] Clinically, it presents as subacute or chronic, painful ulcers, with or without lymphadenopathy. Lupus vulgaris, the most frequent form of reinfection tuberculosis, can affect the penis. The usual picture is of confluent papules leading to a plaque that, viewed by diascopy, shows 'apple-jelly' deposits representing cellular infiltrates. Papulonecrotic tuberculids involving the glans[26] and BCG balanitis following instillation for bladder carcinoma[27] are unusual presentations. (Fig. 2.8)

Syphilis

Primary, secondary, tertiary, and congenital lesions can affect the anogenital area. HIV patients can have unusual lesions and may fail to respond to standard therapy. The primary syphilitic chancre occurs at the site of inoculation 3 weeks after exposure to *Treponema pallidum*. A painless, button-like papule ulcerates centrally. Although often single, it can present as 'kissing' lesions. Commonly, it involves the inner prepuce, coronal sulcus, penile shaft, or anus.[28] (Fig. 2.9)

Untreated, systemic dissemination of the spirochete occurs during the secondary stage, up to 6 months after healing of the primary lesion. Eighty percent of these

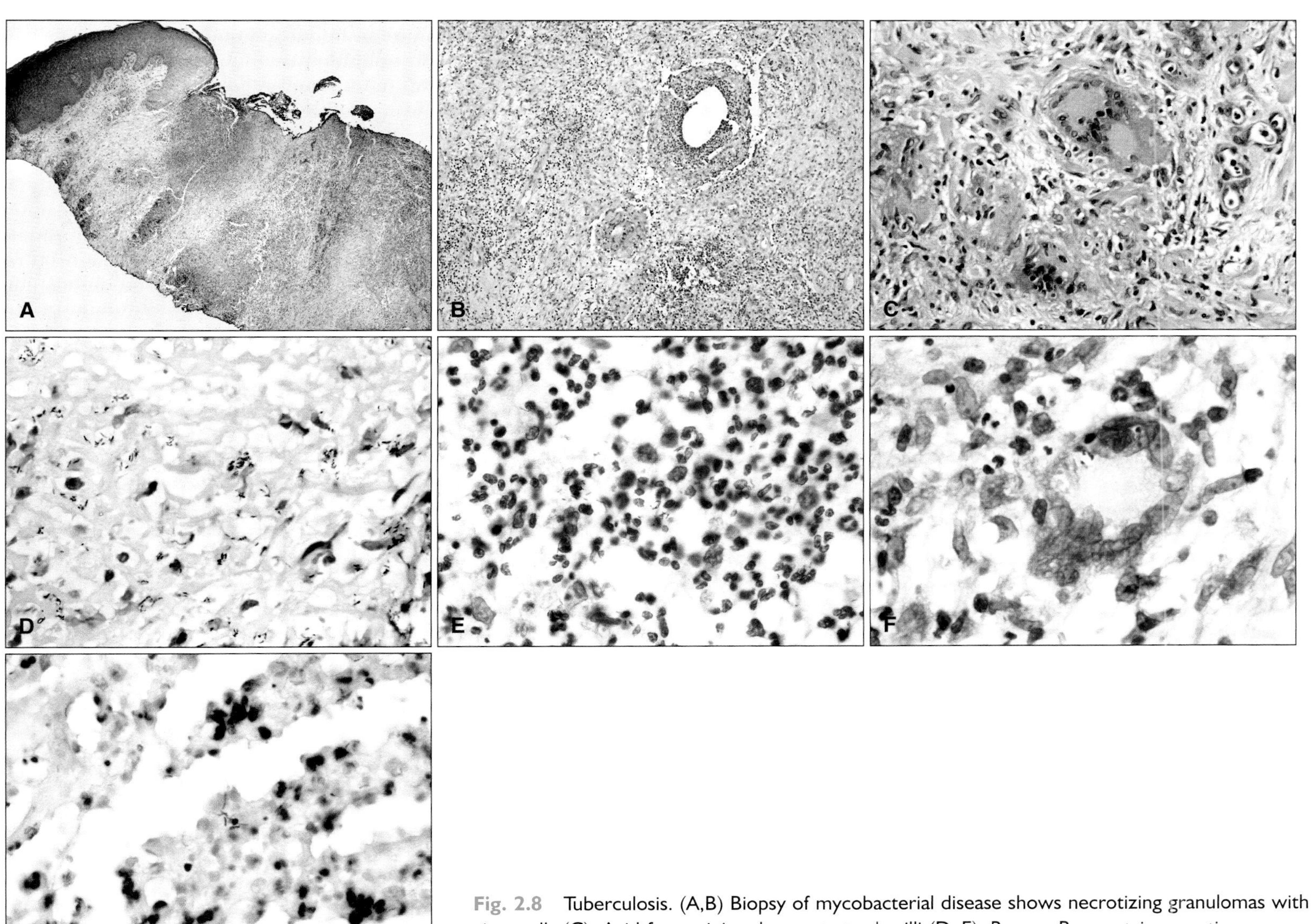

Fig. 2.8 Tuberculosis. (A,B) Biopsy of mycobacterial disease shows necrotizing granulomas with giant cells (C). Acid-fast staining demonstrates bacilli (D–F). Brown–Brenn stain sometimes succeeds in showing the Gram-positive organisms (G).

patients have a non-pruritic papulosquamous eruption. In dark-skinned persons, annular polycyclic lesions may occur. Large verruciform papules may develop in the anogenital region (condylomata lata). (Fig. 2.10)

Tertiary syphilis targets the bones, central nervous system, and cardiovascular system. There are two cutaneous presentations, nodular and ulcerative.

In tertiary syphilis, the classic lesion is the gumma: an area of necrobiosis surrounded by lymphocytes, plasma cells, histiocytes, giant cells, and fibroblasts. A nodular presentation consists of tuberculoid granulomas with mixed inflammatory cell reaction including plasma cells. Silver stains are usually negative. Polymerase chain reaction has been successfully applied.

Chancroid

Chancroid is caused by the sexually transmitted, Gram-negative, facultative anaerobic bacterium *Haemophilus ducreyi*. Transmission is possible while lesions are active (about 6 weeks in untreated patients). One week after exposure, a papule appears at the inoculation site. This develops into a painful ulcer with gray–yellow exudate and sharp, undermined borders.[29] (Fig. 2.11) Autoinoculation can lead to many lesions that may merge with serpinginous borders. Between 1 and 2 weeks later, half of untreated patients develop unilateral painful adenopathy. Inguinal abscesses and draining sinus tracts may result. Diagnosis calls for isolation of *H. ducreyi* on special culture media. (Figs 2.12–2.13)

Lymphogranuloma venereum

Lymphogranuloma venereum is a sexually transmitted disease caused by *Chlamydia trachomatis* serovars L1, L2, and L3. These target lymphatic tissue of the anorectum and genital area.[30]

The primary lesion is an eroded papule or group of small herpetiform ulcers at the inoculation site (coronal sulcus, frenulum, prepuce, shaft, glans, or scrotum). Urethritis with mucopurulent discharge may occur. The initial lesion is

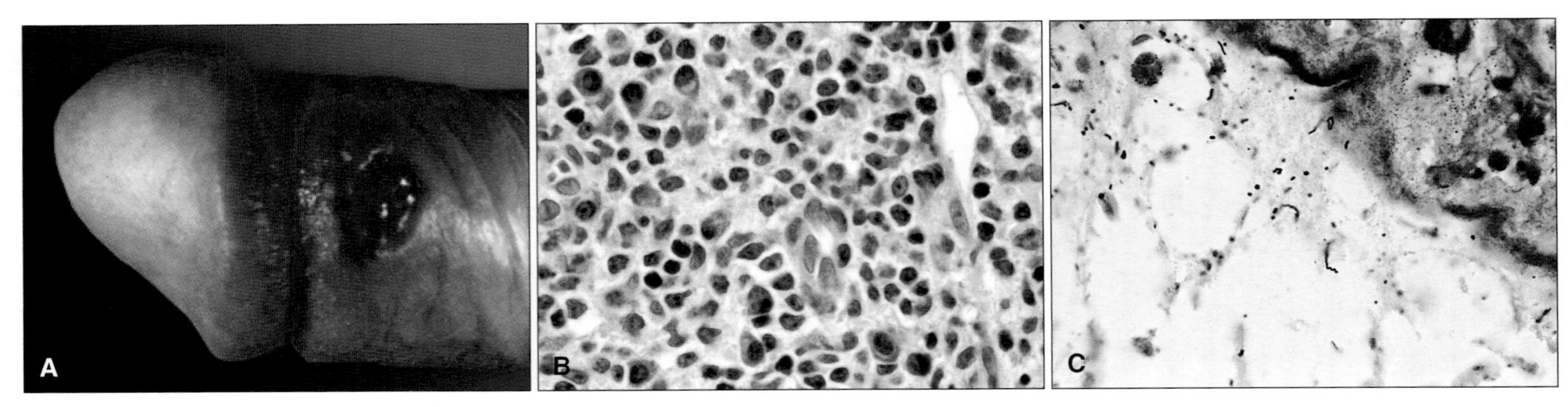

Fig. 2.9 Syphilis. (A) Primary syphilitic chancre presents as a painless button-like eroded nodule. (B) The primary lesion (chancre) of syphilis shows a thinned or ulcerated epidermis with a dense dermal infiltrate rich in plasma cells and lymphocytes. The blood vessels show endarteritis obliterans: marked endothelial swelling and proliferation with infiltration of the vascular wall by inflammatory cells. (C) Silver impregnation stain highlights the spirochetes, spiral organisms 4–15 μm long, around vessels in the epidermis and papillary dermis. Dark-field microscopy of material obtained from the base of the ulcer, immunohistochemical stains and polymerase chain reaction are available tests for identification of the spirochetes.

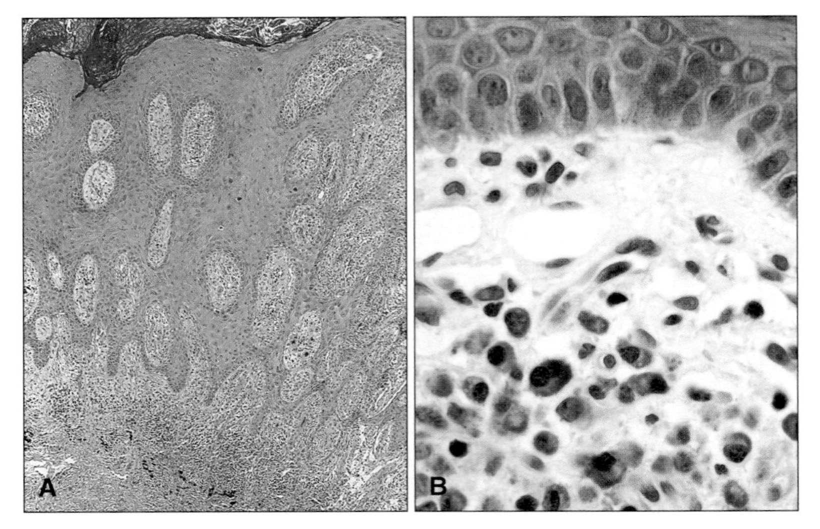

Fig. 2.10 Syphilis. (A,B) The most frequent (80%) clinical presentation of secondary syphilis is a generalized papulosquamous eruption. Secondary mucosal lesions (condylomata lata) appear as soft, moist, red to tan, flat-topped papules, nodules, or plaques. The epidermis may show acanthosis with spongiosis, psoriasiform hyperplasia, interface dermatitis, or pustules. There is a superficial and deep dermal infiltrate composed predominantly of lymphocytes with some admixed histiocytes, and variable numbers of plasma cells.

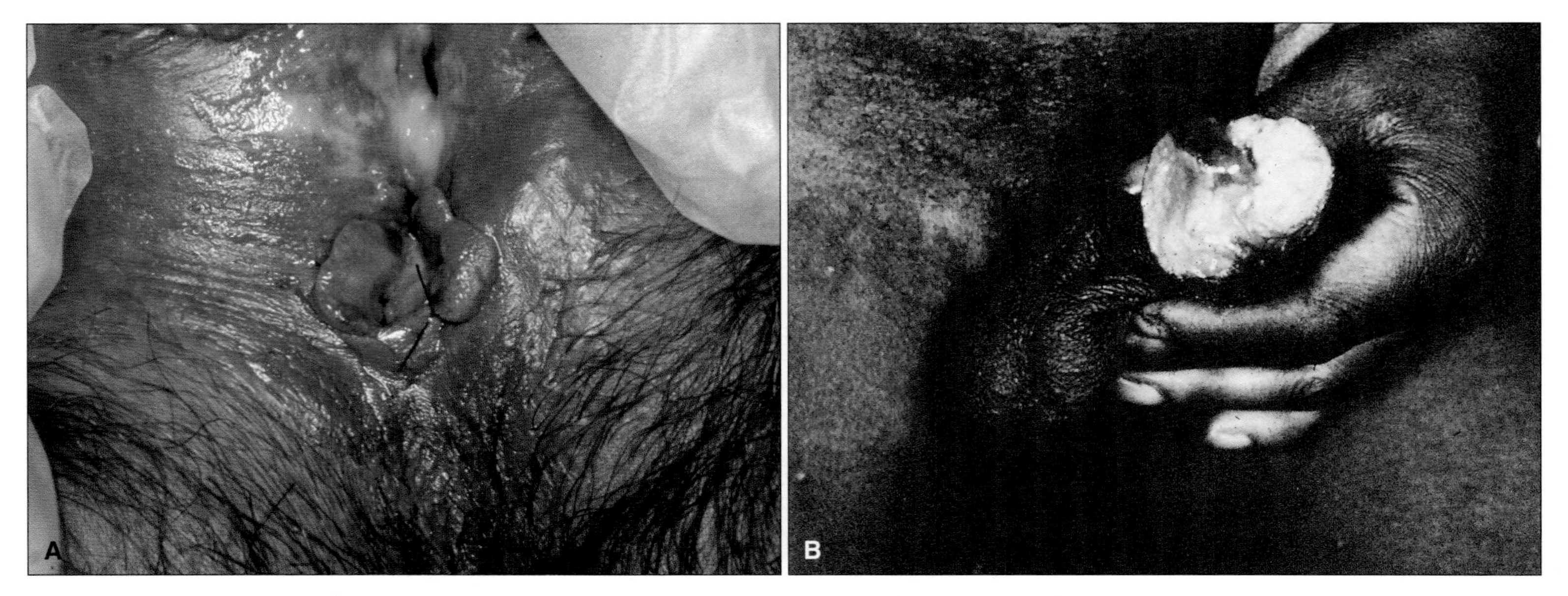

Fig. 2.11 Chancroid. (A,B) Gross appearance of chancroid lesions. These are painful ulcers with yellow–gray exudate and sharp, undermined borders.

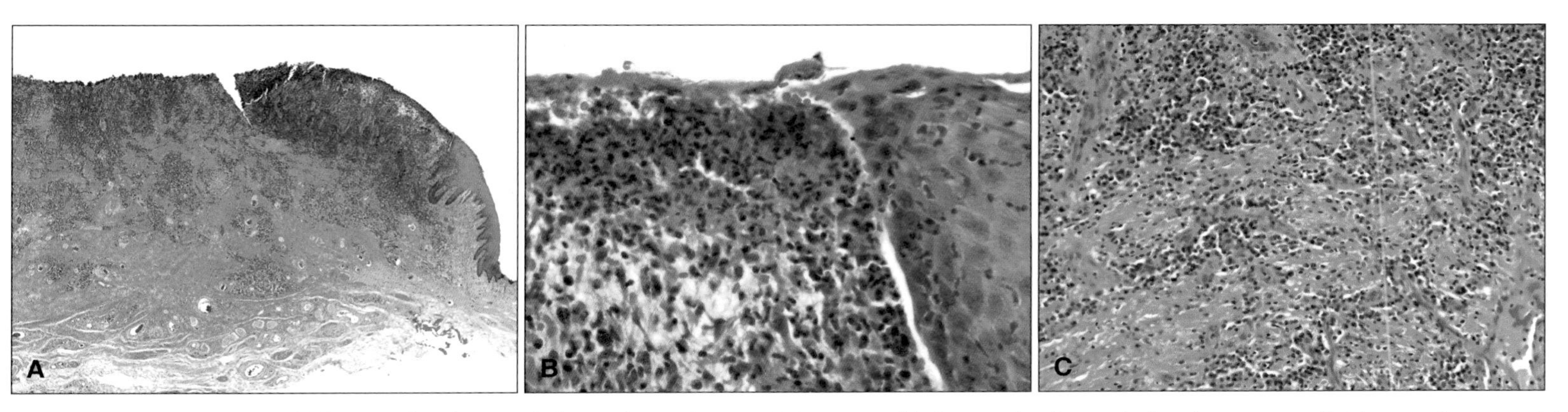

Fig. 2.12 Chancroid. (A–C) Biopsy of a chancroid shows three characteristic zones of inflammation beneath the ulcer: a superficial necrotic zone with fibrin and acute inflammation; a middle zone of granulation tissue; and a deep zone of chronic inflammation.

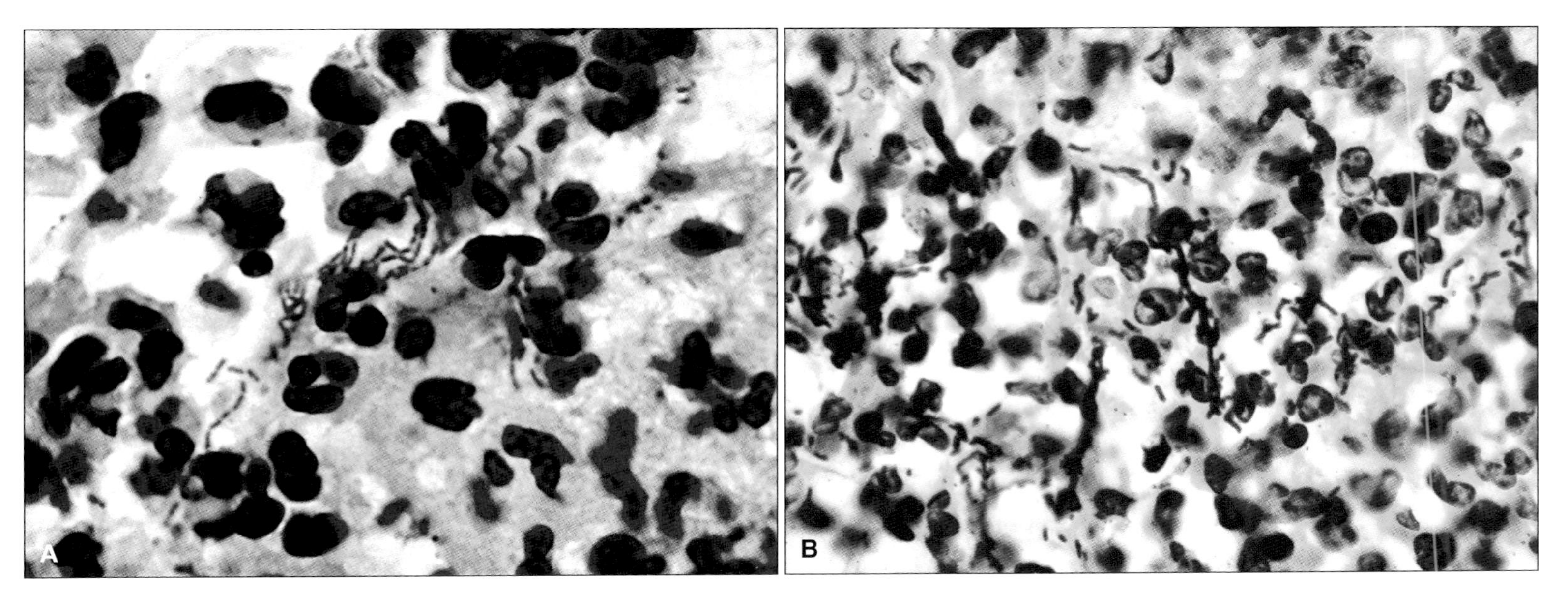

Fig. 2.13 Chancroid. (A) Brown–Brenn stain of a chancroid demonstrates Gram-negative bacilli in chains. (B) Silver impregnation stain on smears can detect the 'railroad track' or 'school of fish' chaining pattern of *H. ducreyi*.

followed several weeks later by inguinal lymphadenitis with bubo formation, often accompanied by proctocolitis. Cord-like lymphangitis of the dorsal penis may accompany femoral and inguinal bubo formation. The cleft due to pressure from the inguinal (Poupart's) ligament between enlarged femoral and inguinal involved lymph nodes is called the groove sign.[31] The third stage includes sequelae from inflammation.

Complications include formation of sinuses and tracts to skin or urethra, and deforming scars of the penis. In the anogenital syndrome, proctocolitis and hyperplasia of perirectal lymph nodes occurs, leading to fistula formation and rectal strictures. (Fig. 2.14)

Donovanosis (granuloma inguinale)

Donovanosis is a chronic, sexually transmitted genital ulcer disease caused by the Gram-negative bacillus *Calymmatobacterium granulomatis*. The primary lesion is a well-defined painless ulcer with beefy red granulation tissue at the base and elevated or hyperplastic borders.[32] Fibrosis occurs with extension of the ulcer. Longstanding untreated disease is associated with lymphedema that in extreme cases can lead to elephantiasis of the penis and scrotum.[33] Lymph node involvement is rare, but subcutaneous nodules (pseudobuboes) can simulate it. Ulcerovegetative, nodular, hypertrophic, and cicatricial forms occur. (Fig. 2.15)

VIRAL INFECTIONS

Herpetic infections

Sexually transmitted genital herpes is primarily caused by type 2 herpes simplex virus (HSV 2). Primary lesions usually consist of a group of clear, fragile vesicles on an erythematous base which quickly rupture, leaving behind superficial erosions. (Fig. 2.16) Lymphadenopathy accompanies primary lesions but usually not recurrences.[34]

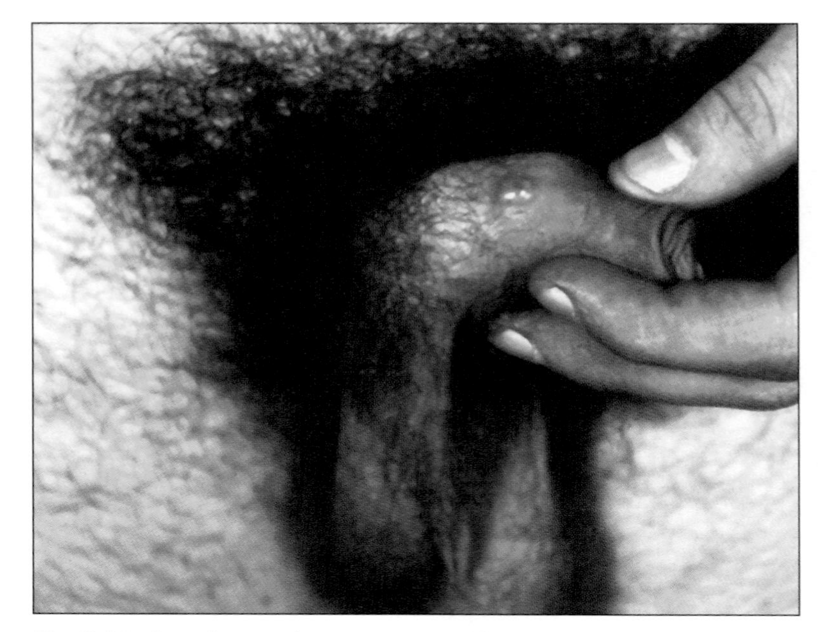

Fig. 2.14 Lymphogranuloma venereum. The inoculation site shows mixed inflammatory reaction. Rare microorganisms are detected within histiocytes by Giemsa staining. Stellate abscesses with an indistinct palisade of histiocytes occur in second-stage nodes.

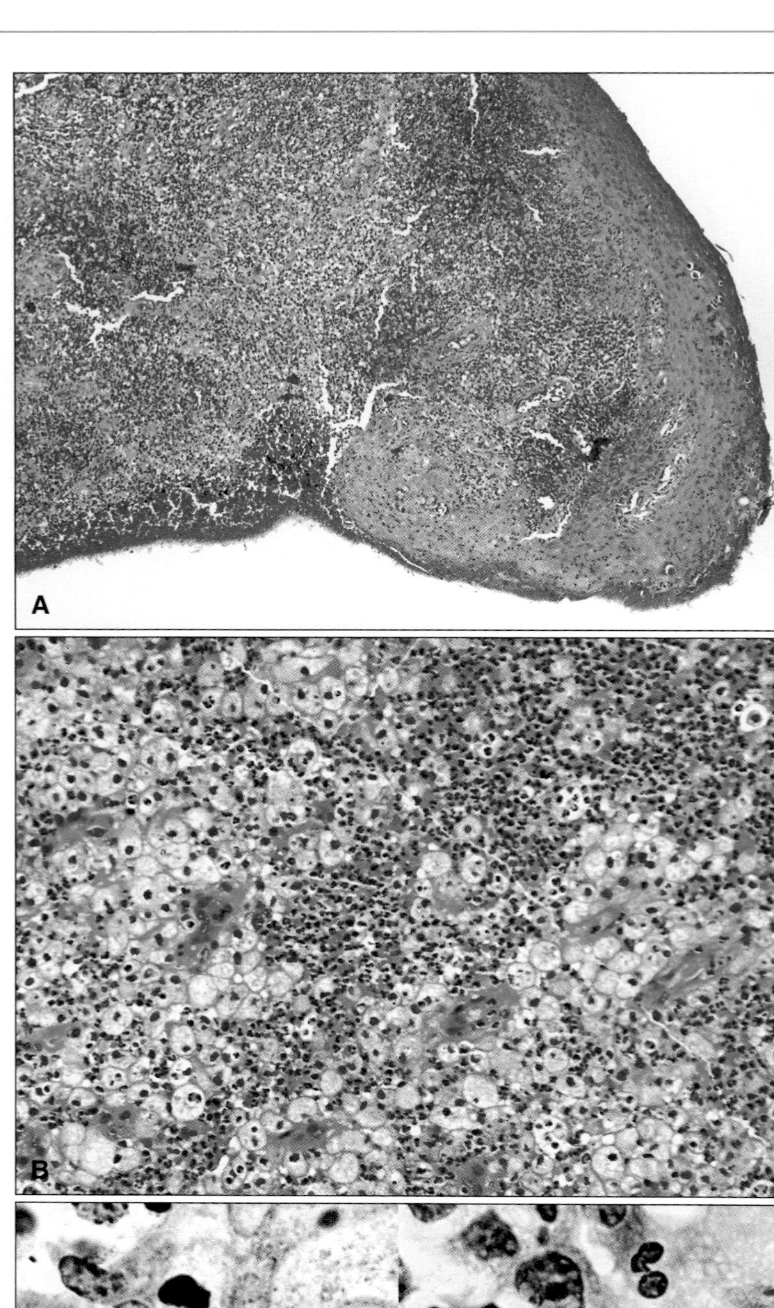

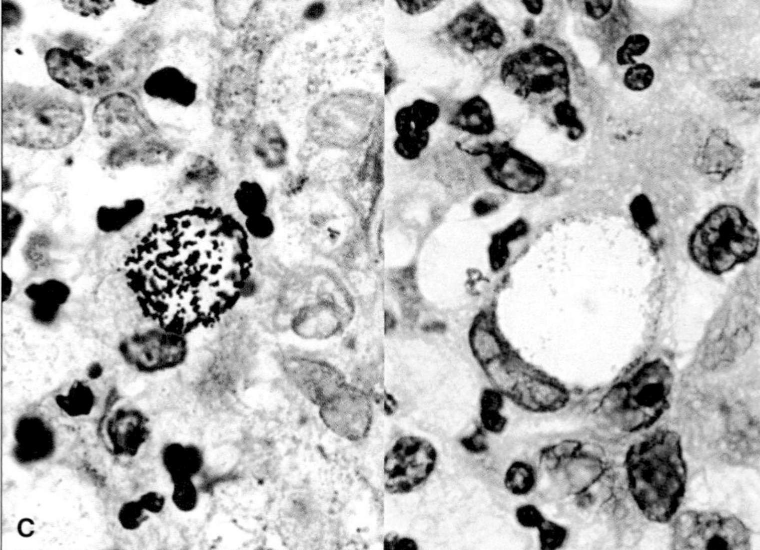

Fig. 2.15 Donovanosis. (A,B) Biopsy of the inoculation site shows an ulcer with pseudoepitheliomatous hyperplasia and granulation tissue. The organism is difficult to find in tissue sections. (C) Giemsa or Warthin–Starry show parasitized histiocytes (Donovan bodies).

Recurrences tend to be less extensive and are preceded by a day or two of tingling and burning (prodrome). Lesions affect the prepuce, glans, and shaft, and are uncommon on the scrotum. Homosexual men may present with perianal lesions. Herpetic urethritis produces scant discharge and dysuria.[35]

Chronic herpetic lesions are painful ulcers with rolled borders. If they persist for more than 1 month, they constitute an AIDS-defining condition.[36] Patients undergoing chemotherapy or transplantation and those with hematologic disorders are also susceptible.[34]

Herpes zoster affects the anogenital area by infecting the third and fourth sacral sensory nerves. It appears as grouped vesicles in a dermatomal distribution. Herpes zoster can be distinguished from herpes simplex with immunoperoxidase stains in biopsy tissue, by cultures, or by molecular probes for viral antigens. (Fig. 2.16)

Human papillomavirus infection

Genital wart (condyloma acuminatum) is one of the most common sexually transmitted diseases, affecting roughly 20 million people in the United States. The most frequent sites in the male are the frenulum, corona, glans, shaft, and scrotum.[37] They may be numerous and confluent with a cobblestone appearance. The high recurrence rate after treatment is attributed to presence of latent human papillomavirus (HPV) in normal-appearing perilesional skin.[38]

HPV is a DNA virus with about 100 genotypes. Types 6 and 11 are often associated with condyloma acuminatum,

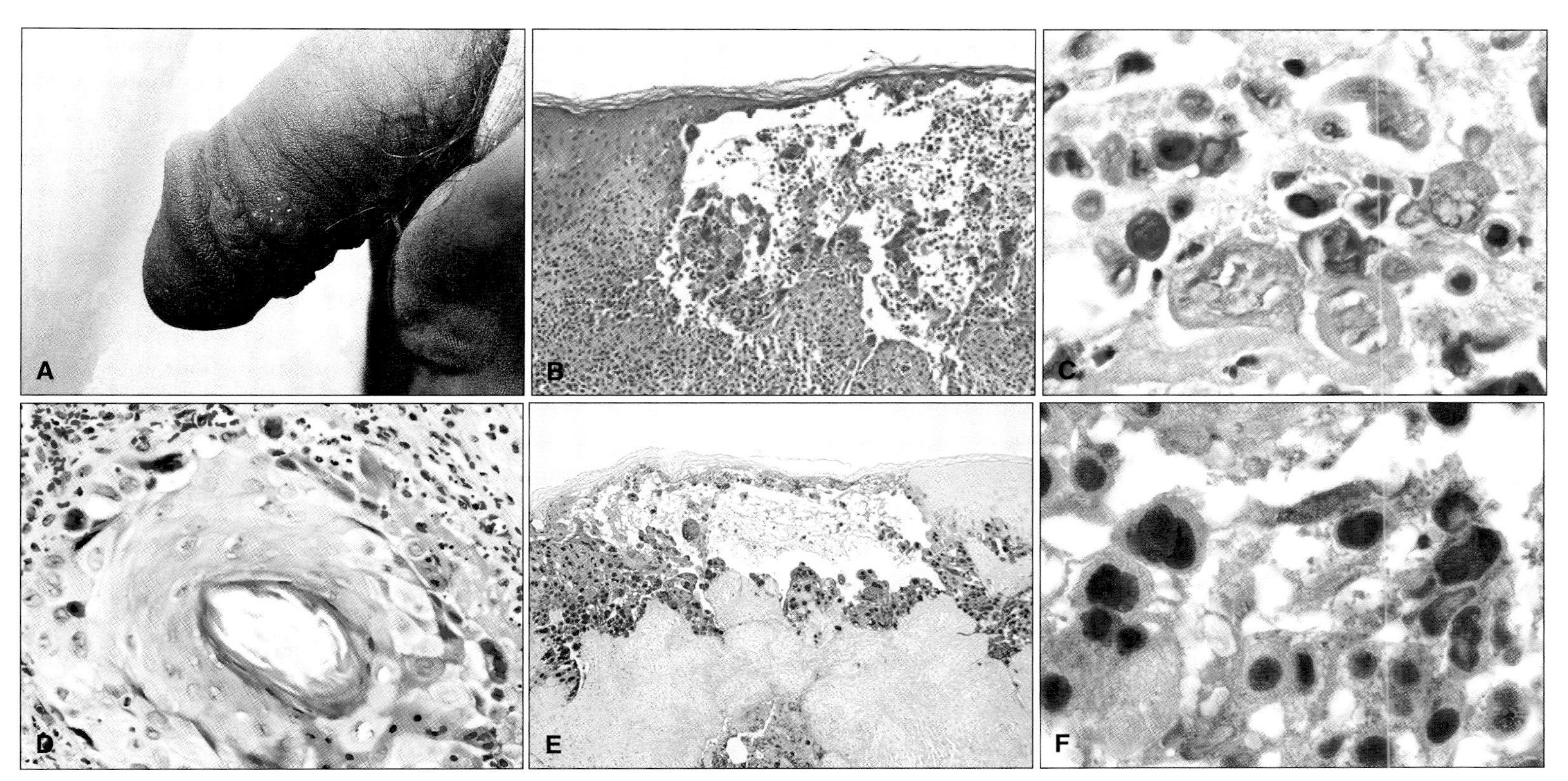

Fig. 2.16 Herpetic infection. (A) Clinically, multiple grouped vesicles appear on an erythematous base. (B) An intraepidermal vesicle is filled with ballooned, acantholyic, infected keratinocytes, serum, and mixed inflammation. (C) The affected keratinocytes show homogeneous, 'ground-glass' nuclei that are multiple (or multilobulated) and exhibit molding and margination of chromatin. (D) Involvement of the pilosebaceous units or eccrine ducts (herpetic syringitis) can occur, especially in recurrences. In herpetic folliculitis, the infected cells are usually in the outer root sheath. (E,F) Immunohistochemical stains decorate the infected cells.

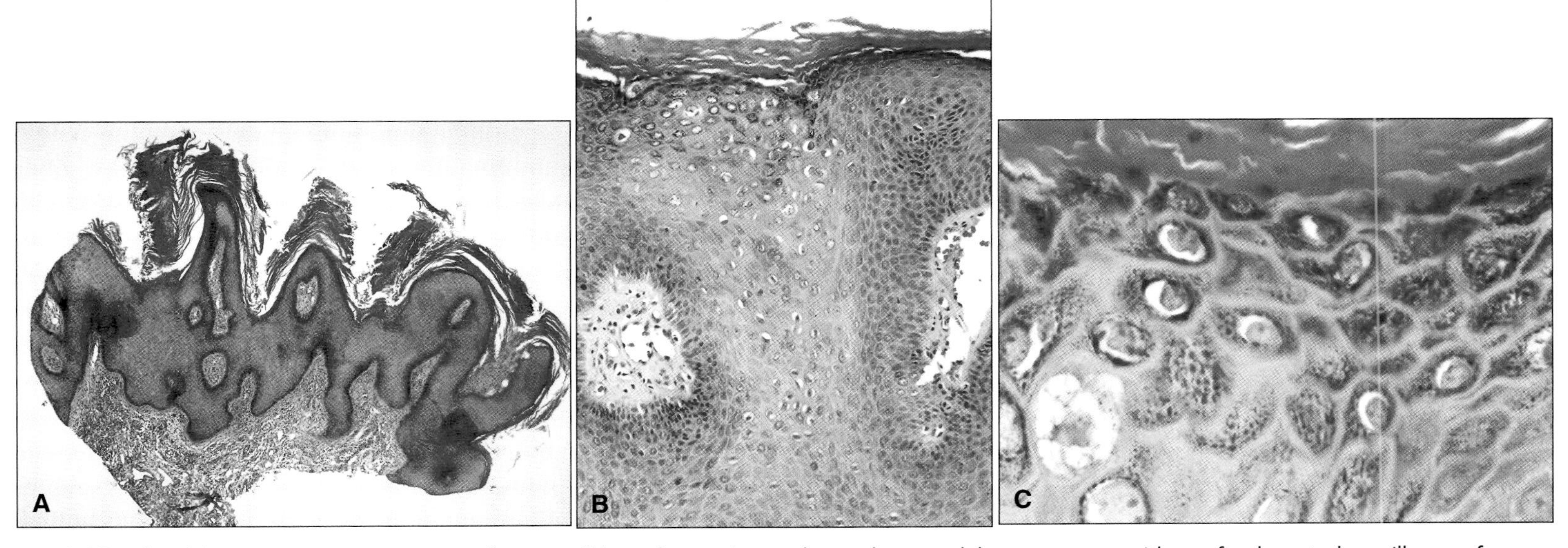

Fig. 2.17 Condylomata acuminata can range from small hyperkeratotic papules, to large nodules, to tumors with a soft, elongated, papillary surface. (A–C) The consistent histologic features of condyloma acuminatum are epidermal hyperplasia presenting as complex papillary infolding, parakeratosis, and koilocytosis (wrinkled, convoluted, moderately enlarged nuclei surrounded by a clear space). Treatment with podophyllotoxin, an agent that affects tubulin function in the mitotic spindle, can produce aberrant mitotic figures that may elicit overdiagnosis of dysplasia.

but confer little risk of subsequent squamous cell carcinoma. 'High-risk' types, especially HPV 16 and 18, are an important cause of anogenital neoplasia (penile squamous cell carcinoma[39]) and their precursor, squamous intraepithelial lesions[40] (SIL). (Fig. 2.17)

Molluscum contagiosum

This cutaneous poxvirus infection presents as clustered, domed-shaped papules with central umbilication. With trauma or irritation, lesions may develop into keratotic

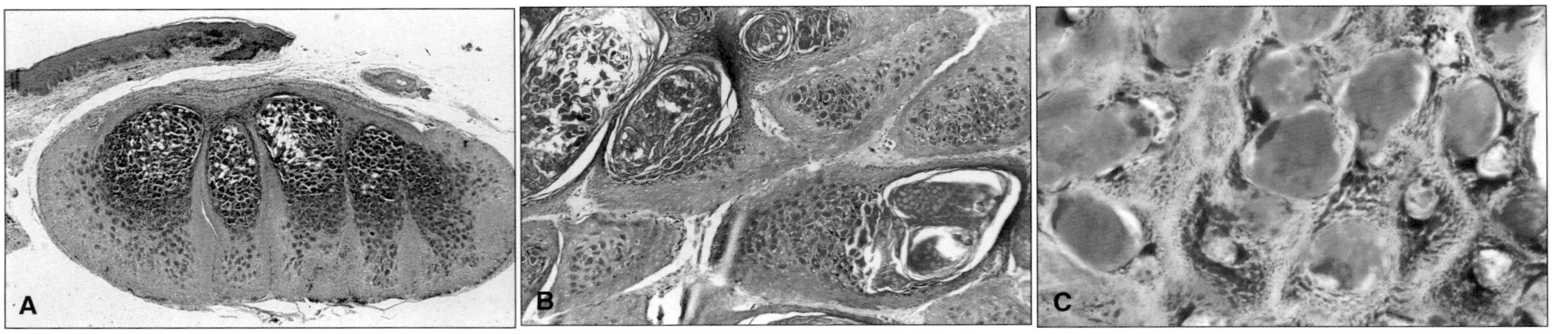

Fig. 2.18 Molluscum contagiosum. (A–C) The lesion consists of endophytic lobules of squamous epithelium separated by a compressed dermis. Infected keratinocytes show round to oval eosinophilc intracytoplasmic inclusions (Henderson–Paterson bodies).

papules indistinguishable from condylomata acuminata.[41] Molluscum contagiosum is favored when white keratin caseum extrudes from the lesion. Primary inoculation and autoinoculation involving the anogenital region is common in children. (Fig. 2.18)

PARASITIC INFESTATIONS

Entamoeba histolytica colitis is particularly common in South America and Southeast Asia. It can affect perineal skin by direct extension from the anus. Males practicing anal intercourse with an affected person may suffer penile involvement.[42] Clinically, it presents as ulcerated painful nodules.[43] Ulcers due to enteric amebiasis start in the anus and extend as large deep painful ulcerations with serpiginous borders. In the tropics, amebic ulcer should be considered when balanoposthitis is resistant to antibiotics.[44]

The filarial worms *Wuchereria bancrofti*, *Brugia malayi*, and *B. timori* lodge in lymphatic vessels, resulting in obstruction, chronic lymphedema, and chronic inflammation. In tropical areas, the disease can affect up to 25% of the male population.[45] In the early stages, the scrotum is swollen, erythematous, and tender. In the chronic phase, thickening of the scrotal skin, elephantiasis, and verruciform epidermal hyperplasia are apparent.[46]

Schistosomiasis

Egg deposition by adult flukes within abdominopelvic veins leads to a florid granulomatous reaction in surrounding tissue that conducts eggs to nearby visceral or cutaneous surfaces. *Schistosoma mansoni* colonizes pelvic veins; its eggs are extruded preferentially into the bladder lumen and are excreted with micturition. Inflammatory masses, sinuses, and fistulas can involve the periurethral tissues and perineum.[47] (Fig. 2.19)

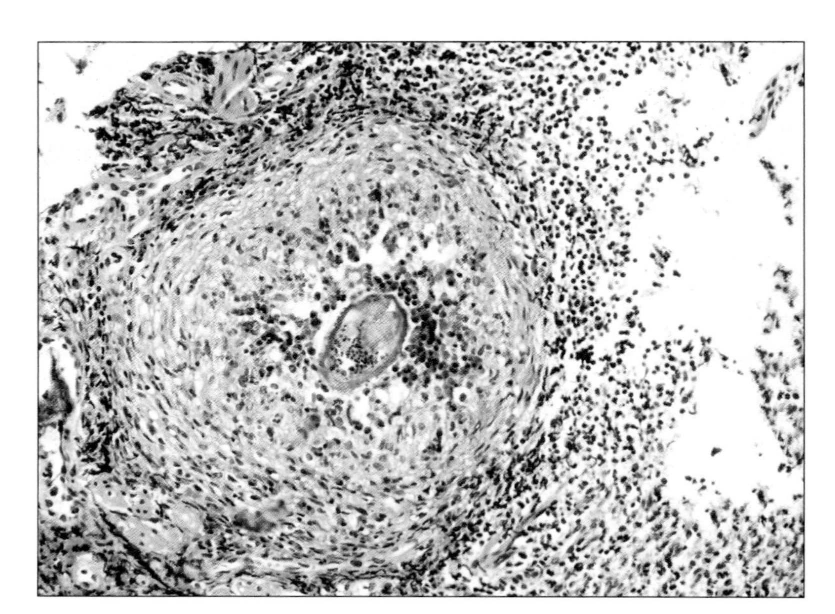

Fig. 2.19 Schistosomiasis. Histologic sections show the dermis containing ova associated with granulomatous reaction. Microabscesses with many eosinophils may sometimes be seen. Ova of *S. mansoni* have a lateral spine.

Scabies

Mites produce tunnels beneath the stratum corneum, on the penis, scrotum, flexor surfaces of the wrist, webspaces, axillae, buttock, and waist. Superimposed eczematous changes are secondary to chronic irritation.[48] (Fig. 2.20) Patients complain of severe pruritus. Scabietic nodules on the glans and scrotum affect a minority of these patients and present as tan to pink papules or nodules. Crusted ('Norwegian') scabies is an uncommon variant affecting immunocompromised patients.[49] Innumerable mites are seen in the stratum corneum of a psoriasiform lesion on the penis, extremities, and at other sites.[50]

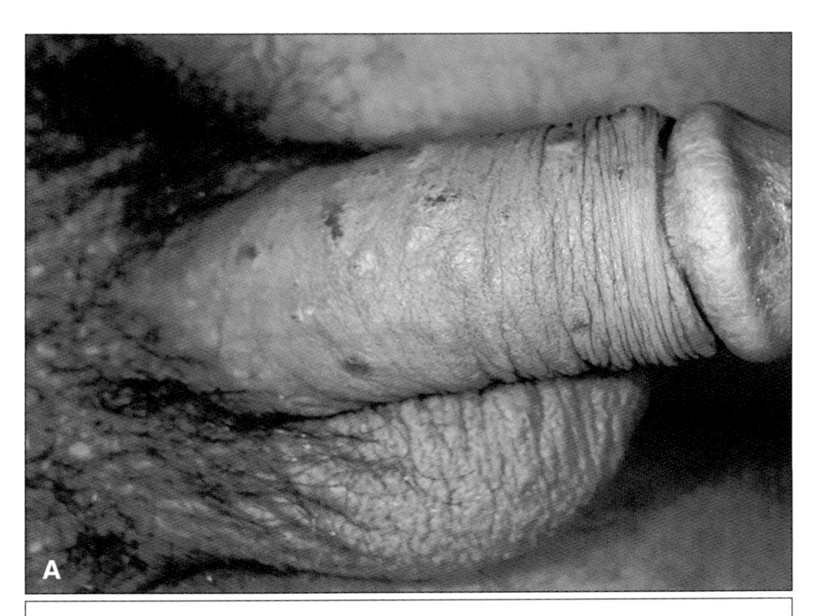

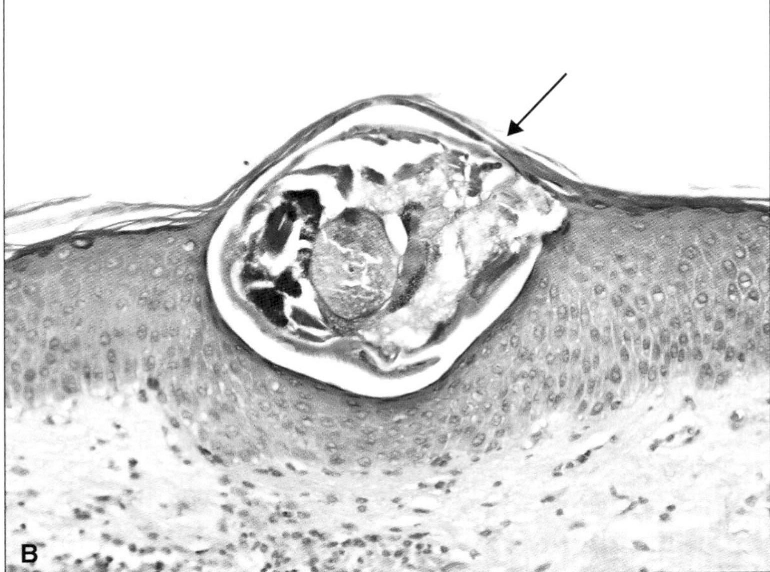

Fig. 2.20 Scabies. (A) Clinically, multiple excoriated papules are noted. (B) There is a superficial and deep infiltrate of lymphocytes, histiocytes and eosinophils. If a burrow is in the biopsy, eggs, larvae, mites (arrow), and excreta (scybala) may be seen.

INFLAMMATORY CONDITIONS

Inflammatory cutaneous disorders of the genitalia can be a diagnostic puzzle. The clinical presentation is frequently non-classical. Warmth and moisture at this anatomic location predispose to secondary infection, further obscuring the diagnosis. Inspection of concomitant lesions from other anatomic locations (nails, scalp, oral mucosa) can facilitate the diagnosis.

SPONGIOTIC AND LICHENOID CONDITIONS

Allergic contact dermatitis

Obvious allergens include latex, rubber additives, topical medications, and spermicides (connubial dermatitis).[39] A mixed etiology is frequent. This is a type IV delayed hypersensitivity reaction. In a non-sensitized person, 5–7 days pass from exposure to clinical onset; the delay decreases to 4–6 hours in a previously exposed person (anamnestic response).

The reaction can be exuberant due to the rich vascularization of this anatomic location.[34,51] Although the reaction originates at the contact site, it may generalize if autoeczematization or id reaction develops. Erythema and marked edema are followed by formation of microvesicles and exudation. (Fig. 2.21) Lichenification accompanies chronic involvement. Secondary bacterial infections are frequent.

Lichen simplex chronicus (circumscribed neurodermatitis)

Lichen simplex chronicus (LSC) lesions are thickened plaques caused by persistent rubbing or trauma.[51] Atopic patients can have an isolated lesion of LSC, e.g. in the scrotum. The differential diagnosis includes psoriasis. (Fig. 2.22)

Prurigo nodularis

Prurigo nodularis is a clinical nodule resulting from longstanding and repeated trauma. The histologic findings are similar to those in LSC, but prurigo nodularis shows greater circumscription and symmetry. The epidermal hyperplasia is not as pronounced and is regular or psoriasiform. (Fig. 2.23)

Seborrheic dermatitis

Seborrheic dermatitis (SD) is a chronic dermatitis that affects skin areas with large numbers of sebaceous glands (scalp, central part of the face, trunk, and flexural areas).[52] It affects 1–3% of the general population. SD is strongly associated with Parkinson's disease, other neurologic conditions, and Down syndrome. SD is also one of the most common cutaneous manifestations of AIDS, in which context it is can be severe and atypically distributed. The pathogenesis is controversial, but association with *Malassezia* is likely. (Fig. 2.24)

Lichen planus

Lichen planus (LP) is a chronic dermatitis characterized by polygonal, violaceous, and flat-topped papules on the skin

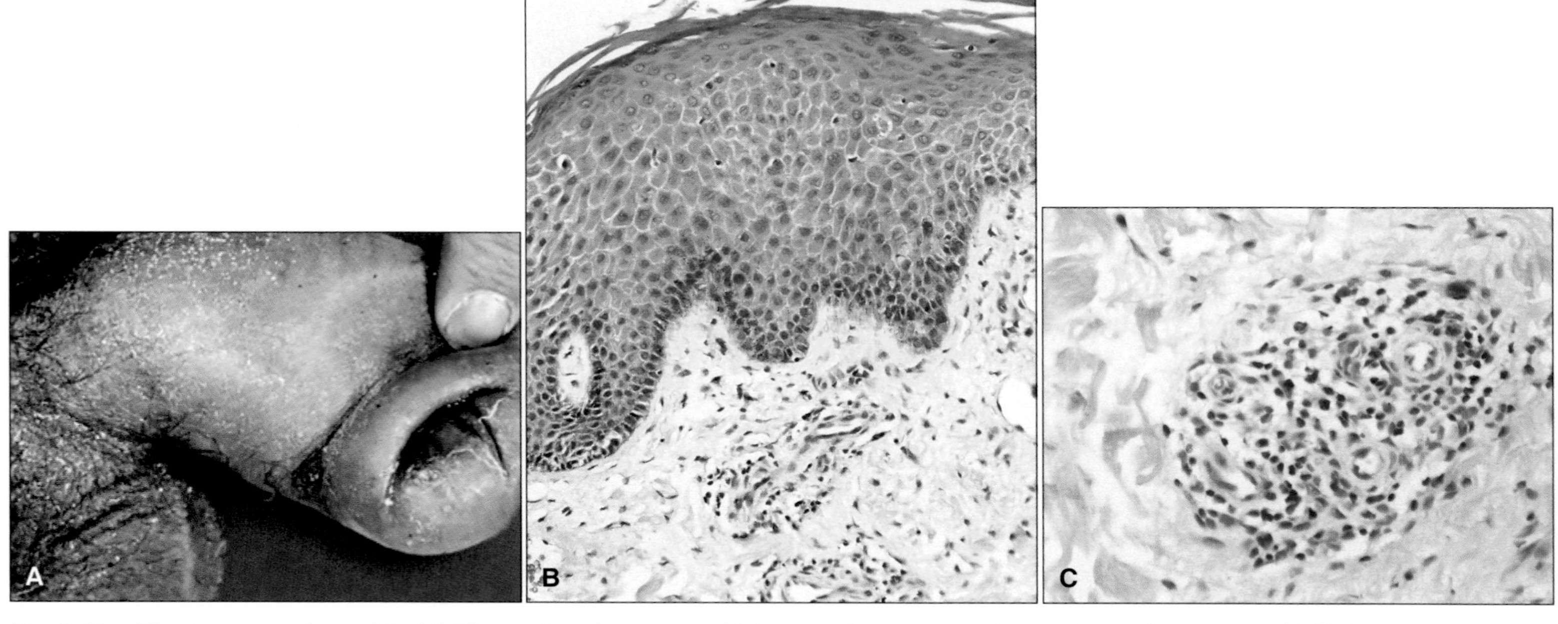

Fig. 2.21 Allergic contact dermatitis. (A) The penis and scrotum exhibit an erythematous, scaly, maculopapular eruption. (B,C) Spongiosis is noted in the epidermis. When it is pronounced in the lower epidermis, formation of spongiotic vesicles in an 'orderly' distribution is seen. Lymphocytes and histiocytes infiltrate about the superficial vascular plexus. Eosinophils are present in the dermis and epidermis. Eventually the epidermis becomes hyperplastic, the dermal inflammatory cell infiltrate becomes denser, and mild fibrosis develops. The differential diagnosis includes other eczematous dermatitides, especially nummular dermatitis. Nummular dermatitis is distinguished by its 'untidy' appearance, conferred by spongiotic microvesicles throughout the epidermis, and irregular acanthosis. In addition, nummular dermatitis has exocytosis of lymphocytes and neutrophils, while allergic contact dermatitis has lymphocytes and eosinophils.

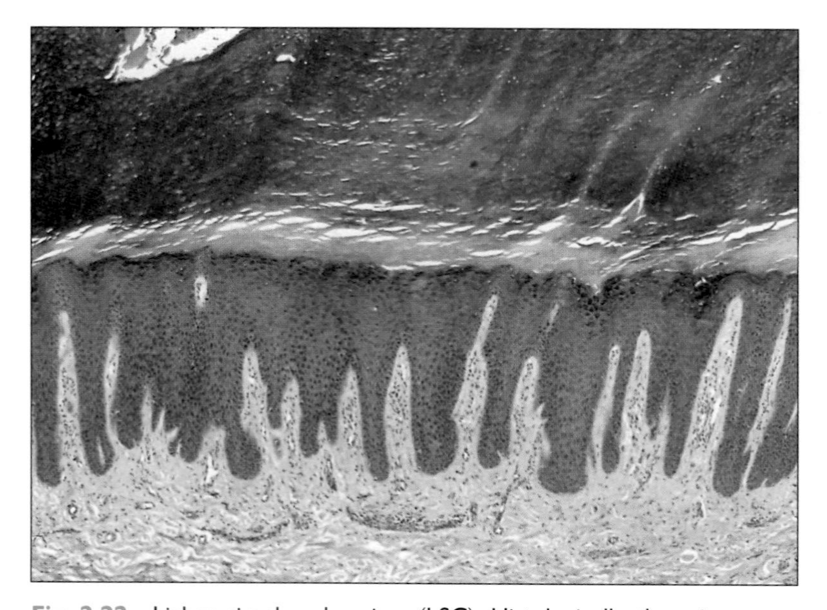

Fig. 2.22 Lichen simplex chronicus (LSC). Histologically, there is epidermal acanthosis with a compact hyperorthokeratosis and hypergranulosis. Collagen fibers in the papillary dermis are arranged perpendicular to the surface. There is chronic perivascular and interstitial inflammation. LSC is favored over psoriasis by hypergranulosis and the absence of neutrophilic intracorneal or intraepidermal microabscesses, or dilated tortuous vessels in the papillary dermis.

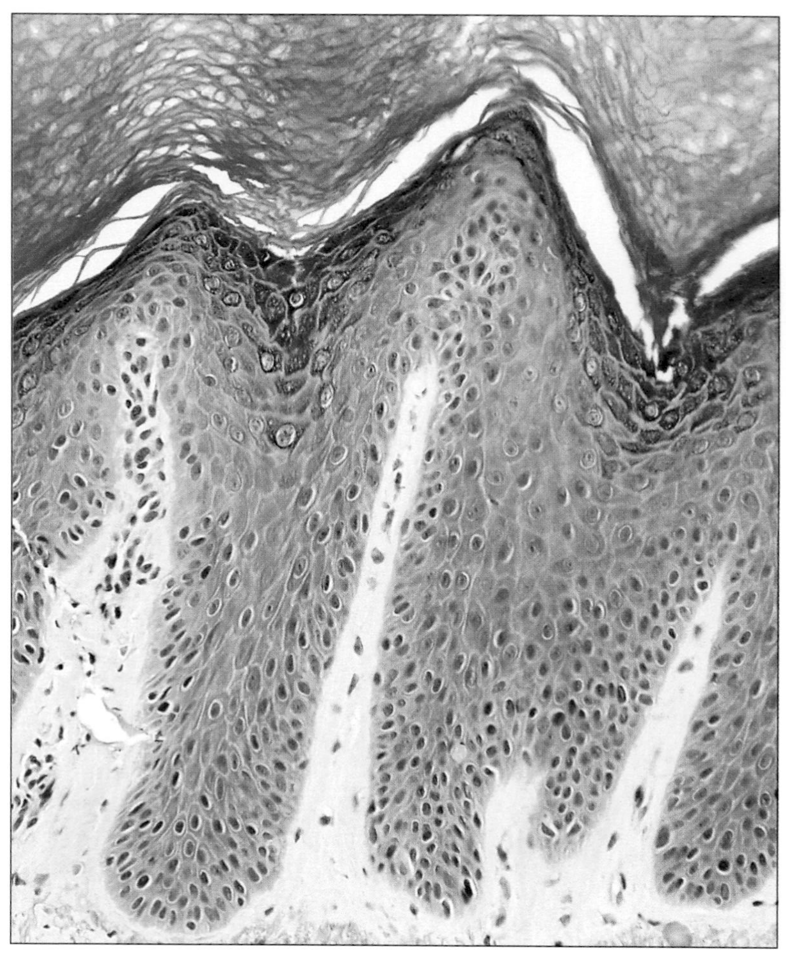

Fig. 2.23 Prurigo nodularis. There is hyperkeratosis with hypergranulosis in a psoriasiform or pseudoepitheliomatous pattern. Mild dermal fibrosis is associated with perivascular inflammation.

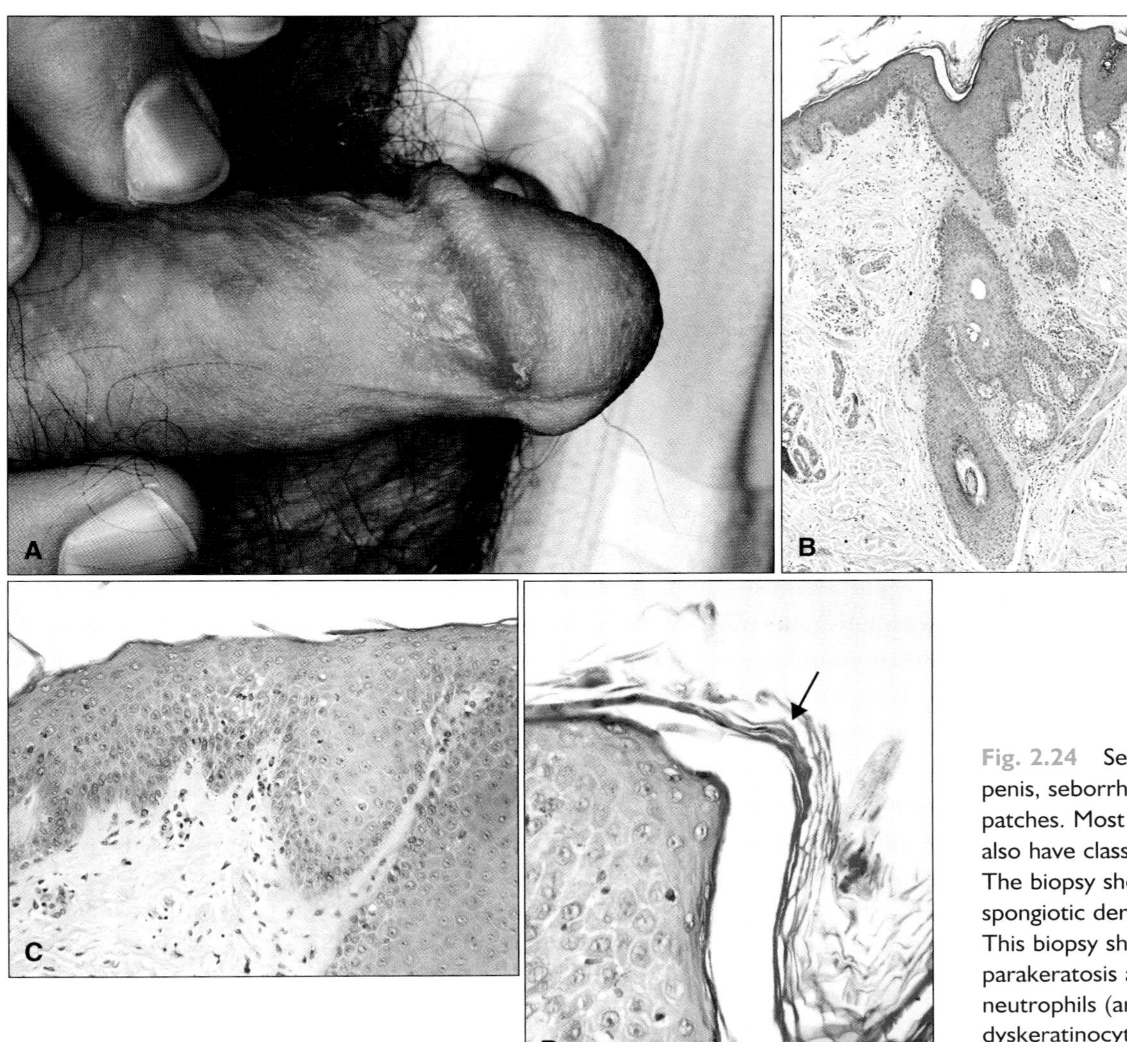

Fig. 2.24 Seborrheic dermatitis. (A) On the scrotum and penis, seborrheic dermatitis presents as greasy, scaly, red patches. Most patients with genital seborrheic dermatitis also have classical lesions in extragenital locations. (B,C) The biopsy shows changes of acute, subacute, or chronic spongiotic dermatitis, depending on the age of the lesion. This biopsy shows subacute spongiosis. (D) There is parakeratosis around hair follicles and exocytosis of neutrophils (arrow). In AIDS patients, scattered necrotic dyskeratinocytes, plasma cells, and neutrophils may be seen in the superficial dermal infiltrate.

and erosive lesions on the mucosa. Cutaneous lesions commonly resolve after several years, leaving postinflammatory hyperpigmentation. Mucosal lesions are more persistent.

Genital LP can present as papules or plaques, hypertrophic lesions, or mucosal erosions. One-quarter of patients with generalized cutaneous LP have genital lesions, usually of the papular type.

On the glans penis, LP presents as violaceous flat-topped papules with a lacy white surface (Wickham's striae).[53] Annular lesions can occur on the shaft or the glans. With time, lesions acquire a grayish hue due to melanin incontinence. Patients complain of pruritus and, when the lesions ulcerate, of pain.

LP is a T cell-mediated disease of unknown etiology. It can be associated with certain medications[54] and chronic liver disease, especially hepatitis C. (Fig. 2.25)

Lichen nitidus

Lichen nitidus is a chronic dermatosis characterized by small, separate, tan, shiny papules affecting the penis,

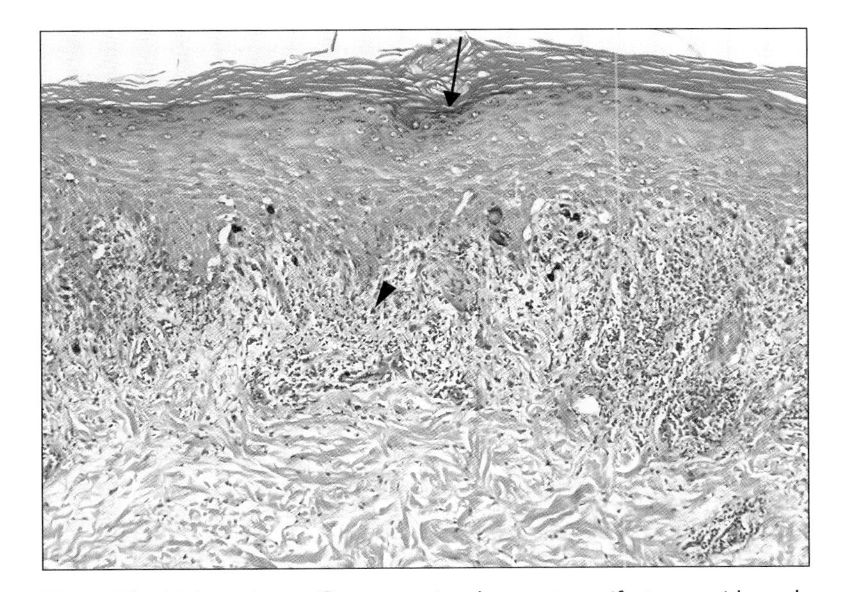

Fig. 2.25 Lichen planus. Cutaneous involvement manifests as epidermal acanthosis with wedge-shaped hypergranulosis (arrow) and hyperkeratosis, without parakeratosis. The dermoepidermal junction shows vacuolar change with Civatte bodies. With time, the rete ridges become pointed (the classic 'sawtooth' appearance) (arrowhead). The dermis shows a band-like lymphohistiocytic infiltrate with colloid bodies and melanophages. Plasma cells are usually present in mucosal lesions.

abdomen, and arms of children and young adults.[52] (Fig. 2.26)

Lichen sclerosus et atrophicus (balanitis xerotica obliterans)

Lichen sclerosus et atrophicus (LSA) is a chronic dermatitis of unknown etiology characterized by atrophic white papules or plaques on anogenital skin.[55] (Figs 2.27 & 2.28) In 15–20% of patients, extragenital involvement occurs (back, periumbilical, neck, and axilla). Involvement of the penis is much more common than perianal involvement in men.[56] In uncircumcised men, a constricted sclerotic band may form 1–2 cm from the distal border of the prepuce, leading to phimosis. Urinary retention may result if the lesion involves the urethral orifice or the phimosis becomes severe. The end stage in uncircumcised males is balanitis xerotica obliterans (BXO), an unretractable thickened foreskin. BXO can also occur because of chronic nonspecific balanoposthitis.

Morphea also shows sclerosis in the reticular dermis and subcutaneous septa, but lacks the elastic fiber destruction seen in LSA. Chronic radiodermatitis also shows epidermal atrophy, papillary dermal edema, and sclerosis. Unlike LSA, however, there is involvement of the reticular dermis, pleomorphic endothelial/fibroblast nuclei, and waxy vessel walls.

Squamous cell carcinoma is a possible complication, occurring in 5.8% of penile LSA.[57,58] Most of these cases have concomitant HPV infection.

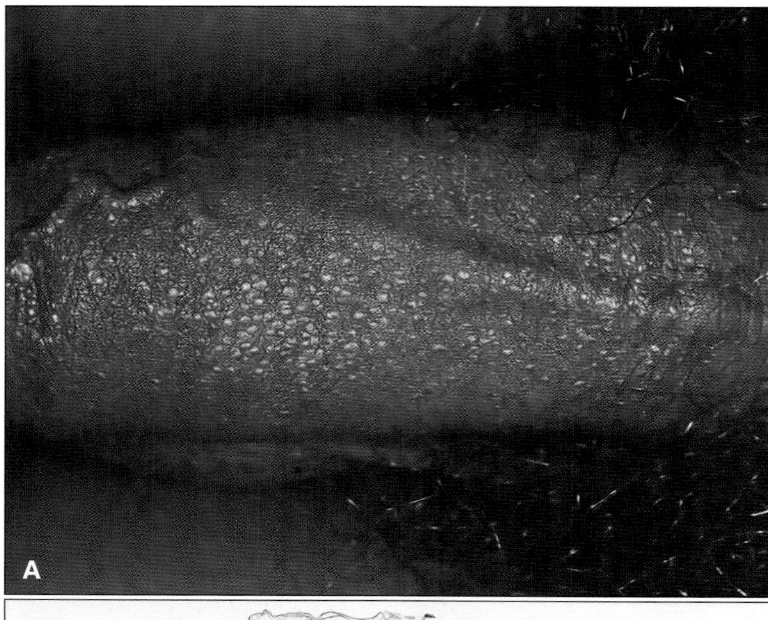

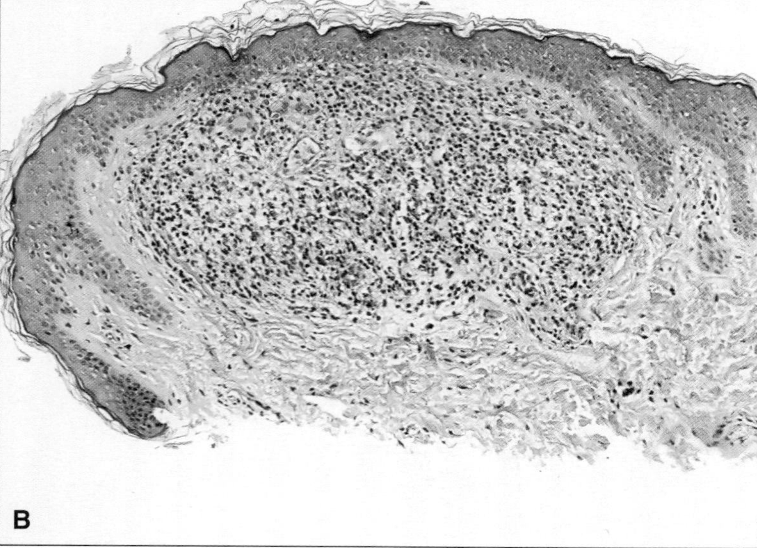

Fig. 2.26 Lichen nitidus. (A) Multiple tiny papules in the penis. (B) The papule is a dermal papilla distended by a lymphohistiocytic infiltrate with giant cells. The overlying epidermis shows basal vacuolization, rare dyskeratinocytes, and parakeratosis. The rete ridges embrace inflammation with claw-like extensions forming a collarette ('ball and claw'). In early lesions, the infiltrate is entirely composed of lymphocytes.

Erythema multiforme

Erythema multiforme (EM), a pleomorphic mucocutaneous hypersensitivity reaction, can be elicited by many immunologic stimuli.[10] Over 100 inciting factors have been reported, including viral, fungal, and bacterial infections, drugs, and neoplasia. Herpesvirus infection is a frequent antecedent to genital EM, and an interval of several weeks may pass between infection and the appearance of EM lesions. Drugs are the most frequent culprit when multiple mucosal sites are involved (Stevens–Johnson syndrome). (Fig. 2.29)

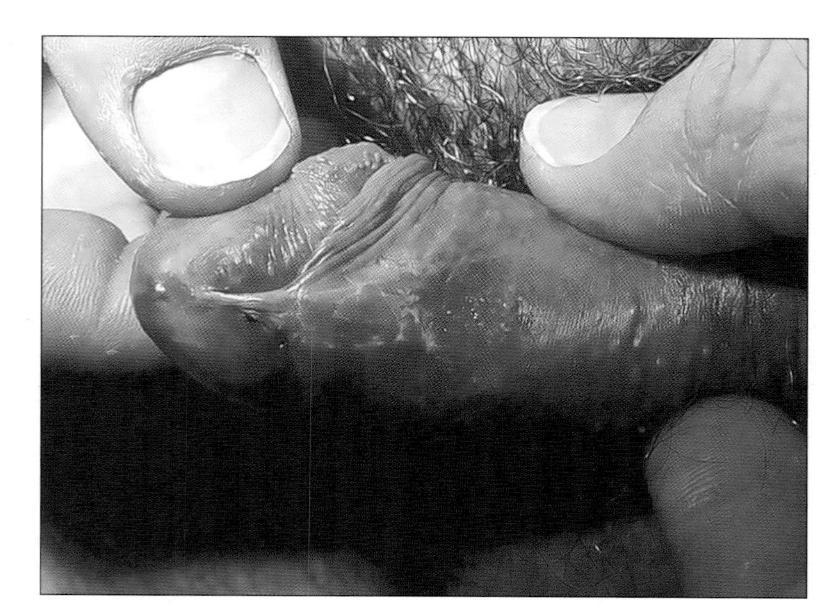

Fig. 2.27 Lichen sclerosus et atrophicus (LSA). On the penis, ivory or porcelain-white macules and plaques occur on the glans and inner aspect of the prepuce. The whitish color of the lesions is due to loss of dermal vasculature and depigmentation. Follicular plugging is frequent within atrophic ('cigarette paper-wrinkled') lesions. The atrophic epidermis of LSA is prone to erosions and fissures. Hemorrhage may lead to ecchymosis.

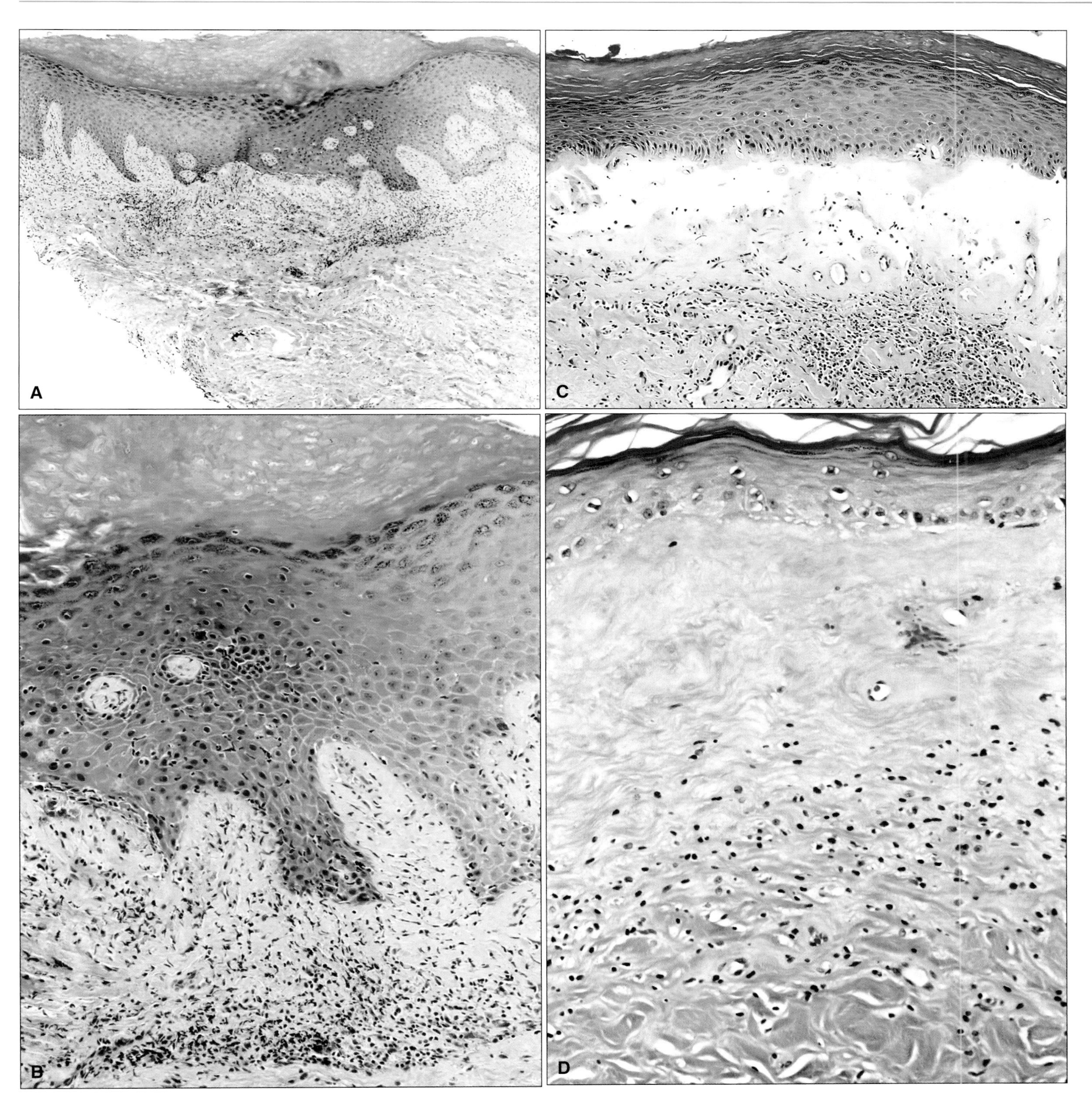

Fig. 2.28 Lichen sclerosus et atrophicus. (A,B) Early histologic findings include epidermis with basal vacuolar changes, dyskeratinocytes, and thickening of the basement membrane associated with a heavy band-like inflammatory infiltrate. The differential diagnosis at this stage includes lichen planus. (C) Established lesions show a hyperkeratotic, atrophic epidermis with vacuolar change of the basal layer. Membrane thickening and keratotic plugging of adnexal ostia occur. A broad zone of dermal sclerosis with dilated thin wall vessels overlies the inflammation. Mild perivascular lymphoplasmacytic infiltration with scattered macrophages and mast cells is noted. The histologic presentation varies with the age of the lesion. The elastic fibers in the dermis are depressed by the dermal edema. Occasionally, the vacuolar change of the epidermis and the dermal edema may produce subepidermal separation and blister formation.[59] (D) End-stage lesions show epidermal atrophy, homogenization of the papillary dermal collagen, and a persistent superficial lymphocytic infiltrate at the upper border of the reticular dermis.

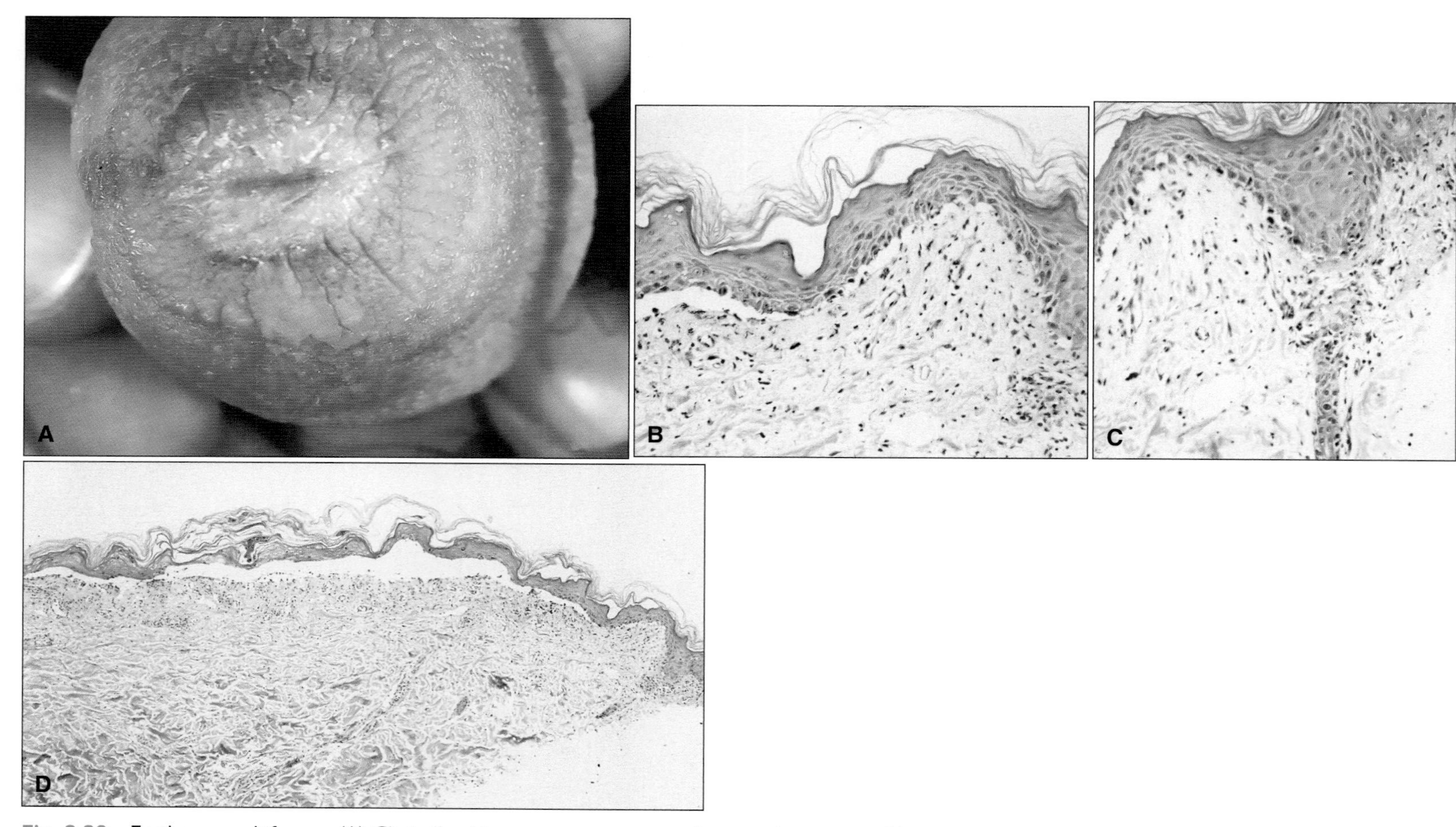

Fig. 2.29 Erythema multiforme. (A) Clinically, this may present as macules, papules, urticarial lesions, plaques, or vesicles. Presentation as a bullous eruption is especially common in the genital area. (B,C) Microscopically, the typical 'targetoid' lesion of erythema multiforme is an area of central necrosis surrounded by circular areas of edema and erythema. Drug hypersensitivity should be suspected when eosinophils are numerous and apoptotic keratinocytes concentrate in the acrosyringium. (D) Established lesions of erythema multiforme (EM) show basal epidermal vacuolar change, many dyskeratinocytes, and a lichenoid chronic inflammatory infiltrate in the upper dermis. EM-like change occurs in paraneoplastic pemphigus. Immunofluorescence studies can separate these disorders.

Fixed drug eruption

Fixed drug eruption is an erythematous, blistered, or eroded cutaneous or mucosal plaque that recurs at the same anatomic location each time the patient is exposed to the inciting compound. The most frequent agents are trimethoprim–sulfamethoxazole, nonsteroidal anti-inflammatory drugs, and chlormezanone.[60,61] The mucous membrane lesions are less symmetric than their cutaneous counterparts and often present as erosions rather than blisters.[62,63] (Fig. 2.30)

IMMUNOBULLOUS AND ACANTHOLYTIC DISORDERS

Autoantibodies can target normal components of the epidermis and basement membrane, leading to blistering disorders. Skin biopsy can define the cleavage and the nature of the inflammatory response. Immunofluorescence tests further distinguish among blistering disorders that overlap clinically and histologically.

Pemphigus vulgaris and its variants

Pemphigus vulgaris has a predilection for mucosal sites. Fragile blisters are characteristic in other parts of the body, but the genitalia show extensive erosions.[64] (Fig. 2.31) Pemphigus vegetans presents as verrucous plaques on intertriginous areas. It can involve only the glans, as a moist, vegetative plaque with erosions.

Bullous pemphigoid

Bullous pemphigoid (BP) is the most frequent blistering disorder of older people. It involves mucosal and flexural sites, so the genital region is a frequent target. Tense blisters – sometimes preceded by urticarial plaques – characterize BP. (Fig. 2.32) Penile lesions often occur together with

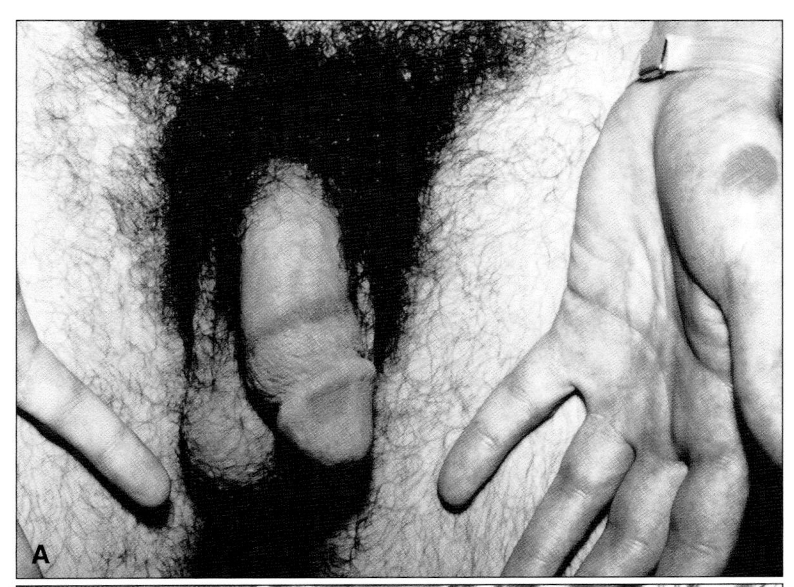

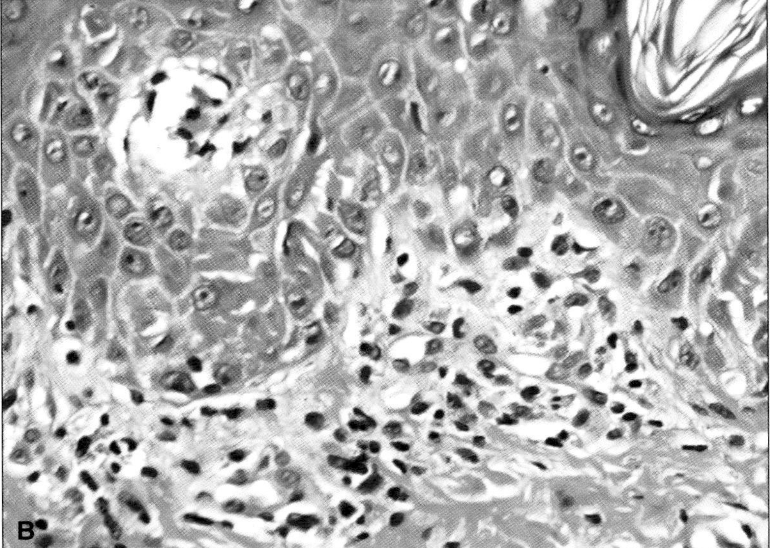

Fig. 2.30 Fixed drug eruption. (A) Although a single lesion is the most frequent clinical presentation, multiple lesions, as in this patient, are also encountered. (B) The basal layer of the epidermis shows vacuolar change and Civatte bodies. An inflammatory dermal reaction tends to obscure the dermal–epidermal junction, as in erythema multiforme. Inflammation can involve the upper epidermis, producing dyskeratinocytes above the basal layer. Prominent melanin incontinence is noted. A deep dermal infiltrate of lymphocytes, neutrophils, and eosinophils is seen.

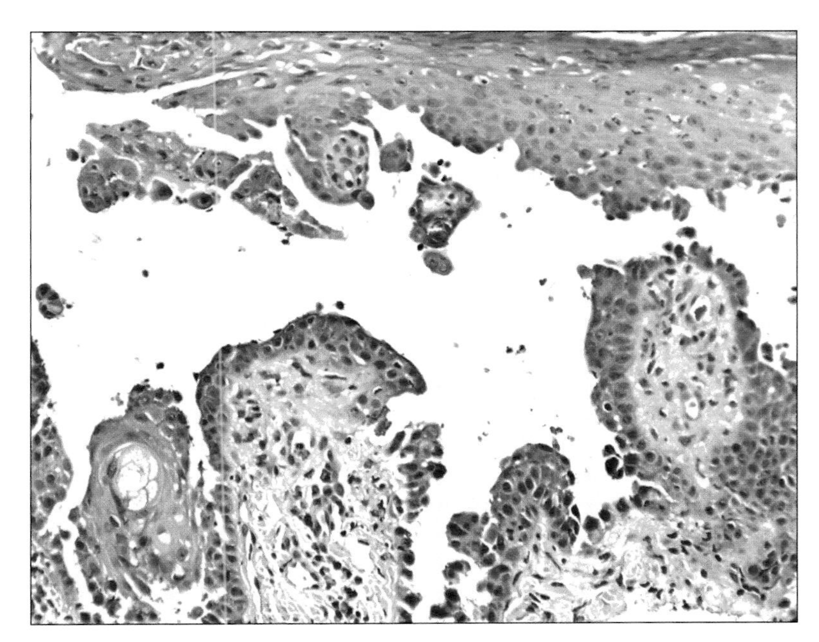

Fig. 2.31 Pemphigus vulgaris. Biopsy shows epidermal acanthosis with suprabasilar clefting with acantholysis. Immunofluorescence examination shows intercellular IgG and C3 in the epidermis.

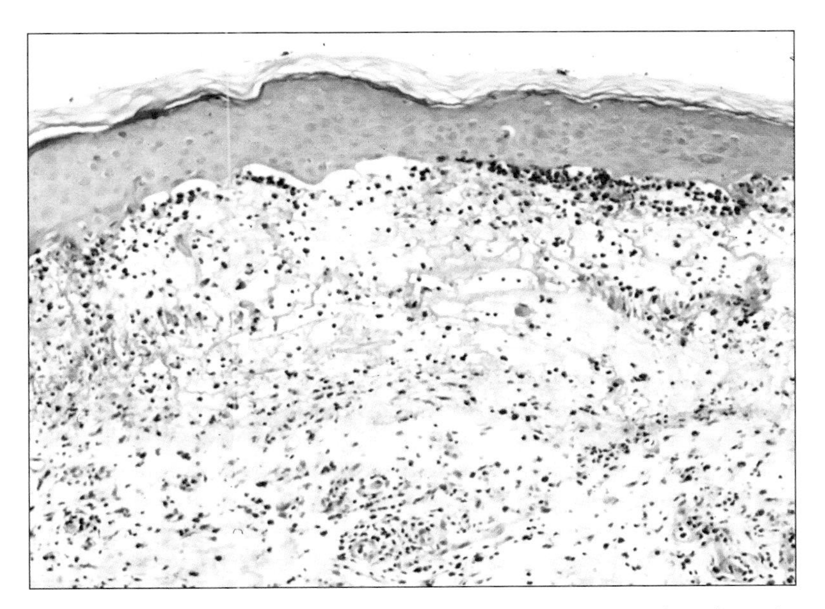

Fig. 2.32 Bullous pemphigoid. The histologic findings are subepidermal blisters with an eosinophilic infiltrate. Immunofluorescence examination shows linear, subepidermal C3 and IgG.

oropharyngeal, nasal, or conjunctival involvement. Chronic cicatricial pemphigoid, a related condition, can cause a low-grade balanoposthitis that leads to phimosis and superimposed BXO.

Dermatitis herpetiformis

Dermatitis herpetiformis (DH) can cause chronic genital ulcers. Immunofluorescence (IF) examination reveals deposition of C3 in the papillary dermis. The differential diagnosis includes IgA dermatitis (IF shows linear IgA deposition), bullous lupus erythematosus (IF shows LE band), and leukocytoclastic vasculitis (shows vascular damage, absent in DH). (Fig. 2.33)

Benign familial pemphigus (Hailey–Hailey disease)

This autosomal dominant disease presents as expanding erythematous plaques in the inguinal creases, scrotum, and perineum, with superimposed erosions, vesicles, and pustules. (Fig. 2.34)

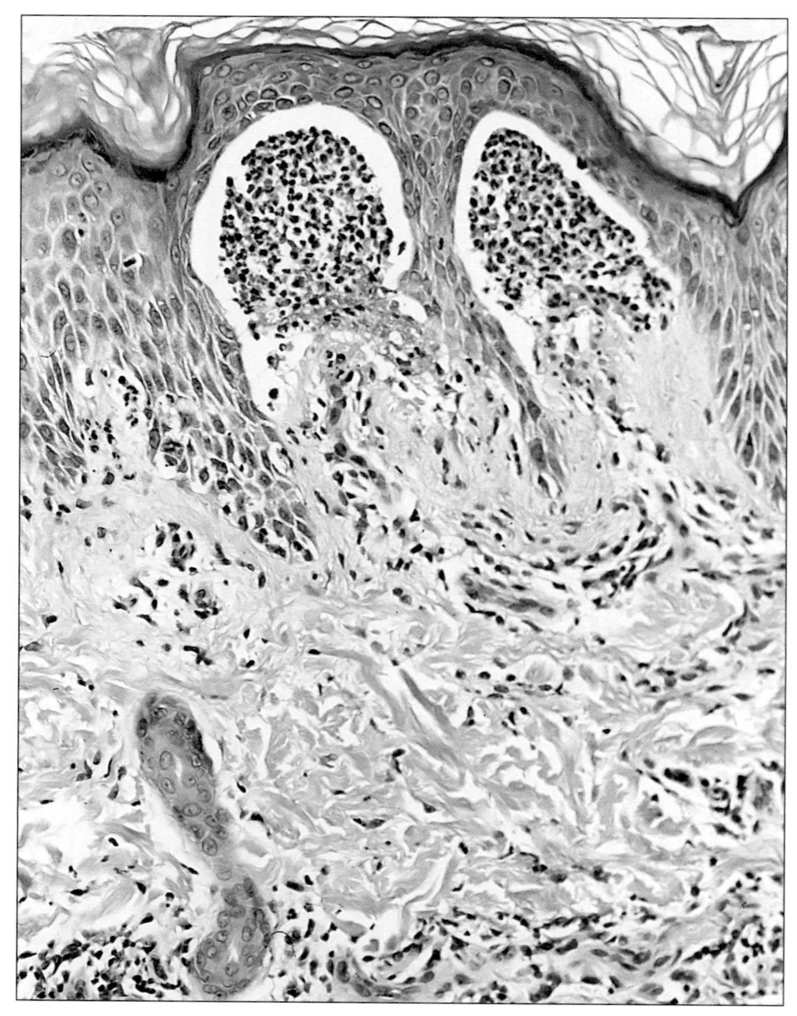

Fig. 2.33 Dermatitis herpetiformis. The histologic presentation is characterized by papillary neutrophilic microabscesses.

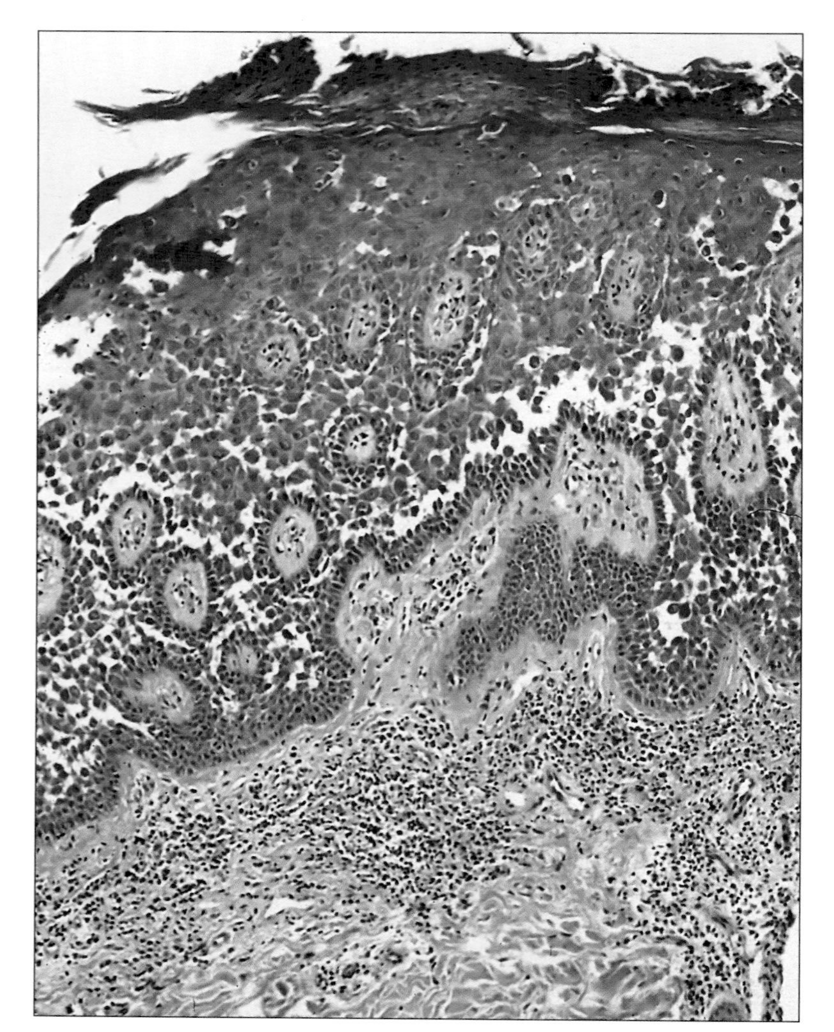

Fig. 2.34 Benign familial pemphigus. Biopsy shows epidermal acanthosis with transepidermal acantholysis. Chronic inflammatory reaction is seen in the upper dermis.

MISCELLANEOUS INFLAMMATORY CONDITIONS

Balanoposthitis

Balanoposthitis is inflammation of the mucosa of the glans (balanitis) and prepuce (posthitis).

Pediatric cases due to chronic, mixed bacterial infection affect young boys (2 to 5 years old) in whom the prepuce is nonretractable. Patients complain of redness, swelling, discharge, and dysuria. Circumcision treats recurrent episodes. Perianal streptococcal cellulitis can accompany childhood acute balanoposthitis.

In adults, balanoposthitis more commonly presents as intertrigo. A specific infectious agent (group B β-hemolytic streptococcus, gonococcus, *Candida albicans*, *Gardnerella vaginalis*, *Trichomonas*, or anaerobes) can sometimes be identified in recurrent cases. Diabetes mellitus is a predisposing factor.

Psoriasis vulgaris

Psoriasis is an epidermal hyperproliferative condition that affects 2% of the US population. Lesions may start at sites of trauma. It is a common noninfectious dermatosis of the glans penis. In occluded skin (preputial sac, inguinal folds, intergluteal cleft, and axilla), the lesion appears as a well-demarcated erythematous plaque without scale (inverse pattern psoriasis).[65] (Fig. 2.35) The diagnosis of genital psoriasis is supported by the presence of psoriasis at other sites (scalp, gluteal folds, and nails). Anogenital psoriasis is commonly a minimally symptomatic disease that waxes and wanes for years.

Plasma cell balanitis (Zoon's balanitis, balanitis circumscripta plasmacellularis)

This lesion affects the glans penis as a solitary, erythematous, discrete, moist plaque with a brown, speckled appearance due to microhemorrhages ('Cayenne pepper').[66,67] (Fig. 2.36) It affects older, uncircumcised men. Contiguous areas are often affected ('kissing lesion'). A tumorous or vegetative type ('plasmo-acanthoma') has been reported. Lesions heal slowly, leaving a rusty macule.

Similar lesions occur in the vulva ('plasma cell vulvitis'), oral mucosa ('plasma cell orificial mucositis', 'plasmocytosis circumorificialis'), and lip ('plasma cell cheilitis').

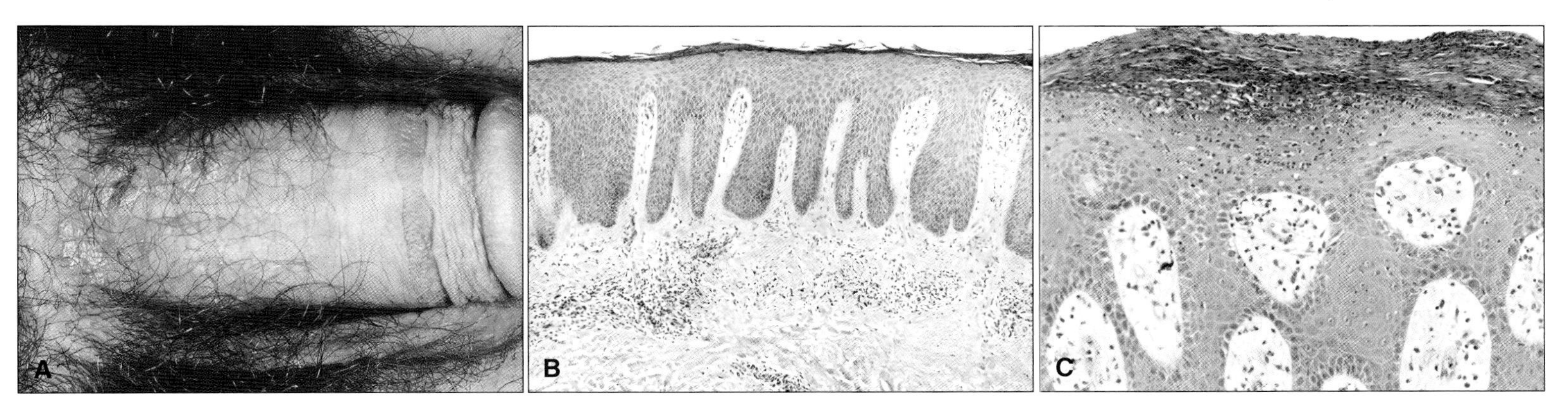

Fig. 2.35 Psoriasis vulgaris. (A) Well demarcated erythematous plaque. (B,C) A well-formed psoriatic lesion shows psoriasiform (regular) epidermal hyperplasia with hyperparakeratosis. Collections of neutrophils can be seen in the stratum corneum (Munro microabscesses) and/or spinosa (spongiform pustules of Kogoj). Thin suprapapillary plates overlie dilated vessels in the papillary dermis. The dermal inflammatory component consists of activated T lymphocytes and neutrophils. Plasma cells can be seen in patients with HIV infection.

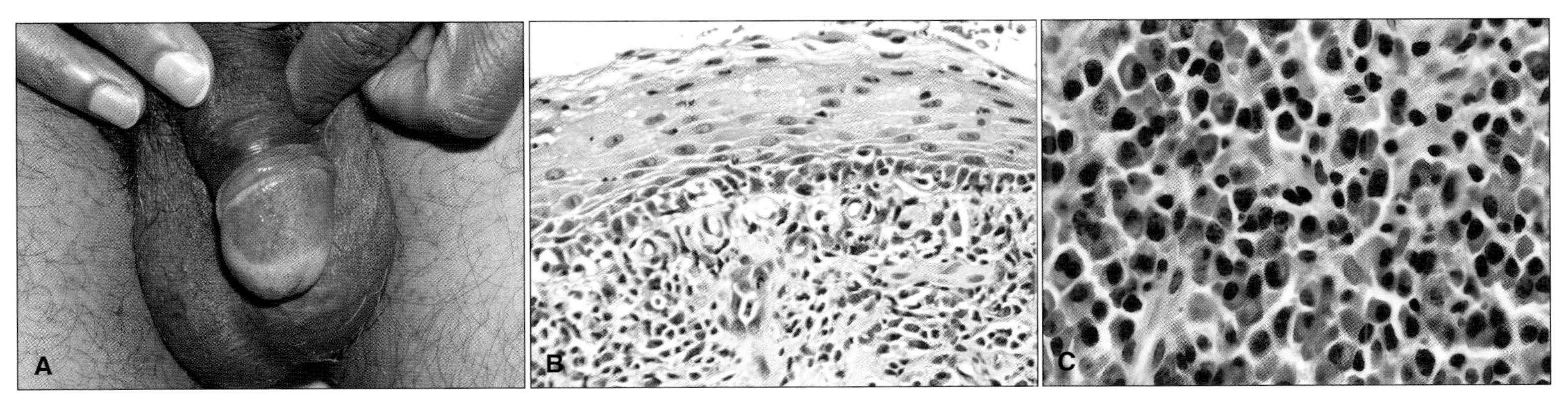

Fig. 2.36 Plasma cell balanitis. (A) Clinically, the lesion is characterized by a well demarcated erythematous moist plaque. (B,C) The epidermis is atrophic, with dense, lichenoid, chronic dermal inflammation. The infiltrate consists mostly of polyclonal plasma cells in the upper and mid dermis.[68] Lymphocytes, mast cells, and scattered neutrophils can be seen. Lymphoid follicles may occasionally be present. Vascular proliferation, red cell extravasation, and hemosiderin are common.[69]

Biopsy is performed to rule out squamous cell carcinoma in situ. Immunohistochemical stains for light chain restriction may be considered to rule out plasma cell neoplasm.

Peyronie's disease (penile fibromatosis)

This disease causes irregular fibrous plaques on the dorsum of the penis, producing distortion or angulation upon erection. Ten percent of these patients also have hand and plantar fibromatosis (Dupuytren's contracture).[70] (Fig. 2.37)

Pyoderma gangrenosum

Pyoderma gangrenosum is an ulcerative reaction pattern that is idiopathic, or associated with diverse disorders including inflammatory bowel disease, chronic active hepatitis, myeloma, rheumatoid arthritis, paraproteinemia, and leukemia. The most frequently affected site is the legs, but the penis, scrotum, and perineum may be involved.[71,72] A hemorrhagic plaque undergoes necrosis with formation of a progressively enlarging ulcer with round borders. The diagnosis is primarily clinical. As with all neutrophilic processes, infection must be ruled out. (Fig. 2.38)

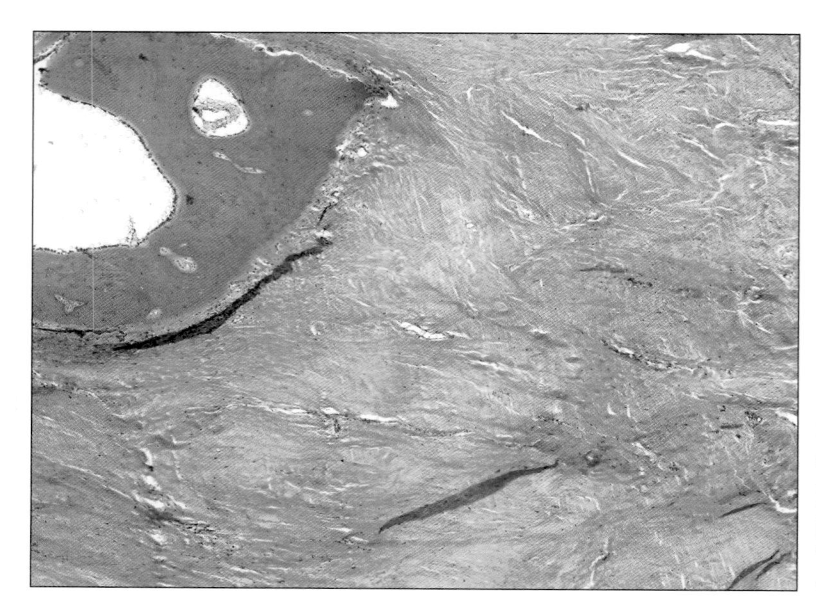

Fig. 2.37 Peyronie's disease. The connective tissue between the tunica albuginea and corpora cavernosa in the dorsum of the penile shaft shows perivascular chronic inflammation, endothelial hyperplasia, and subsequent proliferation of fibroconnective tissue. Changes may also be seen on the ventral aspect of the shaft and in the intercorporeal septum. Calcification or even ossification may occur.

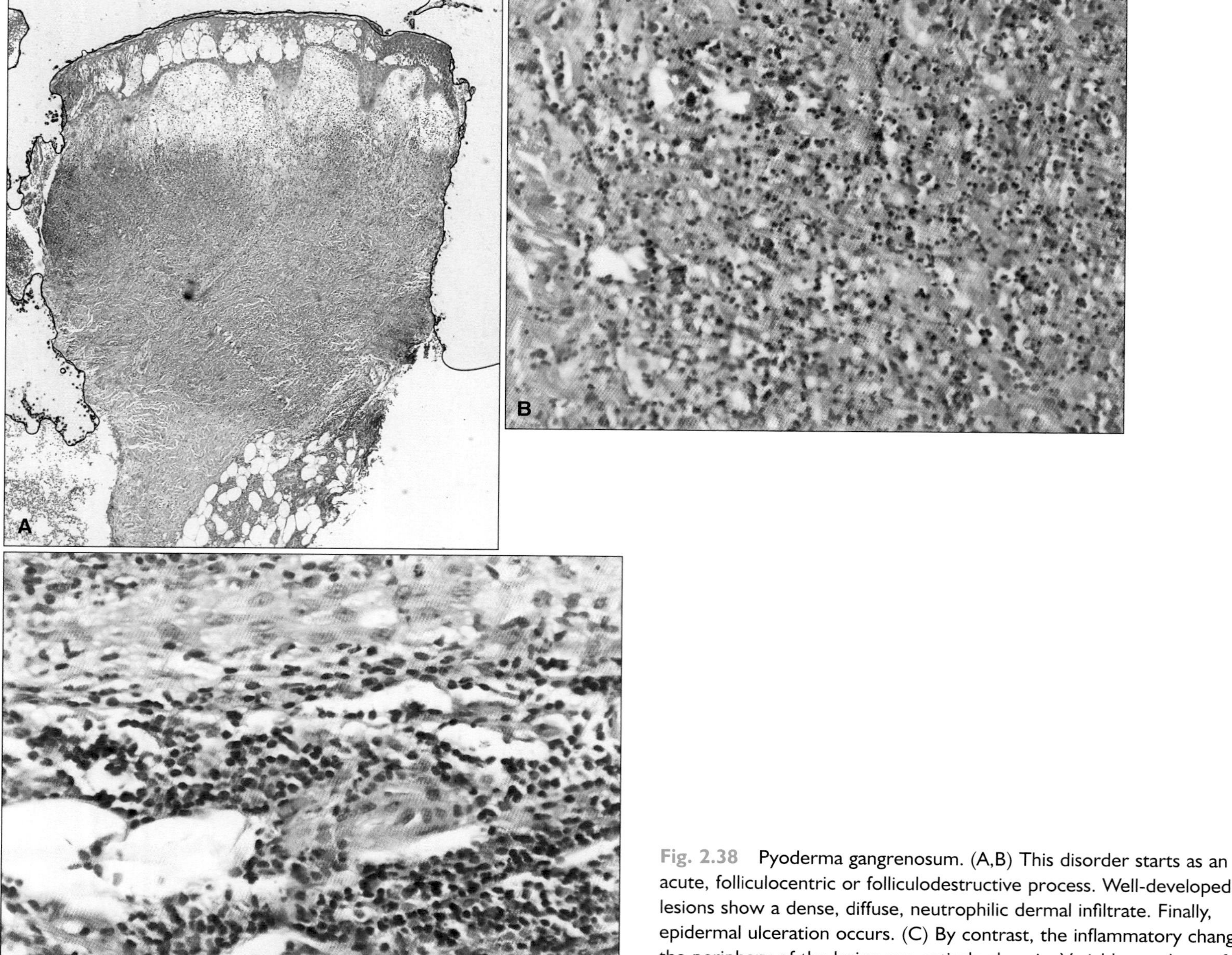

Fig. 2.38 Pyoderma gangrenosum. (A,B) This disorder starts as an acute, folliculocentric or folliculodestructive process. Well-developed lesions show a dense, diffuse, neutrophilic dermal infiltrate. Finally, epidermal ulceration occurs. (C) By contrast, the inflammatory changes at the periphery of the lesion are entirely chronic. Variable numbers of lymphocytes, macrophages, and eosinophils are noted at the periphery. This distinction produces the characteristic 'dichotomous' appearance of the infiltrate.

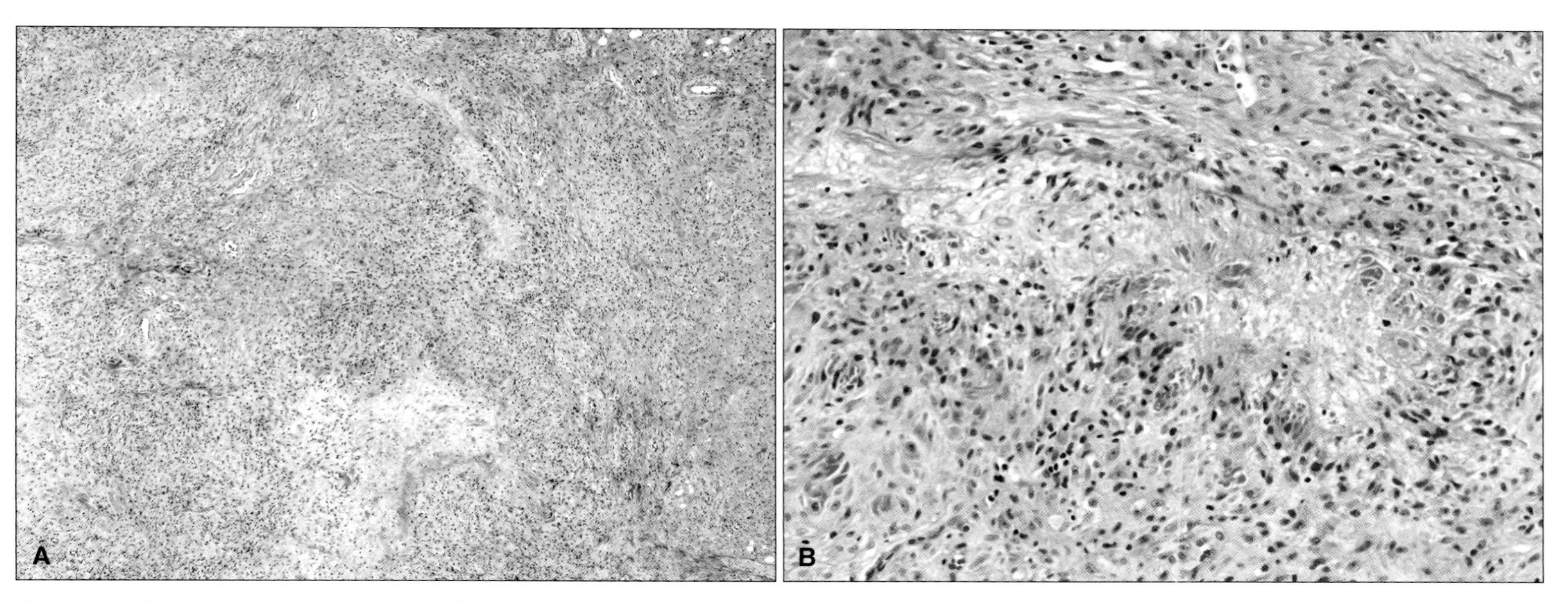

Fig. 2.39 Deep granuloma annulare. (A,B) Biopsy shows deep, palisading granulomas with central, Alcian blue-positive mucinous material.

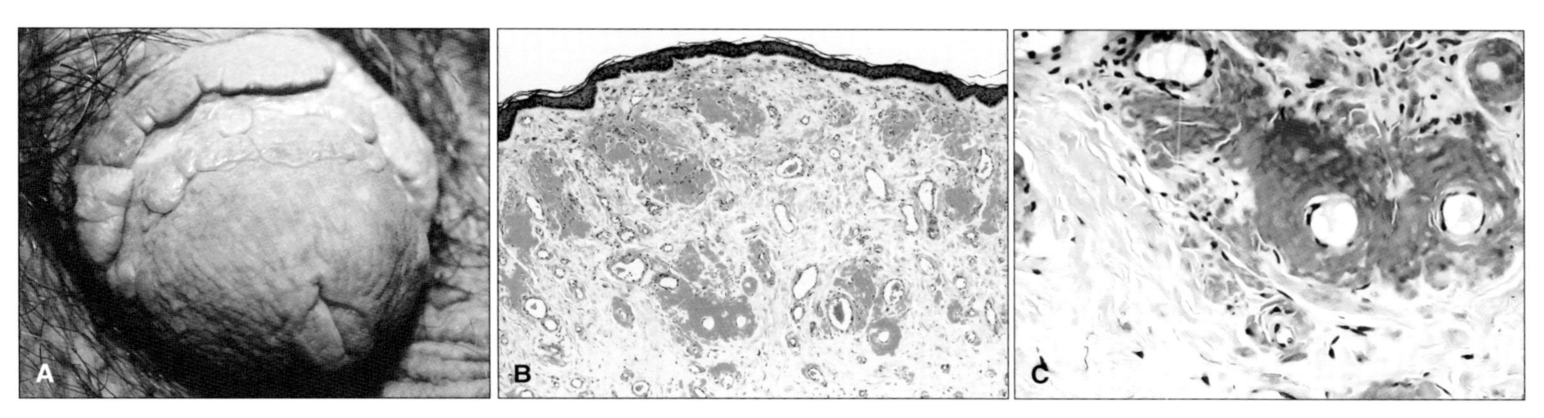

Fig. 2.40 Amyloidosis. (A) Amyloid presents clinically as verrucous papules. (B,C) Homogeneous eosinophilic amorphous deposits around vessels are seen in this lesion. Congo red stains amyloid bright orange. Under polarized light, deposits show the characteristic apple-green birefringence. Electron microscopy shows the β-pleated structure.

Deep granuloma annulare

Granuloma annulare has been reported as small, asymptomatic nodules on the glans penis.[73,74] (Fig. 2.39)

METABOLIC, DEPOSITION, AND MULTISYSTEM DISEASES

AMYLOIDOSIS

Primary amyloidosis has been reported in the penis[75,76] as a subcutaneous mass or verrucous lesions in the glans. Perivascular amyloid deposits may predispose to cutaneous hemorrhage in genital folds. (Fig. 2.40)

IDIOPATHIC CALCINOSIS OF THE SCROTUM

Calcinosis of the scrotum and penis presents as multiple hard, mobile nodules. Transepidermal elimination of chalky white material has been reported. The condition affects males after the third decade. Scrotal calcinosis may be calcification of the dartos similar to calcification of uterine myomas, or it may represent dystrophic calcification of epidermal inclusion cysts.[77] (Fig. 2.41)

POLYARTERITIS NODOSA

Polyarteritis nodosa is a necrotizing vasculitis involving small and medium-sized arteries. Ulcerated subcutaneous nodules or livedo reticularis affect about 15% of patients. Involvement of the testis and epididymis can lead to cutaneous infarcts or painful scrotal swelling. The glans penis can be affected as an isolated nodule.[78] (Fig. 2.42)

WEGENER'S GRANULOMATOSIS

In this systemic disorder, necrotizing granulomas involve cutaneous blood vessels, leading to ulcerative nodules. The most frequently affected organs are the upper airways,

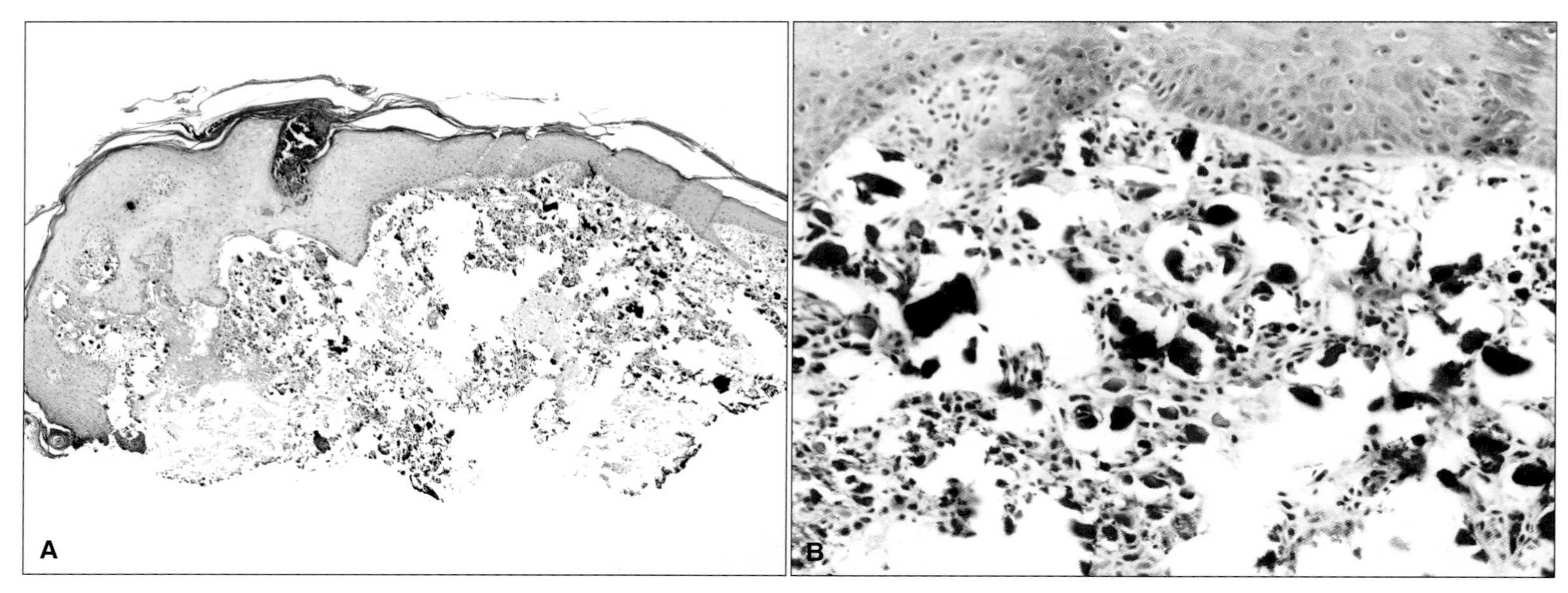

Fig. 2.41 Idiopathic calcinosis of the scrotum. (A,B) Histologically, homogeneous basophilic material is seen. Calcium stains such as von Kossa confirm the diagnosis.

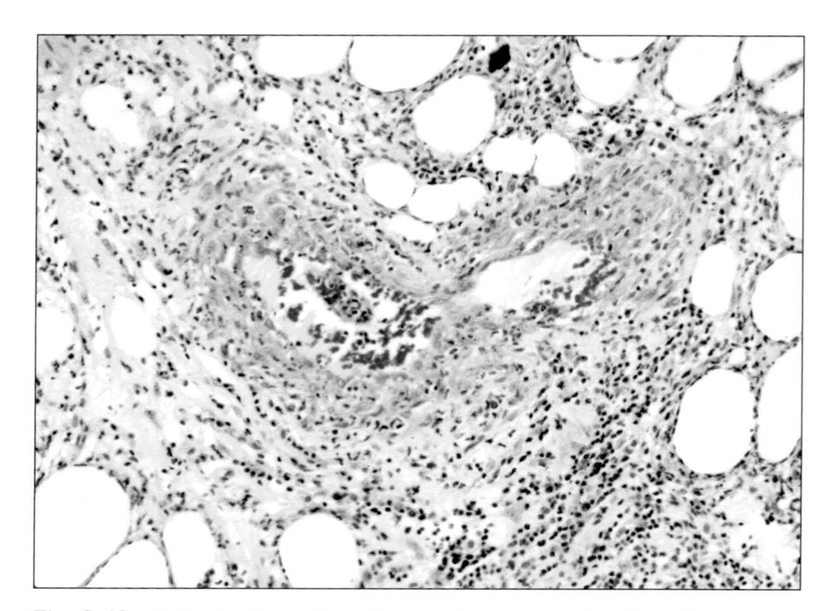

Fig. 2.42 Polyarteritis nodosa. Destruction of vessel walls with acute inflammation and fibrin deposition is seen. Secondary ischemic changes range from pale epidermis to transdermal necrosis.

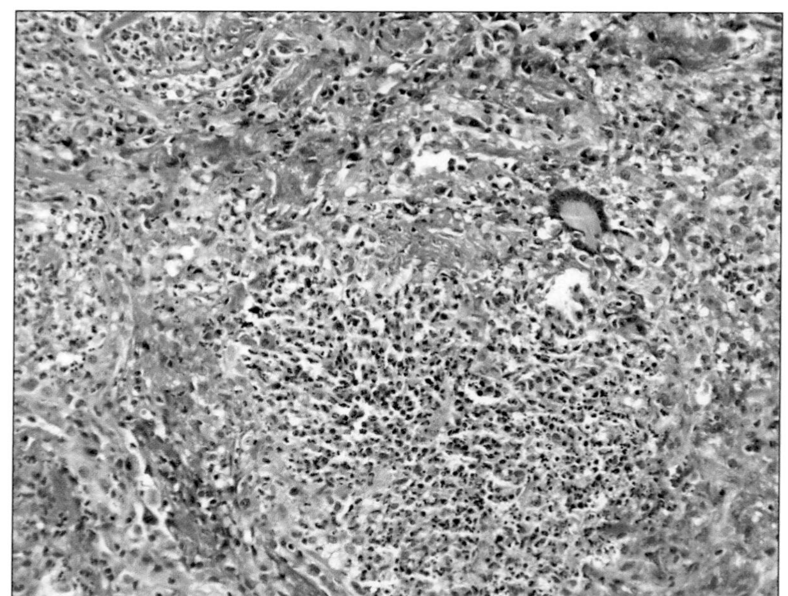

Fig. 2.43 Wegener's granulomatosis. Classic necrotizing vasculitis with granulomatosis is seen in only about 20% of cases. Extravascular changes range from small foci of necrosis with neutrophilic infiltration and palisading histiocytic reaction, to poorly formed granulomas. Occasionally the findings are quite nonspecific, consisting only of chronic inflammation. Vascular involvement is seen as necrotizing vasculitis, granulomatous angiitis, and leukocytoclastic vasculitis.

lungs, and kidneys, but penile necrosis secondary to large vessel vasculitis has been seen.[79,80] (Fig. 2.43)

REITER'S SYNDROME

About one-quarter of men with Reiter's syndrome have balanitis circinata.[34] In uncircumcised men, bright red, exudative plaques with ragged, slightly elevated margins appear around the corona. These are accompanied by small papules that can coalesce. In circumcised men, the lesions are dry and scaly, mimicking psoriasis. The diagnosis is suggested when balanitis circinata occurs with urethritis, conjunctivitis, arthritis, and/or keratoderma blenorrhagica. Concomitant erosive oral mucosal lesions, ocular lesions, bilateral conjunctivitis, and anterior uveitis may be seen.[81] (Fig. 2.44)

SARCOIDOSIS

Sarcoidosis is a chronic granulomatous disorder of unknown etiology. It affects the skin in one-third of cases, as granulomatous dermatitis and erythema nodosum.

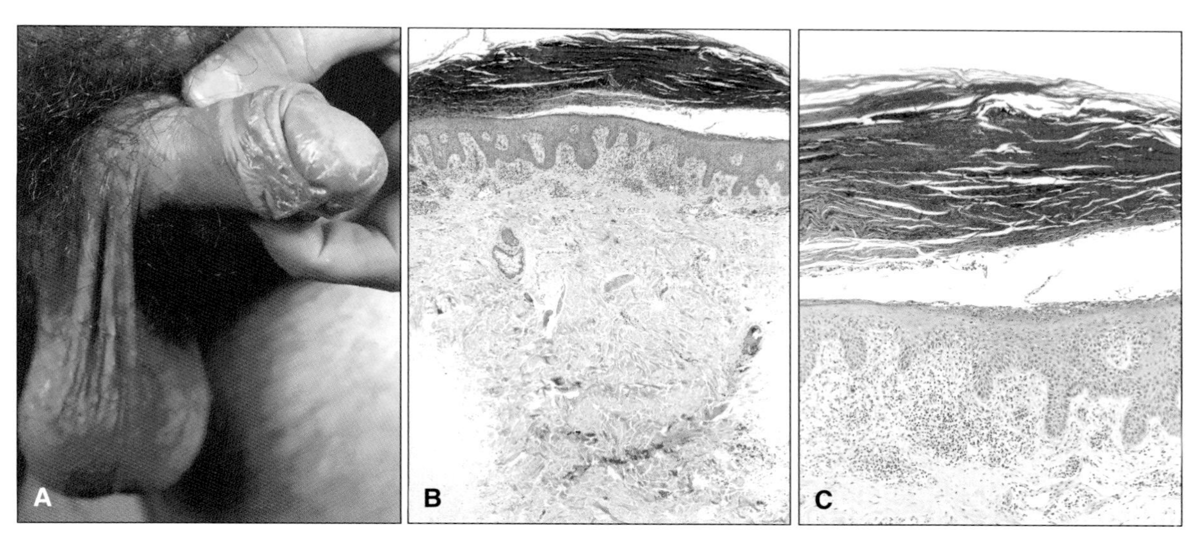

Fig. 2.44 Balanitis circinata. (A–C) Lesions in Reiter's syndrome may be indistinguishable from pustular psoriasis. In buccal and genital lesions, the epidermal psoriasiform hyperplasia and stratum corneum thickening are less prominent.

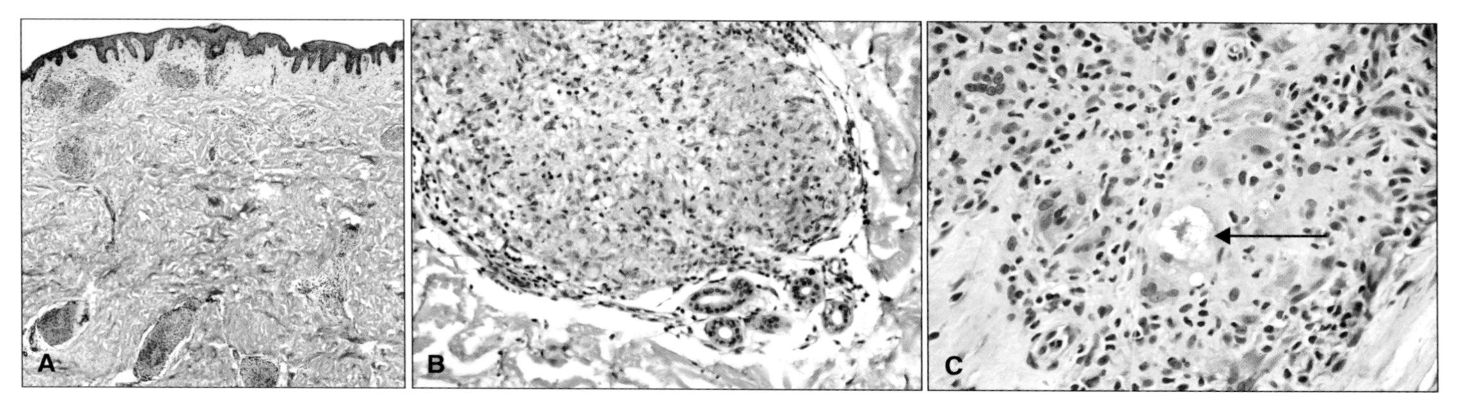

Fig. 2.45 Sarcoidosis. (A–C) The biopsy shows the characteristic noncaseating epithelioid granulomas. The asteroid body (arrow), present in the cytoplasm of the giant cell, is believed by some to be trapped collagen bundles or possibly vimentin intermediate filaments. Asteroid and Schaumann bodies are not specific to sarcoidosis and can be seen in other granulomatous reactions, like tuberculosis. Birefringent calcium salts can be identified in granulomas.

Tender erythematous induration of the distal penile shaft, papules on the penis and scrotum,[82] and yellow plaques on the dorsum of the glans have been reported. Sarcoidosis is a diagnosis of exclusion. Special stains serve to rule out infection, and polarization microscopy to identify foreign material. (Fig. 2.45)

NEUROFIBROMATOSIS

Genital neurofibromas present as skin-colored soft papules, nodules, or plaques. They are often asymptomatic, but large plexiform neurofibromas can alter urinary function. Systemic neurofibromatosis must be considered if the patient also presents with axillary freckling and/or six or more café-au-lait macules larger than 1 cm in diameter.[83,84] (Fig. 2.46)

BEHÇET'S DISEASE

Behçet's (pronounced *beh-'**chets***) disease is a systemic disorder characterized by recurrent oral aphthous ulcers with genital ulceration, synovitis, posterior uveitis, superficial thrombophlebitis, cutaneous pustular vasculitis, and/or meningoencephalitis. Large, deep aphthous ulcerations can affect the scrotum and penis.[85,86] The disease proceeds with multiple flares and remissions. (Fig. 2.47)

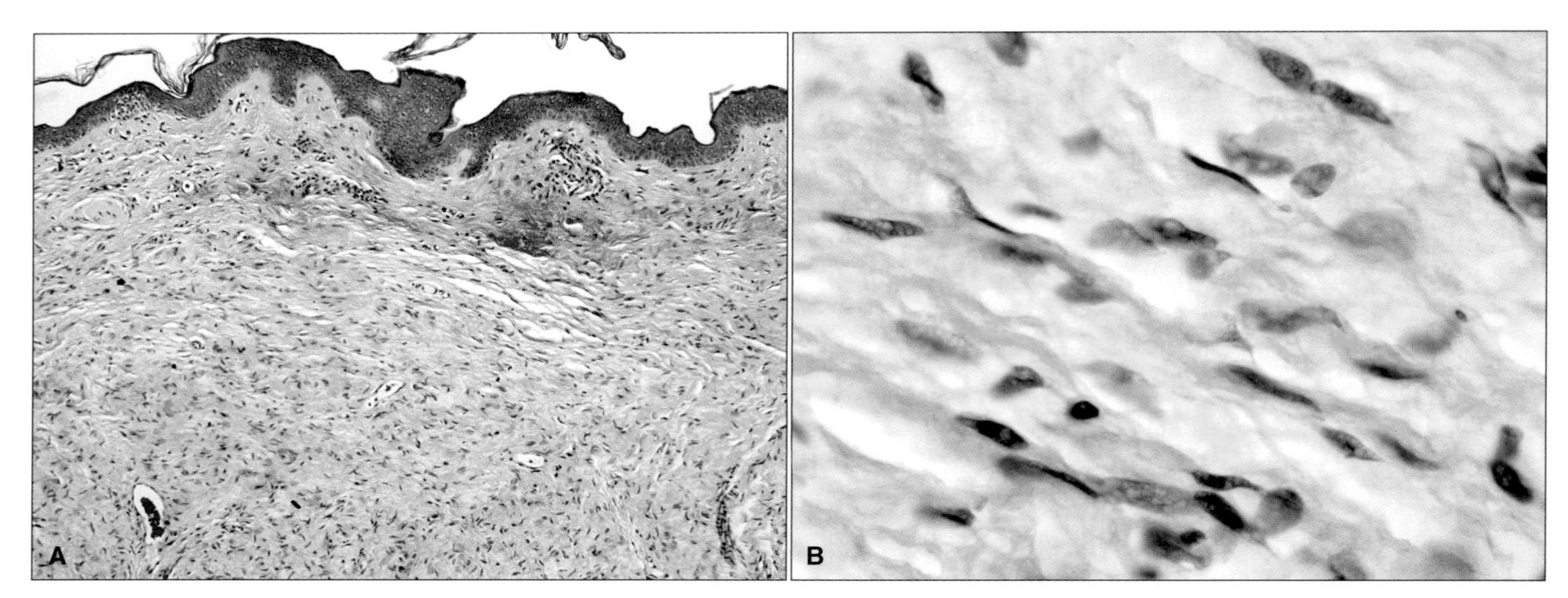

Fig. 2.46 Neurofibroma. (A,B) Histology shows a well-demarcated but non-encapsulated spindle cell proliferation with admixed mast cells.

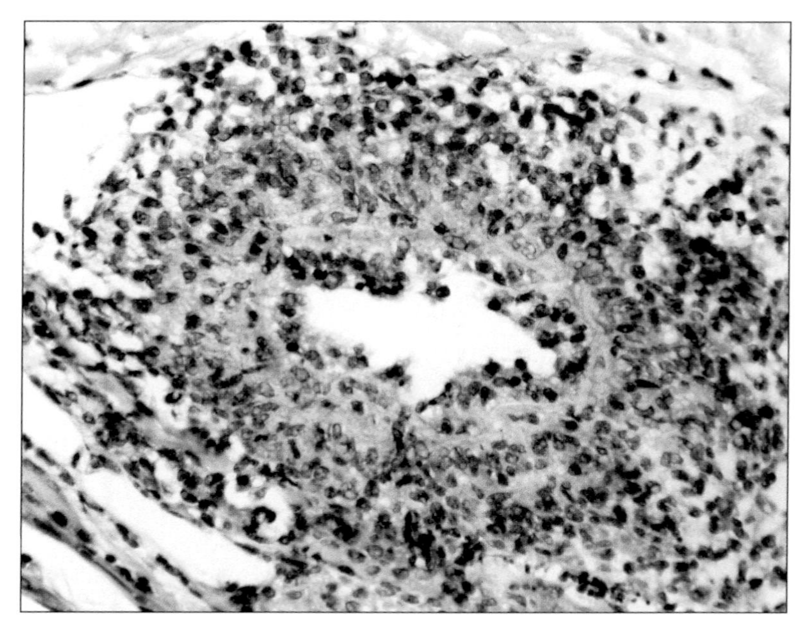

Fig. 2.47 Vascular lesions in Behçet's disease vary from inflammation, to aneurysms, to occlusions. Neutrophilic (as seen in this figure), lymphocytic, and granulomatous vascular reactions are seen.

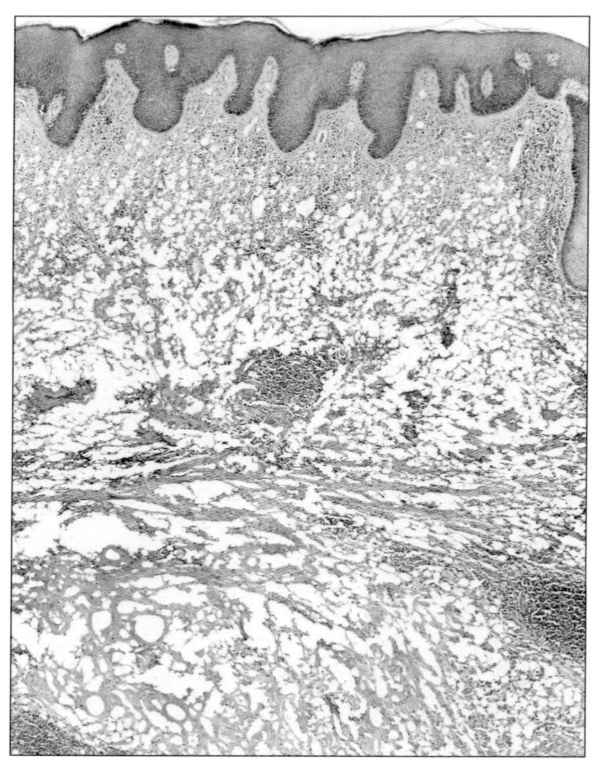

Fig. 2.48 Sclerosing lipogranuloma of the scrotum and penis. Microscopically, foci of fat necrosis with collections of histiocytes, foamy macrophages, and giant cells intermingle with fibrosis and hyalinization. Tissue and blood eosinophilia may occur.

TRAUMATIC DISORDERS

SCLEROSING LIPOGRANULOMA OF THE SCROTUM AND PENIS

This disease presents in otherwise healthy, middle-aged males as a painless mass that involves the scrotum, penile shaft, or suprapubic subcutaneous tissue. These changes are sometimes attributable to self-injection of exogenous material ('paraffinoma'), but reaction to endogenous lipids following breakdown of subcutaneous fat is another postulated cause. Systemic symptoms may occur due to lymphatic transport of lipids to the lungs. (Fig. 2.48)

PIGMENTARY DISORDERS

POSTINFLAMMATORY HYPERPIGMENTATION

Postinflammatory hyperpigmentation (PIH) occurs following inflammatory dermatoses affecting the basal layer, chiefly in darker-skinned people.[87] Fixed drug eruption, lichen planus, and genital herpes are particularly prone to leave residual postinflammatory pigment changes. (Fig. 2.49)

VITILIGO

Vitiligo can affect the penis and scrotum alone or in combination with involvement at other sites. Chemically induced vitiligo of the genitalia has been reported as an occupational leukoderma. Hypopigmentation after inflammation[88] or infection can be differentiated from vitiligo by Wood's lamp examination. (Fig. 2.50)

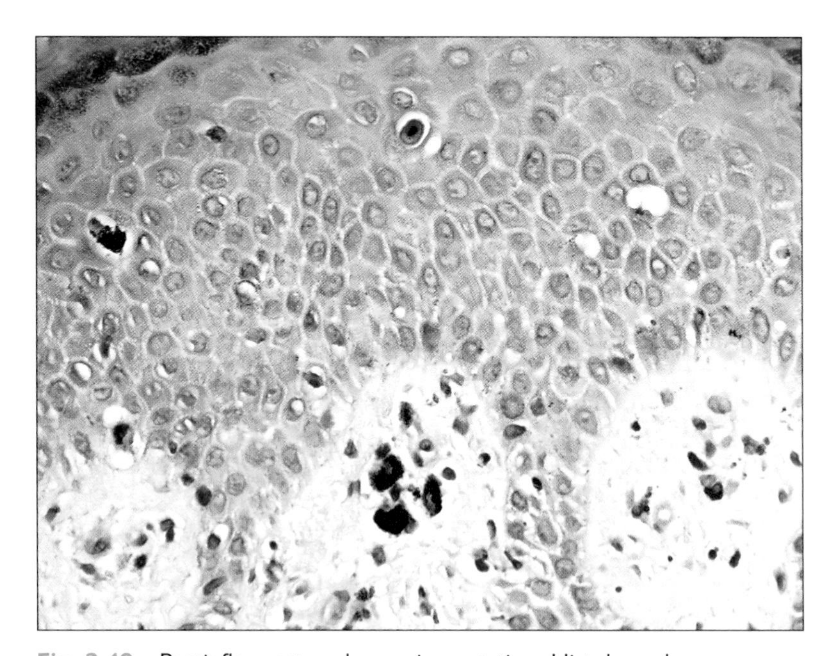

Fig. 2.49 Postinflammatory hyperpigmentation. Histology shows marked melanin incontinence with normal or increased amounts of melanin in the basal layer of the epidermis. The melanin may be contained in macrophages or in deposits in the dermis. Evidence of the inciting inflammatory disorder may include chronic inflammation, dermal fibrosis, and dyskeratinocytes.

GENITAL MELANOCYTIC MACULE/GENITAL LENTIGINOSIS

Genital melanotic macules are large, tan to black, variegated macules with well-defined but irregular borders. Penile lentigines are similar but may appear more variegated. They can be a component of systemic disorders like LAMB syndrome (mucocutaneous lentigines, atrial myxoma, and blue nevi) or LEOPARD (multiple lentigines, congenital cardiac abnormalities, ocular hypertelorism, and retardation of growth).[89] Eruptive crops of melanotic macules raise concern for visceral neoplasia.[90] (Fig. 2.51)

CUTANEOUS CYSTS AND NEOPLASMS

EPITHELIAL AND MELANOCYTIC LESIONS

Seborrheic keratosis

Seborrheic keratoses (SKs) are tan to brown, well-demarcated, raised papules, nodules, or plaques with a hyperkeratotic or verrucous surface. They are common after the third decade. A congenital predisposition has autosomal dominant inheritance. Genital SKs are commonly associated with lesions in the trunk.[92] Heavily pigmented SK may be confused clinically with pigmented basal cell carcinoma

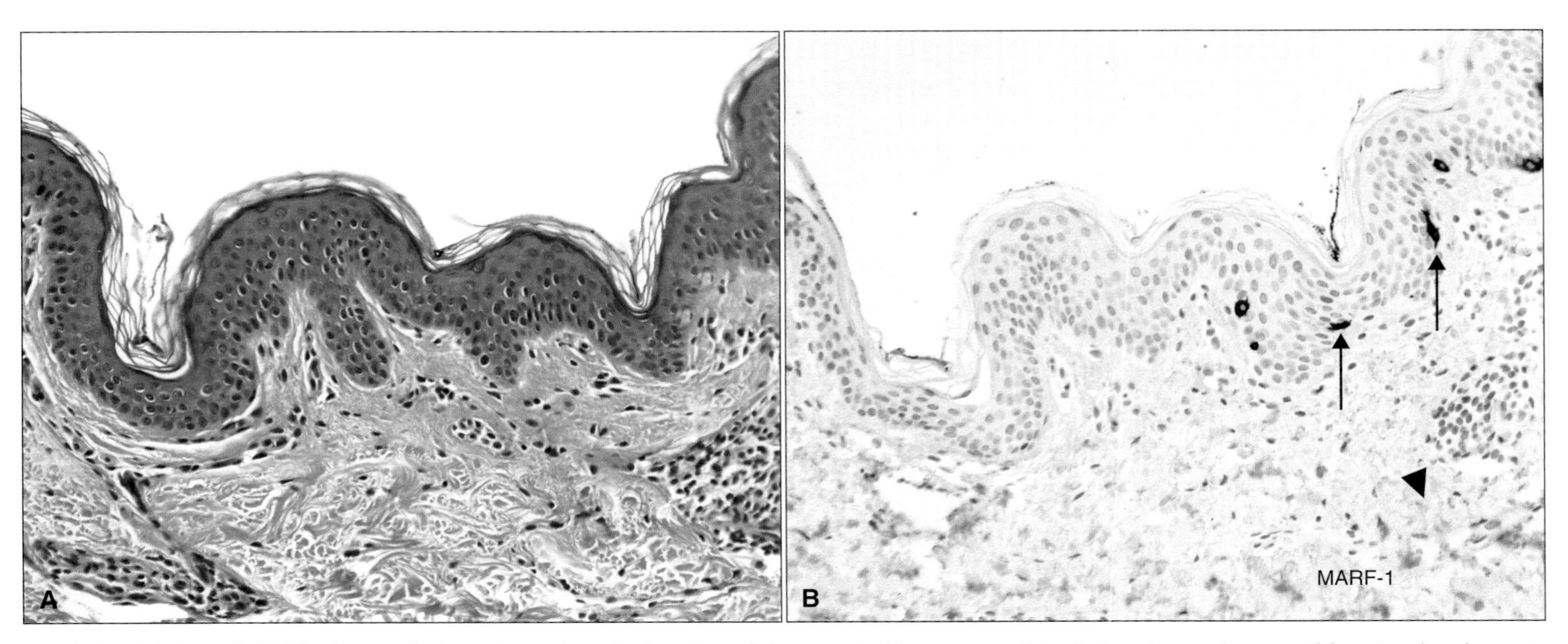

Fig. 2.50 Vitiligo. (A,B) The biopsy findings depend on the location of the sample. The center of the lesion shows absence of functional melanocytes and melanin, as shown in the left half of the H&E and MART-1-stained sections. Marginal skin has melanocytes (arrows) with a sparse lymphocytic infiltrate (arrowhead).

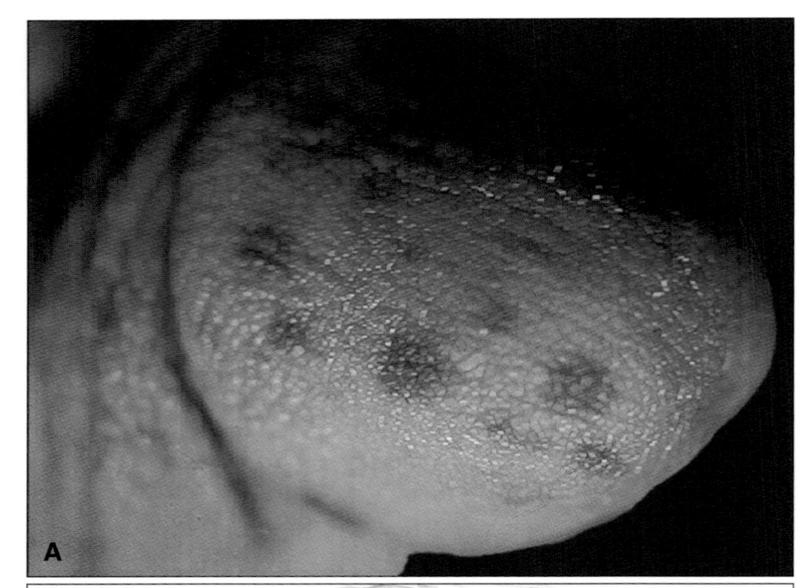

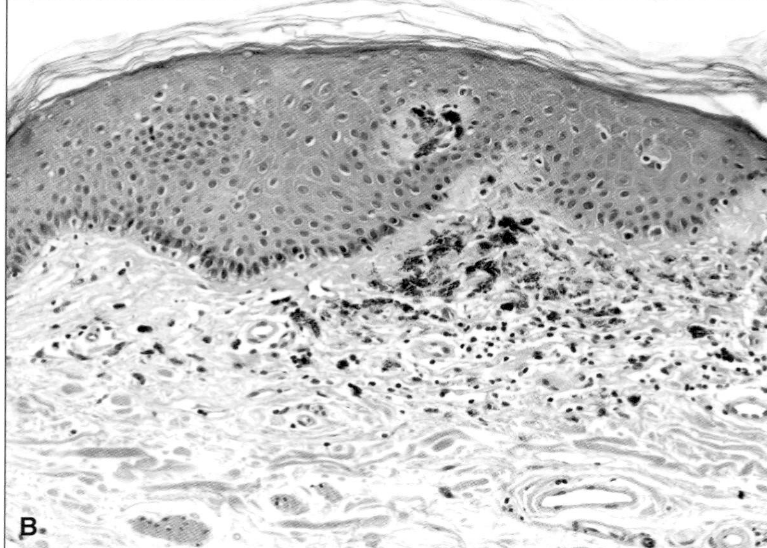

Fig. 2.51 Genital melanocytic macule/genital lentiginosis. (A) Clinically, they present as tan to brown variegated macules. (B) The biopsy is characterized by prominent basal hyperpigmentation, accentuated at the tip of the rete ridges. Although mild acanthosis is noted, the regular elongation of lentigo simplex is not seen. Melanocytes can have normal or increased density.[91] 'Melanotic macule' or 'melanosis' applies to lesions without melanocytic hyperplasia; 'lentigo' is favored when it is present. Melanophages are often seen in the dermis.

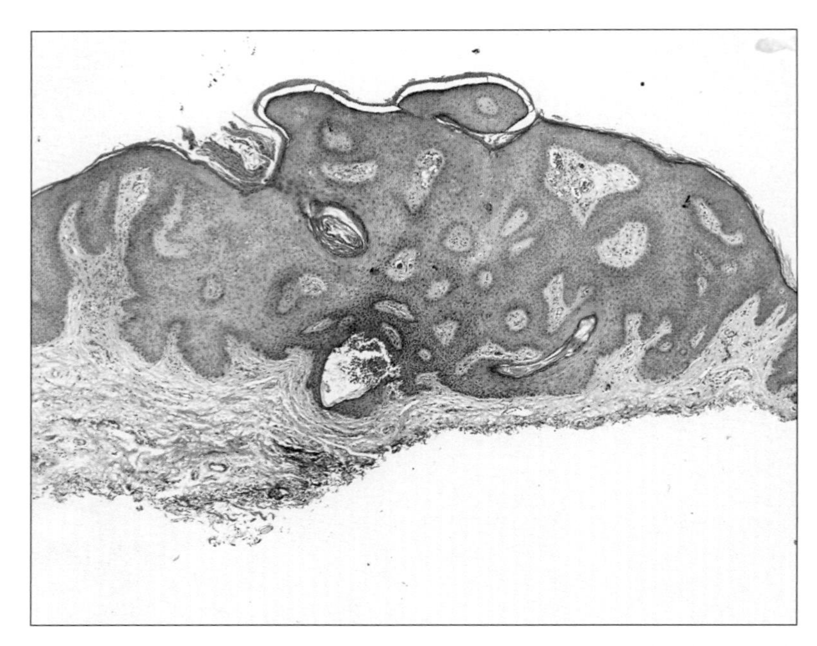

Fig. 2.52 Seborrheic keratoses. They are benign squamoid and basaloid proliferations with acanthosis, hyperkeratosis, and pseudocysts. Papillomatosis and reticulation can occur. Basal layer hyperpigmentation is noted. Inflamed lesions show lymphocytes in dermis and epidermis.

or melanoma. Leser–Trelat's sign is an acute paraneoplastic eruption of multiple SKs with (usually gastrointestinal) malignancy. (Figs 2.52 & 2.53)

Infundibular follicular (epidermoid, epidermal inclusion) cyst

A cyst is a cavity in tissue lined by epithelium and usually containing fluid. A pseudocyst lacks an epithelial lining. Most cutaneous cysts derive from adnexal structures.

This common cyst is lined by epidermis with a granular layer without adnexa. It arises from the infundibulum of the hair follicle. Scrotal cysts may reach massive dimensions.[93,94] Clitoral cysts are a complication of ritual genital mutilation.[95] (Fig. 2.54)

Median raphe cyst

This midline developmental cyst, typically discovered in childhood or young adulthood, may be located anywhere from the anus to the external urethral meatus. The most frequent location is the glans penis. (Fig. 2.55)

Verrucous xanthoma

Penile verrucous xanthoma presents as a hyperkeratotic plaque involving the coronal sulcus. Large lesions can cause phimosis. The etiology is unknown, but epidermal irritation may play a role, causing degeneration followed by a dermal histiocytic response. Patients' lipid metabolism is usually normal. (Fig. 2.56)

Melanocytic nevus

Melanocytic nevi are common in genital skin; a prevalence of 23% has been reported in 17–25-year-olds. Genital nevi can exhibit histologic findings that would be 'atypical' at other body sites. In genital skin, however, these are considered 'site-specific variants', and not indicative of biologic aggressiveness. Junctional or compound nevomelanocytic proliferation is possible. (Fig. 2.57)

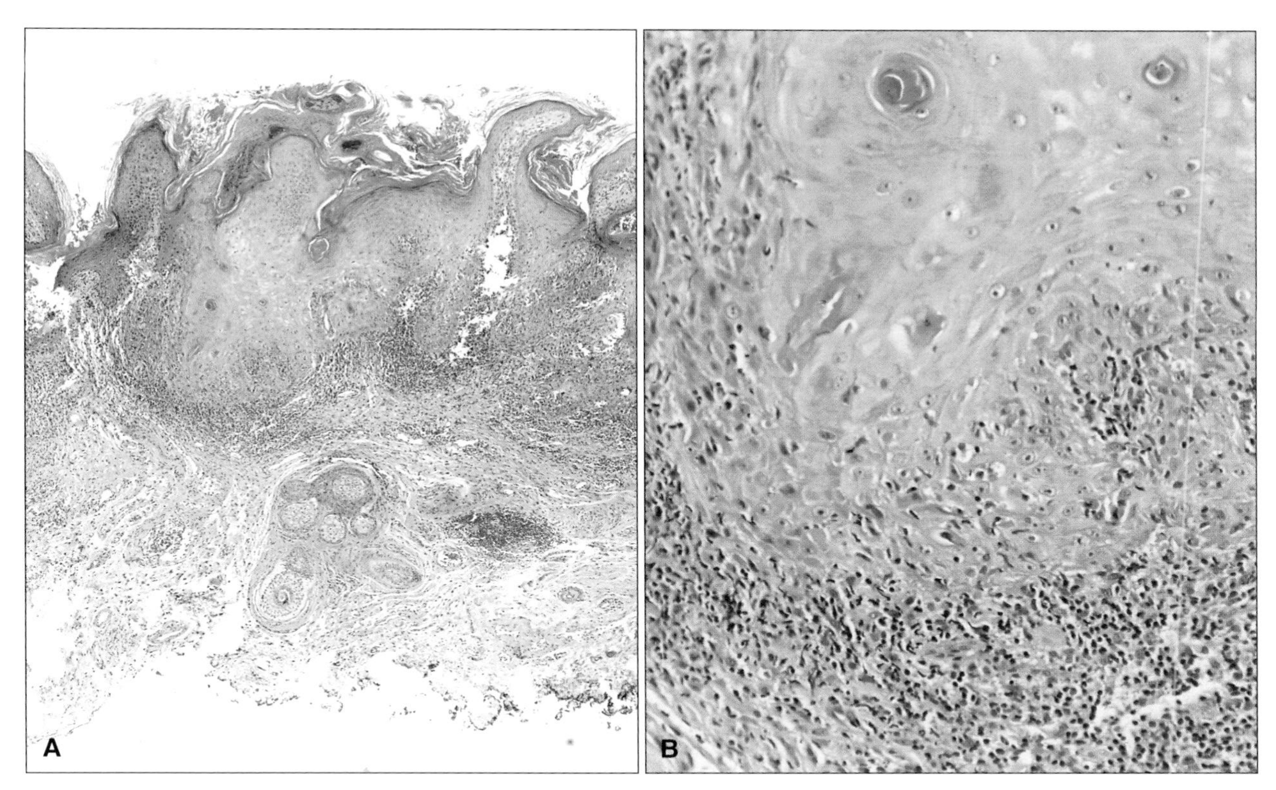

Fig. 2.53 Irritated seborrheic keratosis. (A,B) This lesion may be confused with squamous cell carcinoma. Squamous eddies and absence of pleomorphism or atypical mitosis favors irritated SK. Verrucous lesions in a linear distribution in a young patient are most likely epidermal nevus. It may be impossible to differentiate SK from old condyloma acuminatum if viral cytopathic changes are absent.

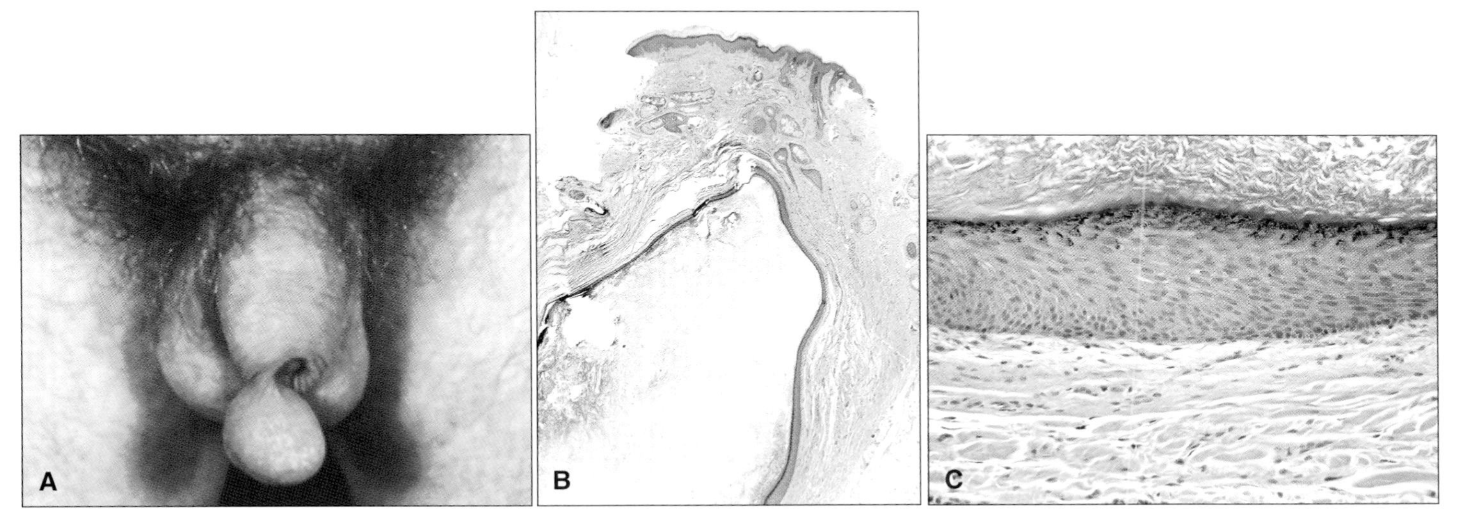

Fig. 2.54 Infundibular follicular cyst. (A) Clinically it presents as a bland, skin-colored nodule or pedunculated mass. (B) Histologically, the sections show a dermal cyst lined by squamous epithelium with a granular layer. (C) The lumen of the cyst is filled by keratin.

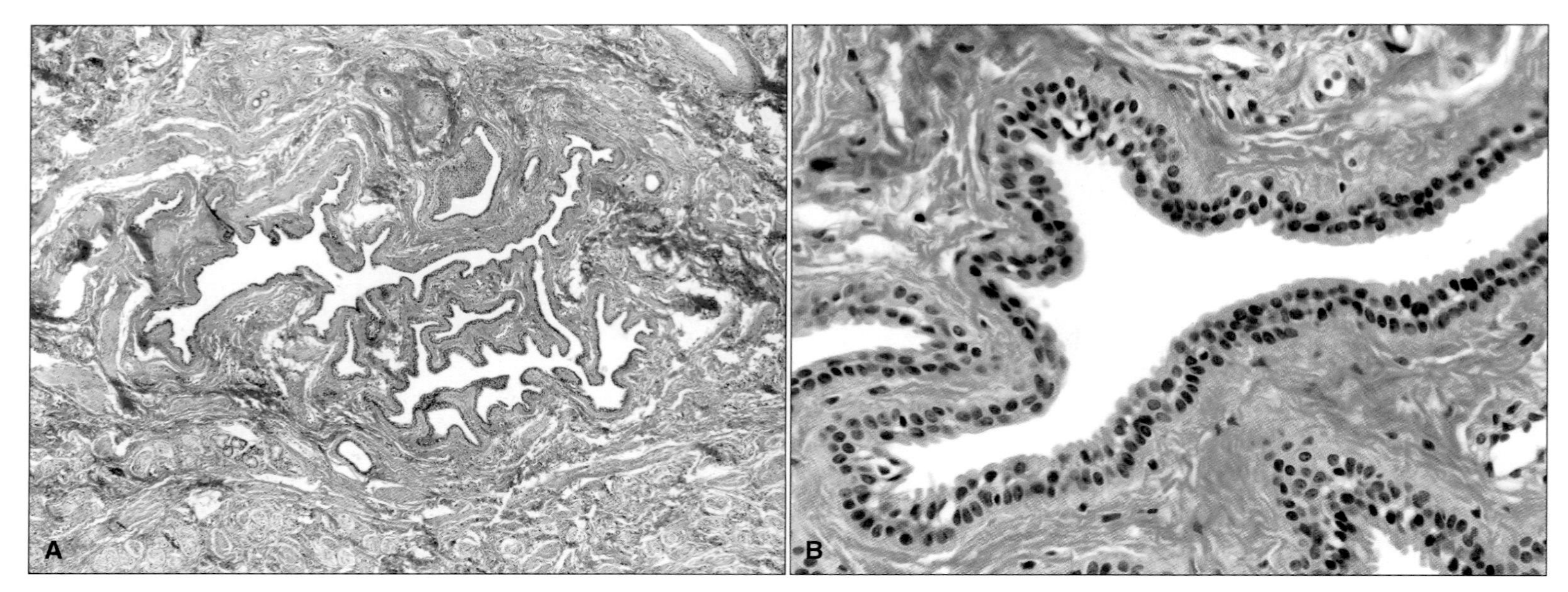

Fig. 2.55 Median raphe cyst. (A,B) The cyst is lined by pseudostratified columnar epithelium (or, near the meatus, with squamous epithelium). Ciliated cells and epithelial cells with neuroendocrine differentiation have been identified.[96,97] Mucous glands have been reported in the wall. The cyst does not communicate with the surface.

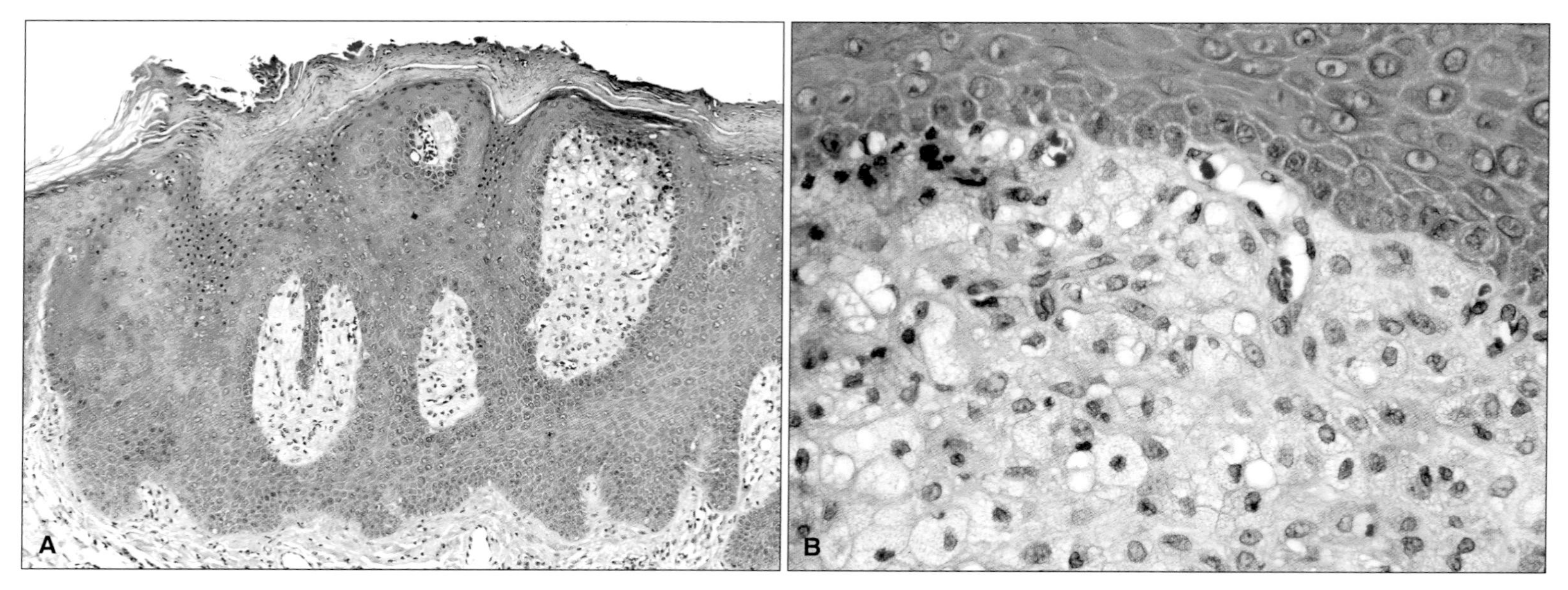

Fig. 2.56 Penile verrucous xanthoma. (A,B) Epidermal acanthosis with papillomatosis is seen. Foamy histiocytes with admixed acute and chronic inflammatory cells infiltrate the dermis. There is often exocytosis of neutrophils into the upper layers of the epithelium and parakeratotic scale. The foamy cells are positive for CD68 and negative for S-100 protein.

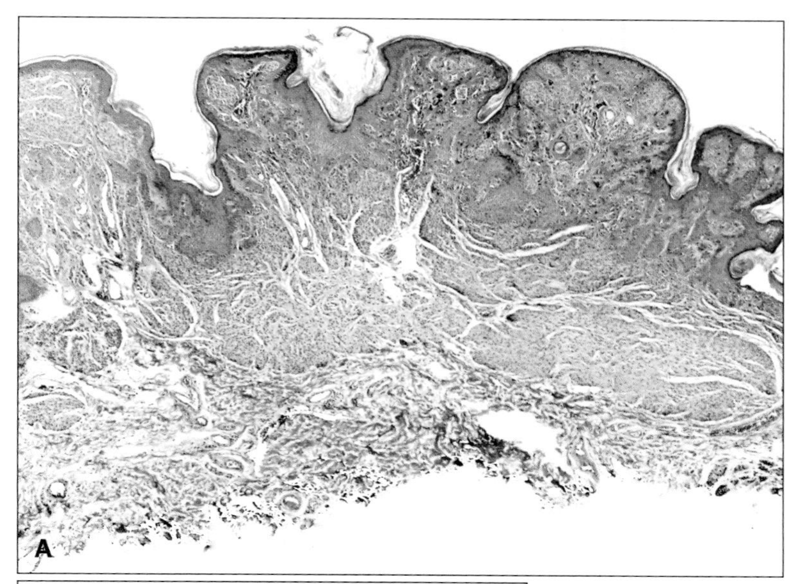

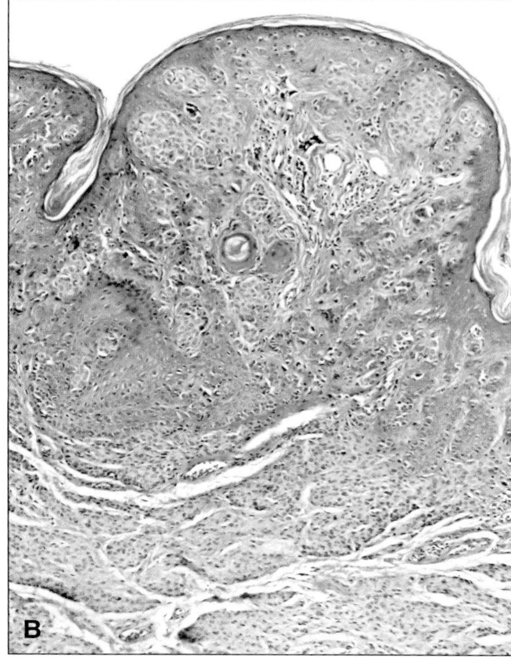

Fig. 2.57 Melanocytic nevus. (A,B) At low power, there is sharp lateral circumscription: the lesion ends in cohesive junctional and dermal nests. The nested pattern of growth with focal confluency can obscure the dermal–epidermal junction. The nests are variably sized and may show dyshesion, leading to distortion of the epidermal architecture. Solitary melanocytes at the periphery do not denote high-grade atypia if they are a minor component. Nevus cell nuclei may be small with uniform chromatin, or may exhibit open chromatin and small amphophilic nucleoli. Transepidermal elimination of nevomelanocytic nests and single cells can be seen.

Malignant melanoma

Malignant melanoma of the male genital tract represents 0.1–0.2% of non-ocular melanomas and 1% of penile neoplasms.[98] The most frequent sites are the glans, prepuce, urethral meatus, shaft, and coronal sulcus. Most present as a macule greater than 1 cm in diameter with variegated color, irregular borders, and areas of ulceration. Malignant melanomas of the scrotum are rare. Penile malignant melanoma has a 5-year survival rate of only 30%. (Fig. 2.58)

Syringoma

This benign tumor arises from eccrine glands. It can affect the dorsal and lateral aspect of the penile shaft as a discrete, skin-colored small papule.[99] (Fig. 2.59)

Basal cell carcinoma

Basal cell carcinoma is rare in genital skin.[100] Clinically, it presents as a pearly papule with telangiectasis. Ulcerative and multicentric presentations have been reported. Recurrence and metastasis are uncommon. (Fig. 2.60)

Extramammary Paget's disease

In males, a pink to red, well-demarcated macule or slightly raised plaque of the perianal skin, scrotum, or penis is the usual presentation of Paget's disease. Isolated scrotal involvement is unusual.

About one-third of cases are associated with an underlying neoplasm. Adnexal adenocarcinoma is the source in 4–7% of patients. Twenty percent have a primary rectal carcinoma. Lesions in the glans suggest an underlying carcinoma of the urethra or bladder.[101] Extramammary Paget's disease can present up to 7 years after treatment for the primary malignancy. (Fig. 2.61)

MESENCHYMAL LESIONS

Angiokeratoma

Angiokeratoma is a proliferation of ectatic superficial vessels with associated epidermal changes that usually arises in the second and third decades. There are five clinical variants, of which the Fordyce (scrotal) type involves the genitalia.[102] The scrotum, penis, upper thigh, and lower abdomen may be involved. Clinically, it presents as multiple red to black papules along the superficial scrotal vessels. (Fig. 2.62) It is associated with varicocele, inguinal hernias, and thrombophlebitis.

Pearly penile papules (hirsuties coronae glandis or hirsutoid papillomatosis)

Pearly penile papules (PPPs) are skin-colored, domed papules arranged circumferentially about the corona and on each side of the frenulum.[103] They are asymptomatic, but are sometimes misdiagnosed as molluscum contagiosum or genital warts. A similar condition in women, papillomatosis labialis, affects the introitus vulvae and labia minora. (Fig. 2.63)

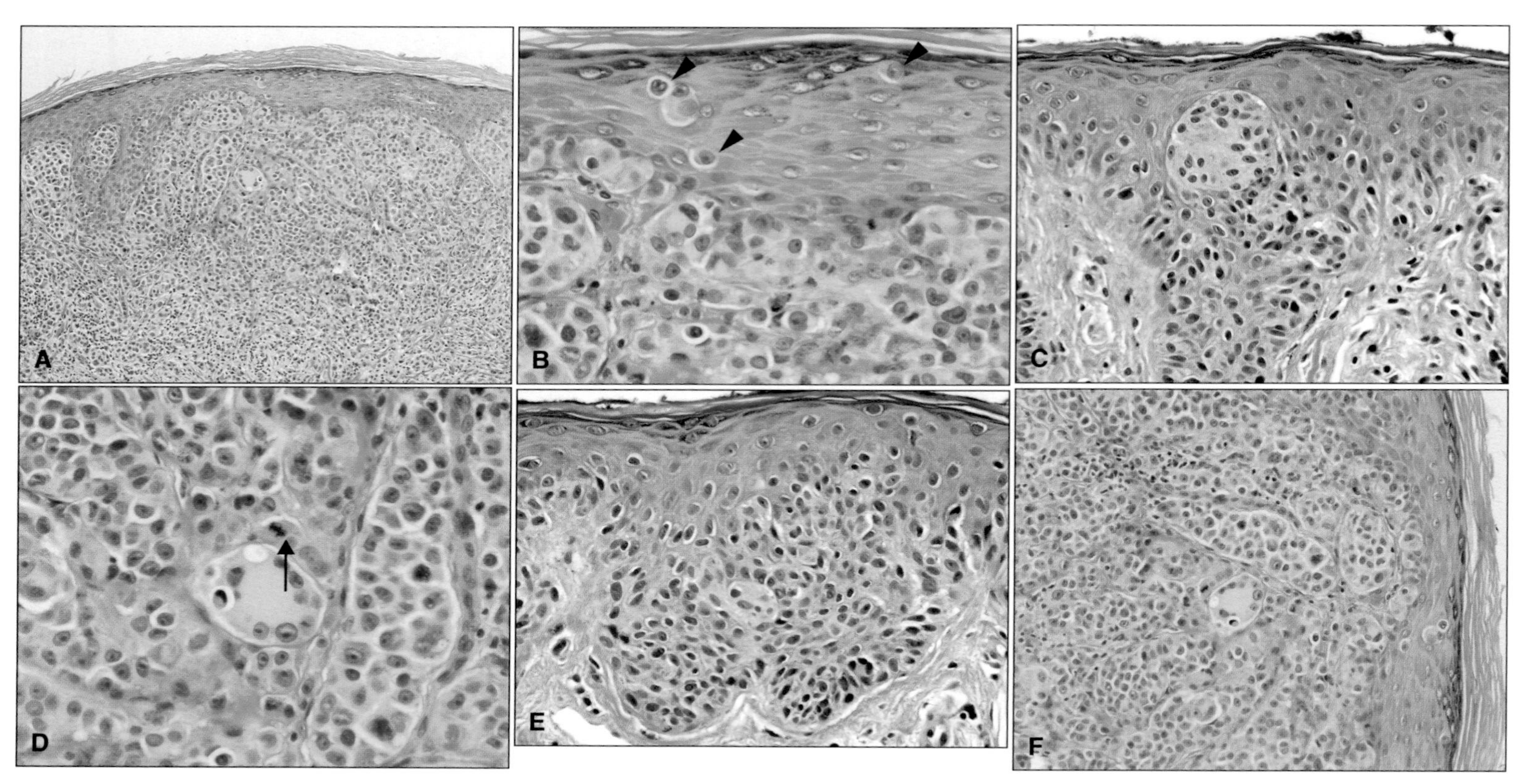

Fig. 2.58 Malignant melanoma. (A) Low power shows an asymmetric proliferation of melanocytes with absence of maturation. (B) High-grade melanocytes are arranged as single cells and nests at the dermal–epidermal junction, with pagetoid spread (arrowheads). (C–F) Mitotic figures (arrow) and vascular and perineural invasion can be seen.

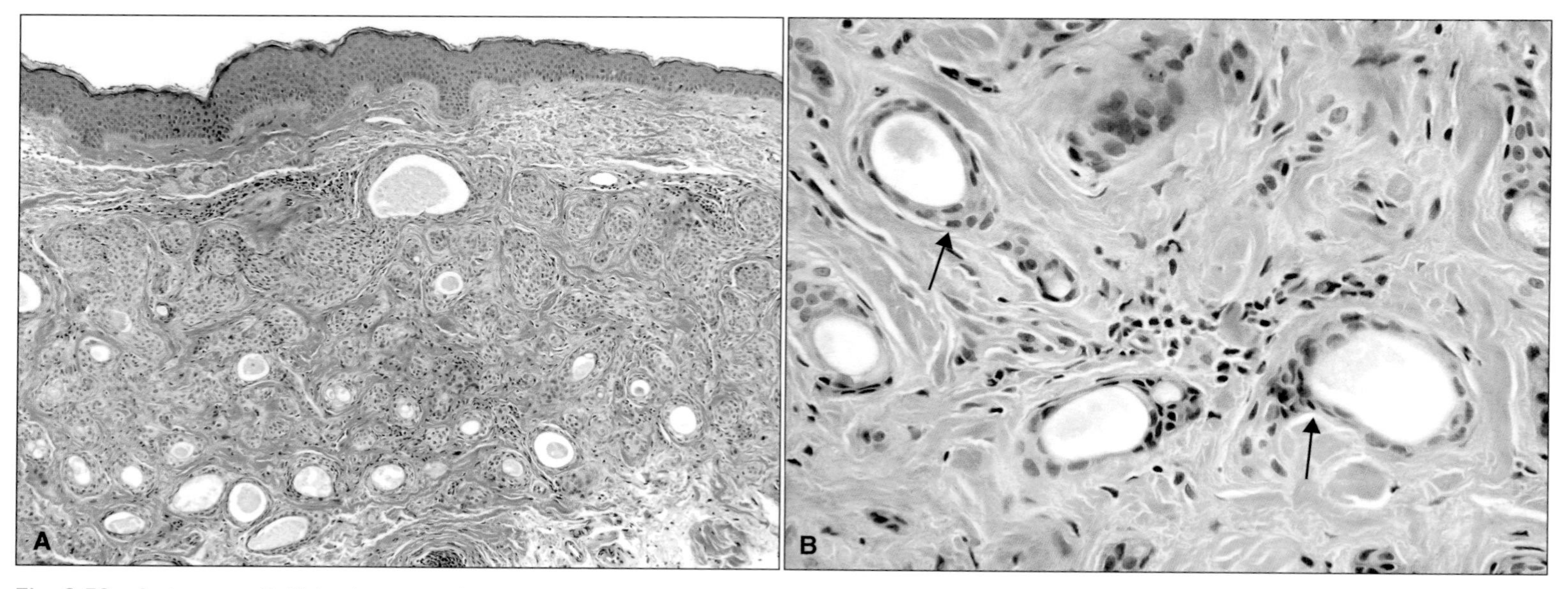

Fig. 2.59 Syringoma. (A,B) In the upper dermis is a well-demarcated proliferation of benign glands. Some show the characteristic 'tadpole' or comma-like structure (arrows).

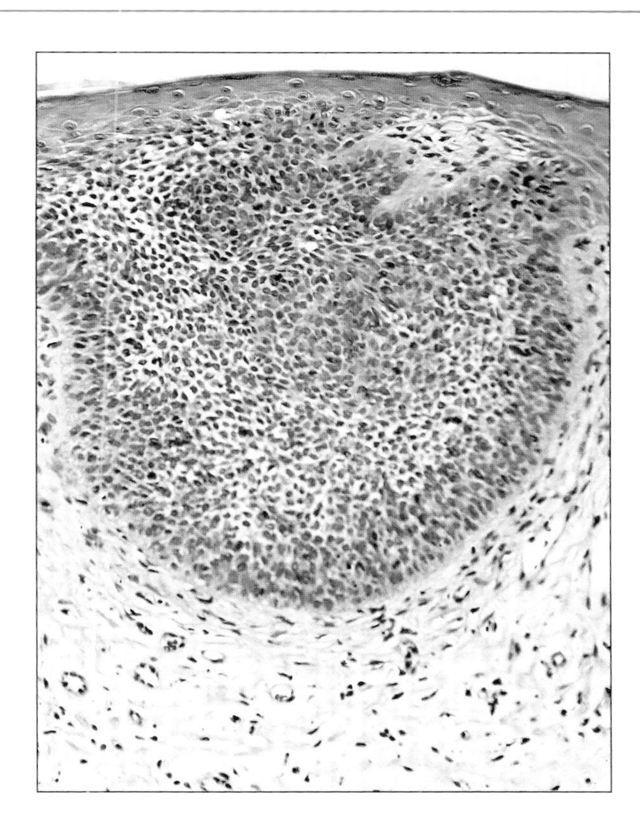

Fig. 2.60 Basal cell carcinoma. The histologic features of basal carcinoma are the same as at extragenital sites. There is a basaloid proliferation of cells with peripheral palisading. Apoptosis and mitotic figures are noted. The stroma is fibrotic and retracts, producing a cleft artifact.

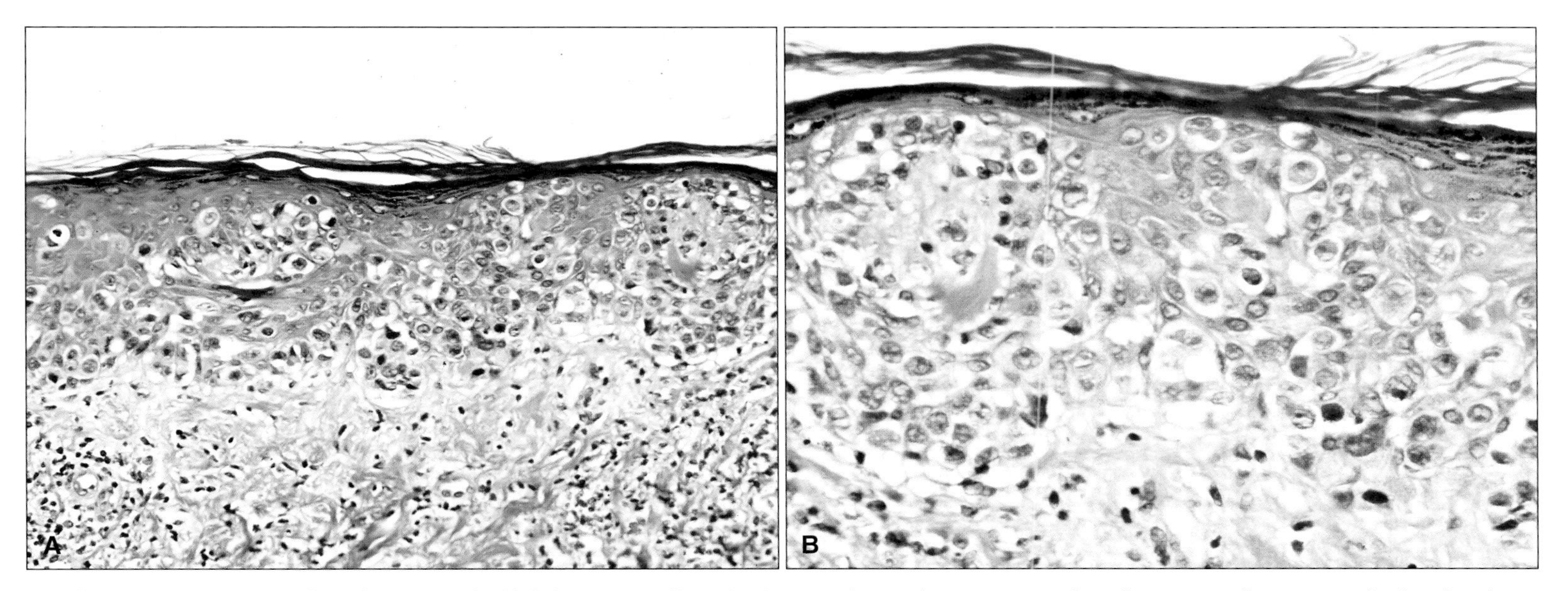

Fig. 2.61 Extramammary Paget's disease. (A,B) Pale tumor cells with pleomorphic nuclei are arranged singly or in small groups in the basal and parabasal epidermis. Gland formation may occur. In advanced stages, the entire thickness of the epidermis may be involved. Adnexal structures (e.g. hair follicles and eccrine ducts) can be affected. Infrequently, Paget's cells can involve the dermis. Melanin colonization can occur. Extramammary Paget's disease has abundant mucin, demonstrable with special stains. Paget's cells stain for carcinoembryonic antigen, CA15.3 and KA-93, low molecular weight keratins, and epithelial membrane antigen (EMA). Most cases are CK7+/CK20–, but some cases secondary to underlying carcinomas are CK20+. The cells do not stain for CD44 or S-100 protein.

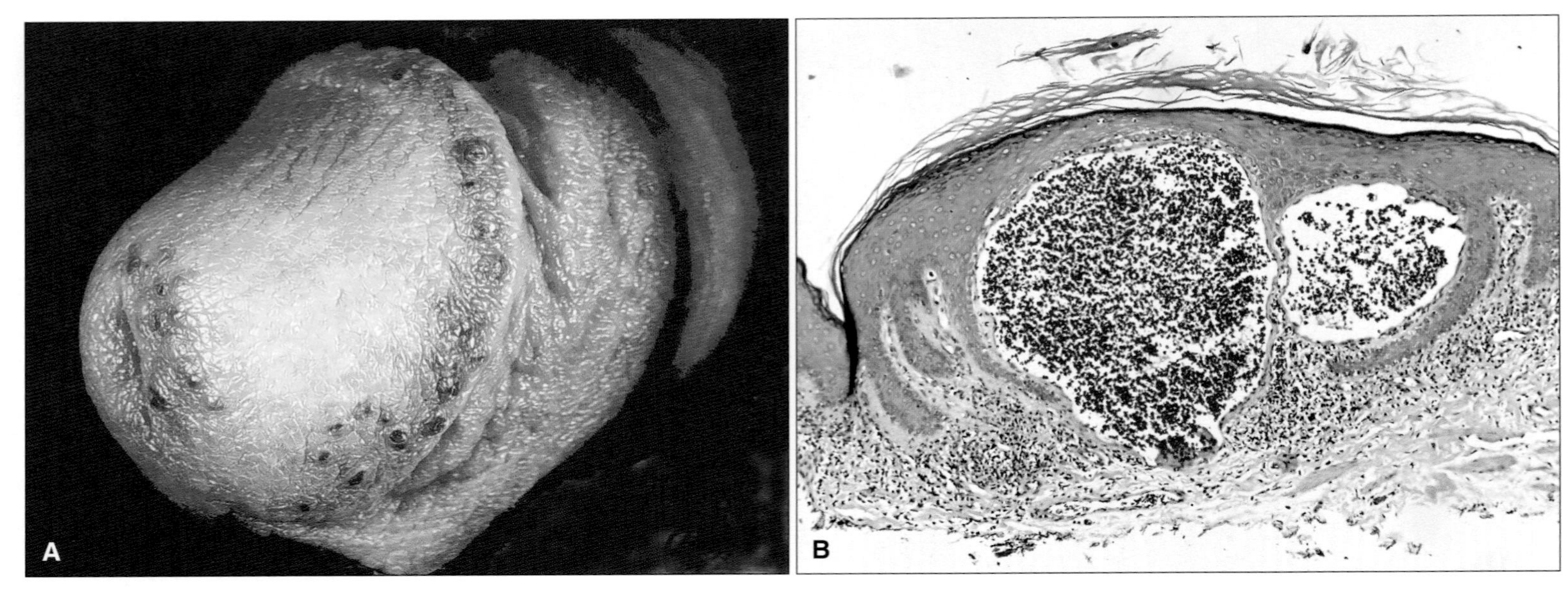

Fig. 2.62 Angiokeratoma. (A) Multiple red to black papules. (B) Dilatation of superficial dermal vessels produces large cavernous channels immediately beneath an acanthotic, hyperkeratotic epidermis. A collarette and thrombosis may be seen.

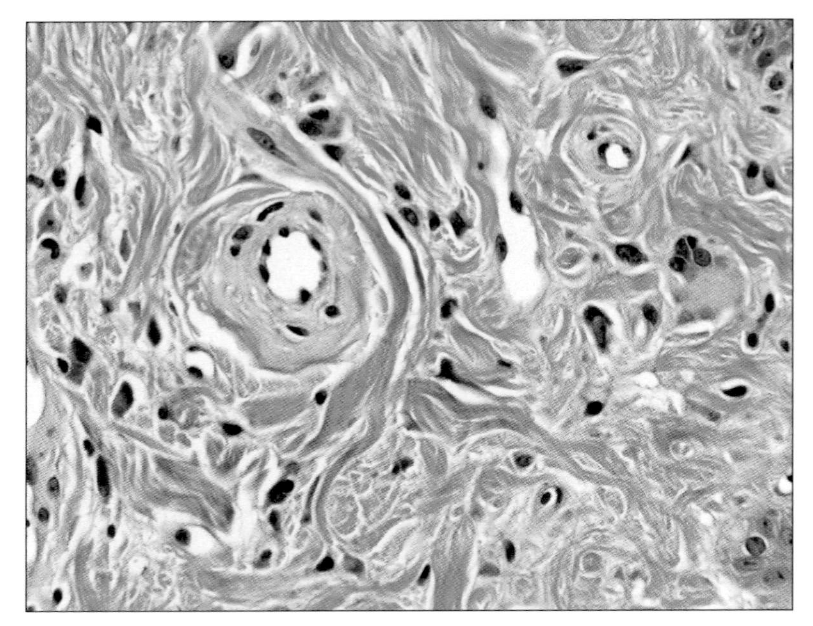

Fig. 2.63 Histologically, pearly penile papules are angiofibromas. Biopsy shows dermal fibrosis, perivascular fibrosis with ectasia, and triangular-shaped bizarre fibroblasts.

Schwannoma (neurilemmoma)

Schwannomas are usually asymptomatic, painless, enlarging tumors involving the penile shaft and frenulum. They can reach large size (20 cm). (Fig. 2.64)

Smooth muscle tumors

Dartic leiomyoma can present as a scrotal mass that contracts upon stimulus by touch or cold. Although often solitary, it can be multiple. Leiomyosarcoma of the penis and scrotum is uncommon, arising from the smooth muscle of the arrectores pilorum in the dermis, muscle in the wall of veins, and dartos.[104] (Fig. 2.65)

Kaposi's sarcoma

Kaposi's sarcoma is a malignant vascular proliferation that presents as confluent violaceous nodules.[105] Lesions in the scrotum and penis are usually asymptomatic, but if the urethra is affected, urinary retention or dysuria can occur. (Fig. 2.66)

Granular cell tumor

Cutaneous granular cell tumor presents as a skin-colored, firm, verrucous, or ulcerated nodule. It can involve the skin and subcutis of the shaft, prepuce, or glans. Deep lesions can occur in the corpus cavernosum.[106] Malignant granular cell tumors occur, with rapid, ulcerating growth and potential for lymphatic dissemination. (Fig. 2.67)

OTHER NEOPLASMS

Lymphoma and leukemia

Mycosis fungoides can involve the ureter, leading to urinary obstruction. Angiocentric T-cell lymphoma can primarily present as ulcerated nodule on the prepuce and coronal sulcus. Cutaneous pseudolymphoma has been reported as part of the clinical spectrum of Lyme borreliosis. (Fig. 2.68)

Metastatic tumors

Urothelial carcinoma, prostatic adenocarcinoma, and rectosigmoid tumors may involve the genital skin by direct extension, or by metastasis. (Fig. 2.69)

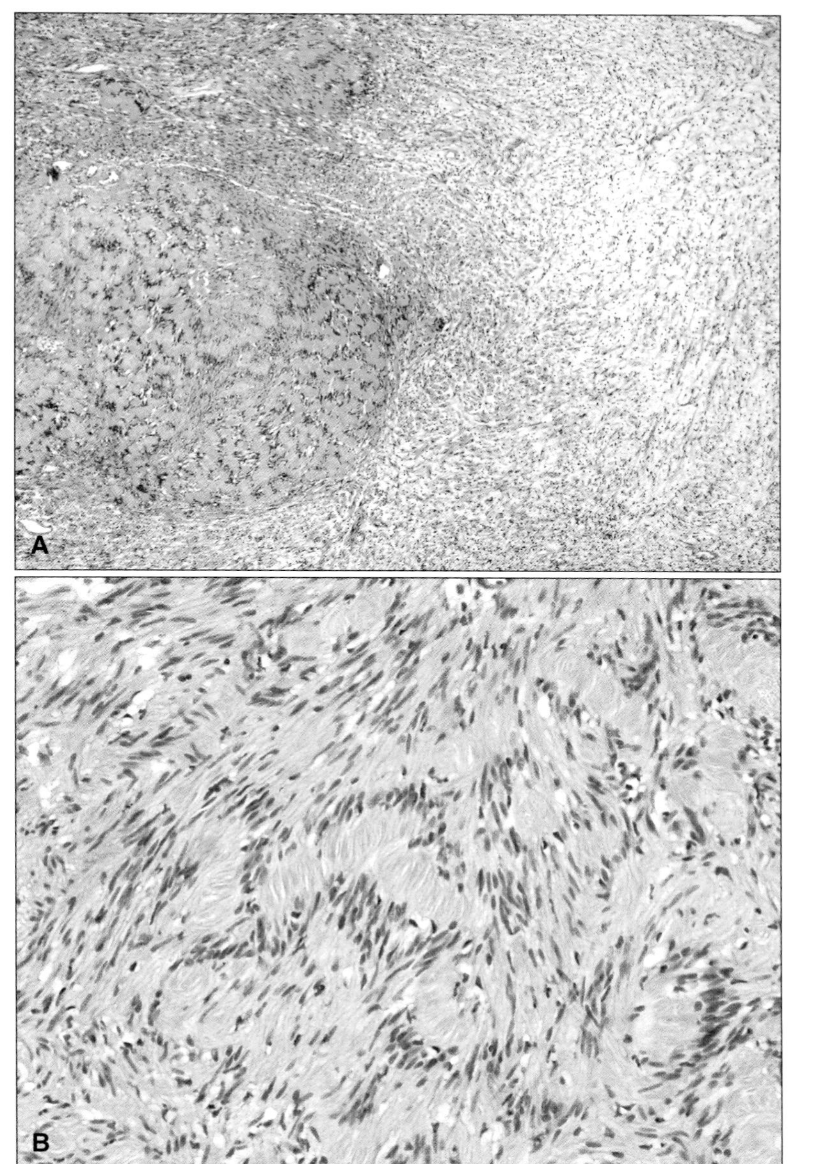

Fig. 2.64 Schwannoma. (A) In the 'Antoni A' regions, spindle-shaped Schwann cells are organized in interlacing fascicles. 'Antoni B' areas consist of widely separated Schwann cells. (B) The nuclei arrange in rows or palisades, forming Verocay bodies. S-100 protein, vimentin, and myelin basic protein are positive. Glial fibrillary acidic protein is only occasionally positive.

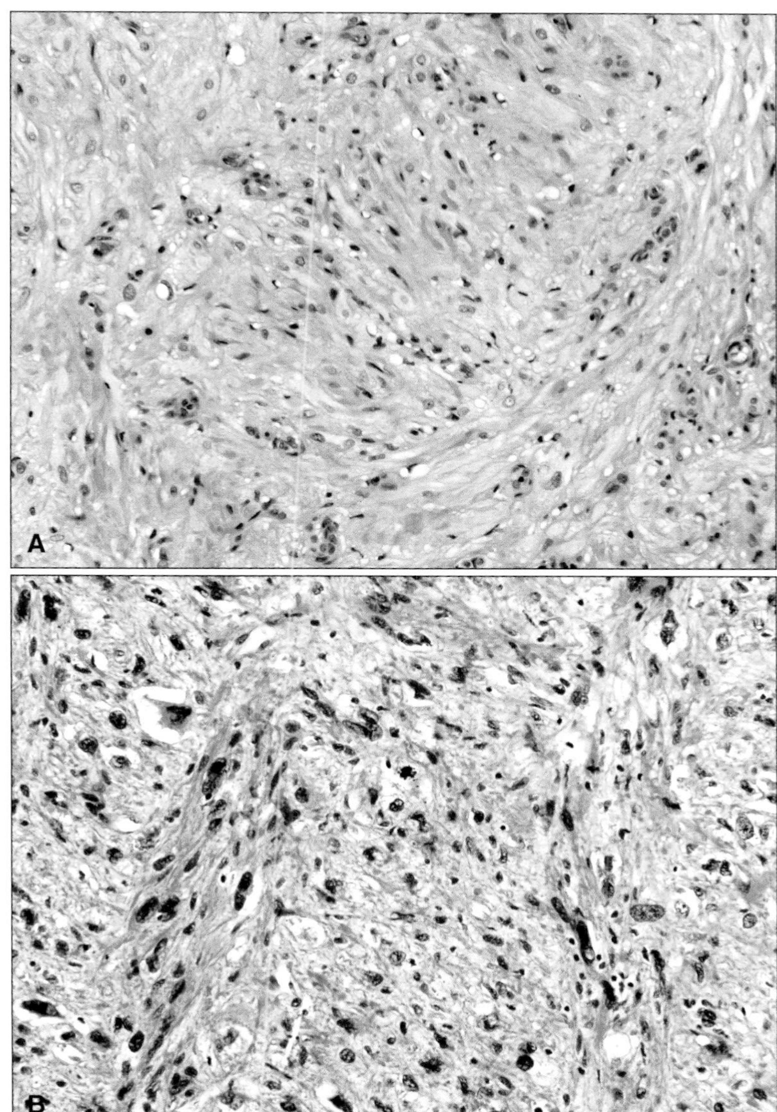

Fig. 2.65 Smooth muscle tumors. (A) In the scrotum, benign leiomyomas can have ill-defined or focally infiltrative margins. They are often cellular and can have rare mitotic figures. Symplastic features may be seen. (B) Leiomyosarcomas consist of interlacing fascicles of spindle-shaped cells with blunt-ended hyperchromatic nuclei. There is at least one mitotic figure per ten high-power fields in cellular areas. Dermal leiomyosarcomas can recur locally (30%) but do not metastasize. Subcutaneous leiomyosarcomas recur frequently (50–70%) and may metastasize to liver, lung, and bone. Deletions in the 13q4–21 region are the most frequent genomic alteration.

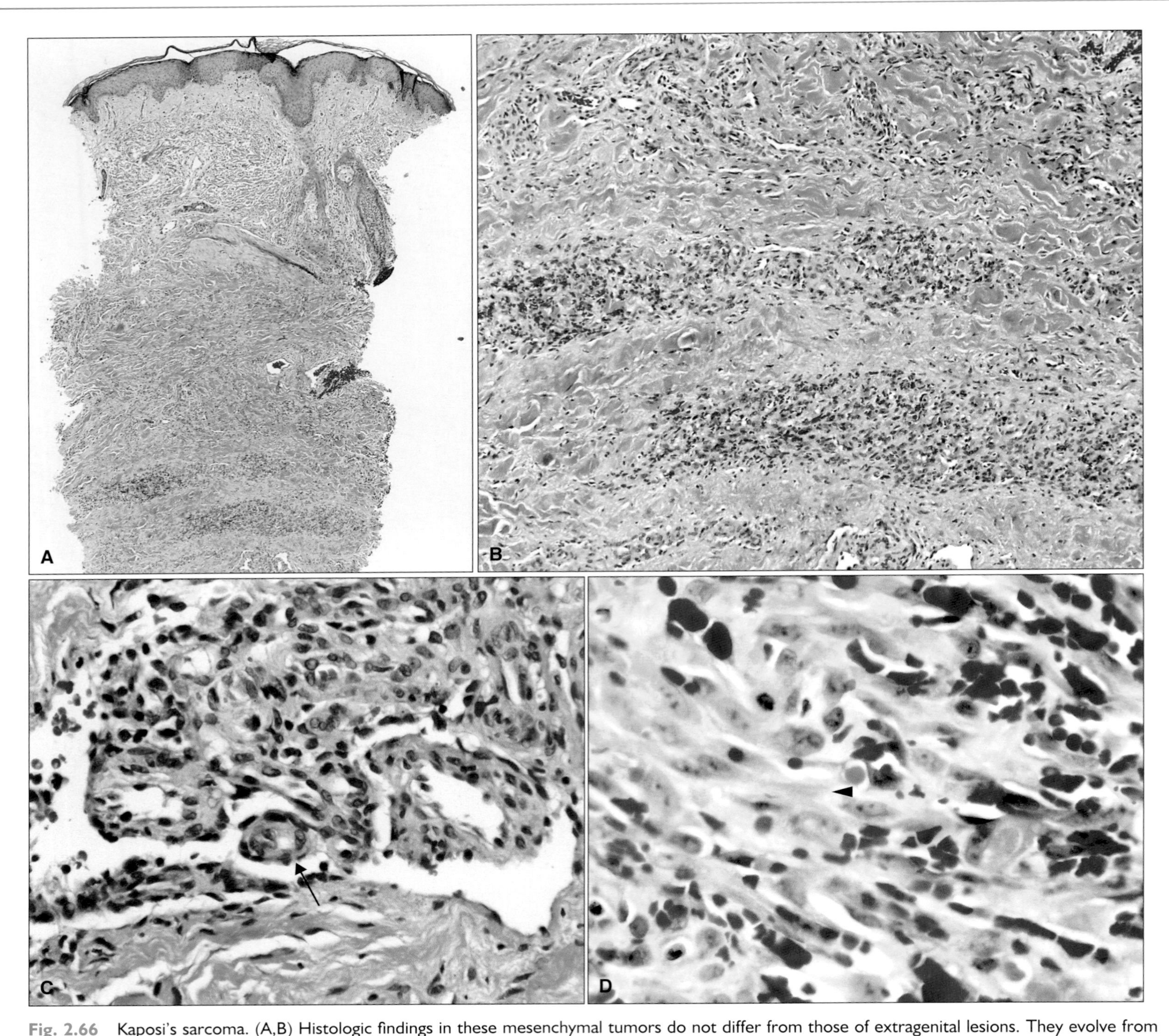

Fig. 2.66 Kaposi's sarcoma. (A,B) Histologic findings in these mesenchymal tumors do not differ from those of extragenital lesions. They evolve from patch through plaque to nodular stages. The flat macule or patch consists of a proliferation of irregular, thin-walled vascular channels. A perivascular lymphoplasmacytic infiltrate is noted. Plaques and nodules combine interlacing spindle cells with poorly defined slit-like vessels. Dilated, thin-walled vessels can be seen at the periphery. (C) When the abnormal proliferating vessels surround dermal structures (vessels or eccrine glands), they form the 'promontory sign' (arrow). Mitotic figures are infrequent. Red cell extravasation, hemosiderin, lymphocytes, and plasma cells are noted. (D) Pink hyaline globules larger than erythrocytes can be seen in spindle cells, macrophages, or the interstitium (arrowhead). They are positive for periodic acid–Schiff, and stain bright red with trichrome stain. They represent phagocytosed red blood cell fragments. Human herpes virus 8 can be detected by polymerase chain reaction or immunohistochemistry. This test is especially useful in difficult lesions or material obtained from needle aspiration.

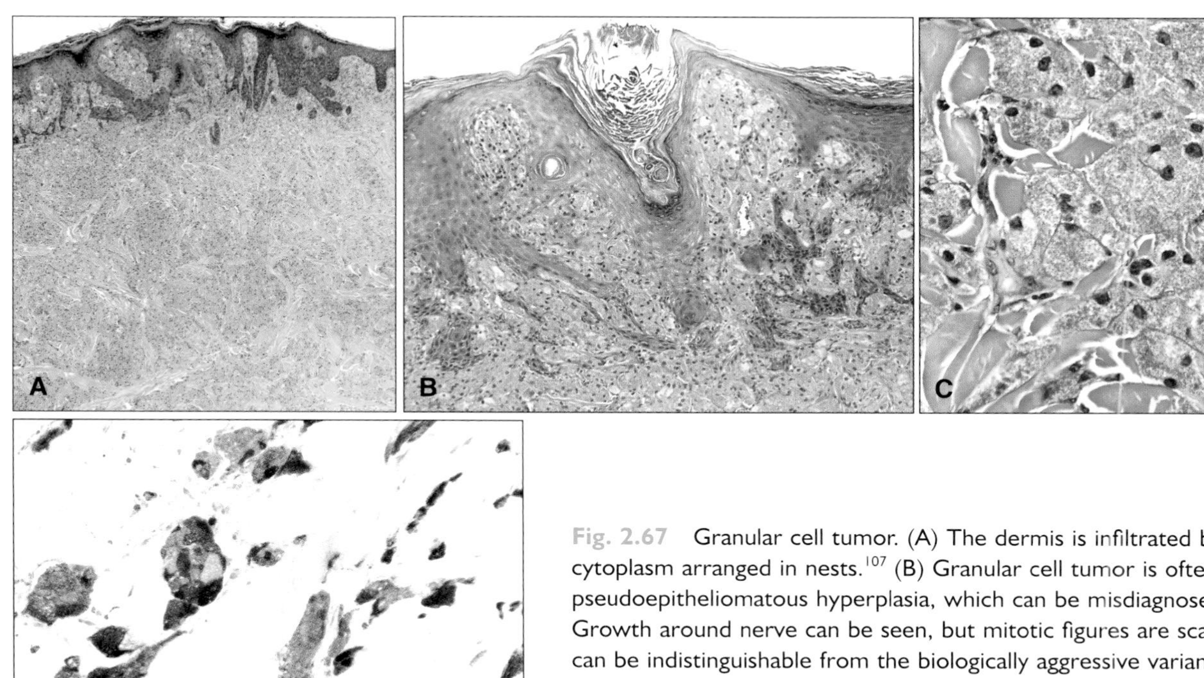

Fig. 2.67 Granular cell tumor. (A) The dermis is infiltrated by large polygonal cells with granular cytoplasm arranged in nests.[107] (B) Granular cell tumor is often associated with pseudoepitheliomatous hyperplasia, which can be misdiagnosed as squamous cell carcinoma. (C) Growth around nerve can be seen, but mitotic figures are scant to nonexistent. The benign lesion can be indistinguishable from the biologically aggressive variant. Increased mitotic activity with atypical forms and necrosis should raise suspicion of malignancy. (D) Other soft tissue tumors may contain cells with granular cytoplasm. Periodic acid–Schiff-positive, diastase-resistant granules differentiate granular cell tumor from xanthoma. The cells are positive for S-100 protein. Electron microscopy shows that the intracytoplasmic granules are membrane-bound lysosomes.

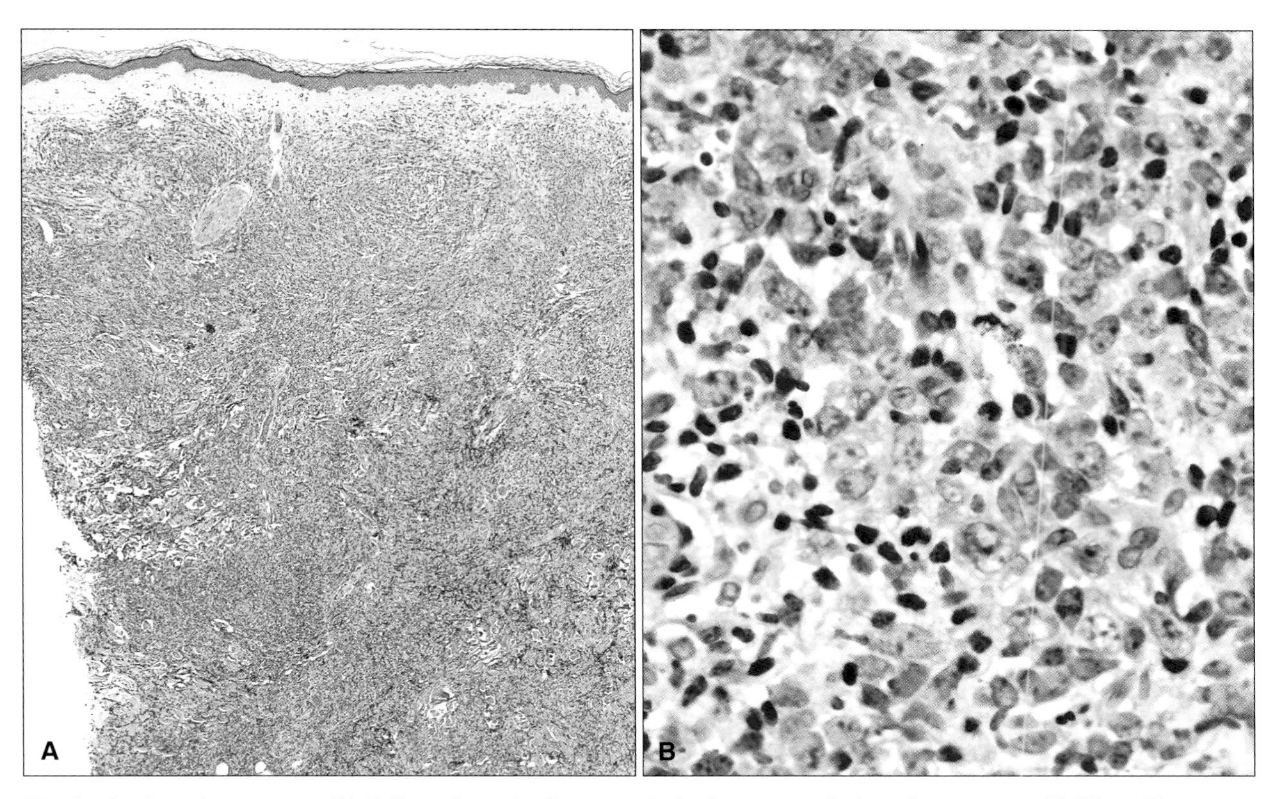

Fig. 2.68 Lymphoma cutis. (A) Diffuse dermal infiltrate with displacement of adnexal structures. (B) The infiltrate consists of large CD20 lymphocytes.

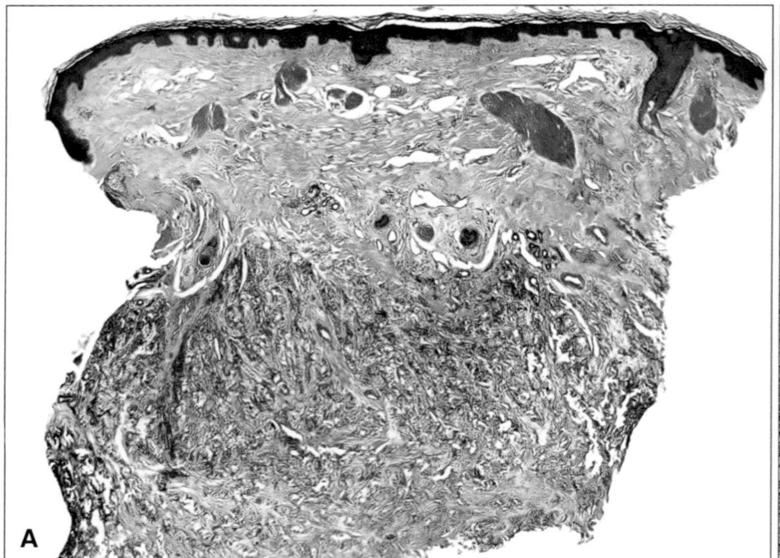

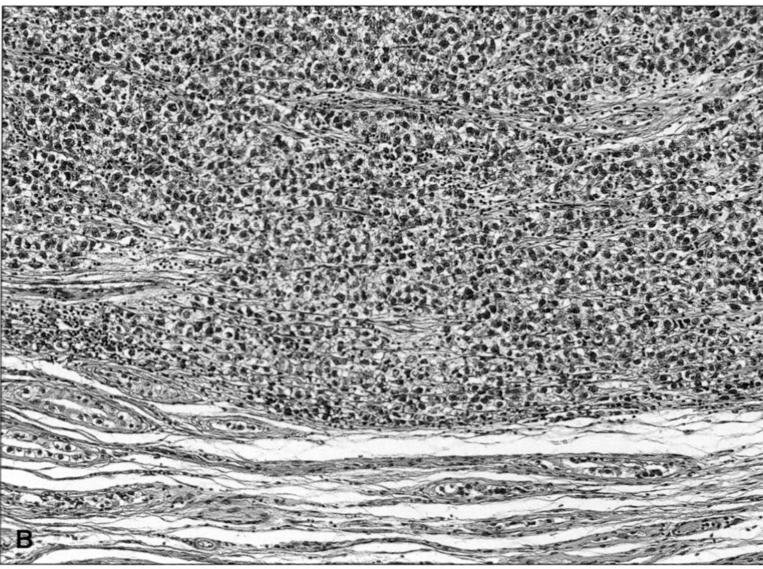

Fig. 2.69 Metastatic tumors. (A) Renal cell carcinoma accounts for 6% of cutaneous metastases in the male. The deposit is usually vascular and can mimic a vascular tumor. The metastasis shows nests of epithelial cells with abundant clear cytoplasm (glycogen and some fat) involving most of the dermis. (B) Metastatic seminoma presents as a collection of round cells with prominent central hyperchromatic nuclei and abundant clear cytoplasm.

REFERENCES

1. Pillai KG, Singh G, Sharma BM. *Trichophyton rubrum* infection of the penis. Dermatologica 1975;150:252–254.
2. Kumar B, Kaur S, Talwar P. Superficial mycotic infection of penis (penile tinea). Indian J Pathol Microbiol 1980;23:196–198B.
3. Pielop J, Rosen T. Penile dermatophytosis. J Am Acad Dermatol 2001;44: 864–867.
4. Dekio S, Qin LM, Jidoi J. Tinea of the glans penis: report of a case presenting as a crop of papules. J Dermatol 1991;18:52–55.
5. Pandey SS, Chandra S, Guha PK, Kaur P, Singh G. Dermatophyte infection of the penis. Association with a particular undergarment. Int J Dermatol 1981;20:112–114.
6. Blumenthal HL. Tinea versicolor of penis. Arch Dermatol 1971;103:461–462.
7. Nia AK, Smith EL. Pityriasis versicolor of the glans penis. Br J Vener Dis 1979;55:230.
8. Mayser P. Mycotic infections of the penis. Andrologia 1999;31(Suppl 1): 13–16.
9. Horowitz BJ, Edelstein SW, Lippman L. Sexual transmission of *Candida*. Obstet Gynecol 1987;72:883–886.
10. Johnson RA. Diseases and disorders of the anogenitalia of males. In: Fitzpatrick TB, Austen KF, Wolff K, Eisen AZ, Freedberg IM, eds. Dermatology in general medicine. New York: McGraw-Hill; 1993: 1993–1442.
11. Eickenberg HV, Amin M, Lich R. Blastomycosis of the genitourinary tract. J Urol 1975;113:650–652.
12. Mankodi RC, Kanvinde MS, Mohapatra LN. Penile histoplasmosis. A case report. Indian J Med Sci 1970;24:354–356.
13. Sills M, Schwartz A, Weg JG. Conjugal histoplasmosis. A consequence of progressive dissemination in the index case after steroid therapy. Ann Intern Med 1973;79:221–224.
14. Allen R, Barter CE, Chachoua LL, Cleeve L, O'Connell JM, Daniel FJ. Disseminated cryptococcosis after transurethral resection of the prostate. Aust NZ J Med 1982;12:296–299.
15. Vapnek JM, McAninch JW. AIDS and the urologist. Infect Urol 1990;3: 101–107.
16. Rudjay AL. Erythrasma with unusual localization. Dermatol Wochenschr 1968;154:994–996.
17. White SW, Smith J. Trichomycosis pubis. Arch Dermatol 1979;115:444–445.
18. Basoglu M, Gul O, Yildirgan I, Balik AA, Ozbey I, Oren D. Fournier's gangrene: review of fifteen cases. Am Surg 1997;63:1019–1021.
19. Kearney GP, Carling PC. Fournier's gangrene: an approach to its management. J Urol 1983;130:695–698.
20. Mouraviev VB, Pautler SE, Hayman WP. Fournier's gangrene following penile self-injection with cocaine. Scand J Urol Nephrol 2002;36: 317–318.
21. Roca B, Cunat E, Simon E. HIV infection presenting with Fournier's gangrene. Neth J Med 1998;53:168–171.
22. Manian FA, Alford RH. Nosocomial infectious balanoposthitis in neutropenic patients. South Med J 1987;80:909–911.
23. Rabinowitz R, Lewin EB. Gangrene of the genitalia in children with pseudomonas sepsis. J Urol 1980;124:431–432.
24. Cunningham DL, Persky L. Penile ecthyma gangrenosum. A complication of drug addiction. Urology 1989;34:109–110.
25. Dahl DM, Klein D, Morgentaler A. Penile mass caused by the newly described organism *Mycobacterium celatum*. Urology 1996;47: 266–268.
26. Nishigori C, Taniguchi S, Hayakawa M, Imamura S. Penis tuberculides: papulonecrotic tuberculides on the glans penis. Dermatologica 1986;172: 93–97.
27. Erol A, Ozgur S, Tahtali N. Bacillus Calmette-Guerin (BCG) balanitis as a complication of intravesical BCG immunotherapy: a case report. Int Urol Nephrol 1995;27:307–310.
28. Mindel A, Tovey SJ, Timmins DJ, Williams P. Primary and secondary syphilis, 20 years' experience. 2. Clinical features. Genitourin Med 1989;65: 1–3.
29. Manget-Velasco CS, Borbujo-Martinez J, Manzano de Arostegui JA, Calderon-Ubeda J, Toribio-Da Pena R, Casado-Jimenez M. [Soft chancroid: 4 clinical cases.] Aten Primaria 1993;12:667–670.
30. Burgoyne RA. Lymphogranuloma venereum. Clinics in Office Practice 1990;17:153–157.
31. Aggarwal K, Jain VK, Gupta S. Bilateral groove sign with penoscrotal elephantiasis. Sex Transm Infect 2002;78:458.
32. Rosen T, Tschen JA, Ramsdell W, Moore J, Markham B. Granuloma inguinale. J Am Acad Dermatol 1984;11:433–437.
33. Sehgal VN, Sharma HK. Pseudoelephantiasis of the penis following donovanosis. J Dermatol 1990;17:130–131.
34. English JC 3rd, Laws RA, Keough GC, Wilde JL, Foley JP, Elston DM. Dermatoses of the glans penis and prepuce. J Am Acad Dermatol 1997;37:1–24; quiz 25–26.
35. Smith MA, Singer C. Sexually transmitted viruses other than HIV and papillomavirus. Urol Clin North Am 1992;19:47–61.
36. Danielsen AG, Petersen CS, Iversen J. Chronic erosive herpes simplex virus infection of the penis in a human immunodeficiency virus-positive man, treated with imiquimod and famciclovir. Br J Dermatol 2002;147: 1034–1036.
37. Cook LS, Koutsdy LA, Holmes KK. Subclinical human papillomavirus infection in male sexual partners of female carriers. J Urol 1993;140: 262–264.

38. Schneider A, Kirchmayr R, De Villiers EM, Gissmann L. Subclinical human papillomavirus infections in male sexual partners of female carriers. J Urol 1988;140:1431–1434.
39. Buechner SA. Common skin disorders of the penis. BJU Int 2002;90: 498–506.
40. Lowhagen GB, Bolmstedt A, Ryd W, Voog E. The prevalence of "high-risk" HPV types in penile condyloma-like lesions: correlation between HPV type and morphology. Genitourin Med 1993;69:87–90.
41. Ayres S Jr, Mihan R. Molluscum contagiosum of the glans penis. Arch Dermatol 1964;89:465–466.
42. Cooke RA, Rodrigues RB. Amoebic balanitis. Med J Aust 1964;1:114–116.
43. Thomas JA, Antony AJ. Amoebiasis of the penis. Br J Urol 1976;48: 269–273.
44. Mhlanga BR, Lanoie LO, Norris HJ, Lack EE, Connor DH. Amebiasis complicating carcinomas: a diagnostic dilemma. Am J Trop Med Hyg 1992;46:759–764.
45. Dissanaike AS, Abeyewickreme W, Wijesundera MD, Weerasooriya MV, Ismail MM. Human dirofilariasis caused by *Dirofilaria* (*Nochtiella*) *repens* in Sri Lanka. Parassitologia 1997;39:375–382.
46. Stayerman C, Szvalb S, Sazbon A. *Dirofilaria repens* presenting as a subcutaneous nodule in the penis. BJU Int 1999;84:746–747.
47. Badejo OA, Soyinka F, Laja AO. Ectopic lesion of schistosomiasis of the penis simulating an early carcinoma. Acta Trop 1978;35:263–267.
48. Elgart ML. Scabies. Dermatol Clin 1990;8:253–263.
49. Burkhart CG. Scabies: an epidemiologic reassessment. Ann Infect Med 1983;98:498–503.
50. Perna AG, Bell K, Rosen T. Localised genital Norwegian scabies in an AIDS patient. Sex Transm Infect 2004;80:72–73.
51. Lynch PJ. Lichen simplex chronicus (atopic/neurodermatitis) of the anogenital region. Dermatol Ther 2004;17:8–19.
52. Horan DB, Redman JF, Jansen GT. Papulosquamous lesions of glans penis. Urology 1984;23:1–4.
53. Reich HL, Nguyen JT, James WD. Annular lichen planus: a case series of 20 patients. J Am Acad Dermatol 2004;50:595–599.
54. Massa MC, Jason SM, Gradini R, Welykyj S. Lichenoid drug eruption secondary to propranolol. Cutis 1991;48:41–43.
55. Meffert JJ, Davis BM, Grimwood RE. Lichen sclerosus. J Am Acad Dermatol 1995;32:393–416; quiz 417–418.
56. Meyrick Thomas RH, Ridley CM, Black MM. Clinical features and therapy of lichen sclerosus et atrophicus affecting males. Clin Exp Dermatol 1987; 12:126–128.
57. Bart RS, Kopf AW. Squamous cell carcinoma arising in balanitis xerotica obliterans. J Dermatol Surg Oncol 1978;4:556–558.
58. Campus GV, Alia F, Bosincu L. Squamous cell carcinoma and lichen sclerosus et atrophicus of the prepuce. Plast Reconstr Surg 1992;89: 962–964.
59. Estcourt CS, Higgins SP, Goorney BP. Recurrent bullous balanitis: an unusual presentation of balanitis xerotica obliterans. Int J STD AIDS 1994; 5:58–59.
60. Pasricha JS. Drugs causing fixed drug eruptions. Br J Dermatol 1979;100: 183–185.
61. Kaupinen K, Stubbs S. Fixed drug eruptions to tetracycline. Br J Dermatol 1985;112:575–578.
62. Dodds PR, Chi TN. Balanitis as a fixed drug eruption to tetracycline. J Urol 1985;133:1044–1045.
63. Sehgal VH, Gangarani OP. Genital fixed drug eruptions. Genitourin Med 1986;62:56–58.
64. Castle WN, Wentzell JM, Schwartz BK, Clendenning WE, Selikowitz SM. Chronic balanitis owing to pemphigus vegetans. J Urol 1987;137: 289–291.
65. Goldman BD. Common dermatoses of the male genitalia. Recognition of differences in genital rashes and lesions is essential and attainable. Postgrad Med 2000;108:89–91, 95–96.
66. Murray WJ, Fletcher MS, Yates-Bell AJ, Pryor JP, Darby AJ, Packham DA. Plasma cell balinitis of Zoon. Br J Urol 1986;58:689–691.
67. Yoganathan S, Bohl TG, Mason G. Plasma cell balanitis and vulvitis (of Zoon). A study of 10 cases. J Reprod Med 1994;39:939–944.
68. Souteyrand P, Wong E, MacDonald DM. Zoon's balanitis (balanitis circumscripta plasmacellularis). Br J Dermatol 1981;105:195–199.
69. Kumar B, Sharma R, Rajagopalan M, Radotra BD. Plasma cell balanitis: clinical and histopathological features – response to circumcision. Genitourin Med 1995;71:32–34.
70. Weiss SW, Goldblum JR. Fibromatosis. In: Weiss SW, Goldblum JR, eds. Enzinger and Weiss's soft tissue tumors. 4th edn. St Louis: Mosby; 2001: 309–346.
71. Gonzalez-Gomez JM, Sierra-Salinas C, Alonso-Usabiaga I, Barco-Galvez A, del Rio-Mapelli L, Garcia-Lorenzo C. [Metastatic Crohn's disease in childhood.] An Esp Pediatr 2001;55:165–168.
72. Lee DK, Hinshaw M, Cripps D, Jarrard DF. Pyoderma gangrenosum of penis. J Urol 2003;170:185–186.
73. Hillman RJ, Waldron S, Walker MM, Harris JR. Granuloma annulare of the penis. Genitourin Med 1992;68:47–49.
74. Narouz N, Allan PS, Wade AH. Penile granuloma annulare. Sex Transm Infect 1999;75:186–187.
75. Leal SM, Novsam N, Zacks SI. Amyloidosis presenting as a penile mass. J Urol 1988;140:830–831.
76. Ritter M, Nawab RA, Tannenbaum M, Hakky SI, Morgan MB. Localized amyloidosis of the glans penis: a case report and literature review. J Cutan Pathol 2003;30:37–40.
77. Sanchez-Merino JM, Bouso-Montero M, Fernandez-Flores A, Garcia-Alonso J. Idiopathic calcinosis cutis of the penis. J Am Acad Dermatol 2004;51(2 Suppl):S118–S119.
78. Kinn AC, Hedenborg L. Polyarteritis nodosa of the penis. Scand J Urol Nephrol 1977;11:289–291.
79. Davenport A, Downey SE, Goel S, Maciver AG. Wegener's granulomatosis involving the urogenital tract. Br J Urol 1996;78:354–357.
80. Vella EJ, Waller DG. Granulomatous vasculitis of the penis with glomerulonephritis. Postgrad Med J 1981;57:262–264.
81. Schneider JM, Matthews JH, Graham BS. Reiter's syndrome. Cutis 2003;71: 198–200.
82. Wei H, Friedman KA, Rudikoff D. Multiple indurated papules on penis and scrotum. J Cutan Med Surg 2000;4:202–204.
83. Kousseff BG, Hoover DL. Penile neurofibromas. Am J Med Genet 1999;87: 1–5.
84. Rodo J, Medina M, Carrasco R, Morales L. Enlarged penis due to a plexiform neurofibroma. J Urol 1999;162:1753–1754.
85. Aksu K, Keser G, Gunaydin G, et al. Erectile dysfunction in Behçet's disease without neurological involvement: two case reports. Rheumatology (Oxford) 2000;39:1429–1431.
86. Ates A, Aydintug OT, Duzgun N, Yaman O, Sancak T, Omur ND. Behçet's disease presenting as deep venous thrombosis and priapism. Clin Exp Rheumatol 2004;22:107–109.
87. Gaffoor PM. Depigmentation of the male genitalia. Cutis 1984;34: 492–494.
88. Osborne GE, Francis ND, Bunker CB. Synchronous onset of penile lichen sclerosus and vitiligo. Br J Dermatol 2000;143:218–219.
89. Barnhill RL, Albert LS, Shama SK, Goldenhersh MA, Rhodes AR, Sober AJ. Genital lentiginosis: a clinical and histopathologic study. J Am Acad Dermatol 1990;22:453–460.
90. Busam KJ, Sachs DL, Coit DG, Halpern A, Hwu WJ. Eruptive melanotic macules and papules associated with adenocarcinoma. J Cutan Pathol 2003;30:463–469.
91. Barnhill RL, Crowson AN. Tumors of melanocytes. In: Barnhill RL, Crowson AN, eds. Textbook of dermatopathology. 2nd edn. New York: McGraw-Hill; 2004:635.
92. Friedman SJ, Fox BJ, Albert HL. Seborrheic keratoses of penis. Urology 1987;29:204–206.
93. Bennett RT, Palmer LS, Kreutzer ER. Massive scrotal epidermal inclusion cysts. Urology 1996;48:781–782.
94. deBoisblanc MW, Robichaux WH, Hellstrom WJ. Large scrotal epidermal inclusion cyst and hydrocele. J La State Med Soc 1995;147:280–281.
95. Hanly MG, Ojeda VJ. Epidermal inclusion cysts of the clitoris as a complication of female circumcision and pharaonic infibulation. Cent Afr J Med 1995;41:22–24.
96. Acenero MJ, Garcia-Gonzalez J. Median raphe cyst with ciliated cells: report of a case. Am J Dermatopathol 2003;25:175–176.
97. Dini M, Baroni G, Colafranceschi M. Median raphe cyst of the penis: a report of two cases with immunohistochemical investigation. Am J Dermatopathol 2001;23:320–324.
98. Crowson AN, Magro CM, Mihm MC. The melanocytic proliferations. A comprehensive textbook of pigmented lesions. New York: Wiley-Liss; 2001.
99. Sola Casas MA, Soto de Delas J, Redondo Bellon P, Quintanilla Gutierrez E. Syringomas localized to the penis (case report). Clin Exp Dermatol 1993;18:384–385.
100. Gibson GE, Ahmed I. Perianal and genital basal cell carcinoma: a clinicopathologic review of 51 cases. J Am Acad Dermatol 2001;45: 68–71.

101. Salamanca J, Benito A, Garcia-Penalver C, Azorin D, Ballestin C, Rodriguez-Peralto JL. Paget's disease of the glans penis secondary to transitional cell carcinoma of the bladder: a report of two cases and review of the literature. J Cutan Pathol 2004;31:341–345.
102. Bechara FG, Huesmann M, Stucker M, Altmeyer P, Jansen T. An exceptional localization of angiokeratoma of Fordyce on the glans penis. Dermatology 2002;205:187–188.
103. Lane JE, Peterson CM, Ratz JL. Treatment of pearly penile papules with CO_2 laser. Dermatol Surg 2002;28:617–618.
104. Fetsch JF, Davis CJ Jr, Miettinen M, Sesterhenn IA. Leiomyosarcoma of the penis: a clinicopathologic study of 14 cases with review of the literature and discussion of the differential diagnosis. Am J Surg Pathol 2004;28:115–125.
105. Micali G, Nasca MR, De Pasquale R, Innocenzi D. Primary classic Kaposi's sarcoma of the penis: report of a case and review. J Eur Acad Dermatol Venereol 2003;17:320–323.
106. Tanaka Y, Sasaki Y, Kobayashi T, Terashima K. Granular cell tumor of the corpus cavernosum of the penis. J Urol 1991;146:1596–1597.
107. Bryant J. Granular cell tumor of penis and scrotum. Urology 1995;45:332–334.

3

DISEASES OF THE SCROTUM

Michael B. Morgan

NORMAL ANATOMY AND FEATURES

- The scrotum is a bilobed pyramidal structure covered with rugose hyperpigmented skin (Fig. 3.1).
- Scrotal skin is copiously endowed with adnexae including sebaceous and apocrine glands.
- An attenuated dermis is contiguous with the dartos muscle, fascial layers, and peritoneal tunica vaginalis reflection.

NON-NEOPLASTIC CONDITIONS

ACANTHOSIS NIGRICANS[1]

- This condition presents as velvety hyperpigmented patches with extension to inguinal creases (Fig. 3.2).
- There is an association with endocrine disturbances including diabetes mellitus, a familial tendency, obesity, various medications, and visceral malignancies.
- Sections show epidermal hyperpigmentation with acanthosis, mild papillomatosis, and hyperkeratosis.

SCROTAL CALCINOSIS[2,3]

- Multiple dermal foci of dystrophic calcification often occur in conjunction with epidermoid cysts (Fig. 3.3).
- Calcific foci may ulcerate the overlying epithelium, simulating carcinoma.

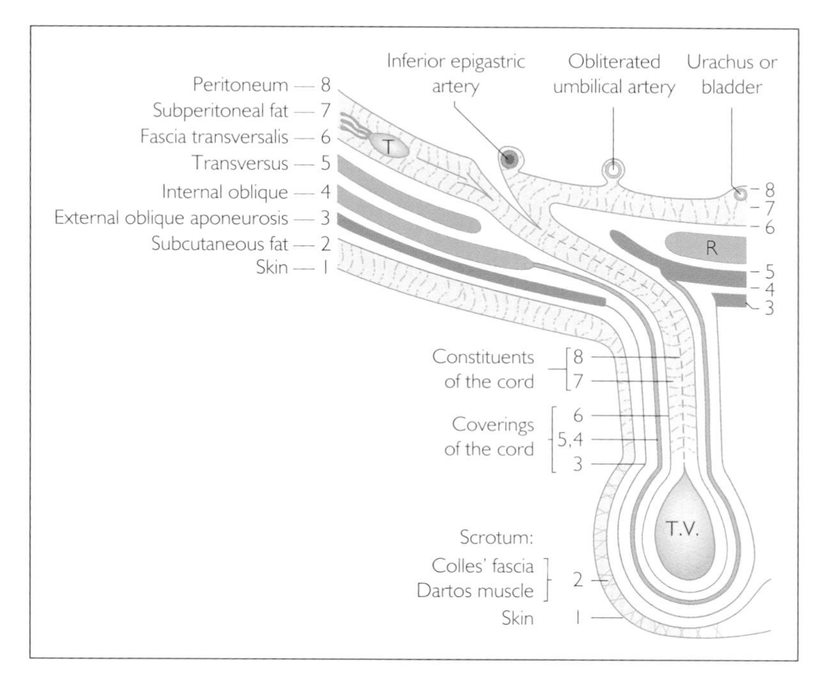

Fig. 3.1 Diagram of the scrotum. T.V, tunica vaginalis; R, rectus abdominis muscle; T, path of testicular descent.

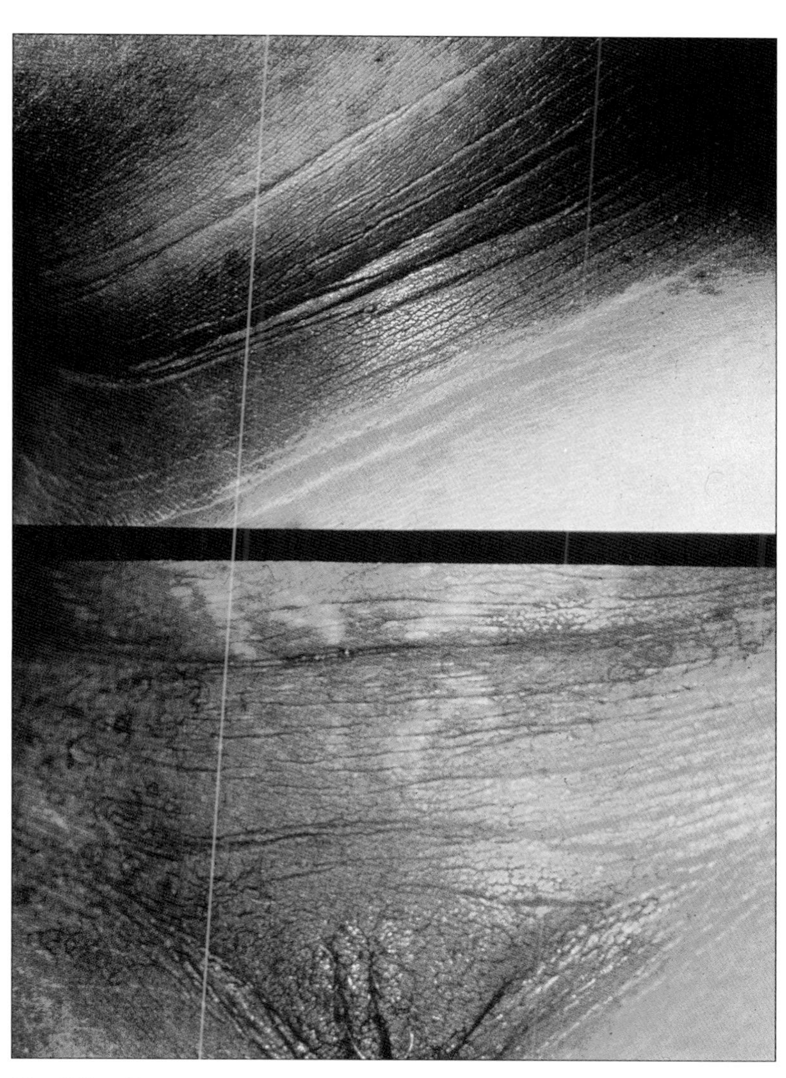

Fig. 3.2 Clinical presentation of acanthosis nigricans.

LICHEN SIMPLEX CHRONICUS[4]

- These hyperpigmented plaques (Fig. 3.4) represent changes following protracted excoriation or manipulation.
- Histology shows epidermal acanthosis and hyperkeratosis with dermal sclerosis.

SCLEROSING LIPOGRANULOMA[5,6]

- These indurated dermal nodules in regions adjacent to the penis represent a granulomatous response to the purposeful or accidental injection of exogenous hydrocarbons or lipids.
- Histology shows foam cells, dermal sclerosis, and macrocyst or microcyst formation resembling 'Swiss cheese' (Figs 3.5 & 3.6).

ELEPHANTIASIS[7]

- Presenting as a pendulous and elongated scrotum with doughy induration, this represents loss or dysfunction of draining lymphatics, seen in the setting of chronic filariasis or, rarely, following inguinal lymphadenectomy.
- Histology shows a variable degree of epidermal hyperplasia with dermal fibrosis and tissue edema (Fig. 3.7).

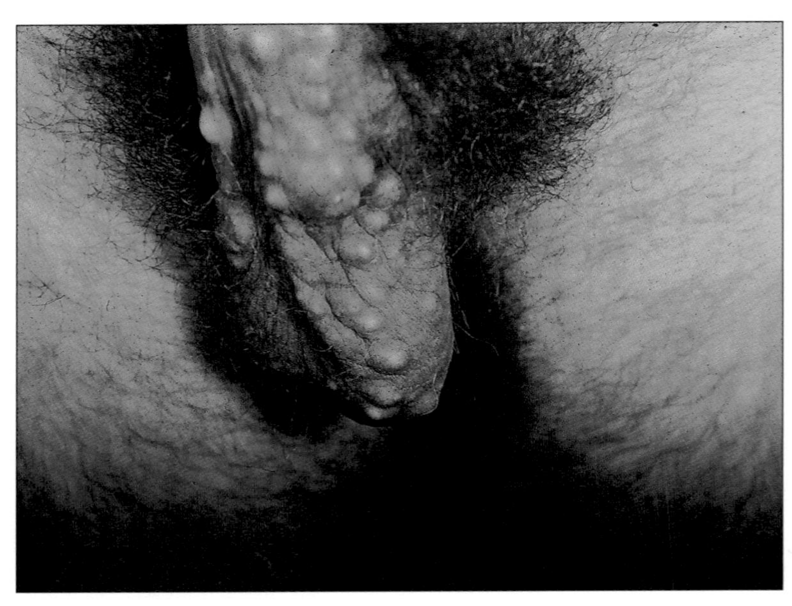

Fig. 3.3 Clinical presentation of scrotal calcinosis.

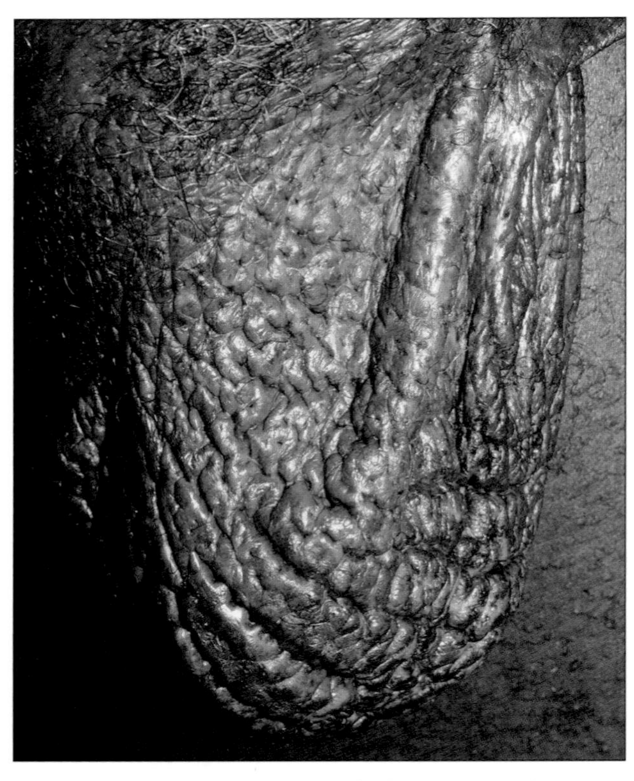

Fig. 3.4 Clinical presentation of lichen simplex chronicus.

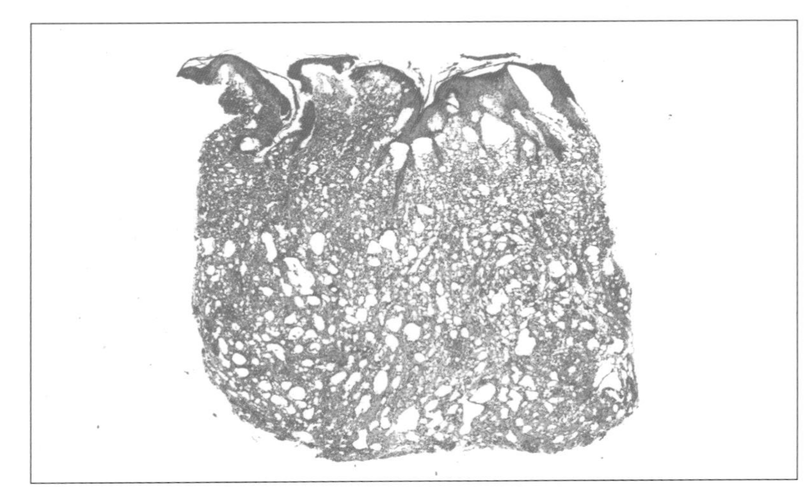

Fig. 3.5 Whole-mount section of sclerosing lipogranuloma.

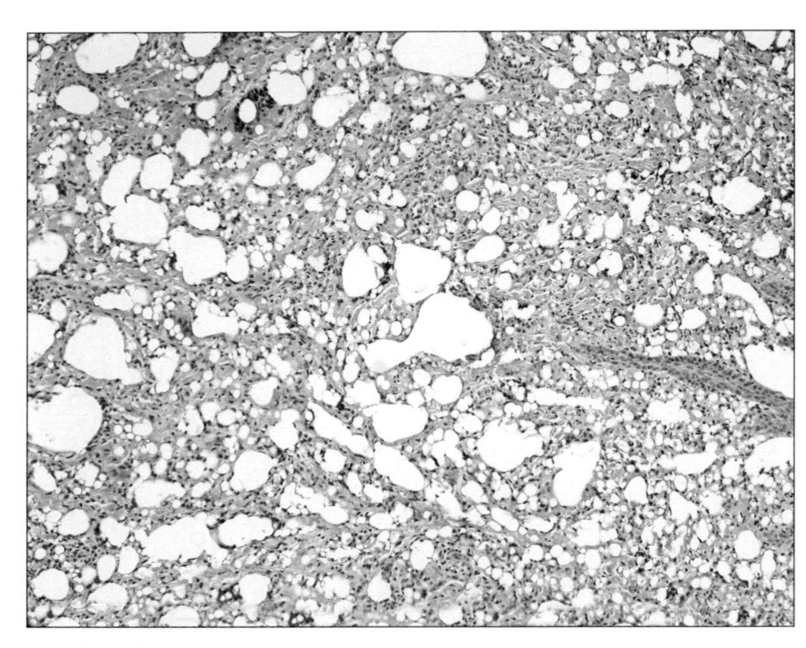

Fig. 3.6 Microscopic features of sclerosing lipogranuloma: note the cysts resembling 'Swiss cheese' (10×).

ANGIOKERATOMA OF FORDYCE[8]

- This lesion appears clinically as multiple erythematous to violaceous papules.
- Histology shows epidermal acanthosis with dilated adjacent endothelium-lined vascular spaces (Figs 3.8 & 3.9).

PEDICULOSIS[9]

- This lice infestation can be caused by two species of insects: *Phthirus pubis* (crab louse) and *Pediculus humanus* (head or body louse).
- Clinically, erythematous papules are seen.
- Handlens shows tiny lice clutching genital hair (Fig. 3.10).

CONDYLOMA ACUMINATUM[10,11]

- Scrotal condyloma acuminatum presents in sexually active males as agminated flesh-colored papules and macerated vegetations (Fig. 3.11).
- It is caused by the human papillomavirus, usually serotypes 6, 11, and 16.
- Histology shows epidermal acanthosis with mild papillomatosis and koilocytic change.
- There is a low risk for malignant degeneration in the immunocompetent host.

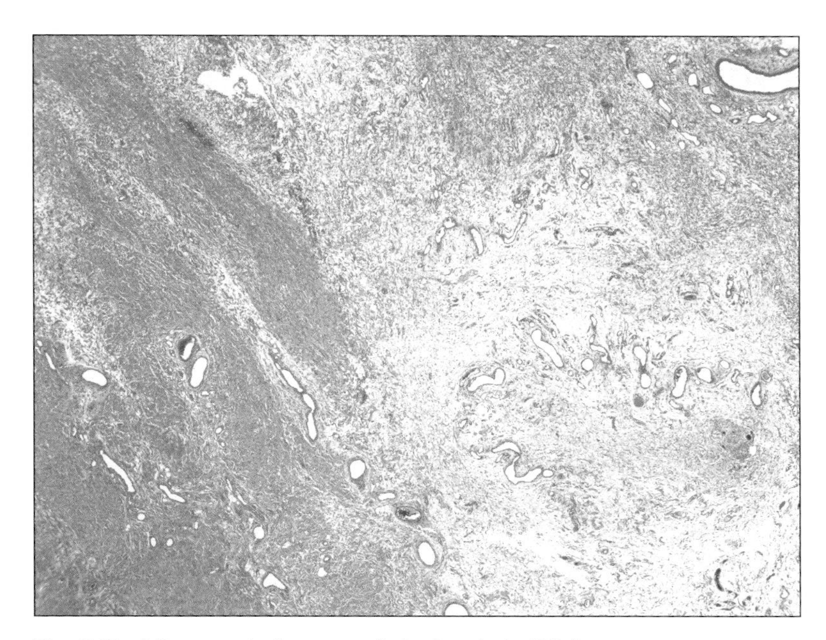

Fig. 3.7 Microscopic features of elephantiasis (10×).

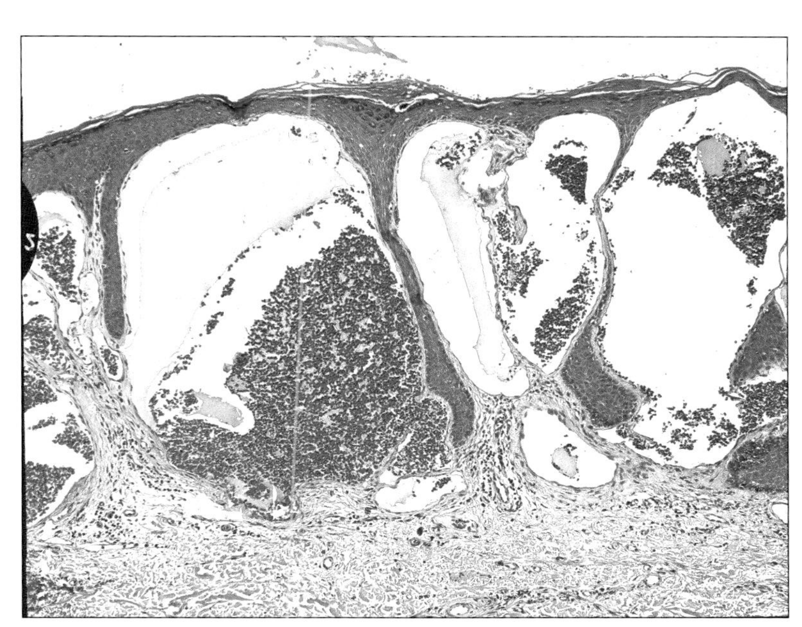

Fig. 3.9 Microscopic features of angiokeratoma: note the close apposition of blood vessels with epithelium (40×).

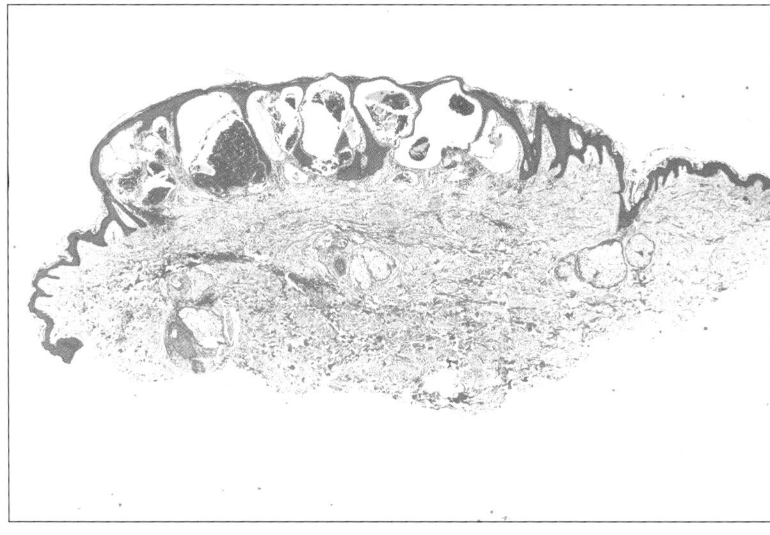

Fig. 3.8 Clinical presentation of angiokeratoma.

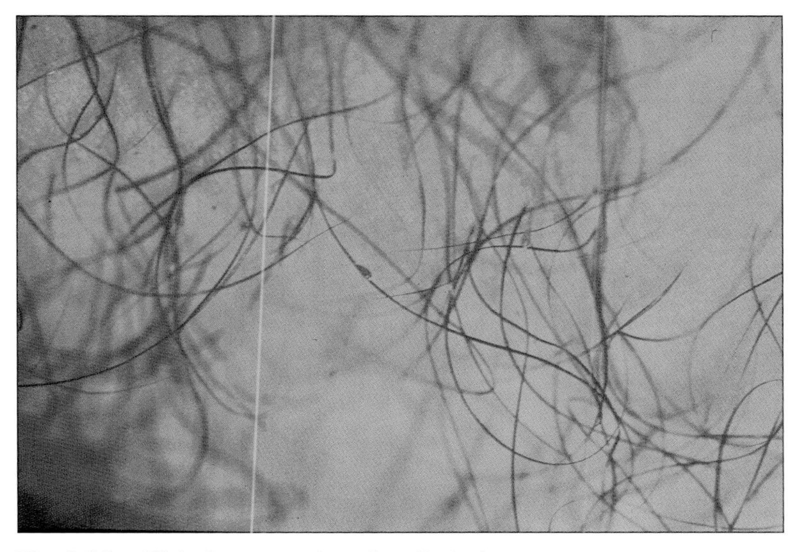

Fig. 3.10 Clinical presentation of pediculosis.

FOURNIER'S GANGRENE[12,13]

- This necrotizing fascitiis is caused by microaerophilic or anaerobic bacteria.
- Predisposing factors include diabetes mellitus and cancer chemotherapy.
- It manifests as a rapidly expanding erythematous patch that evolves to a blackened eschar and bullae.
- Histology shows abundant edema with acute inflammation and necrosis.

NEOPLASTIC CONDITIONS

GIANT CONDYLOMA OF BUSCHKE–LÖWENSTEIN/VERRUCOUS CARCINOMA[14,15]

- This presents as an endophytic/exophytic mass with deeply extending furrows.
- The etiology is infection with oncogenic strains of the human papillomavirus types 16, 18, and 31–35.
- Histology shows deeply infiltrating squamous islands with broad pushing borders comprised of cytologically benign-appearing squamous cells.

CONVENTIONAL SQUAMOUS CELL CARCINOMA[16,17]

- This presents as a variably exophytic or endophytic mass.

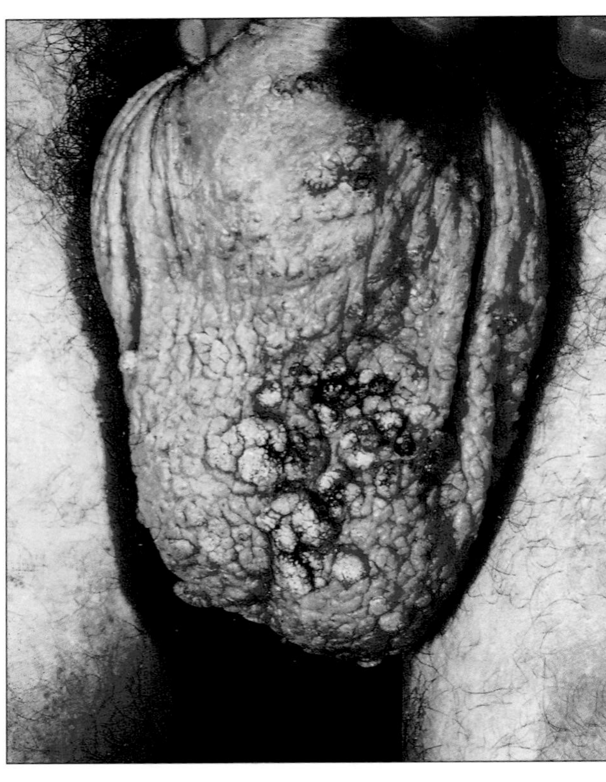

Fig. 3.11 Clinical presentation of scrotal condyloma.

- Contact with petroleum-based tars and oils is a predisposing factor to this lesion traditionally seen in chimney sweeps. It also may occur following long-term ultraviolet exposure, for example in psoriatric patients or nudists.
- Histology shows infiltrating epithelial elements with obvious cytologic atypia.

AGGRESSIVE ANGIOMYXOMA[18,19]

- This presents as a fluctuant ill-defined nodule or mass.
- It affects middle-aged adults, and tends to recur with inadequate re-excision.
- Histology shows variably sized, often hyalinized, blood vessels embedded in a myxoid stroma (Figs 3.12 & 3.13).

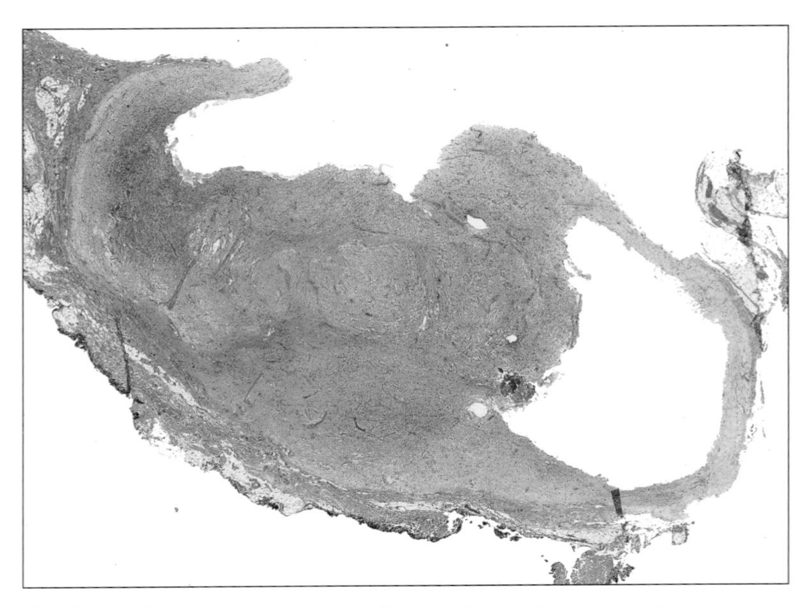

Fig. 3.12 Microscopic features of aggressive angiomyxoma (whole mount).

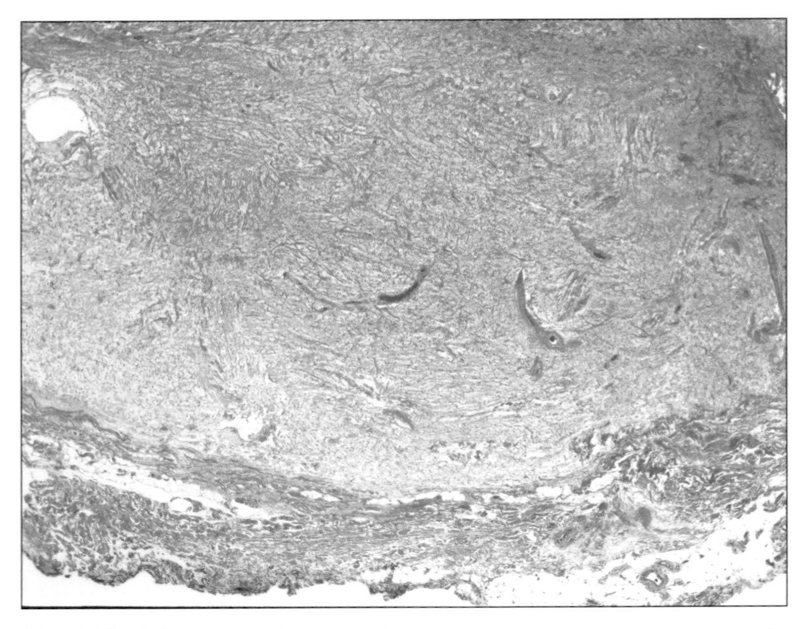

Fig. 3.13 Microscopic features of aggressive angiomyxoma: note vessels (10×).

LEIOMYOSARCOMA[20,21]

- The most common sarcoma of the scrotum this arises within the dartos muscle.
- Clinically, it presents as a rapidly growing, painless mass.
- Histology shows a tumor comprised of sweeping fascicles of cells with blunt-ended nuclei and perinuclear halos, variable nuclear pleomorphism and mitotic activity (Figs 3.14 & 3.15).

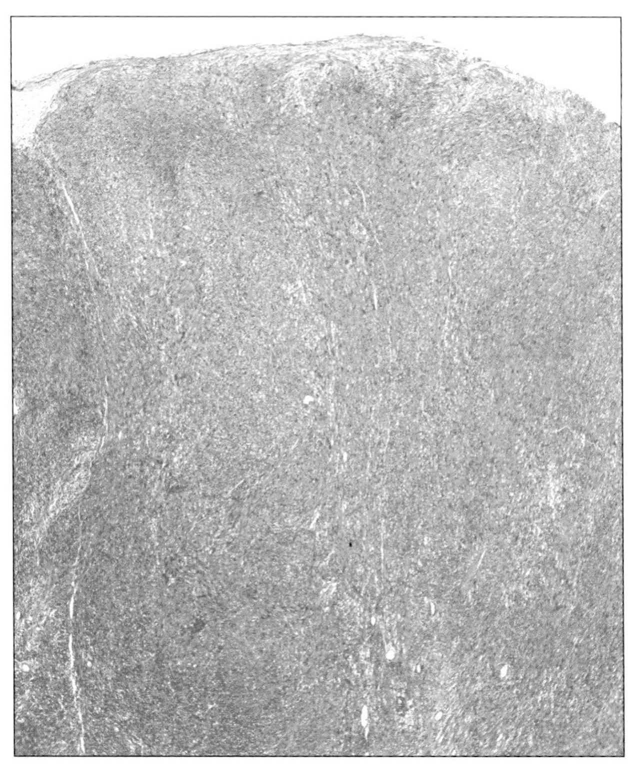

Fig. 3.14 Microscopic features of leiomyosarcoma (whole mount).

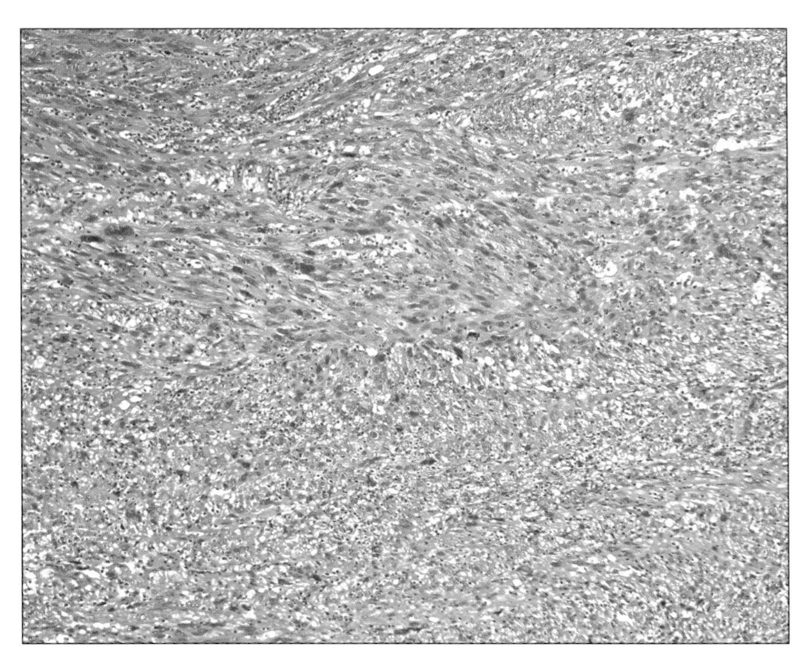

Fig. 3.15 Microscopic features of leiomyosarcoma: note the fascicular growth pattern (100×).

OTHER MALIGNANT TUMORS

- Basal cell carcinoma has been observed following long-term ultraviolet exposure, for example in nudists.
- Paget's disease is a cutaneous adenocarcinoma associated with genitourinary and gastrointestinal adenocarcinomas (Figs 3.16–3.18).
- Malignant mesothelioma is the most common primary tumor of the tunica vaginalis.
- Metastatic carcinoma originates most commonly from the testis, kidney (Figs 3.19 & 3.20), or prostate (Figs 3.21–3.23).

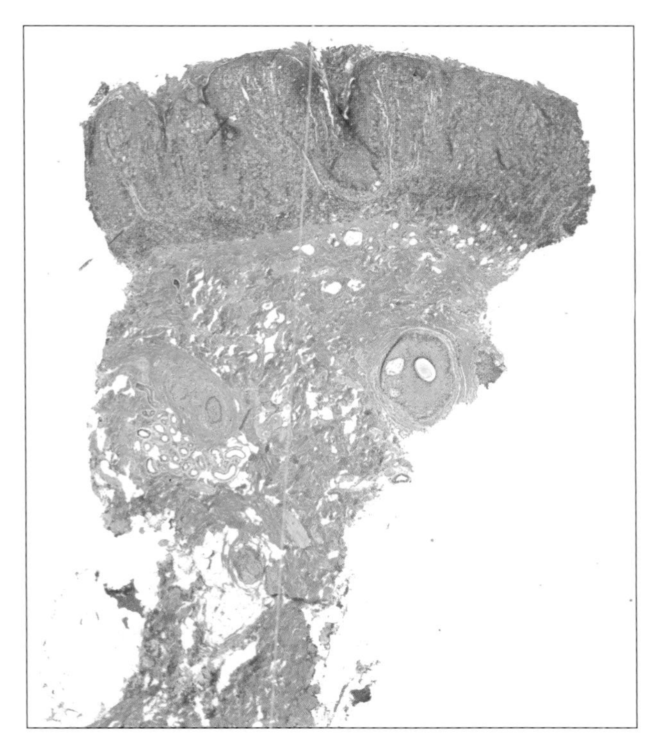

Fig. 3.16 Microscopic features of Paget's disease (whole mount).

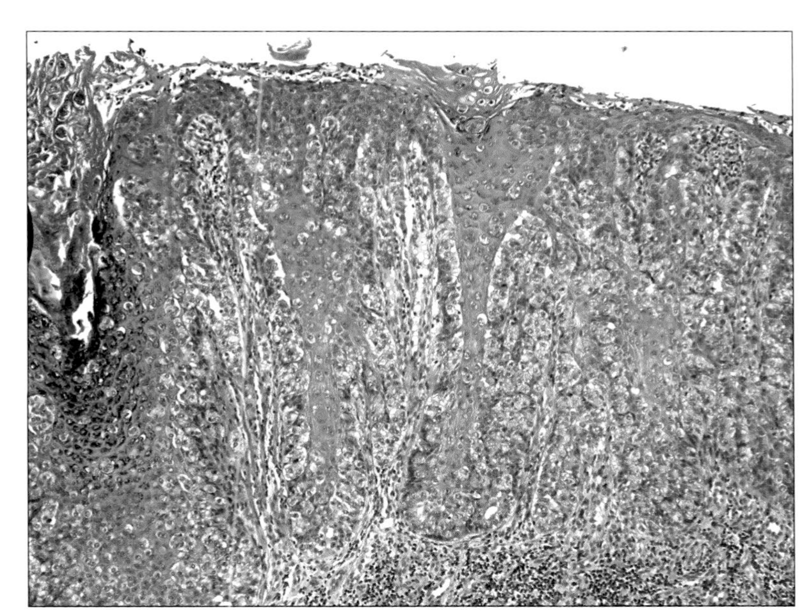

Fig. 3.17 Microscopic features of Paget's disease: note the distinct population of widely scattered malignant epithelioid cells within the epithelium (10×).

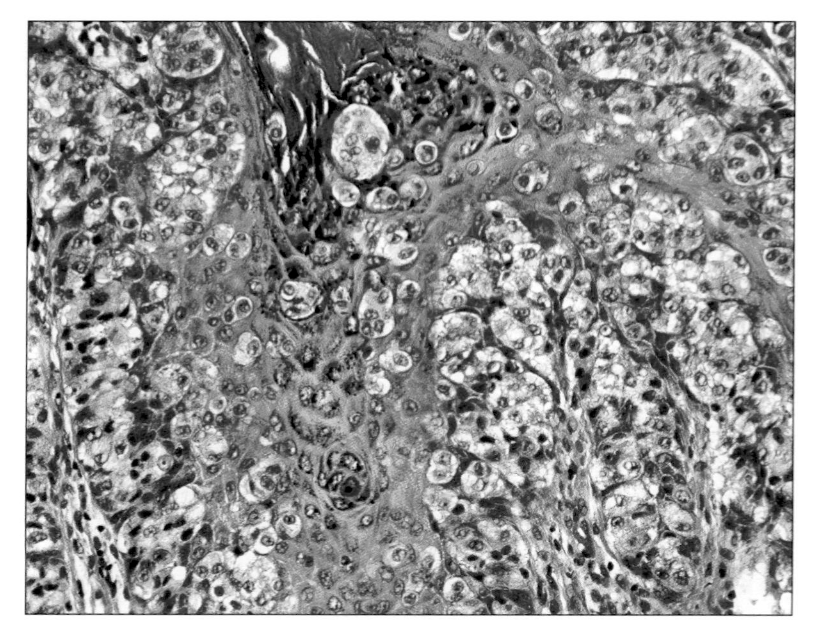

Fig. 3.18 Microscopic features of Paget's disease: note malignant cells with clear cytoplasm and eccentrically placed nuclei (100×).

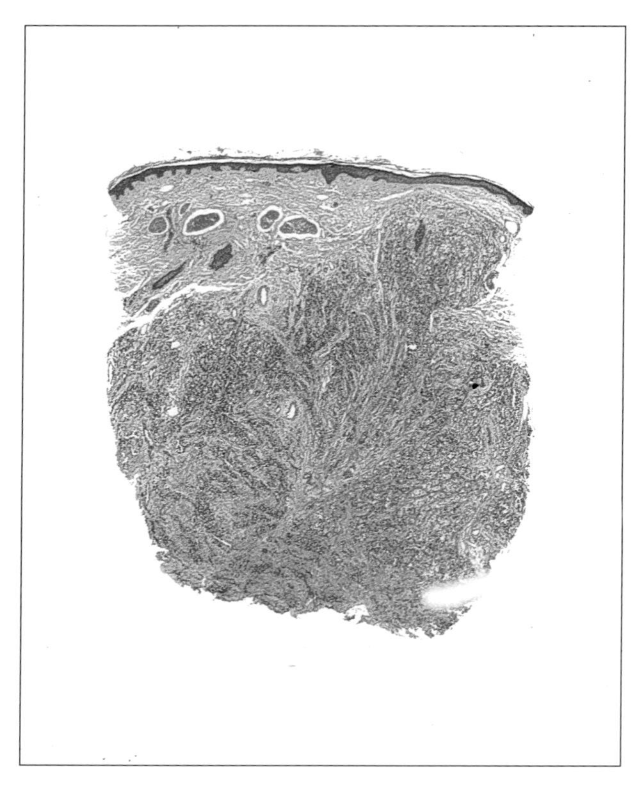

Fig. 3.19 Microscopic features of metastatic renal cell carcinoma to scrotum: note distinct population of clear cells representing the metastases (whole mount).

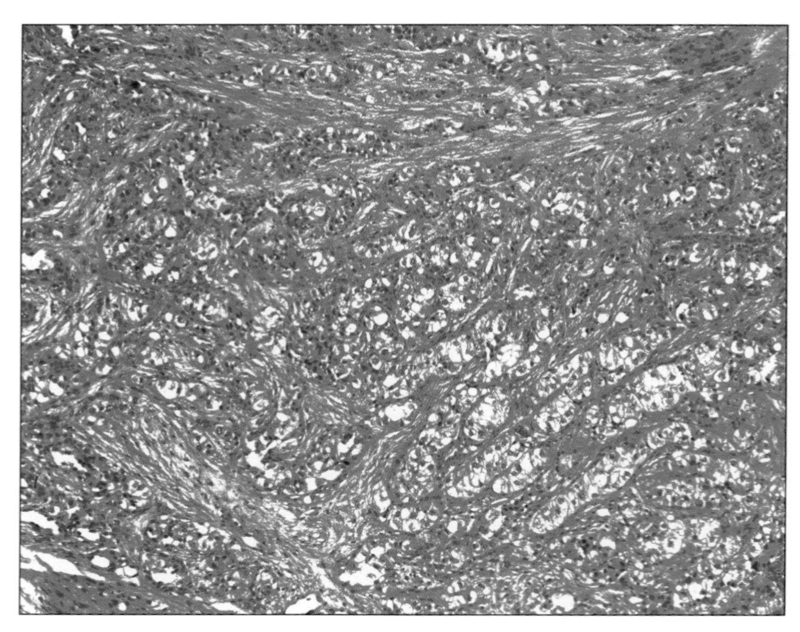

Fig. 3.20 Microscopic features of metastatic renal cell carcinoma: note the cell detail (40×).

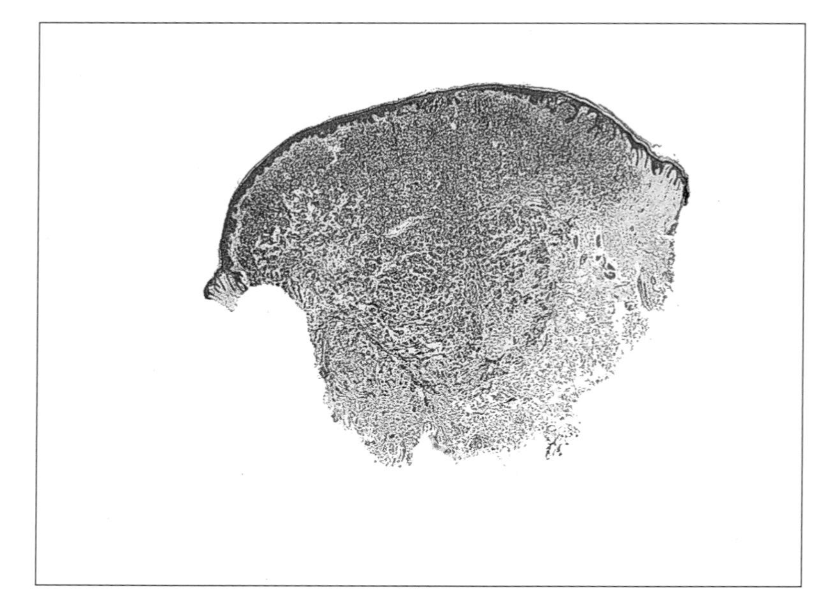

Fig. 3.21 Microscopic features of metastatic prostate carcinoma (whole mount).

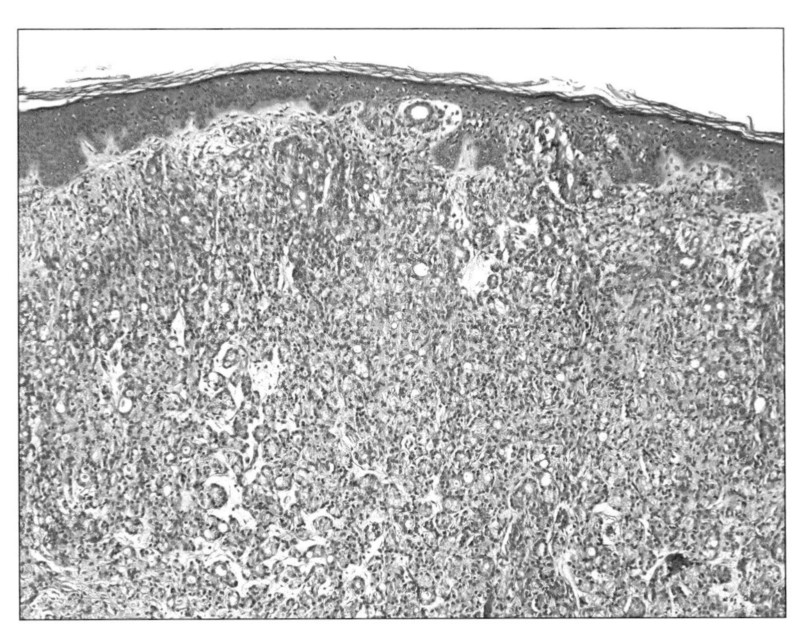

Fig. 3.22 Microscopic features of metastatic prostate cancer: note the closely arrayed collection of tubular glands (10×).

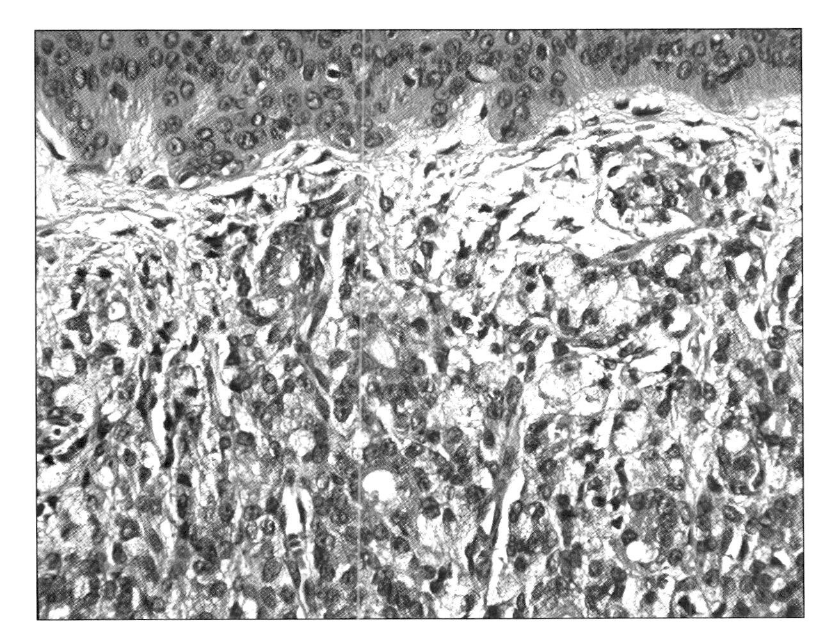

Fig. 3.23 Microscopic features of metastatic prostate cancer: note the cytologic detail of metastatic prostate glands (100×).

REFERENCES

1. Curth H. Classification of acanthosis nigricans. Int J Dermatol 1976;15:592–593.
2. Shapiro L, Platt N, Torres-Rodriguez V. Idiopathic calcinosis of the scrotum. Arch Dermatol 1970;102:199–204.
3. Gormally S, Dorman T, Powell F. Calcinosis of the scrotum. Int J Dermatol 1992;31:75–79.
4. Epstein W. Immunologic (allergic) contact dermatitis. J Dermatol 1975;2:105–110.
5. Oertel Y, Johnson F. Sclerosing lipogranuloma of the male genitalia. Review of 23 cases. Arch Pathol 1977;101:321–326.
6. Smetana H, Bernhard W. Sclerosing lipogranuloma. Arch Pathol 1950;50:296–325.
7. Ottesen E. Wellcome Trust Lecture: Infection and disease in lymphatic filariasis: an immunologic perspective. Parasitology 1984;104:71–76.
8. Imperial R, Helwig E. Angiokeratoma of the scrotum. J Urol 1967;98:379–386.
9. Kim K, Pratt H, Stojanovich C. The sucking lice of North America. University Park, PA: Pennsylvania State Press; 1986.
10. Schlegel R. Papillomavirus and human cancer. Virology 1990;1:297–306.
11. Koronel R, Stefanon B, Pilotti S, Bandieramonte G, Rilke F, De Palo G. Genital papillomavirus infection in males: a clinicopathologic study. Tumori 1991;77:76–82.
12. Radaelli F, Della Volpe A, Colombi M, Bregani P, Polli E. Acute gangrene of the scrotum and penis in four hematologic patients. Cancer 1987;60:1462–1464.
13. Paty R, Smith A. Gangrene and Fournier's gangrene. Urol Clin North Am 1992;19:149–162.
14. Kraus F, Perez-Mesa C. Verrucous carcinoma. Clinical and pathologic study of 105 cases involving the oral cavity, larynx, and genitalia. Cancer 1966;19:26–38.
15. Masih A, Stoler M, Farrow G, Wooldridge T, Johansson S. Penile verrucous carcinoma: a clinicopathologic, human papillomavirus typing and flow cytometric analysis. Mod Pathol 1992;5:48–55.
16. Lowe F. Squamous cell carcinoma of the scrotum. Urology 1985;25:63–65.
17. Castiglione F, Selikowitz S, Dimond R. Mule spinner's disease. Arch Dermatol 1985;121:370–372.
18. Clatch R, Drake W, Gonzalez J. Aggressive angiomyxoma in men. A report of two cases associated with inguinal hernias. Arch Pathol Lab Med 1993;117:911–913.
19. Tsang W, Chan J, Lee K, Fisher C, Fletcher C. Aggressive angiomyxoma. A report of four cases occurring in men. Am J Surg Pathol 1992;16: 1059–1065.
20. Johnson S, Rundell M, Platt W. Leiomyosarcoma of the scrotum. A case report with electron microscopy. Cancer 1978;41:1830–1835.
21. Newman P, Fletcher C. Smooth muscle tumors of the external genitalia. Clinicopathologic analysis of a series. Histopathology 1991;18:523–529.

TESTIS

Aleksander Talerman and Myron Tannenbaum

TESTICULAR TUMORS

Testicular tumors are uncommon, comprising 1–2% of the malignant tumors in the male. Germ cell tumors are by far the most predominant group, comprising approximately 90% of all testicular neoplasms. The incidence of testicular tumors, notably germ cell tumors, shows considerable racial and geographic differences. They are relatively common in Europe and North America and rare in Africa and Asia. In the United States, they are much more common in Caucasians than in blacks. In Europe, the incidence is highest in Scandinavia and lowest in the Mediterranean countries, Hungary, and Finland.[1]

There are considerable differences between ovarian germ cell tumors, which comprise only 20% of ovarian neoplasms, and testicular germ cell neoplasms. In the testis, benign germ cell neoplasms are very rare, occurring only in infancy and early childhood, while in the ovary, approximately 90% of germ cell neoplasms are mature cystic teratomas (dermoid cysts) which are benign and only 6–8% of ovarian germ cell tumors are malignant. Nevertheless, all the histologic types of germ cell tumor occurring in the testis, with the exception of spermatocytic seminoma, are seen in the ovary. This homology also extends to the sex cord stromal tumor group, although the incidence of the various types, as in the case of germ cell tumors, is different.[1]

CLASSIFICATION

A histologic classification of testicular tumors, slightly modified from the amended World Health Organization classification,[1–5] is shown in Table 4.1.

GERM CELL TUMORS

Intratubular germ cell neoplasia

Intratubular germ cell neoplasia (IGCN) is a precursor of invasive germ cell tumors and accompanies virtually all malignant testicular germ cell tumors of adults except spermatocytic seminoma.[6] There is controversy regarding whether lesions of this type occur in infants and children with malignant germ cell tumors.

Clinical findings

- IGCN is seen in 2–8% of males with cryptorchidism and in 0.4–1% of males with a severe degree of oligospermia.[6–10]
- Patients with gonadal dysgenesis or androgen insensitivity syndrome may also develop IGCN.
- Progression to invasive germ cell tumor occurs in approximately 50% of cases and may take 5 years or longer.[7,11,12]
- IGCN has been noted in the contralateral testis in 5% of patients with invasive germ cell tumors.[13]

Pathologic findings

Macroscopic

- In most cases, the testis appears normal.
- In patients with cryptorchidism, the testis is smaller than normal.

Microscopic

- The lesion may be focal or extensive.[6]
- Affected seminiferous tubules show fibrosis, thickening, and decreased diameter.
- Interstitial fibrous tissue may be increased.
- Spermatogenesis is decreased and may be absent in the affected area.[6,9,11,12]
- Large atypical germ cells are, usually located at the periphery of the tubule, often side by side, between or beneath Sertoli cells.
- Atypical germ cells may be occasional or numerous.
- The neoplastic germ cells have clear cytoplasm, atypical nuclei with coarse chromatin, and prominent irregular nucleoli.[6,9,11,12]
- The cytoplasm contains lipid and glycogen, which can be demonstrated histochemically.[6]
- Mitotic figures are often present and may be abnormal.
- Adjacent tubules may be atrophic.
- Occasionally the atypical germ cells may spread in pagetoid fashion into the rete epithelium.[6,9,11,12]
- Sometimes the affected tubules are surrounded by lymphocytes. In such cases, careful examination is mandatory to exclude the presence of microinvasion.[6]

Table 4.1 World Health Organization histologic classification of testicular tumors (slightly modified)

Germ cell tumors
Precursor lesions
Intratubular germ cell neoplasia
Tumors of one histologic type (pure forms)
Seminoma
Variant – seminoma with syncytiotrophoblastic cells
Spermatocytic seminoma
Variant – spermatocytic seminoma with sarcoma
Embryonal carcinoma
Yolk sac tumor
Polyembryoma
Trophoblastic tumors
Choriocarcinoma
Placental site trophoblastic tumor
Teratoma
Mature teratoma
Dermoid cyst
Immature teratoma
Tumors of more than one histologic type
(Mixed germ cell tumors)
Sex cord/gonadal stromal tumors
Pure forms
Leydig cell tumor
Sertoli cell tumor
Variants
Large cell calcifying Sertoli cell tumor
Lipid-rich Sertoli cell tumor
Sclerosing Sertoli cell tumor
Granulosa cell tumor
Adult-type granulosa cell tumor
Juvenile-type granulosa cell tumor (infantile Sertoli cell tumor)
Tumors of the thecoma/fibroma group
Incompletely differentiated sex cord/gonadal stromal tumors
Mixed forms
Unclassified forms
Tumors containing both germ cell and sex cord/gonadal stromal elements
Gonadoblastoma
Mixed germ cell–sex cord/stromal tumor
Miscellaneous tumors
Tumors of ovarian epithelial types
Lymphoid and hematopoietic tumors
Lymphoma
Plasmacytoma
Leukemia
Tumors of the collecting ducts and rete
Adenoma
Carcinoma
Tumors of the tunica, epididymis, spermatic cord, supporting structures, and appendices
Adenomatoid tumor
Mesothelioma
Adenoma
Carcinoma
Melanotic neuroectodermal tumor
Desmoplastic small round cell tumor
Soft tissue tumors
Unclassified tumors
Secondary (metastatic) tumors
Tumor-like lesions
Nodules of immature tubules
Testicular lesions of adrenogenital syndrome
Testicular lesions in androgen insensitivity syndrome
Nodular precocious maturation
Specific orchitis
Nonspecific orchitis
Granulomatous orchitis
Malakoplakia
Adrenal cortical rests
Fibromatous periorchitis
Funiculitis
Residua of meconium peritonitis
Sperm granuloma
Vasitis nodosa
Sclerosing lipogranuloma
Gonadal splenic fusion
Mesonephric remnants
Endometriosis
Epidermal cyst
Cystic dysplasia
Mesothelial cyst
Others

- IGCN must be differentiated from extensive intratubular involvement, by classical seminoma, the so-called intratubular classical seminoma.
- The atypical germ cells are similar in appearance to classical seminoma cells microscopically and ultrastructurally.[6]

Special studies

- IGCN cells stain for glycogen using periodic acid–Schiff (PAS) stain without diastase digestion. They also stain for lipid using frozen material.[6]
- IGCN cells show strong membranous staining with placental alkaline phosphatase (PLAP), a very useful test.[6,9,11,12,14]
- They also stain for ferritin.
- IGCN cells are negative for alphafetoprotein (AFP), human chorionic gonadotropin (HCG), and low molecular weight cytokeratin.[6,9,12]

(Figs 4.1–4.4)

Classical seminoma

Clinical findings

- Classical seminoma is the most common testicular neoplasm. In its pure form, it comprises 40–55% of all testicular germ cell neoplasms. In a further 15% of cases, classical seminoma is one component of a mixed germ cell tumor.[1–6]
- Pure classical seminoma occurs most commonly between the ages of 25 and 50 years. It is rare in children and uncommon after the fifth decade.
- It shows a slight predilection for the right testis and is only occasionally bilateral.[1,6,15]
- In 8.5% of cases, it originates in a cryptorchid testis.[1–6]
- The most common presentation is testicular enlargement (more than 70% of cases), often painless but sometimes associated with slight dragging pain.[1–6,15]
- Gynecomastia is occasionally the presenting sign.[1,6,15,16]
- Some patients may present with signs of metastatic disease.
- Serum PLAP is elevated.[14]
- Serum HCG is elevated in 8–10% of cases.[1–6]
- Classical seminoma is radiosensitive and responds very well to combination chemotherapy.
- Prognosis is very favorable, with more than 95% achieving a complete cure.[1–6,15,16]

Pathologic findings

Macroscopic

- Classical seminoma causes enlargement of the testis, usually without affecting its contour.
- The tumor is solid, well demarcated, and uniform. It varies from white to gray–yellow to tan.

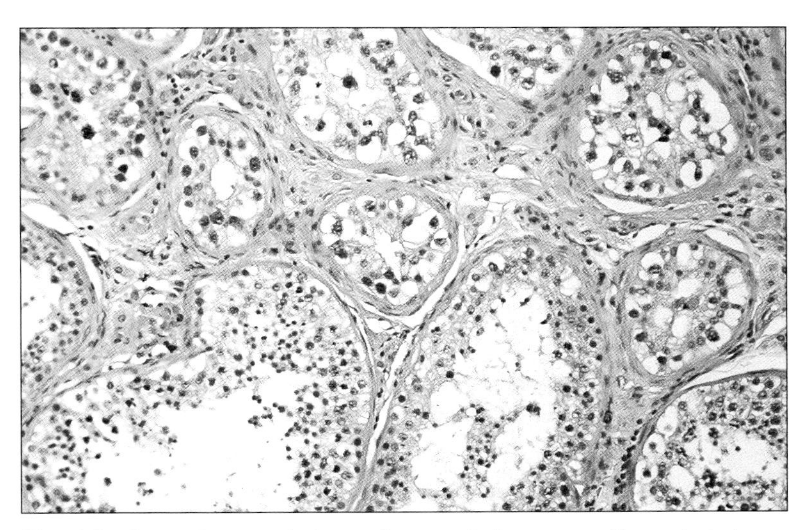

Fig. 4.1 Seminiferous tubules with intratubular germ cell neoplasia have thickened walls and decreased diameter. They are interspersed with unaffected tubules. Note the large atypical germ cells with clear cytoplasm and large prominent atypical nuclei. Mitoses are seen in some cells.

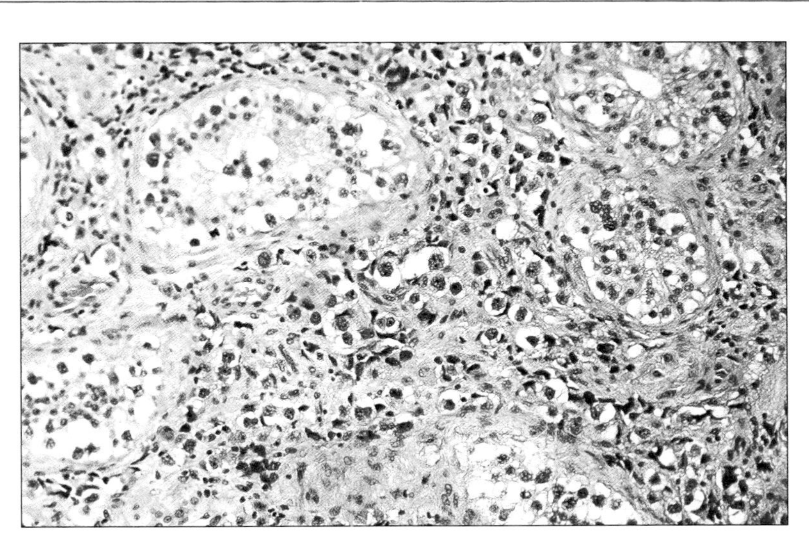

Fig. 4.3 Intratubular germ cell neoplasia and microinvasive classical seminoma. Note the presence of atypical germ cells outside the tubules (center). Also note the lymphocytic infiltration, frequently associated with microinvasion.

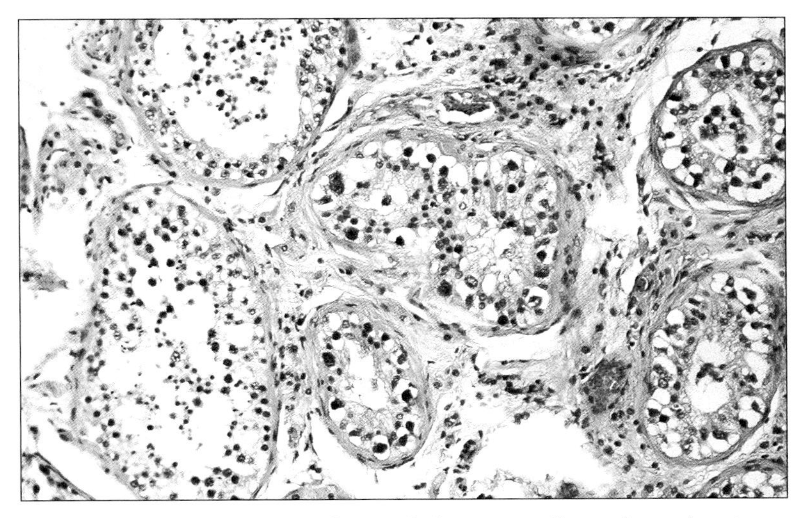

Fig. 4.2 Another example of intratubular germ cell neoplasia, showing similar features to those in Fig. 4.1.

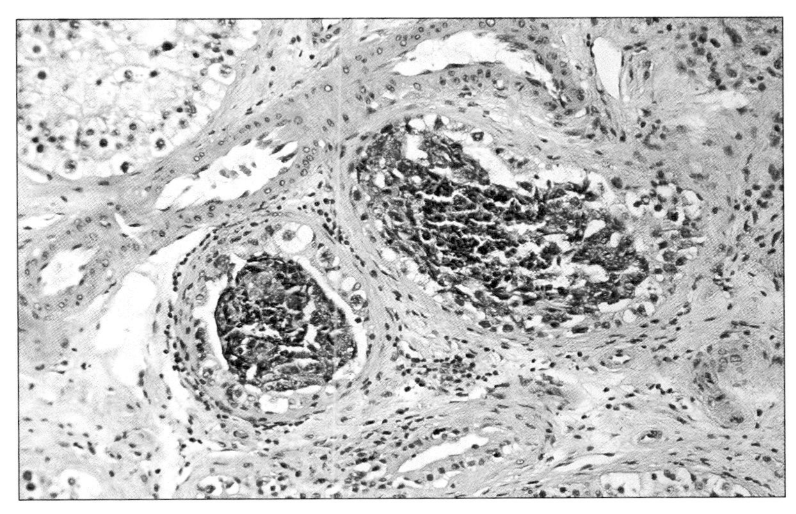

Fig. 4.4 Intratubular germ cell neoplasia associated with intratubular embryonal carcinoma. Note the necrosis within the embryonal carcinoma (center).

- It is bulging and lobulated. Consistency may be soft or firm.
- Hemorrhage and necrosis are uncommon and are seen mainly in large tumors.
- The tumor is usually confined to the testis and only occasionally affects the epididymis and the spermatic cord.[1–6,15,16]

Microscopic

- Classical seminoma exhibits is composed of large uniform cells forming lobules, nests, cords, clusters, and sheets. These are surrounded by fibrovascular tissue that varies from fine delicate septa to dense fibrous bands usually infiltrated by lymphocytes.[1–6,17]
- The lymphocytic infiltrate varies from slight to dense and is composed of T lymphocytes.[6,18]
- Polymorphs, eosinophils, plasma cells, and granulomatous reaction with giant cells are frequently seen.[1–6,17]
- The tumor cells have distinct cellular borders and are uniform, round or oval, with an ample amount of clear or eosinophilic cytoplasm and large, round or polygonal nuclei with one or two distinct nucleoli.
- Mitotic activity is slight to brisk and may vary considerably in different parts of the same tumor.[1–6,17]
- The testis may be markedly fibrotic, and the tumor discernible only with difficulty. Fibrous and even ossified scars may be present in such cases.[1,4–6]
- Syncytiotrophoblastic giant cells are present in 8–10% of cases of classical seminoma. Small hemorrhages and elevated serum HCG are present in such cases. Cytotrophoblastic cells are absent and therefore the

lesion is not a choriocarcinoma. The latter is only occasionally associated with classical seminoma.[1,4-6]
- The syncytiotrophoblastic giant cells must be distinguished from Langhans' and foreign body giant cells associated with granulomatous reaction. These differ from syncytiotrophoblastic giant cells both histologically and immunocytochemically.[1,6]
- Occasionally, classical seminoma may exhibit a prominent tubular pattern and lack lymphocytic infiltration. Such tumors resemble a tubular Sertoli cell tumor or even possibly a metastatic carcinoma. Careful examination may reveal more typical cellular and nuclear features of classical seminoma. PLAP immunohistochemistry can confirm the diagnosis of classical seminoma.[19-21]

Special studies
- Glycogen can be demonstrated in the tumor cells by the PAS stain without diastase digestion.
- Lipid can be demonstrated by special stains in frozen tissue.[6]
- PLAP shows diffusely positive membrane staining, providing confirmation of the diagnosis.[1-6,14]
- HCG is positive in the syncytiotrophoblasts if present, but negative in seminoma cells.
- Ferritin is positive.[6]
- Low molecular weight cytokeratin is negative, although occasional cells may show positive staining. Diffuse positive staining precludes the diagnosis of classical seminoma.[6-22]
- CD30 (Ki-1) is negative.[6]
- Vimentin may be positive.
- AFP is negative.[1-6,22]

(Figs 4.5–4.23)

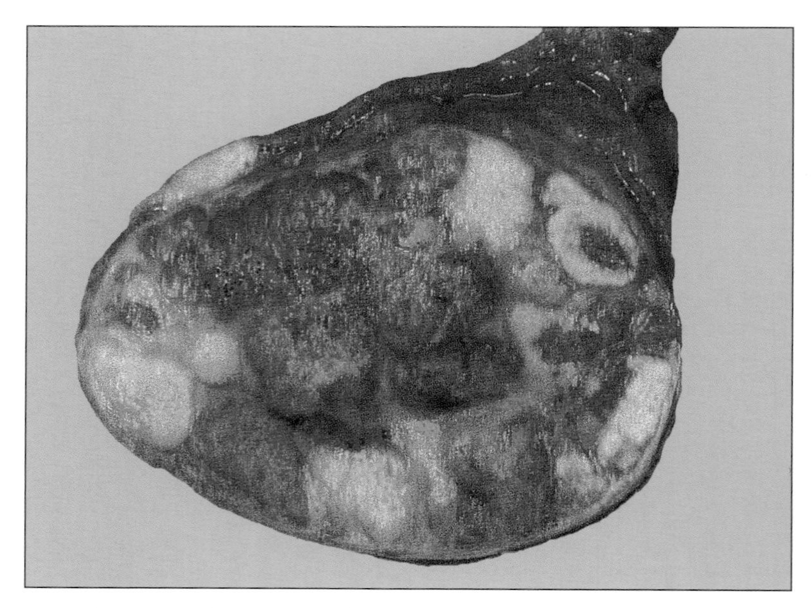

Fig. 4.5 Classical seminoma. Large lobulated tumor causing testicular enlargement without distorting the contour. Note the variegated appearance due to hemorrhage and necrosis associated with large tumors.

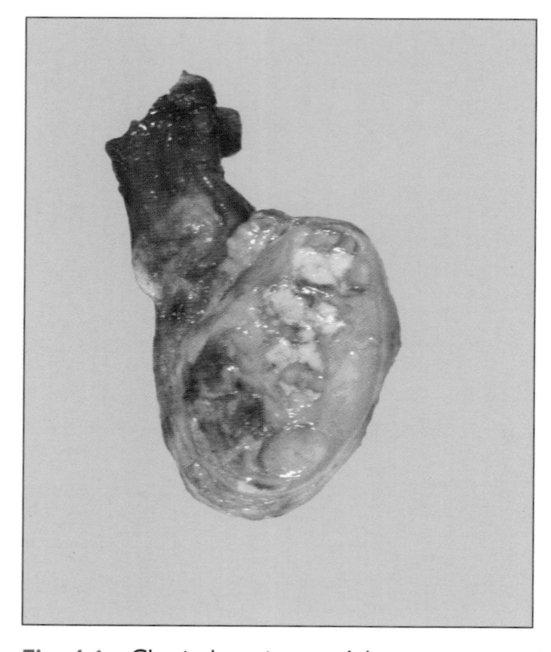

Fig. 4.6 Classical seminoma. A large tumor causing testicular enlargement without distortion of the contour. There is focal hemorrhage and necrosis.

Spermatocytic seminoma

Spermatocytic seminoma is the only germ cell tumor that has no counterpart in the ovary and extragonadal sites.[1,6]

Clinical findings
- Spermatocytic seminoma was formerly considered to be very rare, but more than 200 cases are now on record.[1-6,23-25]
- It comprises approximately 4% (range, 3.5–7.5%) of testicular seminomas.
- It has a wide age range (23–89 years), but most patients are older than 40 years of age.
- It is more often bilateral (range, 4–10%) than classical seminoma (2% of cases). The bilateral involvement tends to be asynchronous but may be synchronous.[1,6,23-25]
- Patients usually present with painless testicular enlargement.
- It has not been associated with maldescent.[1,6,23-25]
- Pure spermatocytic seminoma is indolent. There is only a single well-documented case with metastasis.[29] It is adequately treated by orchiectomy and, like classical seminoma, is highly radiosensitive.[1,6,23-25]
- Rarely there is an admixed mesenchymal malignancy, usually rhabdomyosarcoma or undifferentiated

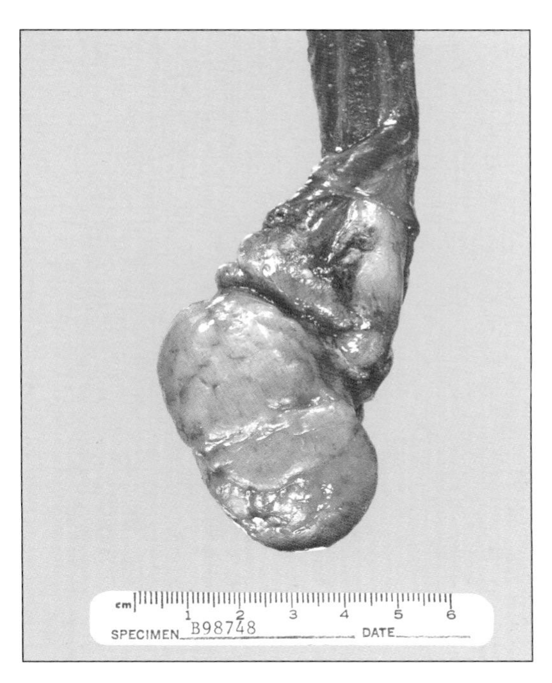

Fig. 4.7 Classical seminoma. The entire testis is replaced by a solid, uniform tumor.

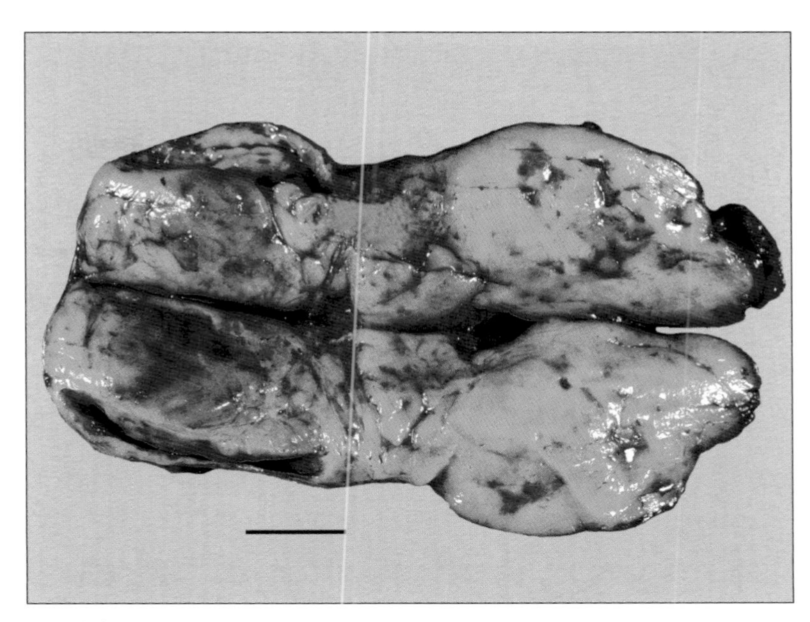

Fig. 4.8 Classical seminoma. A solid tumor replacing the whole testis and showing unusual distortion of the testicular contour.

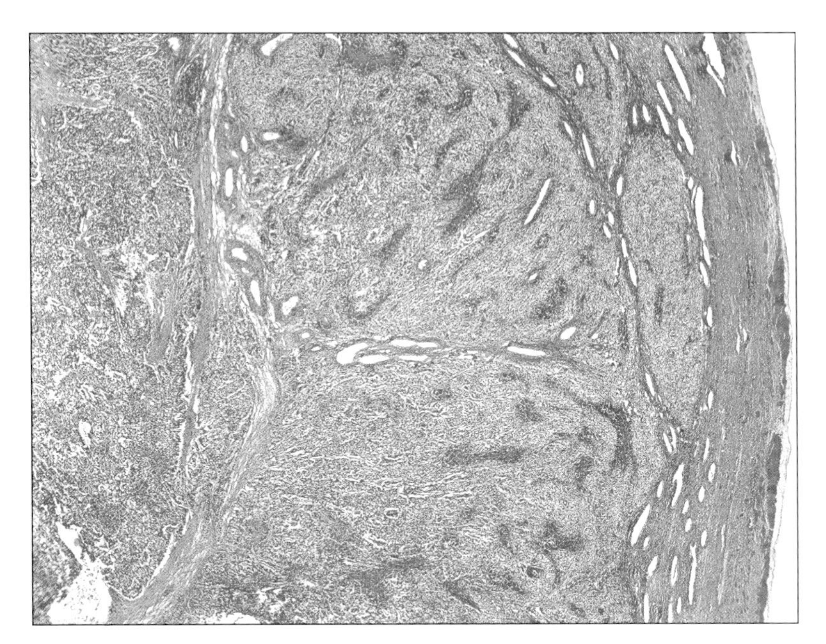

Fig. 4.9 Classical seminoma. Low magnification showing extensive replacement of normal testicular tissue and invasion of the rete testis.

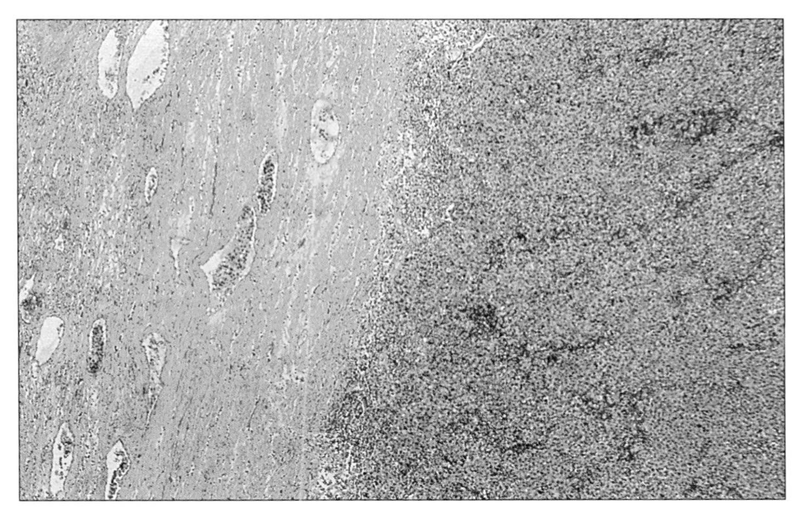

Fig. 4.10 Classical seminoma. Edge of the tumor and vascular invasion.

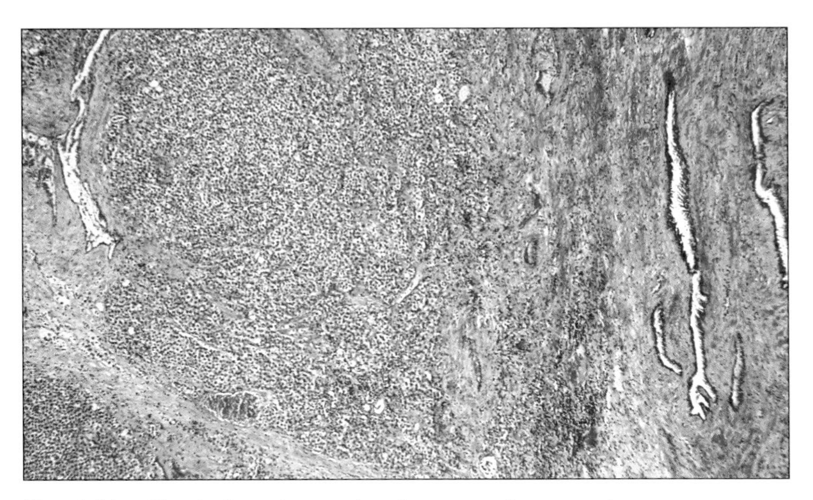

Fig. 4.11 Classical seminoma. Involvement of rete testis.

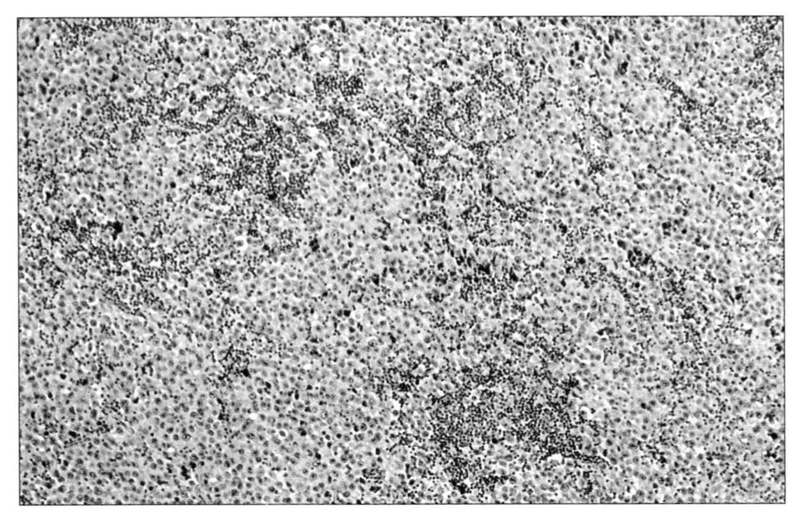

Fig. 4.12 Classical seminoma. A cellular tumor with fine fibrovascular septa and prominent lymphocytic infiltration.

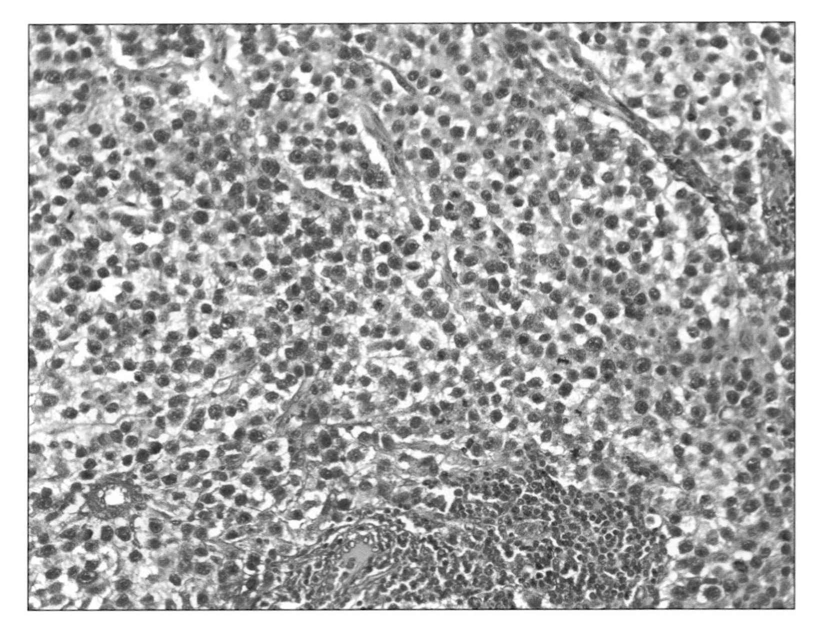

Fig. 4.13 Classical seminoma showing lobular pattern, uniform cells, fibrovascular septa, and a collection of lymphocytes.

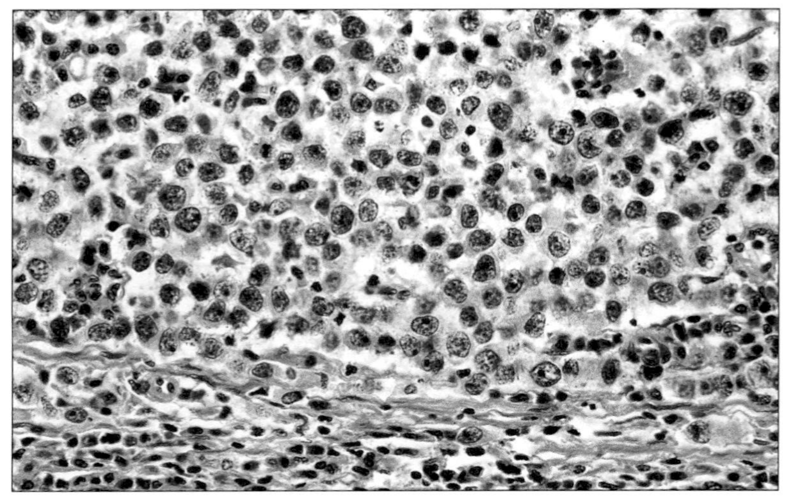

Fig. 4.14 Classical seminoma. Note the uniform cells and the fibrovascular septum infiltrated by lymphocytes.

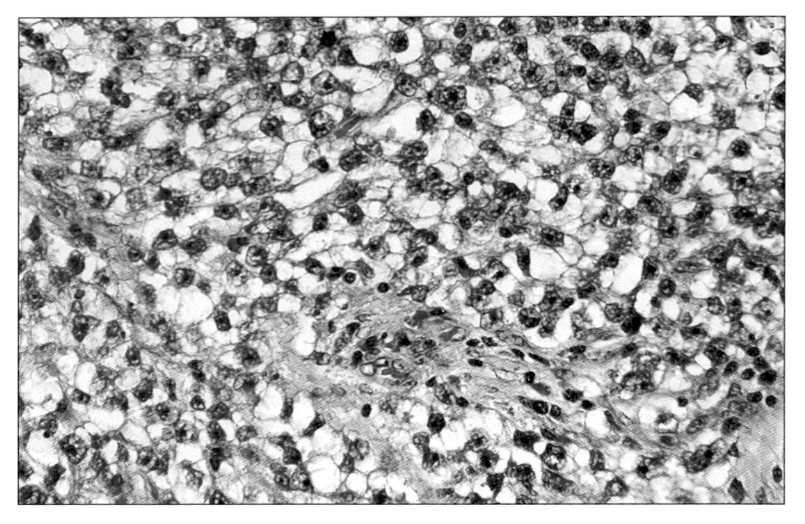

Fig. 4.15 Classical seminoma composed of uniform cells with clear cytoplasm and distinct cellular borders.

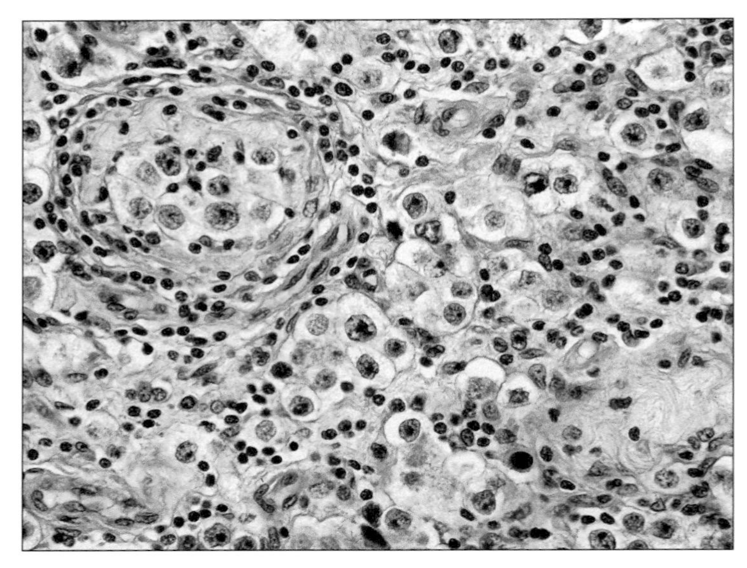

Fig. 4.16 Classical seminoma. The tumor is composed of large, uniform cells with an ample amount of clear, slightly granular cytoplasm and vesicular nuclei with prominent nucleoli.

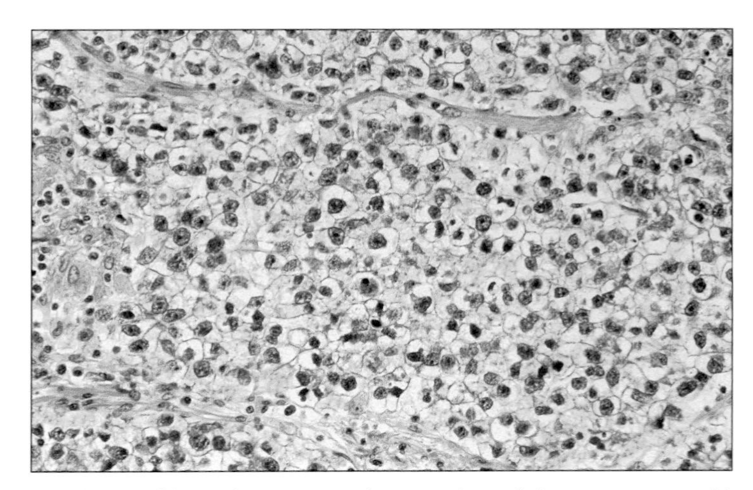

Fig. 4.17 Classical seminoma showing the cellular appearances. Note the distinct cellular borders, clear cytoplasm, and prominent nuclei with nucleoli. A collection of lymphocytes and histiocytes is seen on the left.

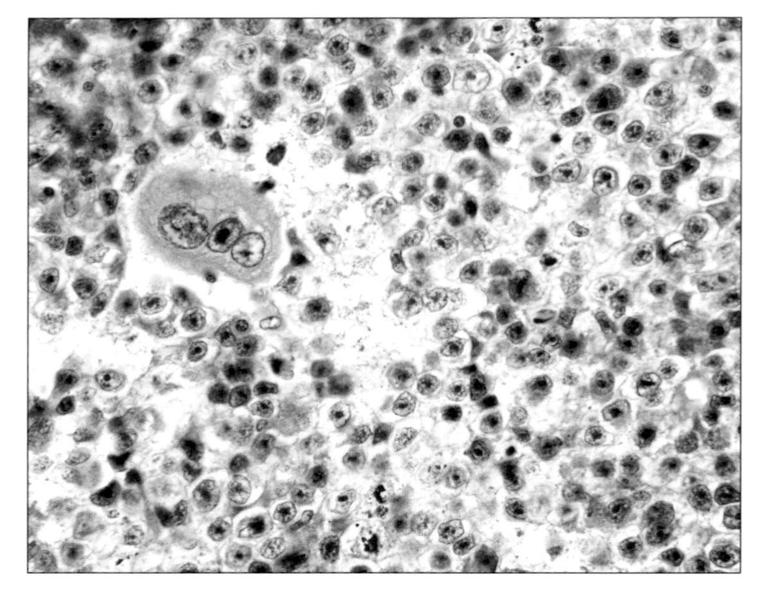

Fig. 4.18 Classical seminoma with syncytiotrophoblastic giant cells (center). Such tumors often show paucity of lymphocytes, as seen here.

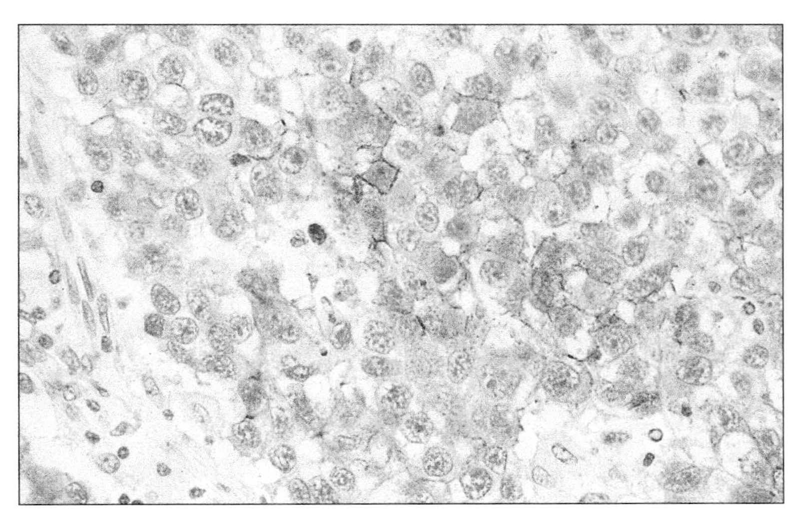

Fig. 4.19 Classical seminoma. Tumor cells show distinct membranous cytoplasmic staining. Placental alkaline phosphatase stain.

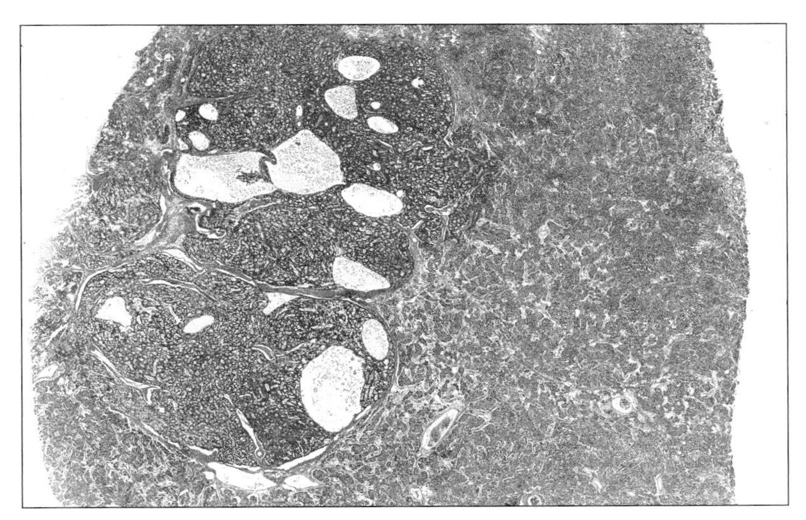

Fig. 4.20 Classical seminoma with distinctive tubular pattern (left). Low magnification.

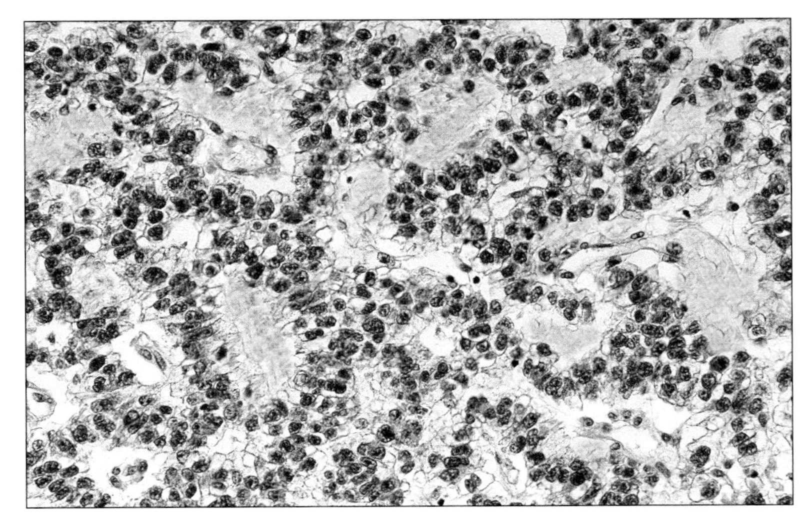

Fig. 4.21 Classical seminoma showing distinctive tubular pattern and designated as tubular seminoma.

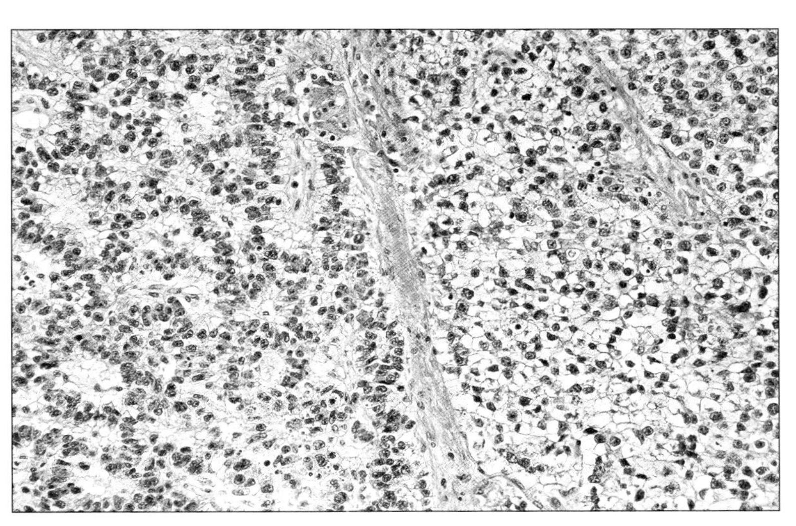

Fig. 4.22 Classical seminoma showing a junction between the tubular pattern (left) and the typical pattern (right).

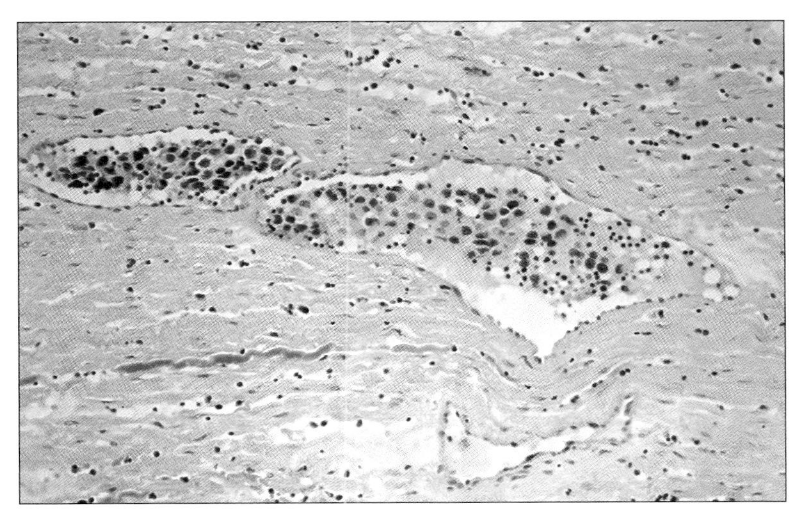

Fig. 4.23 Classical seminoma involving vascular spaces.

sarcoma,[24-28] that can behave aggressively and confer a poor prognosis.

Pathologic findings

Macroscopic findings

- Tumors vary from small nodules to large masses, replacing the testis and invading the epididymis.[1-6,23-25] Typically the testicular contour is undistorted. Satellite nodules may occur.
- Tumors are well circumscribed, solid, gray-yellow, soft, and may be gelatinous or mucoid with small cysts.[1-6,23-25] Hemorrhage can be present in large tumors, but necrosis is rare.

Microscopic findings

- Spermatocytic seminoma is composed of solid sheets of tumor cells with a small amount of fine fibrovascular stroma.

- There is a pronounced intratubular pattern of growth, unlike classical seminoma. An interstitial growth pattern is also seen.[1-6,23-25]
- Numerous seminiferous tubules at some distance from the main tumor mass are distended by tumor cells.[1,6,23-25]
- Spermatocytic seminoma is composed of three types of round or oval cells that differ in size.[1-6,23-25]
- The predominant cell is the intermediate cell, which is medium sized, measuring 15–20 µm. These cells have round nuclei with a fine chromatin pattern and dense, evenly dispersed cytoplasm.
- Intermediate cells predominate. They are medium-sized (15–20 µm), have round nuclei with fine chromatin, and dense, evenly dispersed cytoplasm.
- Small (6–8 µm) lymphocyte-like cells have a round, hyperchromatic nucleus, and a rim of dense, basophilic cytoplasm.
- Giant cells (50–100 µm) are very characteristic of spermatocytic seminoma. They have single or multiple, round or oval nuclei with one of three typical chromatin patterns: 'granular', 'spireme' (long, narrow filaments), or 'even' (very darkly and evenly staining).[1-6,23-25]
- The cytoplasm may be eosinophilic or basophilic and is devoid of glycogen.
- Mitotic activity is frequently brisk.
- Degenerating cells with pyknotic nuclei are often seen, but necrosis is not observed.[1,6,23-25]
- Lymphocytic infiltration is rare and when present is slight. Granulomatous reaction is absent.[1-6,23-25]
- There is no evidence of IGCN.
- Microcysts may occur, and in very edematous tumors may be prominent.[1,4-6,23-25]
- In the small number of cases when the tumor was associated with a single malignant mesenchymal element, the latter was represented most frequently by undifferentiated sarcoma or rhabdomyosarcoma.[26-28]

Special studies
- Spermatocytic seminoma does not stain for PLAP, low molecular weight cytokeratin, vimentin, AFP, or HCG.
- The cytoplasm does not contain lipid or glycogen.[6,30]

(Figs 4.24–4.30)

Embryonal carcinoma

Clinical findings
- Pure embryonal carcinoma is the second most common testicular germ cell neoplasm (15–30%), after classical seminoma.[1-6,31]
- It is also a frequent component of mixed germ cell tumors.[1-6,31-33]

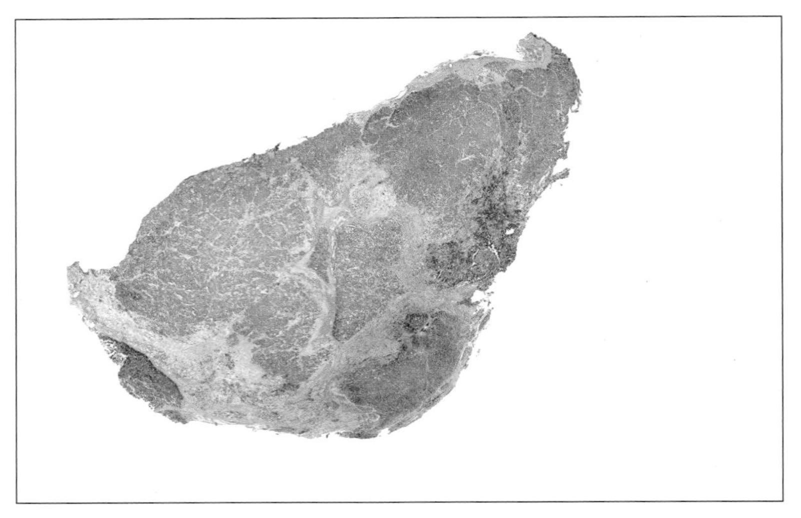

Fig. 4.24 Spermatocytic seminoma replacing testicular tissue. Low magnification.

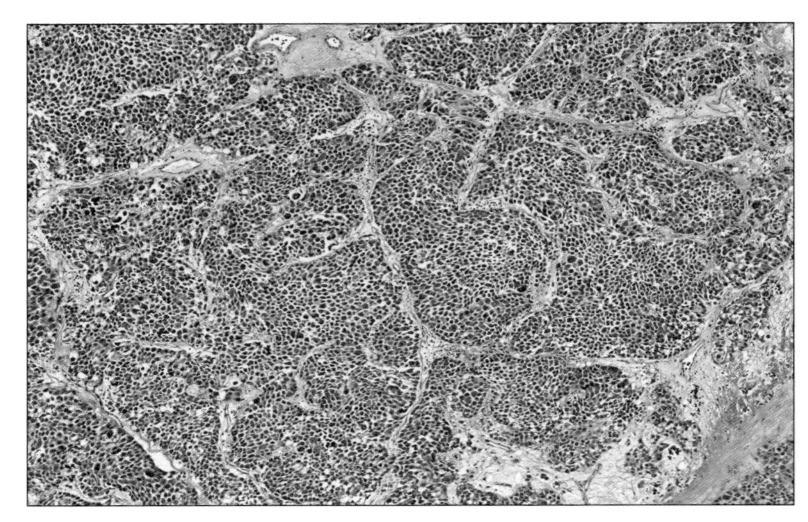

Fig. 4.25 Spermatocytic seminoma showing the pronounced intratubular pattern of growth and lobular appearance.

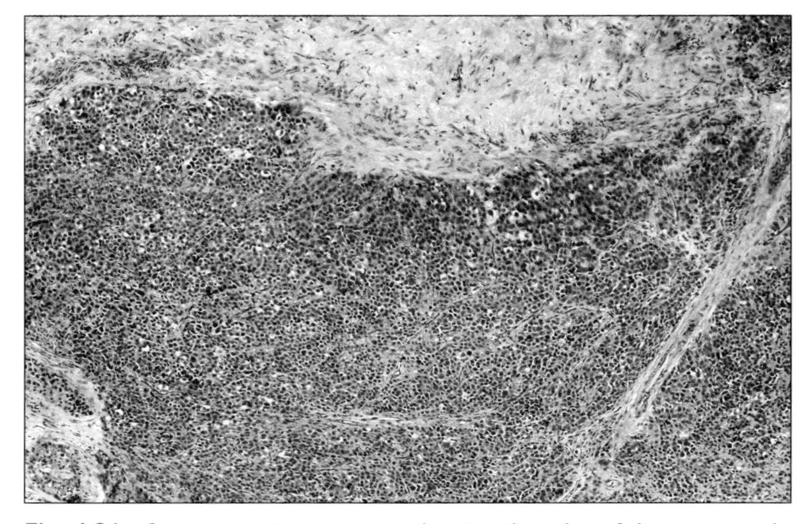

Fig. 4.26 Spermatocytic seminoma showing the edge of the tumor and complete effacement of normal testicular architecture.

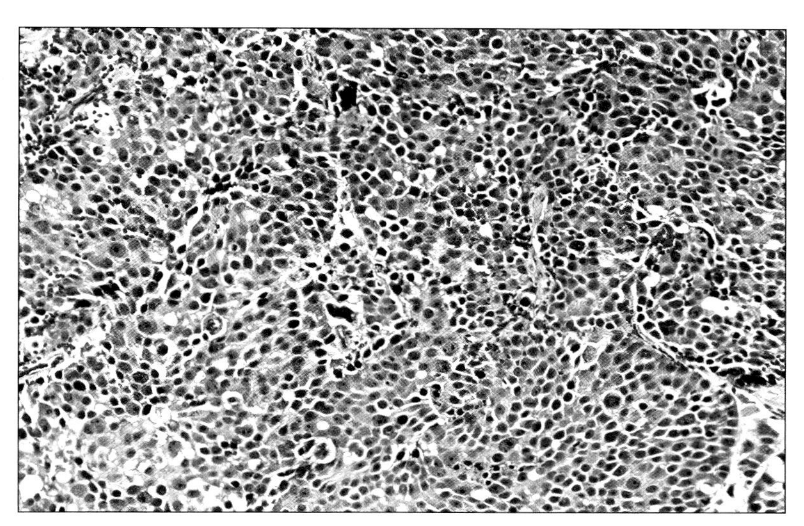

Fig. 4.27 Spermatocytic seminoma showing the marked cellularity and only an imperceptible amount of stroma.

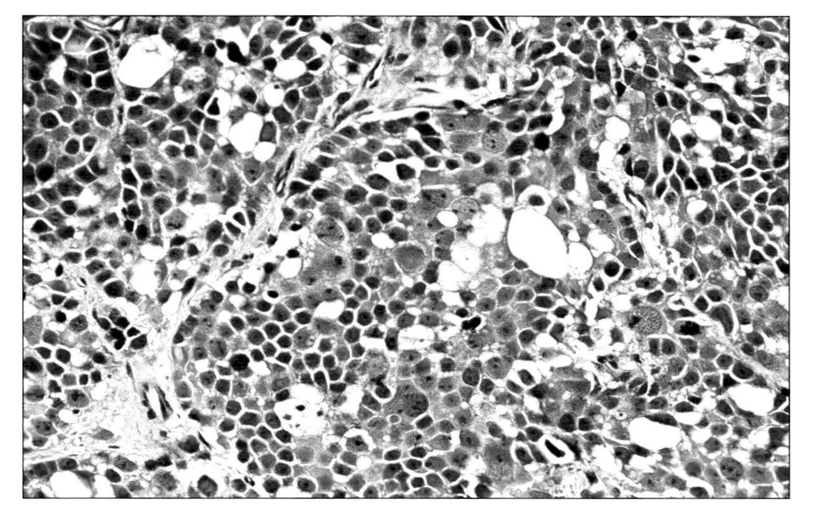

Fig. 4.28 Spermatocytic seminoma showing the cellular composition and a number of microcysts.

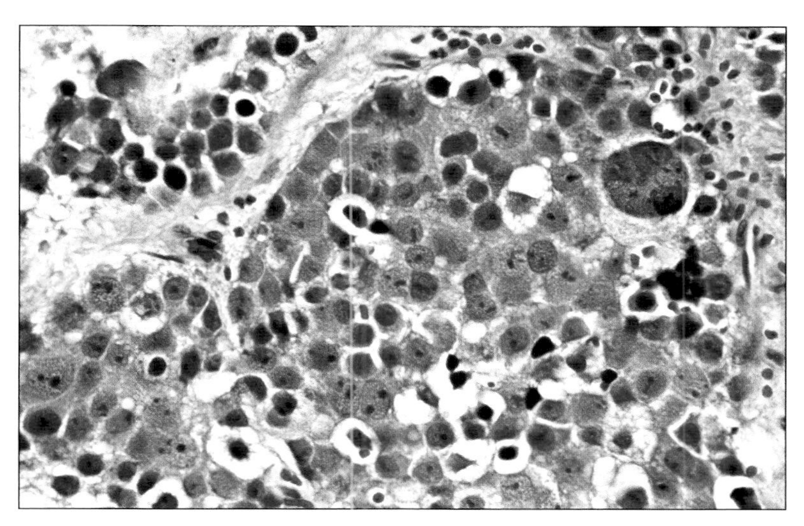

Fig. 4.29 Spermatocytic seminoma composed mainly of intermediate cells with a few small cells and a large multinucleated giant cell.

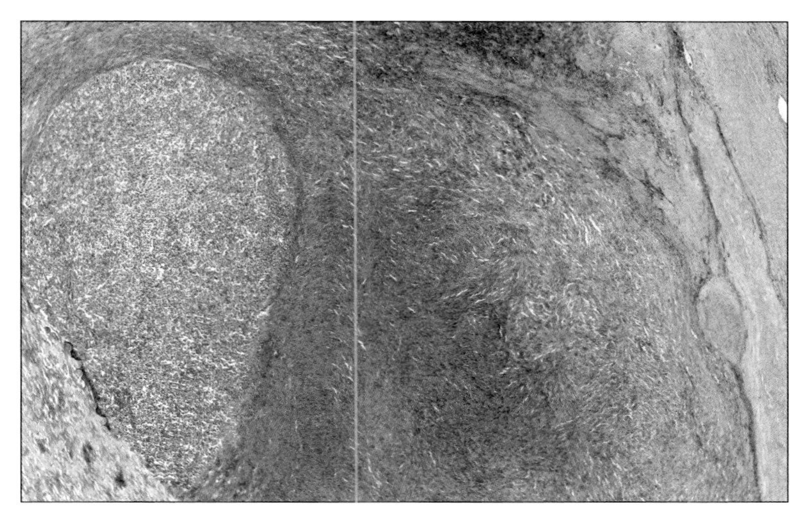

Fig. 4.30 Spermatocytic seminoma and sarcoma. Low magnification.

- The incidence of embryonal carcinoma begins to rise at puberty and peaks in the third decade, 10 years earlier than classical seminoma. In this age group it is the most common testicular tumor.
- Patients present with testicular enlargement, generally painless but sometimes associated with dragging pain.
- The duration of symptoms is usually shorter than in classical seminoma.[1,4–6,31–33]
- Embryonal carcinoma metastasizes to the regional lymph nodes in the parailiac and para-aortic regions.
- Metastatic disease is more common at presentation (30%) than in classical seminoma (10–15%).[1,4–6,31–33] Distant lymph node involvement and hematogenous spread are also more common.[1,4–6,31–33]
- Serum HCG may be elevated due to the presence of syncytiotrophoblastic giant cells. Serum AFP may be elevated, but levels are considerably lower than in choriocarcinoma and yolk sac tumor.[1,6,31]
- Embryonal carcinoma is treated by orchiectomy followed by combination chemotherapy. Complete cure is now achieved in over 80% of cases, including most of those with regional lymph node metastasis.[1,4–6,31,33]

Pathologic findings

Macroscopic findings

- The tumors are usually smaller than classical seminomas, but unlike the latter usually distort the testicular contour.
- On sectioning, the tumors are bulging, irregular, solid, soft, variegated, yellow, white or gray, and often show foci of hemorrhage or necrosis.
- When embryonal carcinoma is mixed with teratoma, cystic areas may be present.[1–6,31–33]
- Invasion of the epididymis and spermatic cord is more common than in classical seminoma.[1,4–6,31–33]

Microscopic findings

- Embryonal carcinoma has solid, papillary, and pseudoglandular patterns. These patterns may be present in pure form, but are often seen in combination.
- The tumor can be very cellular. Some cases may have prominent fibrosis adjacent to the cellular areas.[1,6,31-34]
- Lymphocytic infiltration is seen in 30% of embryonal carcinomas and may be pronounced. Therefore this feature does not distinguish between embryonal carcinoma and classical seminoma.[1,6]
- Granulomatous reaction may be present, but is by far less common than lymphocytic infiltration.
- Embryonal carcinoma with a solid pattern is composed of sheets of tumor cells in a solid or syncytial arrangement with overlapping.[1-6,31-33]
- The cells are large, polygonal, and epithelial-like. The cytoplasm is clear or slightly granular, and eosinophilic.
- Cell boundaries are indistinct and cell membranes, when seen, are fine.[1-6,31-33]
- Nuclei are large and irregular. They may be vesicular with finely dispersed chromatin or hyperchromatic, and may have multiple nucleoli. The nuclear membranes are fine.
- Mitotic figures are abundant, including abnormal forms.
- There is usually considerable cellular and nuclear pleomorphism.[1-6,31-33]
- The papillary pattern has numerous, well-formed papillae of tumor cells.
- The pseudoglandular pattern has cleft-like spaces, but true glandular formation is absent.
- The cells of the papillary and pseudoglandular patterns are less polygonal and more columnar or cuboidal.[1,6]
- Syncytiotrophoblasts, single or in groups, are often seen. They should not be confused with tumor giant cells, which may also be present. The syncytiotrophoblasts are responsible for the elevated serum HCG.[1,4-6,31-33]
- Embryonal carcinoma may show pronounced intratubular involvement with necrosis.[1-6,31,33]
- Hemorrhage and necrosis are common.
- Embryonal carcinoma may show focal yolk sac differentiation, responsible for a slightly elevated serum AFP.[1,6]
- Embryonal carcinoma frequently occurs mixed with teratoma, yolk sac tumor, or other germ cell tumor types (malignant mixed germ cell tumor).[1-6,31-34]

Special studies

- Embryonal carcinoma stains positively for low molecular weight cytokeratin, a useful discriminator from classical or spermatocytic seminoma.[1-6,35,36]
- Embryonal carcinoma showing early differentiation into yolk sac tumor has slight AFP positivity, but pure embryonal carcinoma is AFP-negative.[6]
- Embryonal carcinoma is negative for beta-HCG, but the syncytiotrophoblastic giant cells frequently present show positive staining.
- Embryonal carcinoma shows strong positive staining for CD30 (Ki-1) antigen.[6]

(Figs 4.31–4.45)

Yolk sac tumor

Yolk sac tumor (YST), originally named endodermal sinus tumor,[37] is a malignant germ cell neoplasm differentiating towards vitelline (yolk sac) structures. It produces AFP.[1-6,37]

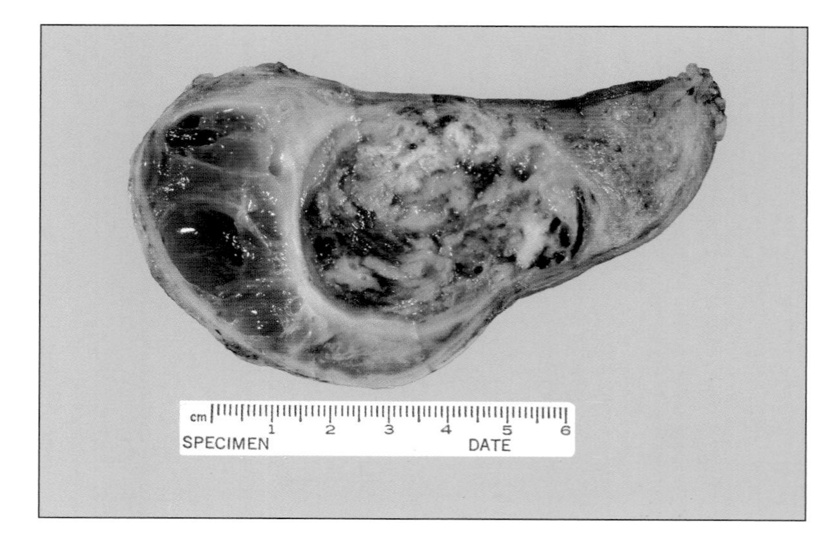

Fig. 4.31 Embryonal carcinoma. The testis shows loss of normal contour and a round, variegated, solid tumor.

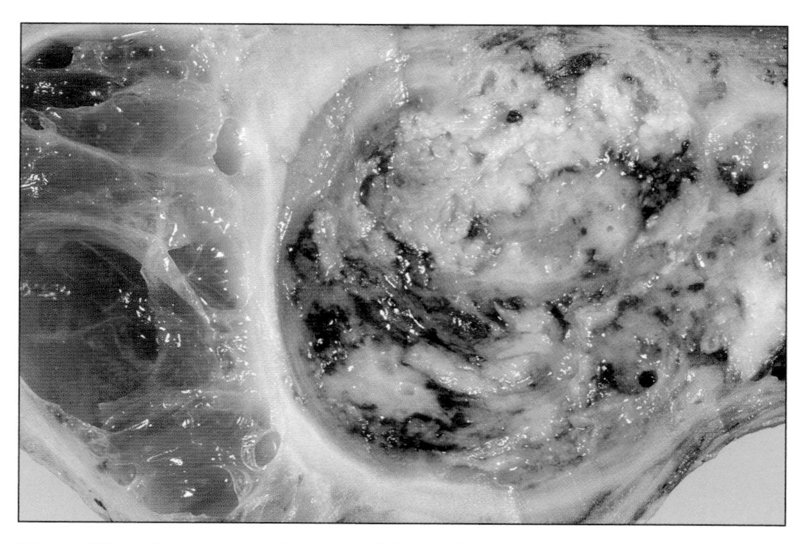

Fig. 4.32 Higher magnification of Fig. 4.31, showing a solid, yellow–gray tumor, well demarcated on the left, but less well in other parts. Note small hemorrhagic foci throughout.

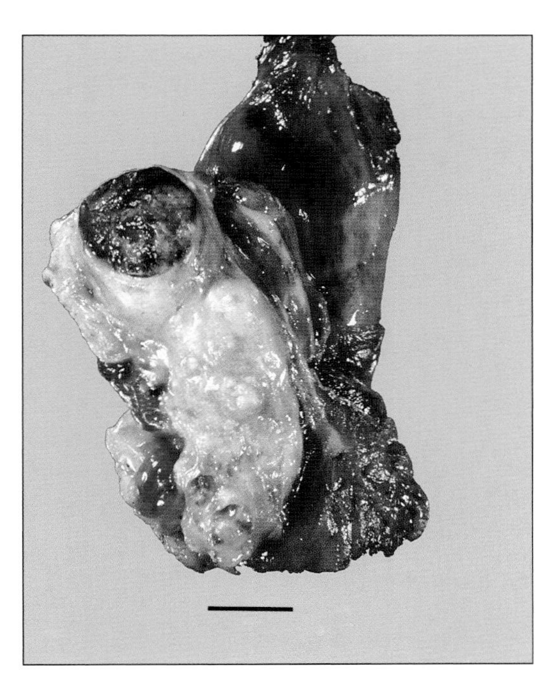

Fig. 4.33 Malignant mixed germ cell tumor composed of embryonal carcinoma and teratoma replacing the testis and distorting the testicular contour.

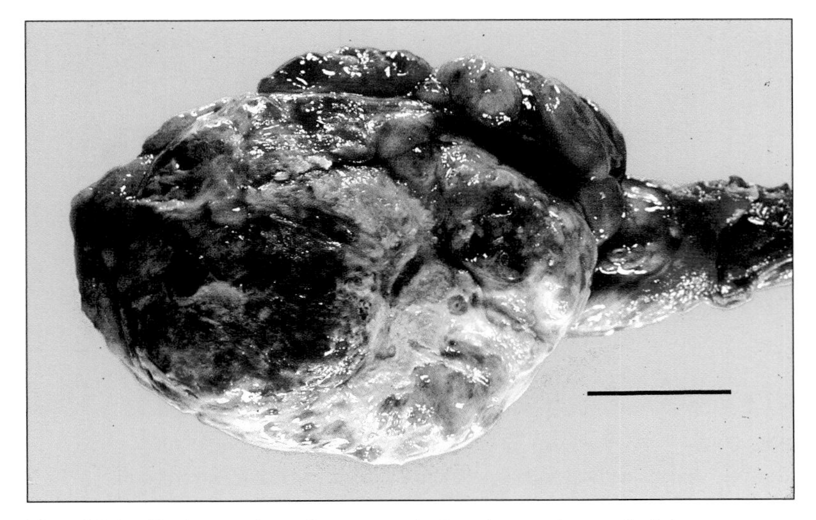

Fig. 4.34 Embryonal carcinoma replacing the testis as a bulging hemorrhagic and necrotic tumor.

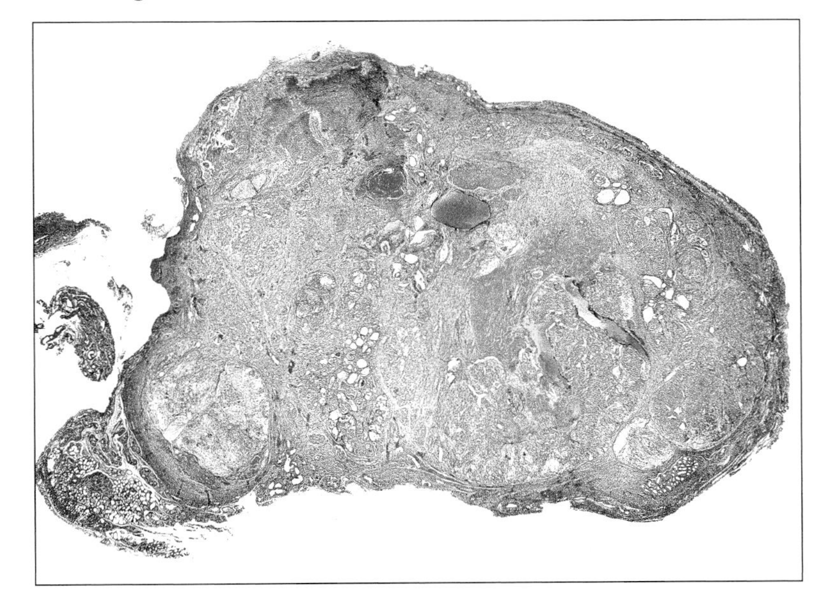

Fig. 4.35 Embryonal carcinoma replacing the whole testis.

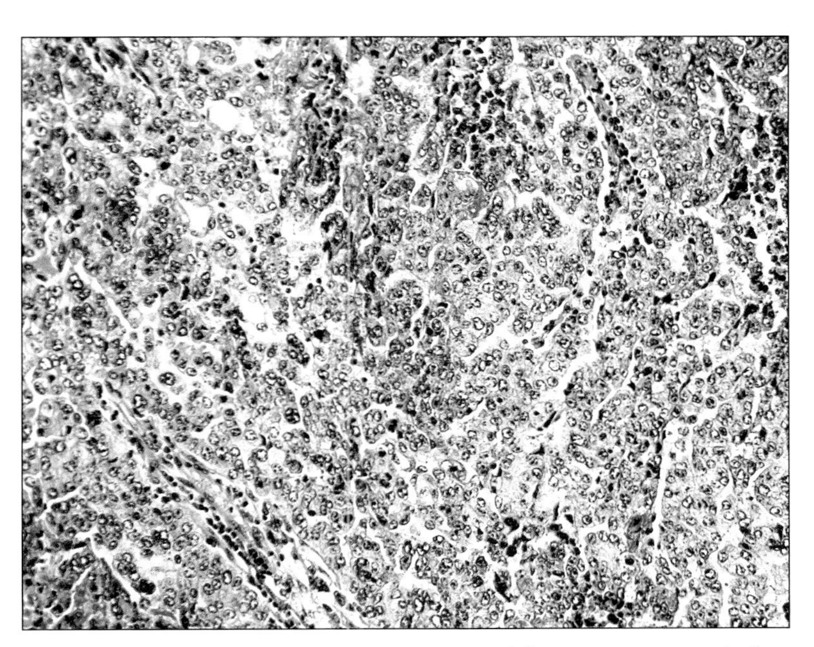

Fig. 4.36 Embryonal carcinoma showing a solid pattern composed of sheets of uniform tumor cells with large prominent nuclei.

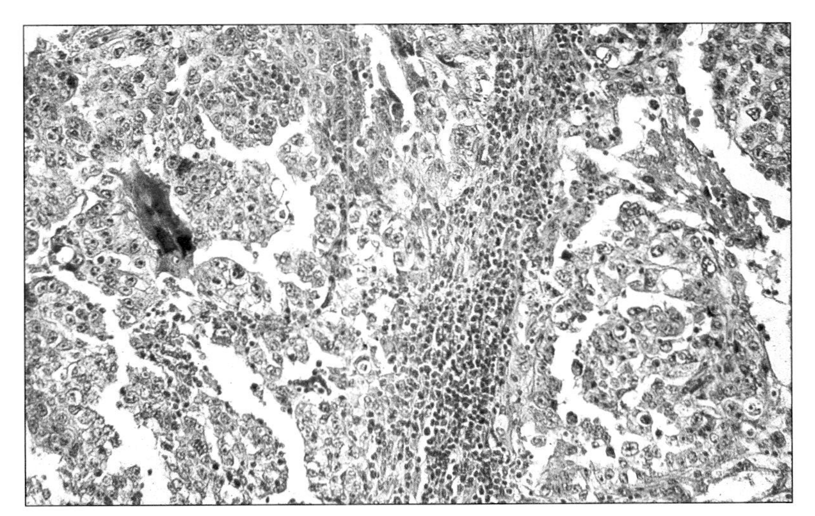

Fig. 4.37 Embryonal carcinoma showing papillary and solid patterns and a syncytiotrophoblastic giant cell (center).

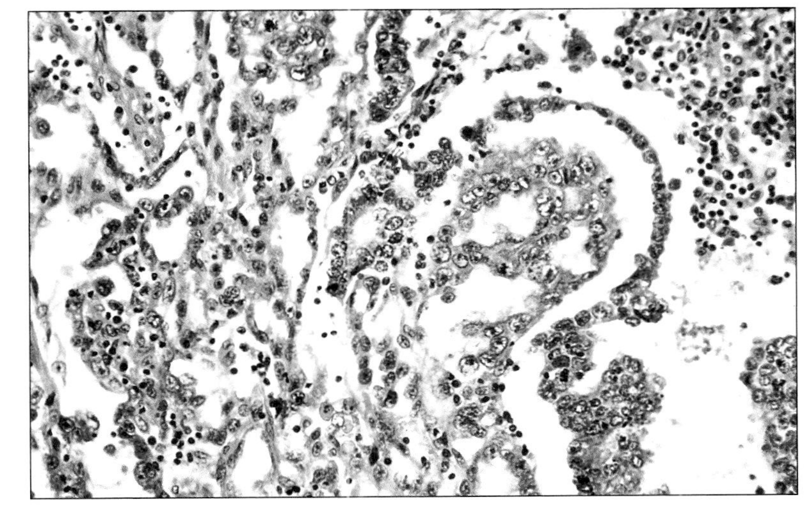

Fig. 4.38 Embryonal carcinoma showing a pseudoglandular pattern. The centrally located structure is composed of tumor cells and does not correspond to a Schiller–Duval body seen in yolk sac tumors.

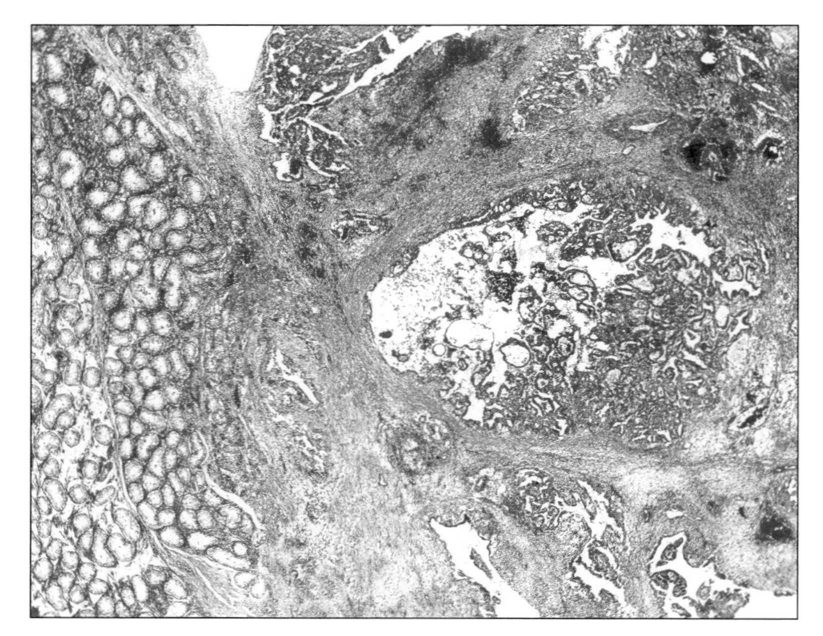

Fig. 4.39 Embryonal carcinoma showing a lobular pattern representing intratubular growth of the tumor, which has undergone extensive necrosis.

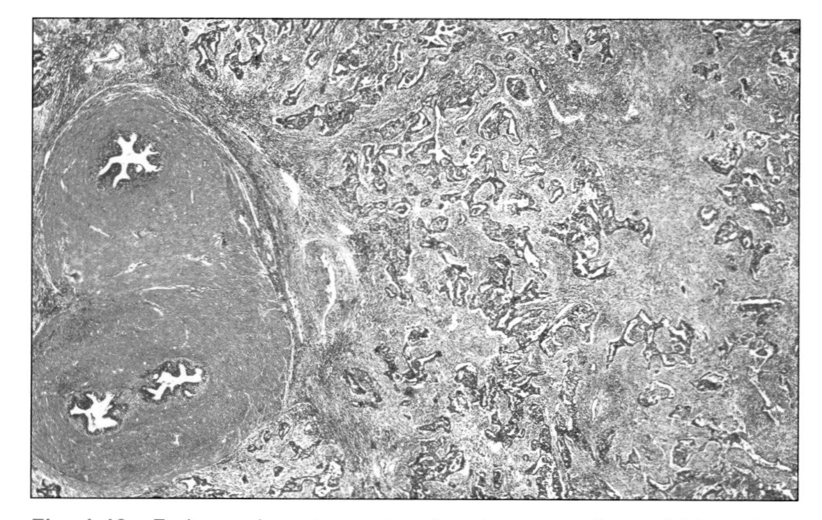

Fig. 4.40 Embryonal carcinoma invading the spermatic cord. Note the pronounced pseudoglandular and papillary patterns.

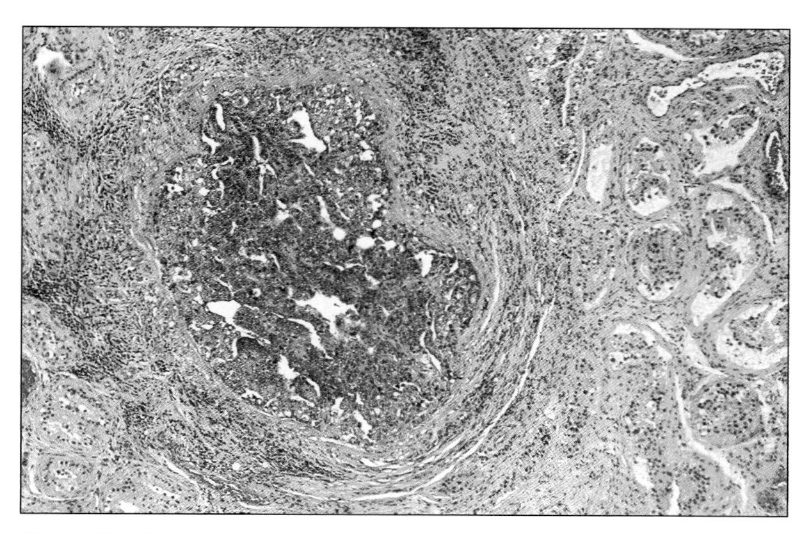

Fig. 4.41 Embryonal carcinoma associated with lymphocytic infiltration.

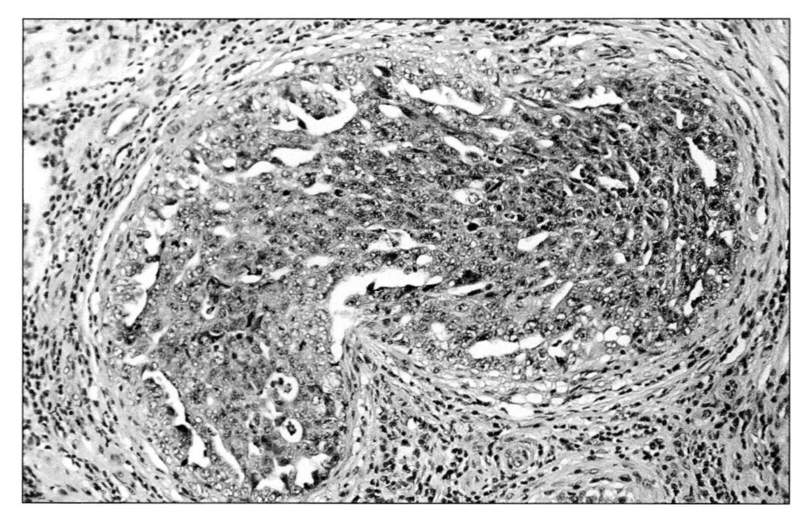

Fig. 4.42 Embryonal carcinoma showing a solid pattern, intratubular involvement, and lymphocytic infiltration.

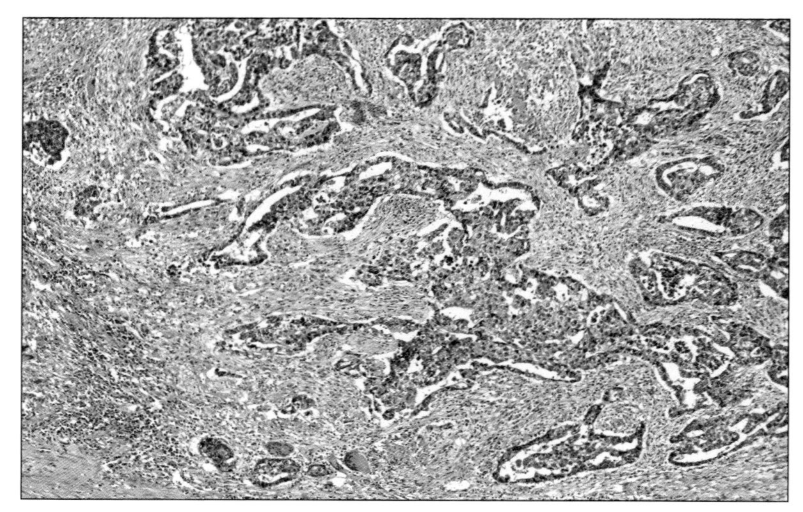

Fig. 4.43 Embryonal carcinoma showing solid, pseudoglandular, and papillary patterns associated with lymphocytic and granulomatous reaction.

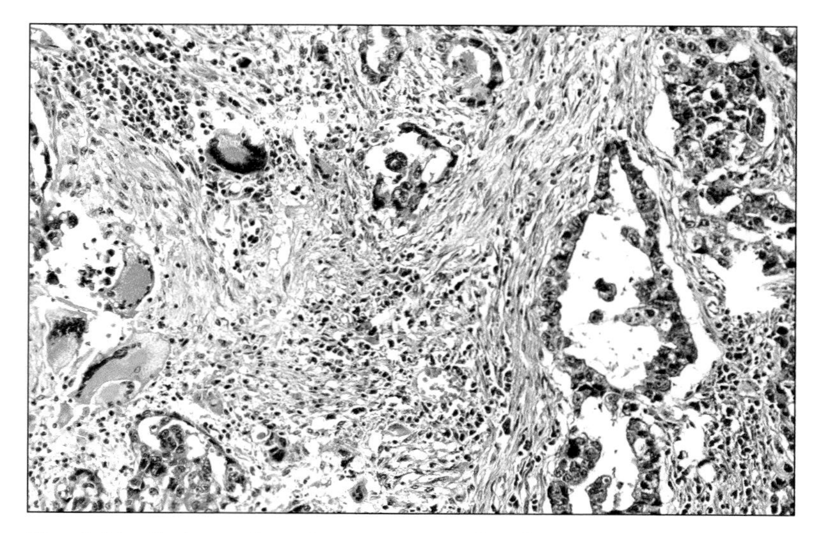

Fig. 4.44 Embryonal carcinoma associated with granulomatous and lymphocytic reaction.

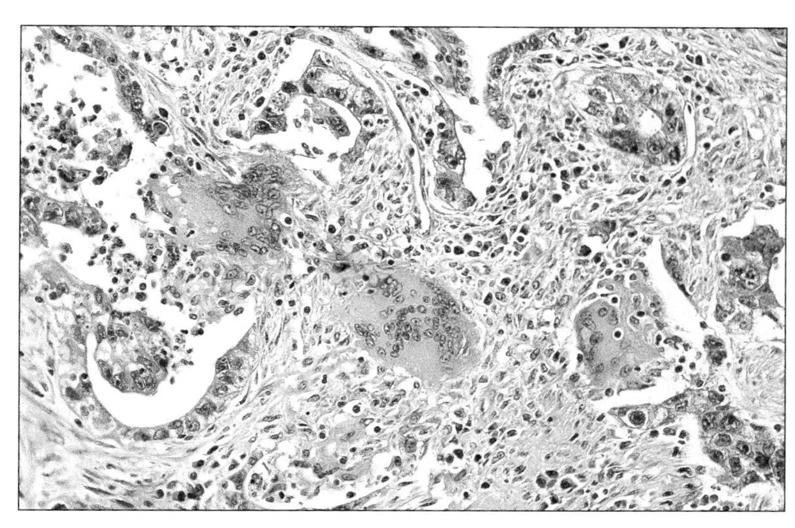

Fig. 4.45 Embryonal carcinoma showing pseudoglandular and papillary patterns and pronounced granulomatous reaction.

Clinical findings

- YST occurs in two age groups: infants and young children,[1,6,38–41] and postpubertal subjects.[1,6,42–44]
- Pediatric YST is seen from birth to 5 years; 74% of tumors occur in boys less than 2 years old.
- In this age group, YST is the most common testicular neoplasm.[1,6,38–40]
- In postpubertal subjects, YST is seen as a component of approximately 40% of testicular mixed germ cell tumors.[1,6,42,43,45]
- The age distribution of adult YST corresponds to that of mixed germ cell tumors, with a peak in the third and fourth decades.[1,6,42,43]
- The primary treatment in both age groups is orchiectomy.[39,40] For metastatic disease, combination chemotherapy yields a very favorable outcome.[6]

Pathologic findings

The appearance of YST is similar in the two age groups. In infants and young children YST occurs invariably in pure form,[1,6,38–40] while in the adult group YST is nearly always mixed with other neoplastic germ cell elements.[1,6,42,43]

Macroscopic findings

- Pure YST is solid, soft, pale gray or gray–white, and gelatinous or mucoid.[1,4–6,37–40,42–44]
- In infants and young children, the tumors vary in size from small lesions affecting part of the testis to larger tumors replacing most of the testicular parenchyma.[1,6,37–40]
- In adults, in whom YST is usually one component of a mixed tumor, the appearance of the tumor depends on the amount and type of neoplastic germ cell elements.[1,6,42–44] The YST component may vary from microscopic to large and predominant, usually the former.
- Tumors with a predominant YST component are usually large, distort the testicular contour, and frequently show hemorrhage and necrosis.

Microscopic findings

- YST has a varied appearance that reflects the presence of its various histologic patterns.[1,4–6,37,42–44]
- The different patterns are usually intimately intermixed. Sometimes one pattern predominates,[1,6,37,42–44] but tumors composed of a single histologic pattern are rare.[1,6,42–44]
- The following histologic patterns are recognized in YST:[6]
  microcytic or reticular;
  macrocystic;
  solid;
  glandular–alveolar;
  endodermal sinus;
  papillary;
  myxomatous;
  polyvesicular vitelline;
  hepatoid;
  primitive intestinal (enteric).

Microcytic or reticular pattern

- This pattern consists of a meshwork of vacuolated cells producing a honeycomb appearance.
- The tumor cells are usually small and may be compressed by the vacuoles, which may contain a pale eosinophilic secretion.[1,6,37]
- The nuclei vary in size but are usually small.
- Mitotic activity is usually brisk.[1,6,37]
- Hyaline globules are present.
- This pattern is the most common in adults, and less frequent in infants and children.[1,6]

Macrocystic pattern

- This pattern consists of thin-walled spaces of varying sizes, adjacent or separated by other histologic patterns.[1,6,37,38]
- This pattern is more frequent in pediatric tumors.

Solid pattern

- This pattern consists of aggregates of epithelial-like, medium-sized polygonal tumor cells with clear cytoplasm, prominent nuclei that usually show brisk mitotic activity.[1,6,37]
- The cells resemble those of classical seminoma and embryonal carcinoma.
- Sometimes the cells may show pleomorphism and giant cells may be present.
- This pattern is more frequently seen in tumors from adults, often combined with the microcystic pattern.[1,6]

Glandular–alveolar pattern

- This pattern consists of irregular alveoli, gland-like spaces, and tubular structures lined by epithelial-like cells varying from flattened to cuboidal or polygonal.[1,6,37]
- The gland-like spaces or clefts form a meshwork of cavities and channels, sometimes interspersed with myxomatous tissue.[1,6,37]
- This pattern is more common in tumors from adults.

Endodermal sinus pattern

- Schiller–Dural bodies, stalk-like perivascular structures that are a hallmark of YST, distinguish this pattern. They consist of a thin-walled blood vessel invested by loose connective tissue; there is an outer layer of cuboidal, epithelial-like cells with clear cytoplasm and prominent nuclei.[1,4–6,37]
- Mitotic activity is usually present and may be brisk.
- They are seen scattered within the tumor in varying numbers.
- Their absence does not preclude the diagnosis of YST.[1–6]

Papillary pattern

- This pattern has numerous fine papillae with connective tissue cores lined by epithelial-like cells. These have prominent nuclei and often show brisk mitotic activity.
- The connective tissue cores may be edematous or fibrous and hyalinized.
- Sometimes deposits of hyaline material form wide, solid, brightly eosinophilic amorphous papillae.[1,6,37,44]

Myxomatous pattern

- This pattern consists of acellular myxomatous tissue containing cords, strands, or collections of individual cells showing prominent nuclei and mitotic activity.[1,6,37]

Polyvesicular vitelline pattern

- This uncommon pattern consists of vesicles or cysts of various shapes and sizes, surrounded by connective tissue cellular and edematous or dense and fibrous.
- The vesicles are lined by columnar or flattened epithelial-like cells.[1,6,37]
- Sometimes the vesicles are small and adhere to each other. Some vesicles may be hourglass shaped.[1,6,37]

Hepatoid pattern

- Collections of primitive hepatoid cells occur in some tumors, mainly from adults.[1,6,44,45]
- The cells show close resemblance to fetal, adult, or neoplastic liver cells.[1,4–6,44,45]
- Cellular and nuclear pleomorphism and mitotic activity are present.
- Hyaline globules are frequently seen.
- Sometimes collections of such cells may be numerous and of considerable size.[6,44,45]

Primitive intestinal (enteric) pattern

- Embryonal intestinal-like glands can occur.[1–6,37,44] They may be confused with intestinal glands of teratoma, but the marked cellular and nuclear pleomorphism and brisk mitotic activity differentiate them.[1,6,44]
- Hyaline globules may be numerous.
- These glands are usually interspersed by other patterns of YST.[1,6,44]

Special studies

- YST shows strong immunohistochemical staining for low molecular weight cytokeratin.[1,6,36,46]
- YST produces AFP, and staining for AFP is helpful in diagnosis.[1,6,36,37,44,46]
- YST stains for ferritin and PLAP.[6]

(Figs 4.46–4.60)

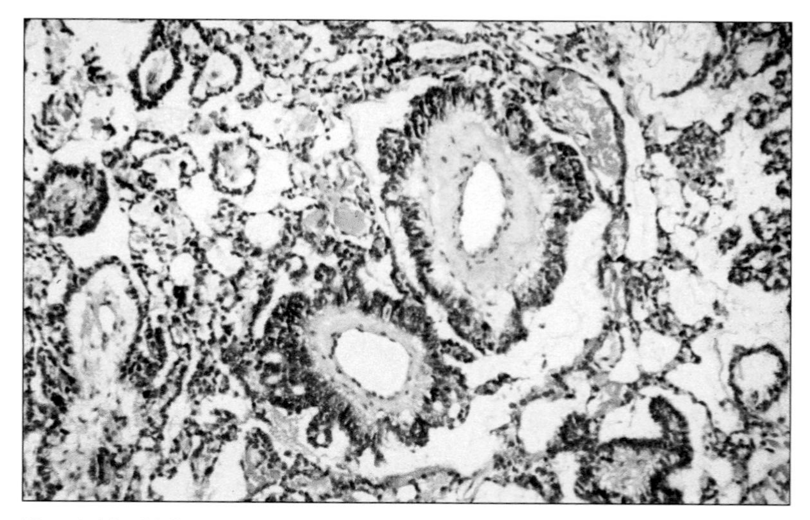

Fig. 4.46 Yolk sac tumor showing perivascular formations (Schiller–Duval bodies) and papillary pattern.

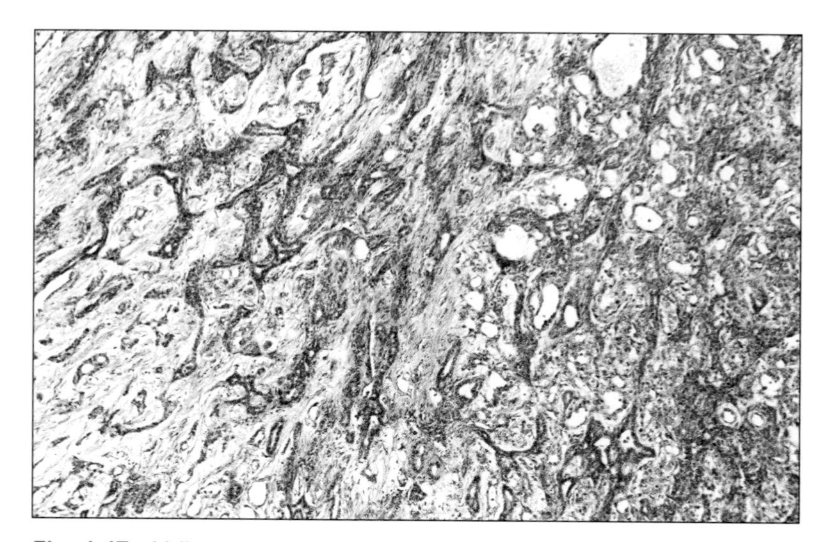

Fig. 4.47 Yolk sac tumor showing glandular–alveolar and myxomatous patterns.

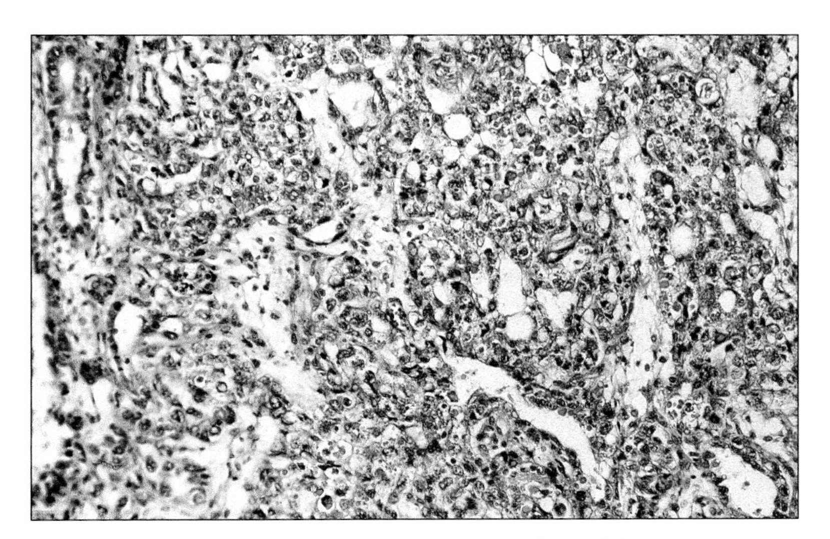

Fig. 4.48 Yolk sac tumor showing predominantly a solid pattern. Numerous hyaline bodies are present.

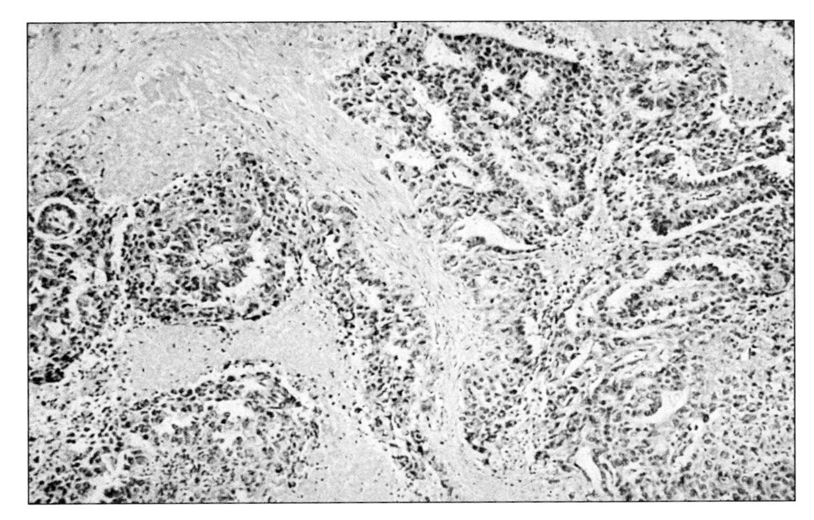

Fig. 4.49 Yolk sac tumor showing endodermal sinus, solid, and glandular patterns and associated with marked necrosis. These features are common in testicular yolk sac tumors in adults.

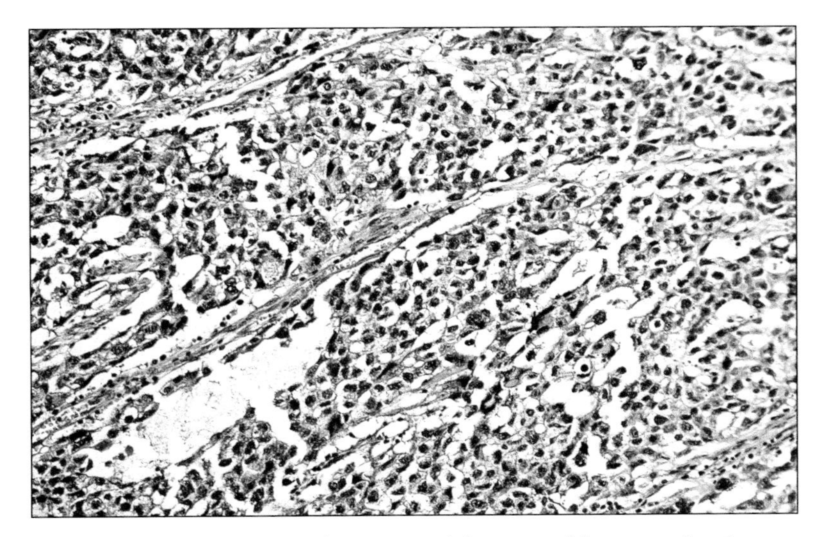

Fig. 4.50 Yolk sac tumor showing a solid pattern. Note occasional microcysts interspersed among the solid sheets of tumor cells.

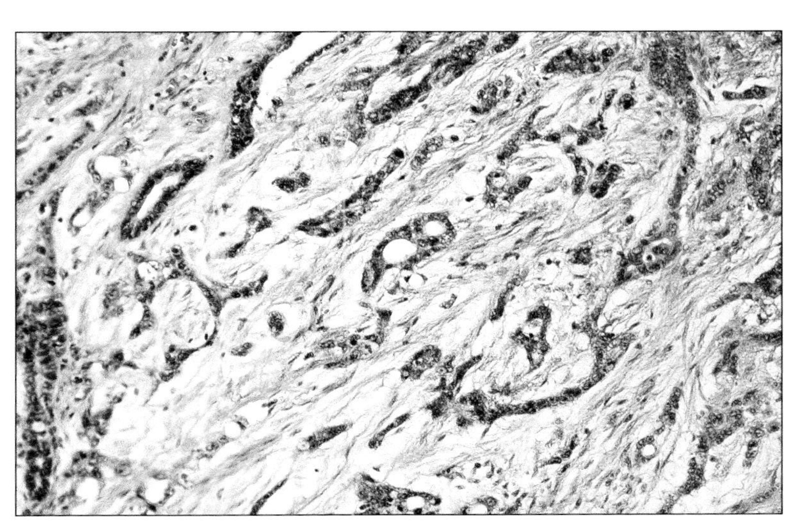

Fig. 4.51 Yolk sac tumor showing a myxomatous pattern with strands, cords, glands, and individual tumor cells interspersed within the myxomatous tissue.

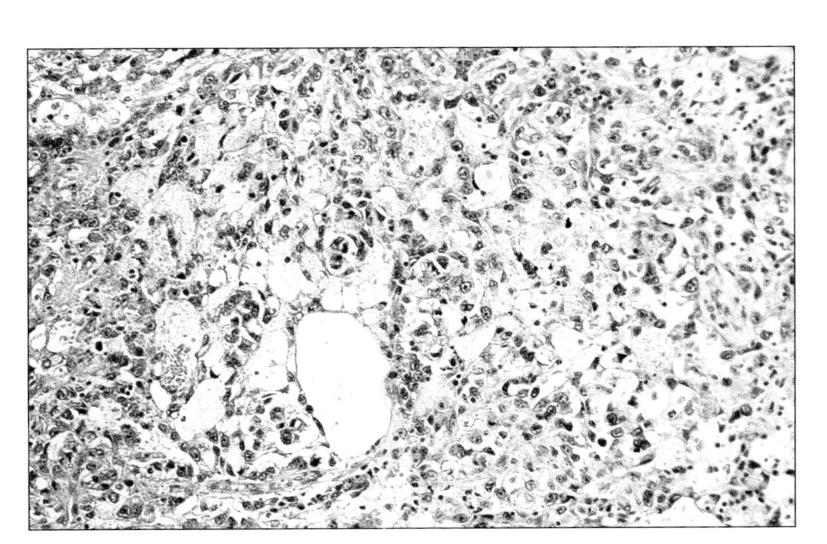

Fig. 4.52 Yolk sac tumor showing solid and microcystic patterns.

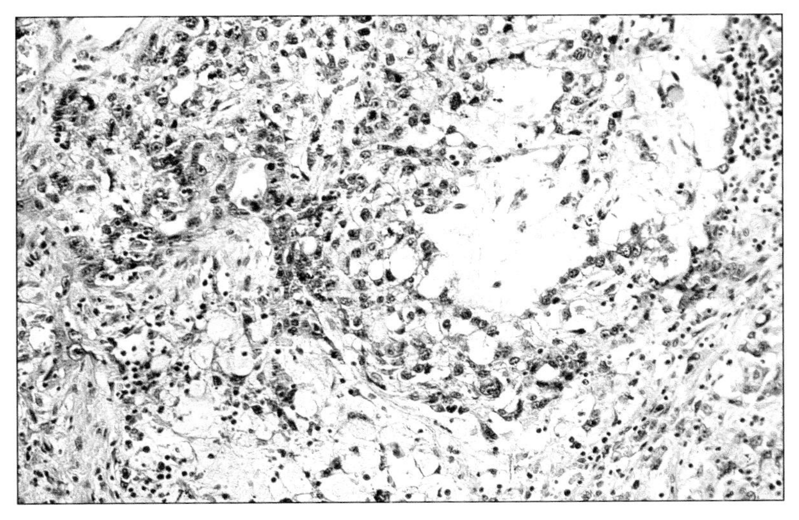

Fig. 4.53 Yolk sac tumor showing solid and microcystic patterns. Note a round hyaline body (top right).

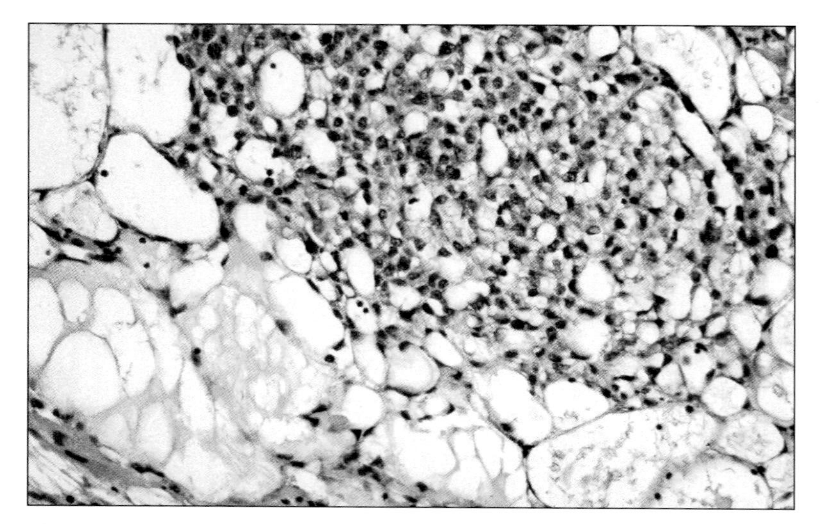

Fig. 4.54 Yolk sac tumor showing solid and microcystic patterns. Macrocystic formations were also present in this tumor.

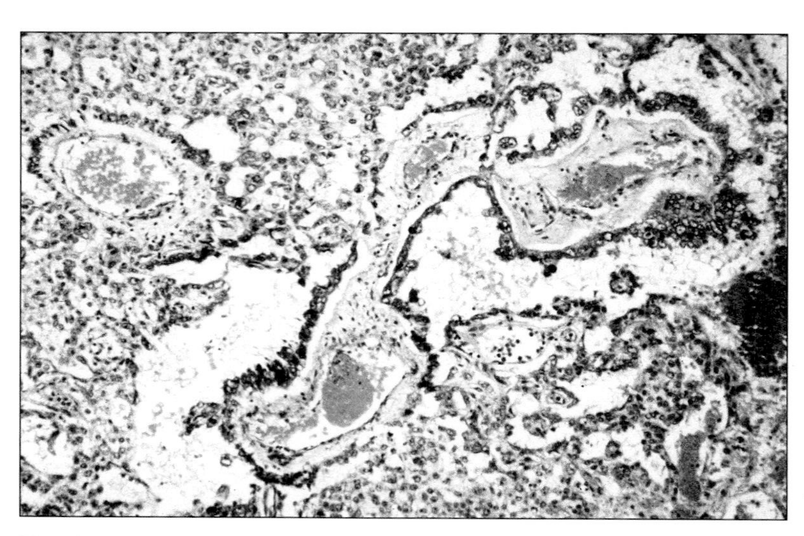

Fig. 4.57 Yolk sac tumor showing endodermal sinus and papillary patterns. Note perivascular formations (Schiller–Duval bodies) sectioned longitudinally and transversely.

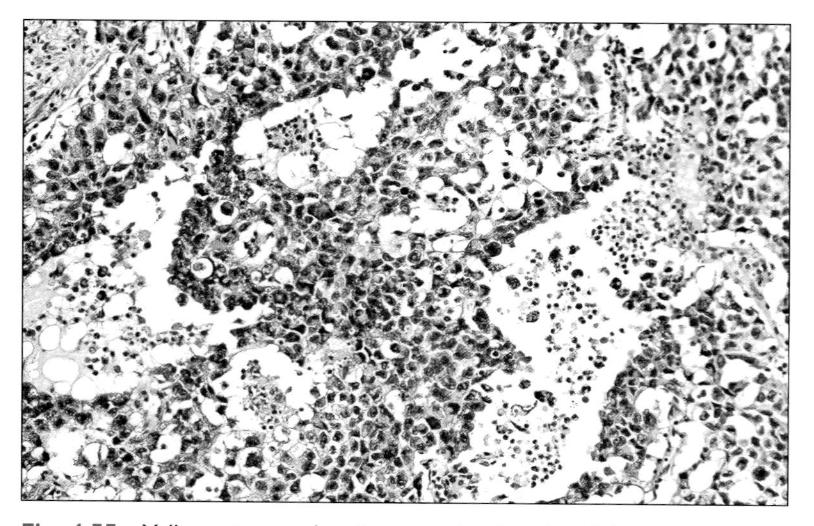

Fig. 4.55 Yolk sac tumor showing a predominantly solid pattern. Microcysts are seen and provide a clue to the diagnosis. The solid pattern is not infrequently confused with embryonal carcinoma or classical seminoma, but microcysts are not seen in the latter tumors.

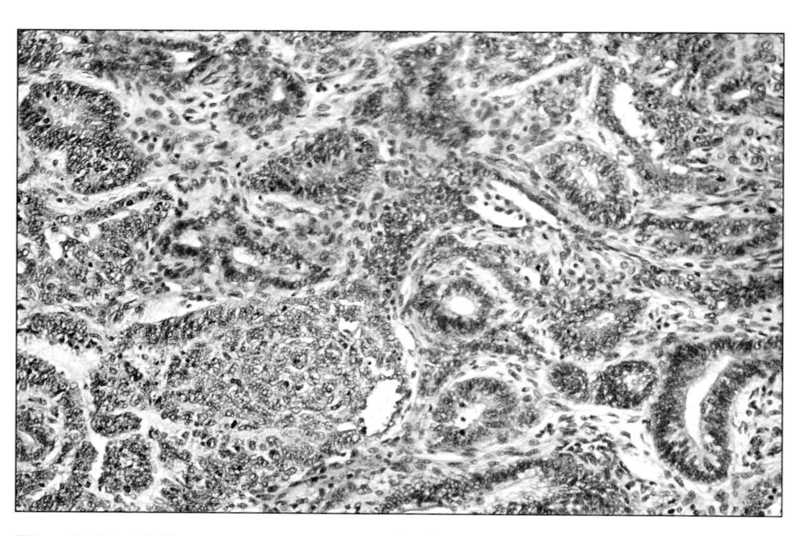

Fig. 4.58 Yolk sac tumor composed of primitive endodermal glands and showing the intestinal or primitive endodermal pattern.

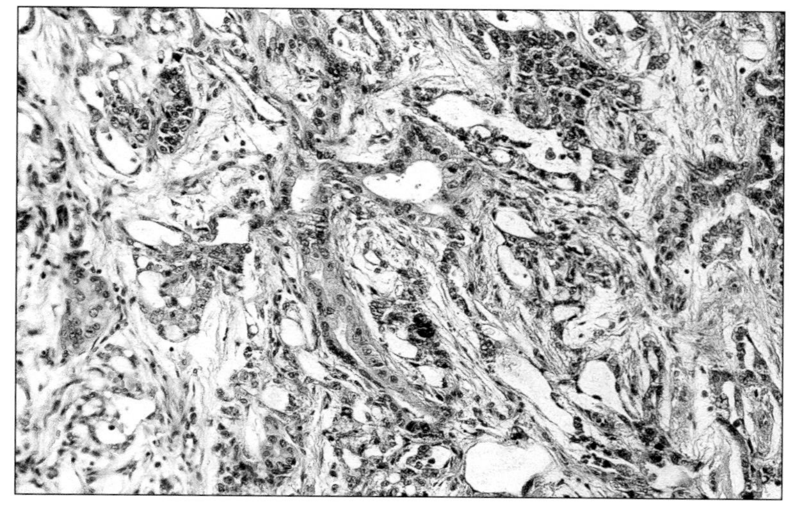

Fig. 4.56 Yolk sac tumor showing a glandular–alveolar pattern.

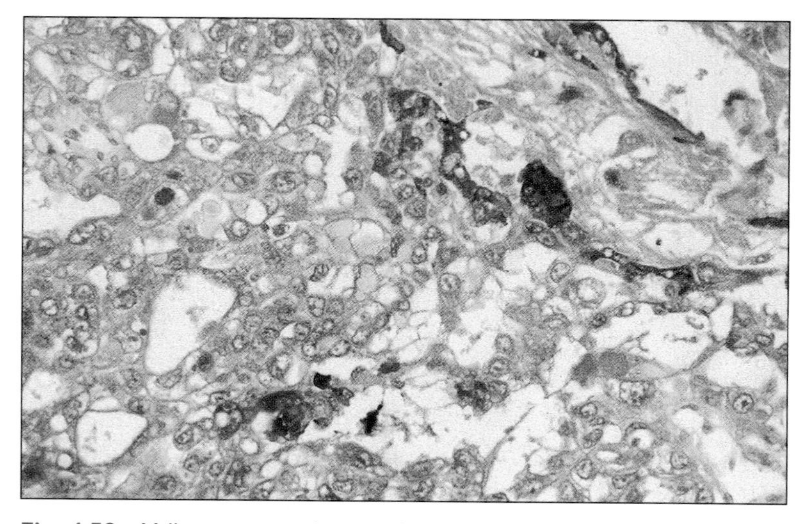

Fig. 4.59 Yolk sac tumor showing focal, intense staining for alphafetoprotein.

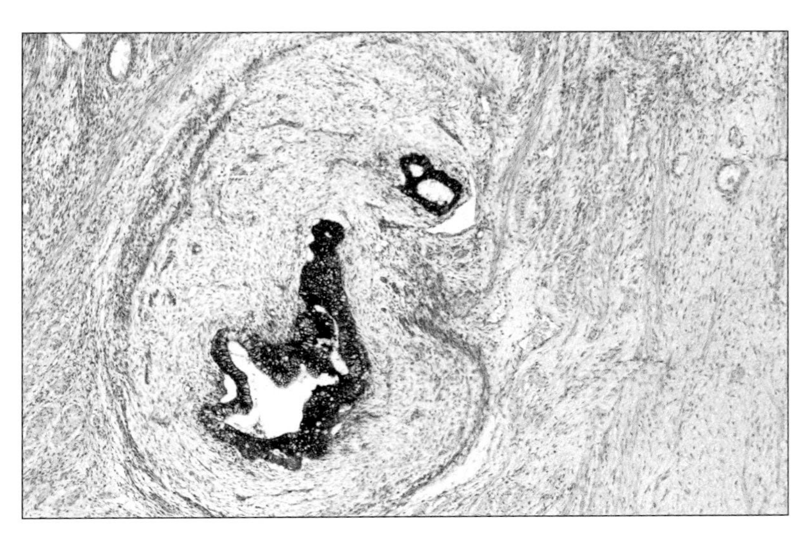

Fig. 4.60 Malignant mixed germ cell tumor containing primitive endodermal glands that show strong alphafetoprotein (AFP) staining. The patient's serum AFP was also considerably elevated.

Choriocarcinoma

Clinical findings

- Choriocarcinoma occurs as a component of mixed germ cell tumors in 8–10% of cases, but is very rare in pure form.[1,4–6,31,47]
- Tumors containing choriocarcinoma are most common between the ages of 15 and 30 years, but may occur from puberty to old age.[1,4–6,31]
- Owing to its early vascular and lymphatic dissemination, it is highly malignant.[1,4–6,31,48]
- Patients present with testicular enlargement and sometimes with metastatic disease.[1,6,31,48,49]
- Occasionally, patients present with gynecomastia due to HCG production.[1,6]
- Elevated serum HCG levels are common due to the synthesis of HCG by the syncytiotrophoblastic component of the tumor.
- Treatment consists of orchiectomy followed by combination chemotherapy.
- Prognosis is favorable even in patients with distant metastases, due to good response to the combination chemotherapy.[4–6]

Pathologic findings

Macroscopic findings

- The testis is at least slightly enlarged, with a distorted contour.
- The tumor is usually hemorrhagic and may be completely obliterated.[1–6]

Microscopic findings

- Choriocarcinoma has two elements, cytotrophoblast and syncytiotrophoblast. The presence of both elements is necessary for diagnosis.
- Isolated syncytiotrophoblastic giant cells do not constitute choriocarcinoma.[1–6]
- Cytotrophoblast is the least differentiated component of the tumor. It gives rise to the syncytiotrophoblast.
- The cytotrophoblast is composed of uniform, medium-sized, polygonal, round, or oval cells with clear cytoplasm and sharp cellular borders.
- The nuclei are centrally located. Some are small and others hyperchromatic, larger and vesicular with prominent nucleoli.[1–6]
- Mitotic activity is usually brisk.
- Cytotrophoblast is HCG-negative.
- Syncytiotrophoblast is composed of large, vacuolated, usually multinucleated cells with a large amount of cytoplasm that varies from eosinophilic to basophilic.
- The syncytiotrophoblastic cells often appear bizarre and the nuclei may be represented by irregular masses of chromatin.[1–6]
- The syncytiotrophoblasts produce HCG and therefore stain positively for HCG and beta-HCG.[1–6,46]
- The syncytiotrophoblasts are located peripherally and often surround the centrally located cytotrophoblasts.[1–6]
- In rare cases, choriocarcinoma may show intermediate trophoblast composed of large polygonal cells with bright eosinophilic cytoplasm and single, round, hyperchromatic nuclei. Such tumors may be associated with an increased secretion of human placental lactogen (HPL) and lower levels of serum HCG.[6,50,51]
- Hemorrhage is usually present and red blood cells are frequently seen within the vacuoles of the syncytiotrophoblast.[1–6]

Special studies

- Syncytiotrophoblasts show intense immunohistochemical staining with HCG and beta-HCG, while cytotrophoblasts are negative.[1,6,46]
- Low molecular weight cytokeratin is positive in both cytotrophoblast and syncytiotrophoblast.[1,6,46]
- HPL is positive in intermediate trophoblastic cells and to lesser extent in syncytiotrophoblasts.[6,50,51]
- Various placental proteins, including PLAP, show staining in syncytiotrophoblasts.[6]

(Figs 4.61–4.68)

Polyembryoma

Polyembryoma is a germ cell tumor composed of embryoid bodies with features of presomite embryos, which have not developed beyond the 18-day stage.[1,6,52–54]

Clinical findings

- Tumors composed entirely of polyembryoma have not been encountered in the testis.[1,6]
- The presence of polyembryoma as a component of a mixed germ cell tumor is rare, but is more common in testicular than in ovarian tumors.[1–6]

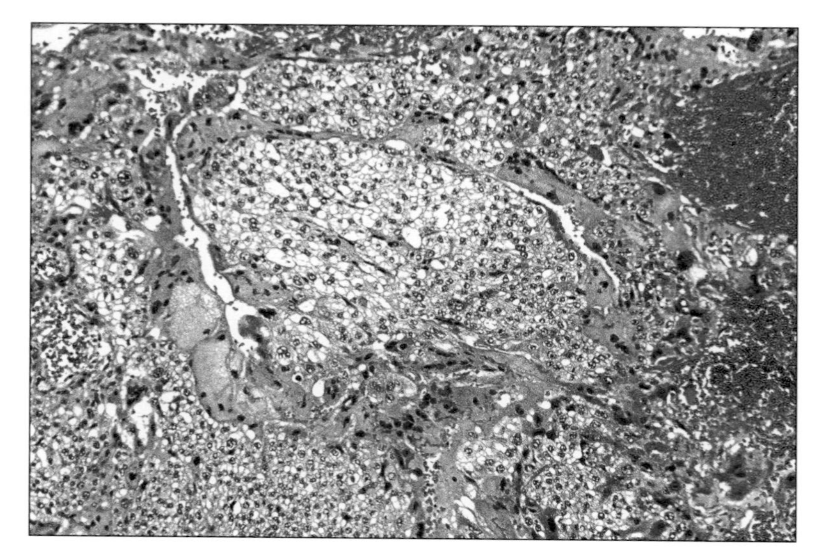

Fig. 4.61 Choriocarcinoma showing central cytotrophoblast and peripheral syncytiotrophoblast composed of large multinucleated cells.

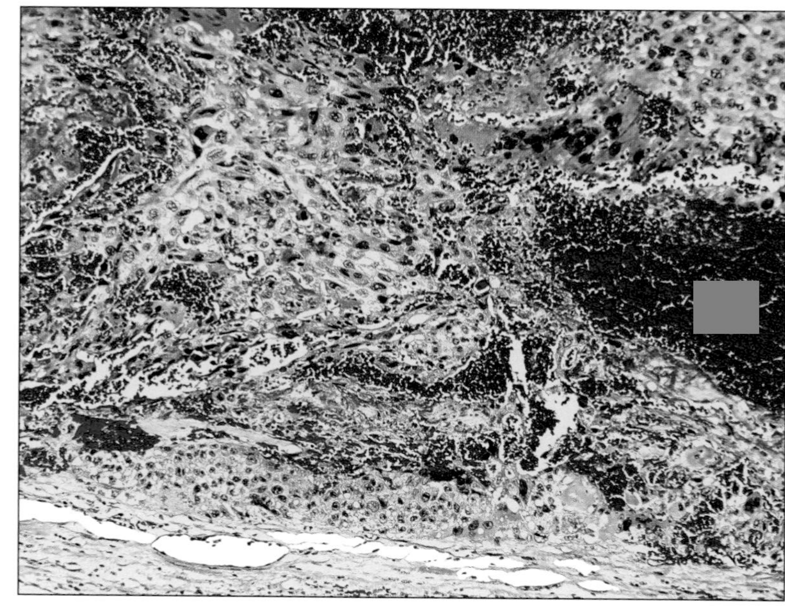

Fig. 4.62 Choriocarcinoma showing marked hemorrhage.

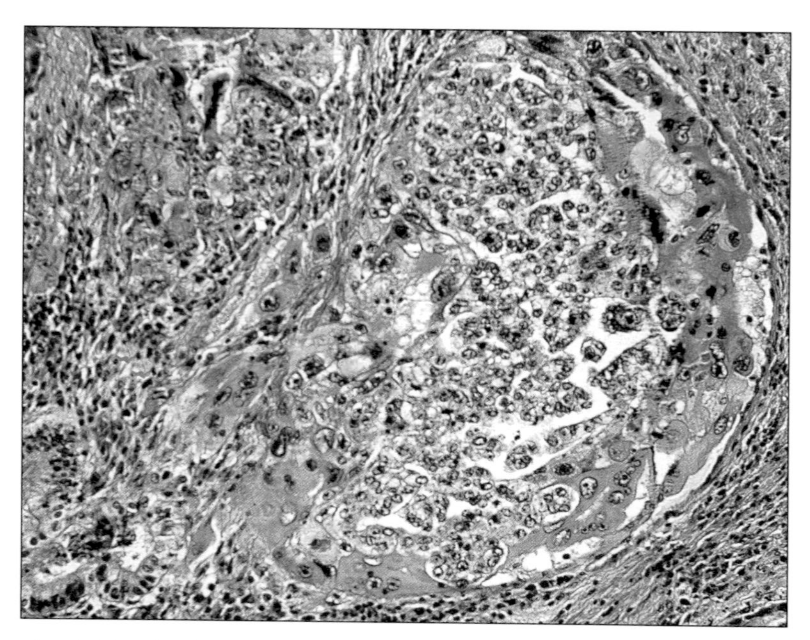

Fig. 4.63 Choriocarcinoma showing centrally located cytotrophoblast surrounded by syncytiotrophoblastic giant cells.

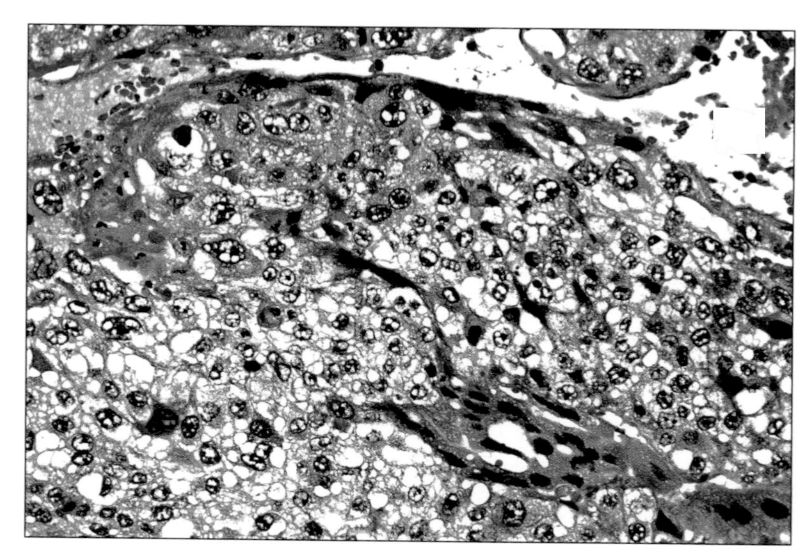

Fig. 4.64 Choriocarcinoma showing cytotrophoblast composed of uniform medium-sized clear cells and syncytiotrophoblast composed of multinucleated and vacuolated giant cells.

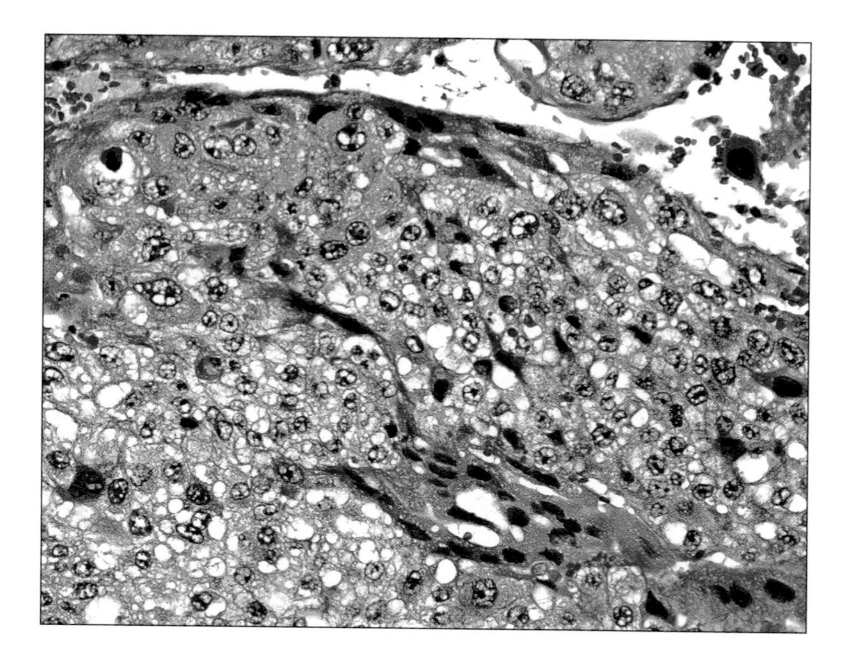

Fig. 4.65 Choriocarcinoma showing intensely basophilic syncytiotrophoblastic giant cells and cytotrophoblast composed of uniform cells with clear cytoplasm.

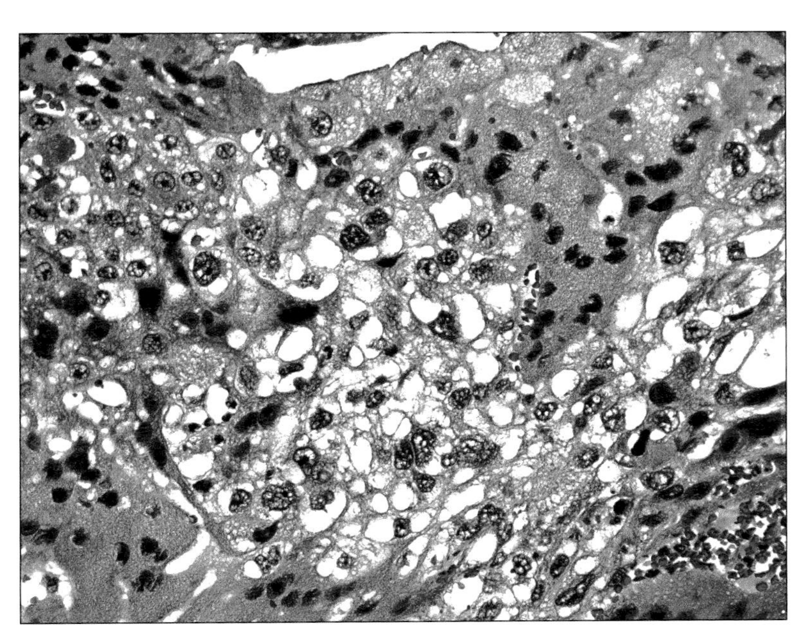

Fig. 4.66 Choriocarcinoma showing centrally located cytotrophoblast composed of clear cells. One of the multinucleated syncytiotrophoblastic giant cells shows hemorrhage (lower right).

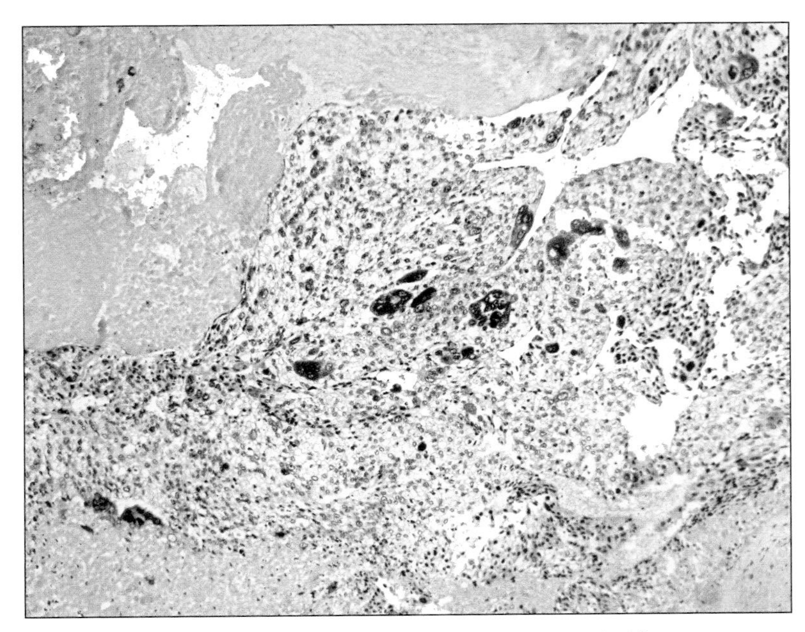

Fig. 4.67 Choriocarcinoma composed of syncytiotrophoblastic giant cells staining positively with beta human chorionic gonadotropin. The cytotrophoblast does not show positive staining. Hemorrhage and necrosis are also in evidence.

- The age range and other features are similar to those observed in other testicular mixed germ cell tumors. This also applies to behavior, prognosis, and therapy.

Pathologic findings

Macroscopic findings
- The tumors show similar appearances to other mixed germ cell tumors.

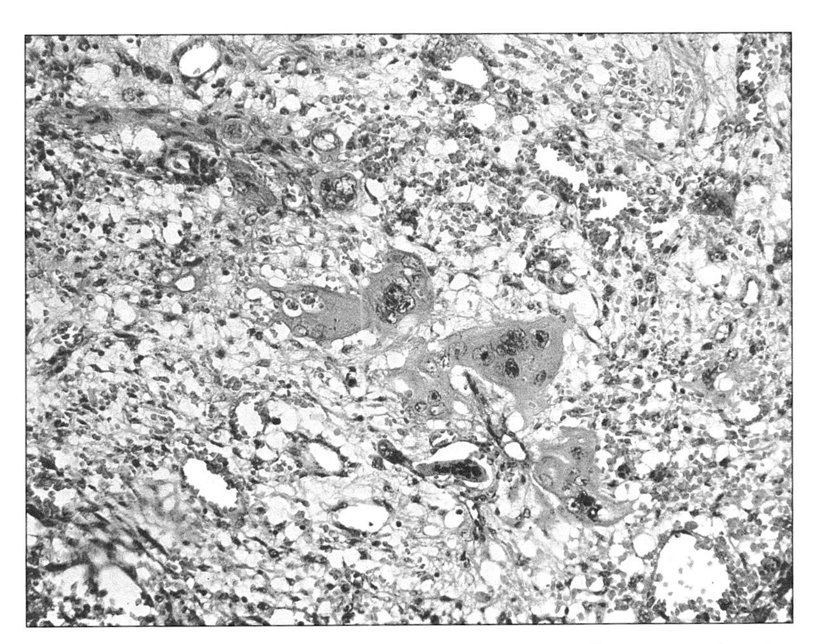

Fig. 4.68 Collection of syncytiotrophoblastic giant cells associated with embryonal carcinoma. There is no cytotrophoblast and therefore this is not a choriocarcinoma.

- They are usually large, soft, and solid, but when associated with teratomatous elements may be partly cystic.
- They often have hemorrhage and necrosis.[1–6]

Microscopic findings
- The embryoid bodies, when well formed, are composed of embryonic disc in the center with amniotic cavity on one side and yolk sac on the other.[1,4–6,52–55]
- The embryonic bodies are surrounded by primitive extraembryonic mesenchyme and myxomatous connective tissue.
- The embryonic disc is usually composed of two cell layers. One layer is made up of tall columnar cells and represents the ectoderm, and the second formed by flattened cells represents the endoderm.[1,4–6,52–55]
- Occasionally, the embryonic disc is composed of three cell layers, with mesenchymal cells interspersed between the other two cell layers.
- The embryoid bodies are frequently less well formed, with absent yolk sac or amniotic cavity, or multiple less well-formed structures.[1,4–6,52–55]
- The embryonic disc may be distorted and may not be composed of two or three cell layers.
- Blastocyst-like structures may be present.[1,6,52–55]
- The surrounding primitive mesenchyme and myxomatous tissue may contain syncytiotrophoblastic giant cells and poorly differentiated teratomatous structures.[1,4–6,52–55]
- The polyembryoma component is usually intimately admixed with other germ cell elements, often in a haphazard pattern.

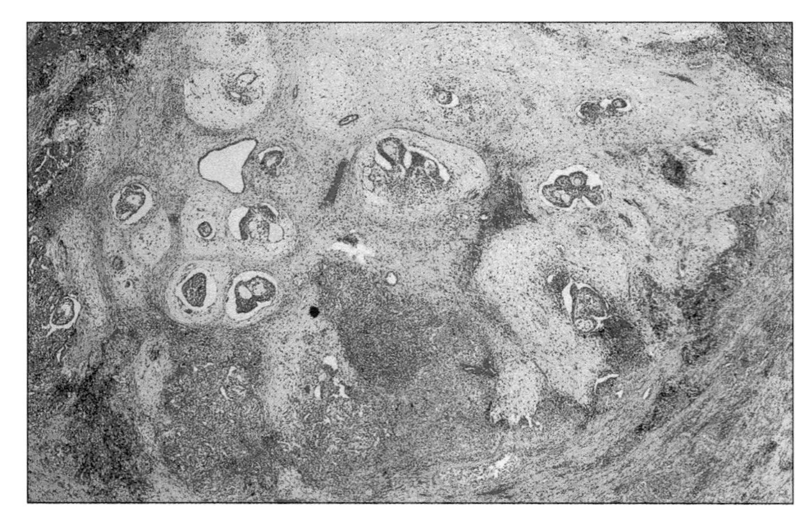

Fig. 4.69 Mixed germ cell tumor showing a large focus of polyembryoma. The embryoid bodies present show atypical features.

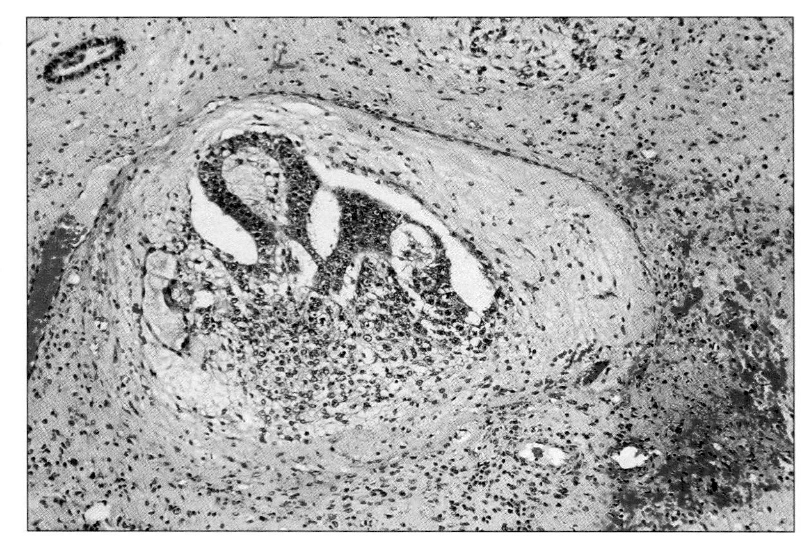

Fig. 4.71 Atypical embryoid body surrounded by myxomatous tissue.

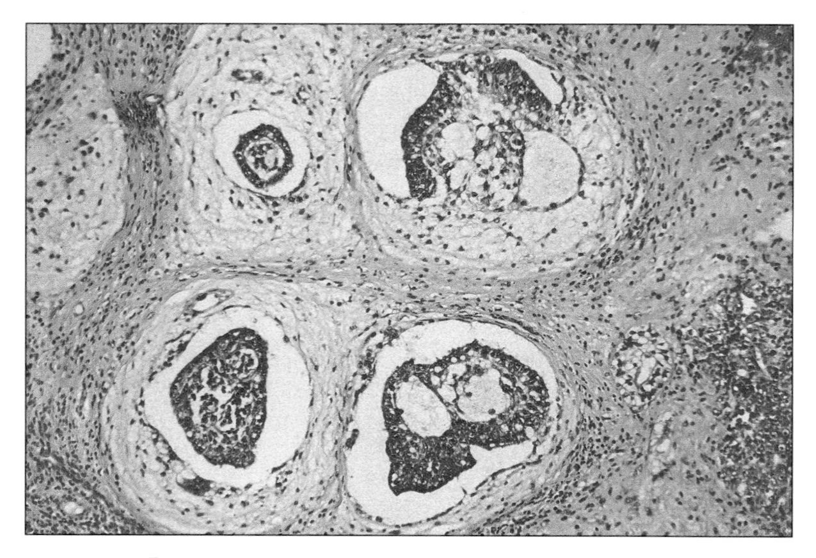

Fig. 4.70 Focus of polyembryoma showing a number of embryoid bodies including one well formed (top right) composed of embryonic disc with amniotic cavity on the left and yolk sac on the right.

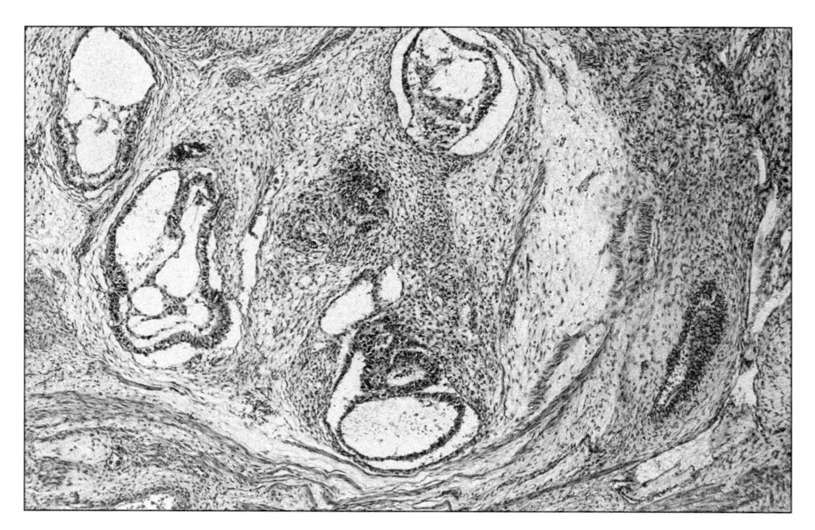

Fig. 4.72 Focus of polyembryoma containing atypical embryoid bodies surrounded by myxomatous tissue and primitive mesenchyme.

Special studies

- Embryoid bodies stain for low molecular weight cytokeratin.
- AFP can be demonstrated within the endodermal cells and within some gland-like structures resembling allantois.
- HCG is present in the syncytiotrophoblastic giant cells seen in the vicinity of the embryoid bodies.[6]

(Figs 4.69–4.72)

Teratoma

- Teratoma is a germ cell neoplasm with differentiation towards somatic structures. These consist of derivatives of the three primitive germ layers: ectoderm, mesoderm, and endoderm.
- These neoplasms show various degrees of differentiation from highly immature to fully mature.[1–6]
- Fully mature tissues are not associated with malignancy;[1–6] immaturity implies the presence of malignant potential.
- The terms immature and mature are preferable to the terms malignant and benign.[1,6]

Clinical findings

- In the testis, the incidence of teratoma shows two peaks, one in infancy and early childhood,[1–6,38,39,56–58] and the other, a higher peak, in early adult life.[1–6,59]
- In infancy and early childhood, teratoma is the second most common testicular tumor after YST.[1–6,38,39,56–58]
- In infancy and early childhood, teratomas occur in pure form, are composed of mature tissues, and are benign. Occasionally, immature elements may be present, but have not been associated with benign behavior.[1,6,38,39,56–58]

- In young adults, teratomas usually have both immature and mature tissues and therefore are malignant.[1-6,59]
- In this age group, teratomas are also frequently mixed with other malignant neoplastic germ cell elements.[1-6,31]
- Pure teratomas are relatively uncommon in young adults.[1-6,31,59]
- In both age groups, the most common presentation is testicular enlargement.
- The initial treatment is orchiectomy.[1-6,39,56-59] In infants and young children, no further therapy is necessary.[1-6,39,56-58] In the adult group, combination chemotherapy has a very positive outcome.[1-6,59]

Pathologic findings

Macroscopic findings

- Pediatric teratomas are usually small.[1-6,39,56-58] In adults, size may vary, but tumors composed mainly of immature elements tend to be larger.[1-6,59]
- The macroscopic findings depend on the composition of the tumor.
- The tumors are usually variegated and may be solid, cystic, or both.[1-6,39,56-59]
- The solid areas may contain spicules of bone and cartilage.
- The cysts may be filled with watery, mucinous, gelatinous, or keratinous material.

Microscopic findings

- Teratoma may contain a great variety of tissues.[1-6,39,56-59]
- Pediatric tumors are composed entirely of mature tissues and show organoid pattern and better organization.[1-6,39,56-58]
- In adults, the tumors tend to be less well organized, with the immature and mature components intermingled haphazardly.[1-6,31,59]
- The immature tissues may show varying degrees of differentiation from highly immature to nearly mature.[1-6,31,59]
- Thyroid, renal, pancreatic, and dental tissues are uncommon in testicular tumors.[1-6,31]

(Figs 4.73–4.75)

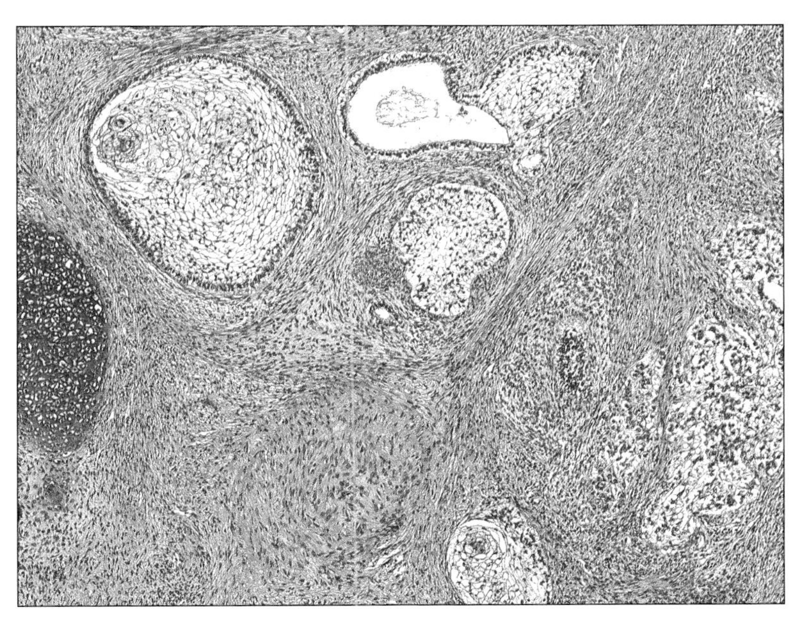

Fig. 4.73 Immature teratoma composed of immature connective tissue, squamous epithelium, and cartilage, showing a haphazard pattern.

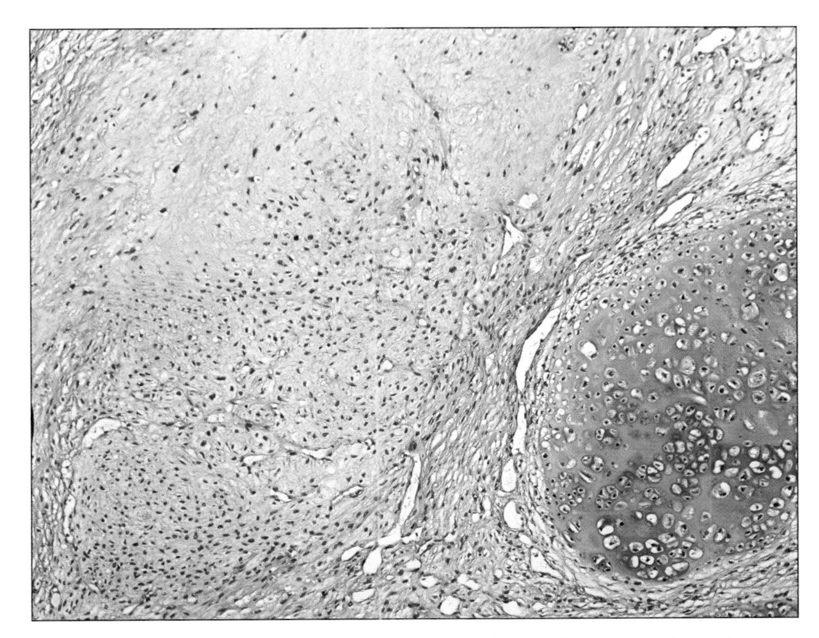

Fig. 4.74 Immature teratoma composed of neural tissue and cartilage.

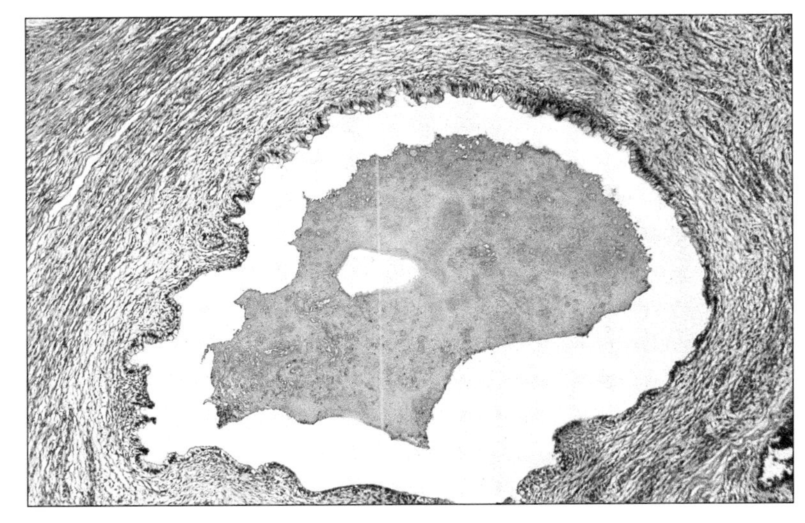

Fig. 4.75 Immature teratoma composed of immature connective tissue surrounding a mature glandular structure.

Mixed germ cell tumors

Mixed germ cell tumors are neoplasms composed of at least two different germ cell tumor types.[1-6]

Clinical findings

- They comprise 35–45% of malignant testicular neoplasms.[1-6]
- The combination of embryonal carcinoma with teratoma is the most common.[1-6,31,46,60]

- Mixed germ cell tumors occur after puberty and are most common in the third and fourth decades. They are rare in infancy and early childhood.[1–6]
- Patients present with testicular enlargement and sometimes pain.
- The primary treatment is orchiectomy followed by combination chemotherapy, with favorable outcome in more than 85% of cases.[1–6,31,60]

Pathologic findings

Macroscopic findings

- The tumors are usually large, variegated, distort the testicular contour, and often show hemorrhage and necrosis.
- They are usually solid but may contain cystic areas.[1–6,31,43,46,60]

Microscopic findings

- Various histologic combinations may be present. Embryonal carcinoma, teratoma, and classical seminoma are the most common components.[1–6,31,60]
- YST elements are seen focally in approximately 40% of cases.[1,6,43,46]
- Choriocarcinoma is less common (10% of cases).[1–6,31,43,46,60]
- Polyembryoma is uncommon.

Special studies

- Histochemical and immunohistochemical studies can be used to confirm various neoplastic germ cell elements.[6,46]

(Fig. 4.76)

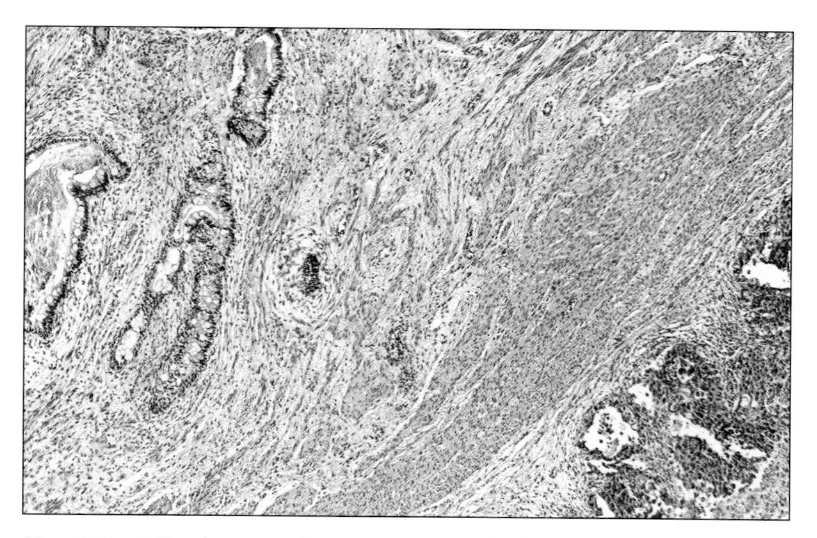

Fig. 4.76 Mixed germ cell tumor composed of teratomatous elements represented by variably differentiated glandular and mesenchymal tissue admixed with embryonal carcinoma.

Primary carcinoid tumor

Clinical findings

- Primary carcinoid tumors are uncommon in the testis.
- Approximately 50 cases have been reported.
- Most patients are 40–60 years old (range, 26–71 years).[61–65]
- The tumor is nearly always unilateral, but bilateral tumors have been reported.
- Patients present with testicular enlargement, which is usually painless.
- The majority of testicular carcinoids occur in pure form, but sometimes the tumor is part of a teratoma.[4–6]
- Primary carcinoid tumors of the testis are usually indolent.[61–65]
- Metastases are rare, occurring in approximately 5% of cases.[62,63]
- Symptoms of carcinoid syndrome have been noted in only a single case.
- The treatment of choice is orchiectomy.
- The prognosis is favorable and most patients are cured.[1–6,61–65]
- The carcinoid produces serotonin, a tumor marker. Its metabolic product, 5-hydroxy-indole acetic acid (5-HIAA), secreted in the urine, can also be used.[6]

Pathologic findings

Macroscopic

- The tumors are solid, yellow to light brown.
- The tumors are usually small (3–5 cm).[1–6,61–65]

Microscopic

- All the primary testicular carcinoids reported have been of the typical insular type, characteristic of midgut derivation.[1–6,61–65]
- The tumor is composed of islands, nests, or aggregates of uniform cells surrounded by connective tissue.
- The connective tissue varies from fine strands to large, dense bands.
- The tumor cells form solid nests and small acini.[1–6,61–65]
- They have ample cytoplasm and oval or round nuclei with finely dispersed chromatin.
- The cytoplasm, especially of cells at the periphery of the nests, contains orange-red granules in the apical part of the cell.
- Ultrastructurally, the cytoplasm shows pleomorphic neurosecretory granules typical of carcinoid tumors of midgut derivation.[64,65]
- Primary carcinoid tumor of the testis must be differentiated from metastasis. The latter is usually bilateral and forms multiple nodules within the testis.[1,4–6,64,65]
- It must also be differentiated from Sertoli cell tumor, Leydig cell tumor, and the rare granulosa cell and Brenner tumor. The typical histologic appearances and

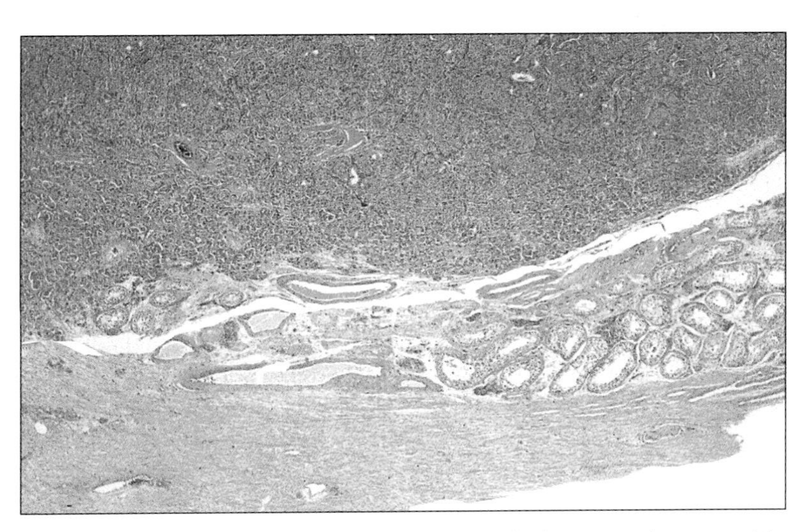

Fig. 4.77 Primary carcinoid tumor. A solid well-demarcated tumor with extensive involvement of the testis.

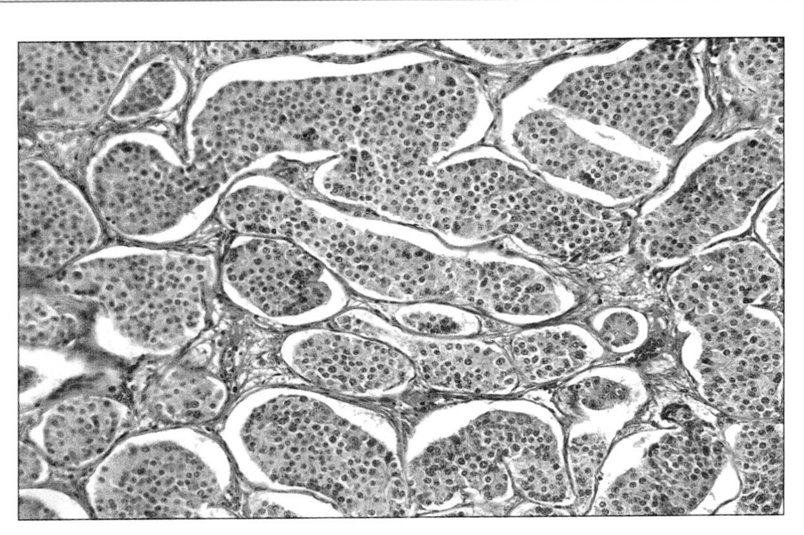

Fig. 4.79 Carcinoid tumor composed of solid nests of uniform polygonal cells with eosinophilic cytoplasm and round nuclei.

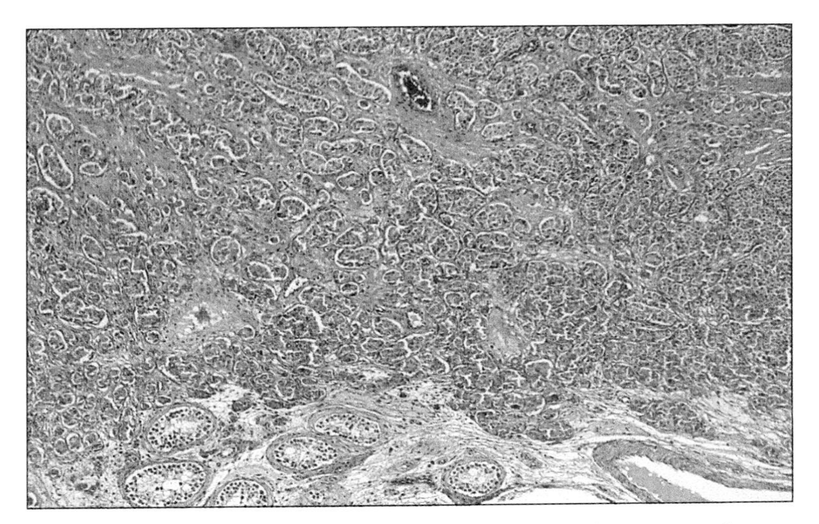

Fig. 4.78 Carcinoid tumor showing the typical nest-like pattern of insular carcinoid tumors.

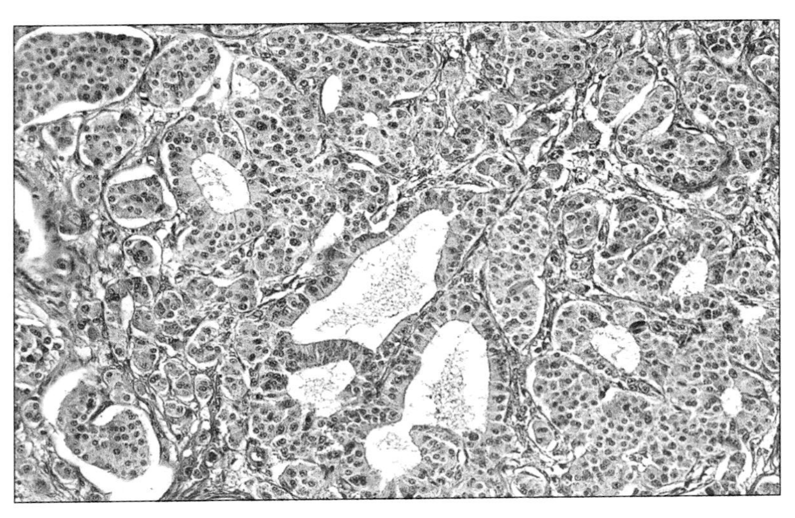

Fig. 4.80 Carcinoid tumor showing solid nest-like and glandular patterns.

histochemical and immunocytochemical reactions are very helpful.

Special studies

- Histochemically, the tumor cells show typical argyrophil and argentaffin reactions with Grimelius and Masson–Fontana stains, respectively.[6,64,65]
- Immunocytochemical studies show low molecular weight cytokeratin positivity, as well as positivity for chromogranin and various other neuroendocrine polypeptides.[6,65]

(Figs 4.77–4.80)

Epidermoid cyst

Most testicular epidermoid cysts are one-sided development of a teratoma and therefore are germ cell neoplasms.

Clinical findings

- Epidermoid cysts account for approximately 1% of enlarged testicles.
- They are encountered at all ages, but are most common from the second to fourth decades.[66–68]
- They are more often found in the right testis.
- They are composed of mature tissue and therefore are benign.[1–6,66–68]
- Orchiectomy or local excision is the treatment of choice.

Pathologic findings

Macroscopic

- Epidermoid cysts average 2 cm in diameter.[66–68]
- They are soft, round or oval, yellow–white, and well demarcated.

- They contain granular, cheesy yellow–white material surrounded by a thin fibrous wall.[1–6,66–68]

Microscopic
- The cyst is lined by laminated squamous epithelium devoid of adnexal structures.[1–6,66–68] It contains keratin and necrotic material.
- Reactive changes may be present with marked foreign body giant cell reaction.[1–6,66–68]
- Parts of the cyst wall may be denuded of squamous epithelium, and focal ulceration may be present.
- Presence of fibrous scars, adnexal structures, teratomatous elements, and IGCN must be carefully excluded by extensive sampling in order to verify the diagnosis.[1,6]

SEX CORD–STROMAL TUMORS

This group comprises approximately 3.5% of testicular neoplasms. It is divided into two main types:

- Leydig (interstitial) cell tumor;
- Sertoli cell tumor (androblastoma).

A few cases of granulosa cell tumor have been reported, but these are rare in the testis.

Leydig cell tumor

Clinical findings
- Leydig cell tumor comprises 1–3% of testicular neoplasms.[69,70]
- It occurs at all ages, including childhood, but is most common from 20 to 50 years.
- In adults, the most common presentation is testicular enlargement, but 15% present with gynecomastia.[69,70]
- Children present with isosexual precocious puberty typically between 5 and 9 years.
- Leydig cell tumor is unilateral in 97% of cases.[69,70]
- In adults, 10% of Leydig cell tumors are malignant.[69–72]
- In patients with gynecomastia, the tumor is usually benign.
- In children, there are no documented cases of malignancy.[69,70]
- The optimal treatment is orchiectomy.
- Presence of metastases is the only definite criterion of malignancy.[69–72]

Pathologic findings

Macroscopic
- The tumors usually measure 3–5 cm in diameter, but may be larger.[69,70]
- Between 10% and 15% of tumors extend beyond the testis.
- The tumors are solid, well circumscribed, sometimes lobulated, and intersected by fibrous septa.
- They are usually uniformly yellow to yellow–tan.
- Hemorrhage and necrosis is seen in 25% of tumors.[69,70]

Microscopic
- The most common pattern is diffuse sheets of neoplastic cells; insular, trabecular, and ribbon-like patterns are also seen.[69,70]
- The stroma is usually inconspicuous. Occasionally it is prominent and hyalinized, forming intersecting broad bands; occasionally the stroma is edematous and myxoid.[69,70]
- The tumor cells are uniform, large, and polygonal, with bright eosinophilic, slightly granular cytoplasm.
- Occasionally the cytoplasm is vacuolated due to lipid accumulation.[69,70]
- The nuclei are round with a single prominent nucleolus.
- In rare cases, the tumor cells may be small, spindle shaped, or both.
- Mitotic activity is usually low and may be absent.[69,70]
- Crystals of Reinke, pathognomonic of Leydig cell tumor, are seen in approximately 33% of cases.
- Lipochrome pigment is seen in 10–15% of cases.[69,70]
- Electron microscopy demonstrates the hexagonal crystalline Reinke crystals, abundant rough endoplasmic reticulum, and membranous whorls.[70]
- There is no single criterion that reliably distinguishes benign from malignant Leydig cell tumor.[69–72] Malignancy is suggested by large tumor size, infiltrative margins, vascular involvement, and focal necrosis.[69–72] Pleomorphism and high mitotic activity (more than 3/10 high-power fields) also suggest malignant behavior.[69,70]

Special studies
- Lipid can usually be demonstrated in tumor cells in frozen tissue.[69,70]
- Vimentin and smooth muscle actin can be demonstrated by immunocytochemical stains.
- Cytokeratin, PLAP, S-100, HMB-45, and lymphoma markers are negative.[69,70]

(Figs 4.81–4.85)

Sertoli cell tumor

Sertoli cell tumor is has the following subtypes:

- typical Sertoli cell tumor;
- large cell calcifying Sertoli cell tumor;
- hyalinizing or sclerosing Sertoli cell tumor;
- lipid-rich Sertoli cell tumor;

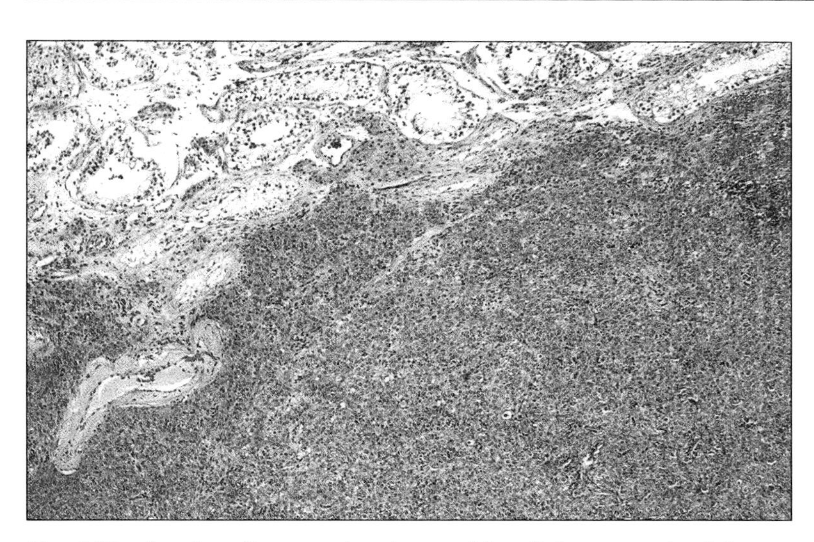

Fig. 4.81 Leydig cell tumor showing a solid well-demarcated cellular tumor replacing testicular tissue.

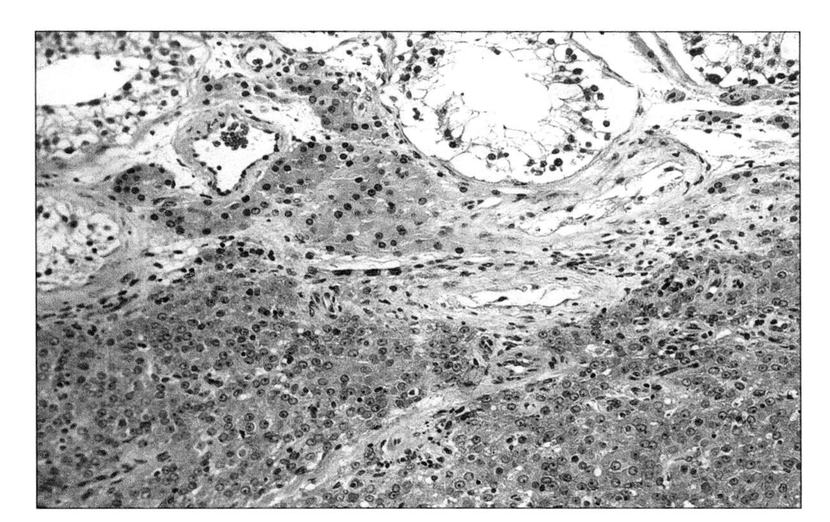

Fig. 4.82 Leydig cell tumor composed of aggregates of uniform polygonal cells with granular basophilic cytoplasm and round vesicular nuclei. A collection of hyperplastic Leydig cells with eosinophilic cytoplasm is also present.

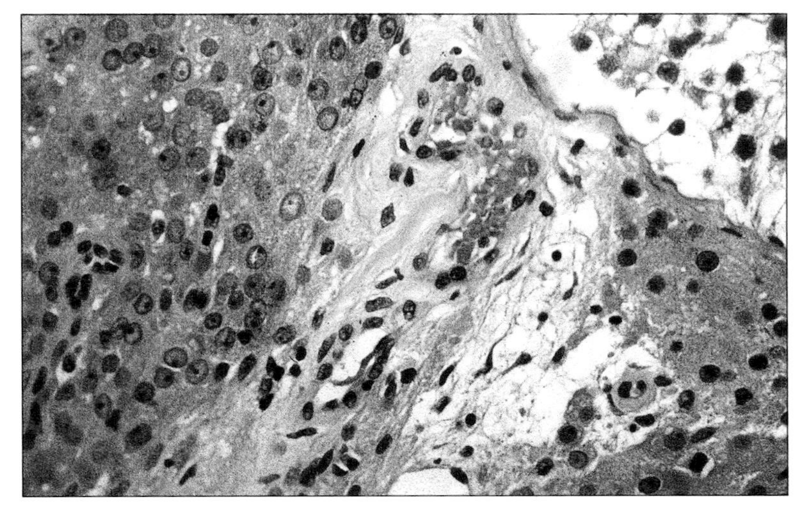

Fig. 4.83 Leydig cell tumor composed of uniform cells with granular cytoplasm and round nuclei with a single prominent nucleolus. There is no mitotic activity.

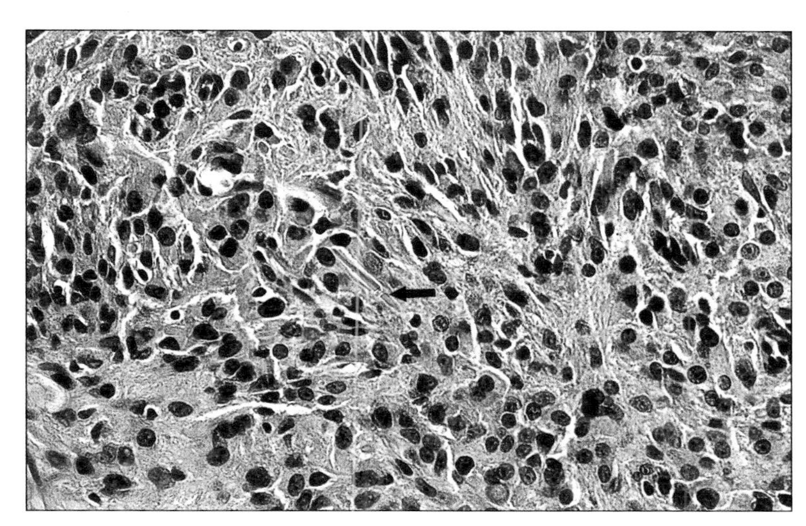

Fig. 4.84 Leydig cell tumor showing Reinke's crystals (arrow).

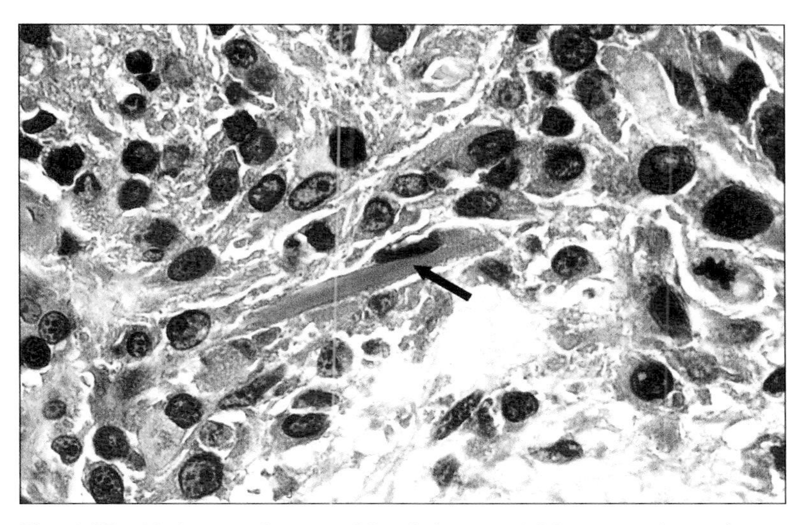

Fig. 4.85 High magnification of Reinke's crystal (Masson trichrome), a diagnostic feature of Leydig cell tumor.

- infantile Sertoli cell tumor (juvenile granulosa cell tumor).

Typical Sertoli cell tumor

Clinical findings

- Sertoli cell tumors are uncommon and comprise less than 1% of testicular neoplasms.[1-5]
- They occur at all ages, with no specific predilection for any age.[1-5]
- Approximately 15% occur in children.[73,74]
- Patients present with testicular enlargement, usually painless.[1-5]
- Patients may also present with gynecomastia.
- Sertoli cell tumor is occasionally associated with testicular feminization or Peutz–Jeghers syndrome.[75]
- The tumor is usually benign in 90% of cases.[1-5,75,76]
- The treatment is orchiectomy.

Pathologic findings

Macroscopic

- The tumor is usually small.[1-5,73,74]
- Malignant variants tend to be larger.[76-78]
- It is well demarcated, sometimes lobulated, and yellow–gray.
- The tumor is usually solid, rarely cystic.[1-5,73,74,76-78]
- Hemorrhage and necrosis are rare, but more common in large tumors.

Microscopic

- The histologic picture can be varied.[1-5]
- Well-differentiated tumors are composed of solid, occasionally hollow, tubules surrounded by fine connective tissue septa.[1-5]
- Sertoli cell tumors associated with testicular feminization syndrome are invariably well differentiated.[1-5]
- Less well-differentiated tumors are composed of cords or nests of tumor cells surrounded by a variable amount of connective tissue.
- Poorly differentiated tumors are composed of sheets or aggregates of tumor cells with only focal nest-like or cord-like pattern.
- The tumor cells resemble normal Sertoli cells, have an ample amount of eosinophilic or clear cytoplasm, and prominent ovoid or spindle-shaped nuclei.[1-5]
- Cellular or nuclear pleomorphism is uncommon.
- Mitotic activity is usually low.
- The connective tissue stroma is usually scanty and fine, but sometimes may be abundant and hyalinized.[1-5]
- Ultrastructurally, the tumor shows basal lamina around the solid tubules, abundant smooth endoplasmic reticulum, lipid droplets, desmosomes, and sometimes Charcot–Böttcher filament bundles.[1-5]
- Presence of metastases is the only definite criterion of malignancy.[1-5,76,77]
- Lack of tubular, nest-like, or cord-like patterns, cellular and nuclear pleomorphism, increased mitotic activity, and vascular invasion are associated with malignancy.[1-5,76]

Special studies

- The tumor cells stain for lipid.[1-5]
- The tumor cells are vimentin-positive and usually cytokeratin-positive.[2]
- PLAP is negative.

(Figs 4.86–4.95)

Large cell calcifying Sertoli cell tumor

Clinical findings

- This is an uncommon subtype of Sertoli cell tumor, with only 60 reported cases.[79]

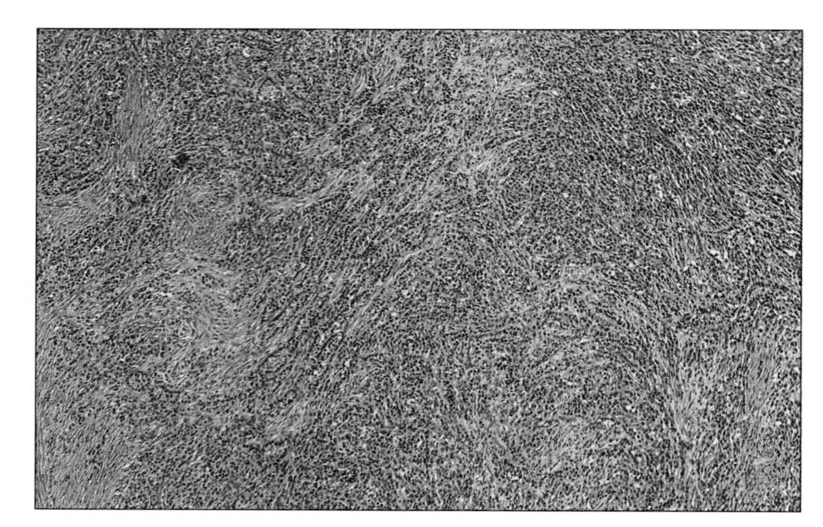

Fig. 4.86 Sertoli cell tumor composed of solid collections of tumor cells showing a solid tubular pattern (center) and a cord-like pattern (right).

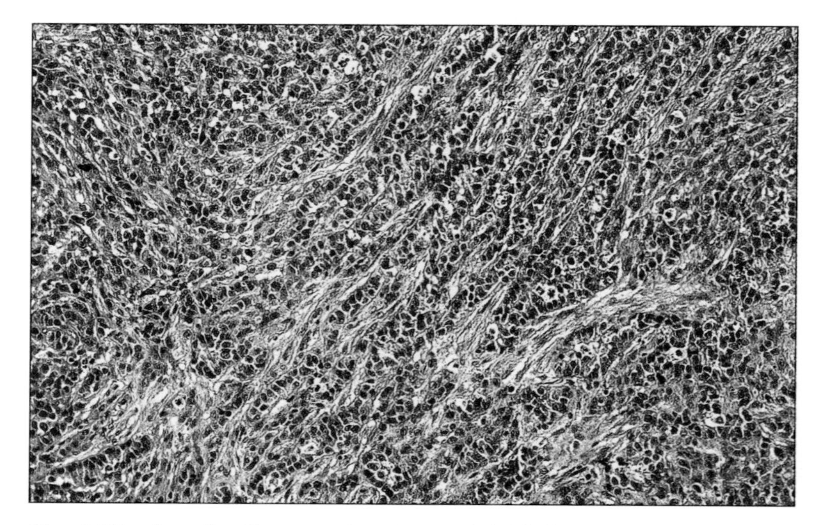

Fig. 4.87 Sertoli cell tumor showing a solid tubular pattern.

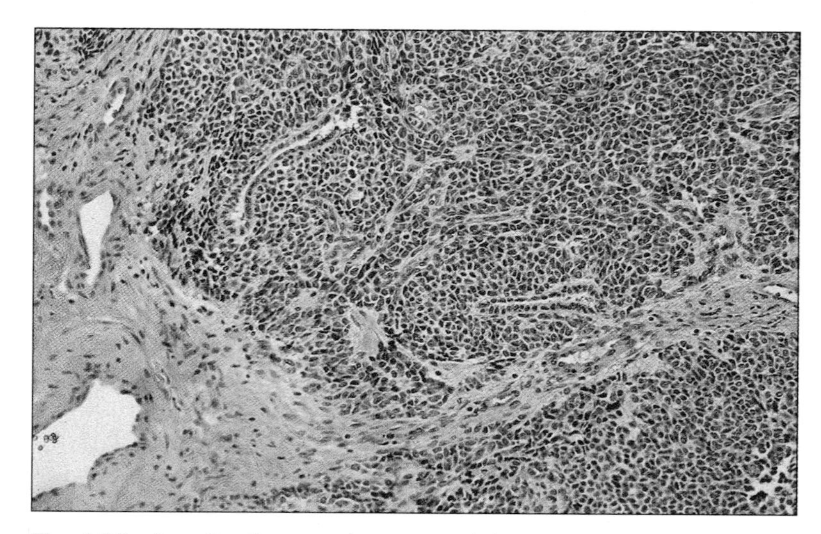

Fig. 4.88 Sertoli cell tumor showing a solid pattern.

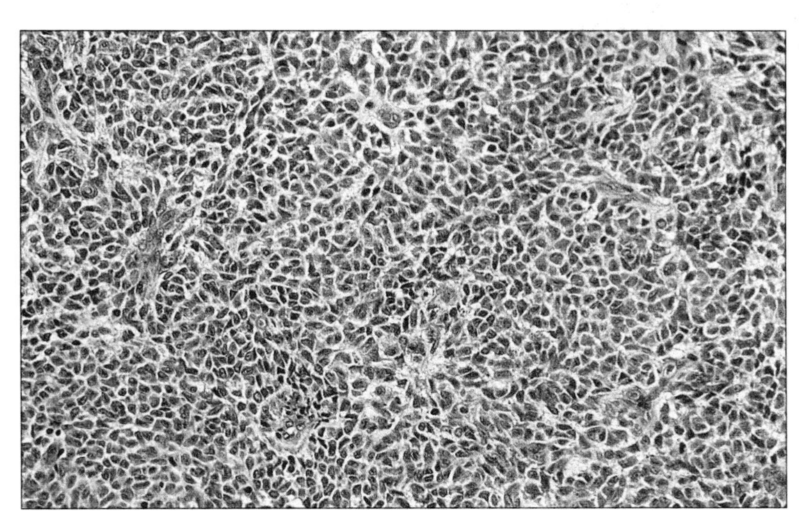

Fig. 4.89 Sertoli cell tumor composed of solid aggregates of ovoid or slightly elongated cells with prominent ovoid or carrot-shaped nuclei.

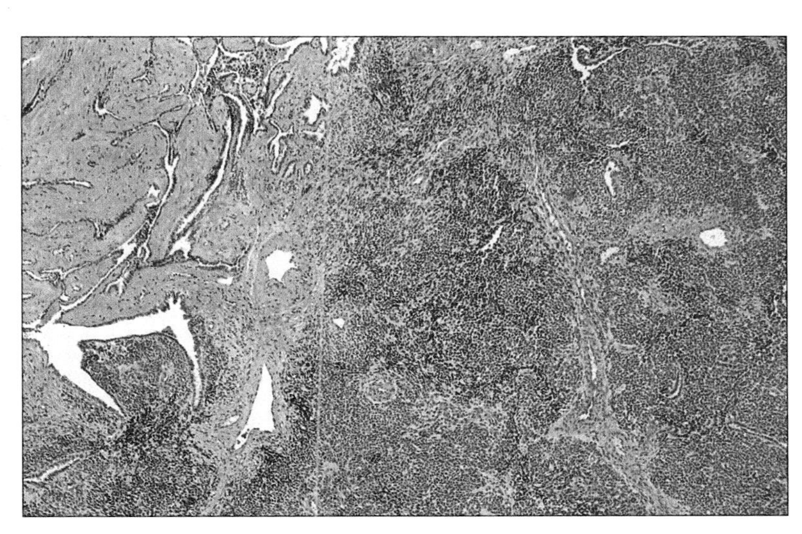

Fig. 4.92 Sertoli cell tumor invading rete testis.

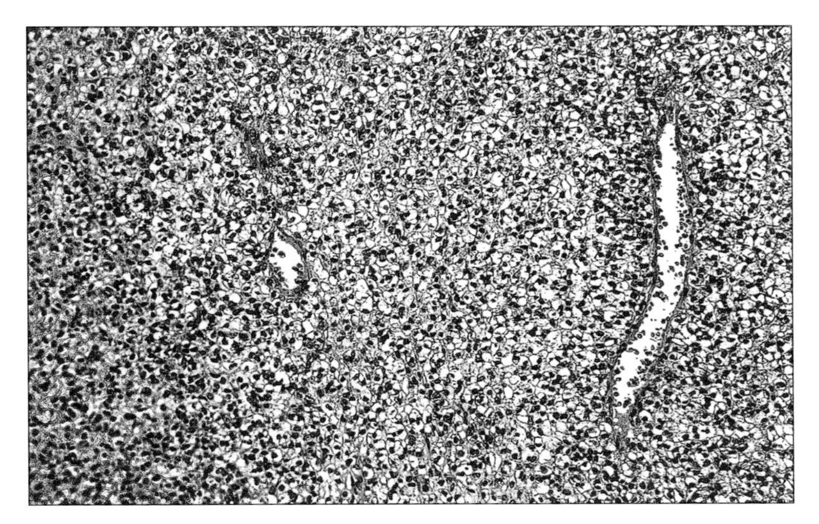

Fig. 4.90 Sertoli cell tumor showing a clear cell pattern.

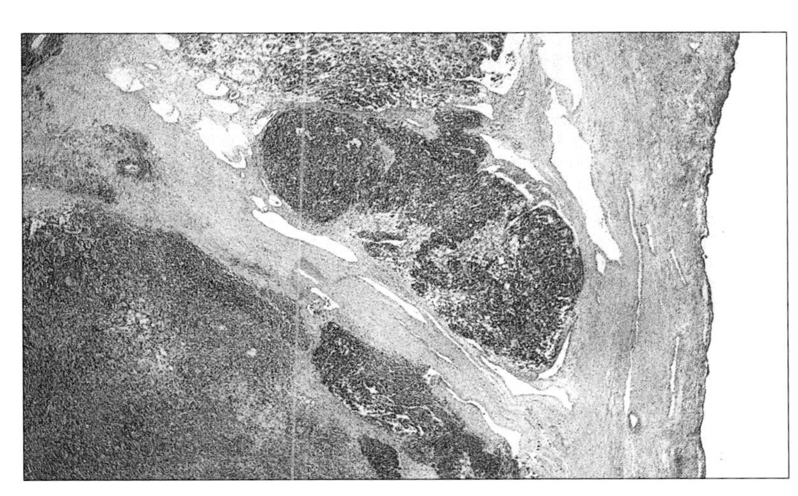

Fig. 4.93 Malignant Sertoli cell tumor invading the testis and reaching close to the tunica albuginea.

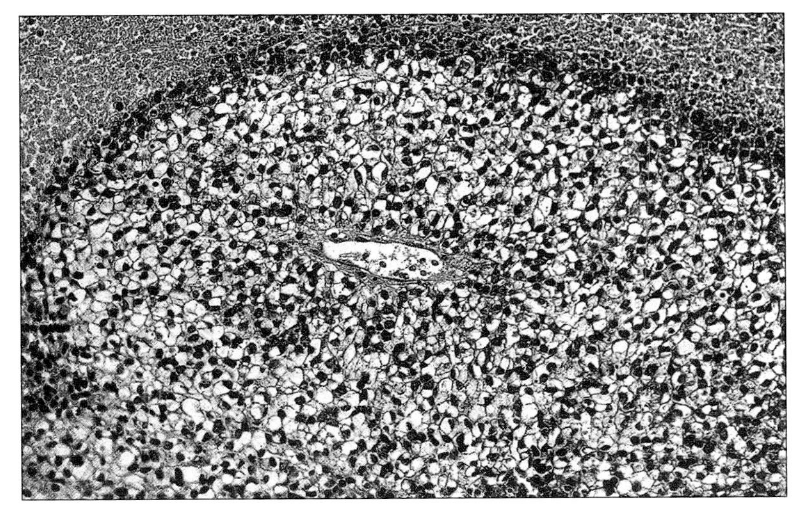

Fig. 4.91 Sertoli cell tumor composed of aggregates of uniform cells with clear cytoplasm. Note the necrosis (top).

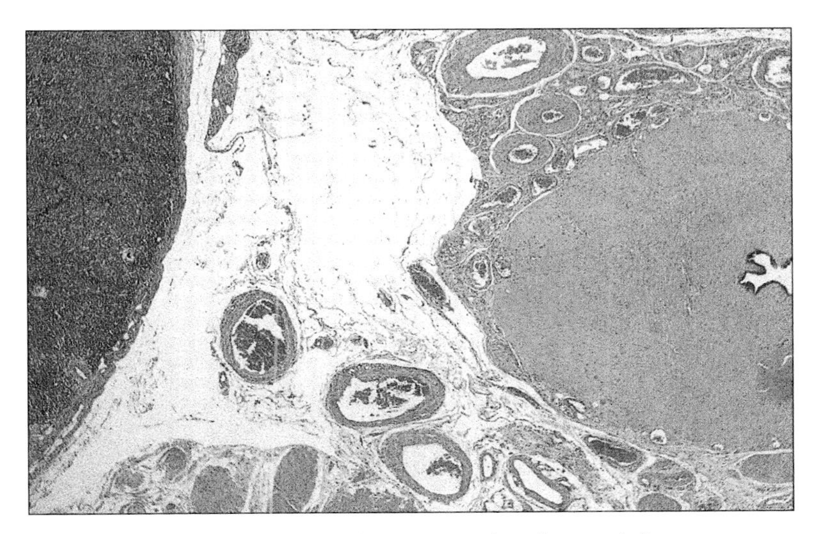

Fig. 4.94 Malignant Sertoli cell tumor invading the vas deferens.

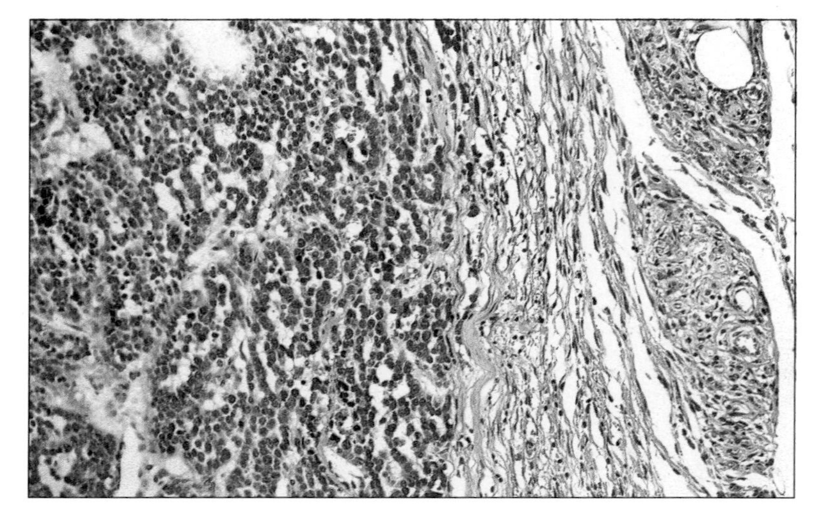

Fig. 4.95 Malignant Sertoli cell tumor showing tubular and solid patterns.

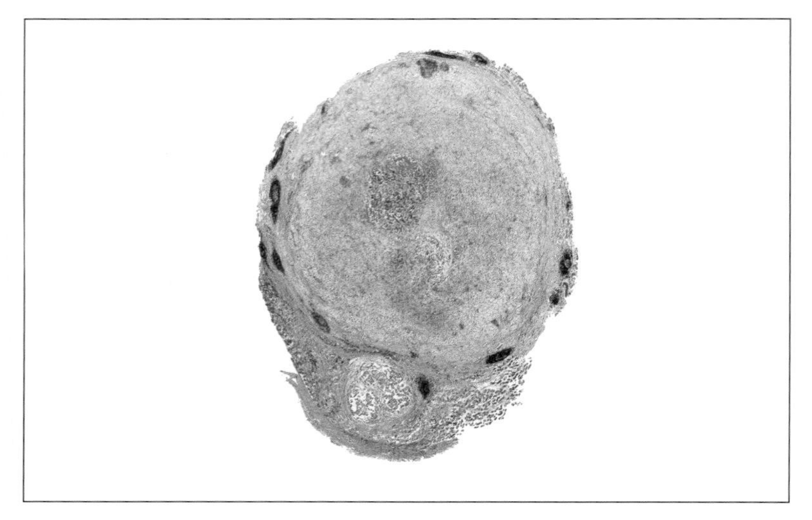

Fig. 4.96 Large cell calcifying Sertoli cell tumor replacing most of the testis. Note the nodularity and large collections of lymphocytes (blue).

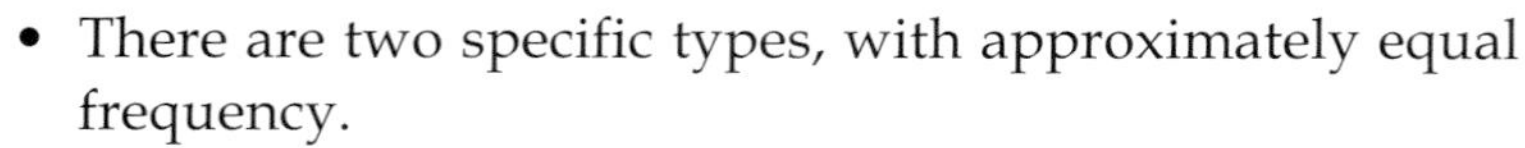

- There are two specific types, with approximately equal frequency.
- One type is frequently bilateral, associated with a variety of abnormalities, and nearly always benign.
- The bilaterality is frequently synchronous, but may be asynchronous.[1-5]
- The associated abnormalities include Carney's complex, gynecomastia, sexual precocity, and Peutz–Jeghers syndrome.[1-5,79-83]
- The other type is unilateral, not associated with any specific abnormalities, but malignant in 15% of cases.[79]
- Patients with benign tumors have ranged from 2 to 38 years of age.[79-83] Malignant tumors have been reported only in adults, with an age range of 28–51 years.[79]
- Patients present with a small, hard or firm testicular mass.
- Excision of the tumor(s) is the treatment of choice. The malignant tumors are usually slow growing and metastasis is a late occurence.[79] Response to radiation and chemotherapy is poor.[79]

Pathologic findings

Macroscopic

- The tumors are usually small, but the malignant variants tend to be large.
- The tumors are frequently multifocal (60%).[79-83]
- They are well circumscribed, firm to hard, yellow to tan, and often gritty due to calcification.[1-5,79-83]

Microscopic[1-5,79-83]

- Architecture is variable. Sheets, nest, trabeculae, or clusters may be seen in addition to tubules.
- Tumor calcification is characteristic and may be massive, occurring as large laminated nodules.
- Cell shape and cytoplasm quality are both variable. Large rounded cells with abundant, eosinophilic,

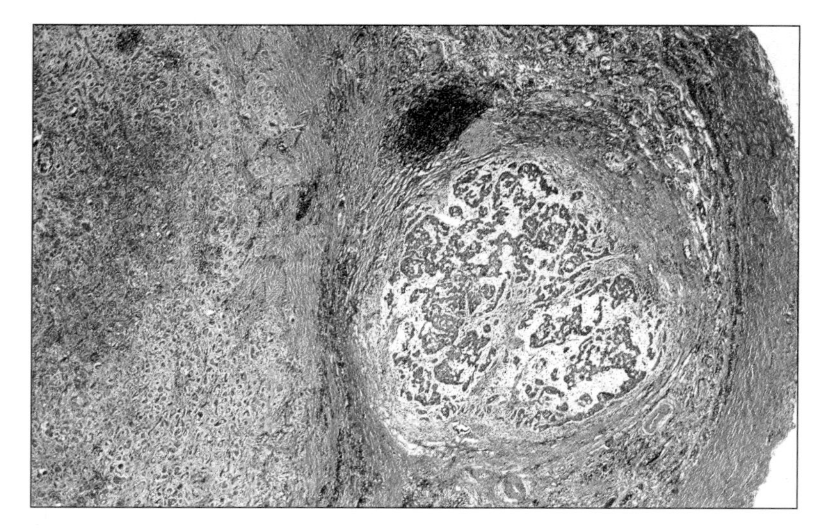

Fig. 4.97 Higher magnification of Fig. 4.96, showing nodularity, dense connective tissue, and lymphocytic aggregates.

granular sytoplasm are typical. Nuclei are small and oval with inconspicuous nucleoli. Mitotic figures are rare.
- A lymphocytic infiltrate is usually present and may be prominent.
- Adjacent foci of intratubular tumor are found in about half of cases.[79]
- Malignant variants show invasive margins, pleomorphism, and mitotic activity.
- Ultrastructurally, tumor cells show features of Sertoli cells. In a few cases Charcot–Böttcher filaments have been identified.[81,82]

Special studies

- Lipid can be demonstrated by histochemical stains.
- The immunohistochemical reactions are similar to those in typical Sertoli cell tumor.

(Figs 4.96–4.99)

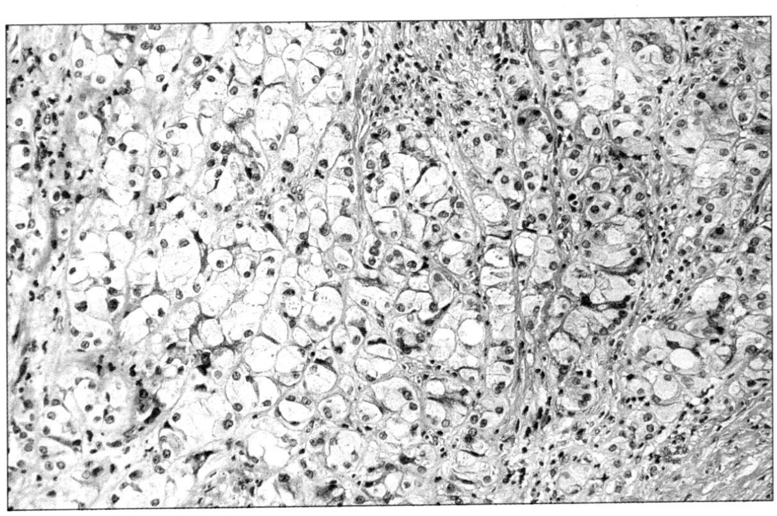

Fig. 4.98 Large cell calcifying Sertoli cell tumor composed of large polygonal cells with clear or slightly granular cytoplasm and small, round nuclei.

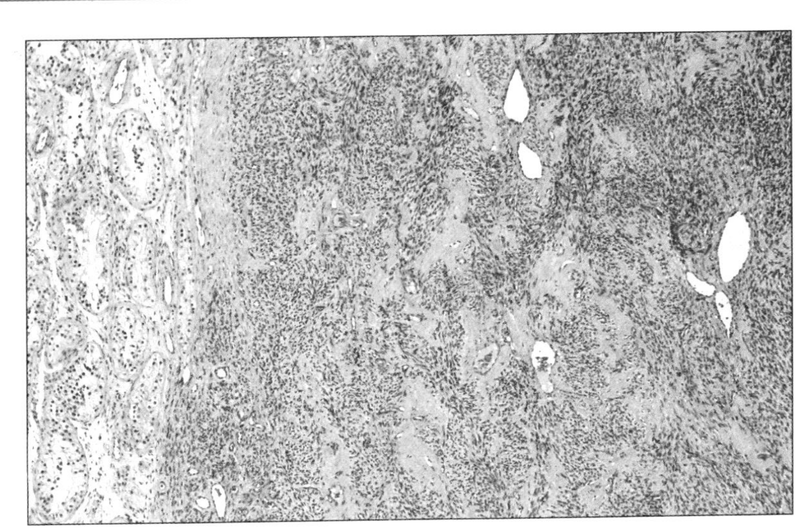

Fig. 4.100 Sclerosing Sertoli cell tumor composed of solid collections of Sertoli cells surrounded by bands of dense hyaline connective tissue.

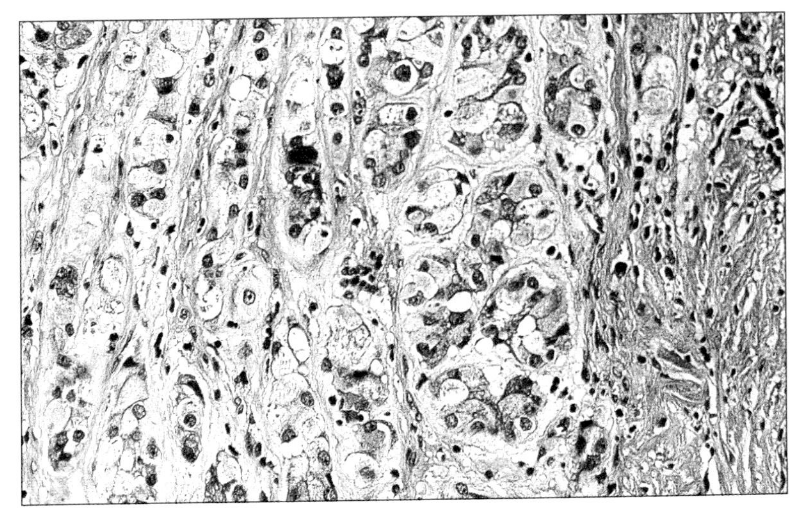

Fig. 4.99 Large cell calcifying Sertoli cell tumor showing the cellular appearances and a calcific concretion (center).

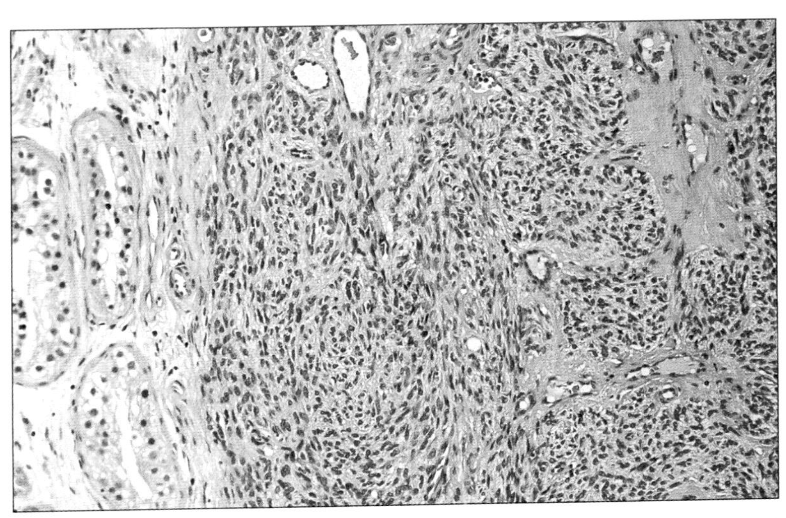

Fig. 4.101 Sclerosing Sertoli cell tumor composed of solid collections of Sertoli cells devoid of specific pattern and surrounded by dense connective tissue.

Sclerosing or hyalinizing Sertoli cell tumor

Clinical findings

- Sclerosing or hyalinizing Sertoli cell tumor is rare.
- There is no specific age predilection.
- Patients present with testicular enlargement.
- The tumor is not associated with endocrine manifestations.
- The clinical course is indolent.
- The tumor is benign.[1-5,84,85]

Pathologic findings

Macroscopic

- The tumor is usually small (less than 1.5 cm in diameter).
- It is solid, firm, white-yellow to tan, and well circumscribed.[84,85]

Microscopic

- It is composed of cords, trabeculae, nests, and tubules, surrounded by dense, fibrous, often hyalinized and hypocellular connective tissue.[84,85]
- The tumor cells have pale eosinophilic cytoplasm and may contain lipid vacuoles.[84]
- The nuclei vary from small hyperchromatic to larger and vesicular.
- Cytologic atypia and mitotic activity are usually present and may be prominent.[84,85]

Special studies

- Immunocytochemical studies show positive staining for vimentin, cytokeratin, and SMA.
- PLAP is negative.[2,84,85]

(Figs 4.100 & 4.101)

Lipid-rich Sertoli cell tumor

Clinical findings

- This is a rare variant of Sertoli cell tumor.
- There is no specific age predilection, but it is seen mainly in adults.
- It is frequently associated with feminizing manifestations.
- Patients present with painless testicular enlargement or feminizing manifestations.
- The tumor has an indolent clinical course.
- The treatment is orchiectomy, which results in disappearance of endocrine manifestations and complete cure.[86]

Pathologic findings

Macroscopic

- The tumors are small, solid, soft, yellow, and well circumscribed.[86]

Microscopic

- The tumor is composed of sheets or aggregates of large uniform cells with clear cytoplasm and small hyperchromatic nuclei.
- Usually there is only a small amount of connective tissue forming fine septa.
- Mitotic activity is low.
- Some cells may be disrupted and small clear cellular lakes may be present.
- The cells contain a large amount of lipid.[86]

Special studies

- Lipid stains are intensely positive.[86]
- Immunocytochemical reactions are similar to those seen in typical Sertoli cell tumor, but may be less intense.

Infantile Sertoli cell tumor (juvenile granulosa cell tumor)

Although this tumor is known as juvenile granulosa cell tumor of the testis, the tumor originates from Sertoli cells and not granulosa cells. This is best seen in areas with intratubular involvement at the edge of the tumor where there is proliferation of immature Sertoli cells. Some of the changes in the tubules are at a slightly later stage, with formation of the cystic spaces so characteristic of this tumor. It is this feature and other similarities to the juvenile granulosa cell tumor of the ovary that has led to the tumor being recognized as a juvenile granulosa cell tumor. Some tumors of this type are admixed with typical clear cell Sertoli cell tumors, further indicating their Sertoli cell origin.

Clinical findings

- Infantile Sertoli cell tumor is rare.[2,87,88]
- It occurs only in newborns and very young infants.
- In this group, it is the most common testicular neoplasm.[2,87,88]
- It may be associated with gonadal dysgenesis and chromosomal abnormalities affecting the Y chromosome.[2,89]
- Patients present with testicular enlargement and may present with maldescent.
- There are no endocrine abnormalities.
- It is benign.
- It is treated by orchiectomy.[87,88]

Pathologic findings

Macroscopic

- The tumor is usually small, but size varies (0.8–6 cm in diameter).
- It is both solid and cystic.
- The cysts contain clear or pale yellow fluid.[87,88]

Microscopic

- At the edge of the tumor are enlarged seminiferous tubules filled with proliferating Sertoli cells.
- Small cystic spaces in the center of the tubule resemble follicles.
- Some of the cystic spaces expand, forming cysts lined by Sertoli cells.
- Partial loss of the cellular lining is seen in some of the cysts.[87,88]
- The fluid within the cyst varies from pale eosinophilic to basophilic.
- The tumor cells form large solid aggregates, which may have a cystic space in the center.[87,88]
- The tumor cells are polyhedral or rounded, with an ample amount of pale eosinophilic or clear cytoplasm.
- The nuclei are round or oval, and hyperchromatic.
- Mitotic activity is evident and may be brisk.
- Cellular and nuclear pleomorphism is absent.
- The solid cellular aggregates are surrounded by connective tissue, which may be prominent, dense, and hyalinized.[87,88]

Special studies

- Immunocytochemical studies show vimentin and SMA positivity.
- Cytokeratin is focally positive in 20–30% of cases.[87,88]

(Figs 4.102 & 4.103)

Granulosa cell tumor (adult granulosa cell tumor)

Clinical findings

- Granulosa cell tumor is rare in the testis.
- There are fewer than 20 well-documented cases.[90,91]
- There is no specific age predominance.
- It is reported in children but not in elderly males.

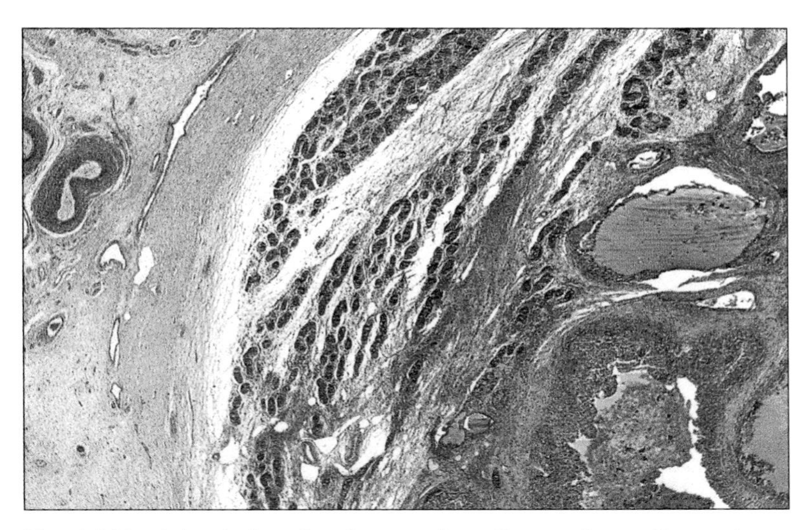

Fig. 4.102 Infantile Sertoli cell tumor (juvenile granulosa cell tumor). There is neoplastic transformation of the seminiferous tubules at the edge of the tumor, with Sertoli cell proliferation, enlargement, and cyst formation. Larger follicle-like cysts, some showing hemorrhage, are present.

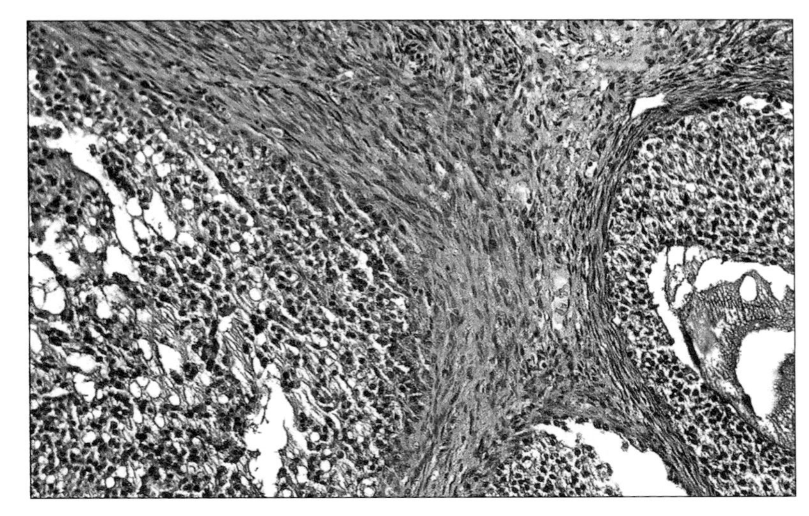

Fig. 4.103 Infantile Sertoli cell tumor showing the follicle-like structures, one solid and one cystic, composed of uniform clear cells similar to those seen in Sertoli cell tumors of the clear cell type.

- Patients present with testicular enlargement or gynecomastia.
- The tumor is usually benign.[90-92]
- Metastasis is rare.[92]
- The treatment is orchiectomy.

Pathologic findings

Macroscopic

- Tumors range from 1.3 to 13 cm in diameter.
- They are well demarcated from surrounding testicular tissue.
- Tumors are solid, homogeneous, yellow to yellow–gray, firm, and somewhat lobulated.[90-92]

Microscopic

- The appearance is similar to that of ovarian adult granulosa cell tumors.[90-92]
- The diffuse and microfollicular patterns with Call–Exner bodies are most common.[90,91]
- Trabecular and cord-like patterns may be present.
- The cells are uniform with scanty cytoplasm and ovoid or rounded nuclei.
- The nuclei may have grooves.
- Occasionally, cytologic atypia may be present.
- Mitotic activity is low.[90,91]

Special studies

- Immunohistochemical studies show inhibin-alpha and vimentin positivity.[2,91]
- Cytokeratin is positive in 20–30% of cases.
- SMA and PLAP are negative.[2,91]

Unclassified and mixed gonadal stromal tumors

This group consists of sex cord stromal tumors that cannot be assigned to any of the previous categories because they either are poorly differentiated or mixed. Although Sertoli–Leydig cell tumor is common in the ovary, combined tumors are rare in the testis.

Clinical findings

- These tumors occur mainly in adults, with no specific age predilection.[87,93]
- Patients present with testicular enlargement.
- Gynecomastia may be present.[87,93]
- The behavior is unpredictable; some are malignant.[87,93,94]
- Orchiectomy is the treatment of choice.
- Long-term follow-up is advisable.
- Malignant variants do not respond well to radiation or chemotherapy.[87,93,94]

Pathologic findings

Macroscopic

- The tumors vary in size from small nodules to large masses replacing the whole testis.
- They are well circumscribed, yellow–white, solid, and lobulated.
- Necrosis and hemorrhage are uncommon but may be seen, especially in large tumors.[87,93,94]

Microscopic

- The unclassified tumors are usually composed of large aggregates of spindle-shaped cells without any specific pattern.
- Some unclassified tumors may be composed of a large number of epithelial-like cells.[87]
- Cellular and nuclear pleomorphism may be evident and may be marked.[87,93,94]
- Mitotic activity is usually evident and may be brisk.
- The mixed tumors, which are uncommon, consist of typical components like Leydig cell tumor, Sertoli cell

tumor, and adult granulosa cell tumor in varying proportions.
- Mixed tumors are usually benign.[87,93]

Special studies
- The findings depend on the composition of the tumor.
- Vimentin and SMA are positive.
- Cytokeratin may be focally positive.
- Inhibin-alpha may be positive.[2]

TUMORS COMPOSED OF GERM CELLS AND SEX CORD DERIVATIVES

Tumors composed of germ cells and sex cord derivatives intimately intermixed are divided into two specific types:

- gonadoblastoma;
- mixed germ cell–sex cord stromal tumor (MGC-SCST).

Gonadoblastoma

Clinical findings
- Gonadoblastoma is uncommon; about 150 cases have been reported.[4–6]
- It usually occurs in dysgenetic gonads, in phenotypic females (80%), less often in male pseudohermaphrodites (20%).[6,95,96]
- The latter usually present with cryptorchidism, hypospadias, and female internal secondary sex organs.[95,96]
- The affected gonads are usually intra-abdominal and are either testes, streak gonads, or indeterminate.
- Gonadoblastoma is occasionally found in true hermaphrodites and rarely in normal ovaries or testes.[6,96]
- All reported cases have been in patients under 30 years of age.[6,95,96]
- It is bilateral in approximately 50% of cases.
- Phenotypically male patients present with developmental abnormalities affecting the genitalia, problems with gender assignment, and abdominal enlargement due to a gonadal tumor.[95,96]
- The majority of patients have 46,XY karyotype or various forms of mosaicism.[95,96]
- Occasionally there is familial incidence.
- Gonadoblastoma proper is benign. However, it is frequently (60%) overgrown by a malignant germ cell neoplasm, most often classical seminoma. In that case, metastases may be present.[6,95,96]
- Gonadoblastoma must be treated by excision of the affected gonad and of the contralateral gonad, which harbors undetected gonadoblastoma in 50% of cases.[6,95,96]

Pathologic findings

Macroscopic
- Gonadoblastoma is small or very small, ranging in size from microscopic to several centimeters in diameter.
- When overgrown by a neoplastic germ cell element, the tumors are larger.
- It is solid, varies from gray to light tan, firm to hard, and is often gritty due to calcification.[1–6,95,96] It may be totally calcified.

Microscopic
- Gonadoblastoma is composed of tumor nests surounded by connective tissue.[1,6,95,96]
- The nests are usually small, solid, and round or oval, and are composed of germ cells and sex cord derivatives resembling immature Sertoli and granulosa cells.
- The germ cells are large and round with clear or slightly granular cytoplasm and large round vesicular nuclei with prominent nucleoli.
- Mitotic activity may be brisk.
- The germ cells show similar histologic, histochemical, and ultrastructural appearances to classical seminoma and normal germ cells.[1,6,95,96]
- The germ cells are intimately intermixed with the sex cord derivatives, which are smaller and epithelioid. They have hyperchromatic, oval, or elongated (carrot-shaped) nuclei. They lack mitotic activity.[1,6,95,96]
- The sex cord derivatives are arranged in three typical patterns:[1,6,95,96]
  lining the periphery of the nests in a coronal arrangement;
  surrounding individual germ cells;
  surrounding small, round spaces containing amorphous, eosinophilic, hyaline, PAS-positive basement membrane material, forming structures resembling Call–Exner bodies. Some of these structures may be calcified.
- The connective tissue surrounding the cellular nests varies from loose and edematous to dense and hyalinized. It may contain luteinized stromal, Leydig-like cells devoid of Reinke crystals.[1,6,95,96]
- The basic appearances of gonadoblastoma may be altered by three processes: hyalinization; calcification; overgrowth by a tumor, most likely a classical seminoma. Any of these processes, when extensive, may lead to obliteration of the gonadoblastoma.[1,6,95,96]

Special studies
- Determination of the karyotype is definitive.[1,6,95,96]
- The tumor cells show reactions typical of germ cells and sex cord derivatives.[2,6]

(Figs 4.104 & 4.105)

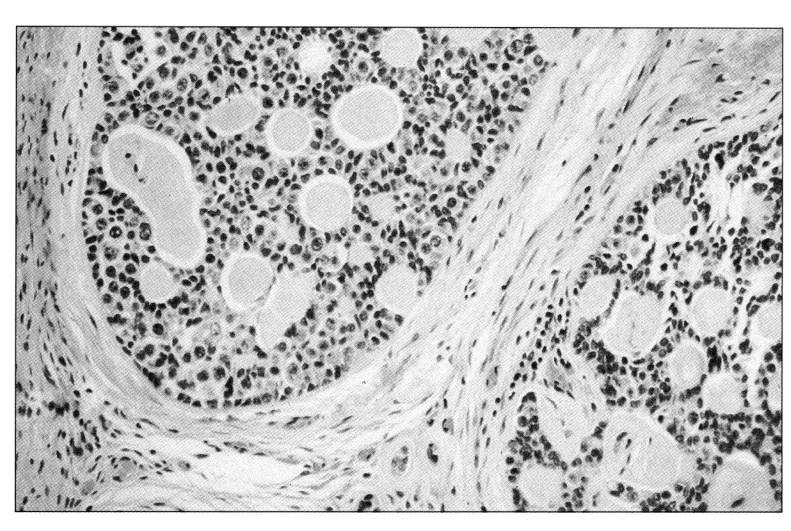

Fig. 4.104 Gonadoblastoma. Two nests composed of germ cells and sex cord derivatives and containing numerous round, eosinophilic, amorphous hyaline bodies.

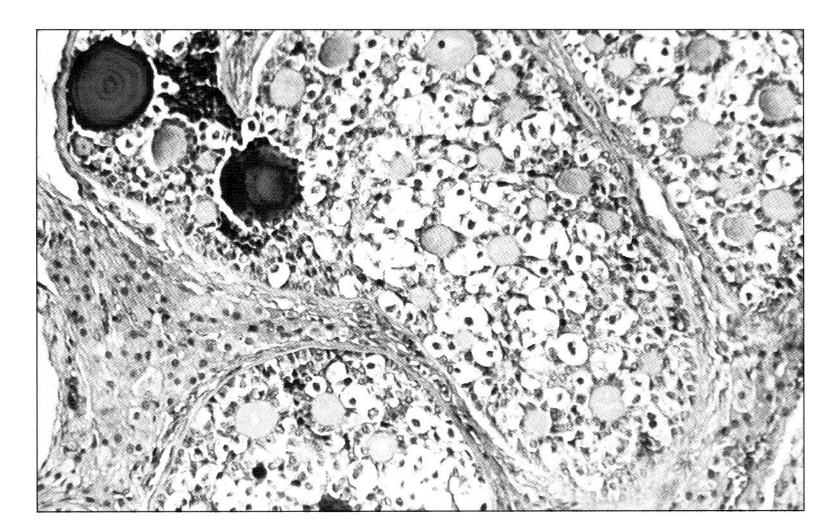

Fig. 4.105 Gonadoblastoma. The tumor nests, in addition to the germ cells, sex cord derivatives, and hyaline bodies, also contain laminated calcific concretions. The surrounding connective tissue contains luteinized stromal Leydig-like cells.

Mixed germ cell–sex cord stromal tumor

Clinical findings

- MGC-SCST is rare as a testicular neoplasm.[6,96]
- It occurs mainly in adults.
- Patients present with testicular enlargement.[6,96–98]
- There is no association with gonadal dysgenesis, anatomic or chromosomal abnormalities.[6,96]
- There are no endocrine abnormalities in males.[6,96,98]
- Fertility is normal.
- In males, all tumors have been benign.[6,96,98]
- Treatment is orchiectomy.

Pathologic findings

Macroscopic

- Tumors vary in size but are much larger than gonadoblastomas.
- They are solid, or partly cystic, gray-white, firm, and well circumscribed.[6,96–98]

Microscopic

- The germ cells and the sex cord derivatives are intimately intermixed.
- Focally, one component may predominate.[6,96,98]
- The germ cells are large, round, with clear or slightly granular cytoplasm and large vesicular nuclei with prominent nucleoli. Mitotic activity varies but is generally low.[96–98]
- The sex cord derivatives resemble immature Sertoli and granulosa cells, and are smaller than the germ cells. The cytoplasm is scanty and the nuclei are large, ovoid, or elongated. Mitotic activity may be brisk.[6,96,98]
- The tumor shows three different histologic patterns:[6,96]
  cord-like or trabecular, composed of large ramifying cords or clusters;
  tubular, composed of solid tubules surrounded by fine connective tissue septa;
  haphazard, composed of aggregates of germ cells and sex cord derivatives devoid of any specific arrangement.
- The haphazard pattern is the most common.
- Sometimes the tumor may contain cystic spaces lined by sex cord cells similar to those seen in cystic sex cord stromal tumors.
- Testicular MGC-SCSTs have been seen only in pure form.[6,96–98]

Special studies

- Karyotyping shows normal male 46,XY karyotype.
- The germ cells and the sex cord derivatives show characteristic histochemical and immunocytochemical reactions.[6,98]

(Figs 4.106–4.109)

HEMATOPOIETIC NEOPLASMS

Malignant lymphoma

Malignant lymphoma of the testis is divided into two main types:

- primary malignant lymphoma of the testis (extranodal malignant lymphoma involving the testis);
- testicular involvement as a secondary manifestation of systemic malignant lymphoma.

Clinical findings

- The primary type is rare.[99]
- The majority of cases are secondary and usually a late manifestation of disseminated disease.[99–105]
- Malignant lymphoma of both types accounts for approximately 5% of testicular neoplasms.[99,100]

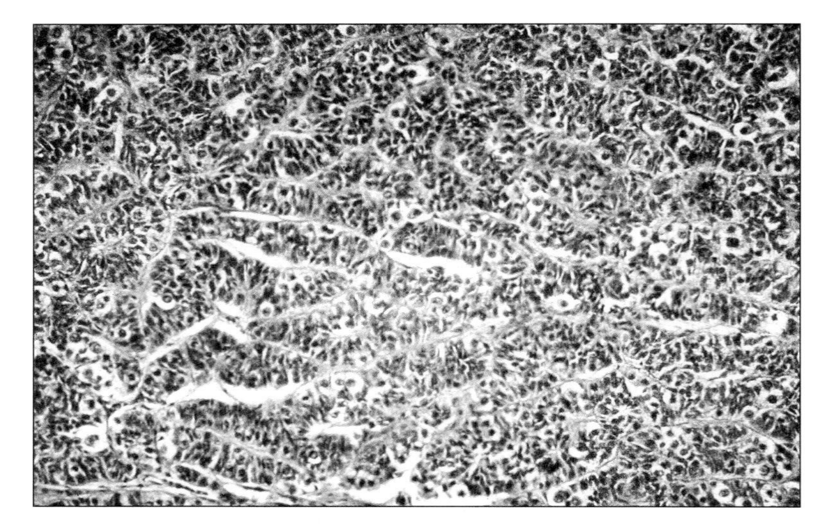

Fig. 4.106 Mixed germ cell–sex cord stromal tumor showing a tubular pattern and composed of solid tubules without a lumen surrounded by fine connective tissue septa.

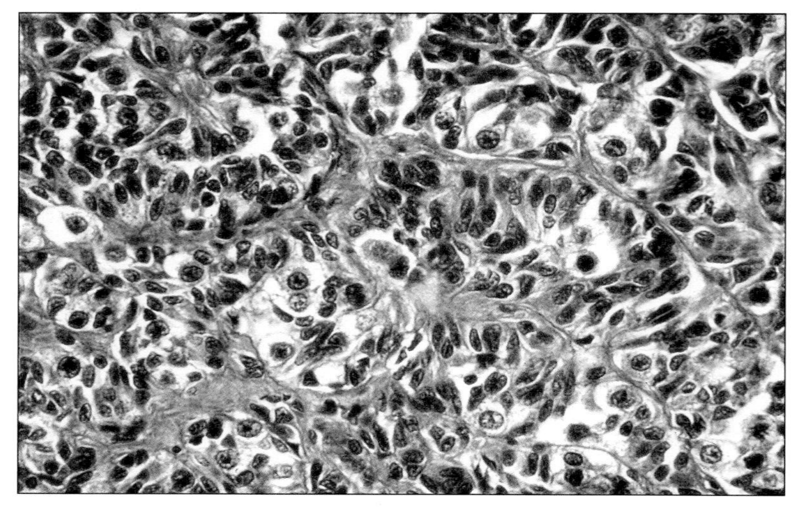

Fig. 4.107 Mixed germ cell–sex cord stromal tumor showing a tubular pattern. The sex cord derivatives composed of ovoid cells with prominent elongated or carrot-shaped nuclei line the periphery of the tubule and surround large round germ cells with prominent round vesicular nuclei.

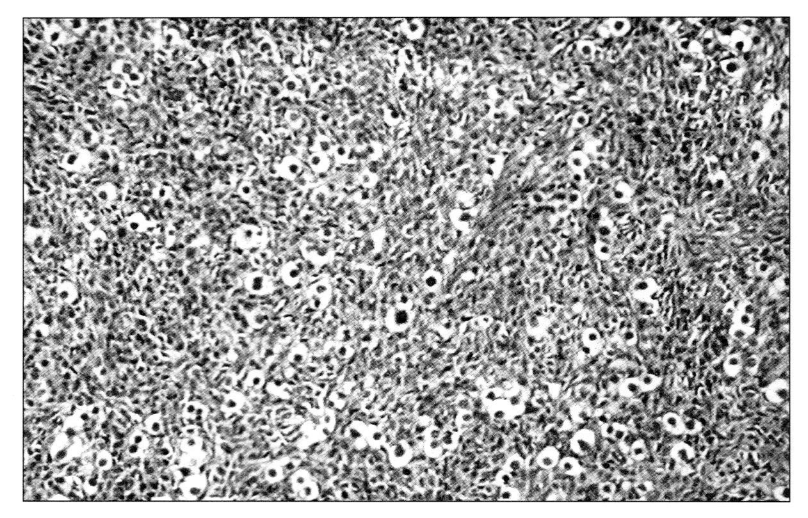

Fig. 4.108 Mixed germ cell–sex cord stromal tumor showing the haphazard pattern. Large aggregates of sex cord derivatives devoid of any specific pattern surround large round germ cells with clear cytoplasm.

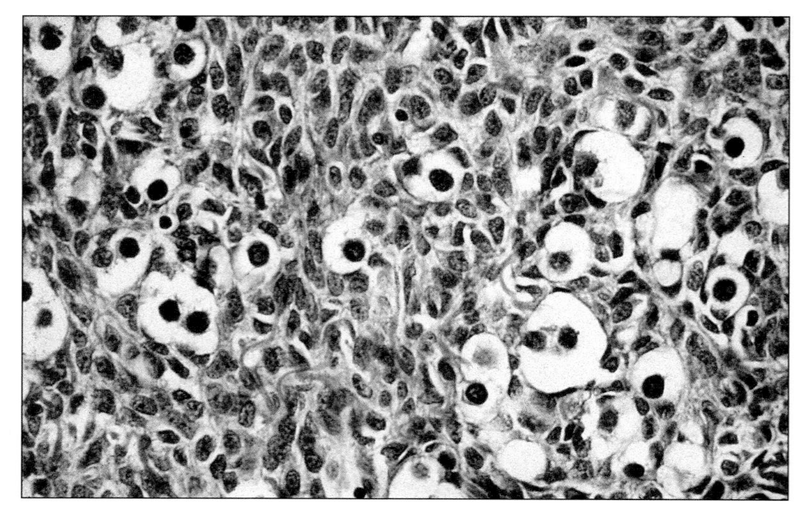

Fig. 4.109 Mixed germ cell–sex cord stromal tumor showing the haphazard pattern. Note the large round germ cells with clear cytoplasm and the more numerous smaller sex cord derivatives.

- It is the most common malignant testicular neoplasm of men over 60 years of age and accounts for 50% of testicular neoplasms in this age group.
- It is bilateral in more than 30% of cases and is the most common bilateral testicular neoplasm.
- The bilaterality may be synchronous or, more often, asynchronous.[99–105]
- The patients present with testicular enlargement, which is usually painless.
- Systemic symptoms are rare in cases of primary testicular type.[99–105]
- The prognosis is much better in the primary type.[98]
- Sclerosis is a favorable prognostic feature.
- There is a 15–30% 2-year survival rate in patients with the secondary type, whereas long-term survival is common in patients with the primary type.[99–105]
- Treatment is orchiectomy followed by appropriate chemotherapy.

Pathologic findings

Macroscopic

- The tumor forms a large mass or, less frequently, multiple nodules, and involves the epididymis in 50% of cases.[99–105]
- The tumor is uniform, white–yellow to tan, fleshy and firm.
- Necrosis is uncommon.[99–105]

Microscopic

- Marked intertubular infiltration by densely packed lymphoma cells is the main finding.
- The lymphoma cells also invade, fill, and efface the seminiferous tubules in at least 35% of cases.[99–105]

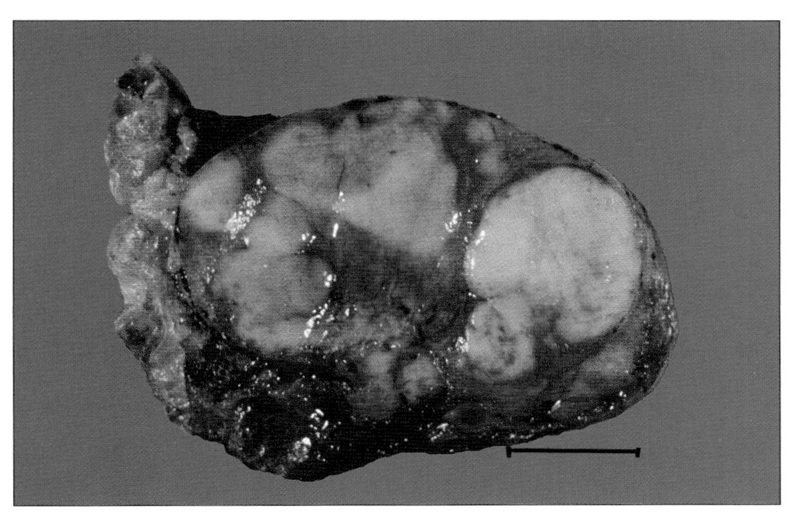

Fig. 4.110 Malignant lymphoma. The tumor shows a nodular pattern and extensive involvement of the testis.

- Discrimination from seminoma is helped by finding unaffected seminiferous tubules within the mass. Reticulin stains highlight the normal distribution of intratubular fibrils, in contrast to their marked condensation in seminoma.
- Sclerosis may be present and may be marked.
- Extratesticular spread is common.[99–105]
- Most testicular lymphomas (over 90%) are of the B-cell type.[104] Diffuse large cell lymphoma is the most common type.[99–105]
- Burkitt's lymphoma frequently affects the testis.
- Hodgkin's disease is very rare.

Special studies
- Tumor cells are positive for lymphocyte common antigen (LCA) and for various B-cell and occasionally T-cell markers.
- Cytokeratin and PLAP are negative.[104]

(Figs 4.110 & 4.111)

Multiple myeloma and plasmacytoma

Clinical findings
- Testicular involvement by multiple myeloma occurs in 2% of cases, but in most of these cases it is recognized only at autopsy.[106–109]
- This occurs usually in older males (most common from the fifth decade onwards).[106]
- Systemic manifestations may be present.
- Bilaterality is seen in 30% of cases.[106]

Pathologic findings

Macroscopic
- The appearance is similar to that of malignant lymphoma, showing a solid mass or nodular involvement.

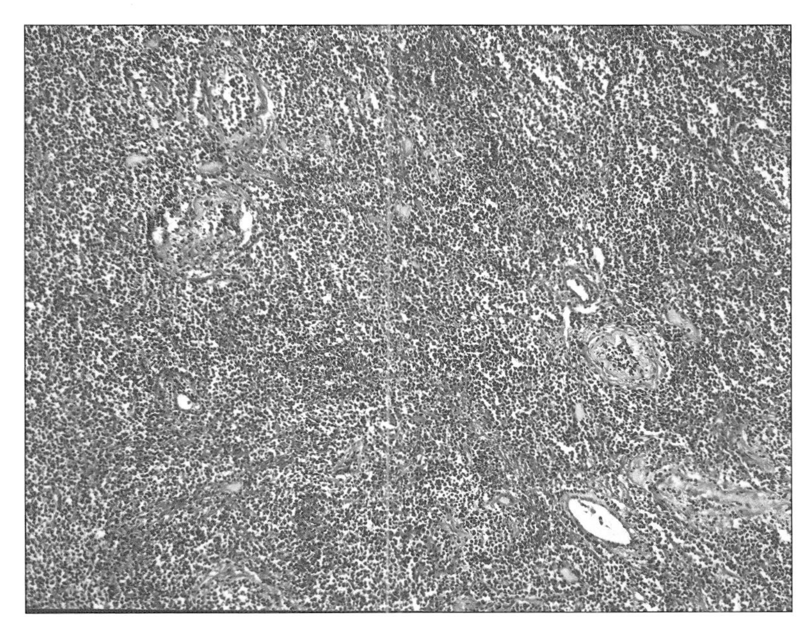

Fig. 4.111 Malignant lymphoma, diffuse large B-cell type. Occasional seminiferous tubules are still visible, but show involvement by the tumor.

- There is a uniform, solid, pink to tan, somewhat lobulated, fleshy to firm mass.[106–109]

Microscopic
- There is proliferation of malignant plasma cells, which vary from mature to highly immature, with giant cells, multinucleated cells, and abnormal forms that invade seminiferous tubules.
- Mitotic activity varies but may be brisk.[106–109]

Special studies
- Serum electrophoresis shows monoclonal gammopathy.
- Bence-Jones protein is usually present in the urine.
- Immunohistochemical staining for immunoglobulins and for kappa and lambda light chains is usually positive.[106–109]
- LCA may be positive, but, in such cases, the tumor is usually a plasmacytoid malignant lymphoma.
- Cytokeratin and PLAP are negative.[106–109]

(Figs 4.112–4.114)

Leukemia

Clinical findings
- Testicular enlargement is seen in 10% of cases of leukemia at autopsy and in 5% of patients with leukemia during life.[110–112]
- It is invariably bilateral and usually asymmetric.[110–112]
- Microscopic leukemic infiltration is seen microscopically at autopsy in 64% of patients with acute leukemia and in 22% of patients with chronic leukemia.

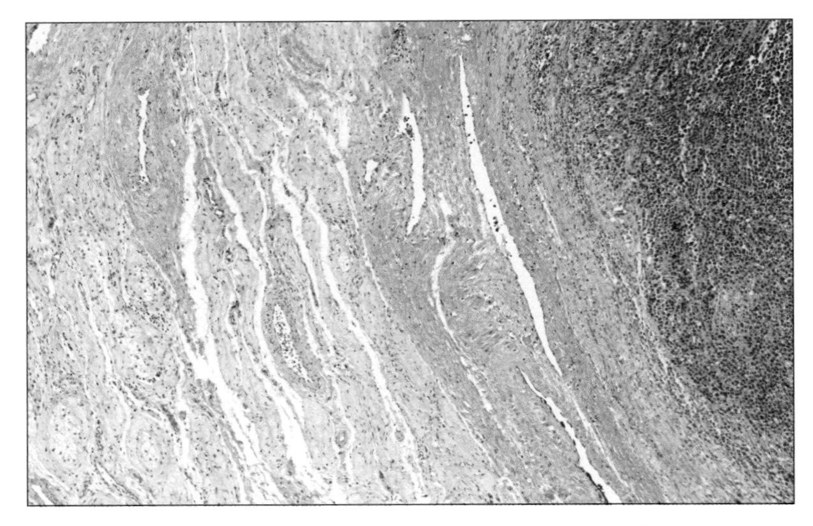

Fig. 4.112 Multiple myeloma involving the testis. Solid cellular tumor replacing testicular tissue.

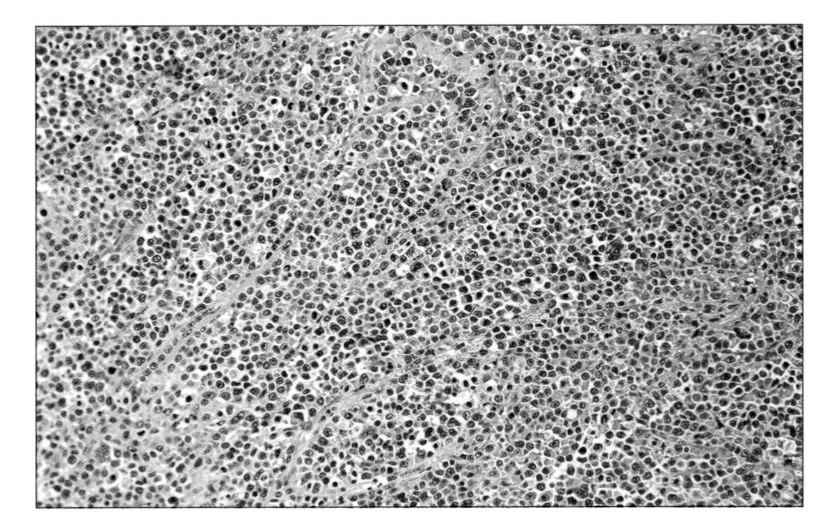

Fig. 4.113 Multiple myeloma involving the testis. The proliferating malignant plasma cells replace testicular tissue.

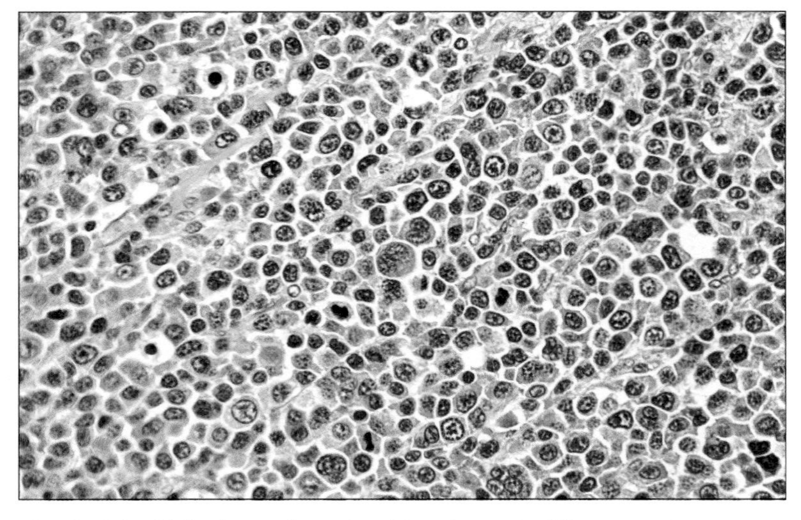

Fig. 4.114 Multiple myeloma involving the testis. The tumor is composed of atypical malignant plasma cells, including binucleated cells and large cells with vesicular nuclei. There is brisk mitotic activity with atypical mitoses.

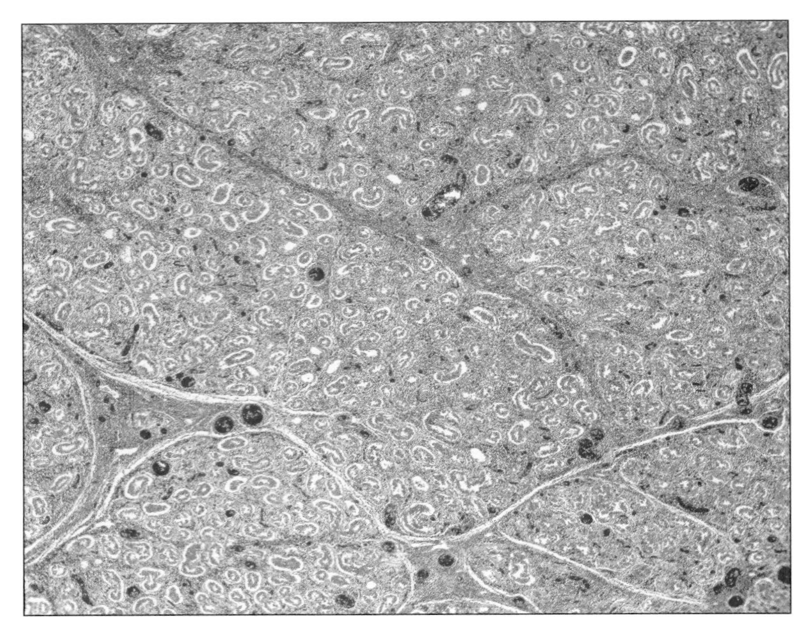

Fig. 4.115 Testis affected by leukemia. Note interstitial involvement and preservation of the seminiferous tubules.

- Testis is an important sanctuary for viable leukemic cells in children treated for lymphoblastic leukemia, and the presence of such cells indicates relapse of the disease.[113]

Pathologic findings

Macroscopic

- Noticeable testicular enlargement is rare.[110–112]

Microscopic

- Interstitial infiltration is the most common finding.
- Involvement of seminiferous tubules occurs but is uncommon.
- The appearance of the neoplastic cells depends on the type of leukemia.[110–112]
- Acute lymphoblastic leukemia occurring in children is most common, as testicular biopsies are performed in order to detect leukemic cells and to diagnose a relapse of the disease at an early stage.[111–113]

Special studies

- Histochemical and immunohistochemical studies should be undertaken to diagnose and confirm the type of leukemia.

(Figs 4.115–4.117)

MISCELLANEOUS NEOPLASMS

Adenomatoid tumor

Adenomatoid tumor is a benign neoplasm of mesothelial origin occurring in the genital tract of both males and females.

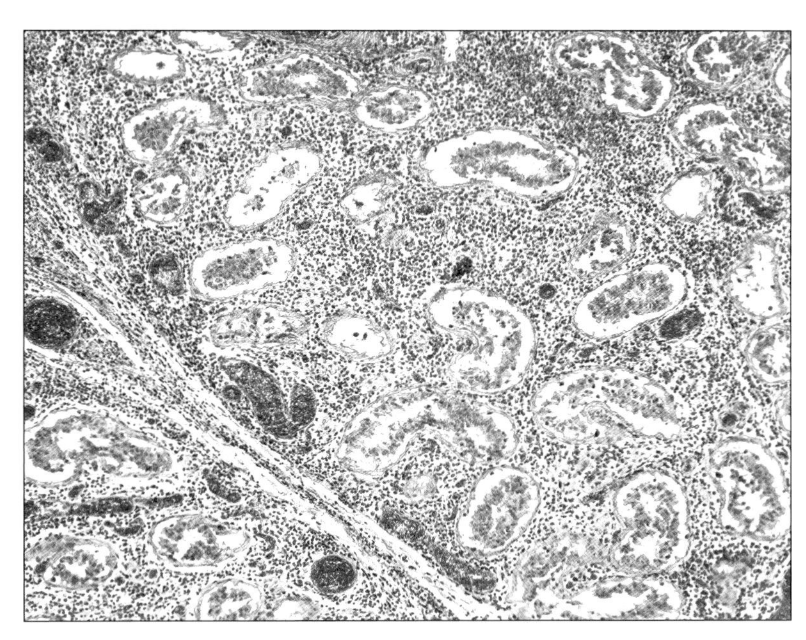

Fig. 4.116 Testis affected by leukemia. Note the dense interstitial infiltration by leukemic cells.

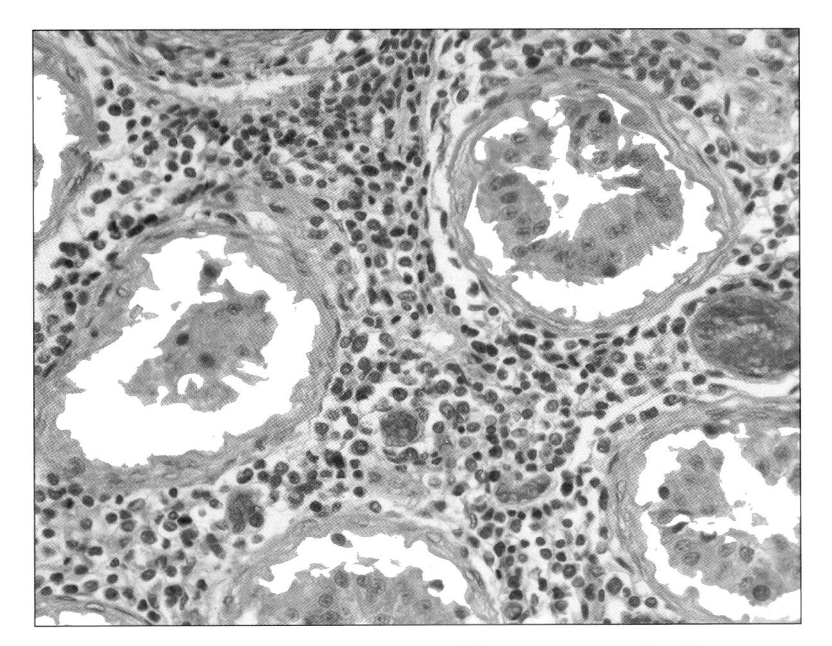

Fig. 4.117 Testis affected by leukemia. There is interstitial infiltration, proliferation of Sertoli cells within the seminiferous tubules, and absence of germ cells.

Clinical findings

- Adenomatoid tumor occurs most frequently in the epididymis, usually at its lower pole.[114,115]
- It may also arise in or beneath the tunica albuginea, within the spermatic cord, or in the testis.
- It is the most common benign neoplasm of the testicular adnexa (60% of cases).
- It is most common from the third to fifth decade, but occurs in all age groups.[114,115]
- Patients present with painless paratesticular enlargement.
- Adenomatoid tumor is invariably unilateral.
- It is benign.
- Treatment is by orchiectomy.[114,115]

Pathologic findings

Macroscopic

- Adenomatoid tumor is solitary, unilateral, and small (usually less than 2 cm, rarely exceeding 5 cm in diameter).
- It is a well-demarcated, gray–white, solid, and firm nodule.[114,115]
- When it involves the testis, it may resemble a classical seminoma.

Microscopic

- The neoplasm is composed of a network of round, oval, or slit-like tubules lined by epithelial-like cells varying from flat to columnar, some of which may contain large intracytoplasmic vacuoles.[114–116]
- Some tumors may show cord-like pattern, cell clusters, and small cysts.
- The cells when columnar may be large and contain an ample amount of dense or vacuolated cytoplasm.
- The nuclei are small and hyperchromatic.
- Mitotic activity is negligible.
- The tubules are surrounded by connective tissue stroma, which is often prominent.[114–116]
- The stroma is usually fibrous and sometimes hyalinized. It may contain smooth muscle.
- Lymphoid aggregates are often seen and may be prominent.
- The tumor may show infiltrative borders.[114–116]
- Ultrastructurally, there are numerous elongated microvilli on the luminal surface and well-developed desmosomes on the lateral cell surface.[116,117]

(Figs 4.118–4.125)

Special studies

- Immunohistochemical staining for cytokeratin is positive.[118]
- Other histochemical stains such as PAS, mucicarmine, and lipid, and immunocytochemical stains such as carcinoembryonic antigen (CEA), S-100, and factor VIII, are negative.[118]

Malignant mesothelioma of the tunica vaginalis

Mesothelioma affecting the tunica vaginalis is invariably malignant,[119] although occasional cases of very well-differentiated benign papillary mesothelioma occurring in this location have been reported.[120]

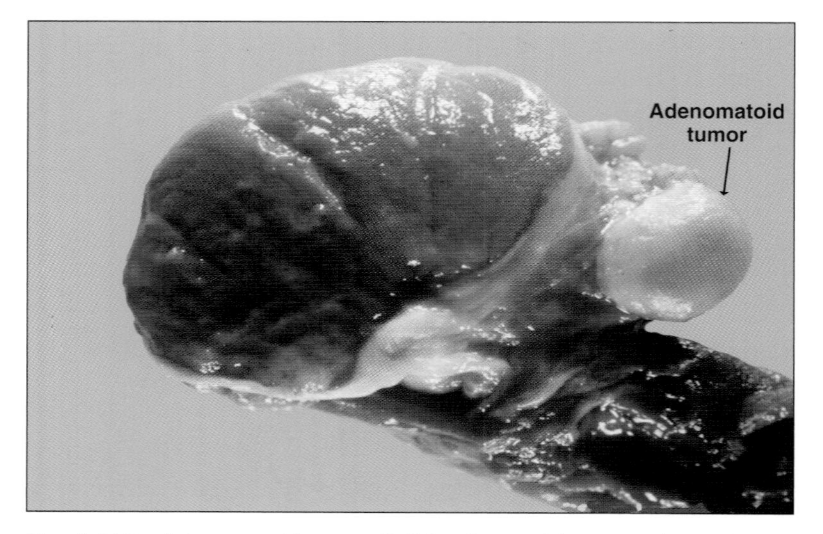

Fig. 4.118 Adenomatoid tumor. Solid, yellow–white tumor located between the testis and the epididymis.

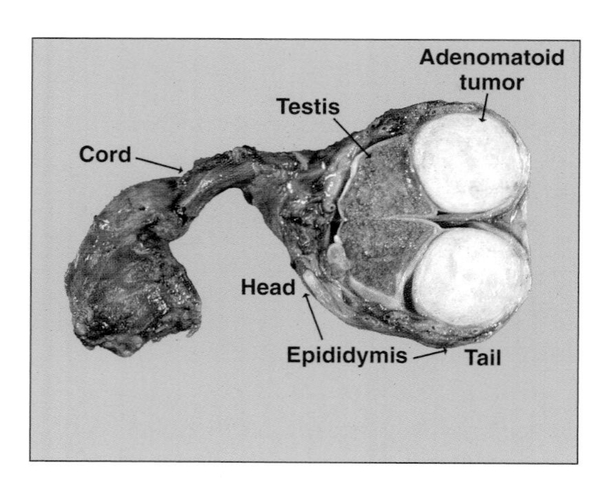

Fig. 4.119 Adenomatoid tumor. Well-demarcated, encapsulated, solid yellow–white tumor compressing the testis.

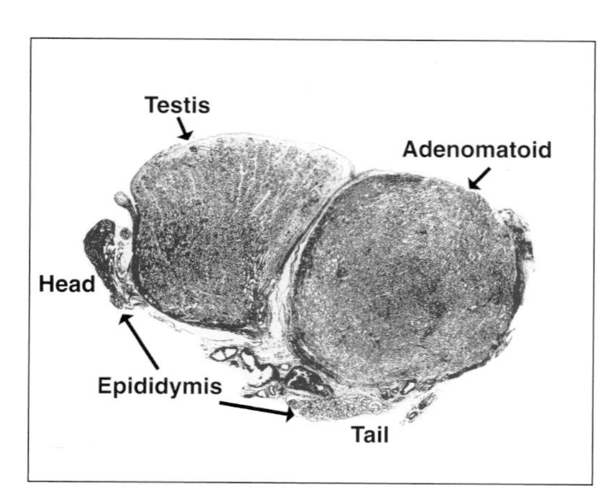

Fig. 4.120 Adenomatoid tumor. Note the relationship to the testis and epididymis.

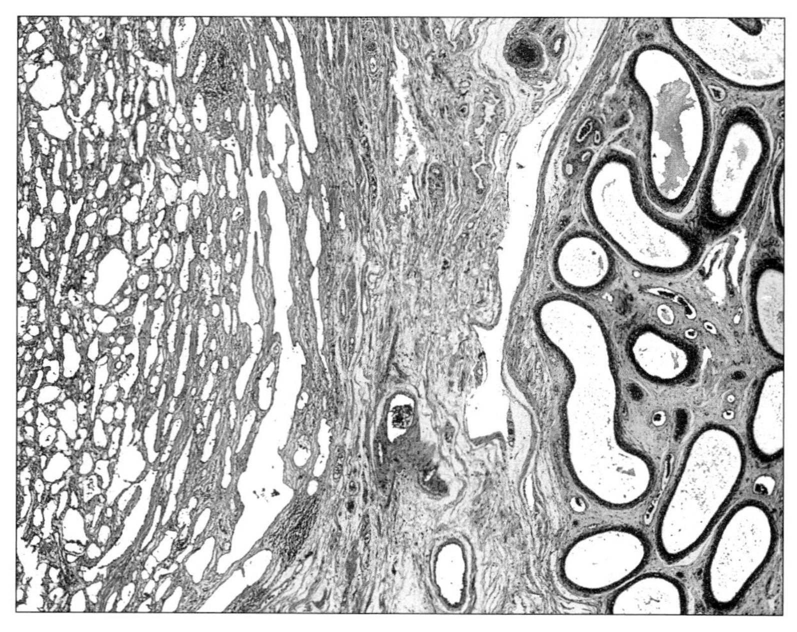

Fig. 4.121 Adenomatoid tumor (left) composed of numerous small spaces, well demarcated from the epididymis (right). Note a few collections of lymphocytes.

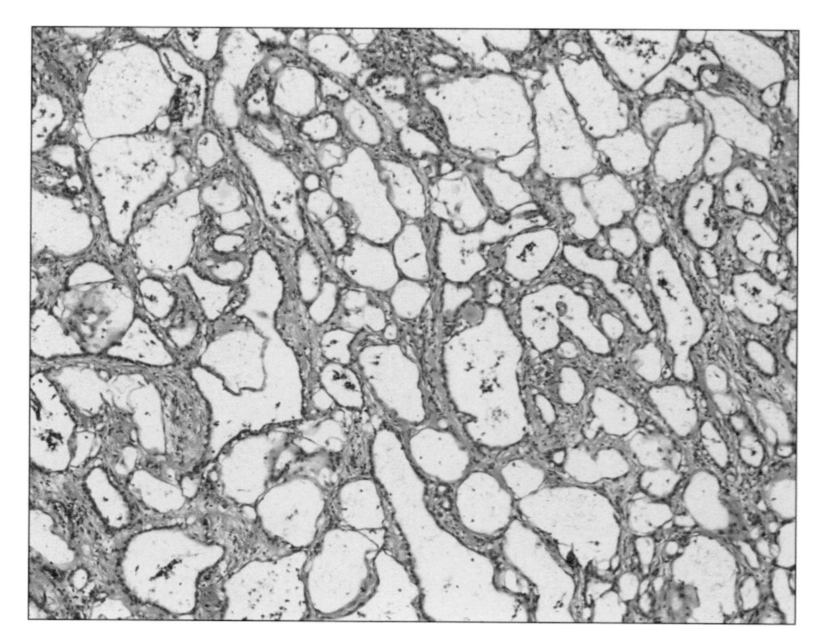

Fig. 4.122 Adenomatoid tumor composed of cystic spaces varying in shape and size surrounded by fibrous connective tissue septa.

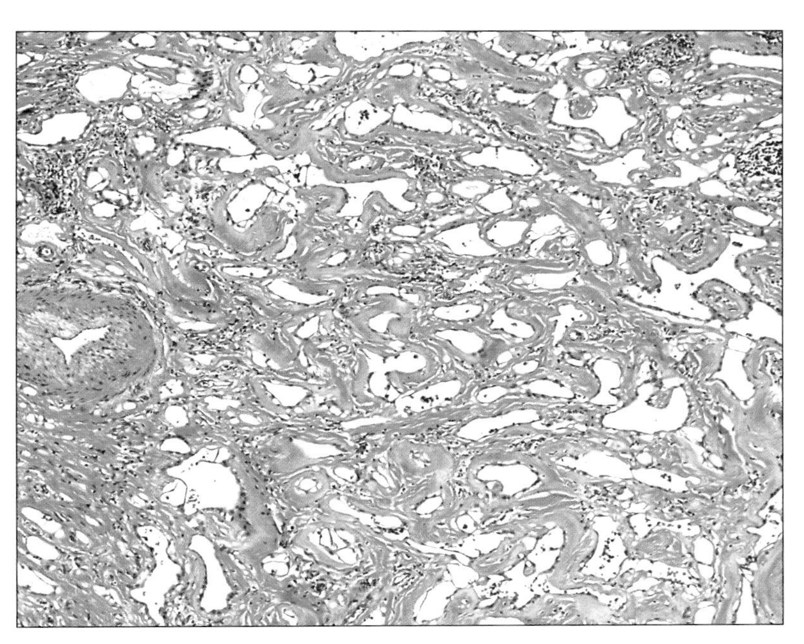

Fig. 4.123 Adenomatoid tumor showing marked hyalinization of the connective tissue surrounding the cystic spaces.

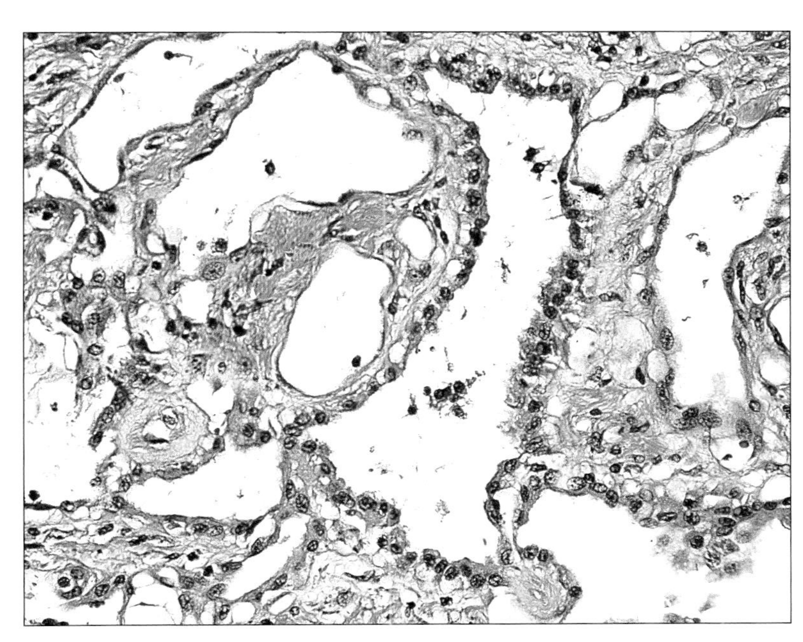

Fig. 4.125 Adenomatoid tumor showing the cystic spaces lined by uniform cuboid cells with granular eosinophilic cytoplasm and uniform round nuclei. Some cells are vacuolated. The surrounding connective tissue is loose and less fibrous.

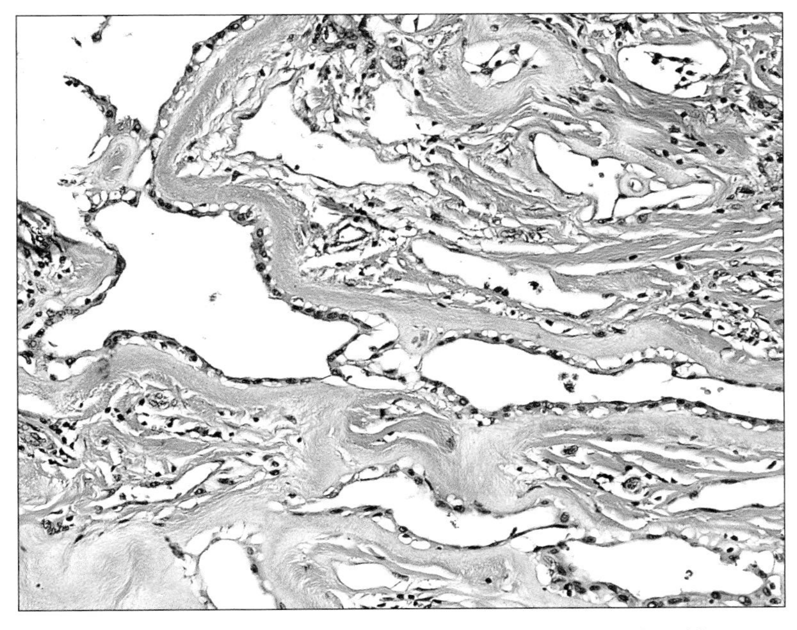

Fig. 4.124 Adenomatoid tumor showing the cystic spaces lined by cuboid cells with vacuolated cytoplasm. There is marked hyalinization of the surrounding connective tissue.

Clinical findings

- This tumor is rare (approximately 30 reported cases).[121-123]
- The age range is from 20 to 75 years, but it is more common in elderly males.
- Patients present with a scrotal mass, often associated with hydrocele, which recurs after tapping.[119,121-123]
- There may be a history of asbestos exposure.[119]

Pathologic findings

Macroscopic

- The tumor forms a partly cystic or solid mass.
- It varies in size (0.6 to 6 cm in diameter).
- Tumor coats the tunica vaginalis or forms numerous nodules on its surface.[119,121-123]

Microscopic

- The tumor has papillary, tubular, diffuse, and, less frequently, biphasic or fibrous patterns, similar to malignant mesotheliomas of the pleural and peritoneal cavities.[119,121-123]
- The cells are typically cuboidal with a moderate amount of eosinophilic cytoplasm and large ovoid vesicular nuclei.
- Sometimes the cells are spindle shaped, with scanty cytoplasm and elongated nuclei.
- Cellular and nuclear pleomorphism, giant cells, and brisk mitotic activity may be present.[119,121-123]
- Invasion of the surrounding structures may be present.[119,121-123]
- Ultrastructurally, the tumor cells show typical features of mesothelioma cells, such as numerous tall slender microvilli, desmosomes, tonofilaments, and mitochondria located near the nucleus.[119]

Special studies

- Immunohistochemical panels used for mesothelioma at other sites are applicable. Useful positive markers include calretinin, WT-1, HBME-1, cytokeratin 5/6, and D2-40.

Tumors of ovarian epithelial types (surface epithelial stromal tumors, Müllerian tumors, excluding Brenner tumor)

Clinical findings

- These tumors are rare.
- They are located either within the testis, in the paratesticular tissue, or involve the tunica vaginalis.
- Age ranges from 14 to 68 years (average, 44 years).[124]

Pathologic findings

Macroscopic

- The tumors form intratesticular or paratesticular solid nodules.
- In one case, the tumor formed multiple nodules on the tunica vaginalis.[124]

Microscopic

- Serous tumor of borderline malignancy is the most common.[124–128]

Special studies

- Immunocytochemical studies show positive staining for cytokeratin.
- CEA and CA-125 may also be positive.[125,127,128]

Brenner tumor

Clinical findings

- Brenner tumor of the testis is very rare.
- It may involve the testis, paratesticular tissue, tunica vaginalis, or tunica albuginea.[129–131]
- All but one[132] reported cases have been benign.[129–131]

Pathologic findings

Macroscopic

- The tumor is small (0.6–2.7 cm in diameter), gray-white to yellow, and solid.[129–131]

Microscopic

- Microscopic evaluation shows well-defined solid or occasionally cystic nests surrounded by dense connective tissue, which may be hyalinized.
- The nests are composed of transitional cells with typical 'coffee bean' nuclei with distinct longitudinal grooves.[129–131]
- The malignant variant shows typical changes, with formation of transitional and squamous cell carcinoma.[132]

Special studies

- Brenner tumors have not been studied with uroplakin antibodies specific for transitional cell epithelium.

(Figs 4.126–4.128)

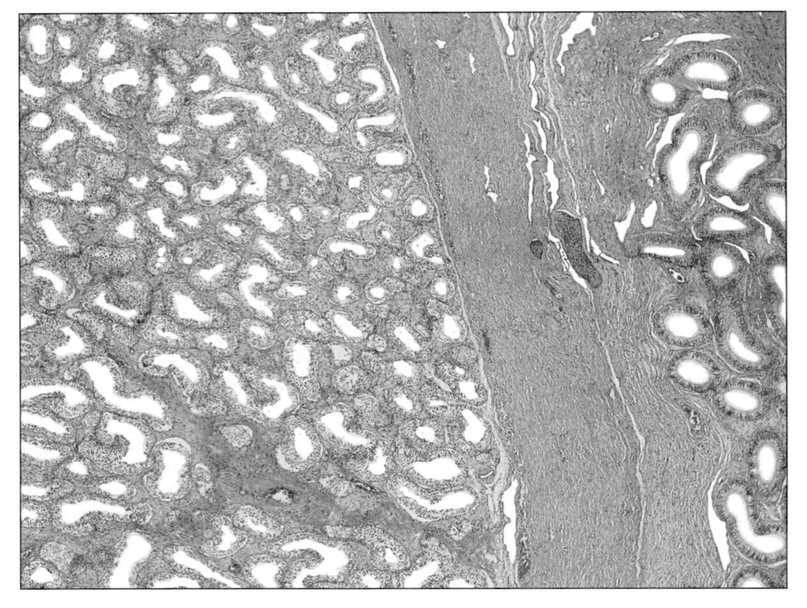

Fig. 4.126 Brenner tumor located between the testis and the epididymis.

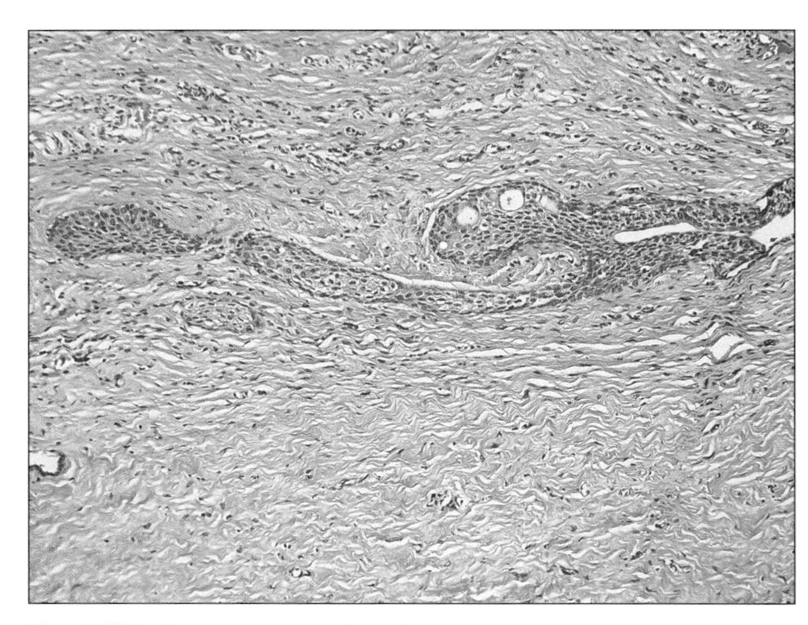

Fig. 4.127 Brenner tumor. Note the typical cellular nests surrounded by dense fibrous connective tissue.

Adenomatous hyperplasia of rete testis

Clinical findings

- This is a rare lesion.
- The age range is 30–44 years.[133–135]
- Most frequently, it is an incidental finding.
- Patients present with a solid or cystic testicular hilar mass.[133–135]
- The lesion is benign and does not recur after excision.

Pathologic findings

Macroscopic

- It is a small (less than 1 cm), round, cystic lesion containing jelly-like material.
- There may be diffuse thickening and calcification.[133–135]

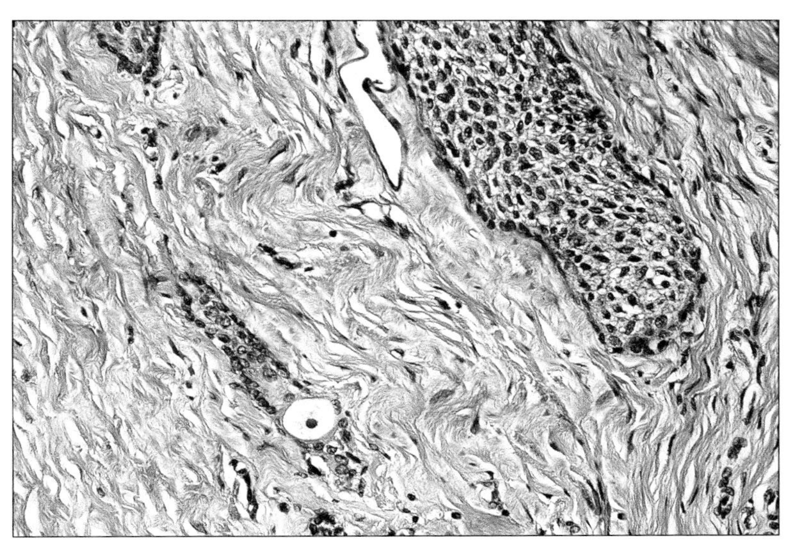

Fig. 4.128 Brenner tumor nests composed of transitional cells with ovoid or elongated nuclei, some showing nuclear grooves. Note the dense connective tissue surrounding the nests.

Microscopic
- There is proliferation of the epithelium lining the rete tubules, with small papillary formations.
- The proliferating cells vary from cuboidal to low columnar.
- There is no mitotic activity and no cellular or nuclear pleomorphism.[133–135]
- Hyaline globules may be present, especially in rete hyperplasia associated with germ cell tumors.

Special studies
- Immunohistochemical studies show staining for cytokeratin and epithelial membrane antigen (EMA).
- Vimentin, SMA, S-100, and desmin are negative.[134,135]

Adenoma, cystadenoma, and adenofibroma of rete testis

Clinical and pathologic findings
- Four tumors have been reported under these designations.[5]
- The tumors were small and either solid or cystic, or both.
- There was continuity with rete testis.[5,136,137]
- The tumors showed papillary and cystic patterns.
- The cysts and papillae were lined by rete epithelium showing minimal cellular and nuclear pleomorphism and absence of mitotic activity.
- The tumors were benign.[5,136,137]

Adenocarcinoma of rete testis

Clinical findings
- This tumor is rare.[138,139]
- It has a wide age range (20–90 years), but is more common after 50 years.
- It is associated with hydrocele in approximately 25% of cases.
- Patients present with a scrotal mass, usually painful.
- The clinical course varies from indolent to highly aggressive.[138,139]

Pathologic findings

Macroscopic
- The tumor is usually located in the hilar region.
- It is a solid, occasionally cystic, gray-white mass.
- It may be affected by hemorrhage or necrosis.[138–142]

Microscopic
- The tumor shows papillary, tubular, and solid patterns.[138–142]
- The tubules are elongated, compressed, and slit-like.
- The papillae project into cystic spaces, and may be small and cellular, or larger with prominent connective tissue cores.
- Transition between normal and neoplastic rete epithelium may be present and is a very useful diagnostic feature.[138,139]
- The surrounding connective tissue may be prominent and is often hyalinized.
- The tumor cells are usually small and cuboidal with scanty cytoplasm.
- The nuclei may show stratification, and usually show moderate pleomorphism and mitotic activity.[138–142]
- Spindle cell pattern suggestive of sarcomatous differentiation may occasionally be seen.[142]

Special studies
- Histochemical studies show PAS, Alcian blue, and mucicarmine positivity.[138,140–142]
- Immunocytochemical studies show cytokeratin and EMA positivity.
- PLAP, HCG, and AFP are negative.[138,140–142]

Papillary cystadenoma and cystadenocarcinoma of the epididymis

Clinical findings
- Papillary cystadenoma is uncommon and cystadenocarcinoma is rare.[5,143,144]
- There is no predilection for a specific age group and the age range is wide.[5,143]
- Cystadenoma is bilateral in 30% of cases.
- Cystadenoma is associated with von Hippel–Lindau disease, especially when bilateral involvement is present.[5,143]
- Cystadenoma is benign and runs an indolent clinical course.[5,143]

Pathologic findings

Macroscopic

- Cystadenoma is small (up to 5 cm in diameter).[5,143,145,146]
- Cystadenoma and cystadenocarcinoma are either cystic or solid, or both.[5,143–146]

Microscopic

- Both tumors show characteristic appearance and are composed of tubules and cysts containing complex papillae.[5,143,144]
- The papillae are lined by uniform, large, clear columnar cells, usually devoid of atypia in cystadenomas,[5,143,145,146] but showing atypical changes in cystadenocarcinomas.[5,144]
- The cytoplasm is rich in glycogen.[5,143]
- The cyst fluid is brightly eosinophilic.
- Presence of metastases is the only definite diagnostic feature of cystadenocarcinoma, as complexity of the papillae and atypical changes may erroneously suggest malignancy.[5,144]

Retinal anlage tumor (melanotic neuroectodermal tumor)

Clinical findings

- This tumor is rare, with fewer than a dozen reported cases.[147]
- Most reported cases affected the epididymis; the remainder occurred in the testis.[147,148]
- Most patients were aged less than 1 year; the oldest was 2 years.[147–150]
- Patients presented with scrotal enlargement.
- The tumor was benign, except for a single case.[147]

Pathologic findings

Macroscopic

- It is a small (usually less than 4 cm in diameter), well-circumscribed, round or oval, solid tumor.
- The cut surface varies from brown or black to predominantly gray–white with dark pigmentation.[147–150]

Microscopic

- The tumor is composed of irregular sheets, cords, nests, clusters, or spaces containing two different types of cells and surrounded by prominent fibrous and hyalinized connective tissue.[147–150]
- The predominant cell type consists of small, undifferentiated, round or oval cells with scanty cytoplasm, small hyperchromatic nuclei, and variable mitotic activity, resembling neuroblastoma.
- The second cell type consists of large, cuboidal or columnar epithelial-like cells with eosinophilic cytoplasm, large vesicular nuclei with small nucleoli and containing melanin pigment.[147–150]
- Rare malignant variants show high mitotic activity.[147]

Special studies

- The larger cells stain for melanin, and Masson–Fontana stain is usually positive, as are HMB-45 and S-100 immunocytochemical stains.
- Neuron-specific enolase (NSE) is usually positive in the smaller cells.
- Cytokeratin is negative.[147–150]

Connective tissue tumors

- Connective tissue tumors, both benign and malignant, are common in the spermatic cord and the epididymis but rare in the testis.
- Of malignant tumors affecting the testicular adnexa, rhabdomyosarcoma occurring in children is most common and will be discussed separately.
- Of benign tumors, leiomyoma is most common and is the second most common tumor of the spermatic cord, after adenomatoid tumor.[2,106]
- In adults, all types of malignant connective tissue tumors have been reported, like liposarcoma, leiomyosarcoma, and malignant fibrous histiocytoma.[2,4,5,151,152]
- The connective tissue tumors affecting the testicular adnexa show similar macroscopic, microscopic, ultrastructural, histochemical, and immunocytochemical features to their counterparts in other locations.[2,4,5,151–154]

(Fig. 4.129)

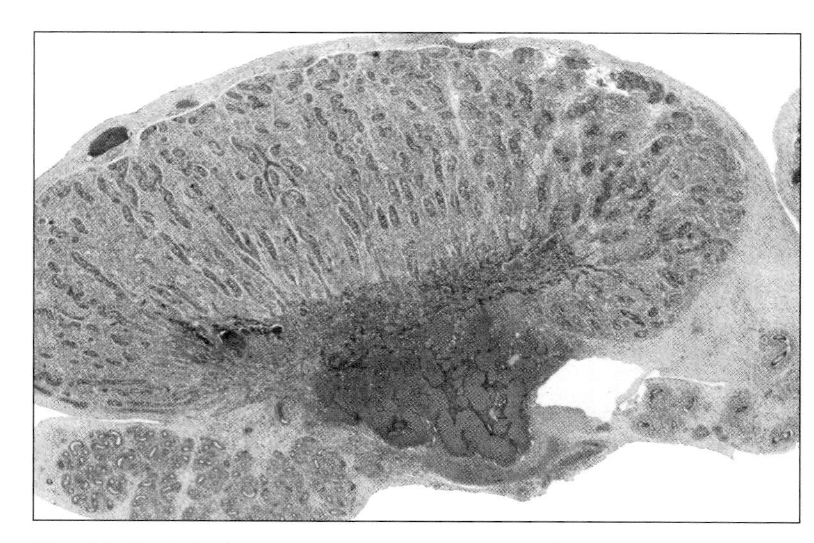

Fig. 4.129 Infant's testis containing a cavernous hemangioma located in the hilum.

Rhabdomyosarcoma

Clinical findings

- Rhabdomyosarcoma affects the spermatic cord (80%) and paratesticular tissue (20%).[155–157]
- It occurs mostly in infants and young children in the first decade, but has been reported in young adults.[155,156,158]
- It is the most common type of sarcoma occurring in children.
- Patients present with a scrotal mass (95%).[155–158]
- Prognosis depends on the type and stage.
- Combined treatment modalities have dramatically improved prognosis (85% 5-year survival rate).[157,159,160]

Pathologic findings

Macroscopic

- It is a gray–white, smooth, lobulated, soft, somewhat glistening and myxomatous mass.
- Usually the testis is not involved.[155–158]

Microscopic[155–159]

- The embryonal type is most common, usually with a myxoid background and variable cellularity.
- The alveolar type is less common.
- A spindle cell pattern is common, with collections of spindle-shaped cells with bright eosinophilic cytoplasm admixed with some large strap-, tadpole-, and racket-shaped cells. These cells may show cross-striations.[159]
- Cellular and nuclear pleomorphism may be marked.
- Mitotic activity may be brisk.[155–159]

Special studies

- Immunohistochemical studies show sarcoma-specific actin, titin, vimentin, desmin, myoglobin, and muscle-specific actin positivity.[155,156]
- Cytokeratin and SMA are negative.
- Ultrastructurally, the presence of sarcomere-related structures like Z-bands, and thick and thin filaments in hexagonal array, confirms the diagnosis.

Metastatic tumors

Clinical findings

- Metastasis to the testis is rare.[161–166]
- They are most common in patients over 50 years of age.
- It usually occurs in patients with known primary cancer but is the initial manifestation in 10% of cases.
- The most common primary sources of testicular metastases are prostate, lung, malignant melanoma of the skin, kidney, colon, pancreas, and stomach, in this order.[161–166]
- Patients present with testicular enlargement, which is bilateral in 15% of cases.
- Prognosis and survival are poor, with the majority of patients surviving less than 18 months.[161–166]

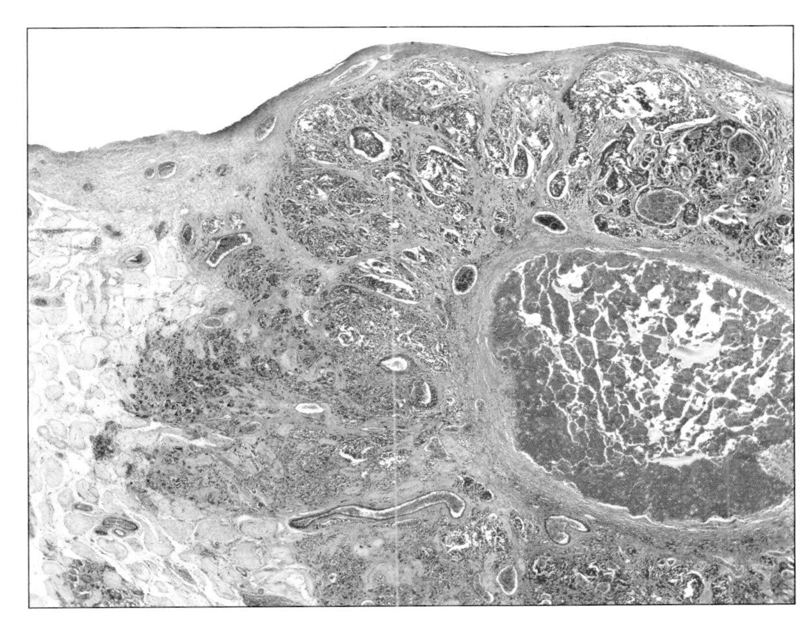

Fig. 4.130 Testis affected by metastatic carcinoma of the prostate, the most common source of metastasis to the testis. Note the numerous tumor nodules and the central necrosis.

Pathologic findings

Macroscopic

- Metastatic tumors form single or multiple nodules.
- Diffuse involvement is occasionally present.[161–166]

Microscopic

- Metastatic tumors usually affect the interstitium, but may invade the tubules and fill them.
- They form single or multiple deposits.[161–166]
- They show frequent vascular involvement.
- They show appearances distinct from primary testicular tumors and similar to the tumor of origin.[161–166]

Special studies

- The findings depend on the primary tumor.[161–166]
- Histochemical stains may show mucin and melanin.
- Immunocytochemical studies may show reactions for cytokeratin, CEA, prostate-specific antigen (PSA), prostate-specific alkaline phosphatase, HMB-45, and S-100.[164–166]

(Fig. 4.130)

NON-NEOPLASTIC LESIONS

CONGENITAL ABNORMALITIES

Anorchia

- Absence of testes is very rare.
- It is sometimes associated with other abnormalities of the urogenital tract.

Supernumerary testes

- This is very rare.
- It may be mistaken macroscopically for a tumor.
- Microscopically, appearances are normal.

Cryptorchidism (maldescent)

Clinical findings

- Cryptorchidism occurs in 0.03–0.4% of male subjects.[167]
- It is usually unilateral.
- There is a slight predilection for the right testis.
- Common locations are upper scrotal (48%), inguinal (42%), and intra-abdominal (10%).[167]
- It is associated with infertility, gonadal dysgenesis, and germ cell neoplasms.[168,169]
- Germ cell neoplasms are 7–35 times more common than in normal males and occur in 5–10% of patients with cryptorchidism.[168,169]
- Torsion may occur and result in infarction.
- The undescended testis may harbor a gonadoblastoma, and in such cases germ cell neoplasms are even more common.[168]

Pathologic findings

Macroscopic

- Testes are smaller and firm.
- They may show fibrous scars.[167]

Microscopic

- There are different findings in prepubertal and postpubertal testes.
- Findings in prepuberal testes include:
  diminished tubular diameter and reduced number of germ cells and Leydig cells;
  edema and early fibrosis of the interstitium;
  presence of microcalcifications in the seminiferous tubules.[167]
- Findings in postpubertal testes include:
  increased fibrosis and decreased number of germ cells;
  reduced tubular diameter and tubular sclerosis;
  thickening of the tunica propria;
  Leydig cell hyperplasia;
  interstitial fibrosis.[167]

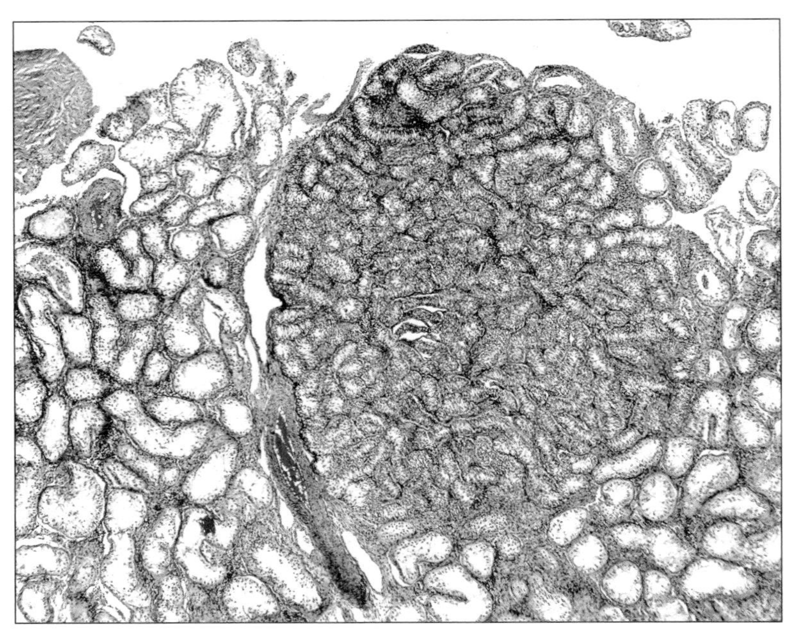

Fig. 4.131 Cryptorchid testis containing a Sertoli cell adenoma (Pick's adenoma) composed of collections of infantile seminiferous tubules.

- Both prepubertal and postpubertal testes frequently contain Sertoli cell adenomas (Pick's adenomas).
- Microcalcifications are more common in prepubertal testes.
- IGCN is much more common in postpubertal testes.[167–169]

(Fig. 4.131)

Klinefelter's syndrome

Clinical findings

- Klinefelter's syndrome consists of gynecomastia, eunochoid habitus, decreased or absent spermatogenesis, apparently normal Leydig cell function, increased follicle-stimulating hormone (FSH) secretion, and abnormal karyotype, usually 47,XXY.[170]
- It occurs in approximately 0.2% of males.
- Patients present with infertility.[170,171]
- It is associated with breast cancer (the same incidence as in normal females).
- It is associated with an increased incidence of mediastinal germ cell tumors.[171]
- Testicular germ cell tumors and sex cord stromal tumors occur, but only occasionally.[171]

Pathologic findings

Macroscopic

- The testes are small.[170,171]

Microscopic

- Germ cells are reduced at birth, show a gradual decrease, and are absent in adults.[170]

- There is tubular fibrosis and sclerosis.
- There is hyperplasia of Leydig cells.[170]

Splenic–gonadal fusion

Clinical findings

- Splenic–gonadal fusion is rare.[172]
- It usually forms a small, discrete nodule.
- Generally, it is an incidental finding.[172–174]

Pathologic findings

Macroscopic

- There is usually a nodule fused to the upper pole of the testis or head of the epididymis.
- The nodule is red–brown in color and resembles splenic tissue.[172–174]

Microscopic

- There is normal splenic tissue attached by a fibrous band to testicular tissue, which may show atrophic changes.[172–174]

Testicular 'tumor' of the adrenogenital syndrome

Clinical findings

- Patients with adrenogenital syndrome (AGS) have increased levels of adrenocorticotropic hormone (ACTH), androstenodione, and 17-hydroxy progesterone in the plasma, and elevated levels of 17-ketosteroids in the urine.[5,175]
- AGS may be associated with undescended testis.
- Patients have an increased risk of germ cell tumors.
- The 'tumors' are rare.[5,175]
- They are found in males with untreated or inadequately treated AGS.[175]
- They occur most often in patients with the salt-losing form (21-hydroxylase deficiency) when untreated or inadequately treated.
- They occur in children and adults.
- There is bilateral synchronous testicular involvement.
- Patients may present with testicular enlargement.[5,175]

Pathologic findings

Macroscopic

- The 'tumors' are found in the hilar region and extend into the testicular parenchyma.
- They measure a few centimeters in diameter (reach up to 10 cm).
- They comprise black to brown, lobulated nodules intersected by fibrous septa.[5,175]

Microscopic

- There is diffuse proliferation of large cells with abundant eosinophilic cytoplasm containing brown lipochrome pigment.
- Nuclear atypia and mitotic activity are rare.[5,175]
- The cells resemble Leydig cells, but there are no crystals of Reinke and the cells are larger and darker due to greater amount of lipochrome pigment.
- The nature of the cells is not known.[5,175]
- The surrounding testicular tissue shows seminiferous tubules decreased in size, decreased spermatogenesis, and dense hyalinized fibrous tissue.
- In some parts of the testis, the seminiferous tubules are widely separated by cellular stroma resembling ovarian stroma, containing collections of Leydig cells.[5,175]

(Figs 4.132–4.134)

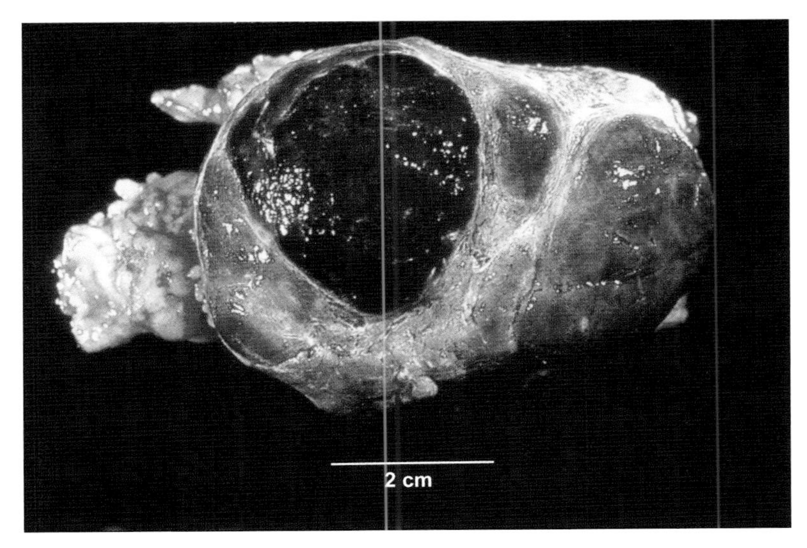

Fig. 4.132 Testicular 'tumor' of adrenogenital syndrome. Note the multiple nodules and the dark color. (Courtesy of R.E. Scully, M.D.)

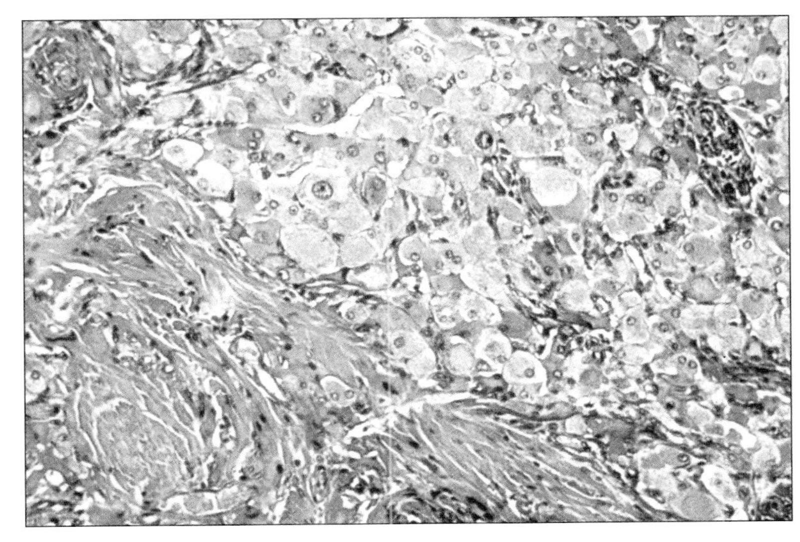

Fig. 4.133 Testicular 'tumor' of adrenogenital syndrome composed of large polygonal cells with granular eosinophilic cytoplasm and round nuclei. The surrounding connective tissue is dense and hyalinized. (Courtesy of R.E. Scully, M.D.)

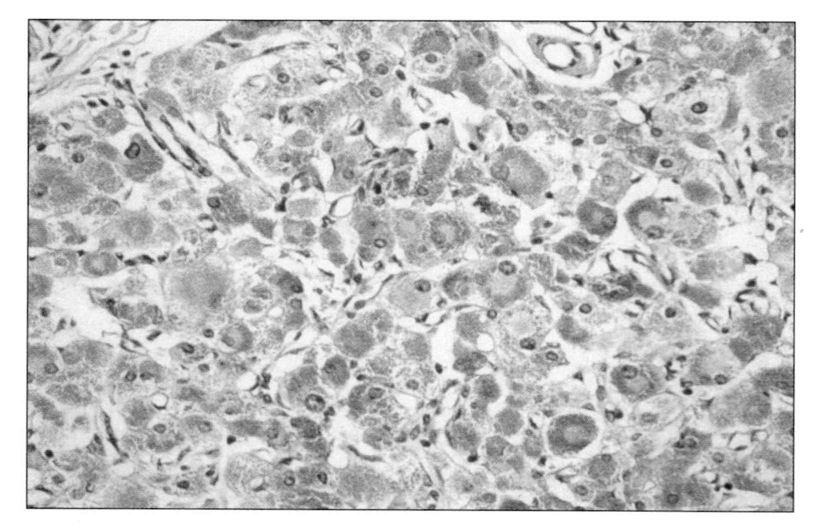

Fig. 4.134 Testicular 'tumor' of adrenogenital syndrome composed of large cells with granular eosinophilic cytoplasm containing a large amount of brown lipochrome pigment. (Courtesy of R.E. Scully, M.D.)

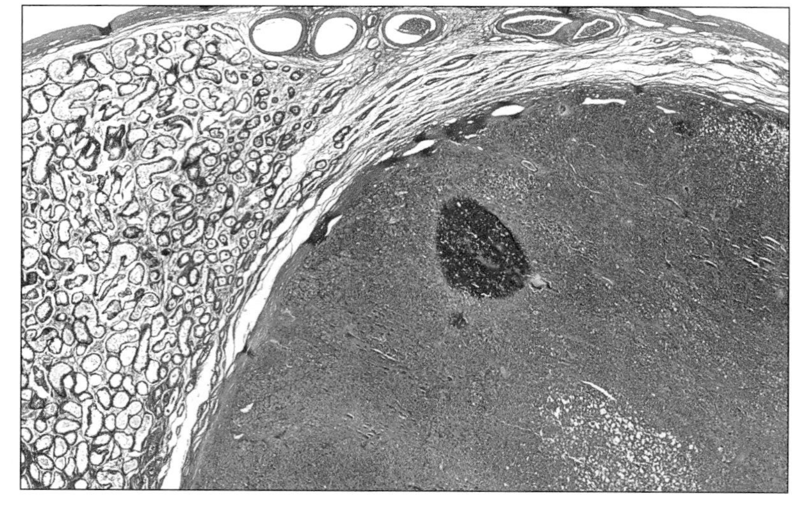

Fig. 4.135 Intratesticular adrenal rest. The well-demarcated lesion is composed of adrenocortical tissue.

Adrenal rests

Clinical findings

- Adrenal rests occur at all ages, but are more frequently found in infants.
- They are found in spermatic cord, epididymis, rete testis, tunica albuginea, and between testis and epididymis.[176,177]

Pathologic findings

Macroscopic

- Small, solid, yellow nodules (usually less than 1 cm in diameter).
- Usually encapsulated.[176,177]

Microscopic

- Usually encapsulated nodule.
- Shows typical appearances of adrenal cortex, including the three layers.
- Absence of adrenal medullary tissue.[176,177]

(Figs 4.135 & 4.136)

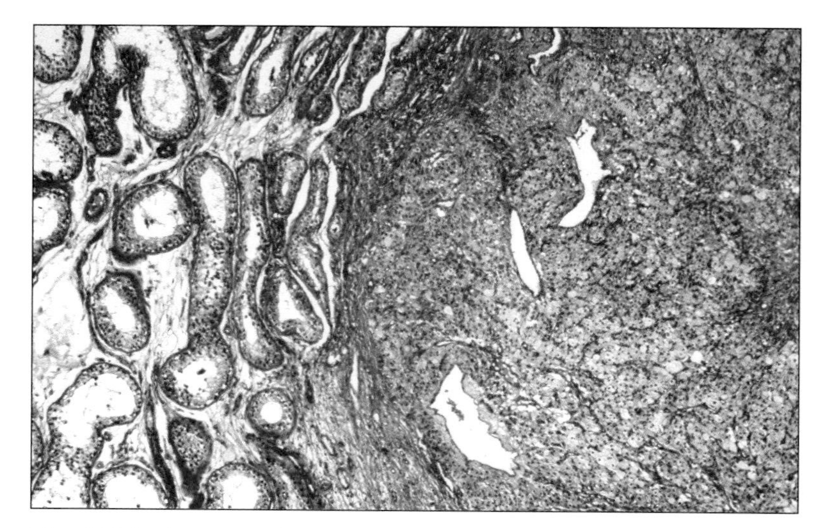

Fig. 4.136 Intratesticular adrenal rest. The lesion shows typical appearances of adrenal cortex.

Cystic dysplasia

Clinical findings

- Cystic dysplasia is rare.
- It occurs in infants and young children.[178]
- Patients present with slight testicular enlargement.
- The condition was bilateral in two of the seven reported cases.[178,179]
- It is associated with renal abnormalities in more than 50% of cases.

Pathologic findings

Macroscopic

- Multicystic mass replacing most of the testis.[178,179]

Microscopic

- Consists of multiple anastomosing cysts varying in size and shape, separated by fibrous septa.[178,179]
- Affects the region of the rete first and then extends into the testicular parenchyma.[178]
- Normal testicular tissue may be compressed by the process, forming a narrow rim.
- The cysts are lined by a single layer of flat or cuboidal epithelial cells, similar to those lining the rete testis.[178,179]

(Fig. 4.137)

VASCULAR LESIONS

Hematomas and infarcts may affect the testis, producing enlargement or a mass. Such lesions must be differentiated from neoplasms, which are the cause of the majority of hemorrhagic testicular lesions.

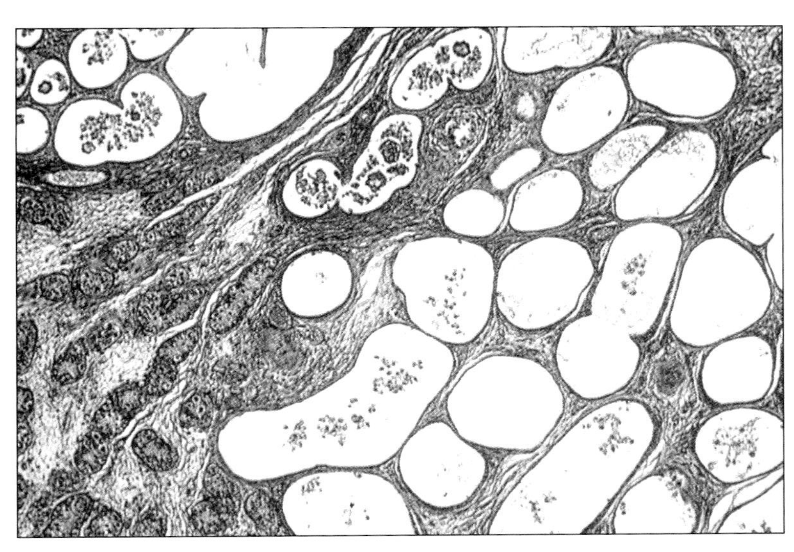

Fig. 4.137 Infant's testis affected by cystic dysplasia. The lesion consists of multiple cysts varying in size and shape, separated by fibrous septa and replacing normal testicular tissue.

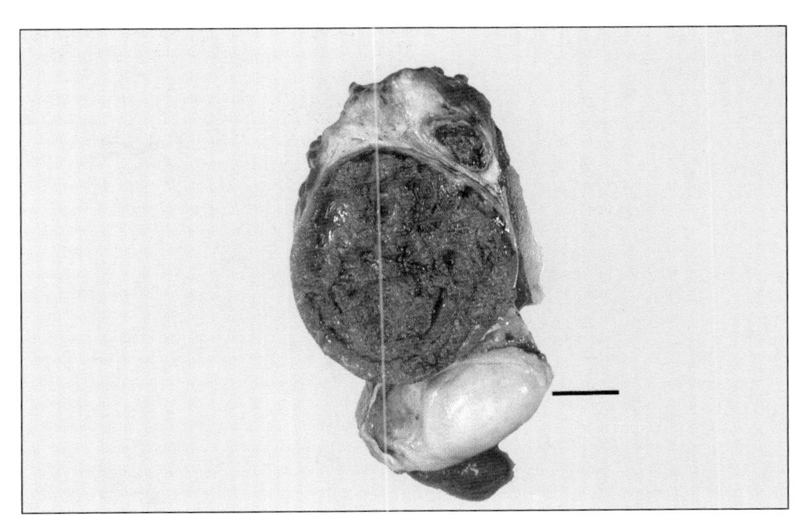

Fig. 4.138 Paratesticular hemorrhage causing a large hematoma. The testis (bottom) is congested, but only slightly affected.

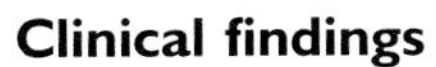

Clinical findings

- A testicular infarct may be caused by torsion or thrombotic occlusion and is commonly seen in periarteritis nodosa.[180,181]
- Testicular hemorrhage may be caused by a rupture of an artery affected by arteritis, producing a hematoma.[180,182]
- Testicular hematoma may be mistaken for a neoplasm, usually a choriocarcinoma.
- Testicular vasculitis is usually associated with systemic vasculitis, but may occur as an isolated lesion.[180,182]

Pathologic findings

Macroscopic

- Appearances vary with the age of the infarct. Early infarcts are intensely hemorrhagic and become paler with age.

Microscopic

- Early infarcts exhibit extensive hemorrhage affecting the testicular tissue. In the later stages, the affected tissue undergoes fibrosis and shrinkage.[180–182]
- Other changes like occlusion of an artery and the presence of periarteritis nodosa may be present.[180,182]

(Fig. 4.138)

INFLAMMATORY DISEASES

Acute orchitis

Clinical findings

- Acute orchitis is uncommon.
- It may be of viral or bacterial origin.[5,183]
- Mumps virus is the most common cause of acute viral orchitis.[184,185]
- Other viruses may also cause acute orchitis, most frequently Coxsackie B virus.[186]
- Mumps virus affects the testis in approximately 25% of adult males with the disease, which is usually associated with epididymitis.[184,185]
- Bilateral involvement is seen in 20% of cases.
- Mumps orchitis affects less than 1% of children with mumps.[184,185]
- Bacterial orchitis is usually seen as a local extension of urogenital tract infection, or septicemia.[183]
- The epididymis is usually affected and the disease presents as epididymo-orchitis.

Pathologic findings

Macroscopic

- Findings are similar in viral and bacterial disease.[5,183]
- The testes are swollen and tender.

Microscopic

- In viral orchitis, the early stages of the disease are characterized by edema, congestion, and lymphocytic interstitial infiltration.
- Interstitial hemorrhage, involvement of the seminiferous tubules by inflammatory cells, and degeneration of the germinal epithelium occur later.
- Healing results in fibrosis and hyalinization, and such areas are present alternating with normal, unaffected areas.[5,183,186]
- In bacterial orchitis, there is congestion and acute inflammatory cell infiltration affecting the interstitium and, in severe cases, the tubules.[5,183,187]
- The process depends on the severity and stage of the disease.
- Abscesses may be present, causing enlargement.[187]

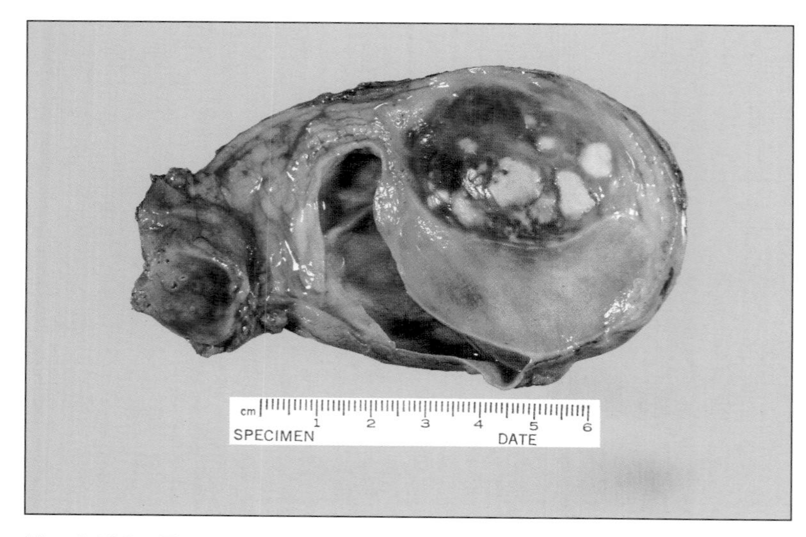

Fig. 4.139 Testis affected by infectious orchitis with necrotic lesions.

- In the later stages, fibrosis and adhesions may be present, causing formation of a mass which may simulate a neoplasm.[5,183]

Special studies

- Viral and bacterial studies make or confirm the diagnosis.

(Fig. 4.139)

Infectious or specific granulomatous orchitis

- This may be caused by syphilis, tuberculosis, leprosy, and various fungal infections.[183,188]
- It is uncommon.
- Congenital syphilis causes bilateral, painless testicular enlargement. Microscopically, there is granulomatous interstitial inflammation, endarteritis, and fibrosis.
- Tertiary syphilis affects the testis, causing similar findings to congenital syphilis, but, in addition, gummata may be present, enhancing the testicular enlargement.[183,188]
- Tuberculosis usually affects the epididymis, and testicular involvement is seen only in late stages. Abscesses and tracts are present. Microscopically, the lesions show the typical picture of tuberculosis.[189–191]
- Lepromatous leprosy affects the testis more frequently than the epididymis. The process is usually bilateral. The testes are usually decreased in size. Microscopically, typical lepromatous lesions are present.[183]
- Fungal infections usually occur as a part of systemic illness. Various organisms are involved like *Blastomyces*, *Cryptococcus*, *Candida*, *Histoplasma*, and *Aspergillus* species. They may affect part of the testis or produce confluent involvement. Microscopically, there is a mixed inflammatory infiltrate and granuloma formation with or without necrosis.[183,188]
- Sarcoidosis rarely affects the testis or epididymis.[192]

Special studies

- Clinical, microbiologic, and serologic correlation is required; biopsy may be needed.

Nonspecific or idiopathic granulomatous orchitis

Clinical findings

- The pathogenesis is not known.
- It accounts for 0.2% of testicular enlargements.
- It occurs most frequently between 50 and 70 years of age.[183,187]
- The onset of disease may be associated with influenza-like illness or urinary tract infection.[183,188,193,194]
- Patients present with unilateral testicular enlargement, which may be associated with some tenderness and pain. The latter usually disappears, resulting in a painless mass.
- In 50% of cases, the epididymis and the spermatic cord are swollen and indurated.[183,188,193,194]

Pathologic findings

Macroscopic

- The tunica albuginea is thickened and swollen, but the testis and epididymis are only slightly enlarged.
- The testis feels rubbery, is paler than normal, and less bulging when sectioned.
- Lobulation may be present.[183,188,193,194]

Microscopic

- Initially there are regressive changes in the seminiferous tubules and chronic inflammatory cell infiltration of the interstitium, which later affects the seminiferous tubules.
- Sertoli cell proliferation and regression of the germinal epithelium occur later.[183,188,193,194]
- In some cases the main inflammatory cells are plasma cells.
- Eosinophils may be well in evidence, but acute inflammatory cells are rare.
- Langhans' giant cells are common.[183,187,193,194]
- In more mature lesions, the seminiferous tubules show sarcoid-like appearance with proliferation of chronic inflammatory cells, histiocytes, and giant cells. Distinct granulomas are absent.
- There is inflammation of the tunica vaginalis, with fibrinous exudate and fibrous thickening.
- Involvement of the epididymis is not uncommon.
- Sperm granulomata may be seen.
- Proliferative endarteritis and organizing thrombosis may be seen.[183,188,193,194]

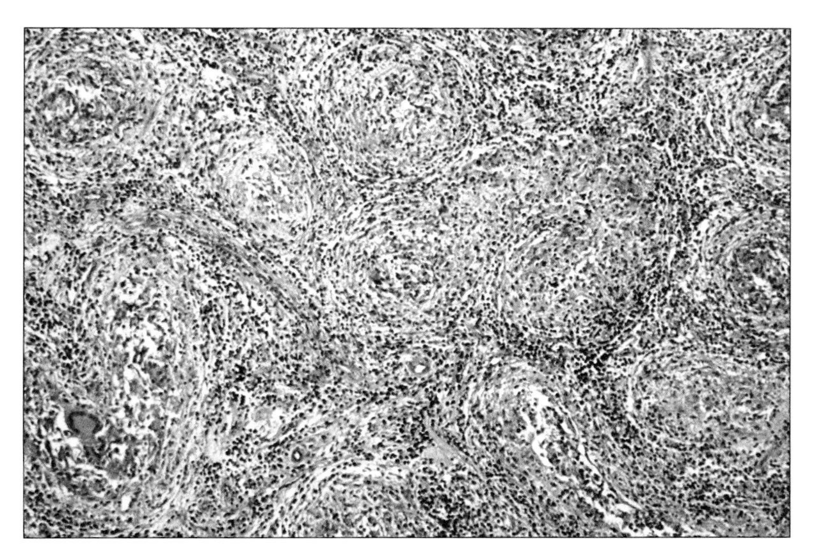

Fig. 4.140 Nonspecific granulomatous orchitis. Note the typical sarcoid-like appearance of the seminiferous tubules.

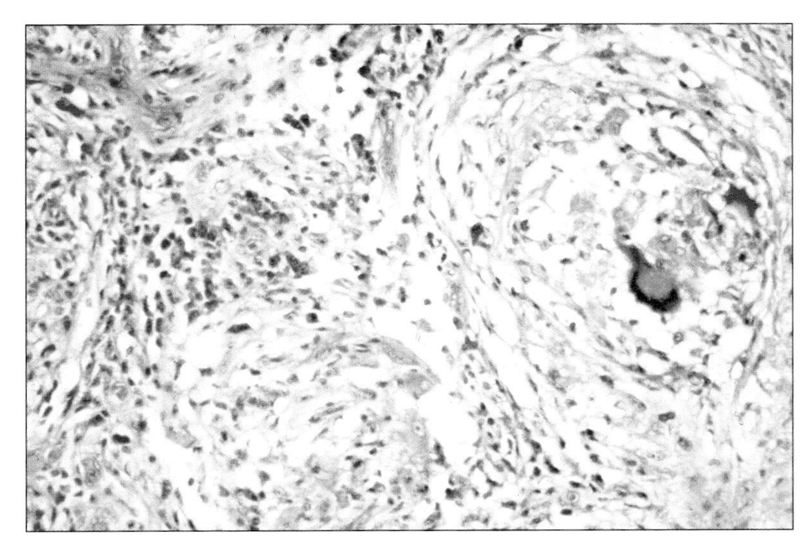

Fig. 4.141 Nonspecific granulomatous orchitis. Seminiferous tubule containing numerous proliferating histiocytes, some lymphocytes, and a Langhans' giant cell. Note the sarcoid-like appearance.

Special studies

- Microbiological, histochemical, and immunocytochemical studies are negative.[183,188,193,194]

(Figs 4.140 & 4.141)

Malakoplakia

Clinical findings

- It affects both the testis and epididymis.[183,188,195–197]
- The testis alone is affected in 66% of cases. Isolated involvement of the epididymis is rare.
- It occurs only in adults at any age but mainly between 40 and 70 years.[183,188,195–197]
- Involvement was unilateral in all reported cases.
- Patients present with testicular enlargement.[183,188,195–197]

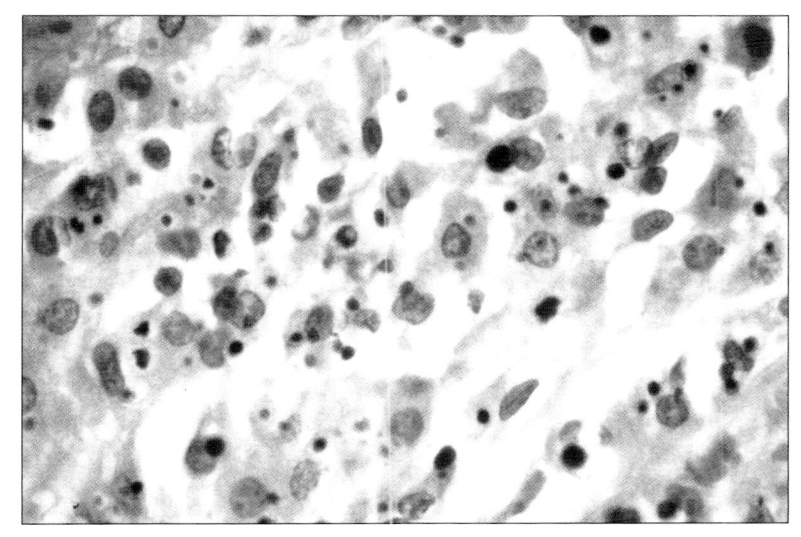

Fig. 4.142 Malakoplakia involving the testis. The lesion is composed of large cells with granular eosinophilic cytoplasm and large round vesicular nuclei. The cells contain small basophilic inclusions (Michaelis–Gutmann bodies).

- Occasionally there is history of urinary tract infection.
- Fibrous adhesions to the surrounding connective tissue are common and cause difficulties at orchiectomy.

Pathologic findings

Macroscopic

- The testicular tissue is replaced by yellow–tan to brown tissue, which may be divided into lobules by fibrous bands.
- Abscesses are frequently present.[183,188,195–197]

Microscopic

- The seminiferous tubules and the interstitium are replaced by collections of large cells with prominent granular eosinophilic PAS-positive cytoplasm (von Hansemann cells), considered to be histiocytes.[183,188,195–197]
- Some of these cells contain small solid or target-like inclusions in the cytoplasm known as Michaelis–Gutmann bodies and considered to represent the breakdown products of bacteria, most frequently *Escherichia coli*.
- Acute and chronic inflammatory cells, granulation tissue, and fibrosis are also present and may obscure the typical appearances of the lesion.
- Abscesses may be present.[183,188,195–197]
- Ultrastructural examination shows ingested breakdown products of bacteria in phagolysosomes.[196]

Special studies

- Histochemical stains like PAS, von Kossa, and Prussian blue are positive in Michaelis–Gutmann bodies, indicating the presence of mucopolysaccharides, calcium, and iron, respectively.[183,188,195–197]

(Fig. 4.142)

Fibromatous periorchitis (fibrous pseudotumor)

Clinical findings

- Fibromatous periorchitis affects the tunica vaginalis or tunica albuginea.[198–200]
- In the diffuse form, it consists of dense fibrous thickening of the tunica vaginalis; in the localized form, single or multiple nodules or plaques affect the tunica.[198]
- There is no specific age predilection (age range of reported cases, 15–70 years).[198–200]
- Patients present with slight scrotal enlargement or induration.
- It is considered a reactive lesion.[198–200]

Pathologic findings

Macroscopic

- There is thickening of the tunica, which may be general in the diffuse form or show nodularity in the localized form.
- The thickened tunica is white and firm.[198–200]

Microscopic

- The lesions may be fibrocollagenous with focal calcification, or, less frequently, cellular, composed of fascicles of uniform spindle cells.[198–200]
- The spindle cells are uniform and devoid of atypical features.
- Mixed inflammatory cell infiltration and granulation tissue may be present in the cellular lesions.
- There is no infiltration of the surrounding tissue.[198–200]

(Fig. 4.143)

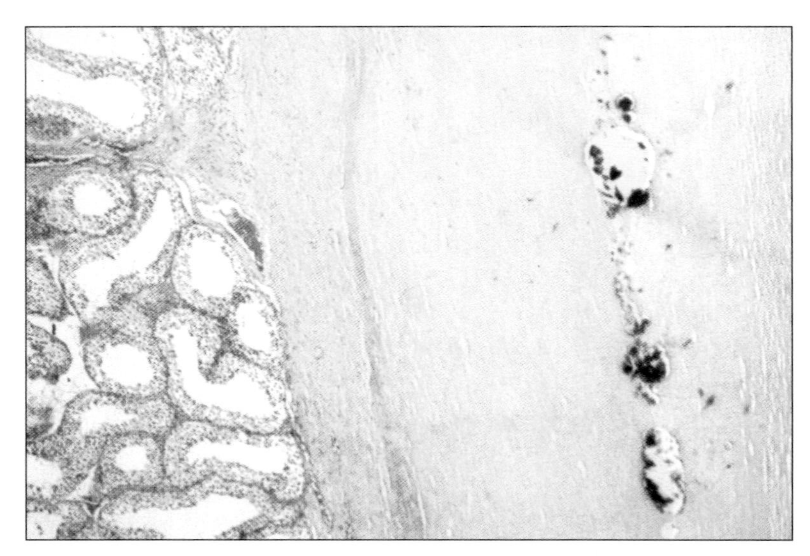

Fig. 4.143 Fibromatous periorchitis. The tunica shows marked thickening. The lesion is fibrocollagenous with focal calcification.

Vasitis nodosa

Clinical findings

- There is nodular thickening of the vas deferens.[201]
- The age range is 18–50 years.[201–204]
- Patients may present with localized pain and tenderness, but more often the lesion is asymptomatic.
- Patients often have a history of vasectomy.
- Sperm granuloma is seen in 30% of patients.
- The condition is bilateral in 16% of cases.[201–204]

Pathologic findings

Macroscopic

- There is a small (0.3–1.0 cm), firm, pale, demarcated nodule located in the spermatic cord.[201–203]

Microscopic

- It is characterized by proliferation of vas deferens epithelium, forming small ductules.
- The walls of the ductules are infiltrated by inflammatory cells, mainly lymphocytes.[201]
- The ductules are usually confined to the wall of the vas deferens, but may extend into the surrounding connective tissue.
- The ductules are lined by cuboidal or low columnar epithelial cells devoid of atypical changes.[201]
- Spermatozoa are present in the lumen of the ductules.
- Perineural and vascular wall involvement is seen in 20% of cases.[202–204]
- The lesion may extend to the skin and form a vasocutaneous fistula.[204]

Sperm granuloma

Clinical findings

- This represents a granulomatous reaction to extravasated spermatozoa.[205–207]
- It has a wide age range (18–74 years), but usually is seen in young adults.[205–209]
- It virtually always involves the epididymis or vas deferens.
- There is a small painful nodule (up to 4 cm in diameter).
- Usually, there is a history of vasectomy, trauma, or epididymitis.[205–209]
- In approximately 90% of cases associated with vasectomy, the lesion involves the vas deferens.[208]
- It is associated with vasitis nodosa in 30% of cases.[207]

Pathologic findings

Macroscopic

- There is a firm, small (1–4 cm), well-demarcated nodule, which may contain soft, yellow–white foci.[205–209]

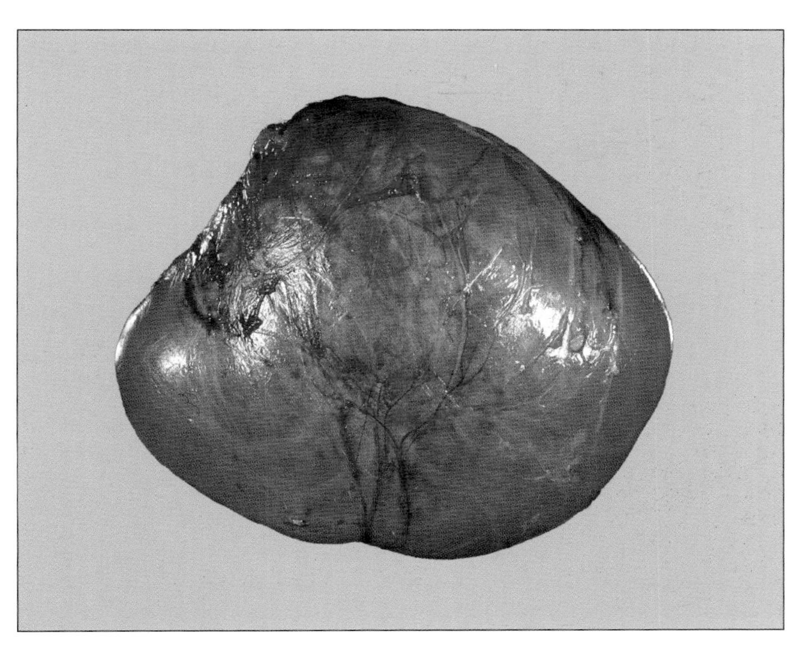

Fig. 4.144 Spermatocele forming a cystic transilluminating mass.

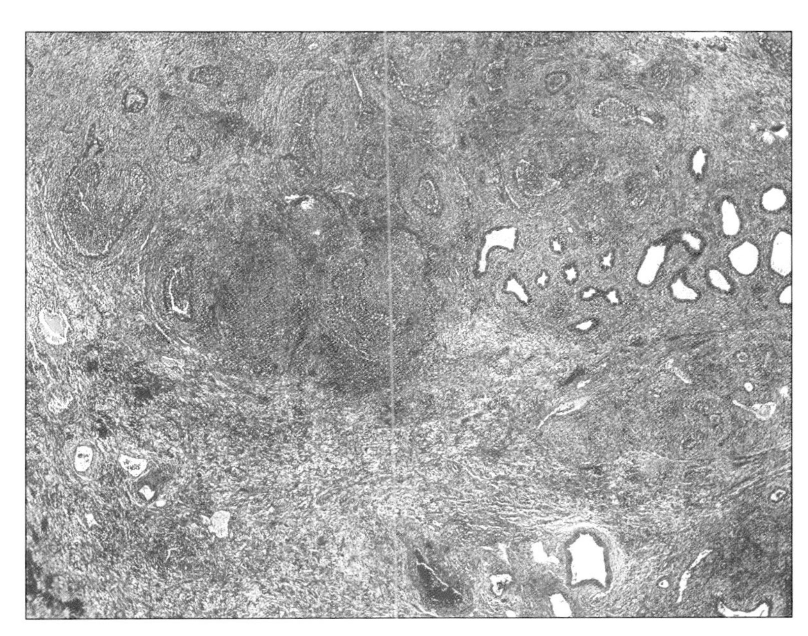

Fig. 4.146 Sperm granuloma. Late stage with extensive inflammation of the epididymis, including the ducts. There is early fibrosis.

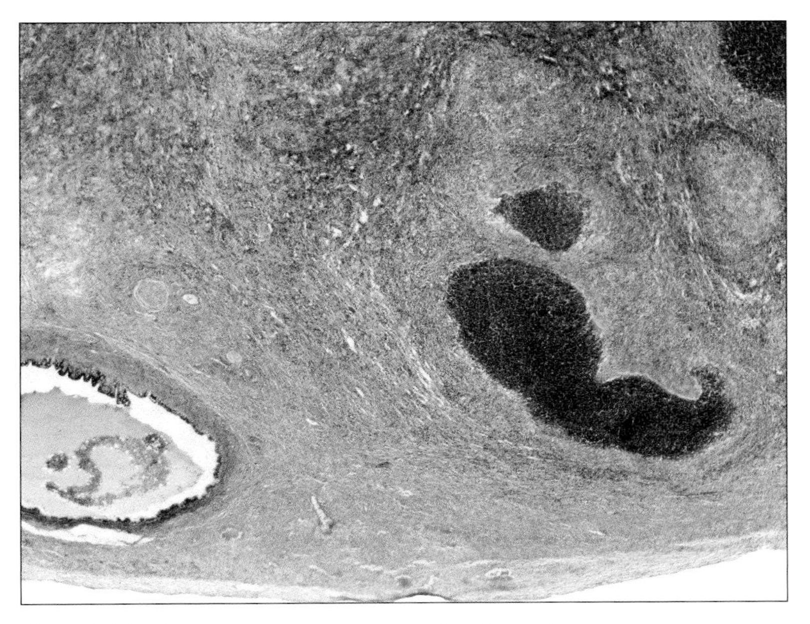

Fig. 4.145 Sperm granuloma. Large collections of spermatozoa surrounded by inflammatory cells are seen in the epididymis.

Microscopic

- The appearances depend on the stage of the process.
- In the early stages, the aggregates of spermatozoa are surrounded by acute inflammatory cells. The latter are gradually replaced by histiocytes with formation of granulomas, mostly devoid of giant cells. There is phagocytosis of the spermatozoa by the histiocytes.
- In the later stages, there is progressive fibrosis and hyalinization, and accumulation of lipofuscin pigment. The ducts show dense infiltration by acute inflammatory cells and histiocytes, with ulceration and necrosis. Occasionally, squamous metaplasia of the ductal epithelium may occur.[205–209]

(Figs 4.144–4.146)

REFERENCES

1. Talerman A, Roth LM. Pathology of the testis and its adnexa. New York: Churchill Livingstone; 1986.
2. Eble JN, Sauter G, Epstein JI, Sesterhenn IA. Tumours of the urinary system and male genital organs. Pathology and genetics. World Health Organization classification of tumours. Lyon: IARC Press; 2004.
3. Mostofi FK, Sesterhenn I. Histological typing of testis tumours. World Health Organization international histological classification of tumours. 2nd edn. Berlin: Springer, 1998.
4. Ulbright T, Amin MB, Young RH. Tumors of the testis, adnexa, spermatic cord, and scrotum. Atlas of tumor pathology. 3rd series, Fascicle 25. Washington, DC: Armed Forces Institute of Pathology; 1999.
5. Young RH, Scully RE. Testicular tumors. Chicago: ASCP Press; 1990.
6. Jacobsen GK, Talerman A. Intratubular germ cell neoplasia. Atlas of germ cell tumours. Copenhagen: Munksgaard; 1989.
7. Skakkebaek NE. Carcinoma-in-situ of the testis: frequency and relationship to invasive germ cell tumours in infertile men. Histopathology 1978;2: 157–170.
8. Pryor JP, Cameron KM, Chilton CP. Carcinoma in situ in testicular biopsies from men presenting with infertility. Br J Urol 1981;55: 780–784.
9. Nistal M, Codesai J, Paniagua R. Carcinoma in situ of the testis in infertile men. A histological, immunocytochemical, and cytophotometric study of DNA content. J Pathol 1989;159:205-210.
10. Berthelsen JG, Skakkebaek NE. Value of testicular biopsy in diagnosing carcinoma-in-situ testis. Scand J Urol Nephrol 1981;15:165–168.
11. Burke AP, Mostofi FK. Intratubular malignant germ cells in testicular biopsies: clinical course and identification by staining for placental alkaline phosphatase. Mod Pathol 1988;1:475–479.
12. Coffin CM, Ewing S, Dehner LP. Frequency of intratubular germ cell neoplasia with invasive testicular germ cell tumors: histologic and immunohistochemical features. Arch Pathol Lab Med 1985;109: 555–559.
13. Von der Maase H, Rorth M, Walbom-Jorgensen S, et al. Carcinoma in situ of the contralateral testis in patients with testicular germ cell cancer. A study of 27 cases in 500 patients. Br Med J 1986;293:1398–1401.

14. Jacobsen GK, Norgaard Pedersen B. Placental alkaline phosphatase in testicular germ cell tumours and in carcinoma in situ of the testis. Acta Pathol Microbiol Scand A 1988;92:323–329.
15. Schultz HP, Von der Maase H, Rorth M, et al. Testicular seminoma in Denmark 1976-1980. Acta Radiol Oncol 1984;23:263–270.
16. Babaian RJ, Zagars GK. Testicular seminoma: the M.D. Anderson experience. An analysis of pathological and patient characteristics and treatment recommendations. J Urol 1988;139:311–314.
17. Ulbright TM. Germ cell neoplasms of the testis. Am J Surg Pathol 1993;17: 1075–1091.
18. Bell DA, Flotte TJ, Bhan AK. Immunohistochemical characterization of seminoma and its inflammatory cell infiltrates. Hum Pathol 1987;18: 511–520.
19. Young RH, Finlayson N, Scully RE. Tubular seminoma: report of a case. Arch Pathol Lab Med 1989;113:414–416.
20. Talerman A. Tubular seminoma. Arch Pathol Lab Med 1989;113:1204.
21. Zavala-Pompa A, Ro JY, El-Naggar AK, et al. Tubular seminoma: an immunohistochemical and DNA flow-cytometric study of four cases. Am J Clin Pathol 1994;102:397–401.
22. Eglen DE, Ulbright TM. The differential diagnosis of yolk sac tumor and seminoma. Usefulness of cytokeratin, alpha-fetoprotein, and alpha-1-antitrypsin immunoperoxidase reactions. Am J Clin Pathol 1987;88: 328–332.
23. Talerman A. Spermatocytic seminoma. Clinicopathological study of 22 cases. Cancer 1980;45:2169–2176.
24. Burke AP, Mostofi FK. Spermatocytic seminoma: a clinicopathologic study of 79 cases. J Urol Pathol 1993;1:21–32.
25. Eble JN. Spermatocytic seminoma. Hum Pathol 1994;25:1035–1042.
26. True LD, Otis CN, Delprado W, et al. Spermatocytic seminoma of testis with sarcomatous transformation. A report of five cases. Am J Surg Pathol 1988;12:75–82.
27. Floyd C, Ayala AG, Logothetis CJ, et al. Spermatocytic seminoma with associated sarcoma of the testis. Cancer 1988;61:409–414.
28. Matoska J, Talerman A. Spermatocytic seminoma associated with rhabdomyosarcoma. Am J Clin Pathol 1990;94:89–95.
29. Matoska J, Ondrus D, Hornak M. Metastatic spermatocytic seminoma: a case report with light microscopic, ultrastructural and immunohistochemical findings. Cancer 1988;62:1197–1201.
30. Talerman A, Fu YS, Okagaki T. Spermatocytic seminoma: ultrastructural and microspectrophotometric observations. Lab Invest 1984;51:343–349.
31. Jacobsen GK, Barlebo H, Olsen J, et al. Testicular tumors in Denmark 1976-1980: pathology of 1,058 consecutive cases. Acta Radiol Oncol 1984;23: 239–247.
32. Pierce GB Jr, Abell MR. Embryonal carcinoma of the testis. Pathol Annu 1970;5:27–60.
33. Vugrin D, Chen A, Feigl P, et al. Embryonal carcinoma of the testis. Cancer 1988;61:2348–2352.
34. Marin-Padilla M. Histopathology of the embryonal carcinoma of the testis. Embryological evaluation. Arch Pathol Lab Med 1968;85:614–622.
35. Battifora H, Sheibani K, Tubbs RR, et al. Antikeratin antibodies in tumor diagnosis. Distinction between seminoma and embryonal carcinoma. Cancer 1984;54:843–848.
36. Mietinen M, Virtanen I, Talerman A. Intermediate filament proteins in human testis and testicular germ cell tumors. Am J Pathol 1985;120: 402–410.
37. Teilum G. Endodemal sinus tumors of the ovary and testis. Comparative morphogenesis of the so-called mesonephroma ovarii (Schiller) and extraembryonic (yolk sac-allantoic) structures of the rat placenta. Cancer 1959;12:1092–1105.
38. Harms D, Janig U. Germ cell tumours of childhood. Report of 170 cases, including 59 pure and partial yolk sac tumours. Virchows Arch (A) 1986; 409:223–239.
39. Hawkins EP. Pathology of germ cell tumors in children. Crit Rev Oncol Hematol 1990;10:165–179.
40. Kaplan GW, Cromie WC, Kelalis PP, et al. Prepubertal yolk sac testicular tumors: report of the testicular tumor registry. J Urol 1988;140: 1109–1112.
41. Hu LM, Phillipson J, Barsky SH. Intratubular germ cell neoplasia in infantile yolk sac tumor. Verification by tandem repeat sequence in situ hybridization. Diagn Mol Pathol 1992;1:118–128.
42. Talerman A. The incidence of yolk sac tumor (endodermal sinus tumor) elements in testicular germ cell tumors in adults. Cancer 1975;36:211–215.
43. Talerman A. Endodermal sinus (yolk sac) tumor elements in testicular germ cell tumors of adults: comparison of prospective and retrospective studies. Cancer 1980;46:1213–1217.
44. Ulbright TM, Roth LM, Broadhecker CA. Yolk sac differentiation in germ cell tumors. A morphologic study of 50 cases with emphasis on hepatic, enteric, and parietal yolk sac features. Am J Surg Pathol 1986;10:151–164.
45. Jacobsen GK, Jacobsen M. Possible liver cell differentiation in testicular germ cell tumours. Histopathology 1983;7:537–548.
46. Mostofi FK, Sesterhenn I, Davis CJ Jr. Immmunopathology of germ cell tumors of the testis. Semin Diagn Pathol 1987;4:320–341.
47. Bredael JJ, Vugrin D, Whitmore WF Jr. Autopsy findings in 154 patients with germ cell tumors of the testis. Cancer 1982;50:548–551.
48. Cajal SRY, Pinango L, Barat E, et al. Metastatic pure choriocarcinoma of the testis in an elderly man. J Urol 1987;137:516–519.
49. Henry SC, Walsh PC, Rotner MB. Choriocarcinoma of the testis. J Urol 1974;112:105–108.
50. Manivel JC, Niehans G, Wick MR, et al. Intermediate trophoblast in germ cell neoplasms. Am J Surg Pathol 1987;11:693–701.
51. Ulbright TM, Loehrer PJ. Choriocarcinoma-like lesions in patients with testicular germ cell tumors. Two histologic variants. Am J Surg Pathol 1988;12:531–541.
52. Evans RW. Developmental stages of embryo-like bodies in teratoma testis. J Clin Pathol 1957;10:31–39.
53. Marin-Padilla M. Origin, nature and significance of the “embryoids” of human teratomas. Virchows Arch (A) 1965;340:105–121.
54. Gaillard JA. Yolk sac tumour patterns and entoblastic structure in polyembryomas. Acta Pathol Microbiol Scand (A) 1972;233:18–25.
55. Nakashima N, Murakami S, Fukatsu T, et al. Characteristics of “embryoid body” in human gonadal germ cell tumors. Hum Pathol 1988;19: 1144–1154.
56. Harms D, Janig U. Immature teratomas of childhood. Report of 21 cases. Pathol Res Pract 1985;179:388–400.
57. Tapper D, Lack EE. Teratomas in infancy and childhood: a 54 year experience at the Children’s Hospital Medical Center. Ann Surg 1983;198: 398–410.
58. Kooijman CD. Immature teratomas in children. Histopathology 1988;12: 491–502.
59. Leibovitch I, Foster RS, Ulbright TM, et al. Adult primary pure teratoma of the testis. The Indiana experience. Cancer 1995;75:2244–2250.
60. Dunphy CH, Ayala AG, Swanson DA, et al. Clinical stage I nonseminomatous and mixed germ cell tumors of the testis. A clinicopathologic study of 93 patients on a surveillance protocol after orchiectomy alone. Cancer 1988;62:1202–1206.
61. Berdjis CC, Mostofi FK. Carcinoid tumors of the testis. J Urol 1977;118: 777–782.
62. Hosking DH, Bowman DM, McMorris SL, et al. Primary carcinoid of the testis with metastases. J Urol 1981;125:255–256.
63. Kaufman JJ, Waisman J. Primary carcinoid tumor of testis with metastasis. Urology 1985;25:534–536.
64. Talerman A, Gratama S, Miranda S, et al. Primary carcinoid tumor of the testis: case report, ultrastructure and review of the literature. Cancer 1978; 42:2696–2706.
65. Zavala-Pompa A, Ro JY, El-Naggar AK, et al. Primary carcinoid tumor of testis: immunohistochemical, ultrastructural, and DNA flow cytometric study of three cases with a review of the literature. Cancer 1993;72: 1726–1732.
66. Price EB. Epidermoid cysts of the testis: a clinical and pathologic analysis of 69 cases from testicular tumor registry. J Urol 1969;102:708–713.
67. Shah KH, Maxted WC, Chun B, et al. Epidermoid cysts of the testis: a report of three cases and analysis of 141 cases from the world literature. Cancer 1981;47:577–582.
68. Dieckmann KP, Loy V. Epidermoid cyst of the testis: a review of clinical and histogenetic considerations. Br J Urol 1994;73:436–441.
69. Kim I, Young RH, Scully RE. Leydig cell tumors of the testis. A clinicopathological analysis of 40 cases and review of the literature. Am J Surg Pathol 1985;9:177–192.
70. Lawrence WD, Young RH, Scully RE. Sex cord-stromal tumors. In: Talerman A, Roth LH, eds. Pathology of the testis and its adnexa. New York: Churchill Livingstone; 1986:67–92.
71. Grem JL, Robins HI, Wilson KS, et al. Metastatic Leydig cell tumor of the testis. Report of three cases and review of the literature. Cancer 1986;58: 2116–2119.
72. Bertram KA, Bratloff B, Hodges JF, et al. Treatment of malignant Leydig cell tumor. Cancer 1991;68:2324–2329.
73. Weitzner S, Gropp A. Sertoli cell tumor of testis in childhood. Am J Dis Child 1974;128:541–543.
74. Kaplan JW, Cromie WJ, Kelalis PP, et al. Gonadal stromal tumors: a report of the prepubertal testicular tumor registry. J Urol 1986;136:300–302.

75. Wilson DM, Pitts WC, Hintz RL, et al. Testicular tumors with Peutz-Jeghers syndrome. Cancer 1986;57:2238–2240.
76. Jacobsen GK. Malignant Sertoli cell tumors. J Urol Pathol 1993;1:233–255.
77. Henly JD, Young RH, Ulbright TM. Malignant Sertoli cell tumors of the testis. A study of 13 examples of a neoplasm frequently misinterpreted as seminoma. Am J Surg Pathol 2002;26:541–550.
78. Young RH, Koelliker DD, Scully RE. Sertoli cell tumors of the testis, not otherwise specified. A clinicopathologic analysis of 60 cases. Am J Surg Pathol 1998;22:709–721.
79. Kratzer SS, Ulbright TM, Talerman A, et al. Large cell calcifying Sertoli cell tumor of the testis. Contrasting features of six malignant and six benign tumors and review of the literature. Am J Surg Pathol 1997;21: 1271–1280.
80. Proppe KH, Scully RE. Large cell calcifying Sertoli cell tumor of the testis. Am J Clin Pathol 1980;74:607–619.
81. Proppe KH, Dickersin GR. Large cell calcifying Sertoli cell tumor of the testis: light microscopic and ultrastructural study. Hum Pathol 1982;13: 1109–1114.
82. Tetu B, Ro JY, Ayala AG. Large cell calcifying Sertoli cell tumor of the testis: a clinicopathologic, immunohistochemical and ultrastructural study of two cases. Am J Clin Pathol 1991;96:717–722.
83. Redgrave NG, Allan P, Johnson WF. Large cell calcifying Sertoli cell tumour of the testis. Br J Urol 1995;75:411–412.
84. Zukerberg LR, Young RH, Scully RE. Sclerosing Sertoli cell tumor of the testis: a report of 10 cases. Am J Surg Pathol 1991;15:829–834.
85. Anderson GA. Sclerosing Sertoli cell tumor of the testis: a distinct histological subtype. J Urol 1995;154:1756–1758.
86. Teilum G. Estrogen producing Sertoli cell tumors (androblastoma tubulare lipoides of human testis and ovary). Homologous ovarian and testicular tumors. III. J Clin Endocrinol 1949;9:301–318.
87. Lawrence WD, Young RH, Scully RE. Juvenile granulosa cell tumor of the infantile testis. A report of 14 cases. Am J Surg Pathol 1985;9:87–94.
88. Harms D, Kock LR. Testicular juvenile granulosa cell and Sertoli cell tumours: a clinicopathological study of 29 cases from the Kiel Paediatric Tumour Registry. Virchows Arch 1997;430:301–309.
89. Tanaka Y, Sasaki Y, Tachibana K, et al. Testicular juvenile granulosa cell tumor in an infant with X/XY mosaicism clinically diagnosed as true hermaphroditism. Am J Surg Pathol 1994;18:316–332.
90. Talerman A. Pure granulosa cell tumor of the testis: report of a case and review of the literature. Appl Pathol 1985;3:117–122.
91. Jimenez-Quintero LP, Ro JY, Zavala-Pompa A, et al. Granulosa cell tumor of the adult testis: a clinicopathologic study of seven cases and a review of the literature. Hum Pathol 1993;24:1120–1126.
92. Matoska J, Ondrus D, Talerman A. Malignant granulosa cell tumor of the testis associated with gynecomastia and long survival. Cancer 1992;69: 1769–1772.
93. Campbell CM, Middleton AW Jr. Malignant gonadal stromal tumor: case report and review of the literature. J Urol 1981;125:257–259.
94. Gohji K, Higushi A, Fujii A, et al. Malignant gonadal stromal tumor. Urology 1994;43:244–247.
95. Scully RE. Gonadoblastoma. A review of 74 cases. Cancer 1970;25: 1340–1356.
96. Talerman A. The pathology of gonadal neoplasms composed of germ cells and sex cord stroma derivatives. Pathol Res Pract 1980;170:24–38.
97. Bolen JW. Mixed germ cell-sex cord stromal tumor: a gonadal tumor distinct from gonadoblastoma. Am J Clin Pathol 1981;75:565–573.
98. Matoska J, Talerman A. Mixed germ cell-sex cord stroma tumor of the testis. A report with ultrastructural findings. Cancer 1989;64:2146–2153.
99. Talerman A. Primary malignant lymphoma of the testis. J Urol 1977;118: 783–786.
100. Duncan PR, Checa E, Gowing NFC, et al. Extranodal non-Hodgkin's lymphoma presenting in the testicle: a clinical and pathologic study of 24 cases. Cancer 1980;45:1578–1584.
101. Paladugu RR, Bearman RM, Rappaport H. Malignant lymphoma with primary manifestation in the gonad. A clinicopathologic study of 38 patients. Cancer 1980;45:561–571.
102. Turner RR, Colby TV, McKintosh FR. Testicular lymphomas: a clinicopathologic study of 35 cases. Cancer 1981;48:2095–2102.
103. Doll DC, Weiss RB. Malignant lymphoma of the testis. Am J Med 1986;81:515–524.
104. Ferry JA, Harris NL, Young RH, et al. Malignant lymphoma of the testis, epididymis and spermatic cord. A clinicopathologic study of 69 cases with immunophenotypic analysis. Am J Surg Pathol 1994;18:376–390.
105. Hyland J, Lasota J, Jasinski M, et al. Molecular pathological analysis of testicular diffuse large cell lymphomas. Hum Pathol 1998;29:1231–1239.
106. Young RH, Scully RE. Miscellaneous neoplasms and non-neoplastic lesions. In: Talerman A, Roth LM, eds. Pathology of the testis and its adnexa. New York: Churchill Livingstone; 1986:103–104.
107. Chica G, Johnson DE, Ayala AG. Plasmacytoma of testis presenting as primary testicular tumor. Urology 1978;11:90–92.
108. Oppenheim PI, Cohen S, Anders KH. Testicular plasmacytoma. A case report with immunohistochemical studies and literature review. Arch Pathol Lab Med 1991;115:629–632.
109. White J, Chan YF. Solitary testicular plasmacytoma. Br J Urol 1995;75: 107–108.
110. Givler RL. Testicular involvement in leukemia and lymphoma. Cancer 1969;23:1290–1295.
111. Eden OB, Hardisty RM, Innes EM, et al. Testicular disease in acute lymphoblastic leukaemia in childhood. Br Med J 1978;1:334–338.
112. Reed H, Marsden HB. Gonadal infiltration in children with leukaemia and lymphoma. J Clin Pathol 1980;33:722–729.
113. Layfield LJ, Hilborne LH, Ljung BM, et al. Use of fine needle aspiration cytology for the diagnosis of testicular relapse in patients with acute lymphoblastic leukemia. J Urol 1988;139:1020–1022.
114. Viprakasit D, Tannenbaum M, Smith AM. Adenomatoid tumor of the male genital tract. Urology 1974;4:325–327.
115. Keily EA, Flanagan A, Williams G. Intrascrotal adenomatoid tumours. Br J Urol 1987;60:255–257.
116. Taxy JB, Battifora H, Oyasu R. Adenomatoid tumors. A light microscopic, histochemical, and ultrastructural study. Cancer 1974;34:306–316.
117. Barwick KW, Madri JA. An immunohistochemical study of adenomatoid tumors utilizing keratin and factor VIII antibodies. Evidence for a mesothelial origin. Lab Invest 1982;47:276–280.
118. Mackay B, Bennington JL, Skoglund RW. The adenomatoid tumor. Fine structural evidence for a mesothelial differentiation. Cancer 1971;27: 109–115.
119. Antman K, Cohen S, Dimitrov NV, et al. Malignant mesothelioma of the tunica vaginalis testis. J Clin Oncol 1984;2:447–451.
120. Chetty R. Well differentiated (benign) papillary mesothelioma of the tunica vaginalis. J Clin Pathol 1992;45:1029–1030.
121. Carp NZ, Petersen RO, Kusiak JF, et al. Malignant mesothelioma of the tunica vaginalis testis. J Urol 1990;144:1475–1478.
122. Reynard JM, Hasan N, Baithun SI, et al. Malignant mesothelioma of the tunica vaginalis testis. Br J Urol 1994;74:389–390.
123. Eden CG, Bettochi C, Coker CB, et al. Malignant mesothelioma of the tunica vaginalis. J Urol 1995;153:1053–1054.
124. Young RH, Scully RE. Testicular and paratesticular tumors and tumor-like lesions of ovarian common epithelial and Mullerian types. A report of four cases and review of the literature. Am J Clin Pathol 1986;86: 146–151.
125. Axiotis CA. Intratesticular serous papillary cystadenoma of low malignant potential: an ultrastructural and immunohistochemical study suggesting Mullerian differentiation. Am J Surg Pathol 1988;12:56–63.
126. Brito CG, Bloch T, Foster RS, et al. Testicular papillary cystadenomatous tumor of low malignant potential. A case report and discussion of the literature. J Urol 1988;139:378–379.
127. Remmele W, Kaiserling E, Zerban U, et al. Serous papillary cystic tumor of borderline malignancy with focal carcinoma arising in testis: case report with immunohistochemical and ultrastructural observations. Hum Pathol 1992;23:75–79.
128. De Nictolis M, Tommasoni S, Fabris G, et al. Intratesticular serous cystadenoma of borderline malignancy. A pathological, histochemical and DNA content study of a case with long-term follow-up. Virchows Arch (A) 1993;423:221–225.
129. Ross L. Paratesticular Brenner-like tumor. Cancer 1968;21:722–726.
130. Goldman RL. A Brenner tumor of the testis. Cancer 1970;26:853-856.
131. Uzoaru I, Ray VH, Nadimpalli V. Brenner tumor of the testis. J Urol Pathol 1995;3:249–253.
132. Caccamo D, Socias M, Truchet C. Malignant Brenner tumor of the testis and epididymis. Arch Pathol Lab Med 1991;115:524–527.
133. Nistal M, Paniagua R. Adenomatous hyperplasia of the rete testis. J Pathol 1988;154:343–346.
134. Ulbright TM, Gersell DJ. Rete testis hyperplasia with hyaline globule formation. A lesion simulating yolk sac tumor. Am J Surg Pathol 1991;15: 66–74.
135. Hartwick RW, Ro JY, Srigley JR, et al. Adenomatous hyperplasia of the rete testis. A clinicopathologic study of nine cases. Am J Surg Pathol 1991; 15:350–357.
136. Altaffer LF, Dufour DR, Castleberry GM, et al. Coexisting rete testis adenoma and gonadoblastoma. J Urol 1982;127:332–335.

137. Murao T, Takahashi T. Adenofibroma of the rete testis. A case report with electron microscopy findings. Acta Pathol Jpn 1988;38:105–112.
138. Nochomovitz LE, Orenstein JM. Adenocarcinoma of the rete testis: consolidation and analysis of 31 reported cases with a review of miscellaneous entities. J Urol Pathol 1994;2:1–38.
139. Stein JP, Freeman JA, Esrig D, et al. Papillary adenocarcinoma of the rete testis: a case report and review of the literature. Urology 1994;44: 588–594.
140. Nochomovitz LE, Orenstein JM. Adenocarcinoma of the rete testis: case report, ultrastructural observations and clinicopathologic correlates. Am J Surg Pathol 1984;8:625–634.
141. Crisp-Lindgren N, Travers H, Wells MM, et al. Papillary adenocarcinoma of rete testis. Autopsy findings, histochemistry, immunohistochemistry, ultrastructure, and clinical correlations. Am J Surg Pathol 1988;12: 492–501.
142. Visscher DW, Talerman A, Rivera LR, et al. Adenocarcinoma of the rete testis with a spindle cell component. A possible metaplastic carcinoma. Cancer 1989;64:770–775.
143. Price EB. Papillary cystadenoma of the epididymis: a clinicopathologic analysis of 20 cases. Arch Pathol 1971;91:456–470.
144. Salm R. Papillary carcinoma of the epididymis. J Pathol 1969;97: 253–259.
145. Calder CJ, Gregory J. Papillary cystadenoma of the epididymis: a report of two cases with an immunohistochemical study. Histopathology 1993;23: 89–91.
146. Kragel PJ, Pestaner J, Travis WD, et al. Papillary cystadenoma of the epididymis: a report of three cases with lectin histochemistry. Arch Pathol Lab Med 1993;114:672–675.
147. Pettinato G, Manivel JC, d'Amore ES, et al. Melanotic neuroectodermal tumor of infancy. A reexamination of a histogenetic problem based on immunohistochemical, flow cytometric and ultrastructural study of 10 cases. Am J Surg Pathol 1991;15:233–245.
148. Ricketts RR, Majmudar B. Epididymal melanotic neuroectodermal tumor of infancy. Hum Pathol 1985;16:416–420.
149. Cutler LS, Chaudhry AP, Topazian R. Melanotic neuroectodermal tumor of infancy: an ultrastructural study, literature review, and reevaluation. Cancer 1981;48:257–270.
150. Johnson RE, Scheithauer BW, Dahlin DC. Melanotic neuroectodermal tumor of infancy. A review of seven cases. Cancer 1983;52:661–666.
151. Yahia P, Auslaender L. Primary leiomyosarcoma of the testis. J Urol 1989; 141:955–956.
152. Eltorky MA, O'Brien TF, Walzer Y. Primary paratesticular malignant fibrous histiocytoma: case report and review of the literature. J Urol Pathol 1993;1:425–429.
153. Hargreaves HK, Scully RE, Richie JP. Benign hemangioendothelioma of the testis: case report with electron microscopic documentation and review of the literature. Am J Clin Pathol 1982;77:637–642.
154. Suriawinata A, Talerman A, Vapnek JM, et al. Hemangioma of the testis: case reports of unusual occurrences of carvernous hemangioma in a fetus, and a capillary hemangioma in an older man. Ann Diagn Pathol 2001;5: 80–83.
155. Loughlin KR, Retik AB, Weinstein HJ, et al. Genitourinary rhabdomyosarcoma in children. Cancer 1989;63:1600–1606.
156. Stewart LH, Lioe TF, Johnston SR. Thirty-year review of intrascrotal rhabdomyosarcoma. Br J Urol 1991;68:418–420.
157. Cecchetto GG, Grotto P, De Bernardi B, et al. Paratesticular rhabdomyosarcoma in childhood: experience of the Italian Cooperative Study. Tumori 1988;74:645–647.
158. Arean VM, Kreager JA. Paratesticular rhabdomyosarcoma. Am J Clin Pathol 1965;43:418–427.
159. Cavazzana AO, Schmidt D, Ninfo V, et al. Spindle cell rhabdomyosarcoma. A prognostically favorable variant of rhabdomyosarcoma. Am J Surg Pathol 1992;16:229–235.
160. Hughes LL, Baruzzi MJ, Ribeiro RC, et al. Paratesticular rhabdomyosarcoma: delayed effects of multimodality therapy and implications for current management. Cancer 1994;73:476–482.
161. Price EB, Mostofi FK. Secondary carcinoma of the testis. Cancer 1957;10: 592–595.
162. Meares EM Jr, Ho TL. Metastatic carcinomas involving the testis: a review. J Urol 1973;109:653–655.
163. Tiltman AJ. Metastatic tumours of the testis. Histopathology 1979;3: 31–37.
164. Haupt HM, Mann RB, Trump DL, et al. Metastatic carcinoma involving the testis. Clinical and pathologic distinction from primary testicular neoplasms. Cancer 1984;54:709–714.
165. Grignon DJ, Shum DT, Hayman WP. Metastatic tumours of the testes. Can J Surg 1986;29:359–361.
166. Almagro UA. Metastatic tumors involving the testis. Urology 1998;32: 357–360.
167. Nistal M, Paniagua R, Diez-Pardo JA. Histologic classification of undescended testes. Hum Pathol 1980;11:666–674.
168. Batata MA, Chu FCH, Hilaris BS, et al. Testicular cancer in cryptorchids. Cancer 1982;49:1023–1030.
169. Muller J, Skakkebaek NE, Nielsen OH, et al. Cryptorchidism and testis cancer. Atypical infantile germ cells followed by carcinoma in situ and invasive carcinoma in adulthood. Cancer 1984;54:629–634.
170. Gordon DL, Krmpotic E, Thomas W, et al. Pathologic testicular findings in Klinefelter's syndrome. 47,XXY vs 46,XY/47,XXY. Arch Intern Med 1972; 130:726–729.
171. Hasle H, Mellemgaard A, Nielsen J, et al. Cancer incidence in men with Klinefelter syndrome. Br J Cancer 1995;71:416–420.
172. Ceccacci L, Tosi S. Splenic-gonadal fusion: case report and review of the literature. J Urol 1981;126:558–559.
173. Andrews RW, Copeland DD, Fried FA. Splenogonadal fusion. J Urol 1985; 133:1052–1053.
174. Knorr PA, Borden TA. Splenogonadal fusion. Urology 1994;44:136–138.
175. Rutgers JL, Young RH, Scully RE. The testicular "tumor" of the adrenogenital syndrome. A report of five cases and review of the literature on testicular masses in patients with disorders of the adrenal glands. Am J Surg Pathol 1998;12:503–513.
176. Dahl EV, Bahn RC. Aberrant adrenal cortical tissue near the testis in human infants. Am J Pathol 1962;40:587–598.
177. Mares AJ, Shkolnik A, Sacks M, et al. Aberrant (ectopic) adrenocortical tissue along the spermatic cord. J Pediatr Surg 1980;15:289–292.
178. Nistal M, Regardera J, Paniagua R. Cystic dysplasia of the testis: light and electron microscopic study of three cases. Arch Pathol Lab Med 1984;108: 579–583.
179. Tesluk H, Blankenberg TA. Cystic dysplasia of testis. Urology 1987;23: 47–49.
180. Dahl EV, Baggenstoss AH, De Weerd JH. Testicular lesions of periarteritis nodosa with special reference to diagnosis. Am J Med 1960;28:222–228.
181. Skoglund RW, McRoberts JW, Ragde H. Torsion of the spermatic cord: a review of the literature and an analysis of 70 new cases. J Urol 1970;104: 604–607.
182. Shurbardji MS, Epstein JI. Testicular vasculitis: implications for systemic disease. Hum Pathol 1998;19:186–189.
183. Morgan AD. Inflammation and infestation of the testis and paratesticular structures. In: Pugh RCB, ed. Pathology of the testis. Oxford: Blackwell; 1976:79–138.
184. Gall EA. The histopathology of acute mumps orchitis. Am J Pathol 1947; 23:637–651.
185. Manson AL. Mumps orchitis. Urology 1990;36:355–358.
186. Craighead JE, Mahoney EM, Carver DH, et al. Orchitis due to Coxsackie virus group B types: report of a case with isolation of virus from the testis. N Engl J Med 1962;267:498–500.
187. O'Hourihane DB. Infected infarcts of the testis: a study of 18 cases preceded by pyogenic epididymo-orchitis. J Clin Pathol 1970;23:668–675.
188. Young RH, Scully RE. Granulomatous orchitis. In: Talerman A, Roth LM, eds. Pathology of the testis and its adnexa. New York: Churchill Livingstone; 1986:110.
189. Christensen WI. Genitourinary tuberculosis. A review of 102 cases. Medicine 1974;53:377–390.
190. Cos LR, Cockett ATK. Genitourinary tuberculosis revisited. Urology 1982; 20:111–117.
191. Ferrie BG, Rundle JSH. Tuberculous epididymo-orchitis. A review of 20 cases. Br J Urol 1983;55:437–439.
192. Amenta PS, Gonick P, Katz SM. Sarcoidosis of testis and epididymis. Urology 1981;17:616–617.
193. Spjut H, Thorpe J. Granulomatous orchitis. Am J Clin Pathol 1956;26: 136–145.
194. Wegner HE, Loy V, Dieckmann KP. Granulomatous orchitis: an analysis of clinical presentation, pathological anatomic features and possible etiologic factors. Eur Urol 1994;26:56–60.
195. McClure J. Malakoplakia of the testis and its relationship to granulomatous orchitis. J Clin Pathol 1980;33:670–678.
196. McClure J. Malakoplakia. J Pathol 1983;140:275–330.
197. Stevens SA. Malakoplakia of the testis. Br J Urol 1995;75:111–112.
198. Young RH, Scully RE. Fibromatous periorchitis. In: Talerman A, Roth LM, eds. Pathology of the testis and its adnexa. New York: Churchill Livingstone; 1986:113–114.

199. Begin LR, Frail D, Brzezinski A. Myofibroblastoma of the tunica testis: evolving phase of so-called fibrous pseudotumor? Hum Pathol 1990;21: 866–868.
200. Parveen T, Fleischmann J, Petrelli M. Benign fibrous tumor of the tunica vaginalis testis. Report of a case with light, electron microscopic, and immunocytochemical study, and review of the literature. Arch Pathol Lab Med 1992;116:277–280.
201. Civantos F, Lubin J, Rywlin AM. Vasitis nodosa. Arch Pathol 1972;94: 355–361.
202. Kovi J, Agbata A. Benign neural invasion in vasitis nodosa. JAMA 1974; 228:15–19.
203. Zimmerman KG, Johnson PC, Paplanus SH. Nerve invasion by benign proliferating ductules in vasitis nodosa. Cancer 1983;51: 2066–2069.
204. Balogh K, Travis WD. Benign vascular invasion in vasitis nodosa. Am J Clin Pathol 1985;83:426–430.
205. Friedman NB, Garske GL. Inflammatory reactions involving sperm and seminiferous tubules: extravasation, spermatic granulomas and granulomatous orchitis. J Urol 1949;62:363–374.
206. Glassy FJ, Mostofi FK. Spermatic granulomas of the epididymis. Am J Clin Pathol 1956;26:1303–1313.
207. Young RH, Scully RE. Sperm granuloma. In: Talerman A, Roth LM, eds. Pathology of the testis and its adnexa. New York: Churchill Livingstone; 1986:121–122.
208. Schmidt SS, Morris RR. Spermatic granuloma: the complication of vasectomy. Fertil Steril 1973;24:941–947.
209. Dunner PS, Lipsit ER, Nochomovitz LE. Epididymal sperm granuloma simulating a testicular neoplasm. J Clin Ultrasound 1982;10:353.

5

FINE-NEEDLE ASPIRATION OF THE PROSTATE

John Maksem and Iqbal Kapadia

In 1930, Russell Ferguson reported the diagnosis of prostate cancer by transperineal fine-needle aspiration (FNA); however, it was not until three decades later that Sixten Franzen of Sweden's Karolinska Institute applied the procedure to diagnostic uropathology. In the United States, urologists perform prostate biopsies with 18-gauge cutting needles using automated biopsy devices. Consequently, most pathologists in the United States have had little opportunity to examine prostate FNAs.

Prostate aspiration biopsy is a sensitive and specific,[1,2] easily performed office procedure requiring no expensive equipment, anesthesia, or antibacterial prophylaxis.[3–5] Some have argued that FNA is most appropriate for repeated follow-up of men managed by watchful waiting, whereas ultrasonography and biopsy should be used in preoperative evaluation when radical prostatectomy is anticipated.[6] Others maintain that FNA is a reasonable initial diagnostic procedure for detecting prostate cancer, and that core biopsy may be reserved for individuals with negative cytology who are clinically suspected of having prostate cancer.[7] We view the two techniques as complementary and synergistic.[8] As recently as 1988, Benson recommended to the National Institutes of Health Consensus Development Panel on the Management of Clinically Localized Prostate Cancer that FNA should be encouraged as a standard part of the urologist's diagnostic armamentarium: performed by urologists; taught to urology residents; and its interpretation learned by pathology residents.[9]

FNA and ultrasound-guided cutting-needle biopsy using automated biopsy devices have a high and equal accuracy in diagnosing prostate cancer. Maksem[8] reported on 228 matched core and FNA specimen pairs among which 90 carcinomas were discovered by either method. Eighty-four (93%) cancers were detected by core biopsy and 86 (96%) by FNA. In a comparable study of 246 matched cases in which 103 carcinomas were discovered, 96 (93%) of cancers were detected by core biopsy and 101 (98%) by FNA.[10]

FNA may be used to detect clinically inapparent prostate carcinomas prior to transurethral resection (TUR). Among 102 men with clinically benign prostates by rectal examination, four-quadrant FNA before TUR correctly identified 17 of 19 T1 cancers. After correcting for adequate diagnostic material, FNA identified all cases of T1b (tumor in >5% of resected tissue) prostate carcinoma but no cases of T1a (tumor in <5% of resected tissue) carcinoma. No false-positive diagnoses were rendered.[1]

BENIGN PROSTATE

Benign prostate epithelium contains ducts and acini. Ducts transform into acini, yielding intermediate-size structures. Ducts are branching, tubular structures consisting of secretory epithelial cells, rare endocrine cells, and a jacket of basal cells. Acini are intermediate to small, regular, bag-like structures consisting of cells identical to those in the ducts.

In elderly men, ductuloacinar glands vary from narrow to wide, sometimes with cystic dilatation owing to prostate hyperplasia, and contain a mixture of columnar and cuboidal cells. In young men there are more glands, more acinar than ductal glands, and a more uniform population of columnar cells.

Nuclei of benign epithelial cells are unilayered, round to oval, regularly distributed, and monotonous. Chromatin is finely granular, and the nuclear size is comparable to that of an erythrocyte. Nucleoli are generally indistinct, except in occasional cases of epithelial hyperplasia, where chromocenters or micronucleoli may be seen. (Figs 5.1–5.7)

CYTOLOGIC ATYPIAS

Cases with cytologic atypia comprise benign, premalignant, and malignant proliferations. Sources of atypical cells include: injury or inflammation; seminal vesicle puncture; putative and confirmed premalignant conditions (atypical small acinar proliferation and prostate intraepithelial neoplasia); and poorly sampled or volumetrically limited well-differentiated prostate adenocarcinomas.

All patients with cytologic atypia must be followed up because, in many cases, atypia is associated with carcinoma. Among 104 men whose initial FNA showed 'severe dysplasia', repeat FNA found 36 (35%) dysplasias and 41 (39%) carcinomas.[12]

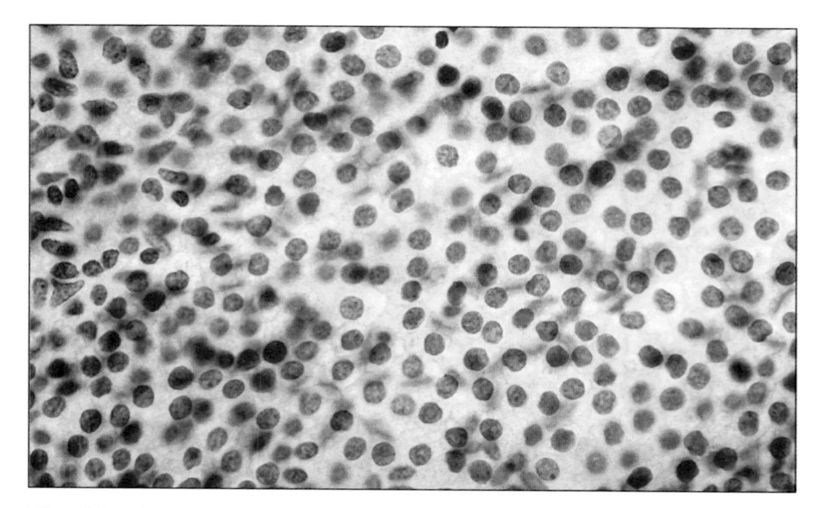

Fig. 5.1 Because ducts are large and mechanically disrupted (opened) by aspiration biopsy, many ducts appear as flat sheets of cells with orderly nuclei. The cell borders within ducts and acini have distinct, hexagonal, honeycomb configurations.

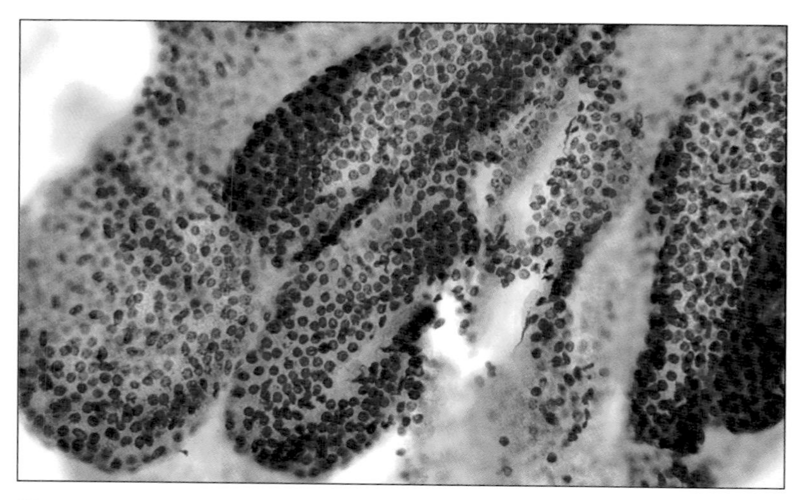

Fig. 5.2 Conversely, acini are unaltered (unopened) by fine-needle aspiration and remain intact because of their small size. Here, a cascade of ductuloacinar structures shows how tubular glands terminate in a flourish of bag-like structures.

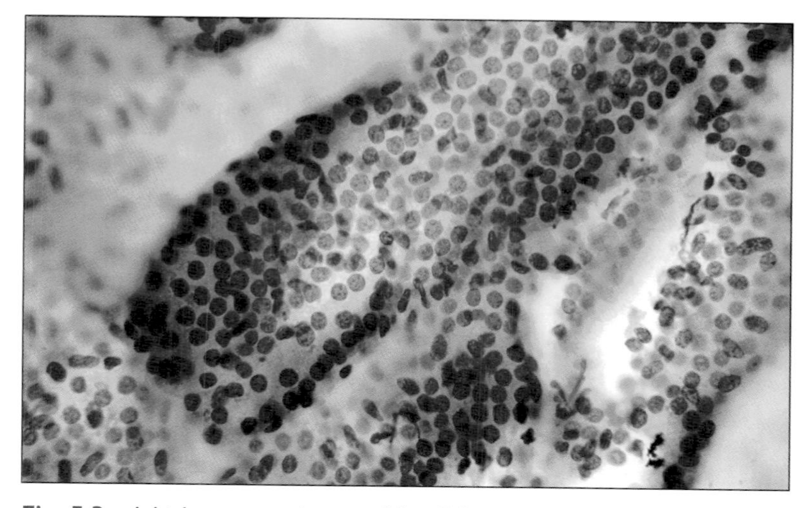

Fig. 5.3 A higher-power image of Fig. 5.2 shows that 3 acinar structures are composed of both secretory and basal cells. The basal cells form a reticulated or basket-weave cytoplasmic pattern in a continuous jacket around benign ductuloacinar glands that is absent in malignancy.

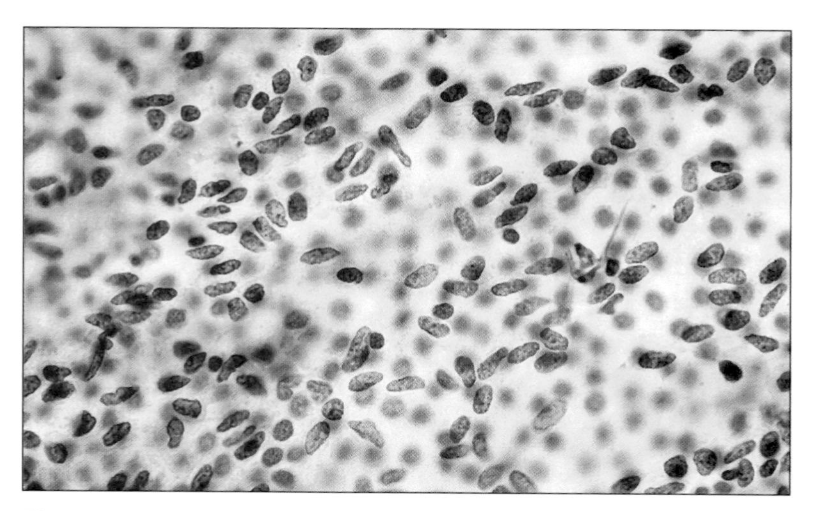

Fig. 5.4 The secretory cells of the prostate are separated from its stroma by a layer of basal cells. Here, the same field as in Fig. 5.1 is refocused to show the underlying basal cells with fusiform nuclei. Basal cells are present in normal, atrophic, and hyperplastic epithelium. They are few or absent in atypical small acinar proliferations and prostate intraepithelial neoplasia; and they are absent in transitional cell and squamous cell metaplasia and in prostate cancer.

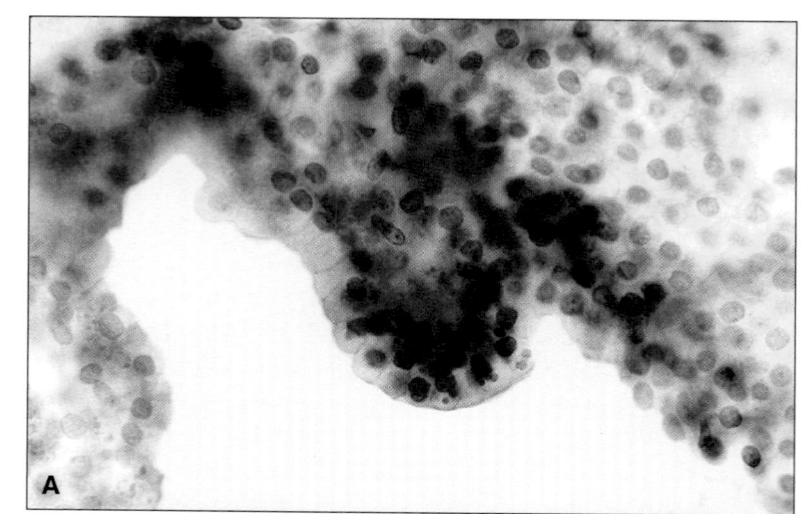

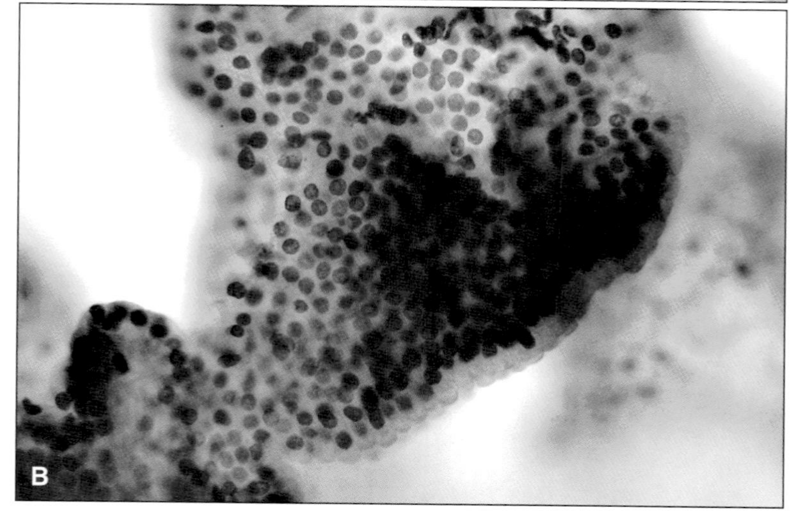

Fig. 5.5 In hyperplasia, epithelial cells are present above the plane of the epithelial cell sheet, forming hills, valleys, and club-like aggregates. (A) A knob of epithelial cells shows an orderly arrangement of secretory cells with a long apex-to-base axis, basally oriented nuclei, perinuclear tertiary lysosomes, and subnuclear basal cells. (B) A partly twisted duct epithelial sheet demonstrates similar features.

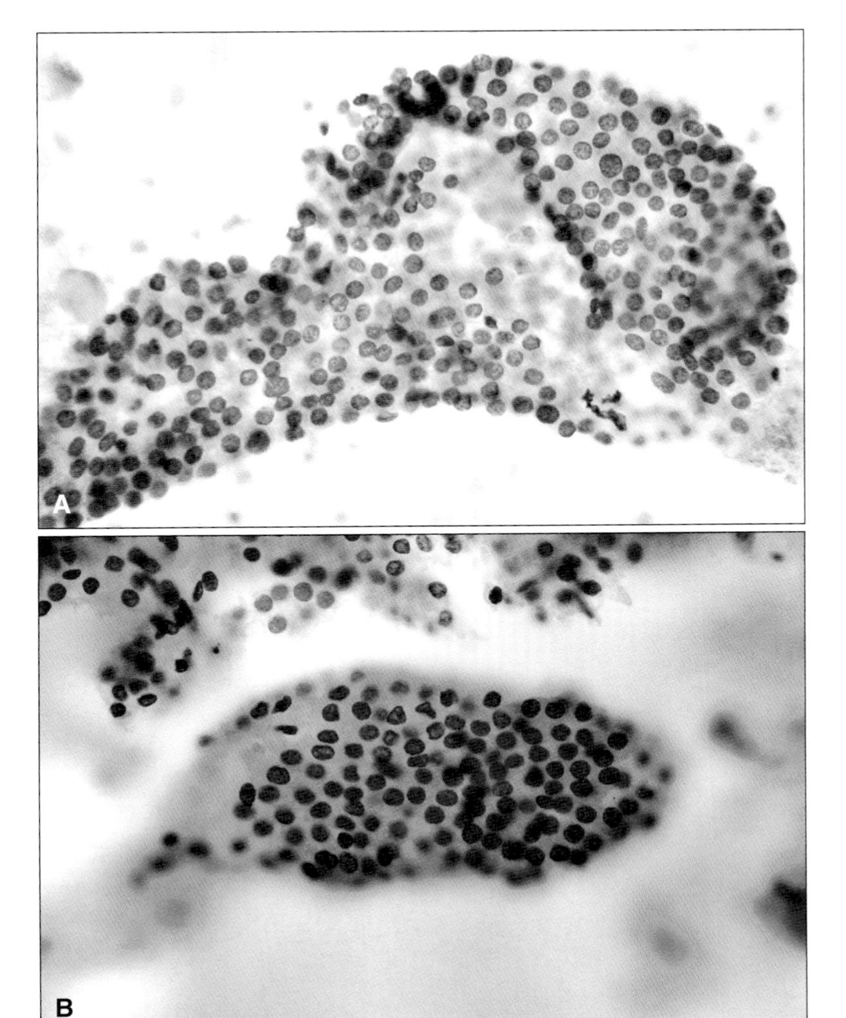

Fig. 5.6 In atrophy, cells are cuboidal, with sharp cell boundaries that lack scalloping of the apical cytoplasm. (A) A somewhat irregularly shaped, atrophic acinar structure shows sparse basal cells and regularly arrayed secretory cells. (B) A much smaller acinar structure appears to be made almost entirely of secretory cells. Atrophic and hyperplastic changes commonly occur together, because hyperplasia and atrophy generally coexist.

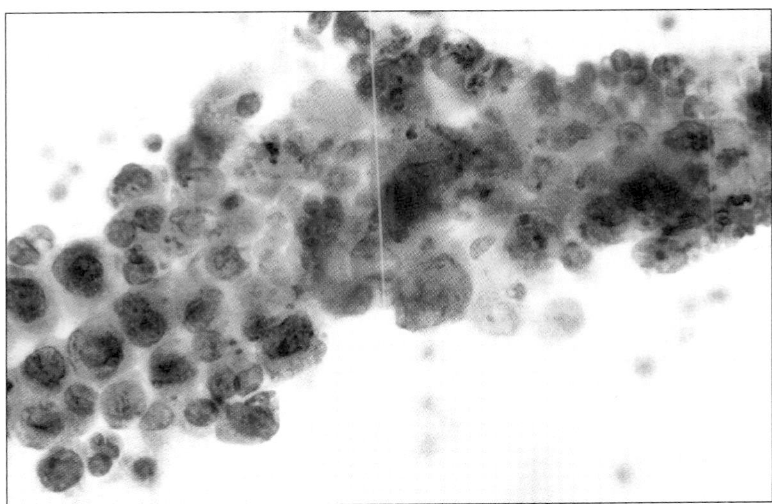

Fig. 5.7 Seminal vesicle punctures may yield bizarre cells that can be misinterpreted as undifferentiated large cell malignant neoplasm.[11] Seminal vesicle epithelium is negative for prostate-specific antigen. Seminal vesicle epithelium has coarse golden pigment, and seminal vesicle puncture often yields blobs and angulated aggregates of waxy eosinophilic substance. Similar epithelium is present in the ejaculatory ducts, but coarse epithelial pigment and amorphous secretory material is not seen.

No good clues reliably separate those atypias with high cancer risk from those without. In a comparison of six smears from histologically proven benign disease and six from cancer, no cytomorphometric criteria were identified that accurately subdivided cases as benign or malignant.[13] On the other hand, silver staining for nucleolar organizing regions in FNAs improved the sensitivity of cancer diagnosis from 87% to 96%,[14] making it a useful and inexpensive tool in routine practice.

It is not the mere presence of nucleoli that is indicative of prostate cancer, but the presence of sizable nucleoli.[15] An analysis of prostatic nucleolar morphometric features revealed a difference in the number of nucleoli between definitely benign samples and other atypia groups. The best feature for distinguishing between atypia groups was nucleolar size.

As with cutting-needle biopsy, if cancer is not found in a prostate gland in which there is a high index of suspicion for cancer, the procedure should be repeated. A frankly benign diagnosis in a clinically suspicious gland carries an approximately 20% chance of malignancy on repeat biopsy.[12] This figure is comparable to a reported 23% transrectal cutting-needle biopsy false-negative rate.[16]

INFLAMMATION

Prostatitis can produce a palpably abnormal – generally doughy – prostate and alter the appearance of the prostate epithelium. The aspirates of prostatitis are abundantly cellular, and inflammatory cells are present in all cases. In uncomplicated cases, epithelial atypia is proportionate to the stage and intensity of the inflammatory process. Inflammatory atypia comprises nuclear enlargement, small to intermediate-size nucleoli, and intracytoplasmic lumens that may indent the regular contour of the nuclear envelope. Various types of metaplasia may be seen.[17]

With inflammation, the architecture of the prostate is altered and individual prostate nuclei may be degenerated and stripped of their cytoplasm. Carcinoma should be diagnosed with caution in the setting of prostatitis.[18] The pathologist must weigh carefully whether the atypia is proportionate to the degree of inflammation, as in repair, or disproportionate, which may tend to suggest a neoplastic basis. (Figs 5.8–5.13)

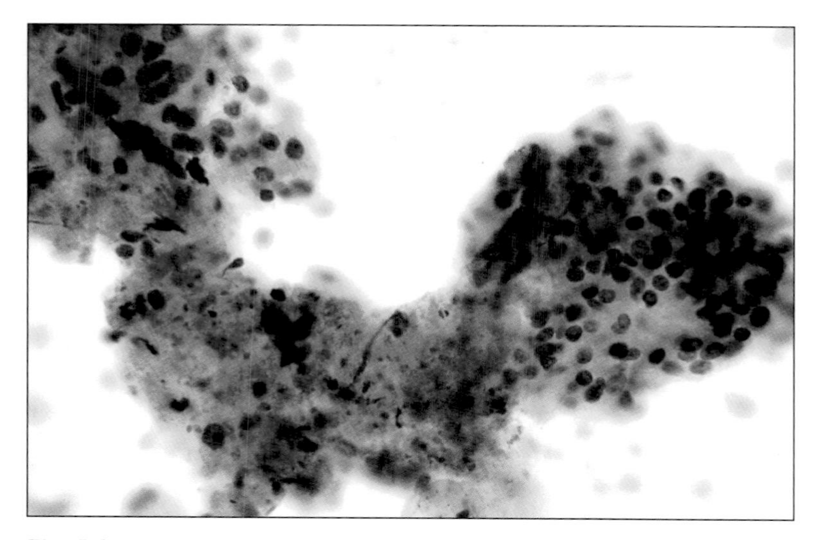

Fig. 5.8 In acute prostatitis, epithelial cells occur as small, sometimes 'exploded', aggregates mixed with the neutrophils. In this example, histiocytes, eosinophils, and bacteria are admixed with necrotic epithelium. There is loss of distinct cell borders, slight to moderate anisonucleosis, small to intermediate-size nucleoli, nuclear crowding, overlapping, and indentation.

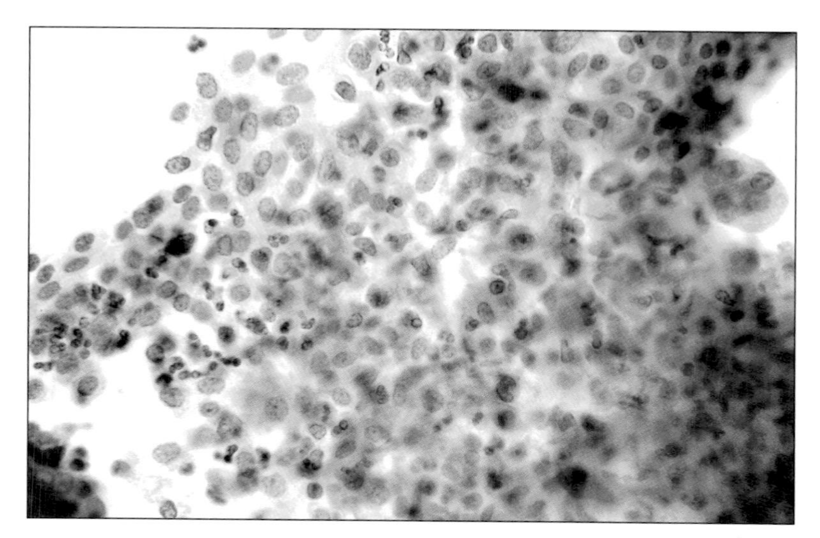

Fig. 5.9 Acute prostatitis shows high numbers of neutrophils. Subacute inflammation both masks and disorganizes associated secretory epithelium.

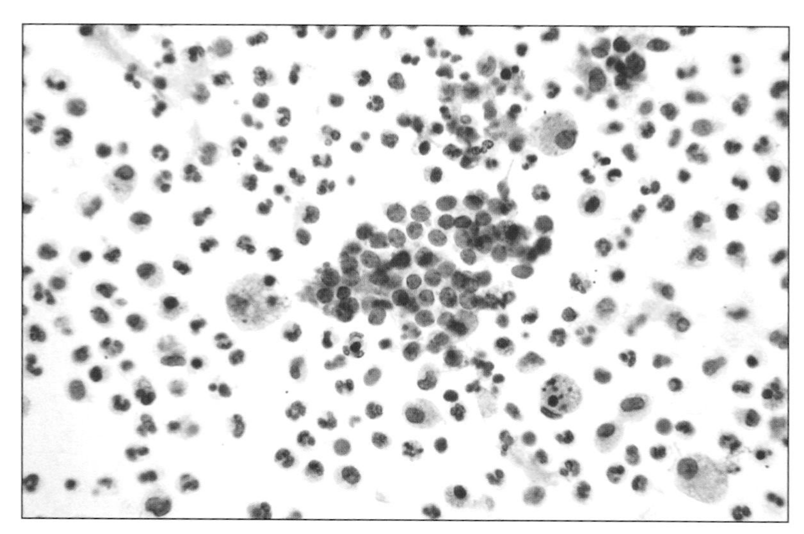

Fig. 5.10 Signature changes of chronic prostatitis comprise histiocytes, with lesser numbers of neutrophils, eosinophils, lymphocytes, giant cells, and plasma cells. Epithelial disorganization and atypia will typically appear less severe than with acute prostatitis. Frequently there is accumulation of intracellular refractive golden-brown pigment (coarse basophilic material in tetrachrome stains), representing constipated tertiary lysosomes.

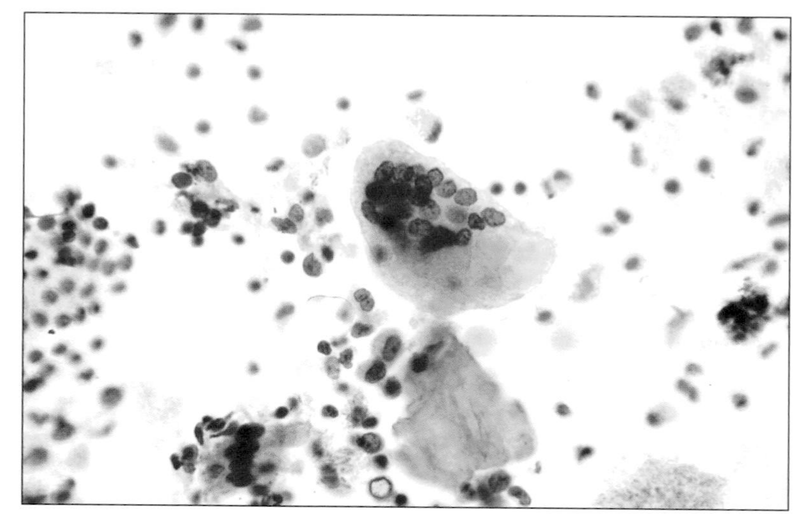

Fig. 5.11 Here, a smooth-contoured multinucleated histiocyte, probably formed within a prostatic duct, lies adjacent to an orangeophilic, angulated prostatic crystalloid.

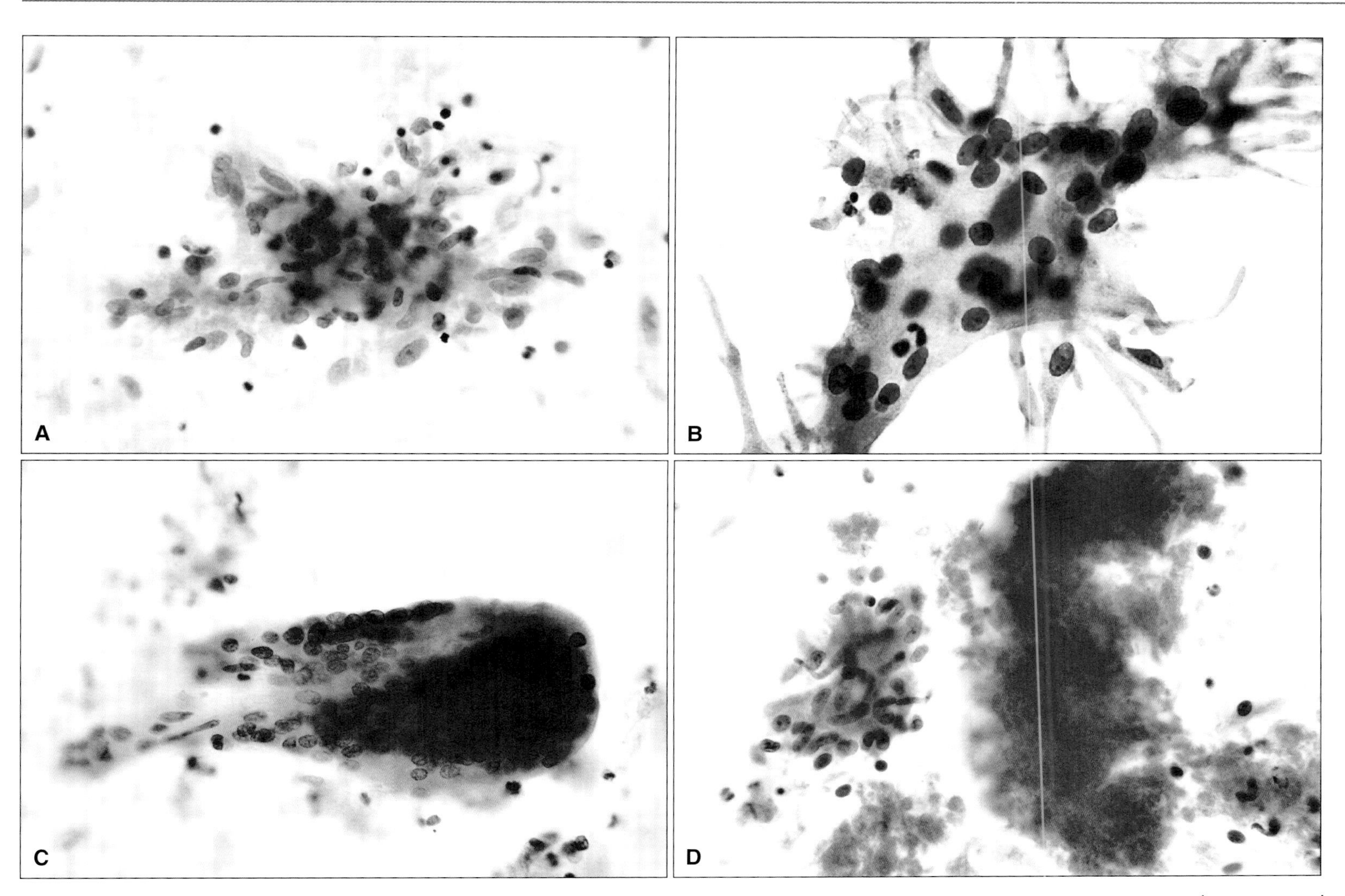

Fig. 5.12 Granulomatous prostatitis feels like prostate cancer to the palpating finger. The most common cause is instrumentation, such as transurethral resection, but infectious etiologies (tuberculosis, blastomycosis) are also possible and can be ruled out by special stains and culture. Fine-needle aspiration shows ill-defined aggregates of immobilized macrophages, some with numerous nuclei and some with dendritic borders, caused by juxtaposition of histiocytes to stromal cells (A,B). Cytoplasmic fusion among adjacent histiocytes leads to the formation of these giant cells with prominent dendritic processes (C). Amorphous necrotic debris may be seen, and epithelial changes are similar to those of chronic prostatitis. Iatrogenic granulomatous prostatitis occur with bacille Calmette-Guérin (BCG) therapy for bladder cancer, accompanied by caseous necrosis (D).

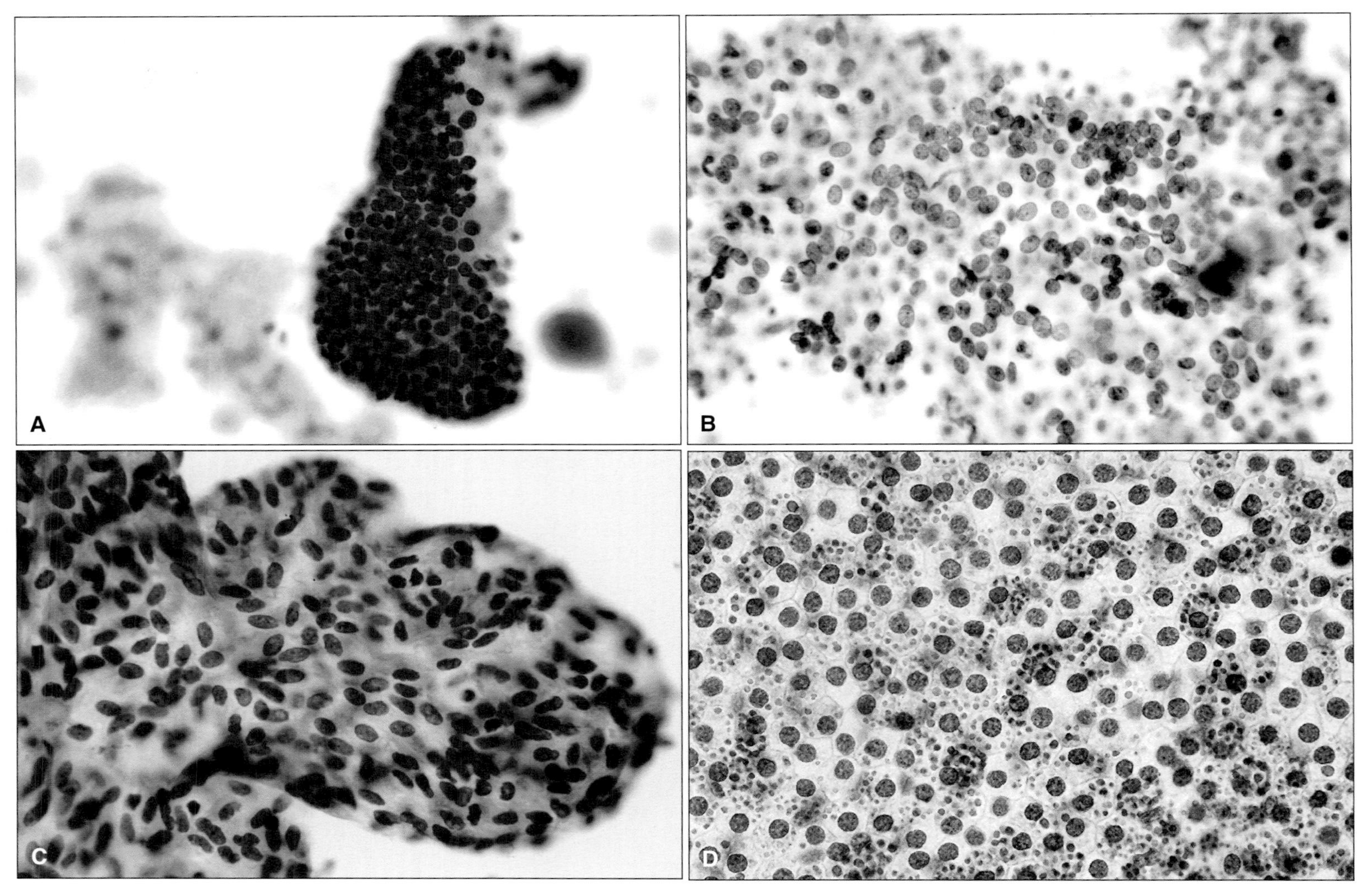

Fig. 5.13 In healed prostatitis, there will be re-establishment of prostatic architecture, with crowding and slight to moderate disorganization of the sheet architecture of epithelial cells. Crowded secretory cells may show minor nuclear shape irregularities (A). There is rounding and irregular proliferation of basal cells (B). Associated epithelial changes include squamous and transitional cell metaplasia. Secretory acini may be replaced by immature metaplastic cells (C). Retention of epithelial pigment in constipated tertiary lysosomes reflects the repair that has occurred within the epithelium (D).

ATYPICAL SMALL ACINAR PROLIFERATION (ASAP)

Histologically, putative premalignant changes are separated into two categories: atypical small acinar proliferation (ASAP) and prostatic intraepithelial neoplasia (PIN), which is a ductal lesion. Prostatic pre-neoplasia is a primary proliferation of abnormal epithelium and not a transient and reversible injury-repair phenomenon or some form of metaplasia.

In cytologic material, ASAP refers to the spectrum of lesions most commonly comprising post-atrophic hyperplasia, adenosis, atypical adenomatous hyperplasia, and well-differentiated small acinar adenocarcinoma.[19] FNAs lack the tissue context that is helpful in deciphering between these lesions in histologic material.[20] Cytologic ASAP is therefore an operational – rather than a biologic – risk factor. The operational risk entails overlooking a carcinoma or overcalling a biologically indolent lesion. (Fig. 5.14)

PROSTATIC INTRAEPITHELIAL NEOPLASIA (PIN)

PIN is a non-destructive intraductal pre-neoplastic epithelial proliferation. PIN is easy to identify in FNA specimens because ducts are seen as sheets of several hundred nuclei laid side to side *en face*. This arrangement exposes aberrations among large numbers of juxtaposed nuclei for which benign epithelium provides excellent internal control to which the eye is exquisitely sensitive. Basal cells are retained and may on occasion be seen in routinely stained cytological preparations or by staining for basal cell-specific

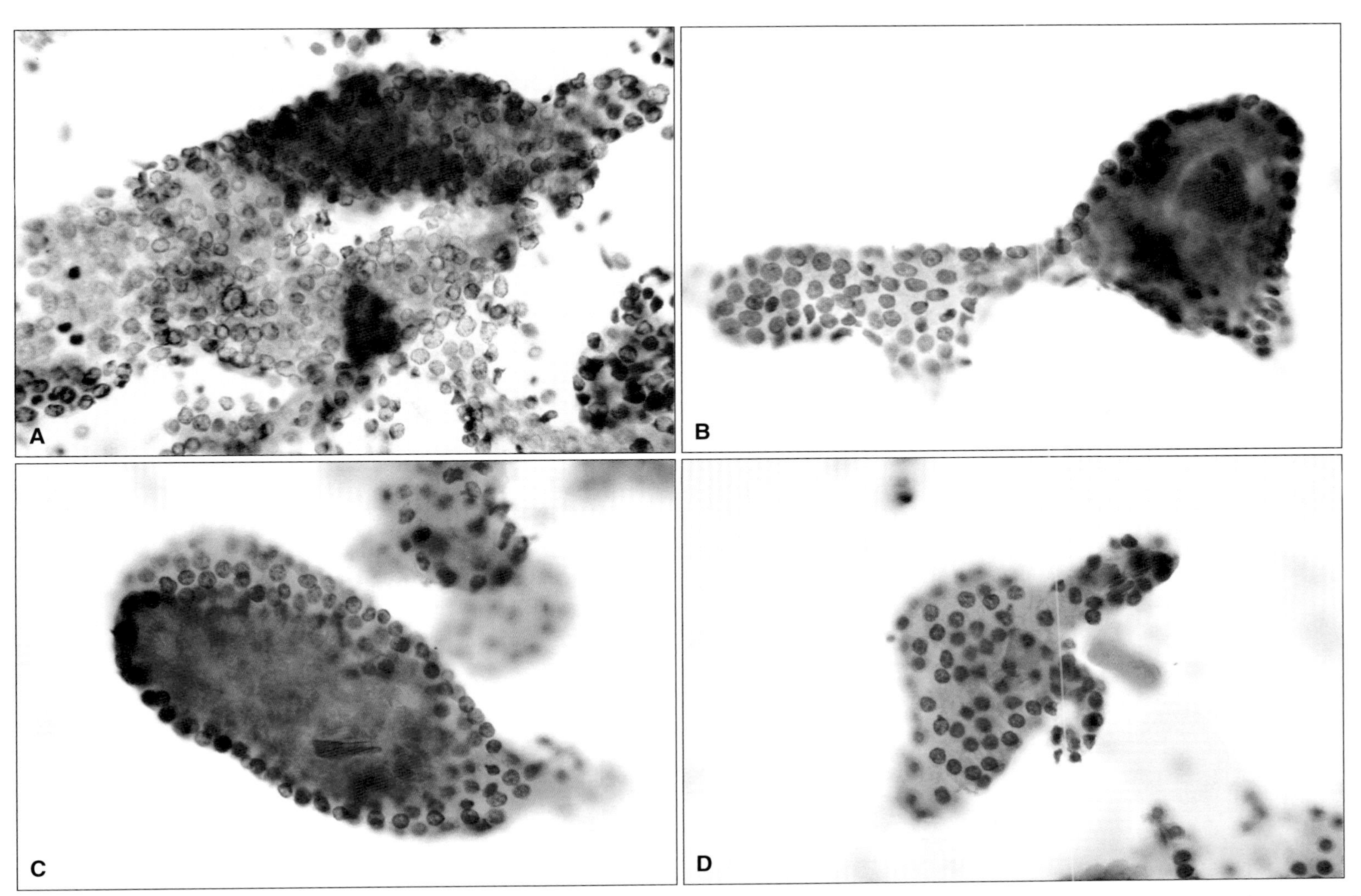

Fig. 5.14 Atypical small acinar proliferations (indeterminate for malignancy) in fine-needle aspiration material are characterized by smooth-contoured, moderate to small acini with somewhat irregularly distributed and irregularly contoured 'billowy' nuclei (A). Cottony, orangeophilic secretion (B) (corresponding to basophilic mucin in hematoxylin–eosin preparations) is seen in an irregularly shaped but smooth-contoured acinus showing a pinched neck, with slightly irregular nuclei featuring small nucleoli. Prostate crystalloids may be seen within the acinar lumen (C) or adjacent (D). Basal cells are reduced in number or absent, but the diagnosis of 'cytologic ASAP' relies on ensuring the absence of frank cancer nuclei and not on demonstrating the presence of basal cells.

keratin. The Gleason system does not specifically recognize large simple ducts among its carcinoma patterns, nor does it recognize well-differentiated ductal adenocarcinoma, but FNA atlases[21] have illustrated these; therefore, it is the presence of basal cells that distinguishes PIN from adenocarcinoma. In practice, these two lesions blend into a differential diagnostic spectrum best reported as 'PIN versus well-differentiated ductal adenocarcinoma'. (Fig. 5.15)

CARCINOMA

Features that differentiate prostate adenocarcinoma from benign epithelium or epithelial atypia include the major criteria applied to most cancers: dyshesion, variation in nuclear size (anisonucleosis), variation in nuclear shape (poikilonucleosis), and nucleolar prominence. The last three features comprise nuclear anaplasia. If three of the four major criteria are present, a diagnosis of cancer can be confidently rendered. For example, nuclear folds, angulations, or hyperchromasia may hide enlarged nucleoli.

CYTOLOGIC IDENTIFICATION OF CARCINOMA

In liquid-fixed FNA collections, glands retain a substantial part of their three-dimensional structure. In tissue, the patterns of cancer include intermediate to small acini, attenuated angulated glands, large ducts with papillary and pseudopapillary excrescences, cribriform glands, and solid or dyshesive epithelial cell groupings. In cytologic preparations, the same patterns are present, but the degree

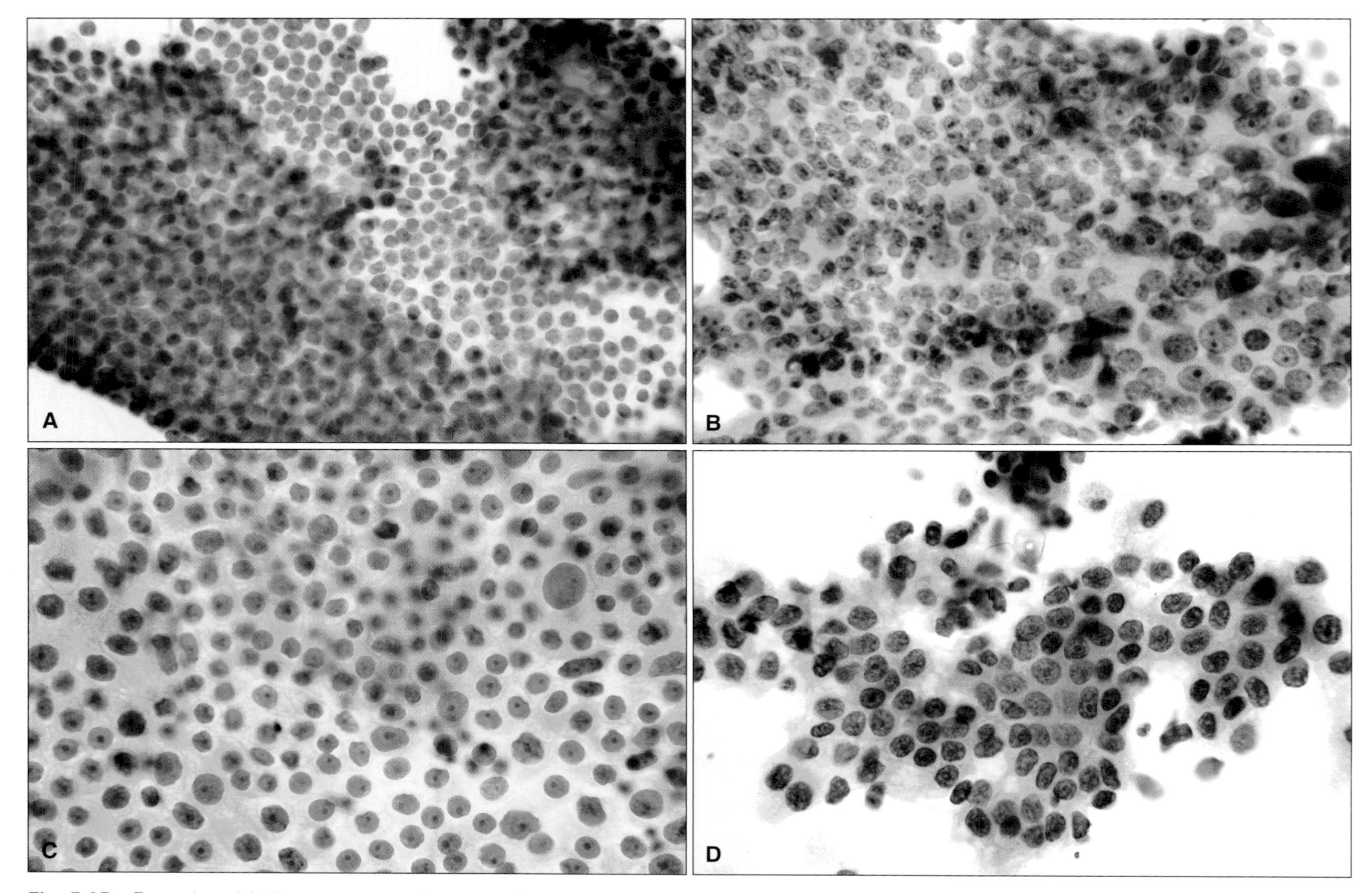

Fig. 5.15 Examples of findings appropriately reported as 'PIN versus well-differentiated ductal adenocarcinoma' are illustrated here. A partly opened duct lined by cells with uniform nuclei having intermediate-sized nucleoli is shown (A). Rare basal cells are evident in the upper right edge of this sheet. An abrupt transition of secretory cell types within an opened duct (B) suggests cancerization versus the onset of PIN. Many basal cells remain along the left side of this sheet. A large opened duct is lined by secretory cells with 'cancer nuclei' (C). A portion of an opened duct displays secretory cells with wrinkles, clefts, and prominent nucleoli (D).

of gland crowding and stromal invasion cannot be assessed. In addition to pattern, the diagnosis of cancer requires the absence of basal cells and the presence of frankly malignant nuclei.

Ductal carcinomas are papillary, pseudopapillary, or cribriform. Excluding the cribriform pattern, the papillary and pseudopapillary duct pattern is separated from PIN by the presence of basal cells in PIN. The Gleason system does not recognize large simple ducts among its carcinoma patterns, nor does it recognize well-differentiated ductal adenocarcinoma, but FNA atlases have illustrated the same.[21] Undifferentiated carcinoma is either solid or dissociated.

GRADING OF ACINAR CARCINOMA

The basis of Gleason grading is differentiation: the resemblance of carcinomatous glands to normal prostate. Increased anaplasia is generally accompanied by decreased differentiation. Gland size roughly determines Gleason pattern. Small, regular and intermediate-size glands correspond to Gleason acinar patterns 1 or 2; small, irregular glands to Gleason acinar pattern 3; and very small, highly irregular or abortive glands to Gleason acinar pattern 4.

Historically, cytologic grading of prostate carcinoma relied on the degree of nuclear anaplasia, with two exceptions: microadenomatous complexes in well-differentiated carcinoma and cellular dyshesion in poorly differentiated carcinoma. In our opinion, the cytologic grading of prostate carcinoma[22] should be akin to breast cancer grading in which nuclear, architectural, and proliferative features are equally weighted but separately evaluated – the latter more so by ploidy and S-phase fraction determination than by mitosis counting, as frequent mitoses are not a characteristic of prostate cancer. The most effective way to measure

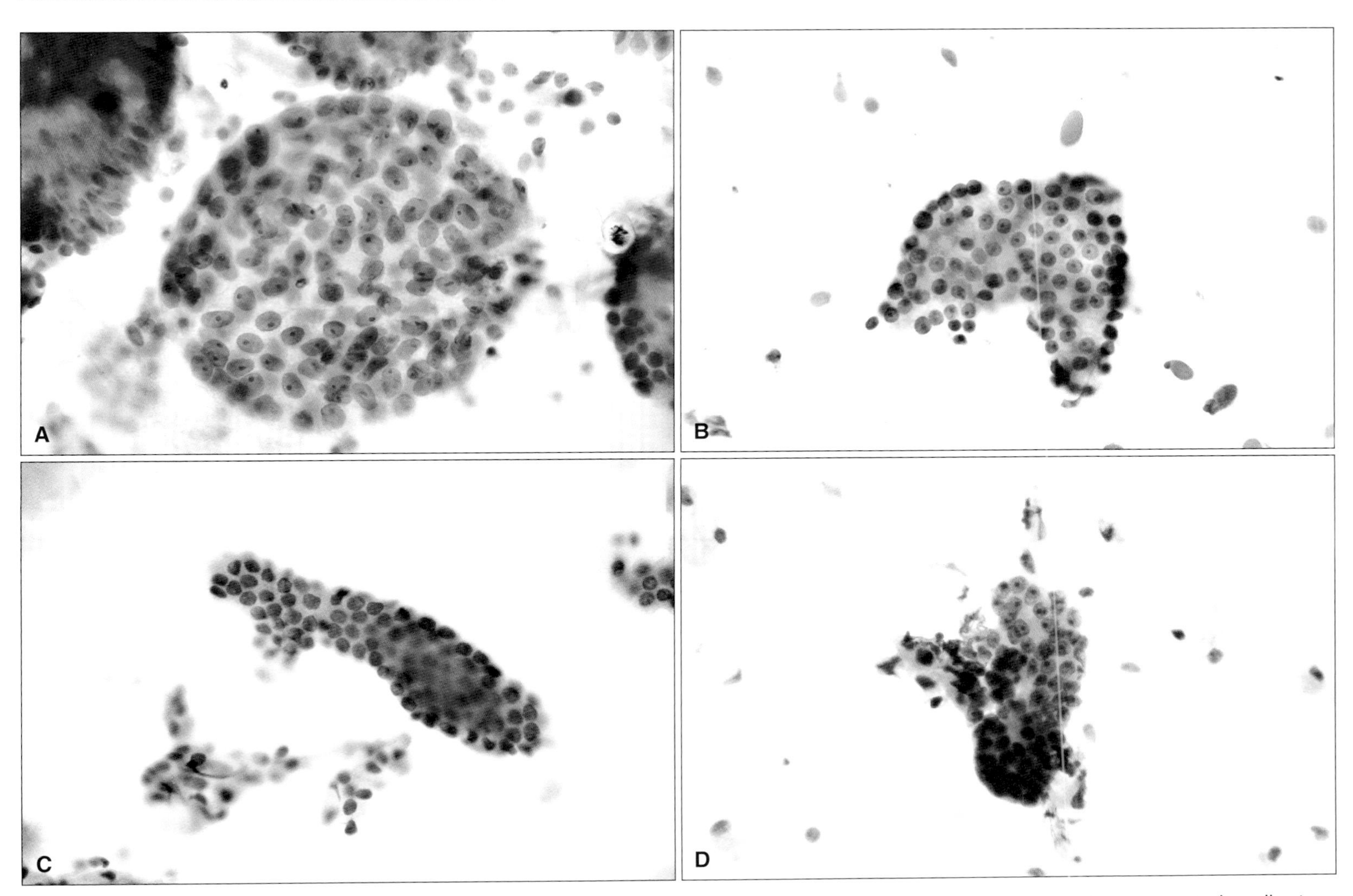

Fig. 5.16 At low magnification, it may be difficult to distinguish well-differentiated acinar carcinoma from normal epithelium or atypical small acinar proliferation when basal cells are not apparent; nuclear anaplasia is mild; or nuclear folds, angulations, or hyperchromasia hide enlarged nucleoli. High magnification becomes necessary with such specimens. Distinction of patterns 1 and 2 is not possible in cytology preparations because the regularity of the gland-to-gland arrangement cannot be assessed. Small or highly attenuated glands with straight or jagged contours, with or without branching, correspond to Gleason pattern 3. These panels illustrate several well to moderately differentiated acinar carcinomas. Secretory cells populating a symmetric, rounded acinar structure without basal cells all bear 'cancer nuclei' (A). A small curvilinear acinus without basal cells exhibits uniform nuclei with regular, intermediate-sized nucleoli (B). One of many irregularly-shaped, smoothly contoured acini with slightly notched hyperchromatic nuclei from an aspirate with low-grade adenocarcinoma is shown (C). A small acinar structure shows prominent nucleoli (D). Note how the nuclei form at least three well-defined microadenomatous arcades.

prostate cancer ploidy may well be by FNA and image analysis.[23] Abnormal DNA histogram patterns are best seen using the disaggregated cells of FNA samplings.[24] (Figs 5.16–5.18)

SPECIAL TYPES OF CARCINOMA

Ductal carcinoma, including endometrioid carcinoma, has a papillary pattern that may be mixed with flat sheets of tumor cells. Isolated pseudopapillae of cancer cannot be differentiated from high-grade PIN; when these occur in the absence of other obvious cancer patterns or without large tumor cell sheets so that basal cells cannot be satisfactorily evaluated, the differential diagnosis of 'PIN versus well-to-moderately differentiated ductal carcinoma' should be offered.

Cribriform carcinoma is either regular or irregular. The regular variety shows smooth, uniformly arborizing

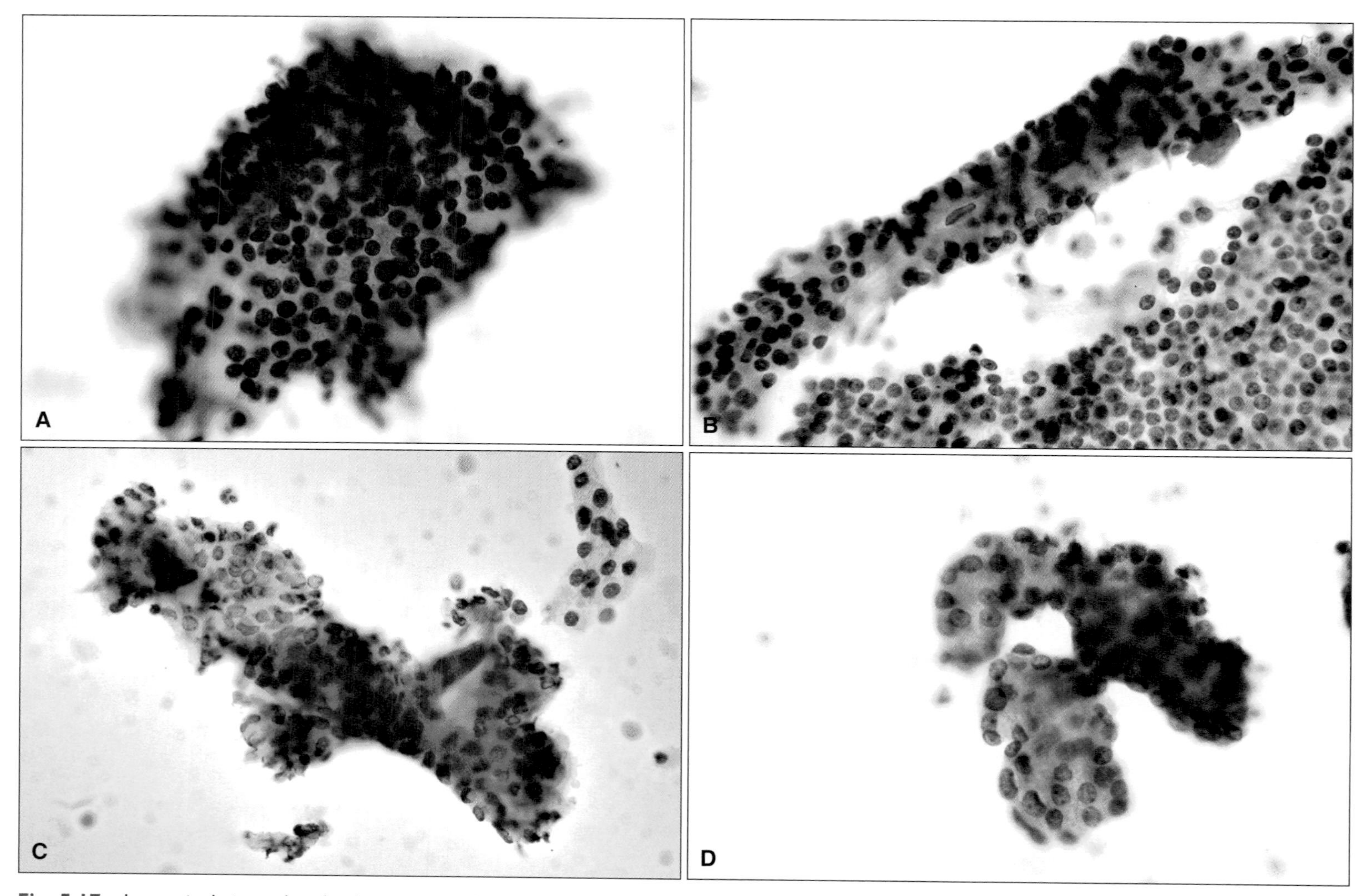

Fig. 5.17 Increasingly irregular gland contours indicate progressively higher architectural grade. In fine-needle aspiration biopsies, Gleason pattern 3 may be underestimated because the infiltration of malignant glands between preformed benign glands cannot be assessed. Evidence of multiple branch points implies 'gland fusion', corresponding to the histologic transition from Gleason grade 3 to grade 4. Very small, highly irregular or abortive glands with branched or fused structures correspond to Gleason acinar pattern 4. Nuclear anaplasia is conspicuous, and is roughly (but not necessarily) proportional to the degree of architectural distortion. Recognition of irregular, small, attenuated glands is never a problem, and their presence even in small numbers is diagnostic of cancer. The accompanying panels illustrate moderately to poorly differentiated carcinoma features. A fragment of a tubuloacinar cancer gland appears very cellular because it contains a 'double-barrel' lumen (A). An attenuated tubuloacinar cancer gland shows a pipe stem lumen that contains a small prostatic crystalloid (B). A ragged, splayed cancer gland exhibits several small branch points (C). A complex cancer gland with several 'pinched neck' points of attenuation and at least three dominant sacs gives the impression of 'gland fusion' (D).

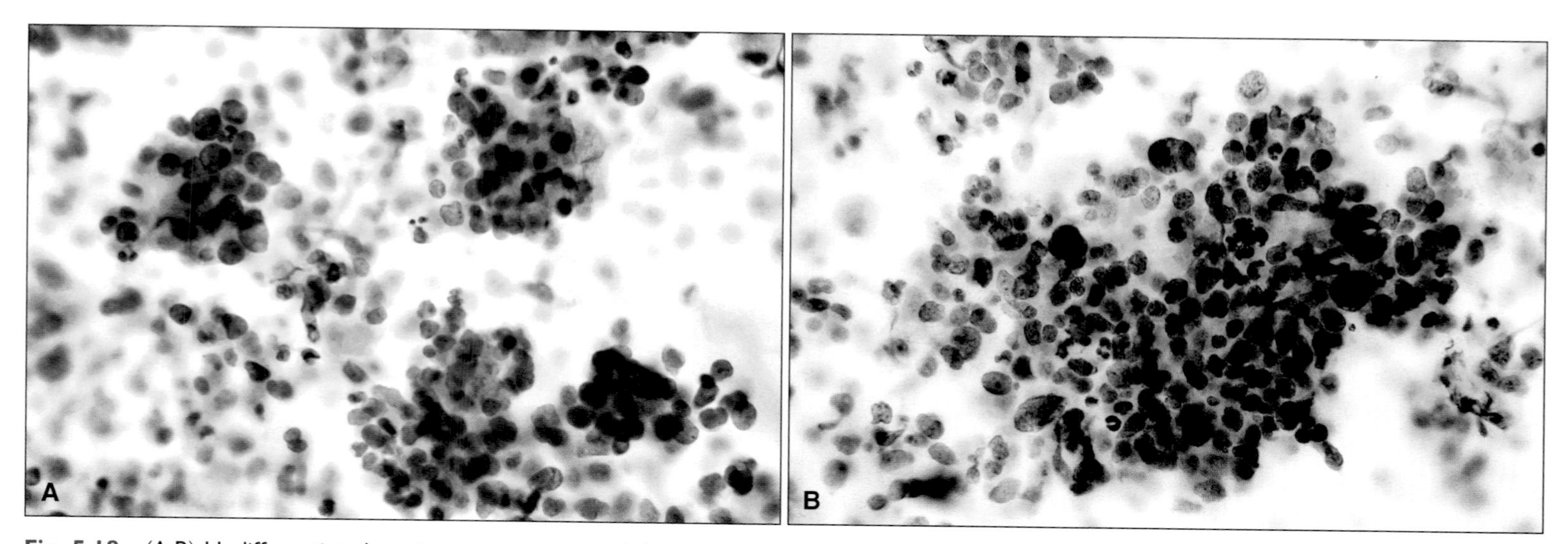

Fig. 5.18 (A,B) Undifferentiated carcinoma appears as solid tumor clusters or dissociated tumor cells and corresponds to Gleason pattern 5 carcinoma. Poorly differentiated invasive transitional cell cancer or large cell lymphoma may be mistaken for this lesion. Immunohistochemical stains for prostate-specific antigen and prostate-specific acid phosphatase are useful in differentiating prostate cancer from other tumor types.

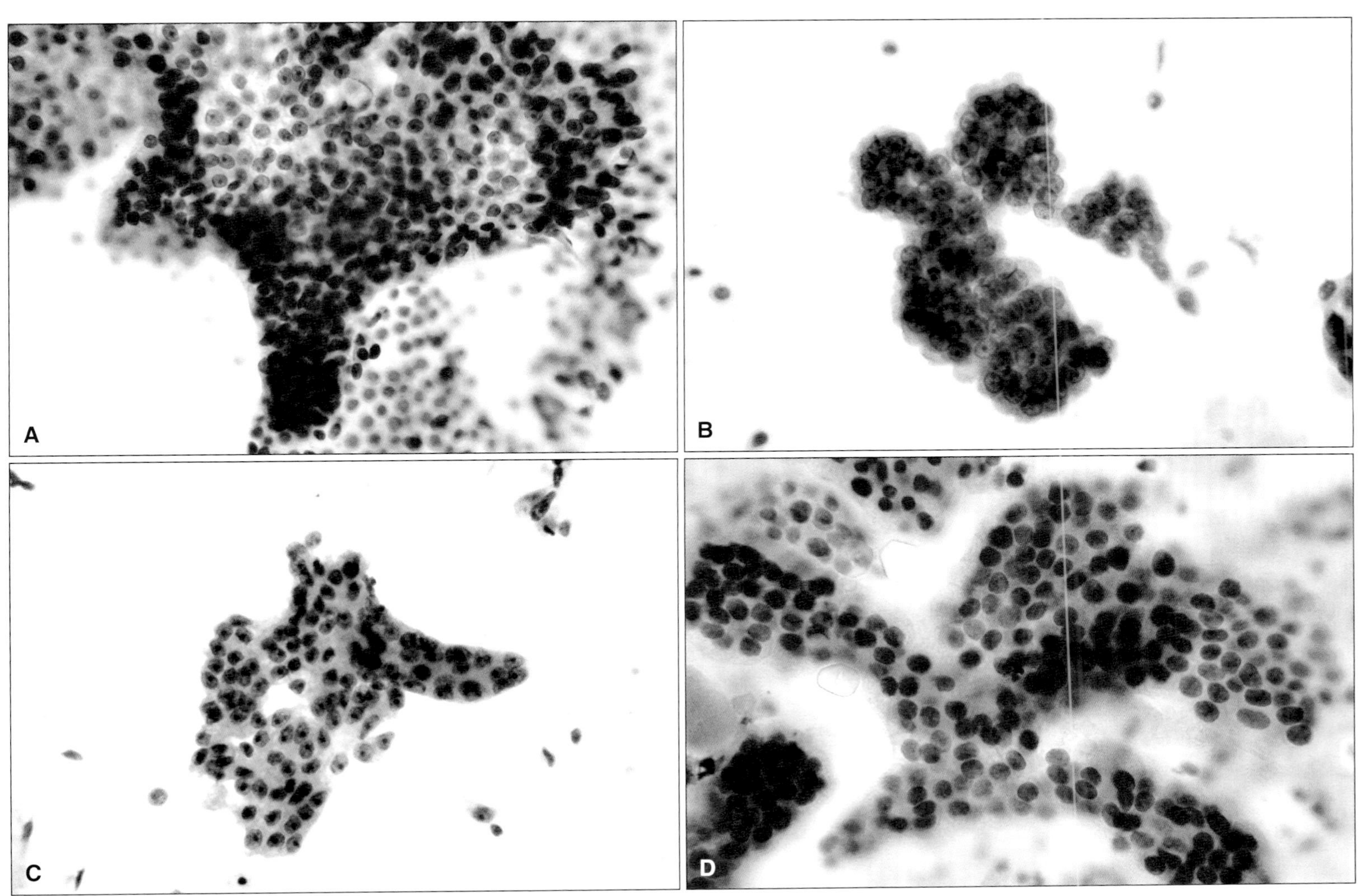

Fig. 5.19 Flat sheets of ductal carcinoma are usually interrupted by pseudopapillae and true papillae which cause clumping and protrusion of cancer nuclei. Ductal carcinomas with papillary and pseudopapillary structures usually correspond to Gleason pattern 3 carcinoma. In (A), a pseudopapilla arises from a flat sheet of secretory epithelial cells with uniform 'cancer nuclei'. A free-floating detached pseudopapilla with 'cancer nuclei' is shown at higher power in (B). A similar fragment of an epithelial sheet (C) has a markedly attenuated pseudopapilla showing uniform 'cancer nuclei'. A multiply branched pseudopapilla with enlarged, hyperchromatic 'cancer nuclei' is seen in (D).

lumens interrupting a solid core of epithelial cells. The irregular variety shows arborization of angulated, variably sized lumens. (Figs 5.19–5.21)

THERAPY-INDUCED CHANGES

Radiation and hormone therapy may cause downgrading or disappearance of cancer in biopsy specimens. Antiandrogen therapy induced regressive changes in secretory cells that included increased apoptotic bodies, and reduced mitotic activity of non-neoplastic prostate, PIN, and prostate adenocarcinoma, the latter effect interpreted as indicating suppressed proliferative activity.[25] In our experience, these changes, which are similar to those induced by Lupron, are now commoner than the more widely described diethylstilbestrol or radiation-induced metaplasias, especially with the use of medical therapy both preoperatively for prostate cancer and for benign prostate enlargement in men with subsequently discovered prostate cancer.

Following antiandrogen therapy, benign epithelium appears simplified with a pronounced basal cell layer. PIN also shows a prominent basal cell layer, yet retains a degree of secretory cell stratification but with less evident nuclear crowding because of therapy-induced cytoplasmic clearing and enlargement. Other effects of therapy include squamous and/or glycogenic metaplasia.

Following androgen deprivation, adenocarcinomas exhibit nuclear and cytoplasmic shrinkage and cytoplasmic clearing. Nucleoli became less conspicuous, chromatin more condensed. Acinar adenocarcinomas (the most differentiated group) are most affected, whereas cribriform, solid, or trabecular adenocarcinomas (the least differentiated group) are less affected or unaffected.

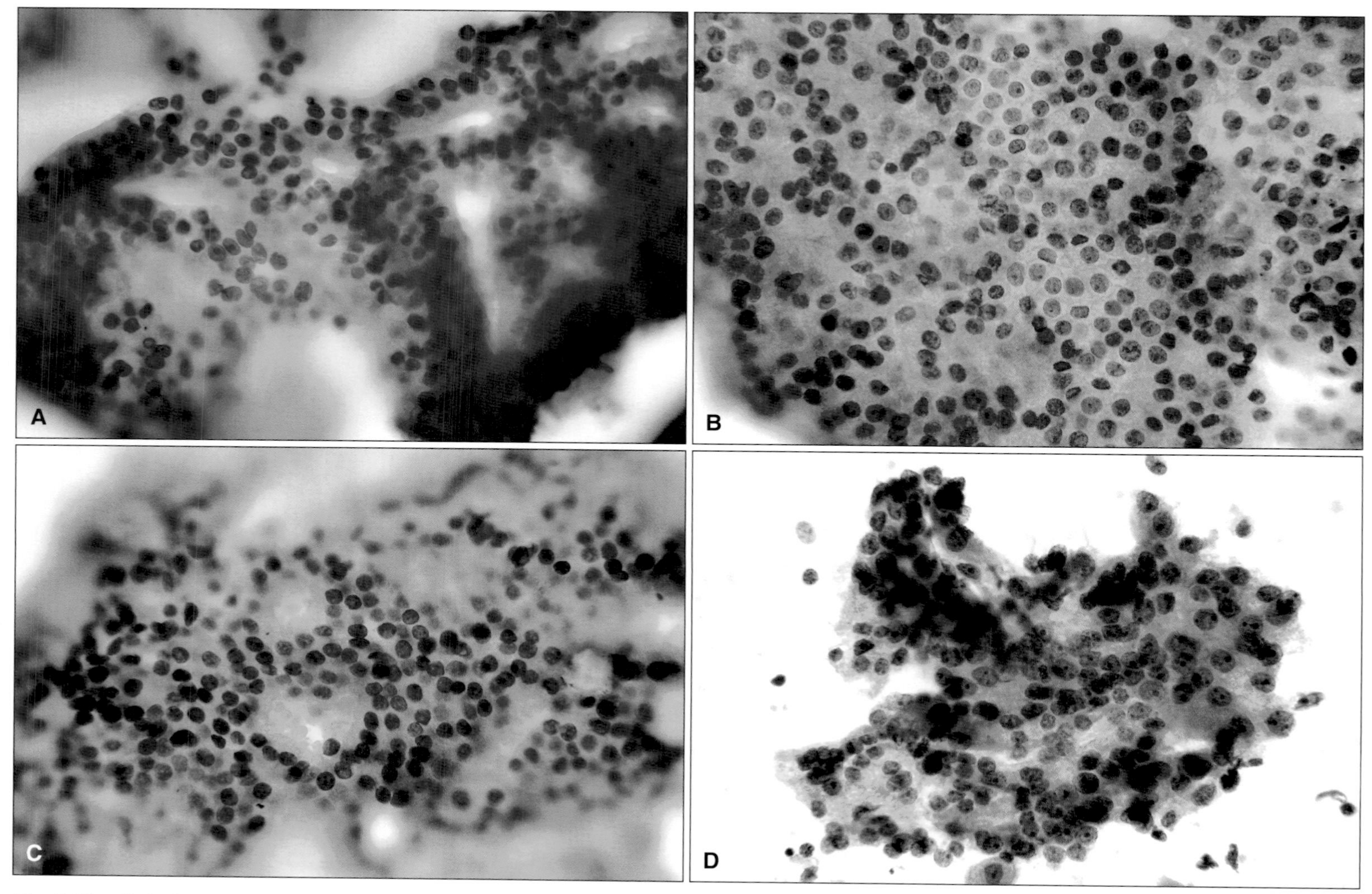

Fig. 5.20 Cribriform carcinoma may be regular or irregular. Regular cribriform carcinoma has smooth, uniformly arborizing lumens interrupting a solid core of epithelial cells, usually with a smooth external surface. Irregular cribriform carcinoma shows arborization of angulated, variably sized lumens and an uneven external surface often associated with smaller more irregularly contoured cribriform tumor cell clusters and dyshesive tumor cells. Cribriform carcinoma on fine-needle aspiration corresponds to a Gleason pattern 4 carcinoma. (A) Broad lumens and narrow bridges of otherwise unsupported secretory cells, some with recognizable intermediate-size nucleoli, characterize this regular cribriform carcinoma. (B) Small, uniform lumens give a nearly solid appearance to this microbiopsy of cribriform carcinoma. (C) Small but well-recognized lumens show the retained polarity of the epithelial cell cytoplasmic axis to the lumens of this cribriform carcinoma. (D) There are repetitive rosettes of nuclei and barely visible lumens in this example of poorly differentiated cribriform carcinoma.

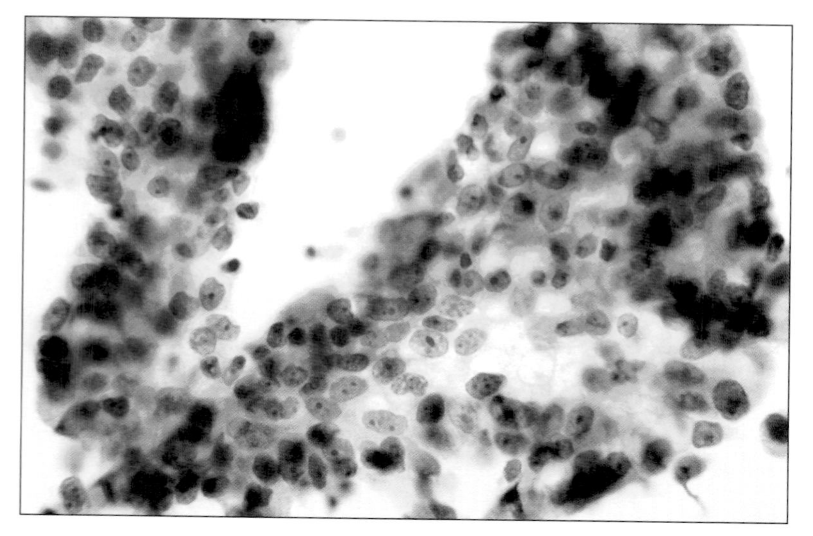

Fig. 5.21 Signet ring cells may be seen among prostate cancers. Mucus-producing tumors do not respond well to hormonal therapy, and their clinical aggressiveness is disproportionately high in relation to their degree of nuclear anaplasia. In the case of mucus-producing tumors, the decoration of tumor cells with prostate-specific antigen excludes secondary tumors such as colonic adenocarcinoma.

DIAGNOSTIC PITFALLS

Excluding technical limitations, the main reasons that cancer is not diagnosed are that: the sample is hypocellular, the tumor is small and not sampled, the tumor is well-differentiated and difficult to distinguish from ASAP or PIN, or the tumor is obscured by inflammation. In our experience, the most common cause for a missed diagnosis of cancer is inadequate cellularity.

False-positive cytologic diagnoses are often due to morphologic patterns that can be confused with carcinoma, such as ASAP, PIN, prostatitis, and seminal vesicle puncture. Trott et al[26] noted only one false positive among 1165 positive aspiration biopsies between 1965 and 1973; the error occurred in a patient with a previous prostate abscess. The proof of a false-positive cancer diagnosis is difficult, and can be verified only by serial sectioning of a radical prostatectomy specimen. Using ex vivo cytologic material prepared from 100 autopsy specimens and 100 surgically removed prostates aspirated prior to formalin fixation, no incorrect diagnoses of carcinoma were rendered.[27]

REFERENCES

1. Agatstein EH, Hernandez FJ, Layfield LJ, Smith RB, deKernion JB. Use of fine needle aspiration for detection of stage A prostatic carcinoma before transurethral resection of the prostate: a clinical trial. J Urol 1987;138:551–553.
2. Conrad S, Hautmann SH, Henke RP, et al. Detection and characterization of early prostate cancer by six systematic biopsies and fine needle aspiration cytology in prostates from bladder cancer patients. Eur Urol 2001;39(Suppl 4):25–29.
3. Maksem JA, Galang CF, Johenning PW, Park CH, Tannenbaum M. Aspiration biopsy of the prostate gland: a brief review of collection, fixation, and pattern recognition with special attention to benign and malignant prostatic epithelium. Diagn Cytopathol 1990;6:258–266.
4. Maksem JA. Technical report. Performance and processing of prostate aspiration biopsies. A strategy to ensure optimum cellularity and fixation. J Urol Pathol 1995;3:347–353.
5. Maksem JA. Cytopathology of the prostate. In: Foster CS, Bostwick D, eds. Pathology of the prostate. Philadelphia: Saunders; 1998:35–55.
6. Andersson L, Hagmar B, Ljung BM, Skoog L. Fine needle aspiration biopsy for diagnosis and follow-up of prostate cancer. Consensus Conference on Diagnosis and Prognostic Parameters in Localized Prostate Cancer. Stockholm, Sweden, May 12–13, 1993. Scand J Urol Nephrol Suppl 1994;162:43–49; discussion 115–127.
7. Engelstein D, Mukamel E, Cytron S, Konichezky M, Slutzki S, Servadio C. A comparison between digitally-guided fine needle aspiration and ultrasound-guided transperineal core needle biopsy of the prostate for the detection of prostate cancer. Br J Urol 1994;74:210–213.
8. Maksem JA. Ultrasound assisted core and aspiration biopsy of the prostate gland: their complementary function in prostate cancer diagnosis. In: Resnick M, Watanabe H, Karr JP, eds. Diagnostic ultrasound of the prostate. Proceedings of the First International Workshop on Diagnostic Ultrasound of the Prostate. New York: Elsevier; 1989:183–185.
9. Benson MC. Fine-needle aspiration of the prostate. NCI Monogr 1988;(7):19–24.
10. al-Abadi H. Fine needle aspiration biopsy vs. ultrasound-guided transrectal random core biopsy of the prostate. Comparative investigations in 246 cases. Acta Cytol 1997;41:981–986.
11. Mesonero CE, Oertel YC. Cells from ejaculatory ducts and seminal vesicles and diagnostic difficulties in prostatic aspirates. Mod Pathol 1991;4:723–726.
12. Park CH, Galang CF, Johenning PW, Maksem JA, Tannenbaum M. Follow up aspiration biopsies for dysplasia of the prostate gland. Lab Invest 1989;60:70A.
13. Layfield LJ, Goldstein NS. Morphometric analysis of borderline atypia in prostatic aspiration biopsy specimens. Anal Quant Cytol Histol 1991;13:288–292.
14. Bittinger A, von Keitz A, Ruschoff J, Melekos MD. Silver staining nucleolar organizer region in prostate cytology. Zentralbl Pathol 1994;140:103–106.
15. Buhmeida A, Collan Y. Improving the value of fine needle aspiration biopsy of the prostate. Pathologica 2001;93:242–243.
16. Rabbani F, Stroumbakis N, Kava BR, Cookson MS, Fair WR. Incidence and clinical significance of false-negative sextant prostate biopsies. J Urol 1998;159:1247–1250.
17. Maksem JA, Johenning PW, Galang CF. Prostatitis and aspiration biopsy cytology of prostate. Urology 1988;32:263–268.
18. Koss LG, Woyke S, Schreiber K, Kohlberg W, Freed SZ. Thin-needle aspiration biopsy of the prostate. Urol Clin North Am 1984;11:237–251.
19. Smith FL, Bibbo M, Schoenberg HW, Chodak GW. Transrectal aspiration biopsy of the prostate: the importance of atypia. J Urol 1988;140:766–768.
20. Ritchie AWS, Layfield LJ, Turcillo P, deKernion JB. The significance of atypia in fine needle aspiration cytology of the prostate. J Urol 1988;140:761–765.
21. Leistenschneider W, Nagel R. Atlas of prostatic cytology: techniques and diagnosis. New York: Springer; 1985.
22. Maksem JA, Johenning PW. Is cytology capable of adequately grading prostate carcinoma? Matched series of 50 cases comparing cytologic and histologic pattern diagnoses. Urology 1988;31:437–444.
23. Hardt NS, Hendricks JB, Sapi Z, et al. Ploidy results in prostatic carcinoma vary with sampling method and with cytometric technique. Mod Pathol 1994;7:44–48.
24. Buhmeida A, Kuopio T, Collan Y. Influence of sampling practices on the appearance of DNA image histograms of prostate cells in FNAB samples. Anal Cell Pathol 1999;18:95–102.
25. Montironi R, Magi-Galluzzi C, Muzzonigro G, Prete E, Polito M, Fabris G. Effects of combination endocrine treatment on normal prostate, prostatic intraepithelial neoplasia, and prostatic adenocarcinoma. J Clin Pathol 1994;47:906–913.
26. Trott PA, Hendry WF, Pugh RC, Williams JP. Franzen-needle transrectal prostatic biopsy. Lancet 1973;2:620.
27. Sunderland H, Lederer H. Prostatic aspiration biopsy. Br J Urol 1971;43:603–607.

6

PROSTATE

John F. Madden, James L. Burchette, and Myron Tannenbaum

RELEVANT ANATOMY AND HISTOLOGY

PROSTATE GLAND

The prostate consists of three embryologically and histologically distinct divisions: the central, peripheral, and transition zones. In addition, there is a distinctive periurethral zone.[1] The gland is surrounded by a variably well-defined intrinsic capsule that merges focally with surrounding fascial and muscular structures. The anatomy of the prostatic neurovascular bundles is particularly relevant, because of the tendency of carcinoma to extend beyond the capsule along perforating nerve branches.[2,3]

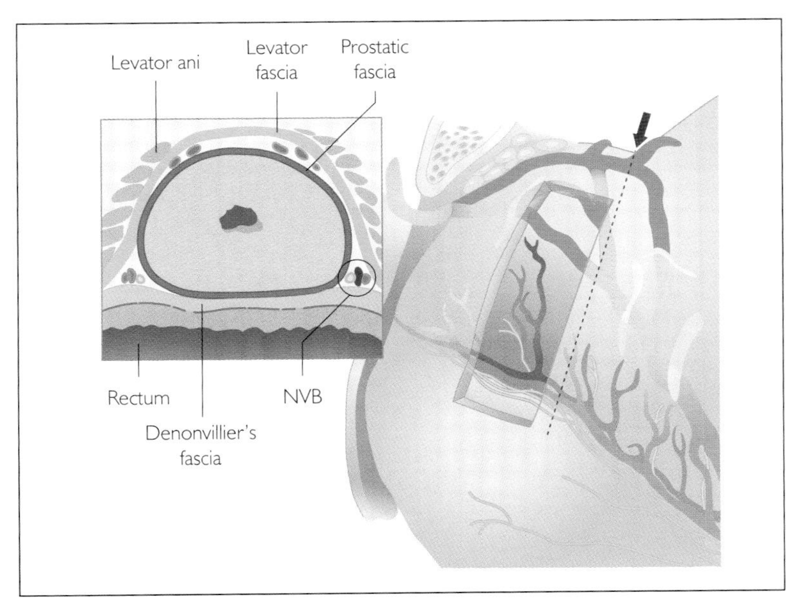

Fig. 6.1 At the flattened posterior (rectal) surface, the prostate capsule merges with Denonvillier's (rectoprostatic) fascia, an anatomic barrier rarely breached by carcinoma. Along the rounded anterior surface, the levator and prostatic fascias circumscribe the periprostatic space. The neurovascular bundles containing the nervi erigentes lie in the posterolateral periprostatic space. The dorsal venous plexus lies in the anterior periprostatic space. NVB, neurovascular bundle.

Anatomy

(Figs 6.1 & 6.2)

Histology

(Figs 6.3–6.18)

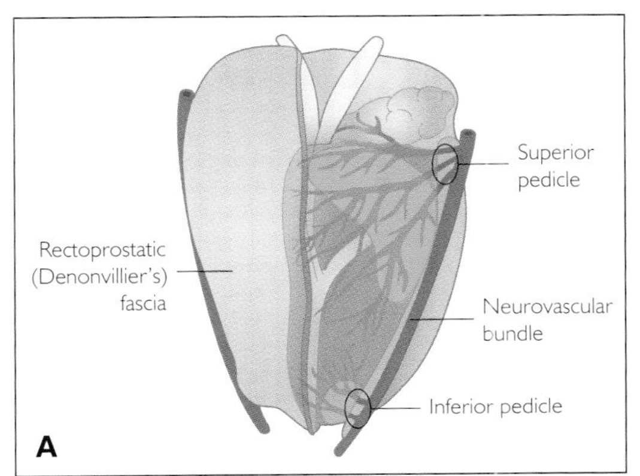

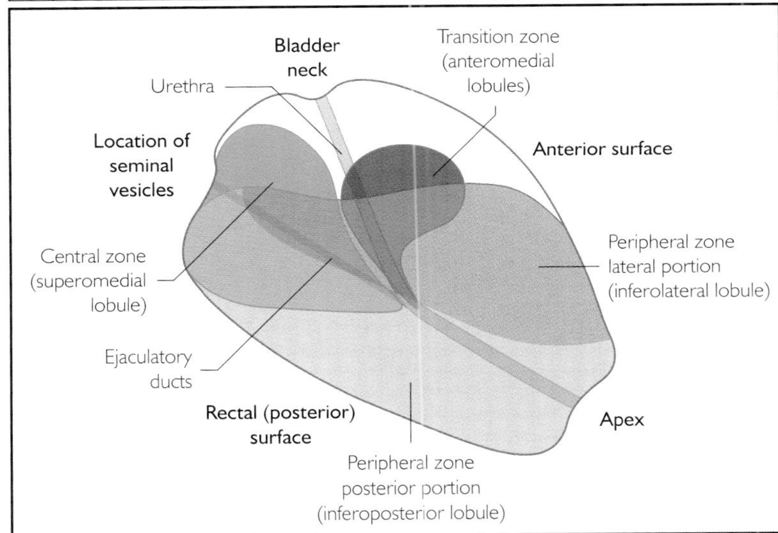

Fig. 6.2 (A) Perforating branches occur throughout the length of contact of the neurovascular bundles with the rectal and lateral surfaces of the prostate. They concentrate in a superior pedicle at the posterior third of the gland and in an inferior pedicle near the apex. These represent common areas for extraprostatic extension by carcinoma. (B) The central zone, about 25% of the prostate volume, approximates a cone with base toward the seminal vesicles, and apex at the verumontanum. The peripheral zone, about 70% of the prostate volume, is a vase-shaped structure that posteriorly enwraps the central zone, and anteriorly enwraps the periurethral and transition zone. The transition zone lies dorsal to the urethra.[1b]

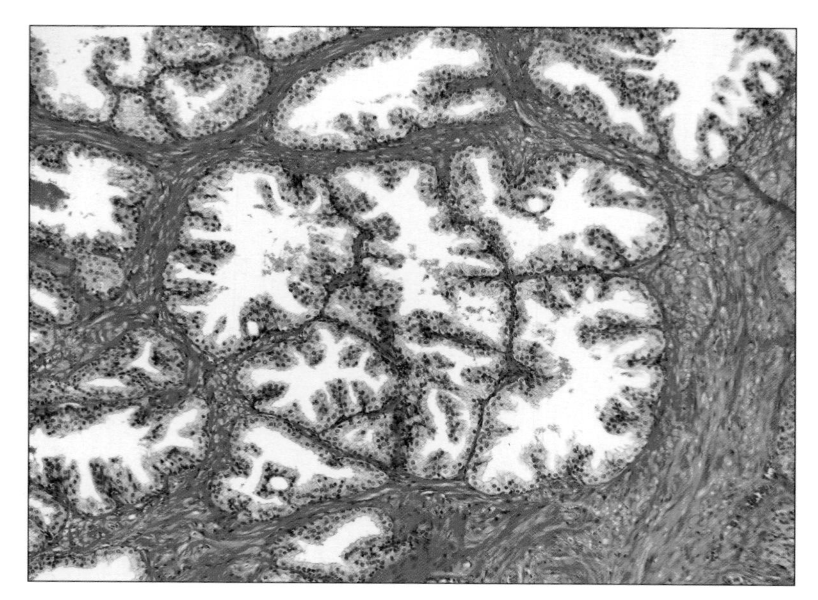

Fig. 6.3 Central zone acini are large (up to 1 mm or more in diameter) and exhibit complex glandular architecture with bridges and fenestrations. Central zone tissue is considered resistant to both carcinoma and inflammatory disease. The pseudopapillary architecture of normal central zone glands should not be mistaken for prostatic intraepithelial neoplasia.

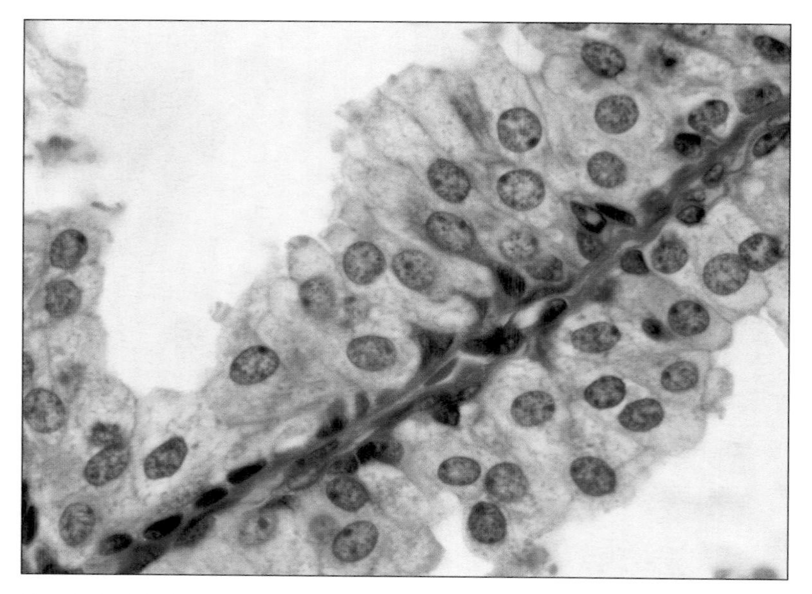

Fig. 6.4 Nuclei in the central zone are crowded and pseudostratified. Small- to medium-sized peripheral nucleoli are present in normal central zone epithelium.[4,5] They should not be misinterpreted as prostatic intraepithelial neoplasia. Secretory cell cytoplasm is darkly staining. This can also convey a mistaken impression of in-situ neoplasia at low power.

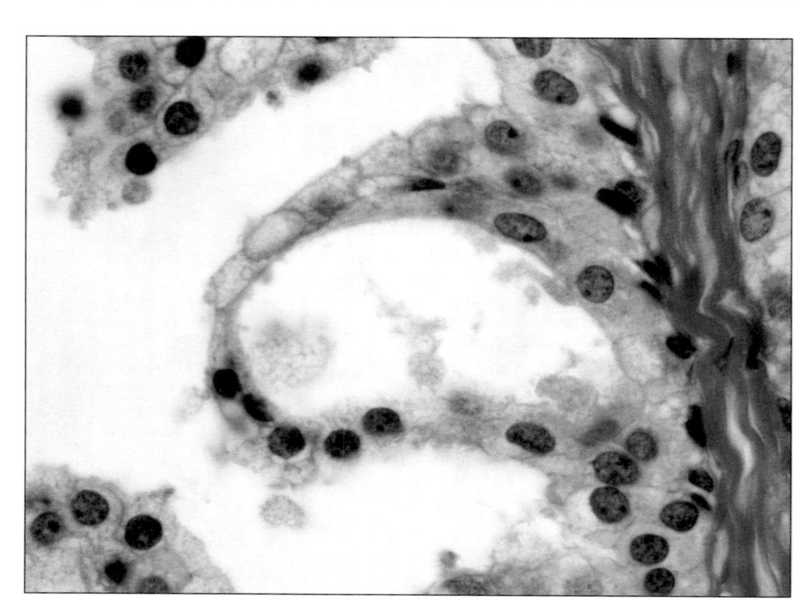

Fig. 6.5 Intraepithelial 'lacunae', associated with secreted lactoferrin,[6] are a normal feature of central zone epithelium and do not represent cribriform prostatic intraepithelial neoplasia.

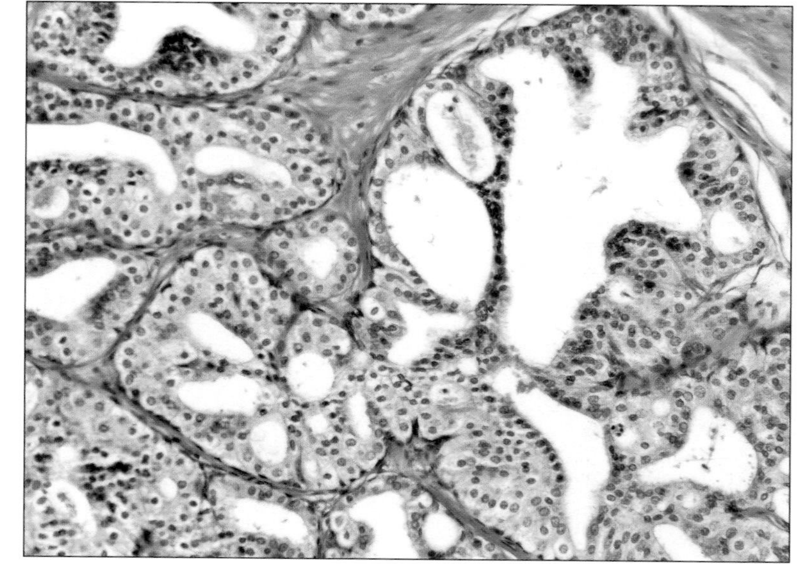

Fig. 6.6 'Clear cell cribriform hyperplasia' is a benign 'proliferation' seen in biopsies from the base of the prostate.[7] Some examples are doubtless fortuitous sections of normal central zone glands with particularly prominent lacunae and infoldings.

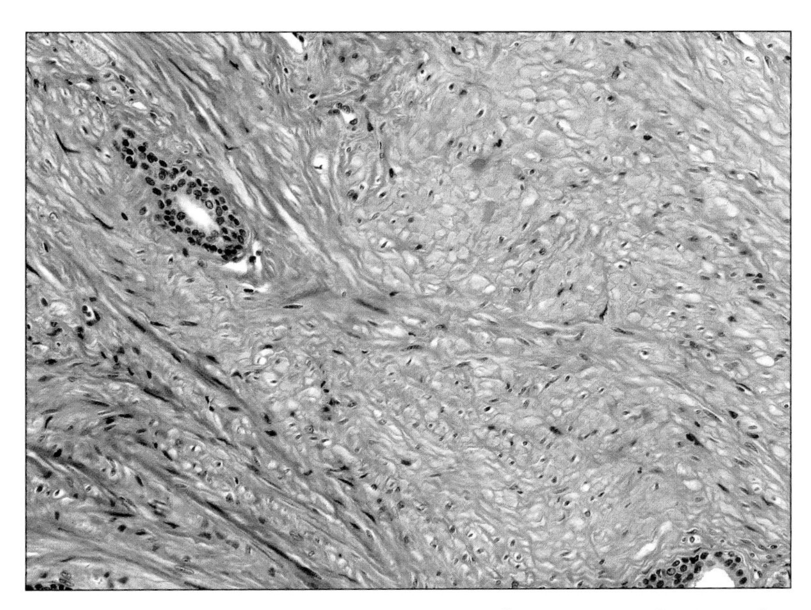

Fig. 6.7 Central zone stroma is compact with crisscrossing laminae of smooth muscle. Stroma is less abundant relative to glands than in other zones.

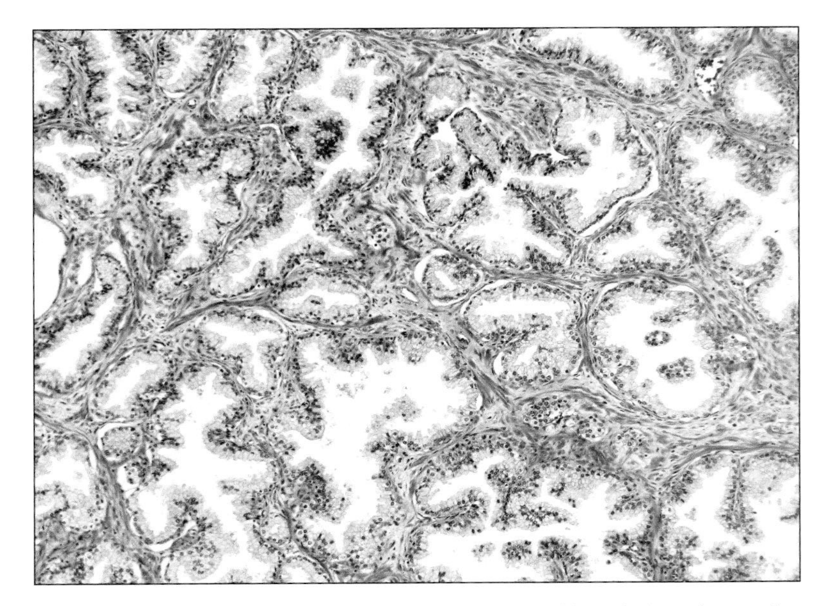

Fig. 6.8 Peripheral zone acini are smaller (150–300 μm) than those of the central zone. Gland contours are corrugated but are less complex than in the central zone. Stroma is loosely and irregularly woven. Gland:stroma ratio is about 1:1. Most needle core biopsies sample this zone.

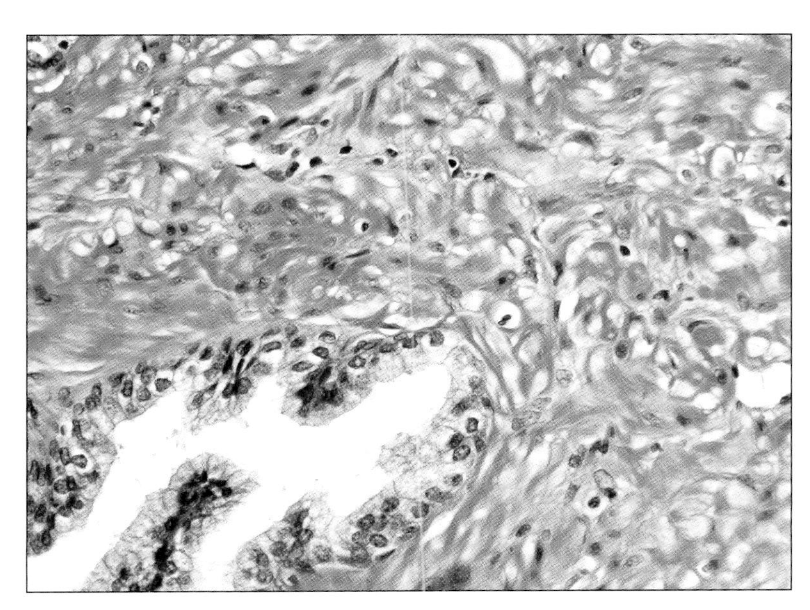

Fig. 6.9 Transition zone acini are indistinguishable from those of the peripheral zone. Stroma of the transition zone is distinctive, with compact, mesh-like, interlacing smooth muscle fascicles. Benign prostatic hyperplasia (see Figs 6.34–6.37) involves this zone, primarily though perhaps not exclusively.[8] Transurethral resection specimens yield most of their tissue from the transition zone.

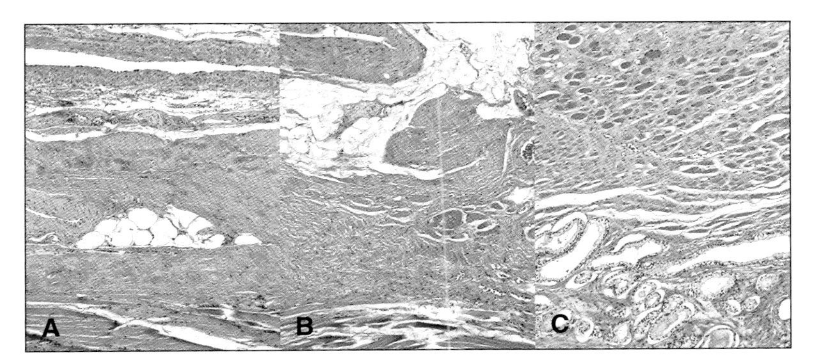

Fig. 6.10 The most exterior, sometimes compressed, smooth muscle layer of the prostate is its capsule (A).[9,10] The capsule, thus defined, merges intimately with Denonvillier's fascia posteriorly (B). It is vague on the posterosuperior surface of the gland[11] and apically merges directly into pelvic striated muscle (C). Fat and ganglia[12] may occur internal to the capsule (D).

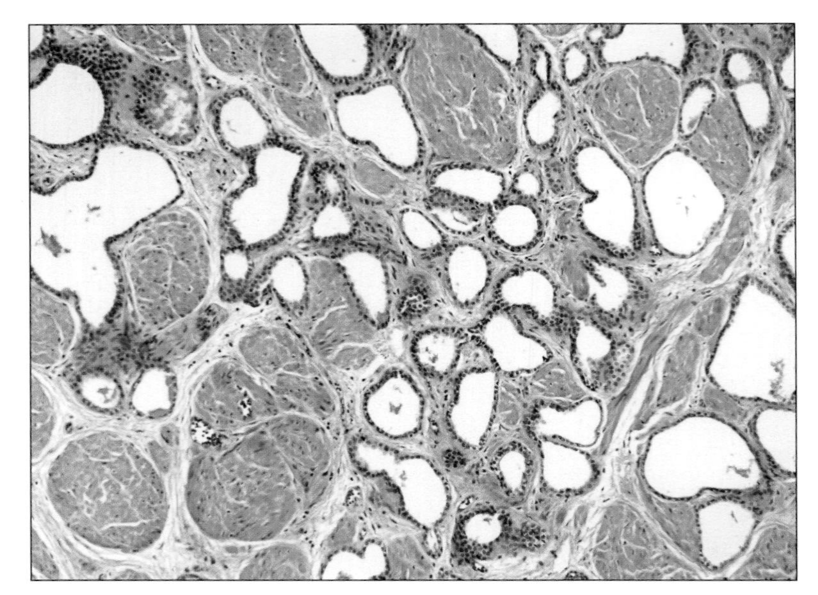

Fig. 6.11 Benign glands among skeletal muscle fibers at the apex can give a false impression of infiltrative growth.

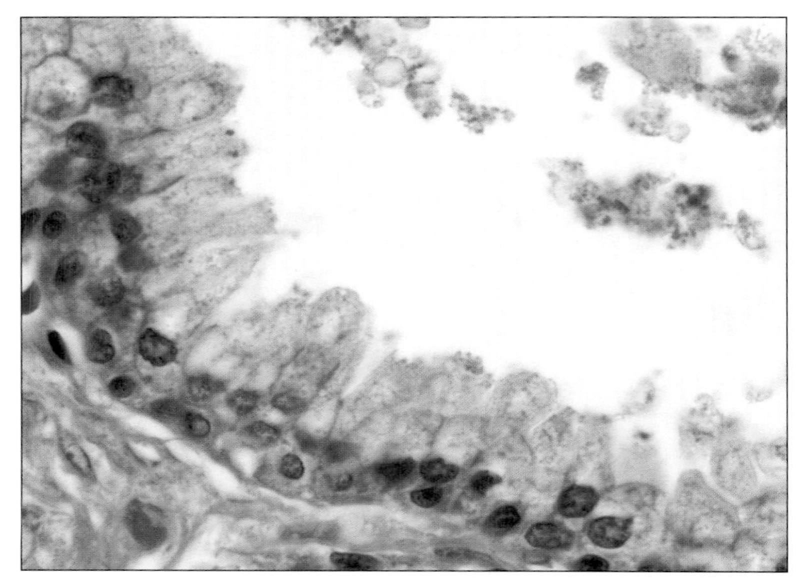

Fig. 6.12 Secretory cells of the peripheral/transition zone exhibit a single layer of basal nuclei. Cytoplasm is 'bubbly' due to the presence of secretory vacuoles. Cohen et al[13] called attention to the 'frayed' appearance of the luminal margin of benign glands, reflecting active apocrine-type secretion.

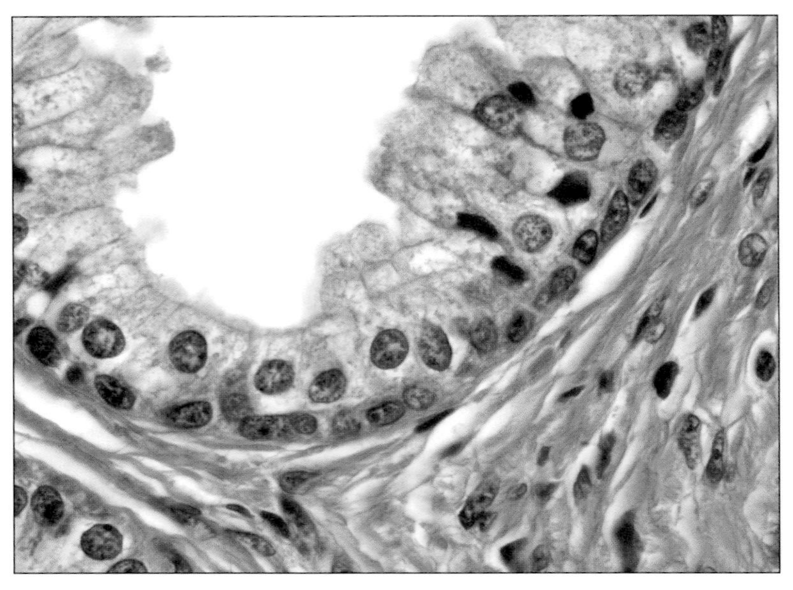

Fig. 6.13 Basal cells have elongated nuclei that are oriented parallel to the basement membrane. Chromatin is uniform. Small chromocenters may be present. Basal cells have scanty cytoplasm and are usually inconspicuous; failure to identify them on routine stains does not imply their absence. A nuclear 'bubble' artifact is often present on formalin-fixed tissue.

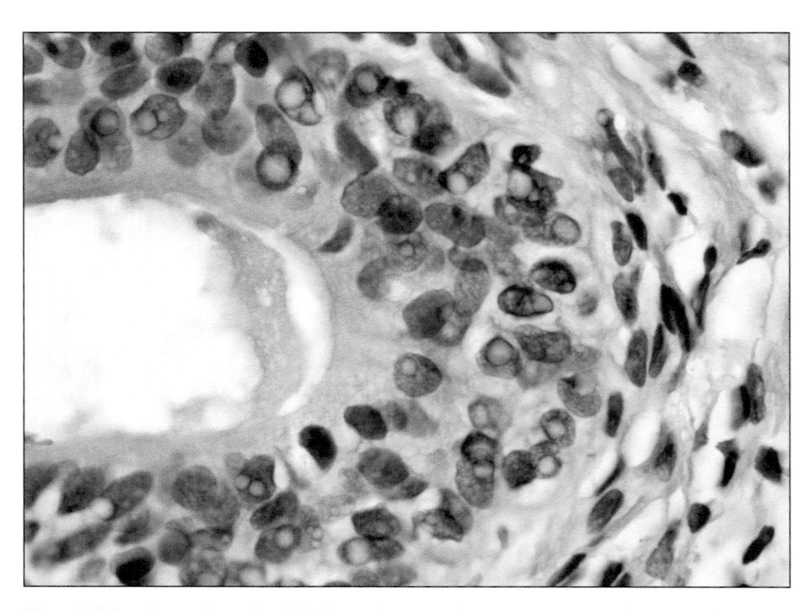

Fig. 6.14 A nuclear 'bubble' artifact is often present on formalin-fixed tissue, demonstrated in this image of basal cell hyperplasia (see Figs 6.44 & 6.45).

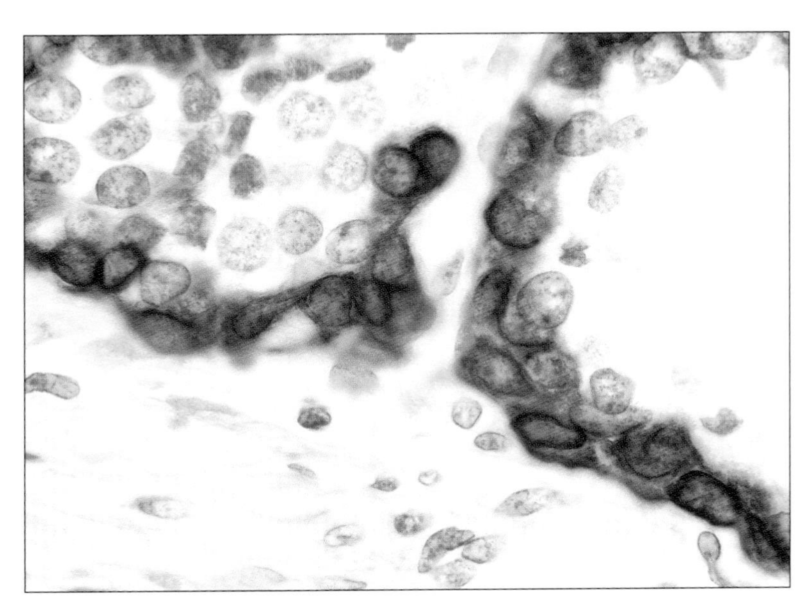

Fig. 6.15 Basal cells stain positively for high molecular weight cytokeratin (34βE12/CK903, cytokeratin 5/6) and for p63 antigen. Unlike myoepithelial cells of breast or salivary glands, prostate basal cells do not exhibit a contractile phenotype and are normally negative for S-100 and muscle markers.

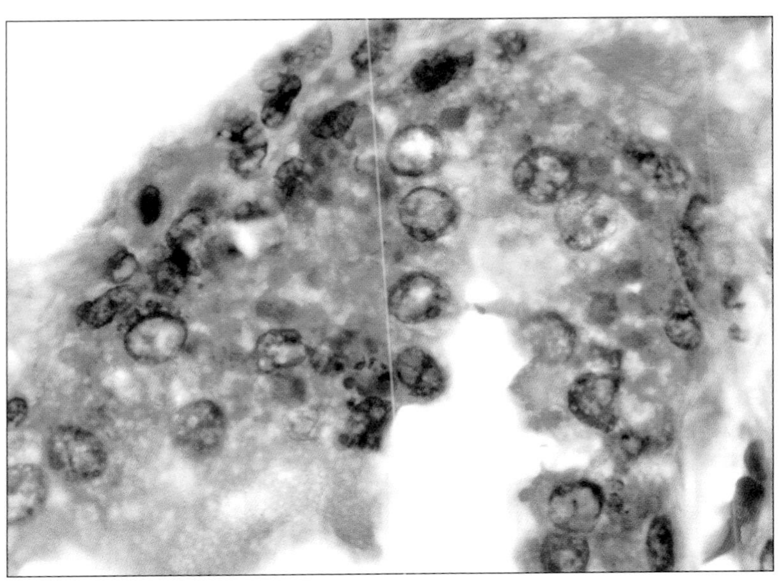

Fig. 6.16 Lipofuscin pigment can occur in prostate glandular cells, but, unlike the pigment of seminal vesicle epithelium, it is typically scant, dusty rather than globular, and is preferentially located in the basal portion of the cells. Pigment may occasionally be seen in prostatic intraepithelial neoplasia or carcinoma.[14]

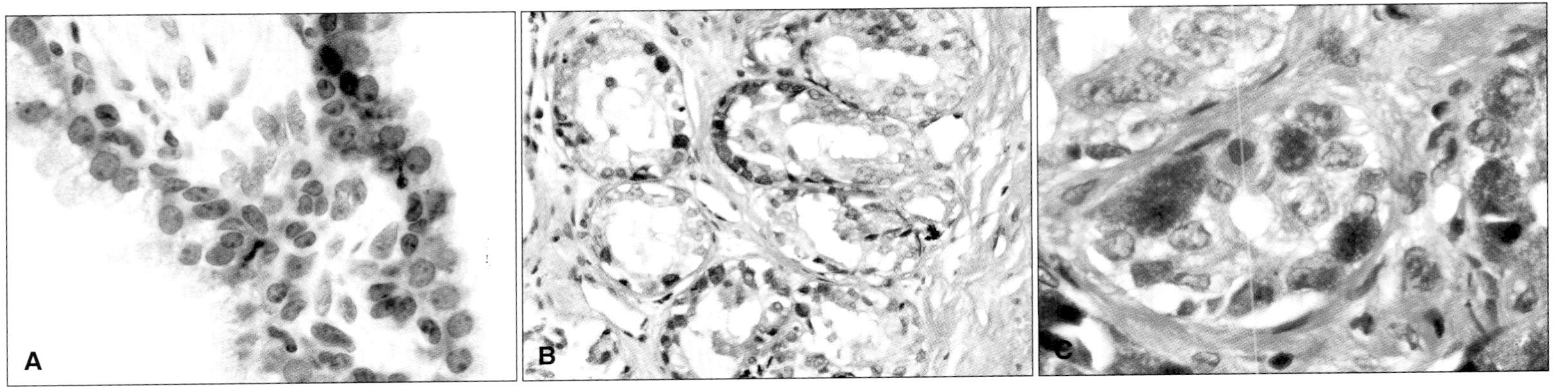

Fig. 6.17 Endocrine-paracrine cells occur as scattered, basally located cells with dendritic processes. Rarely, these cells can be identified on routine stains because of their eosinophilic intracytoplasmic granules. Immunoperoxidase stains for chromogranin (A) and synaptophysin are positive. Proliferation of cells of this type can sometimes be seen in carcinoma ('carcinoma with Paneth cell-like change') (B,C). Immunoperoxidase stains make clear that this finding actually represents neuroendocrine differentiation.[15] The illustrated case was of intermediate grade.

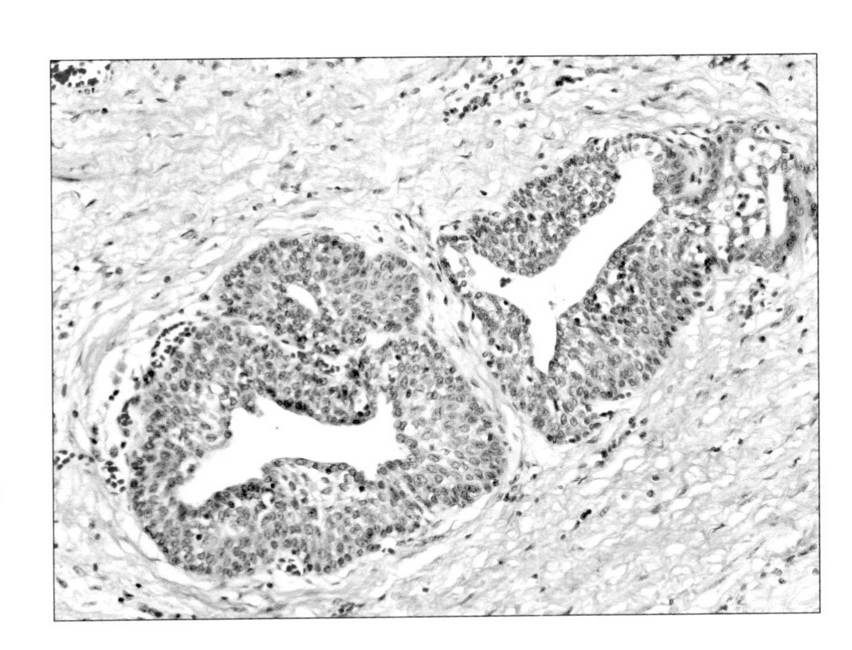

Fig. 6.18 Periurethral zone has distinctive histologic features. Periurethral ducts normally exhibit a composite epithelium consisting of a basal layer of epithelium (variously believed to be urothelial or prostatic basal cell type) with a luminal layer of prostatic ductal cells. 'Cancerization' of these ducts by urothelial carcinoma occurs in carcinoma of the urethra.

PROSTATIC ADNEXA

Bulbourethral glands

The bulbourethral (Cowper's) glands are the male homolog of the female vestibular (Bartholin's) glands. The glands in humans are small. (They are relatively larger by far in many mammals; in others, absent entirely.) They lie superolateral to the membranous urethra and are enclosed by fibers of the urethral sphincter. (Figs 6.19 & 6.20)

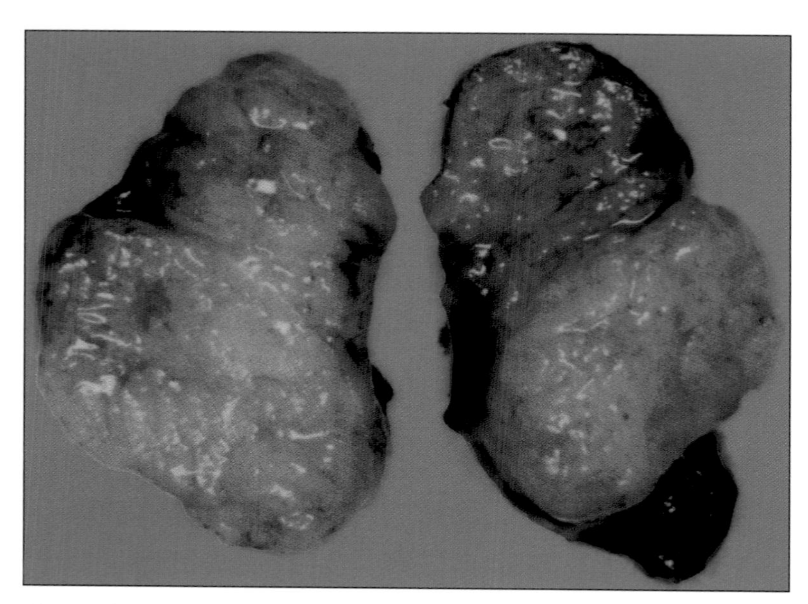

Fig. 6.19 The bulbourethral glands themselves are less than 1 cm in diameter, but their ducts are of substantial length (3 cm), and open into the penile urethra distal to the bulb.

Verumontanum (colliculus seminalis) and prostatic utricle

The verumontanum is a projection on the posterior wall at about the midpoint of the prostatic urethra, near its angulation. The ejaculatory ducts empty through this structure.

The prostatic utricle, a cul-de-sac about 5 mm in length, projects posteriorly from the apex of the verumontanum into the substance of the central zone prostate. The utricle is a remnant of the müllerian duct, and has been variously considered a homolog of the vagina or uterus (hence the name). It can give rise to cysts. (Fig. 6.21)

Ejaculatory ducts

(Fig. 6.22)

Seminal vesicles

(Fig. 6.23)

BENIGN ALTERATIONS

ATROPHY

Atrophy is a common finding. Most cases are postinflammatory; other causes include local ischemia,[21] hormone deprivation therapy, and irradiation. The main value of subclassifying atrophy patterns is to facilitate its distinction

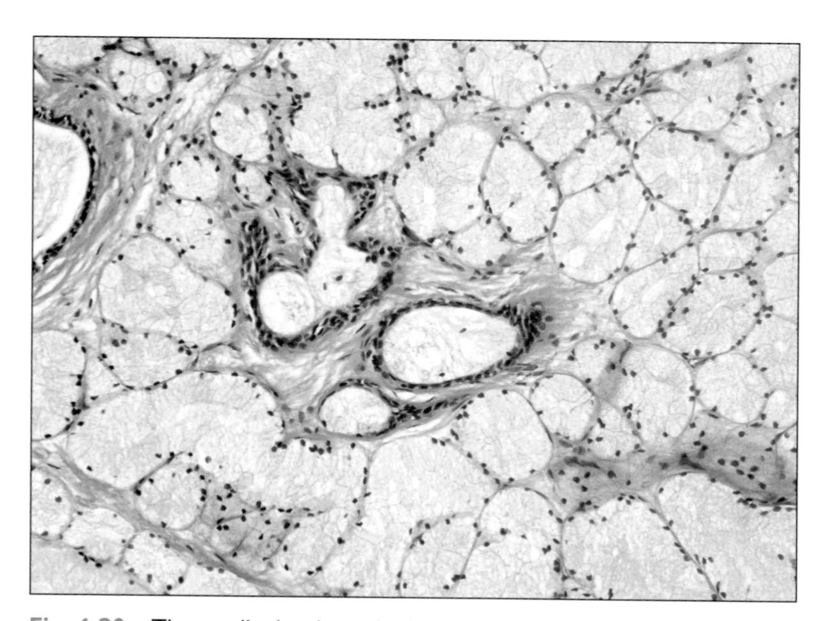

Fig. 6.20 The small, closely packed, mucinous glands of this organ should not be mistaken for Gleason grade 1–2 adenocarcinoma when it is coincidentally sampled in a needle biopsy. Bulbourethral gland epithelium is immunohistochemically positive for prostate-specific antigen, contributing to potential for misinterpretation.[16] Attention to the minuscule basal nuclei, 'clear cell' cytoplasm, and the presence of ducts and lobules will yield the proper diagnosis.

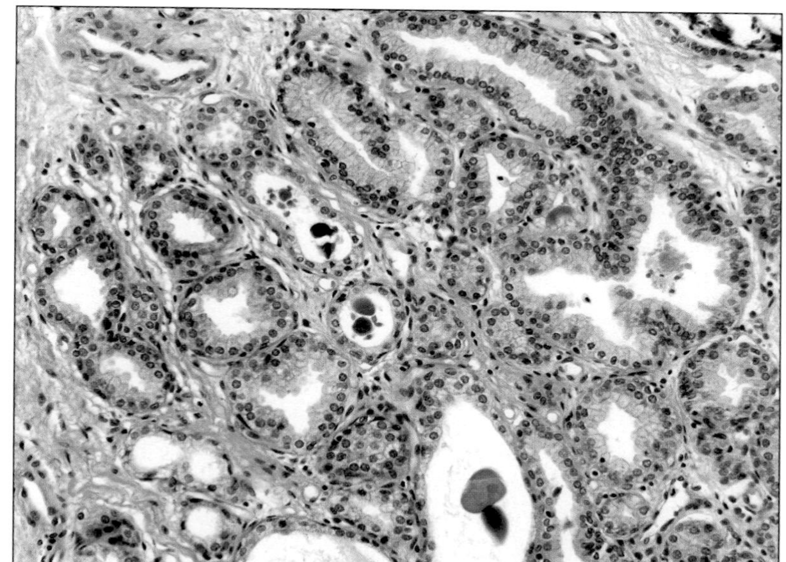

Fig. 6.21 The communicating acini of the verumontanum often appear irregularly crowded. On a small biopsy, this can give an erroneous impression of proliferation. The term 'verumontanum mucosal gland hyperplasia' has been applied.[17–19] The lining epithelium of the utricular ducts does not actually differ structurally or immunohistochemically from prostate epithelium elsewhere in adults, except in its higher concentration of neuroendocrine cells.[20]

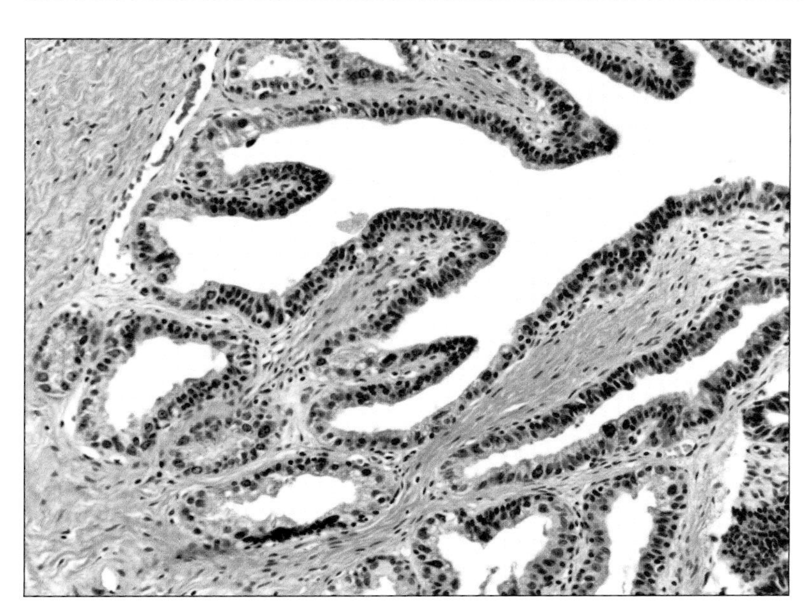

Fig. 6.22 The ejaculatory ducts are lined by epithelium of the seminal vesicle type.

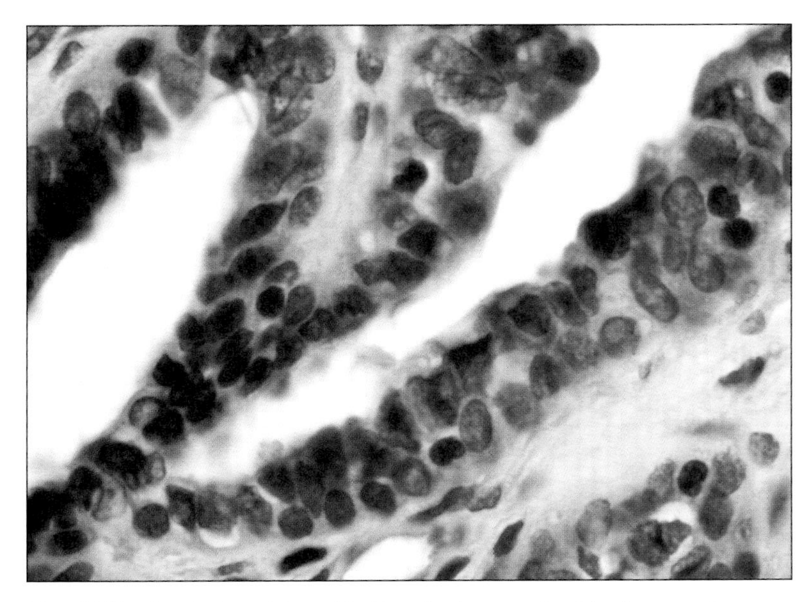

Fig. 6.23 Seminal vesicle epithelium is characterized by large and occasionally bizarre nuclei. Green–golden pigment in coarse granules is characteristic; attention to its presence should avert misinterpretation in small biopsies. Prostate epithelium can contain lipofuscin pigment, in smaller amounts and typically in fine granules.

from carcinoma, which, like atrophy, typically presents as a collection of small acini. (Figs 6.24–6.27)

INFARCT

Prostatic infarcts are common, occur spontaneously in the context of benign prostatic hyperplasia (BPH), may be related to vascular compression, and can cause a spike in serum prostate-specific antigen (PSA). (Fig. 6.28)

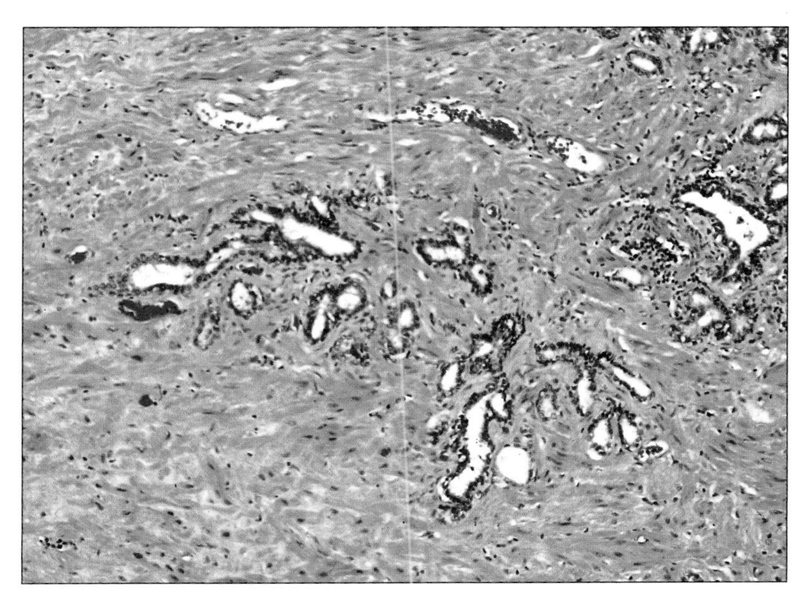

Fig. 6.24 Simple (lobular) atrophy presents as a discrete focus of small glands with increased nuclear:cytoplasmic ratio. Medium-power examination reveals the pre-existing radial acinar architecture. A central duct may be evident. Gland profiles are typically teardrop or star shaped.

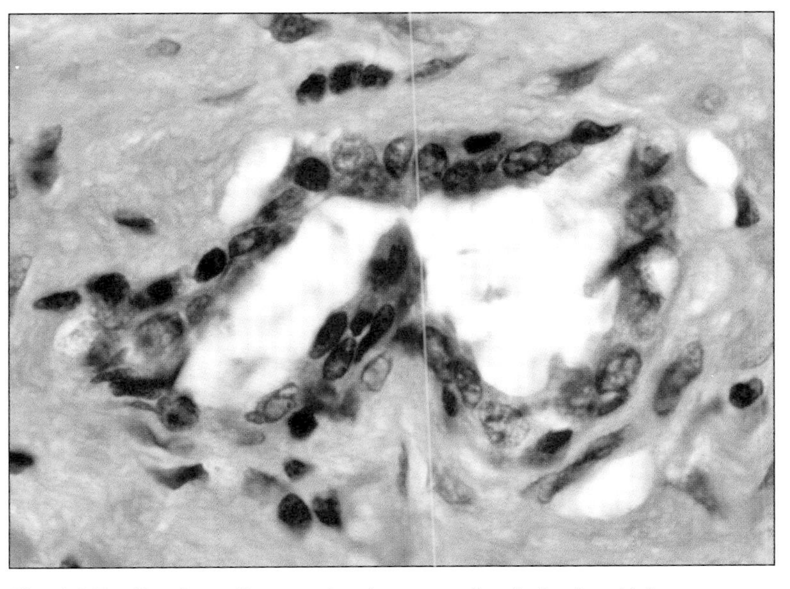

Fig. 6.25 Cytologically, atrophy shows small cell size but high nuclear:cytoplasmic ratio. Nuclei are round and uniform, with darkly staining chromatin. Atrophic epithelium is typically cuboidal but may be flattened (cf. cystic atrophy, below). High-power examination should disclose the presence of basal cells, which often stain more darkly than the atrophic glandular cells, and exhibit nuclear 'bubble' artifact.

GRANULOMATOUS PROSTATITIS

(Fig. 6.29)

METAPLASIAS

(Figs 6.30 & 6.31)

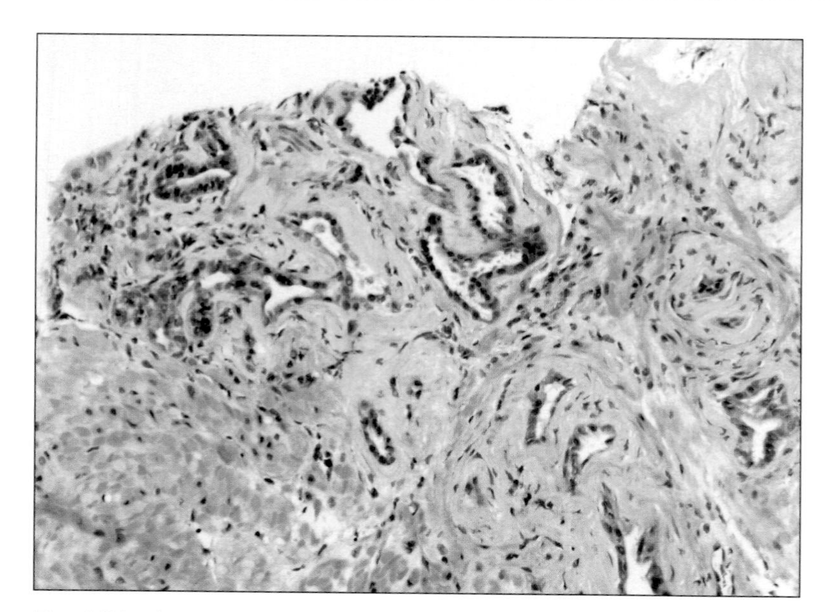

Fig. 6.26 In sclerotic atrophy, glands with staghorn profiles are embedded in a pale, myxoid, reactive stroma. The differential diagnosis includes carcinoma with desmoplastic stroma. However, prostate adenocarcinoma does not typically elicit significant stromal reaction. Accompanying inflammation is typical and should dissuade from precipitate diagnosis of neoplasia.

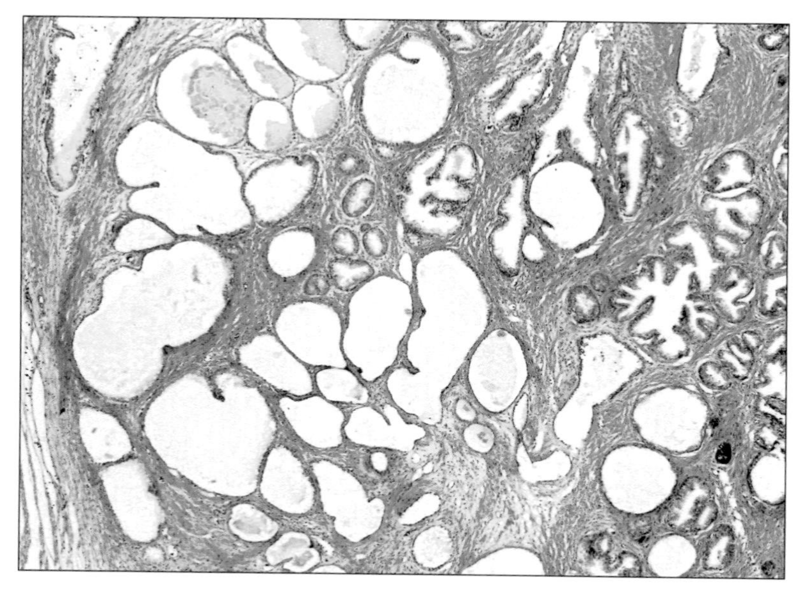

Fig. 6.27 Cystic atrophy is characteristic of the peripheral zone. Dilated, rounded acini, sometimes with a recognizable residual radial acinar arrangement, have scant flocculent eosinophilic content.

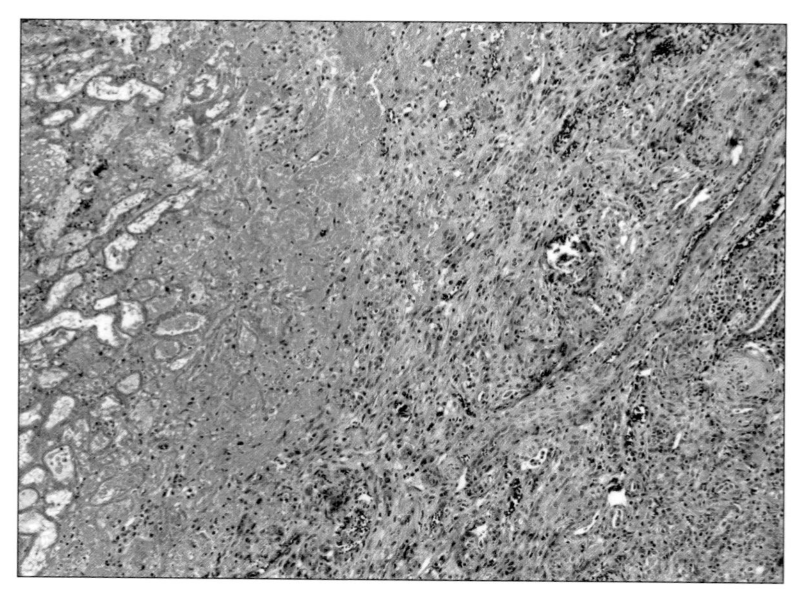

Fig. 6.28 Coagulative necrosis, hemorrhage, and inflammatory infiltration are followed by fibrosis. Squamous metaplasia is common in glands at the periphery of the infarct. Infarcts are rarely biopsied, but in limited samples reactive atypia and mitotic activity can yield a mistaken impression of glandular or stromal neoplasia.[22]

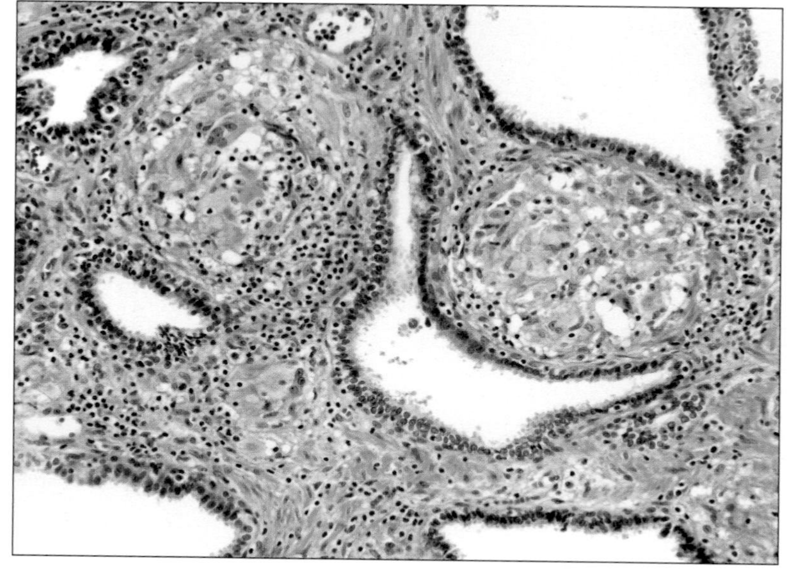

Fig. 6.29 Prostate granulomas are most commonly due to previous instrumentation (biopsy, transurethral resection). Infectious causes include blastomycosis, tuberculosis, and BCG infection (following bladder instillation).

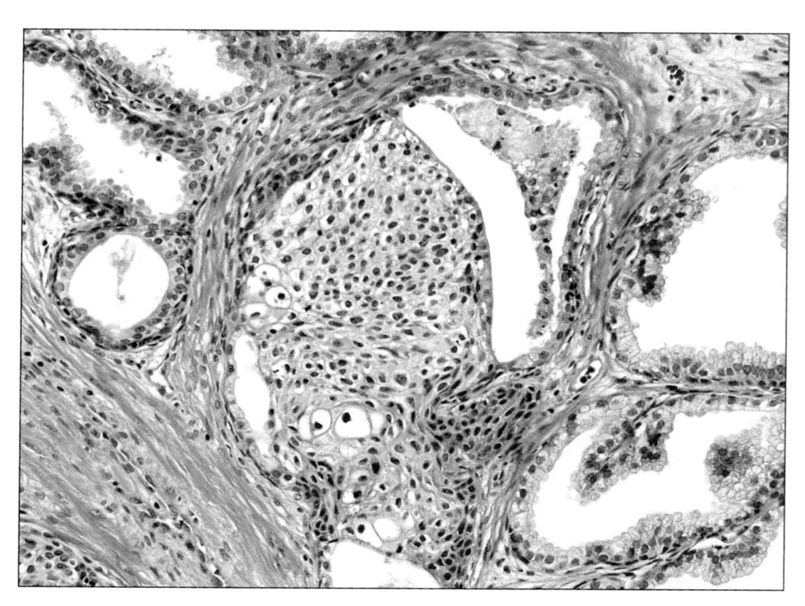

Fig. 6.30 Squamous metaplasia occurs in association with chronic prostatitis, but is especially pronounced in the irradiated prostate,[23] in association with prostatic infarcts,[22] and following androgen deprivation therapy.[24] Loss of prostate-specific antigen expression is characteristic.[25]

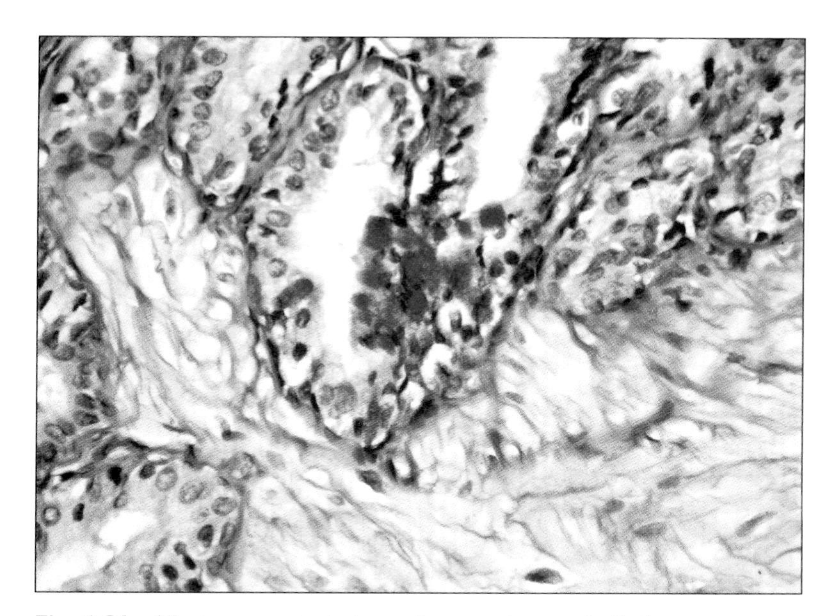

Fig. 6.31 Mucinous metaplasia can be seen in over half of prostatectomy specimens, usually in the inferior periurethral area.[26] It often occurs in association with atrophy or basal cell hyperplasia. Tall columnar cells stain intensely for neutral and acidic mucins (PAS stain). Loss of immunoreactivity for prostate-specific antigen and prostatic acid phosphatatse has been reported.[27]

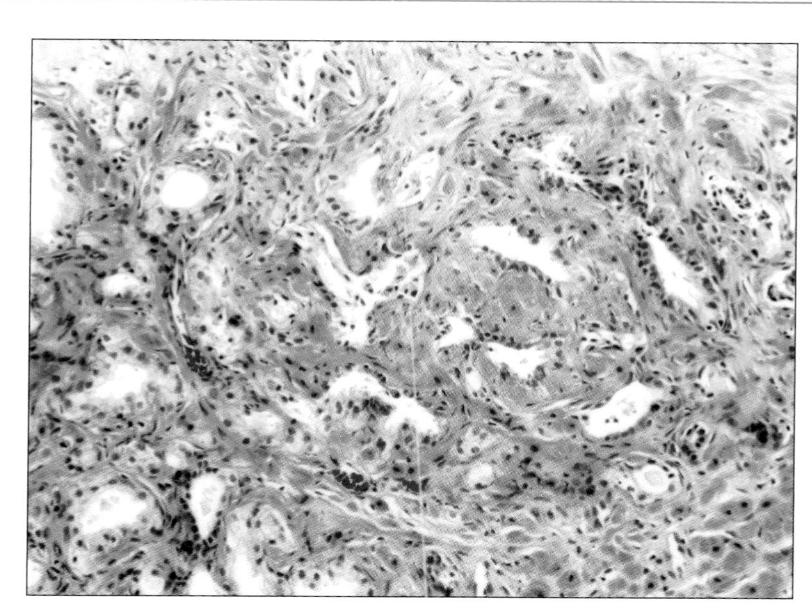

Fig. 6.32 Sclerosing adenosis. Lesions vary in size from a few millimeters up to a centimeter. The myoepithelial proliferation and thickened basement membrane about some of the glands elicit comparison with the identically named breast lesion. Occasional mild cytologic cellular atypia compounds the potential for confusion with neoplasia.

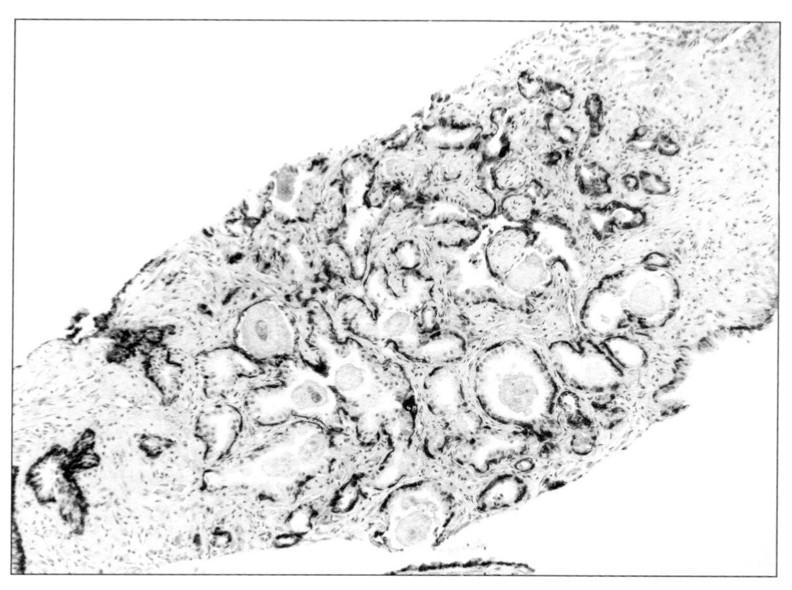

Fig. 6.33 Sclerosing adenosis. The accompanying stroma is cellular and includes single or small clusters of epithelial and basal cells embedded in an often myxoid stroma. In a small biopsy, this appearance could conceivably suggest high-grade (Gleason 4–5) adenocarcinoma. The basal cells exhibit a metaplastic myoepithelial immunophenotype (positive for cytokeratin, S-100, and muscle-specific actin).[28–30]

SCLEROSING ADENOSIS

These uncommon (about 2% of prostate specimens[28]), well-circumscribed lesions are composed of 'variably sized and shaped, often compressed, glands' [29] with a thickened, periodic acid–Schiff (PAS)-positive basal membrane. Most are incidental findings in transurethral resection (TUR) chips. (Figs 6.32 & 6.33)

BENIGN PROSTATIC HYPERPLASIA

(Figs 6.34–6.37)

RADIATION EFFECT

Biopsies of previously irradiated prostate are frequently obtained to investigate biochemical (PSA) recurrence in

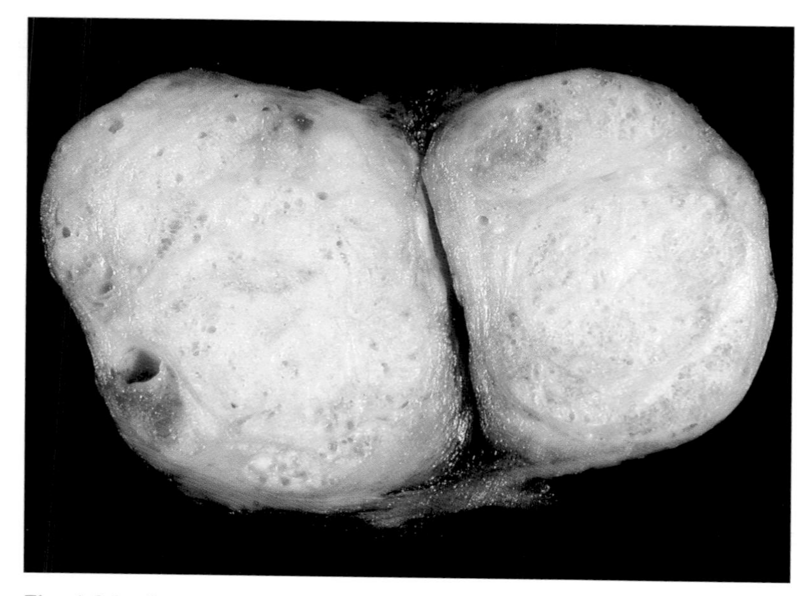

Fig. 6.34 Benign prostatic hyperplasia is a multinodular transformation involving exclusively the transition zone and the periurethral stroma.[31] It is therefore more pronounced in the more anterior portion of the prostate. The hyperplastic transition zone, normally 5% of the volume of the gland, may come to constitute most of the prostatic mass. Hyperplastic nodules may be predominantly stromal (characteristic of periurethral zone), mixed stromal and glandular, or predominantly glandular.

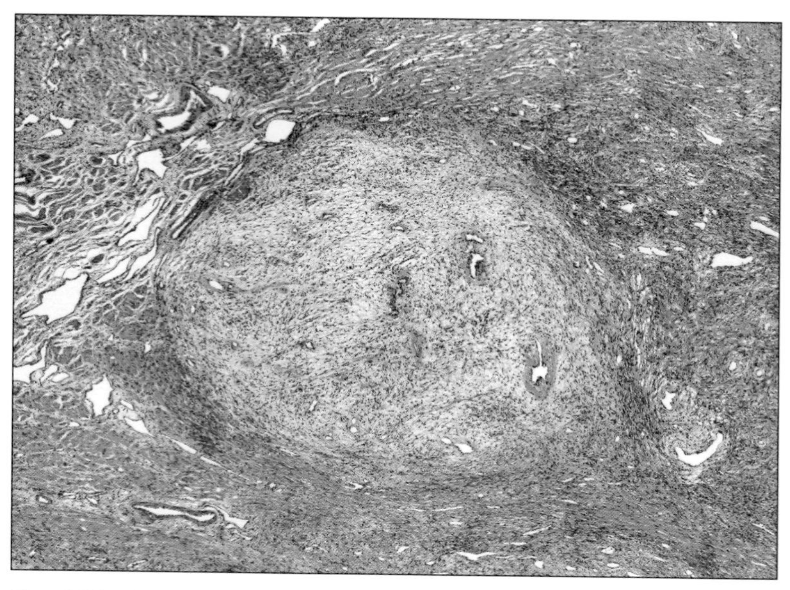

Fig. 6.36 Stromal nodules exhibit a spectrum of fibroblastic, fibromuscular, and muscular types. In addition, Benz et al[32] distinguished an embryonal-mesenchymal form that may be the immature precursor of the other types. Mature stromal nodules exhibit an infiltrate of T lymphocytes. Biochemical studies show increases in a variety of peptide growth factors and interleukins.

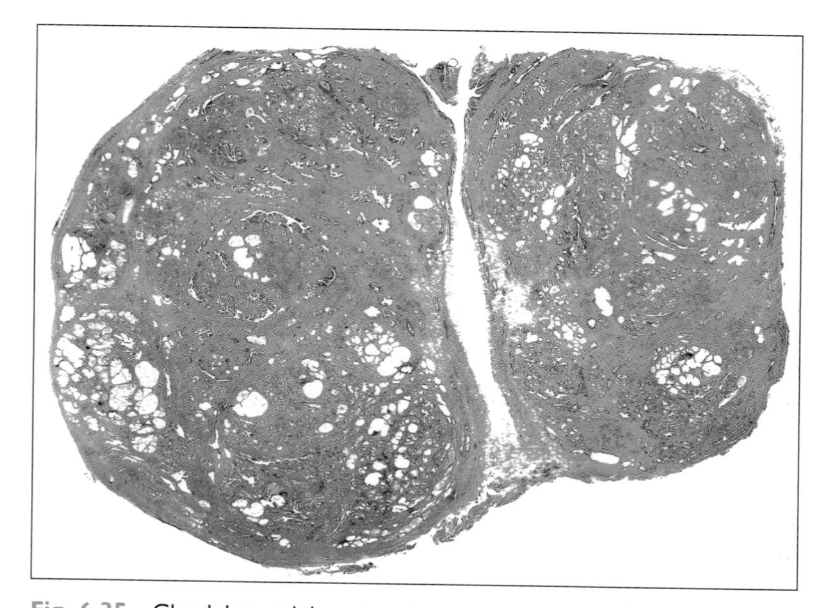

Fig. 6.35 Glandular nodules arise due to increased budding and branching of ductuloacinar units. Acini are commonly cystic and lined by a flattened epithelium. Immunostaining demonstrates attenuation and partial loss of the basal cell layer in many of these glands.

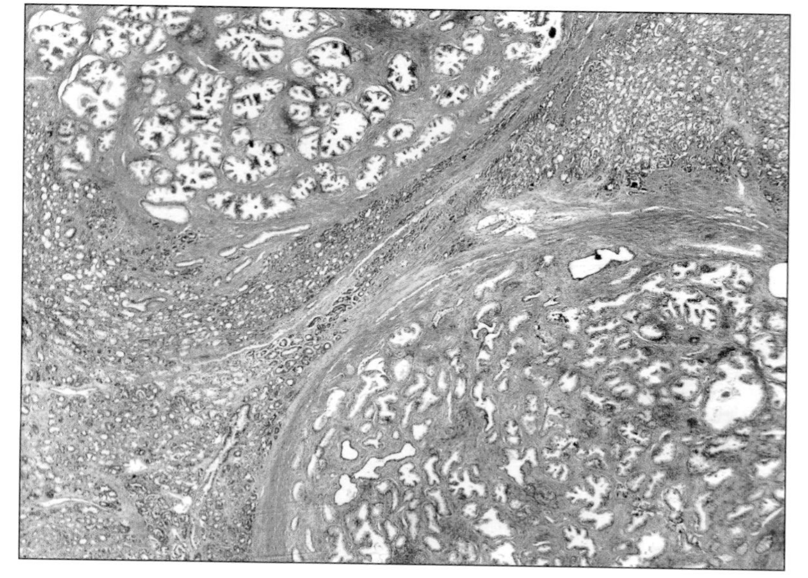

Fig. 6.37 Benign prostatic hyperplasia nodules are relatively resistant to invasion by carcinoma.

patients treated with external beam or brachytherapy. Bostwick and co-workers emphasized the danger of overdiagnosis of carcinoma in benign irradiated prostate because of radiation-induced cytologic atypia and prevalence of atrophic small glands.[23,33] Underdiagnosis of cancer may occur because of the decreased number of tumor glands relative to stroma. (Figs 6.38–6.40)

ANDROGEN DEPRIVATION EFFECT

Androgen deprivation therapy affects both benign and neoplastic prostate tissue.[34] There is atrophy of epithelial cells, stromal edema and/or fibrosis, a decrease in nuclear diameter, and cytoplasmic clear cell change. (Figs 6.41–6.43)

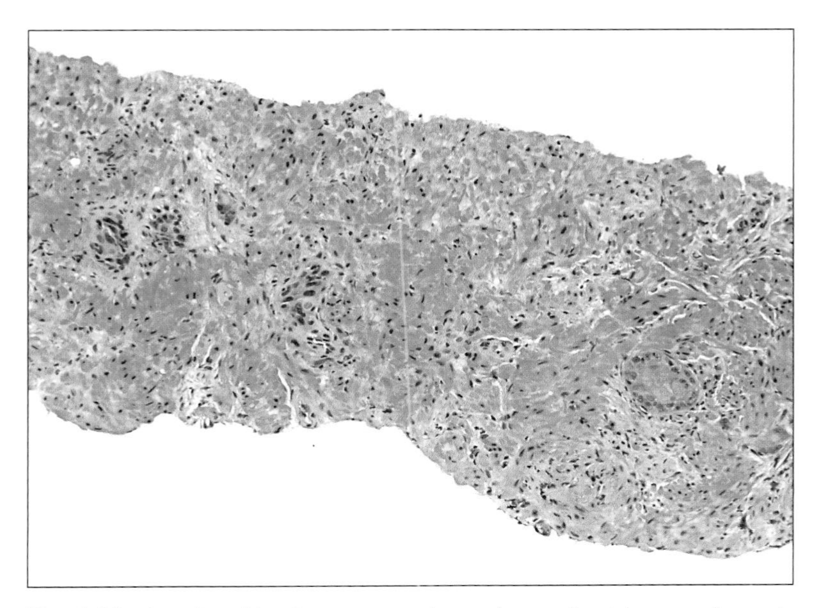

Fig. 6.38 Irradiated benign prostate tissue shows glandular atrophy and stromal fibrosis. Squamous metaplasia is common. Vascular changes include myointimal 'foamy cell' proliferation.

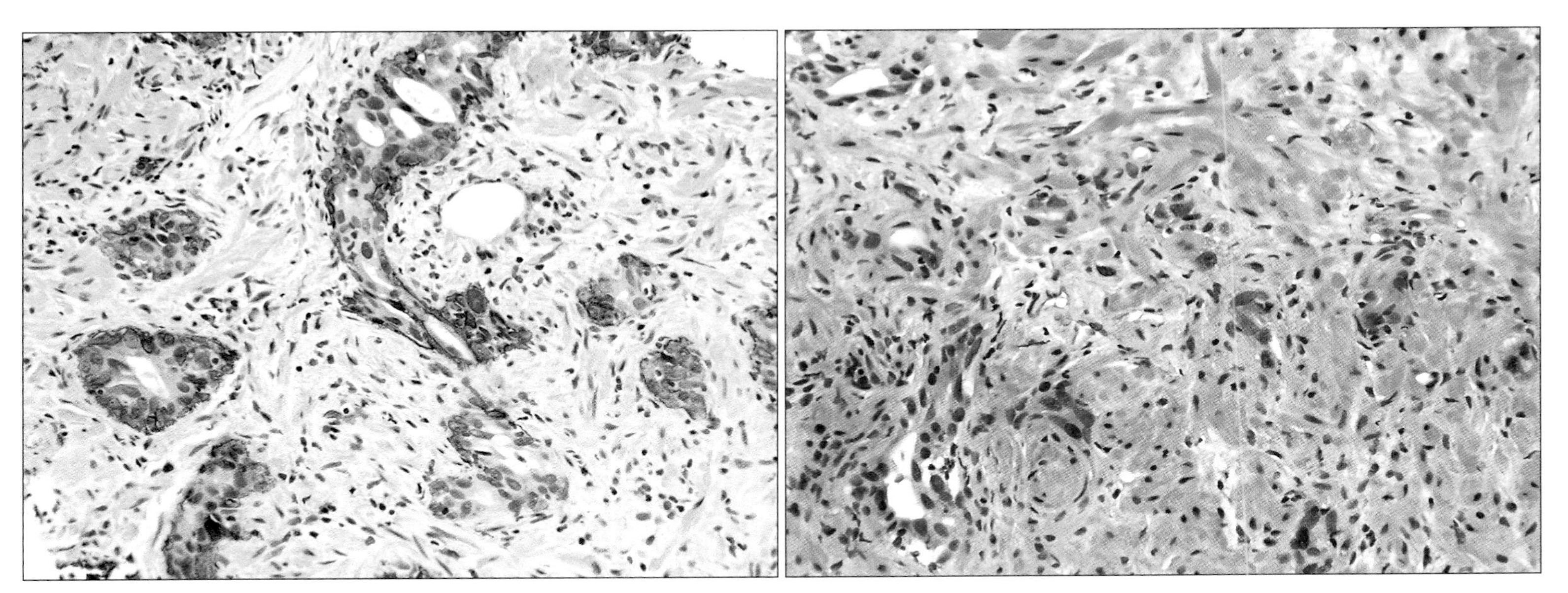

Fig. 6.39 Benign irradiated epithelium may exhibit marked cytologic atypia, including nuclear enlargement and prominent nucleoli. Architectural pattern is preserved. Low-power appreciation of lobular character can help to avoid overdiagnosis of cancer. Basal cell cytokeratin staining is extremely helpful in 'ruling out' carcinoma in atypical small glandular proliferations in the prostate.

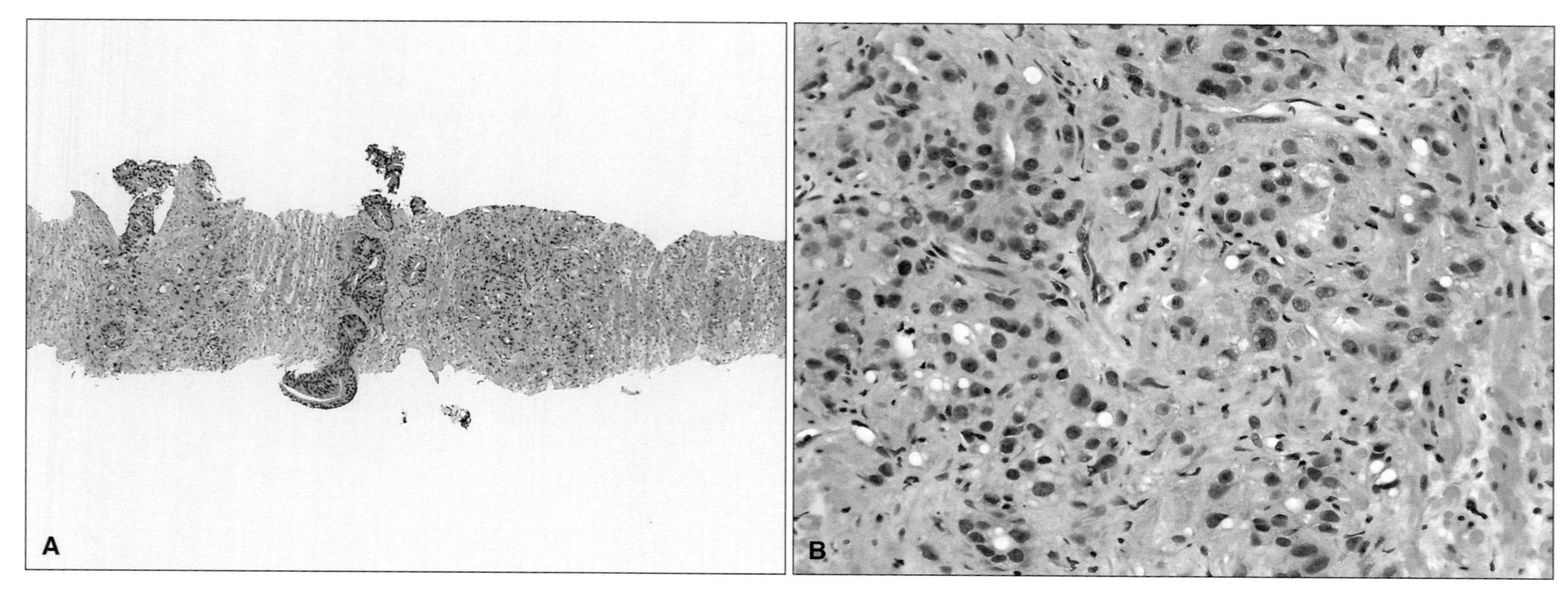

Fig. 6.40 (A,B) Irradiated prostate carcinoma shows a decreased ratio of tumor glands to stroma. Histologic features helpful in the diagnosis of cancer include: infiltrative growth, perineural invasion, intraluminal crystalloids, blue mucin secretions, absence of corpora amylacea, and the presence of coexistent high-grade prostatic intraepithelial neoplasia.[33] Grading is less reliable in irradiated prostate. Both under- and overgrading can occur.

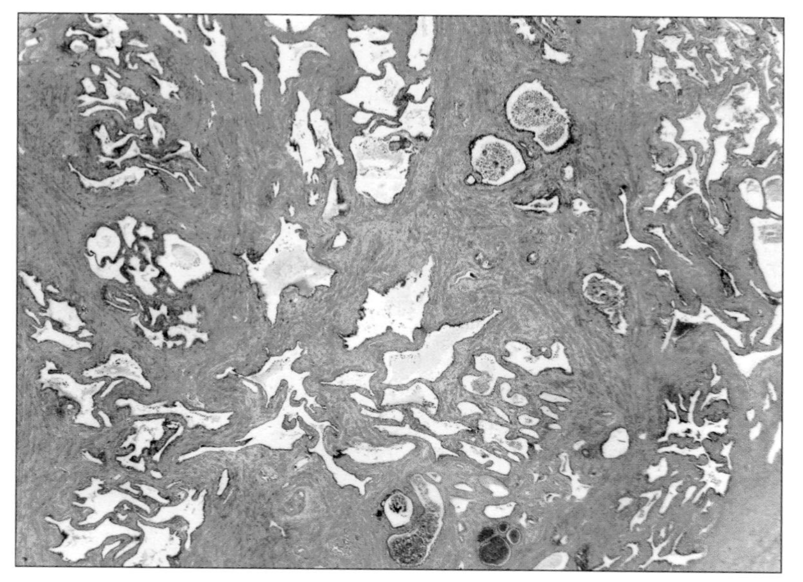

Fig. 6.41 Irradiated prostate. Benign prostate tissue shows marked acinar atrophy and a decreased gland:stroma ratio. Architecture is preserved. Basal cell hyperplasia and squamous metaplasia are seen. Stromal edema is noted early in therapy, followed by fibrosis. Epithelial cells are decreased in size, cytoplasm becomes 'clear', and nuclei are small and hyperchromatic.

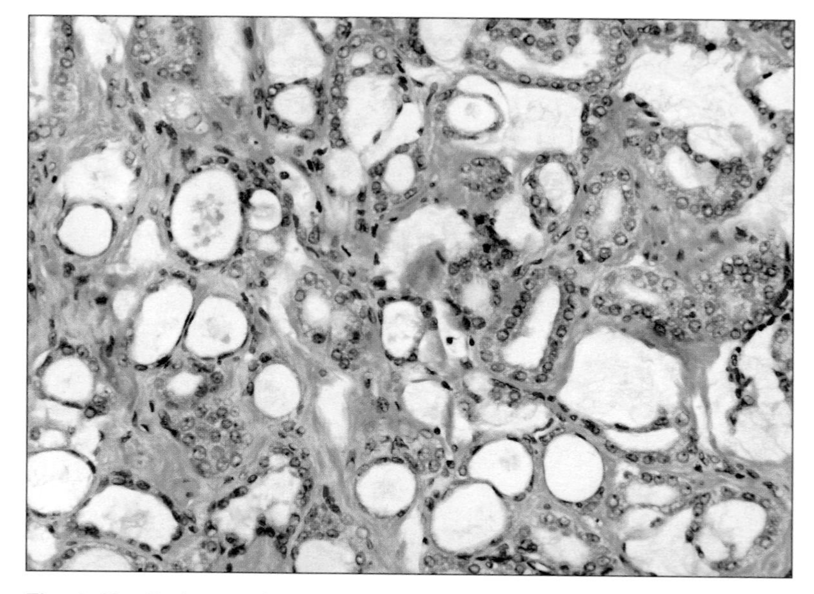

Fig. 6.42 Early in androgen deprivation therapy, there is flattening of the neoplastic epithelium, giving carcinomatous glands an appearance that may be mistaken for benign atrophy on a small biopsy with limited context. A similar focal finding may be seen in patients without a prior history of hormonal therapy ('atrophic carcinoma', see below).[35]

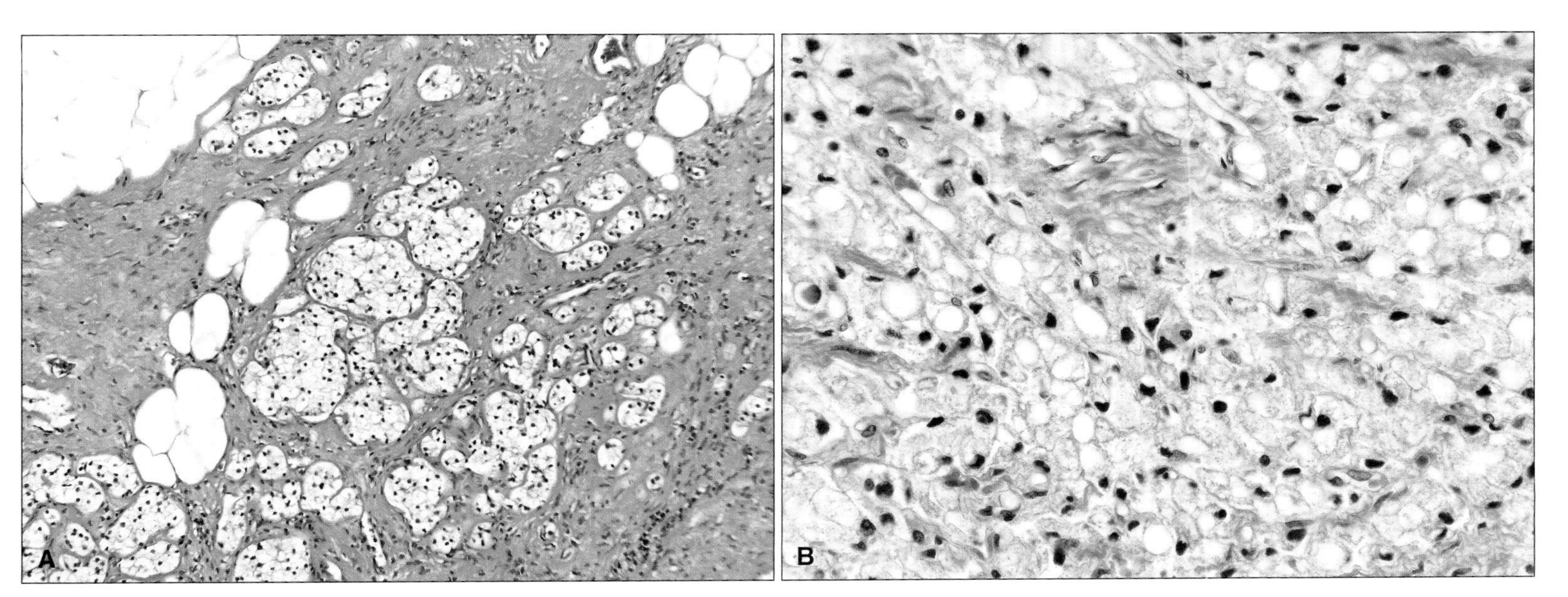

Fig. 6.43 (A,B) Under the influence of androgen deprivation therapy, carcinomatous glands decrease in size. There is prominent clear cell change; nuclei shrink, nucleoli become inconspicuous, and chromatin condenses. Grading of carcinoma under these circumstances is problematic. Overgrading of moderately differentiated carcinoma can occur when some combination of clear cell change and miniaturization of acini leads to a false impression of Gleason 4B or even 5B carcinoma. Undergrading can occur when loss of nucleolar prominence and cytoplasmic changes misleadingly suggest a well-differentiated tumor.

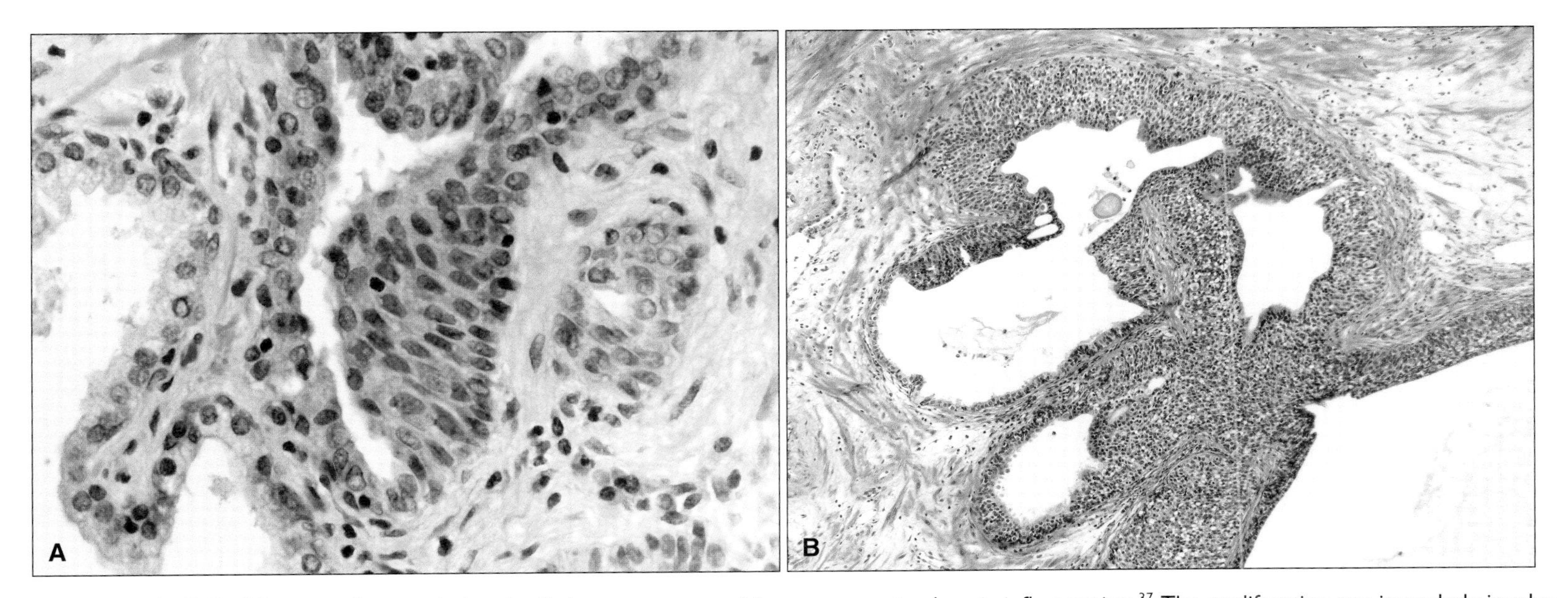

Fig. 6.44 (A,B) Proliferation of prostatic basal cells is common, possibly a response to chronic inflammation.[37] The proliferation can irregularly involve the periphery of the gland, leading to eccentric tufts. Alternatively, involvement can be circumferential. The long axis of the basal cell nucleus, ordinarily parallel to the basement membrane, is often oriented vertically. In formalin-fixed material, the nuclear 'bubble' artifact of basal cell nuclei is prominent. Basal cell hyperplasia occurs in all zones of the prostate. In tangential sections, the proliferation can simulate solid or cribriform architectural patterns.

BASAL CELL HYPERPLASIA[36]

(Figs 6.44 & 6.45)

POSTATROPHIC HYPERPLASIA[15,33,38–42]

This mimic of carcinoma consists of 'microscopic lobular cluster[s] of small acini with irregular atrophic-appearing contours, [yet] lined by cuboidal cells with mild nucleomegaly and micronucleoli'.[39,43] It thus combines the architecture of atrophy with 'reactive' cytologic atypia. Some contend that postatrophic hyperplasia is a pre-neoplastic condition, related to prostatic intraepithelial neoplasia.[37,41] (Figs 6.46 & 6.47)

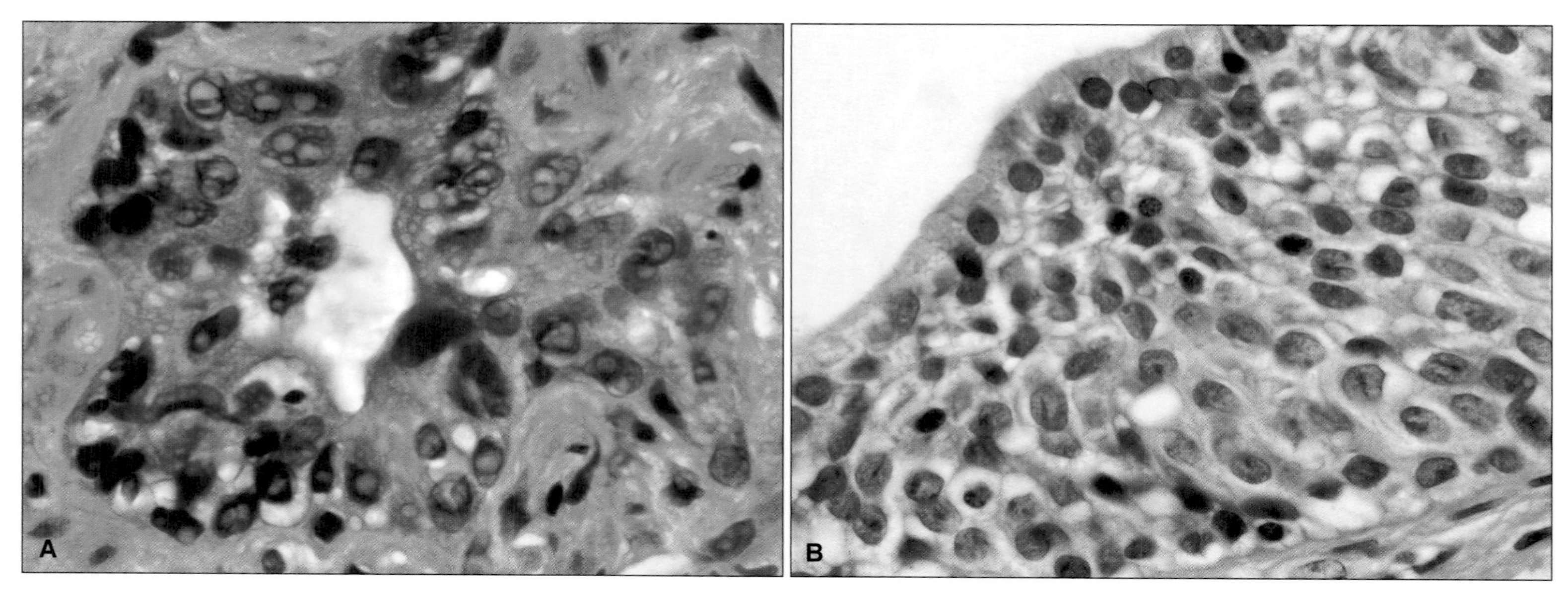

Fig. 6.45 (A,B) Inflammatory stimulus can result in significant nuclear atypia, including prominent nucleoli. Other atypical basal cell proliferations include the rare adenoid cystic-like tumors of the prostate.

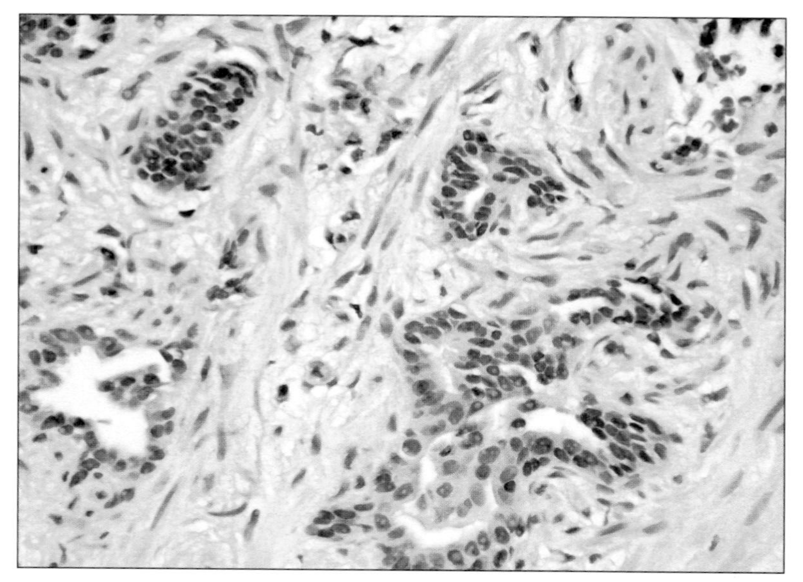

Fig. 6.46 Postatrophic hyperplasia. Small glands lined by flattened to cuboidal epithelial cells lie in a cluster within variably sclerotic stroma, often with a recognizable larger dilated central duct. Patchy chronic inflammation is present. The surrounding acini are lined by high cuboidal epithelium with clear cytoplasm and moderately enlarged, round nuclei. In some cases, mildly enlarged nucleoli may be present. A basal cell layer is present but inconspicuous.

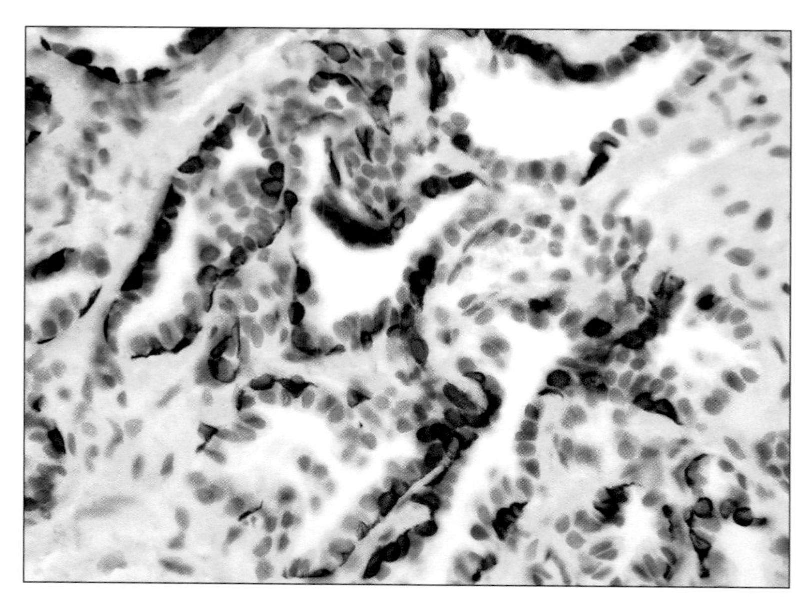

Fig. 6.47 Postatrophic hyperplasia. The basal cell layer may be focally incomplete; cytokeratin 34βE12 staining is positive. Ancillary findings of malignancy (intraluminal basophilic mucin, crystalloids) are absent. Concomitant focal involvement by high-grade prostatic intraepithelial neoplasia may complicate diagnosis.

ATYPICAL ADENOMATOUS HYPERPLASIA

Atypical adenomatous hyperplasia (AAH) is a term that has seen a variety of uses. Here it is used to refer to a limited proliferation of small glands occurring within a hyperplastic nodule. Since hyperplastic nodules are a transition zone phenomenon, AAH is seen most often in TUR specimens. The epithelium is cuboidal, with 'clear' cytoplasm and relatively bland nuclei. Glands are typically crowded.

The morphologic features of AAH resemble those of low-grade carcinoma (Gleason grade 1–2). McNeal[44] described the pattern as a putative pre-neoplastic alteration that contrasted with (what later became known as) prostatic intraepithelial neoplasia (PIN) in the peripheral zone. AAH may well be a precursor of well-differentiated transition zone carcinoma,[45] from which it is distinguished by preservation of an at least partially intact basal cell layer, but the association is not as thoroughly documented as that of PIN with peripheral zone carcinoma. (Figs 6.48 & 6.49)

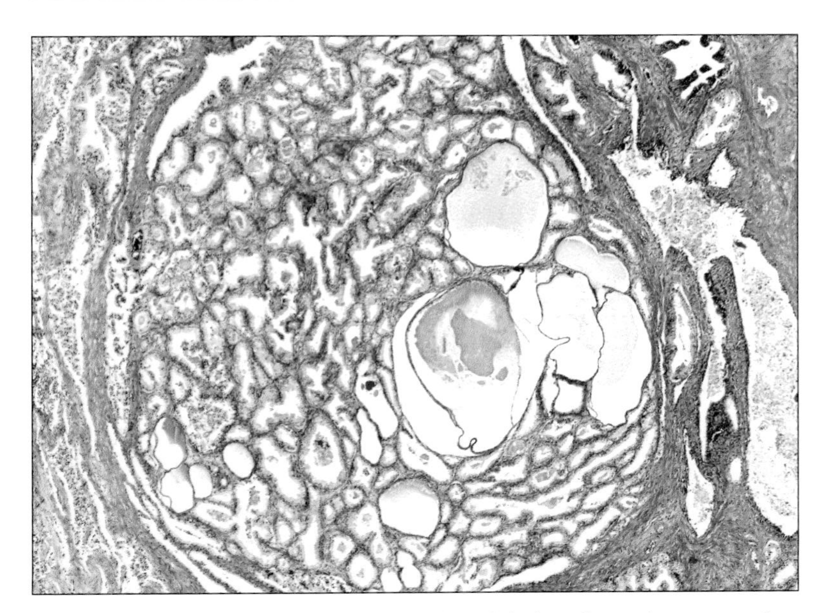

Fig. 6.48 At low power, a periurethral nodule has the architecture of benign prostatic hypertrophy, but areas appear crowded and mildly hyperchromatic.

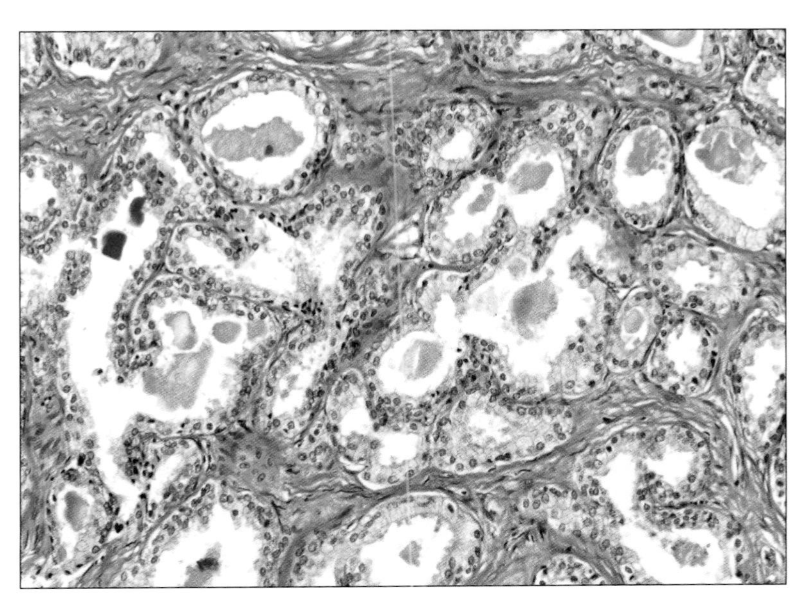

Fig. 6.49 A higher-power view of a periurethral nodule shows separate glands, many with complex profiles. A basal cell layer can be visualized in many glands. In some areas, simple-appearing glands lie back to back. A number of glands contain 'malignant' crystalloids. Cytoplasm is foamy and clear; there is active apocrine secretion. Nuclei are mildly enlarged, but conspicuous nucleoli are not seen.

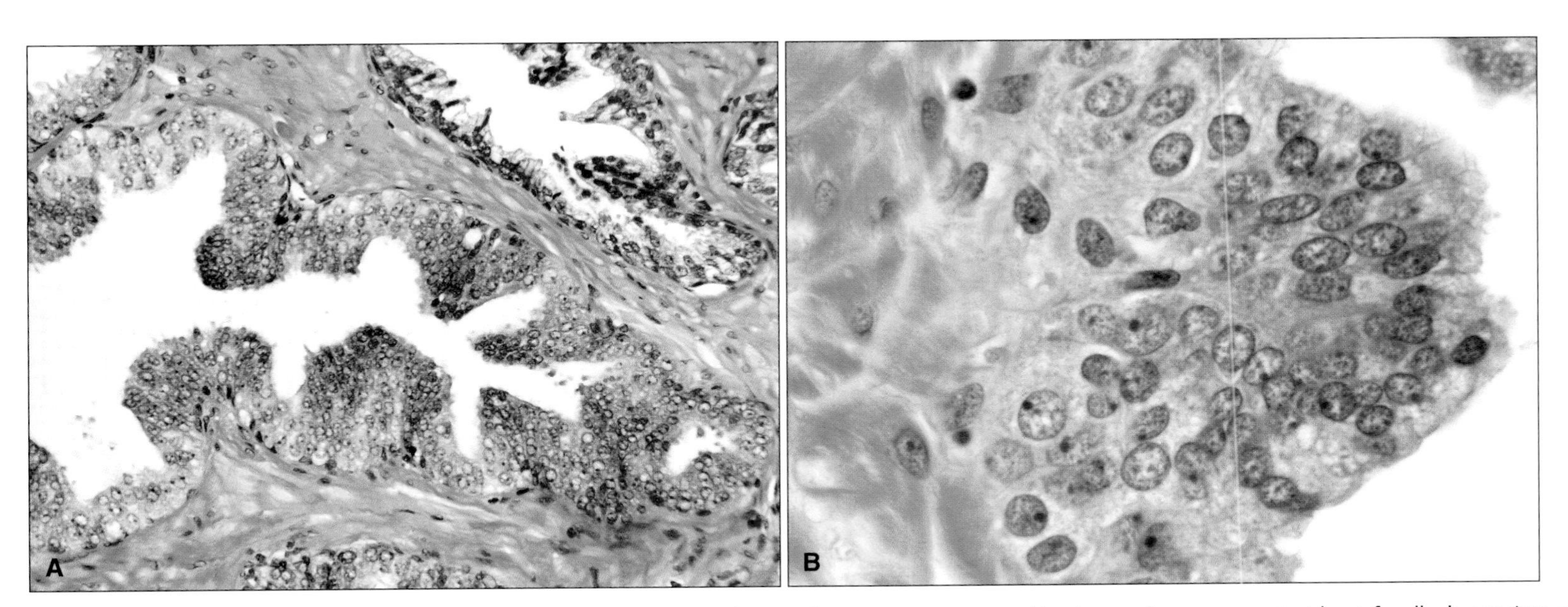

Fig. 6.50 (A,B) The 'tufting' pattern of prostatic intraepithelial neoplasia is the most common and is almost always present at least focally. It consists of glands with scalloped, undulating epithelial profiles due to hillocks of 'heaped-up' epithelium. This pattern in reminiscent of the 'clinging carcinoma' pattern in the breast.

ADENOCARCINOMA AND PRECURSOR LESIONS

PROSTATIC INTRAEPITHELIAL NEOPLASIA[46–48]

High-grade PIN is a precursor of prostatic adenocarcinoma. Histologic features include:

- uniformly enlarged nuclei;
- at least occasional (and typically frequent) macronucleoli, sometimes multiple;
- coarsely clumped and darkly staining chromatin;
- nuclear crowding and stratification;
- tufted architecture, with areas of micropapillary, cribriform, or flat architecture. (Figs 6.50–6.54)

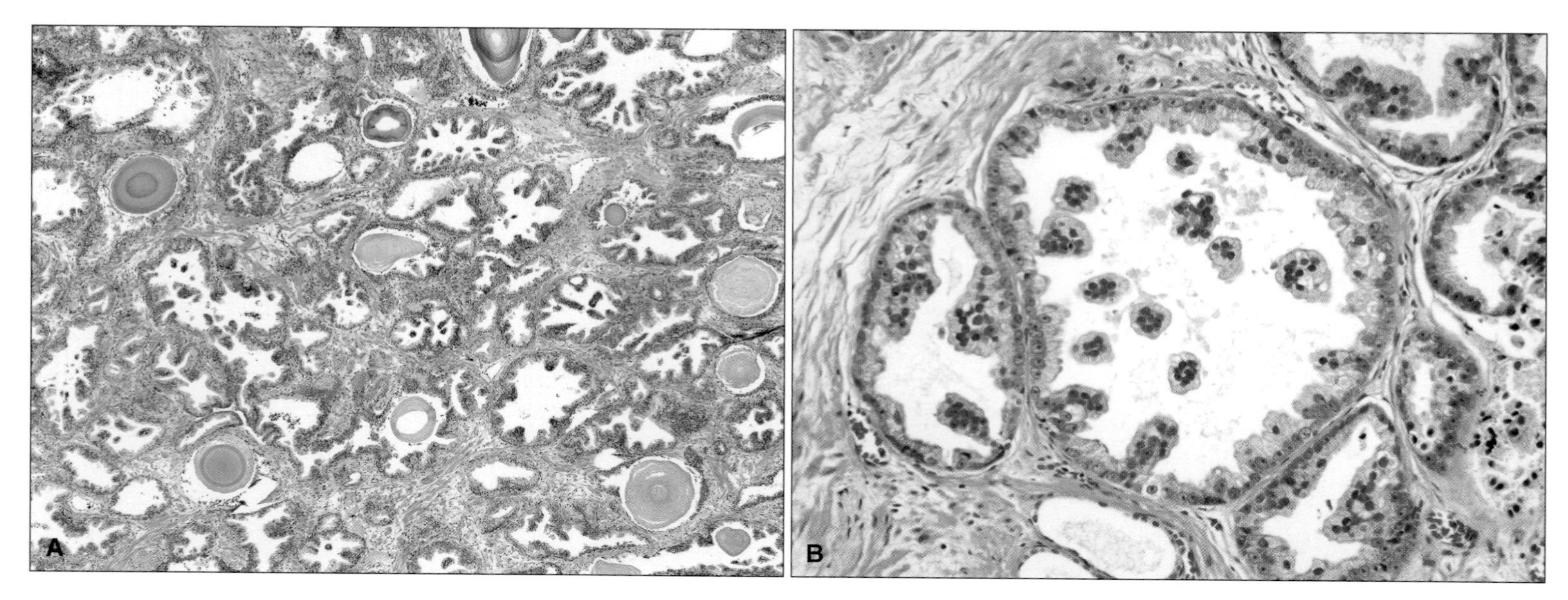

Fig. 6.51 The micropapillary pattern of prostatic intraepithelial neoplasia (PIN) is the second-most common pattern. Finger-like projections of atypical epithelium exhibit more recognizable nuclear atypia at the base than at the tips. Complex budding may occur. Absence of a true fibrovascular core is a helpful feature; a delicate capillary core may be present. Normal central zone epithelium shares a focally micropapillary architecture, some nuclear overlap, and small, peripheral nucleoli that must not be mistaken for PIN. A higher power view of the micropapillary PIN.

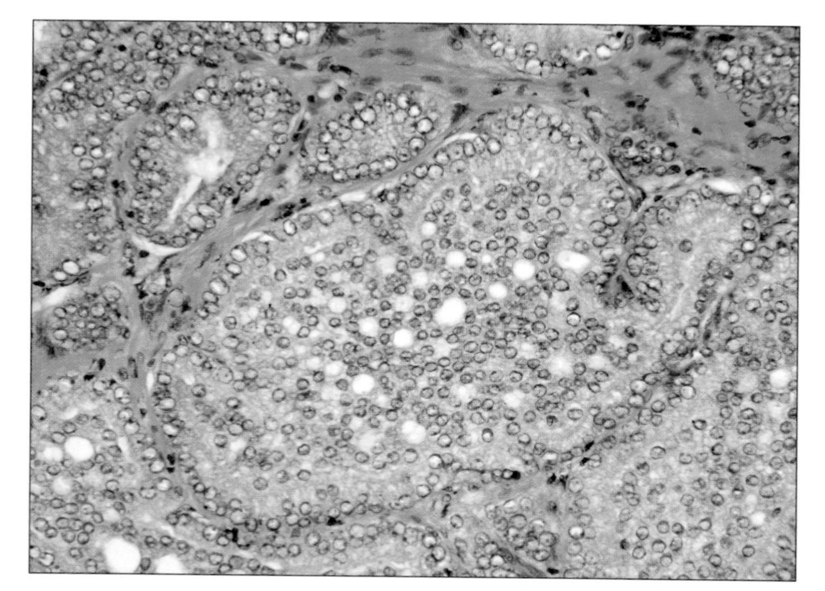

Fig. 6.52 Cribriform prostatic intraepithelial neoplasia (PIN) shows sieve-like spaces that are often elongated; typically, nuclear atypia is more pronounced peripherally. In cribriform PIN, the basal cell layer is at least partially preserved, demonstrable by basal cell cytokeratin stains. However, confident distinction between pure cribriform PIN and cribriform adenocarcinoma may be impossible in a small biopsy, because of the tendency of the latter to spread intraductally by 'cancerization' of adjacent pre-existing spaces (see below).[7,37,49–52]

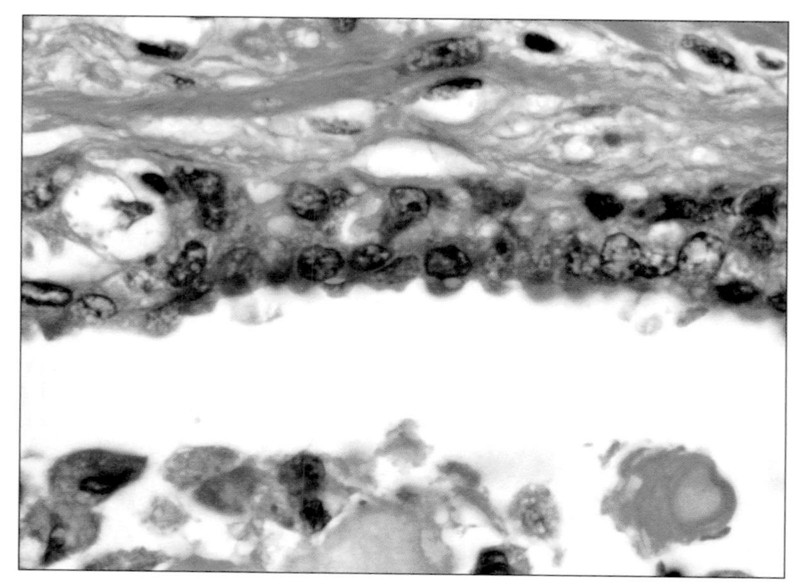

Fig. 6.53 Flat prostatic intraepithelial neoplasia is an unusual pattern. Traces of apocrine secretion may be preserved, in contrast to most carcinomas, in which apocrine activity is diminished or absent.

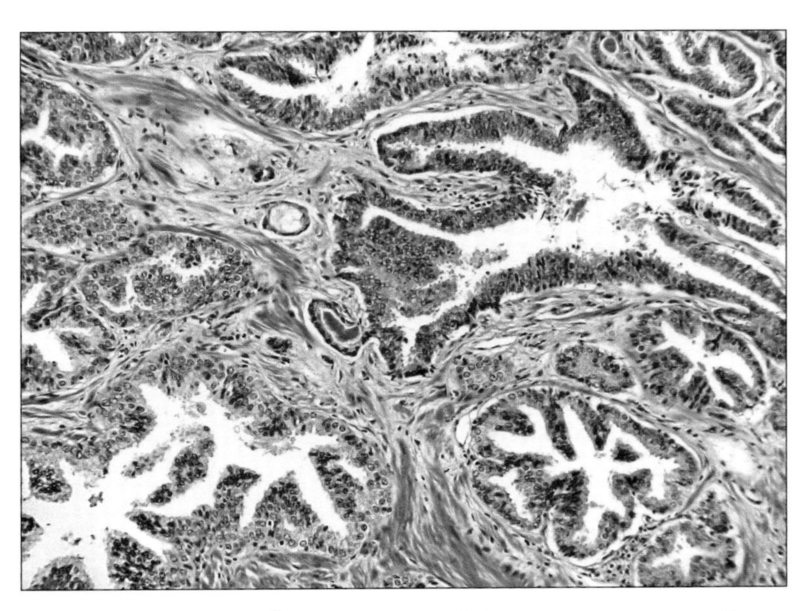

Fig. 6.54 Epstein et al[53] have emphasized that carcinoma is more likely the correct diagnosis in equivocal small glandular foci if the atypical small glands occur in the setting of adjacent prostatic intraepithelial neoplasia.

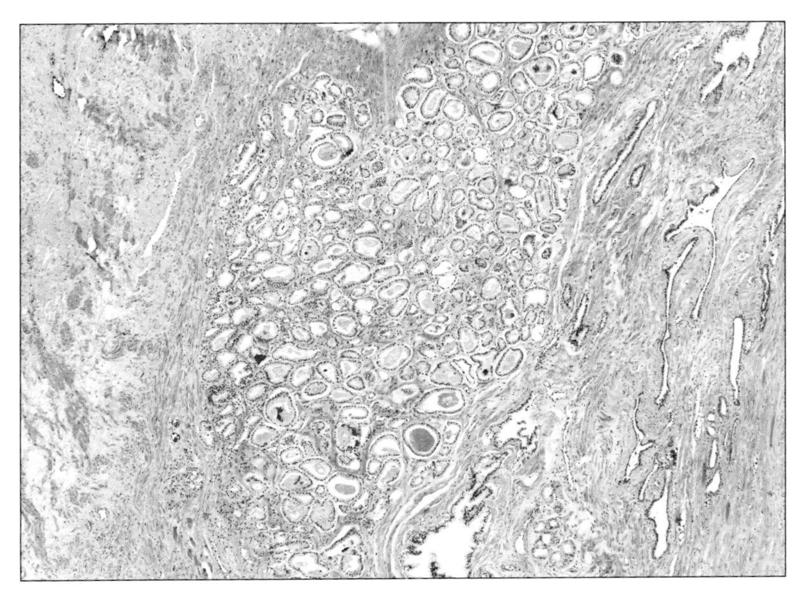

Fig. 6.55 The acini of low-grade (Gleason 1–2) carcinoma are of medium size, simple, and round. There is little intervening stroma. Uniform, closely packed acini distinguish grade 1 from the slightly less monotonous architecture of grade 2. By definition, low-grade carcinoma forms a discrete nodule, with a smooth, expansile peripheral border. Infiltration into the surrounding stroma does not occur.

ADENOCARCINOMA

Gleason grades 1 and 2

The defining feature of grade 1–2 (low-grade) adenocarcinoma is growth as a discrete nodule, without infiltration of the surrounding benign prostate. The presence in a biopsy of malignant glands intimately intermixed with benign glands is incompatible with a diagnosis of low-grade carcinoma.

Gleason described grade 1 cancers as 'single, separate, uniform glands, closely packed, with a definite edge';[54] these accounted for <5% of his original series. Grade 1 cancer occurs primarily in the transition zone, is usually small (<1 cm^3), and is the predominant pattern only in incidentally discovered carcinoma, as occurs in transurethral resections or autopsy prostates. It is almost never encountered in needle core biopsies.

Grade 2 carcinoma comprised about 5% of tumors in Gleason's series.[54] Grade 2 carcinoma occurs as a discrete nodule, although the border with the adjacent prostate is slightly ragged. Distinction of this grade from other carcinoma patterns among specialist[55] and non-specialist[56] pathologists is inconsistent. Like grade 1, most grade 2 carcinomas occur in the transition zone and it is not usually the primary grade encountered in needle biopsies.[57] Some pathologists might cite pattern 2 secondarily in needle biopsies with primary pattern 3 (viz. 3 + 2 = 5) to characterize a particularly orderly and circumscribed focus with moderately differentiated cancer.

Distinguishing features favoring low-grade carcinoma over benign glandular proliferations include:[58]

- extreme uniformity of gland size and shape;
- sharp luminal border;
- extremely close packing of glands with little intervening stroma;
- small lumen;
- absence of benign 'parent' gland;
- absence of corpora amylacea;
- presence of 'significant' nucleolar prominence;
- absence of cytokeratin 34βE12 immunoreactive basal cell layer.

No single criterion is absolute. Basal cell layer is typically discontinuous in AAH, so negative basal cell immunohistochemistry can be misleading.

Distinction from 'clear cell' carcinomas of higher grade (e.g. 4B), deceptively incomplete biopsy samplings of cribriform carcinomas, or better-differentiated, large cell Gleason 3 carcinomas may be an issue in small biopsies. By no means are all transition zone cancers low grade.[59] (Figs 6.55 & 6.56)

Gleason grade 3

This is the most commonly diagnosed pattern in needle biopsy specimens. The essential characteristic that distinguishes moderately differentiated (grade 3) from

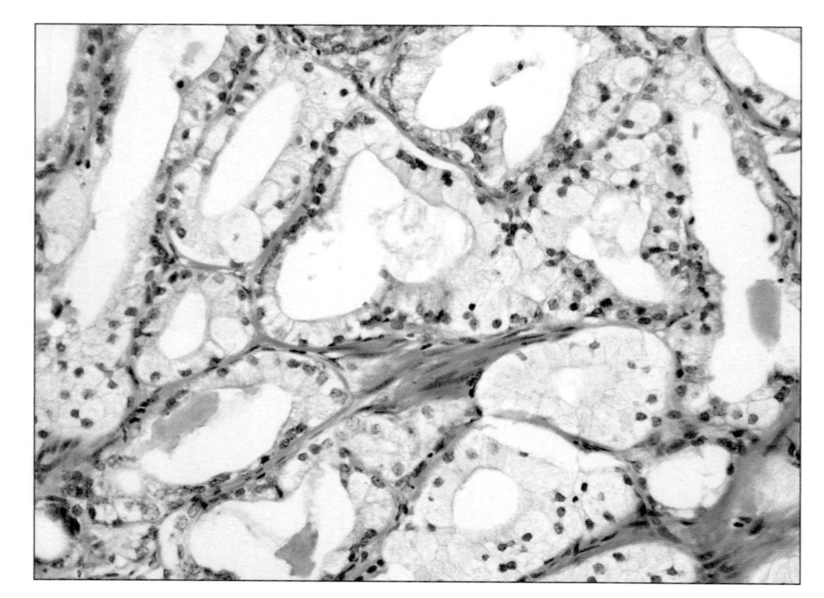

Fig. 6.56 Gleason grade 1–2 adenocarcinoma. The cytoplasm is 'clear' and faintly eosinophilic due to intracytoplasmic accumulation of abnormal, lipid-containing vacuoles.[13] Normal apocrine secretion may be diminished or absent, and, as a result, the normally frayed apical cytoplasmic border is sharply defined. Cytoplasm is abundant. Since nuclei are not enlarged, the nuclear:cytoplasmic ratio may actually be lower than that of adjacent benign acinar cells.

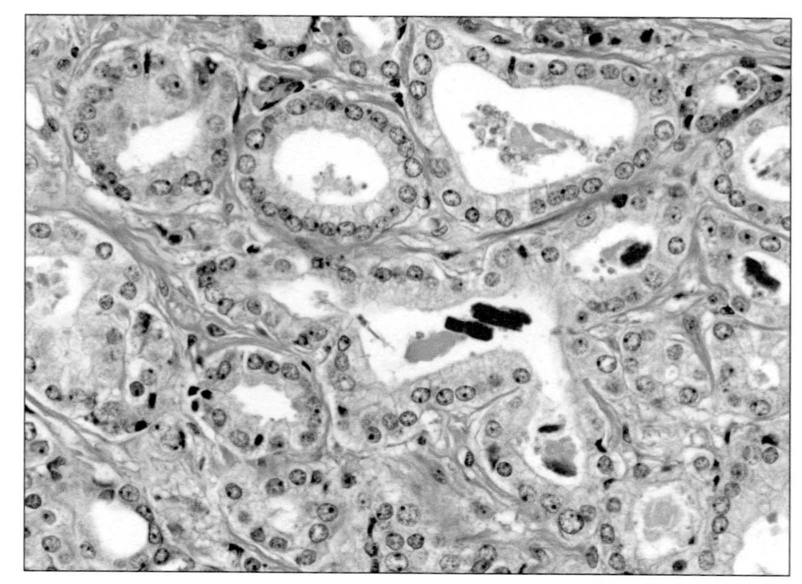

Fig. 6.57 Gleason grade 3 adenocarcinoma. Acini are separated by stroma, with a spacing that is of the order of one gland diameter. The glands often appear to 'split' the pre-existing stromal fibers without eliciting any response. The stroma is typically unreactive. 'Desmoplasia' (e.g. stromal basophilia, fibroblast proliferation, stromal nuclear enlargement, and fibrosis) is more typical of reactive proliferations than of grade 3 carcinoma.

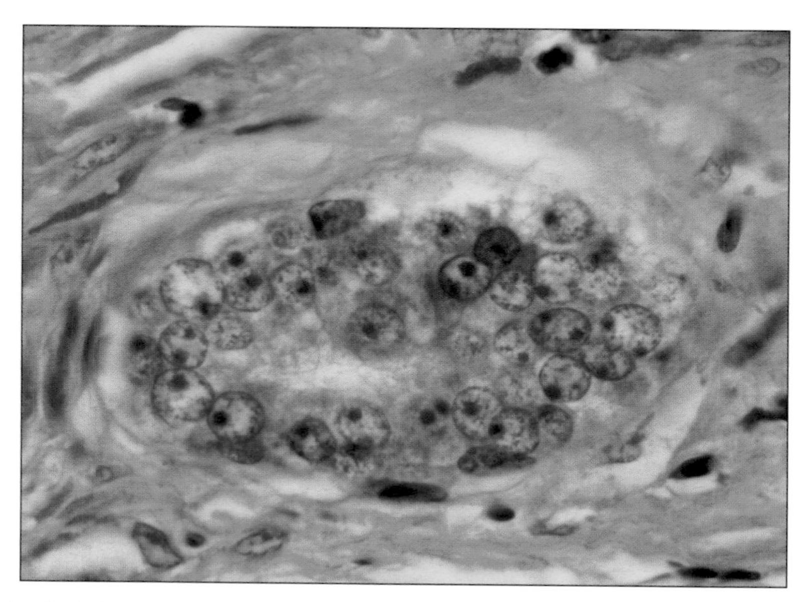

Fig. 6.58 A progressive decrease in luminal diameter is seen in small acinar ('3B') carcinomas. In less well-differentiated examples, the lumen may be altogether absent. This does not raise the grade to 4.

well-differentiated (grade 1–2) carcinomas is absence of clear circumscription, i.e. an infiltrative margin with respect to benign glands and stroma. On needle core biopsy specimens, the presence of malignant glands insinuating among benign glands implies at least a grade 3. In addition, acini of grade 3 carcinoma show variability in size, shape, and spacing.

Grade 3 encompasses a range of acinar architecture. Gleason distinguished three major patterns ('A', 'B', and 'C').[54] Medium to large acinar carcinoma ('large gland carcinoma') is 3A. Carcinoma with a relatively uniform population of small (~0.1 mm or less) acini (the classic 'small glandular proliferation') is 3B. Cribriform carcinoma is 3C. (Figs 6.57–6.65)

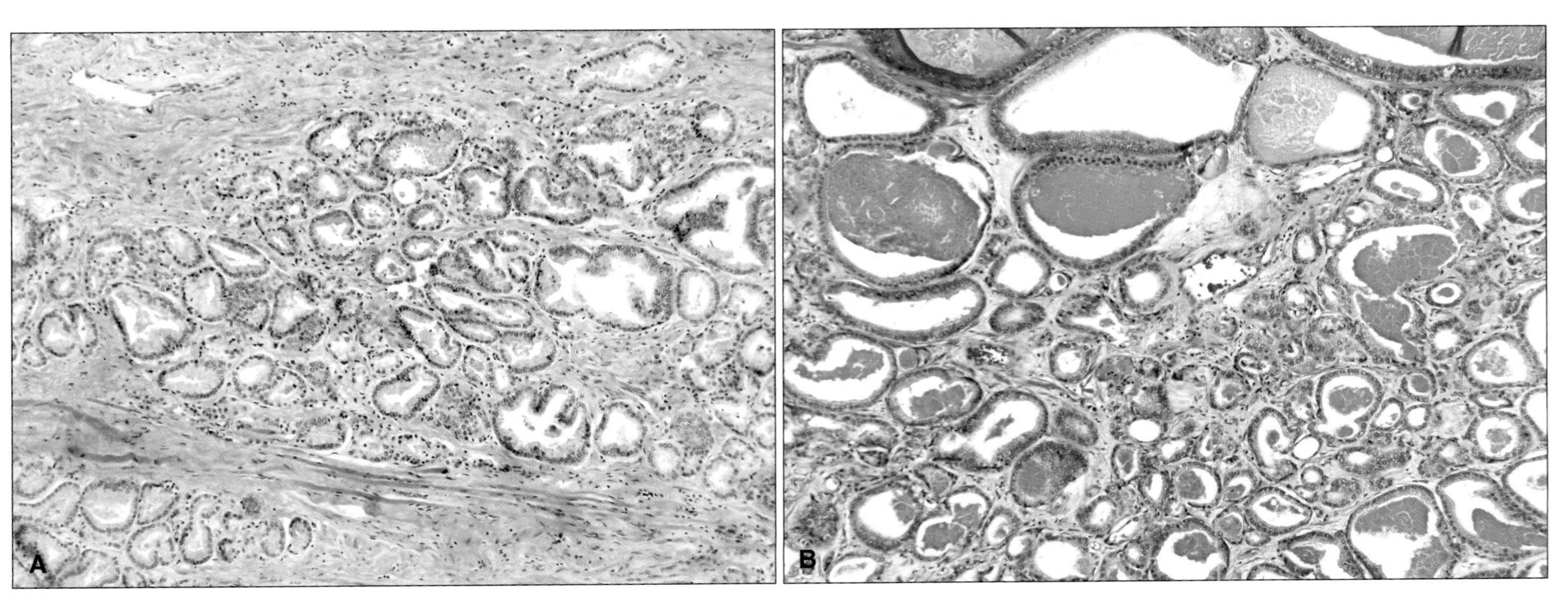

Fig. 6.59 (A,B) In large gland ('3A') carcinoma, lumina are preserved and glands may appear elongated, angulated, and even branching. It may be difficult to distinguish the large glandular variant of grade 3 from high-grade prostatic intraepithelial neoplasia. The presence of plentiful interglandular stroma facilitates the distinction from true glandular fusion, as in grade 4.

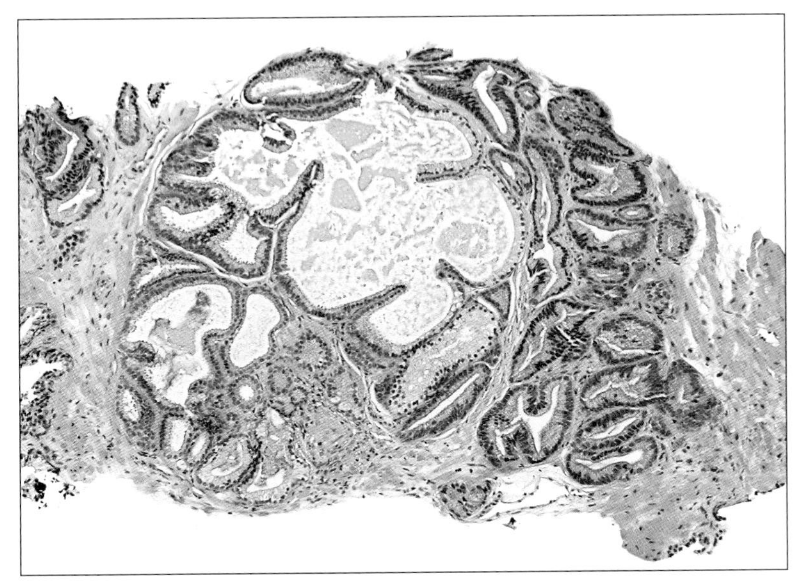

Fig. 6.60 The 'pseudohyperplastic' variant of grade 3 carcinoma has large, cystically dilated glands that are often filled with flocculent secretion.[60] Deceptively benign features may be present, including papillary infoldings, branching, and corpora amylacea. The diagnosis relies on recognition of nuclear enlargement, frequent nucleoli, and crystalloids. Basal cell cytokeratin stain is usually required to substantiate the diagnosis. More easily recognizable 'classic' carcinoma usually accompanies pseudohyperplastic carcinoma.[60]

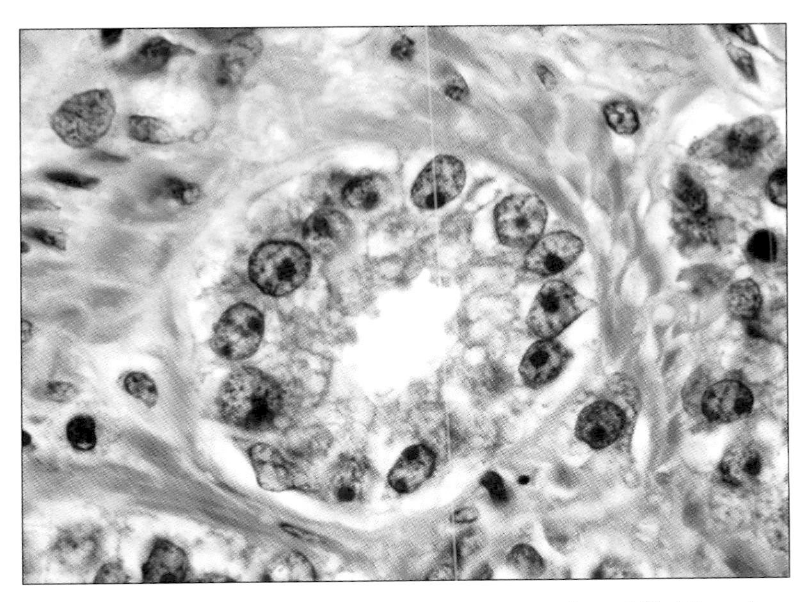

Fig. 6.61 Nuclei in grade 3 adenocarcinoma are enlarged (5–10 μm in diameter, typically 1–2 times the size of adjacent benign nuclei), and the nuclear:cytoplasmic ratio is generally noticeably increased. Nuclei are round, the nuclear envelope is regular, and chromatin is not clumped. The typical 'eosinophilic macronucleolus' in carcinoma exceeds 2 μm in diameter, is reddish in a well-balanced hematoxylin–eosin section, and tends to be located more eccentrically as grade increases.

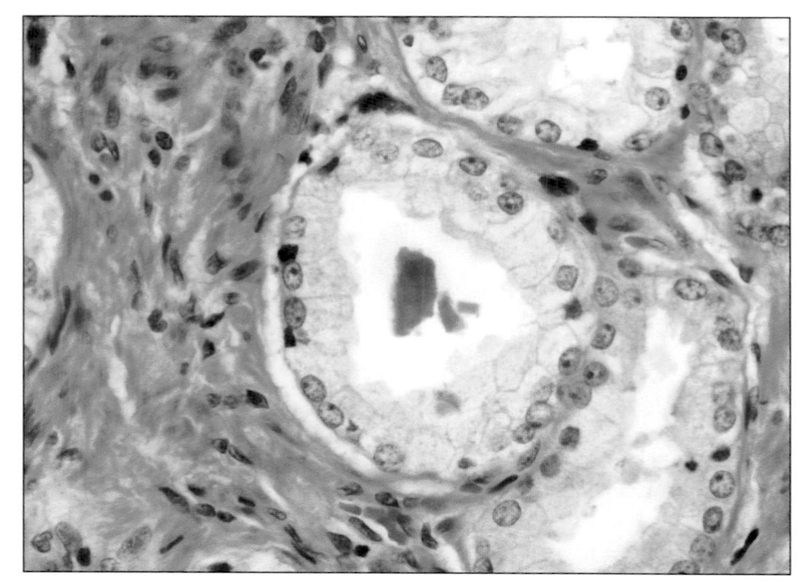

Fig. 6.62 Eosinophilic crystalloids can be seen in atypical adenomatous hyperplasia and in low- and moderate-grade prostatic adenocarcinoma.[38] This finding is nonspecific for cancer, and evidently can be seen in biopsies from benign prostates.[38,61,62]

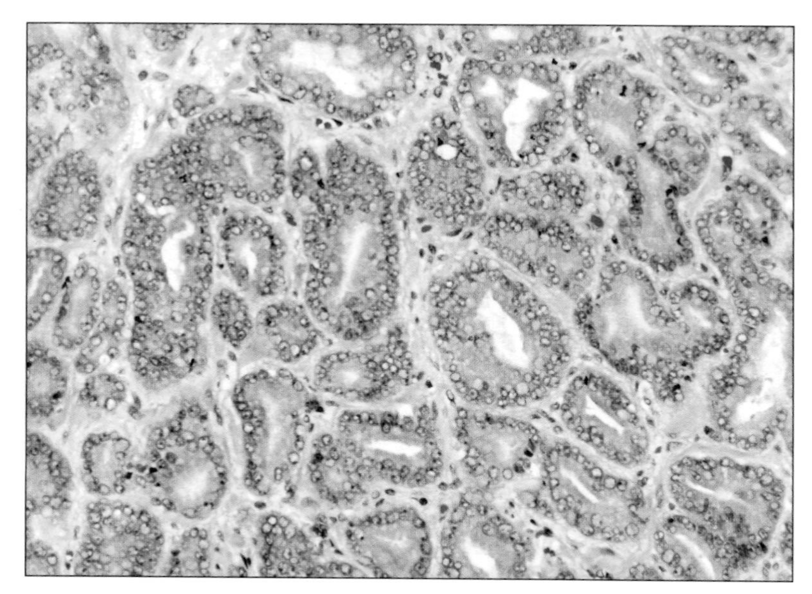

Fig. 6.63 Many grade 3 carcinomas have uniform, glassy, amphiphilic cytoplasm. In such cases, the lilac color of the carcinoma cell cytoplasm contrasts strikingly with the pale, foamy cytoplasm of adjacent benign glands, and provides a low-power clue to the diagnosis of carcinoma.

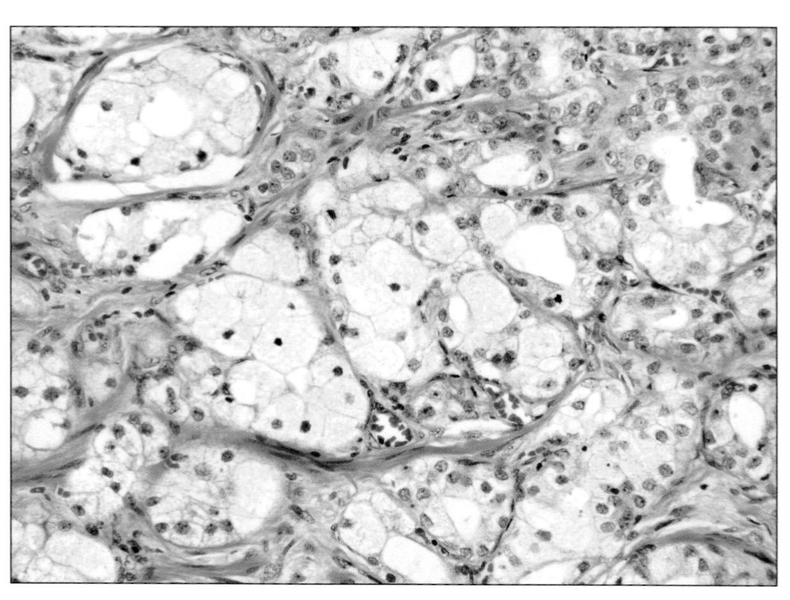

Fig. 6.64 The cytoplasm of grade 3 carcinoma may be clear, like that of grade 2. A cytologic variant of intermediate-grade carcinoma, the 'foamy gland' type,[63] contains abundant xanthomatous cytoplasm. It is frequently one component of a more cytologically conventional carcinoma.[64]

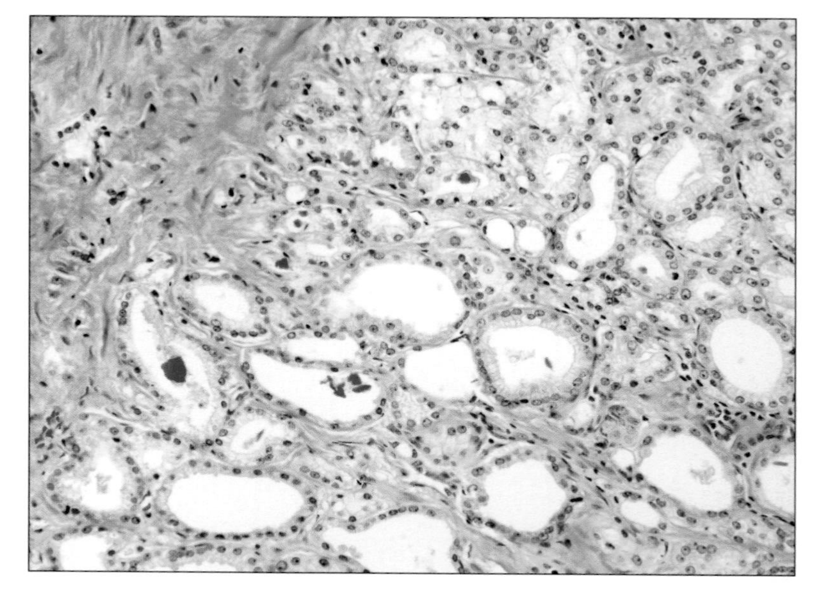

Fig. 6.65 Limited context makes grading difficult. There is an edge to the lesion, relatively clear cytoplasm, and abundant crystalloids, at first suggesting a low grade. However, there is too much variation in gland size. Closer examination shows atrophic features in some large glands at the bottom. Near the top of the field, some cribriform areas are present. Most of the lesion is probably Gleason 3 with clear cell and atrophic features. A few areas are even worrisome for Gleason 4.

Cribriform neoplasia

Gleason included cancers with cribriform features in his depiction of grade 3, grade 4, and grade 5. Grade 3 cribriform lesions had few peripheral lumens, with diameters that were large relative to the height of the epithelium, and relatively simple overall lesion profiles. Grade 4 cribriform lesions had apertures of comparable width to the height of their lining epithelium, with loss of peripheralization, and irregular lesion edges with infiltrative margins. Grade 5 lesions had a few apertures in an otherwise solid mass of cancer cells, or foci of necrosis.

Subsequently, McNeal and co-workers pointed out that some high-grade cribriform lesions retained peripheral basal cells ('carcinoma in situ').[65,66] However these cases were invariably associated with Gleason 4 frankly invasive carcinoma elsewhere in the gland and high tumor volumes.[52] This was later confirmed by Rubin et al, who concurred that high-grade cribriform prostatic intraepithelial carcinoma (McNeal's 'carcinoma in situ') should be interpreted as a 'late event in tumor progression', akin to ductal cancerization rather than intraductal dysplasia.[67]

The practical implications are that: (1) there is some subjectivity in drawing the line between grade 3 and grade 4 cribriform proliferations, less so between grade 4 and grade 5; (2) high-grade cribriform proliferations acceptable by traditional criteria as Gleason 4 may in many cases prove to be cancerization of pre-existing ducts, but their presence is anyway strong evidence of 'classic' invasive high-grade carcinoma nearby. How to inerrantly distinguish 'preinvasive' cribriform PIN from cancerization in small biopsies remains open. (Fig. 6.66)

Gleason grade 4

The cardinal feature of grade 4 adenocarcinoma is often expressed as increasing 'glandular fusion'. Yet three-dimensional reconstructions clearly show that even the apparently separate glands of grade 3 carcinoma actually form a densely interconnected network of tubular acini.[69] The impression of 'fusion' in two-dimensional sections of grade 4 carcinoma more accurately manifests an agglomerative habit of cancer cell growth, independent of any obligatory support by a stromal substratum. The topological derangement could also reflect progressive loss of 'contact inhibition' or decreasing functional anisotropy of cancer cells.

Grade 4 carcinoma, whether as a primary or secondary pattern, confers a markedly worse prognosis than grade 1–2. Accurate distinction between grade 3 and grade 4 carcinoma is consequently an important task. (Figs 6.67–6.79)

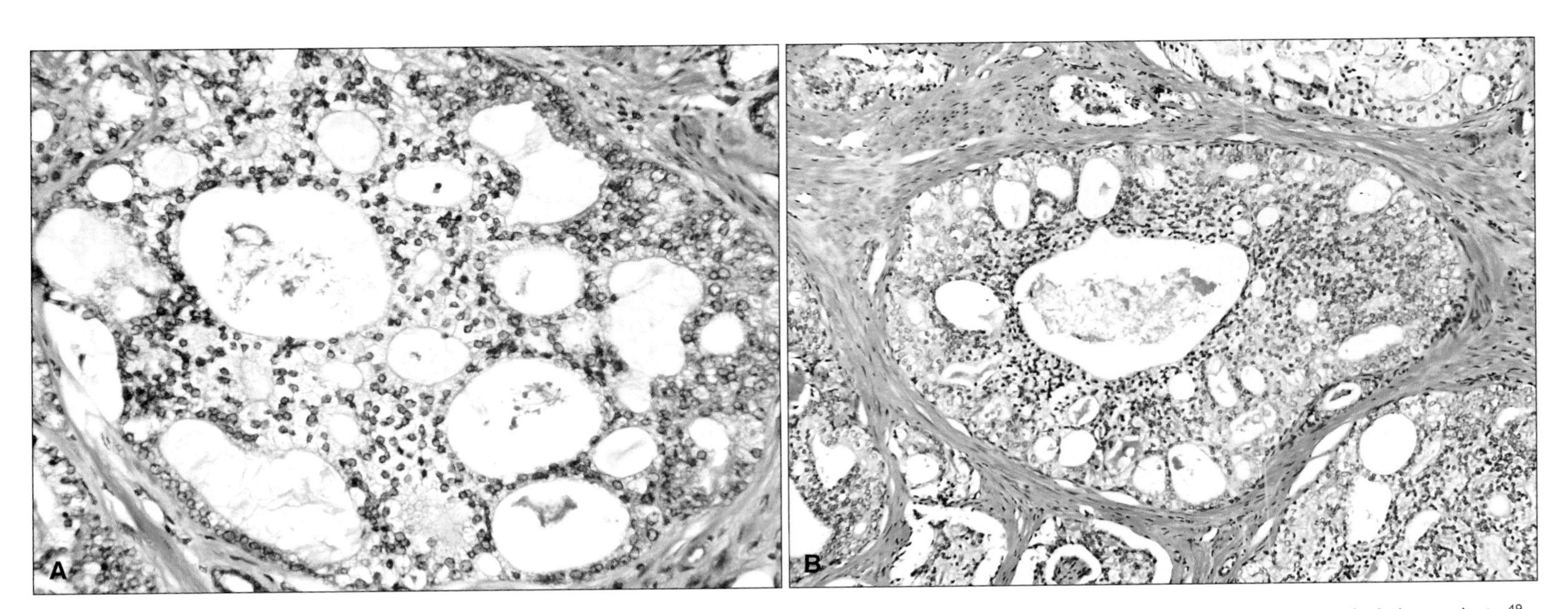

Fig. 6.66 (A,B) The cribriform–papillary type ('3C') must be distinguished from other cribriform proliferations, prostatic intraepithelial neoplasia,[49] grade 4 carcinoma, and benign mimics. When a small cribriform focus has fully patent, evenly spaced lumina, but basal cells are unreactive with cytokeratin 34βE12, then tumor can be interpreted as grade 3C carcinoma.[68]

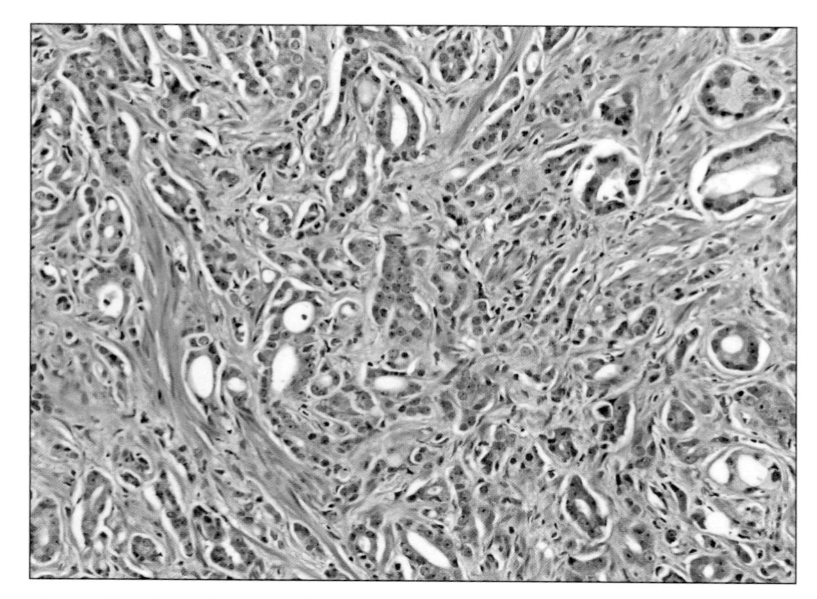

Fig. 6.67 The absence of any intervening stroma between adjacent glands, together with the absence of any clear 'edge' to the proliferation with respect to the adjacent prostate, defines grade 4. 'Fusion' is considered present even if found in a single dimension, i.e. train of glands.

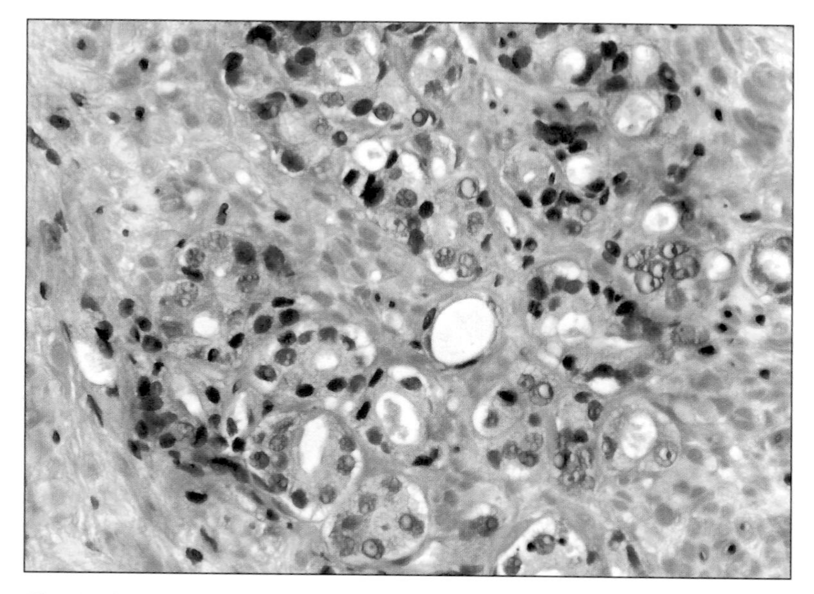

Fig. 6.68 In a small biopsy focus, it may be difficult to distinguish this minimal form of grade 4 carcinoma from a longitudinally sectioned focus of grade 3 carcinoma. If the focus is sufficiently large, irregular epithelial cross-bridges forming multiple distinct lumina and at least focal evidence of lateral budding and branching should be apparent.

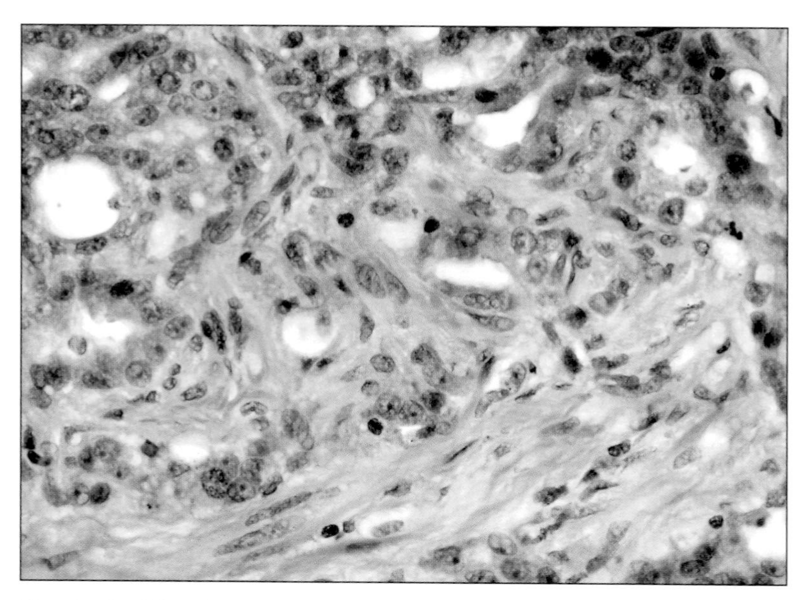

Fig. 6.69 'Glandular fusion' is easily perceived when it encompasses two dimensions, giving rise to irregular aggregations of malignant gland-like structures.

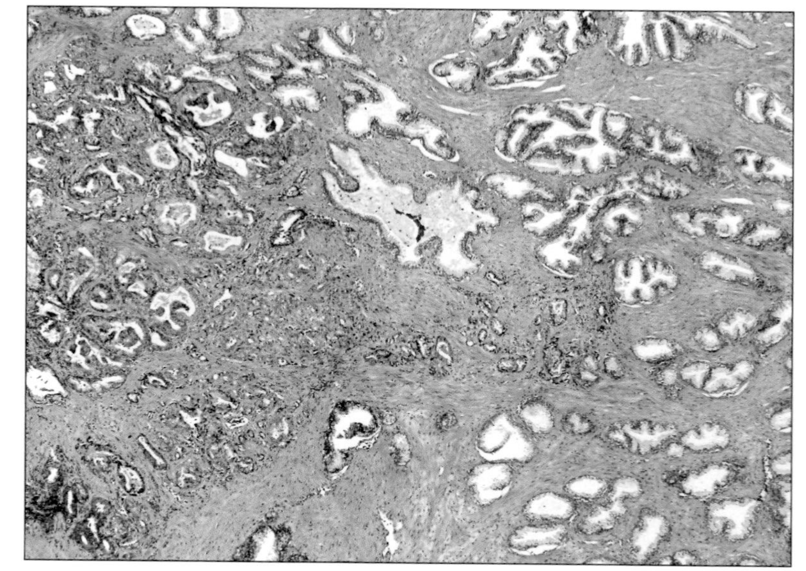

Fig. 6.70 The margins of these neoplastic aggregates are ill defined, stellate, or antler-like. The diagnosis of grade 4 should be avoided if it is possible to draw an imaginary boundary about the proliferation.[68]

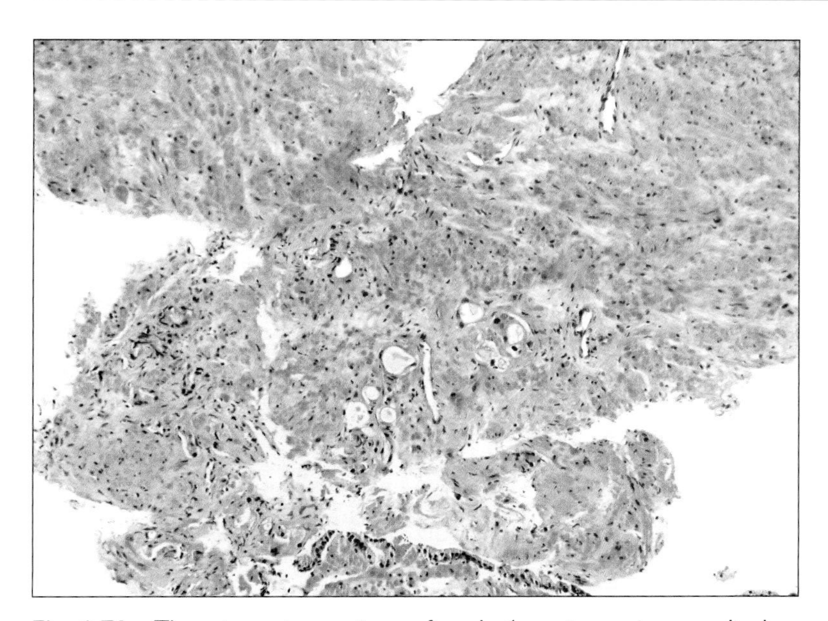

Fig. 6.71 The microacinar pattern of grade 4 carcinoma is exceedingly difficult to distinguish from grade 3 in tiny biopsy foci. In this form, balls of malignant cells with pinpoint to absent lumina raggedly infiltrate the stroma. When only a few such glands are present and the low-power pattern is not evident, such cases are often undergraded.

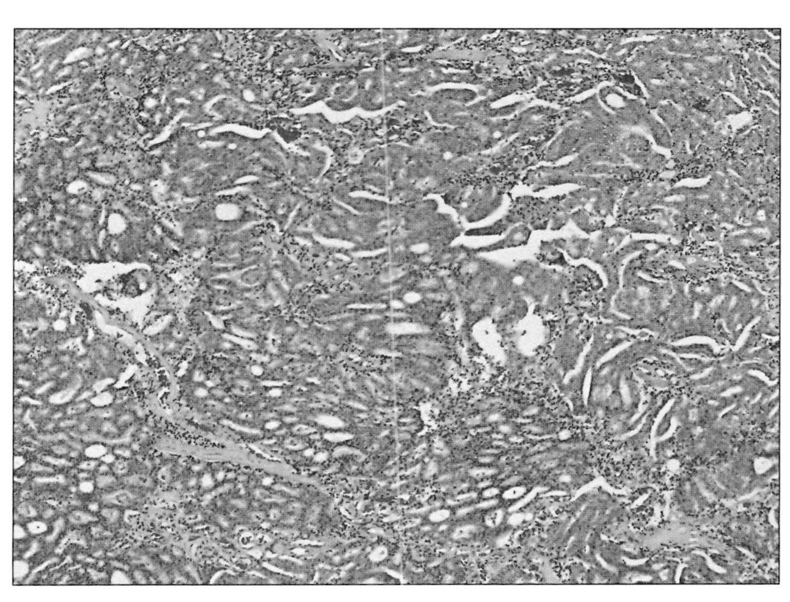

Fig. 6.73 'Endometrioid' or 'prostatic duct' carcinoma is a variant of Gleason 4 carcinoma characterized by extensive papillary or cribriform growth with tall columnar cytology. Most no longer consider this a distinct entity, but a morphologic variant seen focally or extensively in many high-grade cancers.[70]

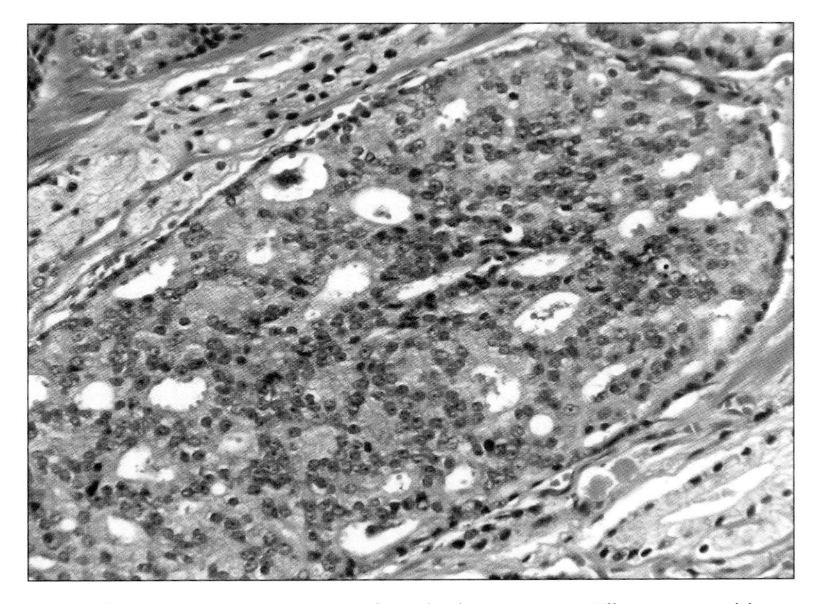

Fig. 6.72 Increasing expanses of grade 4 tumor are still punctuated by occasional persistent lumina in this cribriform focus.

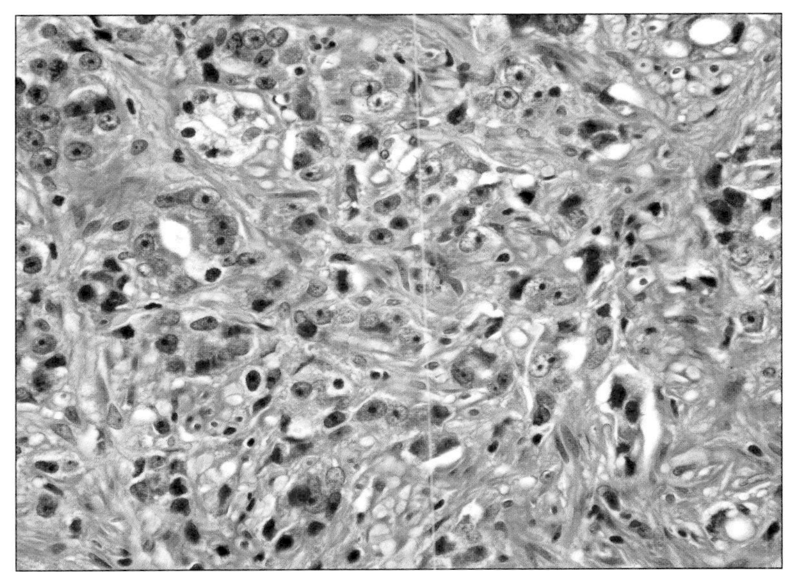

Fig. 6.74 The cytoplasm of grade 4 carcinoma is variable. Indeed, Gleason's two subtypes, ordinary ('4A') and 'hypernephroid' ('4B'), differ chiefly in cytology rather than architecture. Type 4A exhibits a glassy, amphiphilic cytoplasm resembling that of many grade 3 carcinomas. Common variations include cells with prominent, single vacuoles.

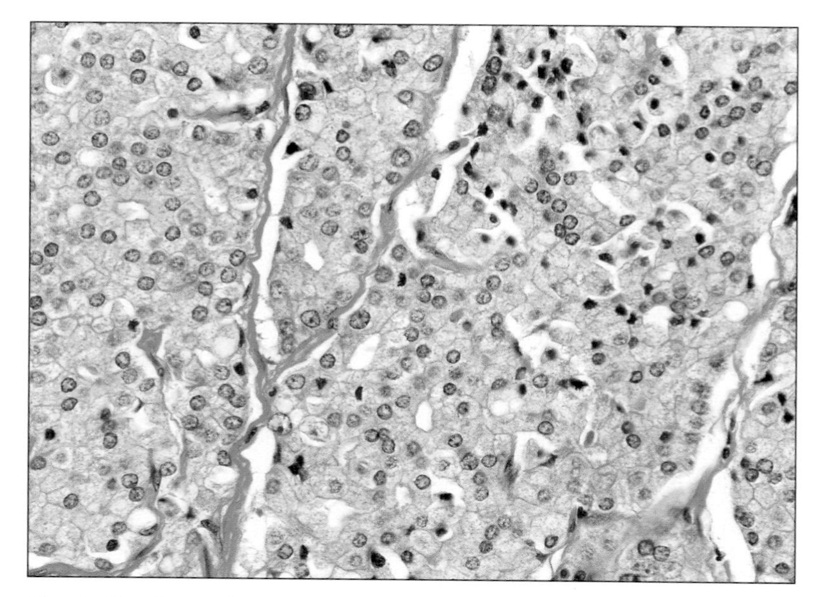

Fig. 6.75 Grade 4A 'hypernephroid' carcinoma exhibits clear cytoplasm and relatively inconspicuous nuclei, resembling renal cell carcinoma. It is rare in a pure form. More commonly it occurs in association with grade 4 carcinoma exhibiting more conventional cytology.

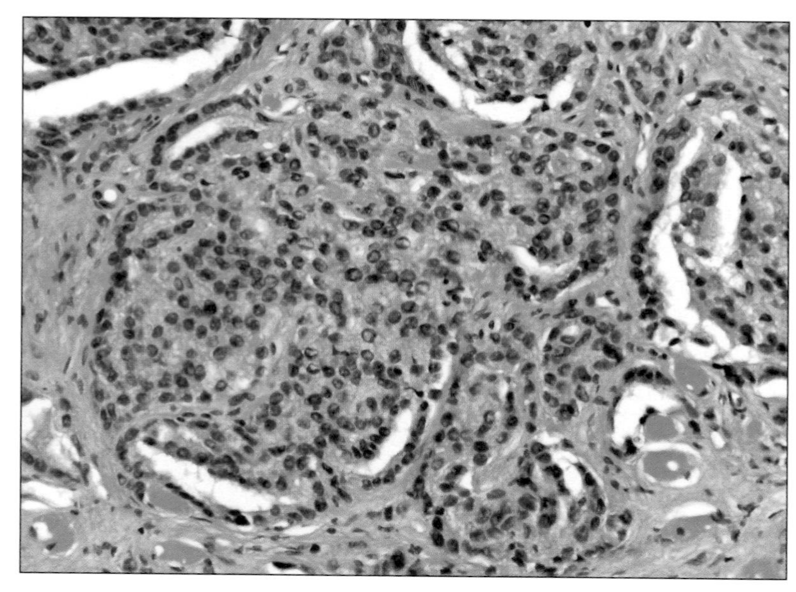

Fig. 6.76 Glomeruloid bodies are found in association with some grade 4 carcinomas.[71] These structures may be diagnostically helpful if encountered on small biopsies.

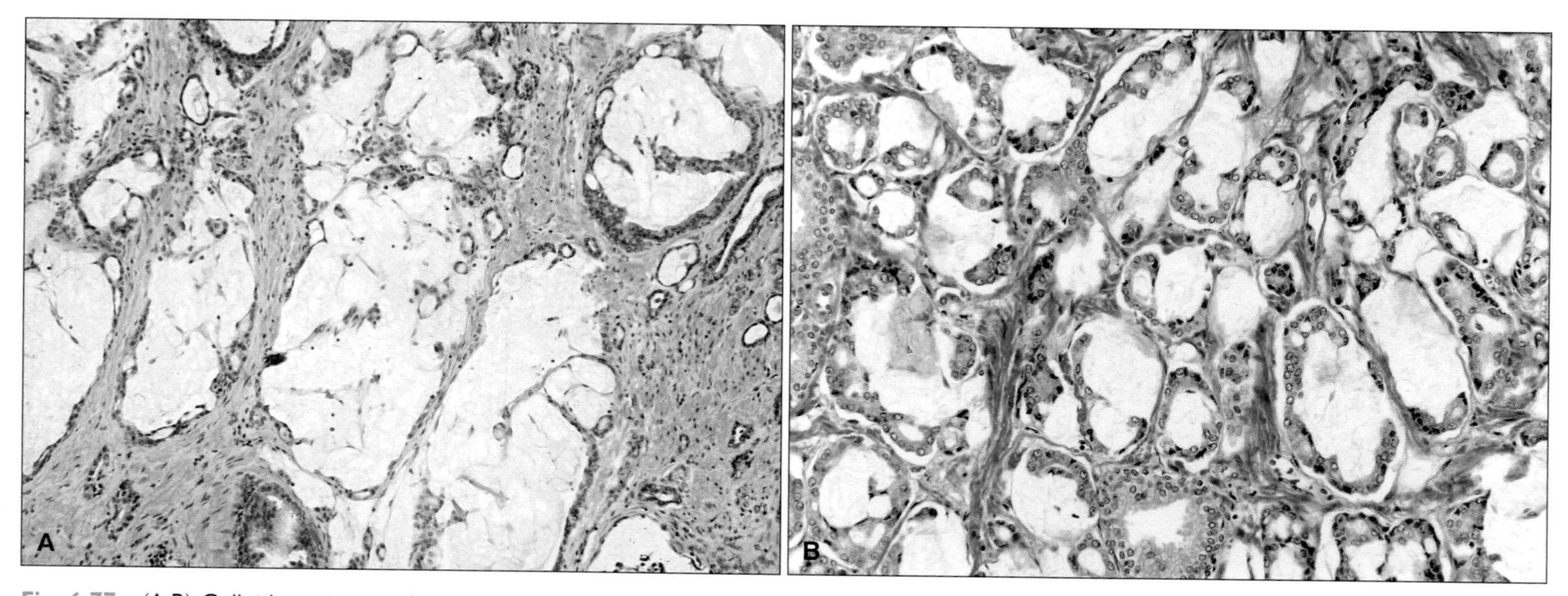

Fig. 6.77 (A,B) Colloid carcinoma of the prostate is a morphologic variant that should be assigned to grade 4.[72–74]

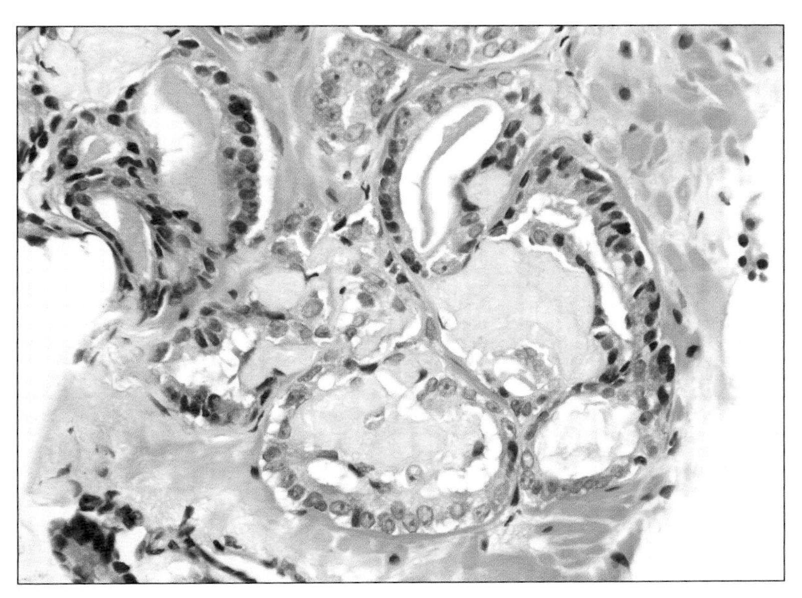

Fig. 6.78 Collagenous micronodules are seen most often in association with mucin-secreting adenocarcinomas.[75,76] They represent fibrous organization of the luminal secretions. Well-developed collagenous micronodules are sufficiently specific to be virtually diagnostic of carcinoma in a small sample.[77,78]

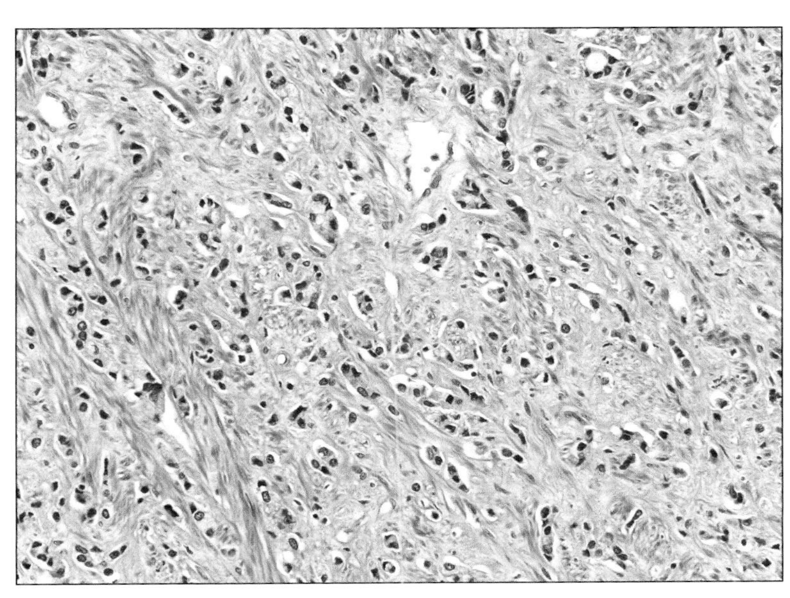

Fig. 6.80 Single cell infiltration is sometimes a focal feature of lower-grade cancers, but even a small focus may be prognostically significant.

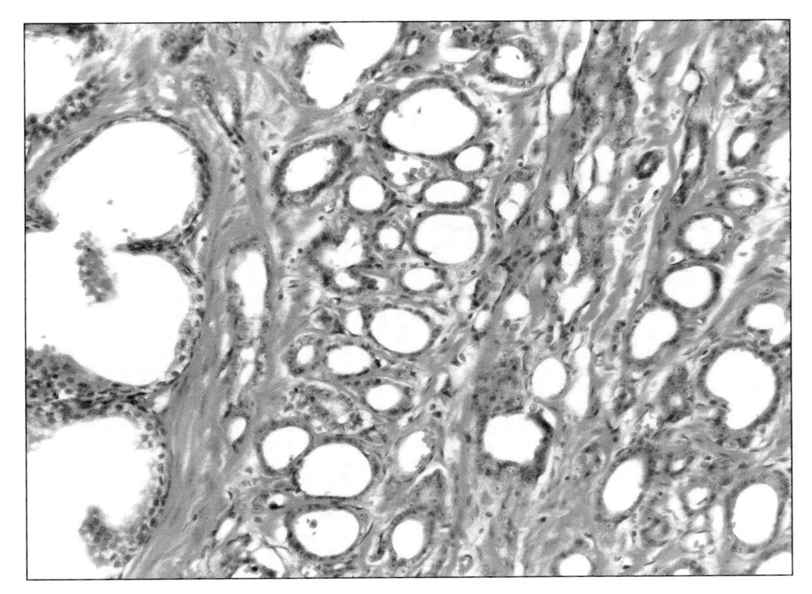

Fig. 6.79 Focal regions of carcinoma with atrophic features resembling hormonally treated carcinoma may frequently be seen in untreated acinar adenocarcinomas of various grades. This may present a diagnostic challenge on a small biopsy.[35] This focus in a prostatectomy for Gleason 3+4 adenocarcinoma shows focal atrophic carcinoma.

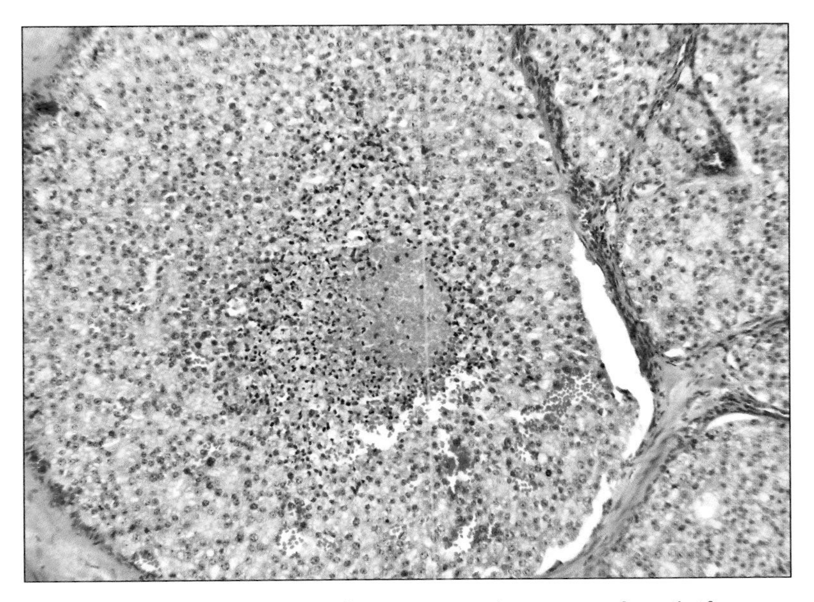

Fig. 6.81 Comedonecrosis often occurs at the center of a cribriform gland, but may occur on a background of a solid proliferation.

Gleason grade 5

Grade 5 carcinoma is defined by loss of glandular differentiation and/or spontaneous necrosis. Three patterns may be distinguished: solid masses, infiltrative single cells (both '5B'), and comedocarcinoma ('5A'). Grade 5 carcinoma has significantly worse prognostic implications than grade 4 carcinoma. A diagnostic comment should indicate the presence of Gleason 5 pattern if it is not the primary or secondary grade. Some experts advocate reporting the primary grade and the highest subsidiary grade. (Figs 6.80–6.83)

STROMAL NEOPLASMS

(Figs 6.84–6.86)

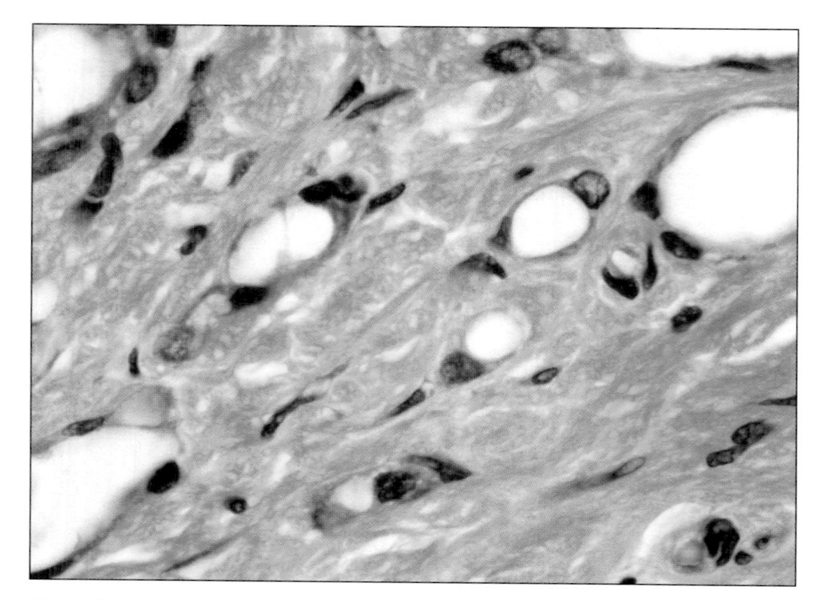

Fig. 6.82 Signet ring cell carcinoma can rarely occur as a pure type, but most often signet ring cell carcinoma areas are present as one component of more conventional acinar adenocarcinoma.[79,80] The signet ring vacuoles contain acidic mucin, stainable with Alcian blue. Signet ring cell carcinoma often has a grade 5 pattern, with single cell infiltration.

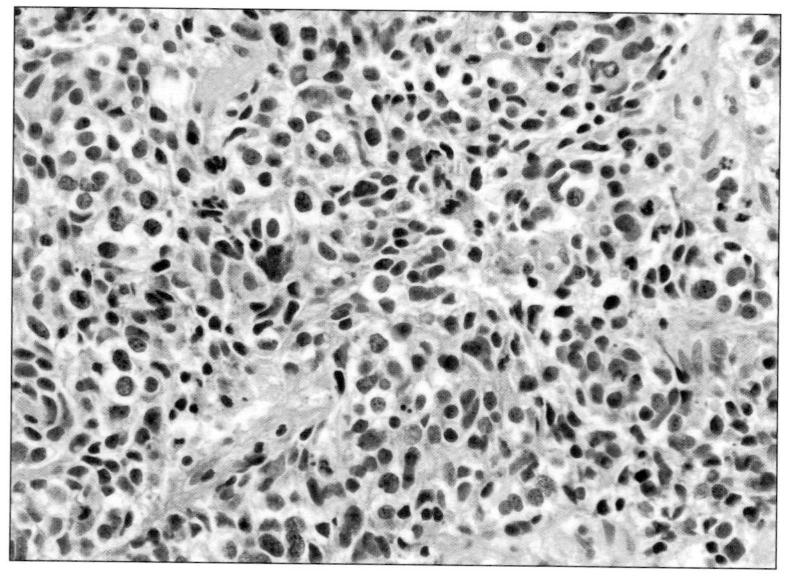

Fig. 6.83 Small cell carcinoma of the prostate is an unusually aggressive subtype that may supervene following androgen deprivation therapy.[81–83] The neuroendocrine phenotype is demonstrable using the usual immunohistochemical stains.

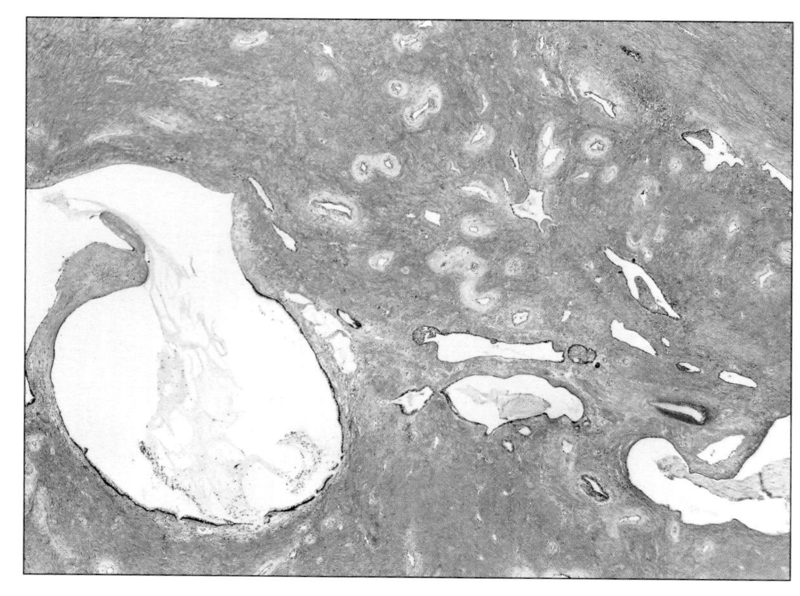

Fig. 6.84 Stromal neoplasia of the prostate often presents as a biphasic, phyllodes tumor-like neoplasm. Tumors can be graded, as in breast, into benign, of uncertain malignant potential, and malignant.[84,85]

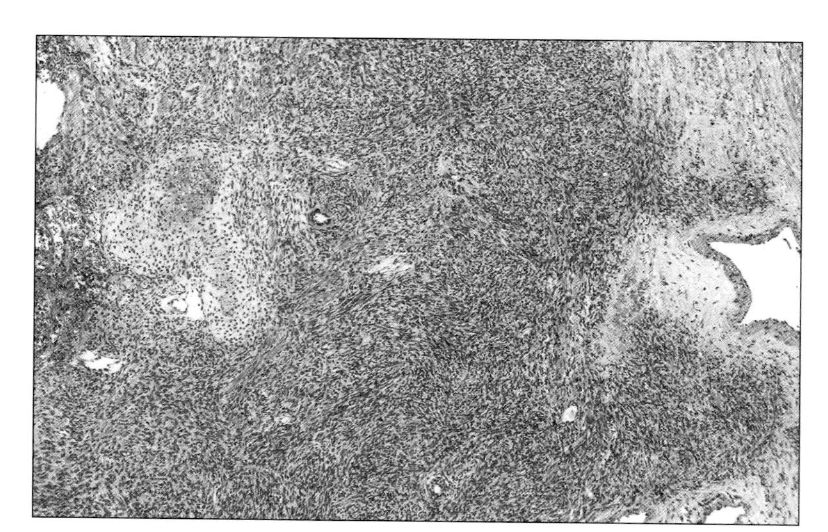

Fig. 6.85 Adult primary sarcomas of the prostate can exhibit a variety of types. Leiomyosarcomatous differentiation is the most common. Many other types have been reported, including chondrosarcoma,[86] synovial sarcoma,[87] osteosarcoma,[88] malignant fibrous histiocytoma,[89] and others.

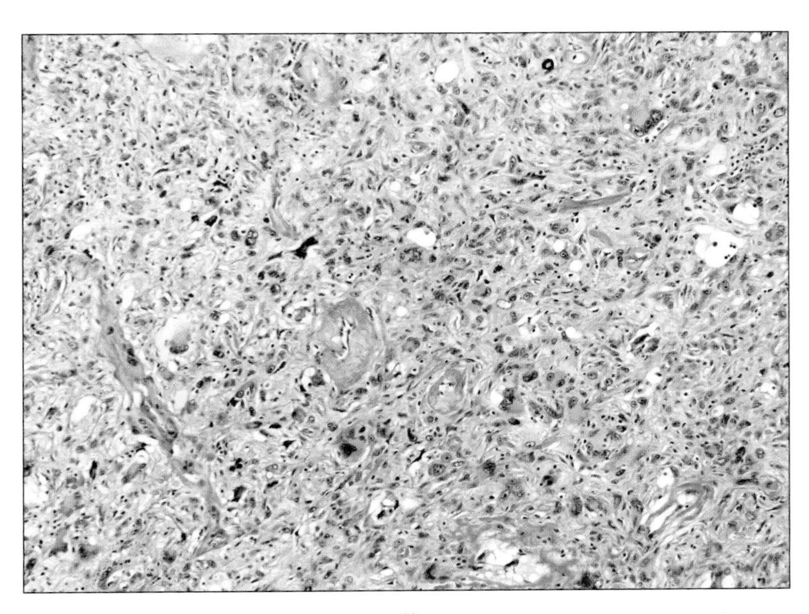

Fig. 6.86 Prostatic carcinosarcoma[90] is a highly aggressive tumor that may arise de novo or following radiation or hormonal therapy for conventional carcinoma. Tumor contains a high-grade adenocarcinoma component together with a sarcoma component that is also usually poorly differentiated. Osteosarcoma and leiomyosarcoma are the most frequent heterologous sarcoma types.

REFERENCES

1. McNeal JE. Prostate. In: Sternberg SS, ed. Histology for pathologists. 2nd edn. Philadelphia: Lippincott-Raven; 1997:997–1017.

1b. Wendell-Smith C. Terminology of the Prostate and Related Structures. Clin Anat 2000;13:207–213.

2. Lepor H, Gregerman M, Crosby R, et al. Precise localization of the autonomic nerves from the pelvic plexus to the corpora cavernosa: a detailed anatomical study of the adult male pelvis. J Urol 1985;133: 207–212.
3. Walsh PC, Lepor H, Eggleston JC. Radical prostatectomy with preservation of sexual function: anatomical and pathological considerations. Prostate 1983;4:473–485.
4. Egevad L. Cytology of the central zone of the prostate. Diagn Cytopathol 2003;28:239–244.
5. Srodon M, Epstein JI. Central zone histology of the prostate: a mimicker of high-grade prostatic intraepithelial neoplasia. Hum Pathol 2002;33: 518–523.
6. Reese JH, McNeal JE, Goldenberg SL, et al. Distribution of lactoferrin in the normal and inflamed human prostate: an immunohistochemical study. Prostate 1992;20:73–85.
7. Ayala AG, Srigley JR, Ro JY, et al. Clear cell cribriform hyperplasia of prostate. Report of 10 cases. Am J Surg Pathol 1986;10:665–671.
8. Gjengsto P, Halvorsen OJ, Akslen LA, et al. Benign growth of different prostate zones in aging men with slightly elevated PSA in whom prostate cancer has been excluded: a prospective study of 510 patients. Urology 2003;62:447–450.
9. Ayala AG, Ro JY, Babaian R, et al. The prostatic capsule: does it exist? Its importance in the staging and treatment of prostatic carcinoma. Am J Surg Pathol 1989;13:21–27.
10. Sattar AA, Noel JC, Vanderhaeghen JJ, et al. Prostate capsule: computerized morphometric analysis of its components. Urology 1995;46:178–181.
11. Di Lollo S, Menchi I, Brizzi E, et al. The morphology of the prostatic capsule with particular regard to the posterosuperior region: an anatomical and clinical problem. Surg Radiol Anat 1997;19:143–147.
12. Sakamoto N, Hasegawa Y, Koga H, et al. Presence of ganglia within the prostatic capsule: ganglion involvement in prostatic cancer. Prostate 1999; 40:167–171.
13. Cohen RJ, McNeal JE, Edgar SG, et al. Characterization of cytoplasmic secretory granules (PSG), in prostatic epithelium and their transformation-induced loss in dysplasia and adenocarcinoma. Hum Pathol 1998;29: 1488–1494.
14. Amin MB, Bostwick DG. Pigment in prostatic epithelium and adenocarcinoma: a potential source of diagnostic confusion with seminal vesicular epithelium. Mod Pathol 1996;9:791–795.
15. Adlakha H, Bostwick DG. Paneth cell-like change in prostatic adenocarcinoma represents neuroendocrine differentiation: report of 30 cases. Hum Pathol 1994;25:135–139.
16. Cina SJ, Silberman MA, Kahane H, et al. Diagnosis of Cowper's glands on prostate needle biopsy. Am J Surg Pathol 1997;21:550–555.
17. Gagucas RJ, Brown RW, Wheeler TM. Verumontanum mucosal gland hyperplasia. Am J Surg Pathol 1995;19:30–36.
18. Gaudin PB, Wheeler TM, Epstein JI. Verumontanum mucosal gland hyperplasia in prostatic needle biopsy specimens. A mimic of low grade prostatic adenocarcinoma. Am J Clin Pathol 1995;104:620–626.
19. Muezzinoglu B, Erdamar S, Chakraborty S, et al. Verumontanum mucosal gland hyperplasia is associated with atypical adenomatous hyperplasia of the prostate. Arch Pathol Lab Med 2001;125:358–360.
20. Wernert N, Kern L, Heitz P, et al. Morphological and immunohistochemical investigations of the utriculus prostaticus from the fetal period up to adulthood. Prostate 1990;17:19–30.
21. Meirelles LR, Billis A, Cotta AC, et al. Prostatic atrophy: evidence for a possible role of local ischemia in its pathogenesis. Int Urol Nephrol 2002; 34:345–350.
22. Milord RA, Kahane H, Epstein JI. Infarct of the prostate gland: experience on needle biopsy specimens. Am J Surg Pathol 2000;24:1378–1384.
23. Bostwick DG, Egbert BM, Fajardo LF. Radiation injury of the normal and neoplastic prostate. Am J Surg Pathol 1982;6:541–551.
24. Das DK, Hedlund PO, Lowhagen T, et al. Squamous metaplasia in hormonally treated prostatic cancer. Significance during follow-up. Urology 1991;38:70–75.
25. Lager DJ, Goeken JA, Kemp JD, et al. Squamous metaplasia of the prostate. An immunohistochemical study. Am J Clin Pathol 1988;90: 597–601.
26. Gal R, Koren R, Nofech-Mozes S, et al. Evaluation of mucinous metaplasia of the prostate gland by mucin histochemistry. Br J Urol 1996;77: 113–117.
27. Grignon DJ, O'Malley FP. Mucinous metaplasia in the prostate gland. Am J Surg Pathol 1993;17:287–290.
28. Grignon DJ, Ro JY, Srigley JR, et al. Sclerosing adenosis of the prostate gland. A lesion showing myoepithelial differentiation. Am J Surg Pathol 1992;16:383–391.
29. Jones EC, Clement PB, Young RH. Sclerosing adenosis of the prostate gland. A clinicopathological and immunohistochemical study of 11 cases. Am J Surg Pathol 1991;15:1171–1180.
30. Luque RJ, Lopez-Beltran A, Perez-Seoane C, et al. Sclerosing adenosis of the prostate. Histologic features in needle biopsy specimens. Arch Pathol Lab Med 2003;127:e14–e16.
31. McNeal JE. Anatomy of the prostate and morphogenesis of BPH. Prog Clin Biol Res 1984;145:27–53.
32. Benz M, Giefer T, Bierhoff E, et al. Morphologische Klassifikation und Vergleich der unterschiedlichen Stromaknotentypen in der hyperplastischen Prostata. Verh Dtsch Ges Pathol 1993;77:111–116.
33. Cheng L, Cheville JC, Bostwick DG. Diagnosis of prostate cancer in needle biopsies after radiation therapy. Am J Surg Pathol 1999;23: 1173–1183.
34. Bostwick DG, Ramnani D, Cheng L. Treatment changes in prostatic hyperplasia and cancer, including androgen deprivation therapy and radiotherapy. Urol Clin North Am 1999;26:465–479.
35. Kaleem Z, Swanson PE, Vollmer RT, et al. Prostatic adenocarcinoma with atrophic features: a study of 202 consecutive completely embedded radical prostatectomy specimens. Am J Clin Pathol 1998;109:695–703.
36. Thorson P, Swanson PE, Vollmer RT, et al. Basal cell hyperplasia in the peripheral zone of the prostate. Mod Pathol 2003;16:598–606.
37. Rioux-Leclercq NC, Epstein JI. Unusual morphologic patterns of basal cell hyperplasia of the prostate. Am J Surg Pathol 2002;26:237–243.
38. Luna-More S, Florez P, Ayala A, et al. Neutral and acid mucins and eosinophil and argyrophil crystalloids in carcinoma and atypical adenomatous hyperplasia of the prostate. Pathol Res Pract 1997;193: 291–298.
39. Cheville JC, Bostwick DG. Postatrophic hyperplasia of the prostate. A histologic mimic of prostatic adenocarcinoma. Am J Surg Pathol 1995;19: 1068–1076.
40. Ruska KM, Sauvageot J, Epstein JI. Histology and cellular kinetics of prostatic atrophy. Am J Surg Pathol 1998;22:1073–1077.

41. Shah R, Mucci NR, Amin A, et al. Postatrophic hyperplasia of the prostate gland: neoplastic precursor or innocent bystander? Am J Pathol 2001;158: 1767–1773.
42. Anton RC, Kattan MW, Chakraborty S, et al. Postatrophic hyperplasia of the prostate: lack of association with prostate cancer. Am J Surg Pathol 1999;23:932–936.
43. Franks LM. Atrophy and hyperplasia in the prostate proper. J Pathol Bacteriol 1954;68:617–621.
44. McNeal JE. Morphogenesis of prostate carcinoma. Cancer 1965;18: 1659–1666.
45. Helpap B, Bonkhoff H, Cockett A, et al. Relationship between atypical adenomatous hyperplasia (AAH), prostatic intraepithelial neoplasia (PIN) and prostatic adenocarcinoma. Pathologica 1997;89:288–300.
46. Bostwick DG. Prostatic intraepithelial neoplasia is a risk factor for cancer. Semin Urol Oncol 1999;17:187–198.
47. Bostwick DG, Sakr W. Prostatic intraepithelial neoplasia. In: Foster CS, Bostwick DG, eds. Pathology of the prostate. Philadelphia: WB Saunders; 1998:95–113.
48. Sakr WA, Partin AW. Histological markers of risk and the role of high-grade prostatic intraepithelial neoplasia. Urology 2001;57(4 Suppl 1): 115–120.
49. Amin MB, Schultz DS, Zarbo RJ. Analysis of cribriform morphology in prostatic neoplasia using antibody to high-molecular-weight cytokeratins. Arch Pathol Lab Med 1994;118:260–264.
50. Frauenhoffer EE, Ro JY, el-Naggar AK, et al. Clear cell cribriform hyperplasia of the prostate. Immunohistochemical and DNA flow cytometric study. Am J Clin Pathol 1991;95:446–453.
51. Kronz JD, Shaikh AA, Epstein JI. Atypical cribriform lesions on prostate biopsy. Am J Surg Pathol 2001;25:147–155.
52. McNeal JE, Reese JH, Redwine EA, et al. Cribriform adenocarcinoma of the prostate. Cancer 1986;58:1714–1719.
53. Kronz JD, Shaikh AA, Epstein JI. High-grade prostatic intraepithelial neoplasia with adjacent small atypical glands on prostate biopsy. Hum Pathol 2001;32:389–395.
54. Gleason DF. Classification of prostate carcinoma. Cancer Chemother Rep 1966;50:125–128.
55. Allsbrook WC Jr, Mangold KA, Johnson MH, et al. Interobserver reproducibility of Gleason grading of prostatic carcinoma: urologic pathologists. Hum Pathol 2001;32:74–80.
56. Allsbrook WC Jr, Mangold KA, Johnson MH, et al. Interobserver reproducibility of Gleason grading of prostatic carcinoma: general pathologist. Hum Pathol 2001;32:81–88.
57. Epstein JI. Gleason score 2-4 adenocarcinoma of the prostate on needle biopsy: a diagnosis that should not be made. Am J Surg Pathol 2000;24: 477–478.
58. McNeal JE, Cohen RJ, Brooks JD. Role of cytologic criteria in the histologic diagnosis of Gleason grade 1 prostatic adenocarcinoma. Hum Pathol 2001; 32:441–446.
59. Noguchi M, Stamey TA, Neal JE, et al. An analysis of 148 consecutive transition zone cancers: clinical and histological characteristics. J Urol 2000;163:1751–1755.
60. Levi AW, Epstein JI. Pseudohyperplastic prostatic adenocarcinoma on needle biopsy and simple prostatectomy. Am J Surg Pathol 2000;24: 1039–1046.
61. Anton RC, Chakraborty S, Wheeler TM. The significance of intraluminal prostatic crystalloids in benign needle biopsies. Am J Surg Pathol 1998;22: 446–449.
62. Henneberry JM, Kahane H, Humphrey PA, et al. The significance of intraluminal crystalloids in benign prostatic glands on needle biopsy. Am J Surg Pathol 1997;21:725–728.
63. Nelson RS, Epstein JI. Prostatic carcinoma with abundant xanthomatous cytoplasm. Foamy gland carcinoma. Am J Surg Pathol 1996;20:419–426.
64. Tran TT, Sengupta E, Yang XJ. Prostatic foamy gland carcinoma with aggressive behavior: clinicopathologic, immunohistochemical, and ultrastructural analysis. Am J Surg Pathol 2001;25:618–623.
65. Cohen RJ, McNeal JE, Baillie T. Patterns of differentiation and proliferation in intraductal carcinoma of the prostate: significance for cancer progression. Prostate 2000;43:11–19.
66. Dawkins HJ, Sellner LN, Turbett GR, et al. Distinction between intraductal carcinoma of the prostate (IDC-P), high-grade dysplasia (PIN), and invasive prostatic adenocarcinoma, using molecular markers of cancer progression. Prostate 2000;44:265–270.
67. Rubin MA, de La Taille A, Bagiella E, et al. Cribriform carcinoma of the prostate and cribriform prostatic intraepithelial neoplasia: incidence and clinical implications. Am J Surg Pathol 1998;22:840–848.
68. Young RH, Srigley JR, Amin MB, et al. Tumors of the prostate gland, seminal vesicles, male urethra, and penis. Third Series. Washington, DC: Armed Forces Institute of Pathology; 2000.
69. Boag AH, Kennedy LA, Miller MJ. Three-dimensional microscopic image reconstruction of prostatic adenocarcinoma. Arch Pathol Lab Med 2001;125: 562–566.
70. Bock BJ, Bostwick DG. Does prostatic ductal adenocarcinoma exist? Am J Surg Pathol 1999;23:781–785.
71. Pacelli A, Lopez-Beltran A, Egan AJ, et al. Prostatic adenocarcinoma with glomeruloid features. Hum Pathol 1998;29:543–546.
72. Lopez JI, Laforga JB. Mucinous (colloid) adenocarcinoma of the prostate. Br J Urol 1995;76:805–806.
73. Randolph TL, Amin MB, Ro JY, et al. Histologic variants of adenocarcinoma and other carcinomas of prostate: pathologic criteria and clinical significance. Mod Pathol 1997;10:612–629.
74. Saito S, Iwaki H. Mucin-producing carcinoma of the prostate: review of 88 cases. Urology 1999;54:141–144.
75. Arangelovich V, Tretiakova M, SenGupta E, et al. Pathogenesis and significance of collagenous micronodules of the prostate. Appl Immunohistochem Mol Morphol 2003;11:15–19.
76. Bostwick DG, Wollan P, Adlakha K. Collagenous micronodules in prostate cancer. A specific but infrequent diagnostic finding. Arch Pathol Lab Med 1995;119:444–447.
77. Epstein JI. Diagnosis and reporting of limited adenocarcinoma of the prostate on needle biopsy. Mod Pathol 2004;17:307–315.
78. Thorson P, Vollmer RT, Arcangeli C, et al. Minimal carcinoma in prostate needle biopsy specimens: diagnostic features and radical prostatectomy follow-up. Mod Pathol 1998;11:543–551.
79. Fujita K, Sugao H, Gotoh T, et al. Primary signet ring cell carcinoma of the prostate: report and review of 42 cases. Int J Urol 2004;11: 178–181.
80. Torbenson M, Dhir R, Nangia A, et al. Prostatic carcinoma with signet ring cells: a clinicopathologic and immunohistochemical analysis of 12 cases, with review of the literature. Mod Pathol 1998;11:552–559.
81. Abrahamsson PA. Neuroendocrine differentiation in prostatic carcinoma. Prostate 1999;39:135–148.
82. Bostwick DG, Grignon DJ, Hammond ME, et al. Prognostic factors in prostate cancer. College of American Pathologists Consensus Statement 1999. Arch Path Lab Med 2000;124:995–1000.
83. Helpap B, Kollermann J. Undifferentiated carcinoma of the prostate with small cell features: immunohistochemical subtyping and reflections on histogenesis. Virchows Arch 1999;434:385–391.
84. Bostwick DG, Hossain D, Qian J, et al. Phyllodes tumor of the prostate: long-term followup study of 23 cases. J Urol 2004;172:894–899.
85. Gaudin PB, Rosai J, Epstein JI. Sarcomas and related proliferative lesions of specialized prostatic stroma: a clinicopathologic study of 22 cases. Am J Surg Pathol 1998;22:148–162.
86. Dogra PN, Aron M, Rajeev TP, et al. Primary chondrosarcoma of the prostate. BJU Int 1999;83:150–151.
87. Iwasaki H, Ishiguro M, Ohjimi Y, et al. Synovial sarcoma of the prostate with t(X;18)(p11.2;q11.2). Am J Surg Pathol 1999;23:220–226.
88. Nishiyama T, Ikarashi T, Terunuma M, et al. Osteogenic sarcoma of the prostate. Int J Urol 2001;8:199–201.
89. Miro AG, De Seta L, Lizza N, et al. Malignant fibrous histiocytoma after radiation therapy for prostate cancer: case report. J Chemother 1997;9: 162.
90. Dundore PA, Cheville JC, Nascimento AG, et al. Carcinosarcoma of the prostate. Report of 21 cases. Cancer 1995;76:1035–1042.

7

FINE-NEEDLE ASPIRATION OF KIDNEY TUMORS

Ruth L. Katz

INTRODUCTION

Fine-needle aspiration (FNA) of kidney masses is performed mainly for the pathologic identification of mass lesions, non-surgical confirmation of advanced neoplasia, confirmation of metastases, staging of tumors, and, in some cases, therapeutic aspiration of cystic lesions.[1] However, in the majority of patients with discrete renal lesions, the decision to perform a nephrectomy is based on radiographic features, precluding the use of FNA.[2]

Specific situations in which renal FNA is of particular clinical value include radiologically indeterminate, small, cystic lesions, and cases in which partial nephrectomy is preferable to radical nephrectomy.[2,3] The latter group includes patients with tuberous sclerosis, patients with unilateral or bilateral benign tumors such as oncocytomas, patients who have already received a contralateral nephrectomy, and patients who may not be able to tolerate loss of renal function. Aspiration is also useful to obtain tissue for ancillary studies, such as cytogenetic or molecular studies.

In patients with irresectable renal neoplasms or with metastases, FNA is the method of choice to confirm tumor type and allow for institution of non-surgical therapy.

TECHNIQUE

Accuracy of FNA of kidney in diagnosing tumors is high, ranging from 73% to 94%.[2] However, there are several challenges in diagnosis: identifying well-differentiated renal cell carcinomas (RCC); differentiating between oncocytoma and chromophobe RCC; and differentiating between high-grade papillary RCC, urothelial carcinoma, and collecting duct carcinomas. Another potential problem is the necrotic, hemorrhagic, or cystic tumor, which provoke a false-negative diagnosis.

Rare complications of kidney FNA include perirenal hemorrhage, pneumothorax, infection, arteriovenous fistula, and urinoma. Fatalities are very rare, as is needle-tract seeding.[4,5]

Ultrasound guidance is commonly used. This method permits the point of entry, angle of incidence, and depth to be defined in absolute terms. Computed tomography localizes smaller lesions, but lacks speed and scanning flexibility. It is used when ultrasound guidance is difficult, as in the morbidly obese.

CYTOLOGY OF THE NORMAL KIDNEY

(Figs 7.1–7.3)

RENAL CYSTS

Of renal mass lesions, 70–80% are cysts.[2] Most are benign, acquired, and solitary. Most solitary simple cysts are clinically insignificant and are discovered during radiologic studies performed for unrelated reasons. It is controversial

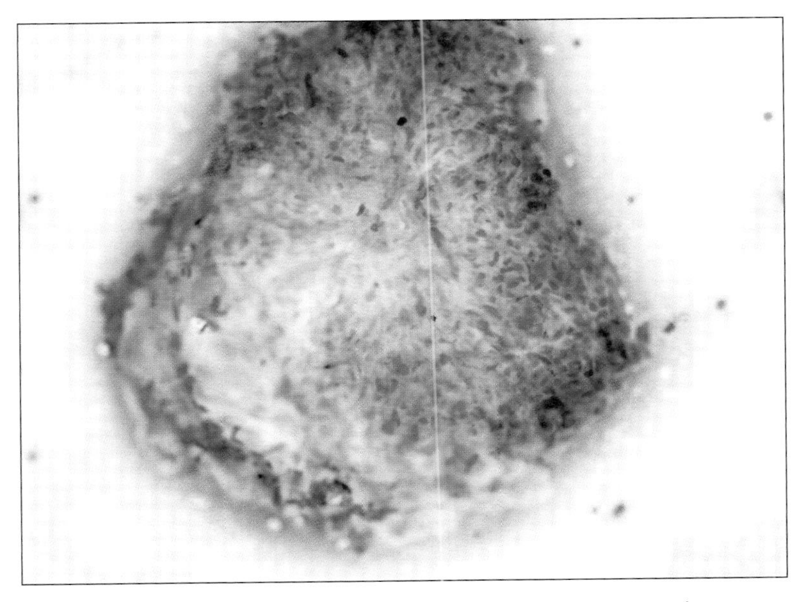

Fig. 7.1 Normal glomeruli appear as large, sharply demarcated, multilayered clusters of epithelial and endothelial cells with a knobby profile. They may be continuous with a short segment of the proximal convoluted tubule. They are distinguished from papillary carcinoma by the presence of two different cell types (endothelial and epithelial) and the absence of atypia and fibrovascular cores.

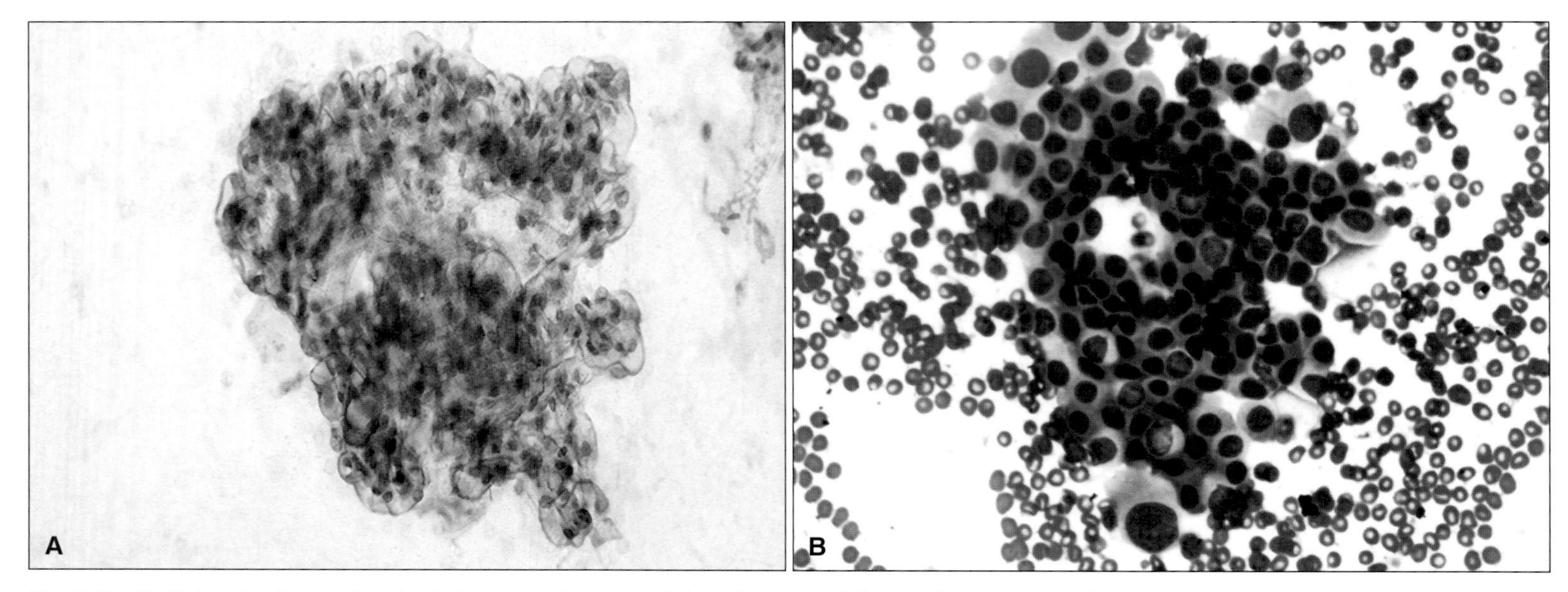

Fig. 7.2 (A,B) Proximal convoluted tubules comprise most of the substance of the renal cortex. Abundant pink granular cytoplasm, resembling oncocytoma, is present. Unlike oncocytoma, cytoplasm is ill defined, with granules spilling out. The nuclear:cytoplasmic ratio is low. Proximal tubular epithelium may also be mistaken for a low-grade, clear cell, renal cell carcinoma (RCC). However, clear cell RCC contains cells with vacuolated clear cytoplasm, unlike proximal tubular epithelium. Both entities, however, may contain cells with nuclei that display small nucleoli.

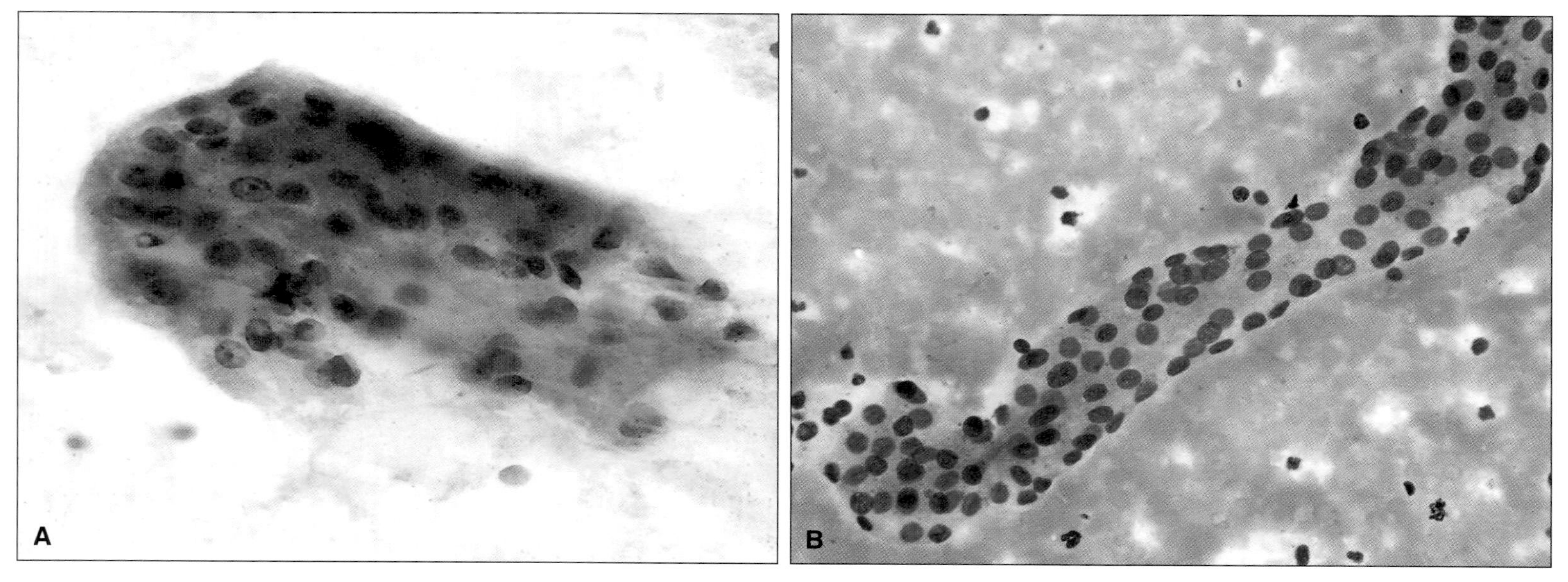

Fig. 7.3 (A,B) Distal convoluted tubules may appear multilayered. Epithelial cells are small and flatter than proximal tubular cells. Nuclei are conspicuous.

whether to perform FNA on simple cysts. While some believe that all simple cysts should be aspirated, some aspirate cysts only if they are radiologically classified as indeterminate or suspicious for malignancy. Only 1–7% of cysts are cystic RCC.

When cysts are multiple, the differential diagnosis is different. Long-term dialysis or transplantation can lead to development of multiple cysts that have a 9% chance of developing RCC. Adult (autosomal dominant) polycystic disease of the kidney leads to development of multiple cysts, and, owing to variable penetrance, age at presentation varies widely. Cytology shows clear, pale amber fluid containing a few foamy macrophages. (Fig. 7.4)

Bloody aspirates occasionally occur in benign cysts, but the presence of blood should suggest possible malignancy. Hemorrhagic cysts very rarely contain Liesegang rings, which are spherical, double-walled structures with radial striations, ranging from 8 to 200 μm. These structures may resemble parasitic ova such as *Dioctophyme renale*, but are cytokeratin negative, unlike the parasite.

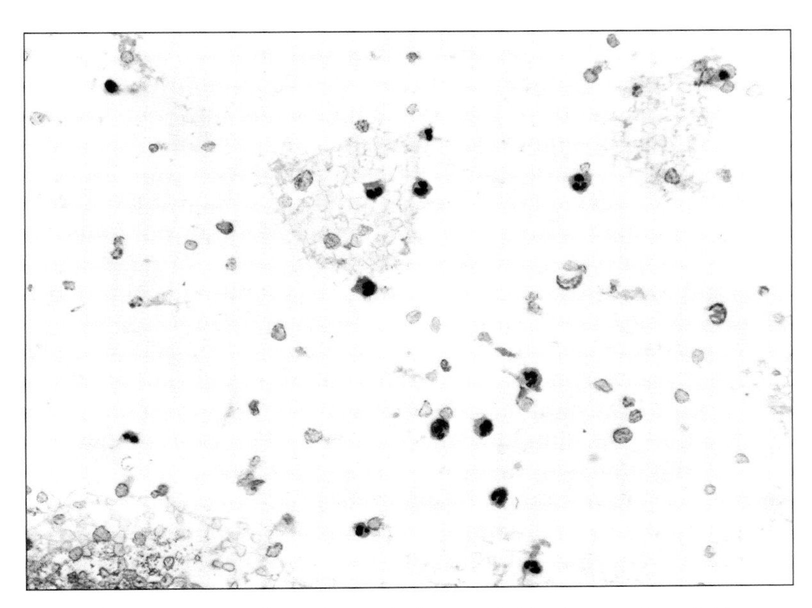

Fig. 7.4 Aspiration of simple cortical cysts yields clear, amber fluid. Benign cyst fluid is sparsely cellular, with a few macrophages and rare epithelial lining cells. There is no atypia. Fragments of degenerated epithelial cells should not be mistaken for carcinoma.

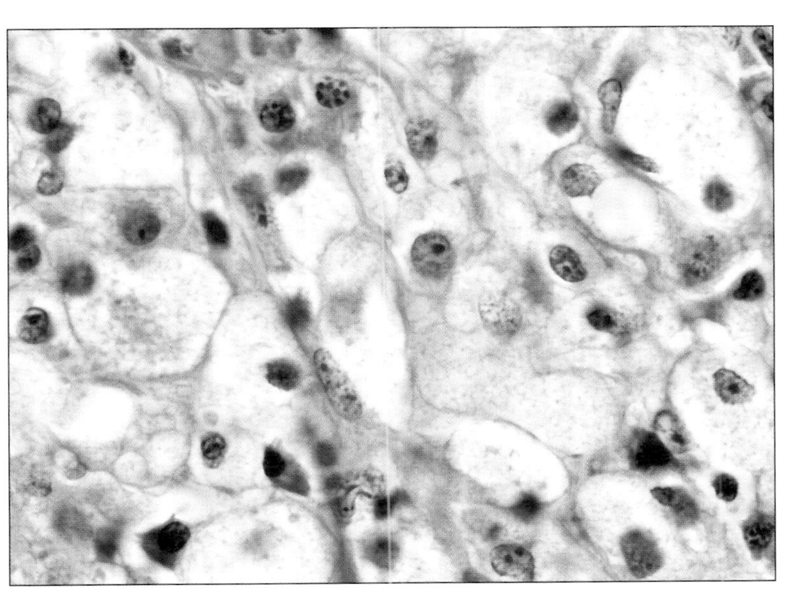

Fig. 7.5 Specimens of xanthogranulomatous pyelonephritis show proliferation of histiocytes with a lymphocytic infiltrate, and areas of necrosis. Degenerated histiocytes should not be confused with renal cell carcinoma. Histiocytes are CD68-positive and CD10-negative.

INFLAMMATORY CONDITIONS

XANTHOGRANULOMATOUS PYELONEPHRITIS

Xanthogranulomatous pyelonephritis is a chronic inflammatory disease of the kidney associated with recurrent urinary tract infections, flank pain, renal mass, or renal calculus. The most common causative organisms are *Escherichia coli*, and *Pseudomonas* and *Proteus* species. Because it sometimes presents as a localized mass, RCC may be in the differential diagnosis. (Fig. 7.5)

RENAL ABSCESS AND INFARCT

Abscess aspirates are cloudy, and white to yellow. Cytology shows acute inflammatory cells. Gram stain of the smear and bacteriologic cultures confirm the diagnosis. Gram-negative organisms are the most common cause. Percutaneous drainage, in conjunction with antibiotic therapy, is both diagnostic and therapeutic.

Renal infarcts are usually due to emboli. Radiographically, they present as wedge-shaped lesions with the apex toward the medulla and the base toward the surface of the kidney. Aspiration of renal infarcts discloses necrotic glomeruli and tubules. Regenerating tubular cells with atypia, occasional cytoplasmic vacuolization, prominent nucleoli, and pleomorphism may lead to a mistaken impression of malignancy.[6]

RENAL EPITHELIAL NEOPLASMS

BENIGN RENAL NEOPLASMS

Renal cortical (papillary) adenoma

Small papillary renal cell tumors occur commonly, and rarely become malignant. In the recent consensus classification, papillary renal cell neoplasms <0.5 cm in diameter and lacking infiltration into the surrounding parenchyma, whether or not encapsulated, are considered renal adenoma.[7]

Metanephric adenomas are unusual tumors that may arise from renal tubular epithelium. Tumors with a cellular stromal component are termed metanephric adenofibroma. Most are small, but size ranges up to 15 cm. Occasionally lymph node metastases have been reported.[2] Metanephric adenoma is composed of aggregates of small tubules and glomeruloid papillae. Cells lack anaplasia. Foci of necrosis may be present.

Oncocytoma

Oncocytoma is a benign renal cortical neoplasm thought to derive from the mitochondria-rich principal cells of the collecting duct. It accounts for 5% of all renal neoplasms, is more frequent in males, and has a peak incidence in the sixth to eighth decade of life. Radiographically, oncocytoma is a well-demarcated, encapsulated tumor, with a characteristic central scar.

Differential diagnostic considerations on FNA include granular RCC, chromophobe RCC, renal cortical cells, and hepatocytes. Special stains may be of assistance in the distinction of oncocytoma from cytologically similar tumors. Unlike conventional RCC, oncocytoma is pancytokeratin positive, vimentin negative, and CD10 negative. Hale's colloidal iron can show apical positivity in oncocytoma, complicating distinction from chromophobe RCC.[8] Cytoplasmic CD3 may be a good marker for oncocytoma.[9] (Figs 7.6 & 7.7)

Angiomyolipoma

Angiomyolipoma is a neoplasm composed of smooth muscle, adipose tissue, and vessels. About 20% of cases are associated with the tuberous sclerosis complex. It may be large and appear destructive on radiographs; because of its high vascularity, it may be confused with RCC on angiography.

Staining for HMB-45, with no staining for CD10, is diagnostic for angiomyolipoma. (Figs 7.8 & 7.9)

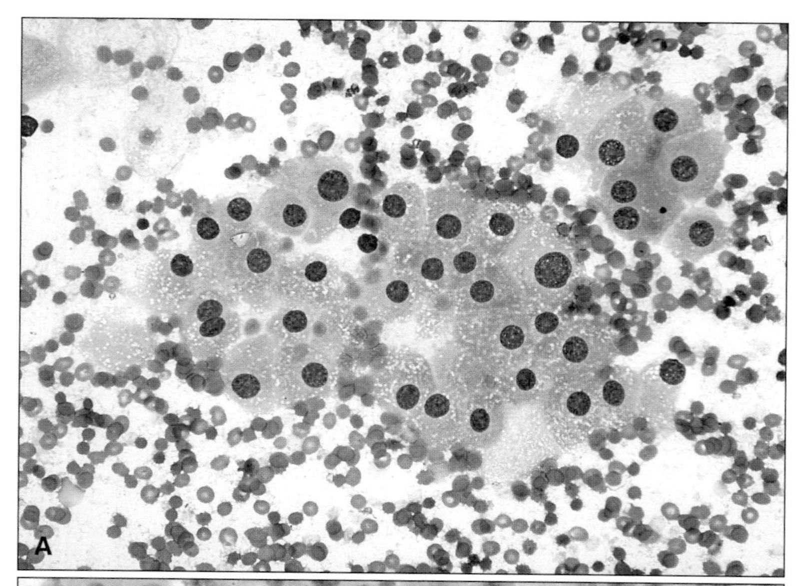

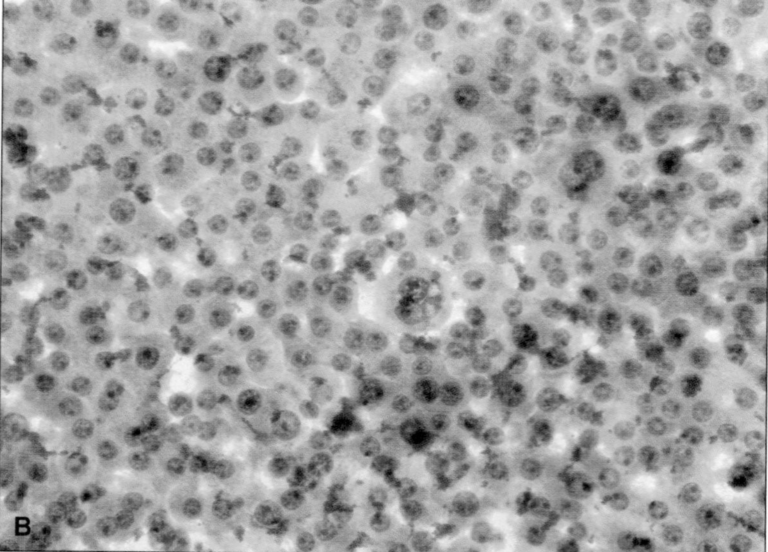

Fig. 7.6 (A,B) Fine-needle aspiration of oncocytoma yields a monotonous population of polygonal cells with abundant granular cytoplasm and well-defined cell borders. The nuclei are small, round, and bland, with inconspicuous nucleoli (similar to the nuclei of Fuhrman grade 1–2 renal cell carcinoma). Mitotic figures are not seen. Cytologic atypia ('degenerative atypia') may sometimes be observed.

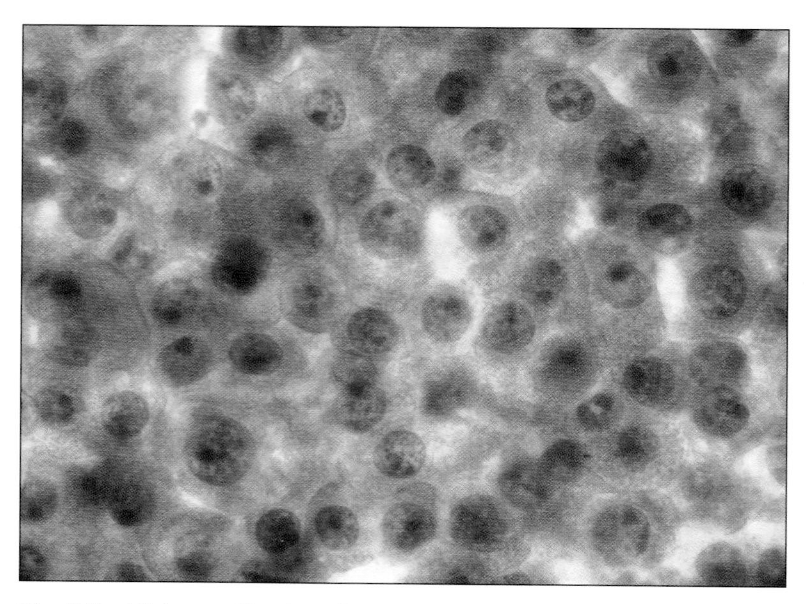

Fig. 7.7 High-magnification of oncocytoma shows granular cytoplasm due to innumerable, morphologically abnormal mitochondria. Electron microscopy shows double-walled mitochondria in the case of oncocytoma, versus single-walled microvesicles in the case of chromophobe renal cell carcinoma.

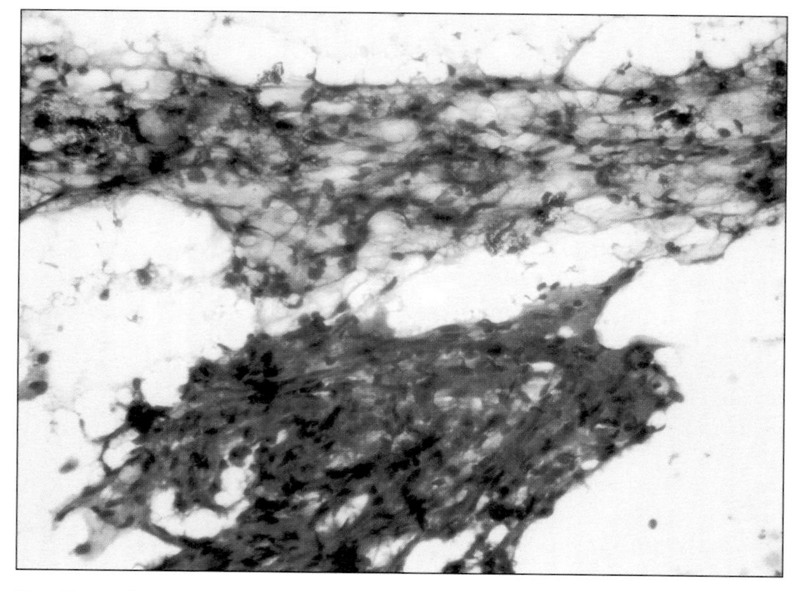

Fig. 7.8 Cytology of angiomyolipoma may show any or all of the three components. Syncytial clusters of mostly spindled mesenchymal cells with delicate ample cytoplasm represent the smooth muscle component. Thick-walled blood vessels lined by endothelial cells may be sampled. The fatty component presents as mature adipose tissue, sometimes with areas of fat necrosis.

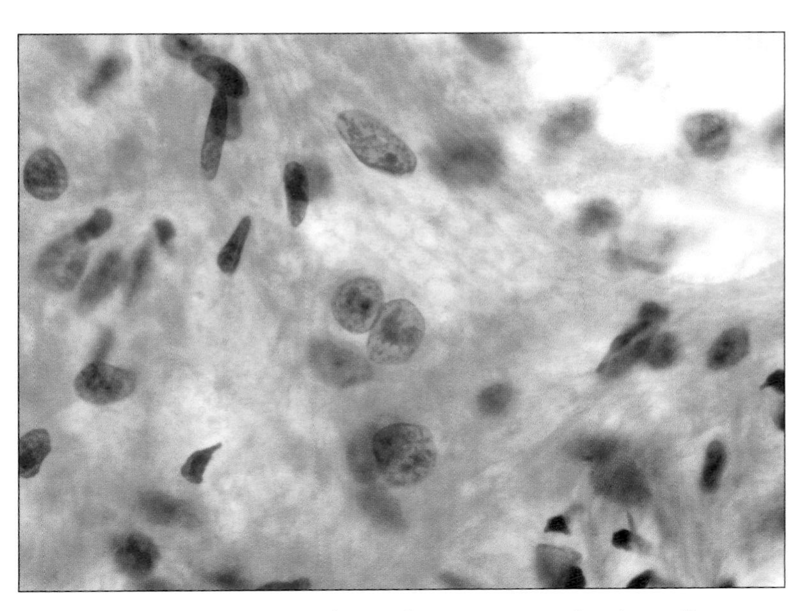

Fig. 7.9 Nuclei of the smooth muscle component of angiomyolipoma are often mildly enlarged and variable, with moderate-sized nucleoli. If the leiomyomatous component is very atypical, it may suggest sarcomatoid renal cell carcinoma. Very cellular smooth muscle with a predominant round cell pattern can be mistaken for a granular renal cell carcinoma.

MALIGNANT RENAL EPITHELIAL NEOPLASMS

RENAL CELL CARCINOMA

RCC is the most common renal tumor, with 28 000 new cases diagnosed per year in the USA (SEER 2002 estimate). Peak incidence occurs in the fifth to seventh decade of life, and males are affected about twice as frequently as females. Risk factors include smoking, obesity, phenacetin or acetaminophen use, industrial chemical exposure, and kidney stones. (Tables 7.1 & 7.2)

Conventional (clear cell) renal cell carcinoma

Conventional (clear cell) RCC accounts for about 75% of all RCCs. The tumor originates from cells of the proximal tubule. In the World Health Organization (WHO) 2002 classification, clear cell renal tumors, regardless of size, are considered carcinoma; hence, the term 'clear cell adenoma' is

Table 7.1 Differential cytologic features of renal cell carcinoma subtypes

	Background	*Arrangement*	*Cytoplasm*	*Nuclei*	*Nucleoli*
Clear cell RCC	Necrotic or clean	Large clusters	Abundant foamy, clear or granular	Round, uniform size	Variable, prominent in high-grade tumors
Low-grade papillary RCC	Foamy macrophages, necrosis	Papillae, occasionally isolated cells	Intracellular hemosiderin, rare nuclear grooves	Small, uniform	Inconspicuous
Chromophobe RCC	Clean	Small groups, isolated cells	Fluffy, clear, granular, thickened cell membrane	Variable size, irregular outline, intranuclear inclusions	Variable
Sarcomatoid RCC	Necrotic or clean	Groups and isolated cells	Elongated spindle cells	Pleomorphic	Prominent
Collecting duct carcinoma	Necrotic or clean	Groups and isolated cells	Scant cytoplasm	Hyperchromatic	Prominent
Urothelial carcinoma	Necrotic or clean	Papillae in low-grade lesions, isolated cells with occasional clusters in high-grade lesions	Scant dense cytoplasm that might contain vacuoles, bizarre cells	High N:C ratio, hyperchromasia	Indented nuclei

Adapted from Renshaw et al.[2]
RCC, renal cell carcinoma; N:C, nuclear:cytoplasmic.

Table 7.2 Immunohistochemistry of renal epithelial neoplasms

	CK7	*CD10*	*EMA*	*LMW keratin*	*HMW keratin*	*Vimentin*	*Ulex lectin*	*CEA*	*Mucin*	*Hale's colloidal iron*	*c-kit (CD117)*
UC	+	–	+	+	+	–	–	±	–	–	NE
PRCC	+	+	+	+	–	+	–	–	–	–	–
CDC*	+	–	+	+	+	+	+	+	+	–	NE
RCC	–	+	+	–	–	+	–	–	–	–	–
CRCC	–	–	+	–	–	–	–	–	–	+	+
ONC	–	–	+	NE	–	–	–	–	–	±	+

UC, urothelial carcinoma; PRCC, papillary renal cell carcinoma; CDC, collecting duct carcinoma; RCC, renal cell carcinoma; CRCC, chromophobe renal cell carcinoma; ONC, oncocytoma; CK7, cytokeratin 7; EMA, epithelial membrane antigen; LMW, low molecular weight; HMW, high molecular weight; CEA, carcinoembryonic antigen; NE, not evaluated.
*Renal medullary carcinoma shows a staining profile similar to that of CDC.

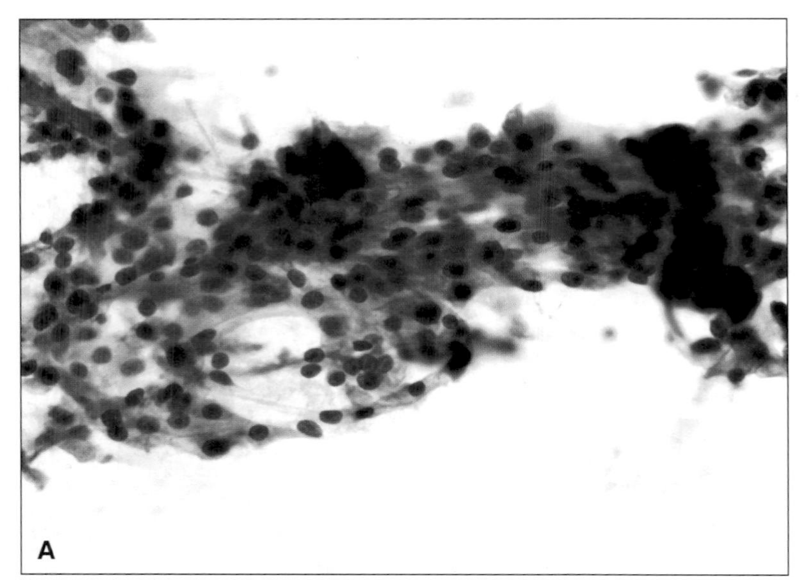

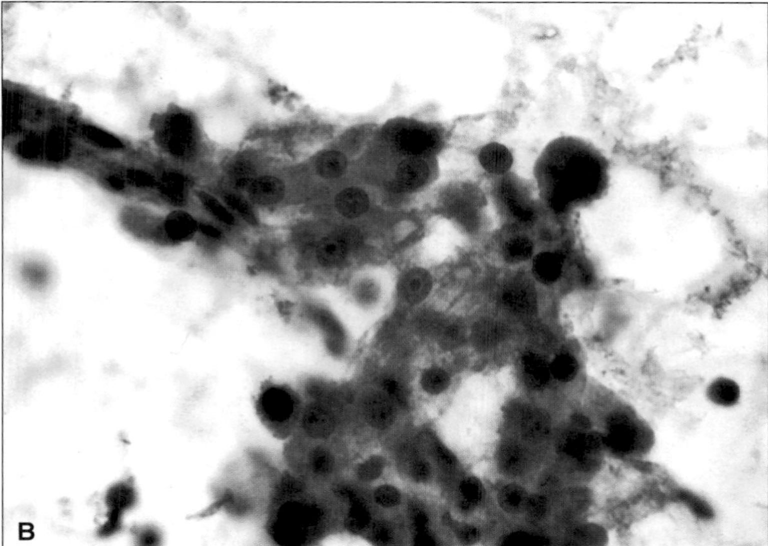

Fig. 7.10 (A,B) Conventional (clear cell) renal cell carcinoma aspirates show large clusters of cells with abundant, vacuolated cytoplasm. The nuclear:cytoplasmic ratio is low, the nucleus eccentric.

obsolete. The term 'granular cell carcinoma' is also no longer used; tumors that contain an admixture or even a predominance of 'granular'-appearing cells are still considered conventional RCC as long as the typical clear cell cytology is represented in any amount, and the tumor is not one of the other special types (see below). CD10 (common acute lymphocytic leukemia antigen; CALLA) is expressed on the brush border of renal tubular epithelial cells. CD10 is also expressed in over 90% of clear cell RCC and in papillary RCC, but not chromphobe RCC and oncocytoma.[10,11] (Figs 7.10 & 7.11)

Chromophobe renal cell carcinoma

Chromophobe RCC accounts for 3–5% of all RCCs. The prognosis is somewhat better than that of conventional RCC. In the classic subtype, the cytoplasm is predominantly

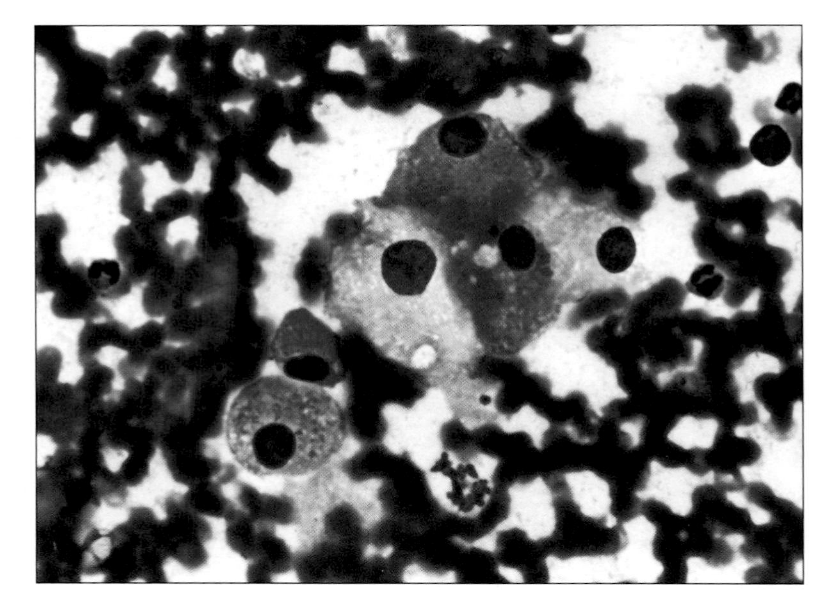

Fig. 7.11 Grading of renal cell carcinoma in fine-needle aspirates is performed as in surgical pathology.[12,13] Differential diagnosis includes benign tubular cells, macrophages, adrenocortical cells, and hepatocytes.

clear. In the eosinophilic subtype, the cytoplasm is filled with eosinophilic granular cytoplasm similar to oncocytoma, with focal vacuoles or clear areas in a subpopulation of 'oncocytic'-like cells. The differential diagnosis includes oncocytoma and conventional RCC. (Figs 7.12–7.14)

Papillary (chromophil) renal cell carcinoma

Papillary renal cell carcinoma (PRCC) accounts for 7–15% of all RCC. PRCC is frequently multifocal and bilateral (ranging from 41% to 80%) and is sometimes associated with renal adenoma.[14] The overall prognosis is better than that of the conventional type of RCC, and multifocality is not associated with a poor prognosis.

At least half of these tumors have true papillae with fibrovascular cores. Two major subtypes are recognized. Type 1 tumors consist of small basophilic cells; type 2 tumors contain large eosinophilic cells. There is some evidence that type 2 tumors may tend to be of higher stage and grade.[15]

The differential diagnosis of PRCC on FNA includes papillary urothelial carcinoma (PUC), and several other subtypes of RCC. PUC usually has a highly multilayered epithelium (>5 cell layers), whereas PRCC typically has fewer (<3) cell layers. Urothelial carcinoma, unlike PRCC, is positive for high molecular weight (34βE12) cytokeratin and negative for vimentin. Conventional RCC tends to have a less vacuolated cytoplasm and central nuclei. It lacks papillae and fibrovascular cores. Unlike PRCC, it is negative for cytokeratin 7 (CK7). Collecting duct carcinoma can have papillae, but is usually of higher grade and positive for *Ulex europaeus* lectin and for mucin.

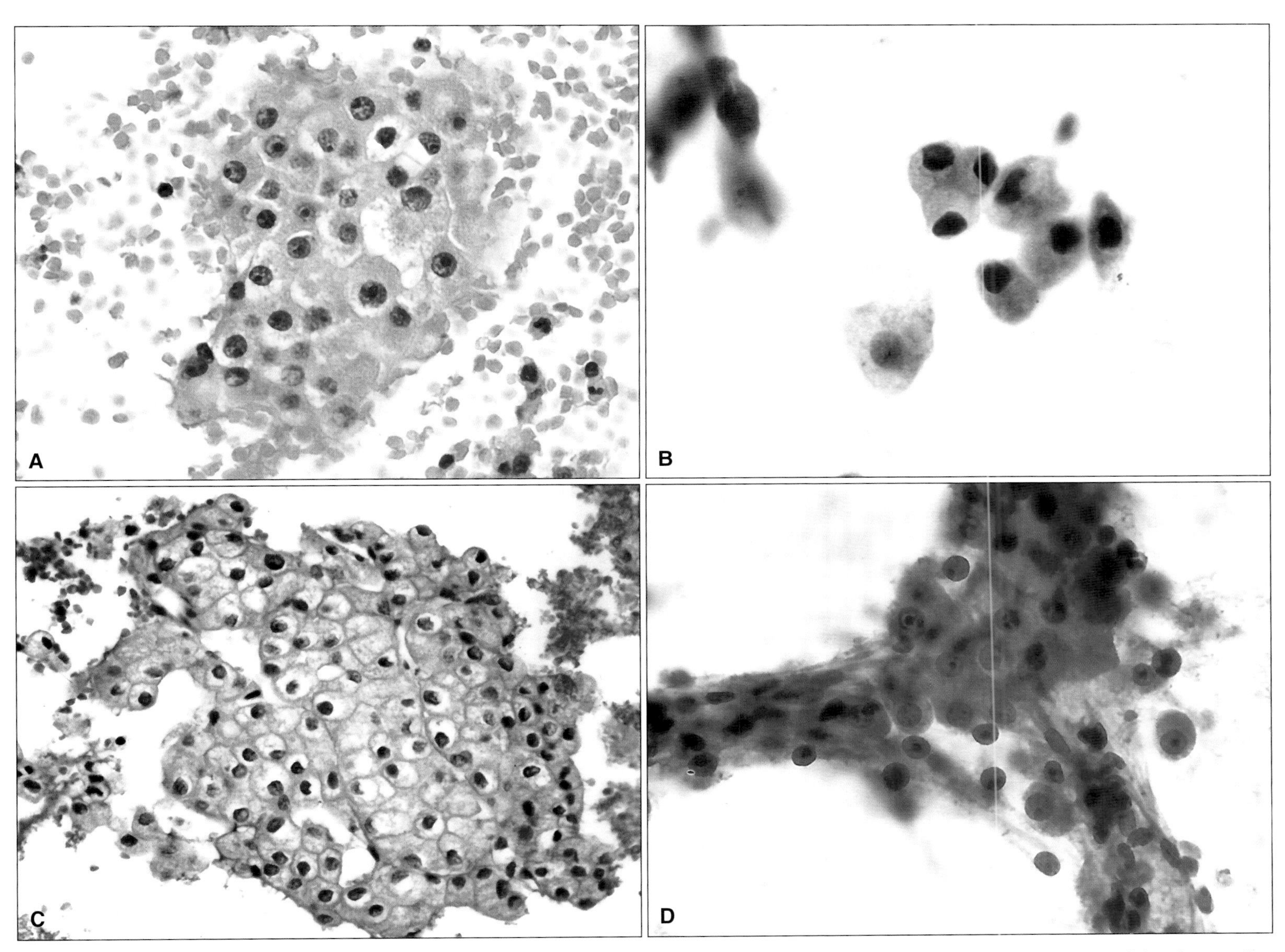

Fig. 7.12 (A–D) Chromophobe renal cell carcinoma displays broad ribbons of cells with 'fluffy' or flocculent cytoplasm, distinct cell borders, and frequent binucleation. The cells are less cohesive than those of clear cell renal cell carcinoma. Diff-Quik stain shows a perivascular reticulated zone.

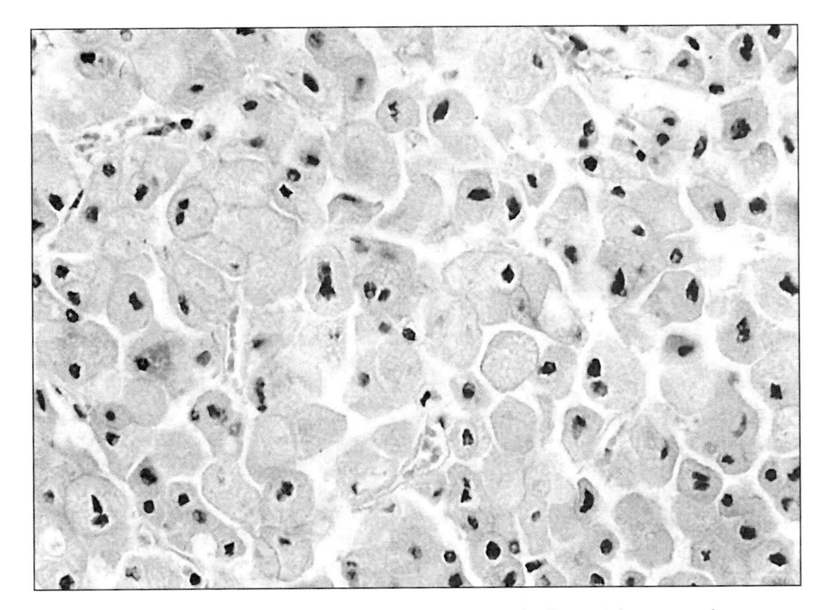

Fig. 7.13 Hale's colloidal iron stain reacts with the acid mucosubstances within the cytoplasmic vesicles of chromophobe renal cell carcinoma. However, this is not a completely reliable criterion; an apical staining pattern occurs in oncocytomas.[8]

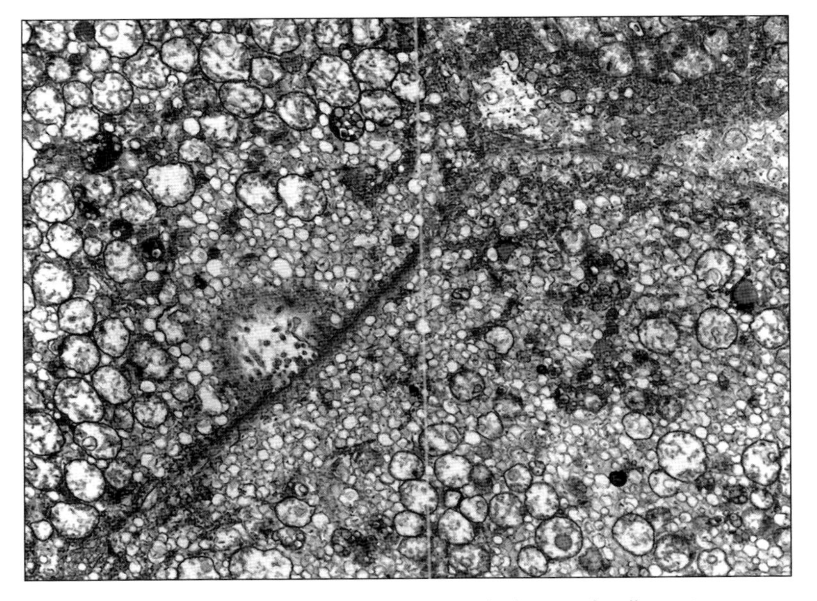

Fig. 7.14 Electron microscopy of chromophobe renal cell carcinoma shows that the cytoplasm is packed with irregularly sized microvesicles.

FNA may sometimes be requested to distinguish metastatic from primary renal carcinoma. The tumors most commonly responsible for metastases to the kidney are lung, stomach, pancreas, breast, and contralateral kidney.[16] None of these is positive for alpha-methylacyl-CoA racemase (AMACR), in contrast to PRCC.[17] Papillary adenocarcinoma of lung (bronchiolar–alveolar type) is positive for thyroid transcription factor-1 (TTF-1). Metastases from breast carcinoma may be positive for estrogen and/or progesterone receptors. (Fig. 7.15)

Sarcomatoid renal cell carcinoma

Sarcomatoid renal cell carcinoma (SRCC) accounts for 3–5% of RCC. SRCC is defined by the presence of a high-grade spindle cell component, with or without epithelioid differentiation.

Formerly considered an independent subtype, SRCCs are now considered extremely dedifferentiated examples of one of the other recognized RCC types, most often conventional RCC of high nuclear grade. Yet the atypical appearance and aggressive clinical behavior warrants retention of the category. Median survival is only 6.6 months, as opposed to that of other RCCs of 19 months. Prognostic factors include stage, presence of tumor necrosis, and percentage of tumor with sarcomatoid histology.[18]

FNA diagnosis may be helpful in irresectable disease to initiate adjuvant therapy with chemotherapy and interferon.

The differential diagnosis is optimally made on smears and cell block preparations and includes clear cell or papillary RCC, when undersampling fails to detect a small component with sarcomatoid dedifferentiation. When adequately sampled, other high-grade neoplasms such as large cell lymphoma, adrenal cortical carcinoma, or the rare primary renal sarcomas may be considered.[19] Immunocytochemistry is positive for epithelial membrane antigen (EMA), cytokeratin, and vimentin. (Fig. 7.16)

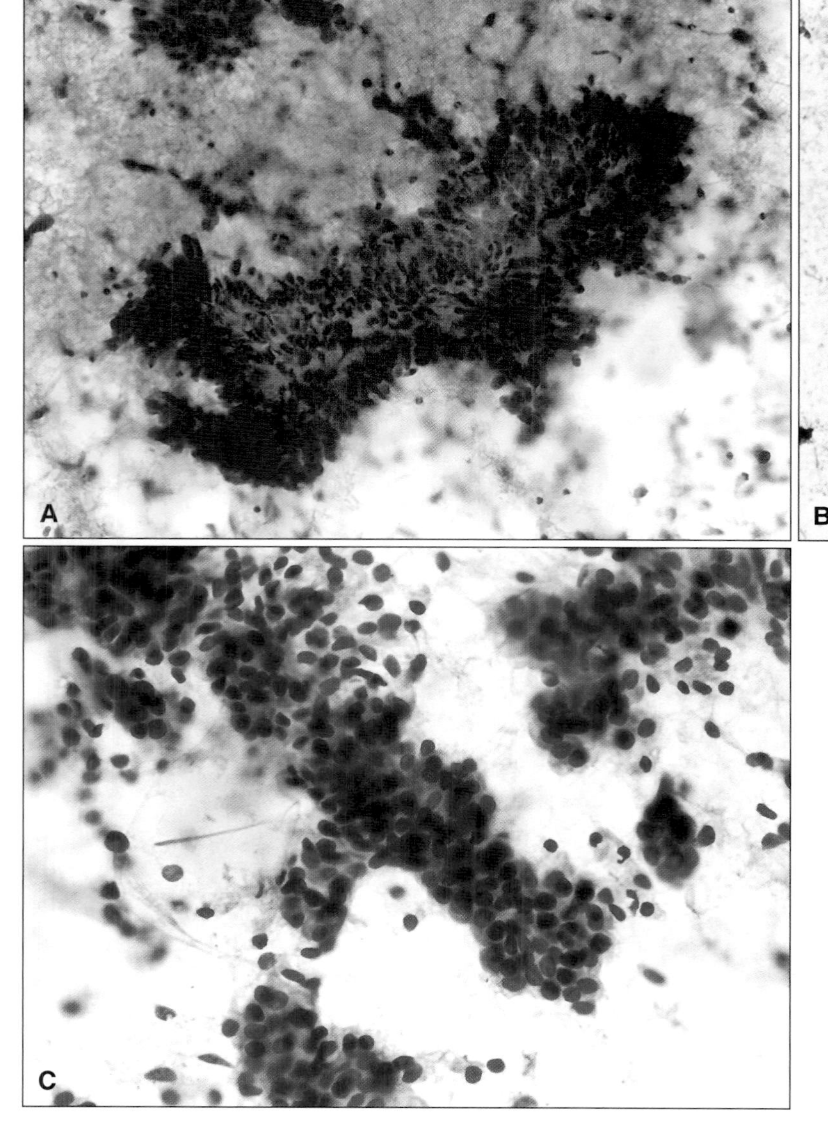

Fig. 7.15 (A–C) Psammoma bodies are seen in 10% of papillary renal cell carcinoma. The cytoplasm is often 'hemosiderin laden', granular, or vacuolated. Nuclei are uniform and pleomorphism is rare. The nuclear:cytoplasmic ratio is high.

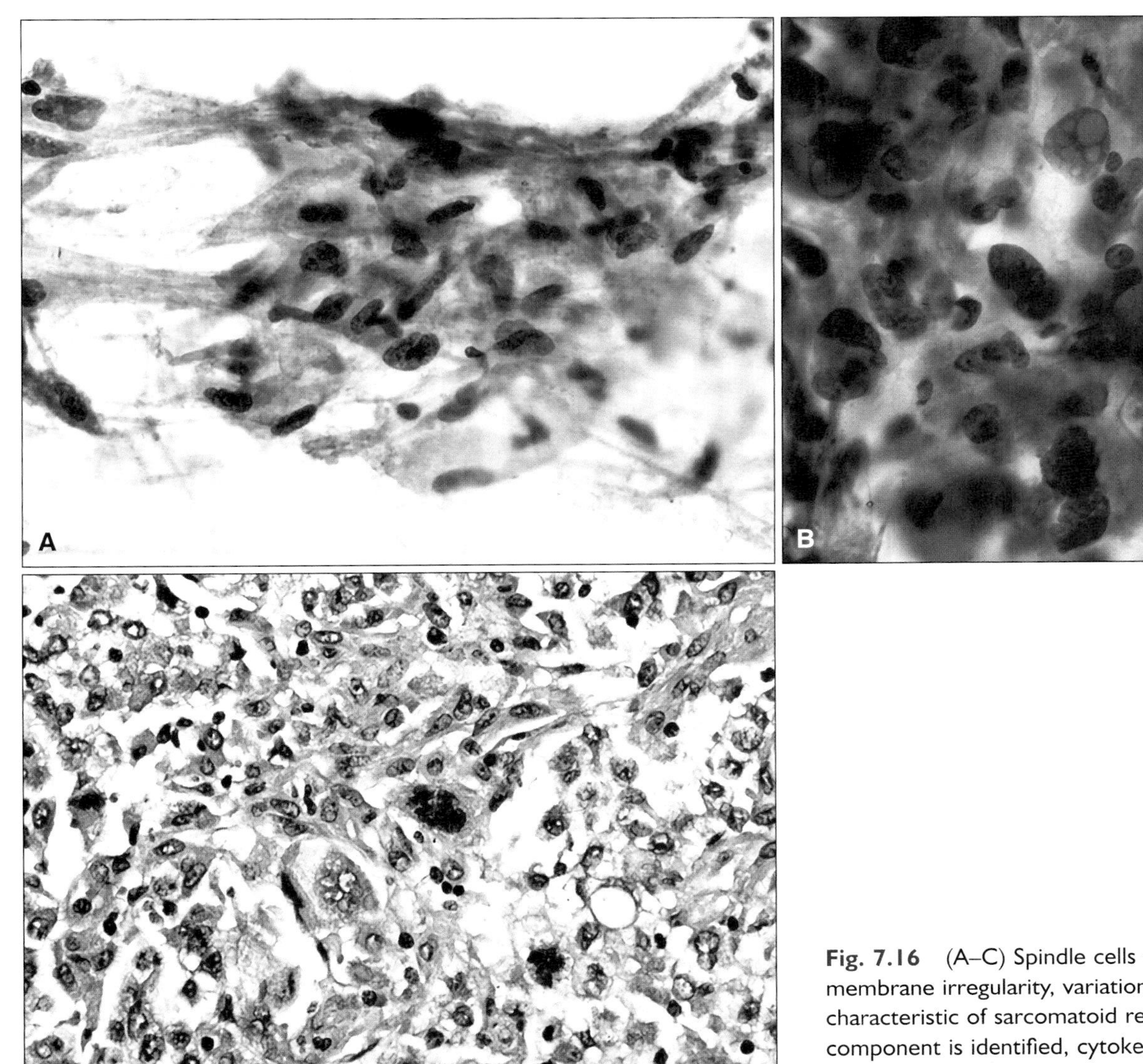

Fig. 7.16 (A–C) Spindle cells with large nuclei, marked nuclear membrane irregularity, variation in size, and prominent nucleoli are characteristic of sarcomatoid renal cell carcinoma. If no epithelioid component is identified, cytokeratin positivity is required for the diagnosis. Morphologic appearance may resemble malignant fibrous histiocytoma, fibrosarcoma, or unclassified sarcoma.

Collecting duct carcinoma (Bellini tumor)

Collecting duct renal cell carcinoma (CDRCC) is rare, comprising approximately 1% of all renal tumors.[20] CDRCC arises in the renal medulla from collecting duct epithelium, unlike other kinds of RCC, which arise from proximal tubule.

Differential diagnosis on FNA includes other renal carcinomas with papillary architecture. PRCC is usually of lower grade and lacks immunoreactivity for *Ulex europaeus* agglutinin. CDRCC, with its medullary location, may radiographically mimic PUC of the renal pelvis. The latter, however, has opaque non-vacuolated cytoplasm and large hyperchromatic nuclei. Furthermore, PUC lacks immunoreactivity for *Ulex europaeus* agglutinin, and unlike CDRCC expresses cytokeratins 7 and 20. Renal medullary carcinoma (RMC) may simulate CDRCC; however, it occurs in a demographically distinctive population, namely young adolescents of African descent who harbor the sickle-cell anemia trait.[21] (Fig. 7.17)

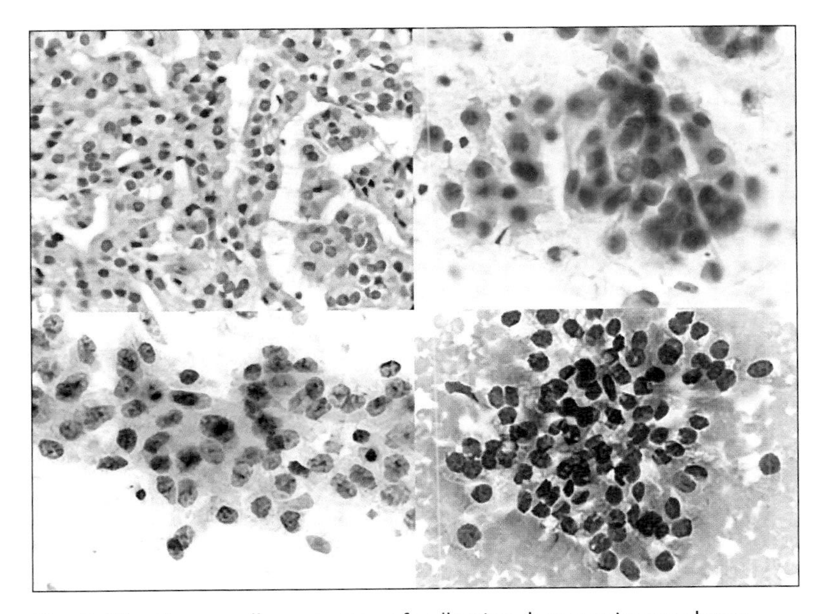

Fig. 7.17 Fine-needle aspiration of collecting duct carcinoma shows cohesive groups arranged in papillary tubular structures, some with scattered single cells.[20,22,23] Cells exhibit finely vacuolated cytoplasm, eccentric nuclei, and occasional mitotic figures.

TUMORS OF THE RENAL PELVIS

Cytologic examination of voided urine may be insensitive for low-grade urothelial carcinoma, due to accompanying ureteropelvic obstruction and to the bland cytology of most low-grade urothelial neoplasms. Diagnostic accuracy is higher with ureteral catheter lavage and (especially) with renal pelvis brushings. Ancillary studies using DNA image analysis for cells with DNA content >5c or multi-probe fluorescence in situ hybridization (FISH) for chromosomes 3, 7, 17, and 9p21.3 to demonstrate chromosomal aneusomies are extremely helpful in distinguishing reactive urothelial cells from carcinoma. FNA is indicated for diagnosis of a renal pelvis lesion if urinary tract cytology findings are negative.

Urothelial carcinoma

Urothelial carcinoma is the most common tumor of the renal pelvis. It accounts for 5–10% of all renal malignant tumors and 5% of all urothelial tumors. It is predominantly seen in the elderly male population, with a peak incidence in the seventh decade. The risk factors (heavy smoking, aniline dye exposure, etc.) are similar to those for urothelial carcinoma at other sites, and, just as for urinary bladder carcinomas, there is a significant association with synchronous or metachronous urothelial tumors at other sites. The most common presentation is painless hematuria. Accompanying stones are found in 10% of cases.

Survival is correlated with stage and tumor grade. Metastasis occurs to lungs, liver, regional lymph nodes, and bone.

The accuracy of FNA for urothelial carcinoma in the renal pelvis is 85%. Low-grade urothelial neoplasia can be confused with PRCC (Table 7.3). Tumors metastatic to the kidney are a pitfall, especially papillary carcinoma of the thyroid or lung. Differential diagnosis of high-grade papillary tumors at this site includes collecting duct carcinomas, metastatic papillary neoplasms, and PRCC. Accurate diagnosis may require immunohistochemistry (see Table 7.2). (Figs 7.18 & 7.19)

Table 7.3 Diagnostic features distinguishing papillary urothelial carcinoma from papillary renal cell carcinoma

	Papillary urothelial carcinoma	*Papillary renal cell carcinoma*
Cellularity	+++	+ to +++
Fibrovascular cores	Abundant	Rare
Epithelial thickness	>5 cell layer	<3 cell layer
Cytoplasm	Vacuolated	Vacuolated, clear, or granular
Stripped nuclei	+	+++
Nuclei	Hypochromatic, fine powdery chromatin, grooves	Open chromatin
Nucleoli	Small	Prominent in higher grades
N:C ratio	Moderate to high	Low

N:C, nuclear:cytoplasmic.

Other carcinomas

Squamous cell carcinoma is the second most frequent malignancy of the renal pelvis. It affects the sexes equally and peaks in the sixth and seventh decades of life. Associated renal calculi are seen in over 50% of cases in some series. Prognosis is poor, with a median survival of less than 5 months. Squamous cell carcinoma of the renal pelvis shows irregular clusters of malignant squamous cells.

Adenocarcinoma and adenosquamous carcinoma are rare in the renal pelvis. Adenocarcinoma exhibits single or clustered malignant glandular cells, resembling colonic adenocarcinoma. Signet ring cells may be seen. Adenosqua-

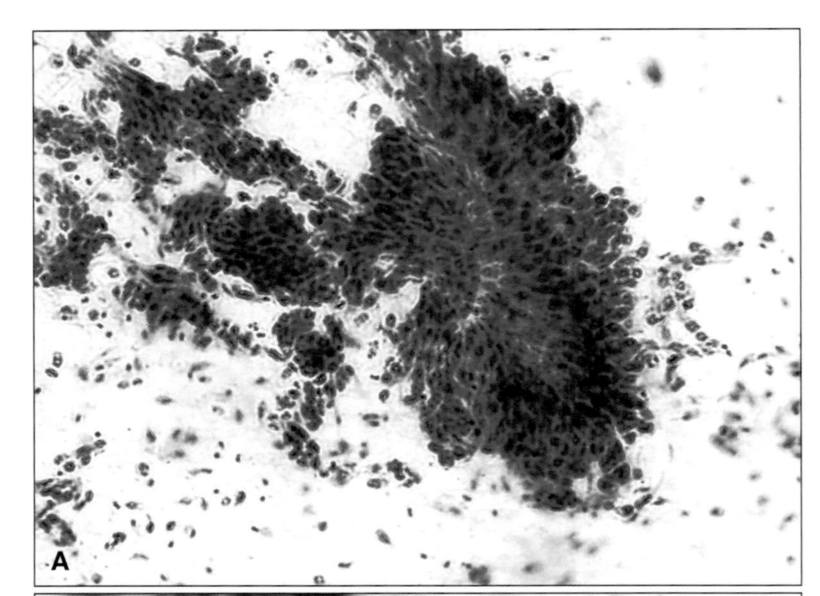

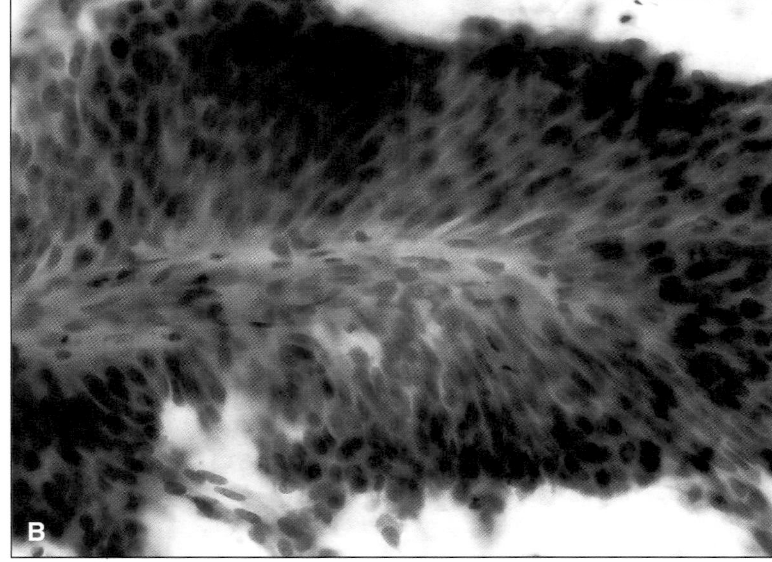

Fig. 7.18 (A,B) Cytology of urothelial carcinoma is identical to that of urinary bladder carcinomas. Low-grade urothelial carcinoma is composed of papillary aggregates of columnar and polygonal urothelial cells with minimal nuclear atypia and slight nuclear membrane irregularity.

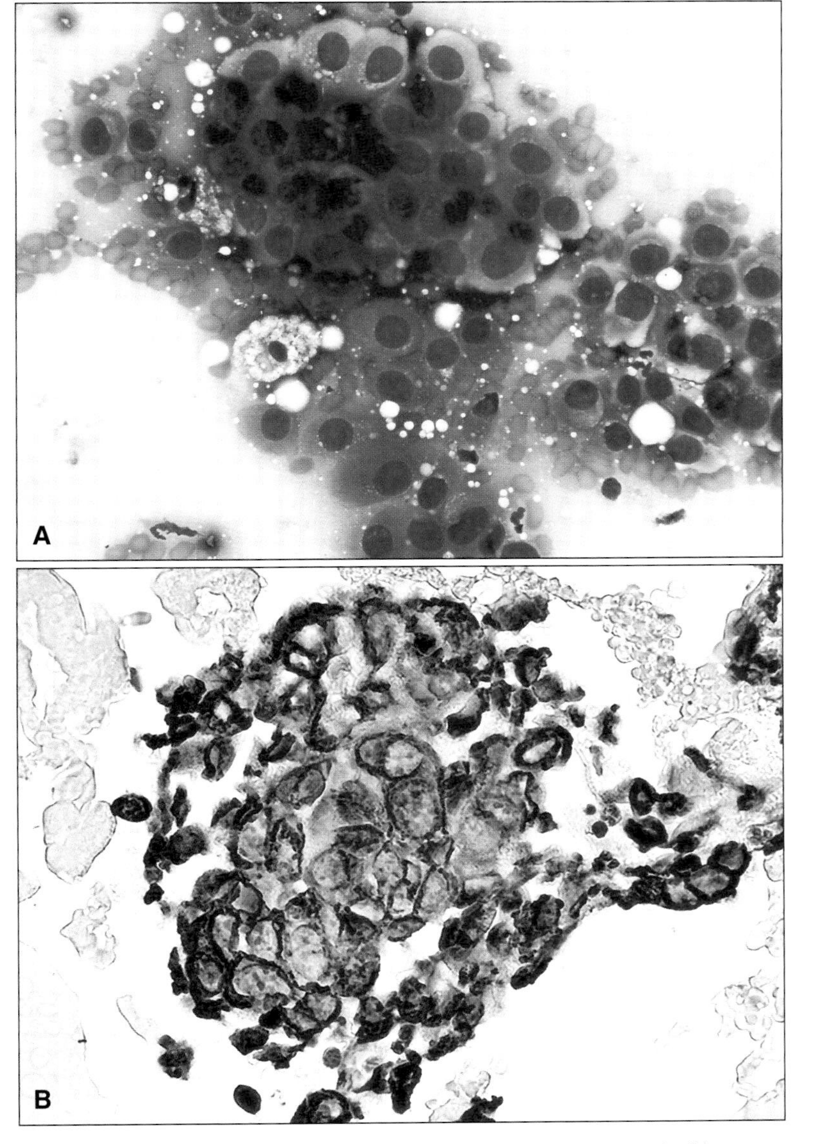

Fig. 7.19 (A,B) High-grade urothelial carcinoma is composed of large columnar or polygonal urothelial cells with well-defined borders, dense cytoplasm, and scattered vacuoles. The nuclei are large and hyperchromatic, with coarse chromatin, and a high nuclear:cytoplasmic ratio. Bizarre multinucleated cells, squamous cells, and even mucin-positive glandular cells may also be seen.

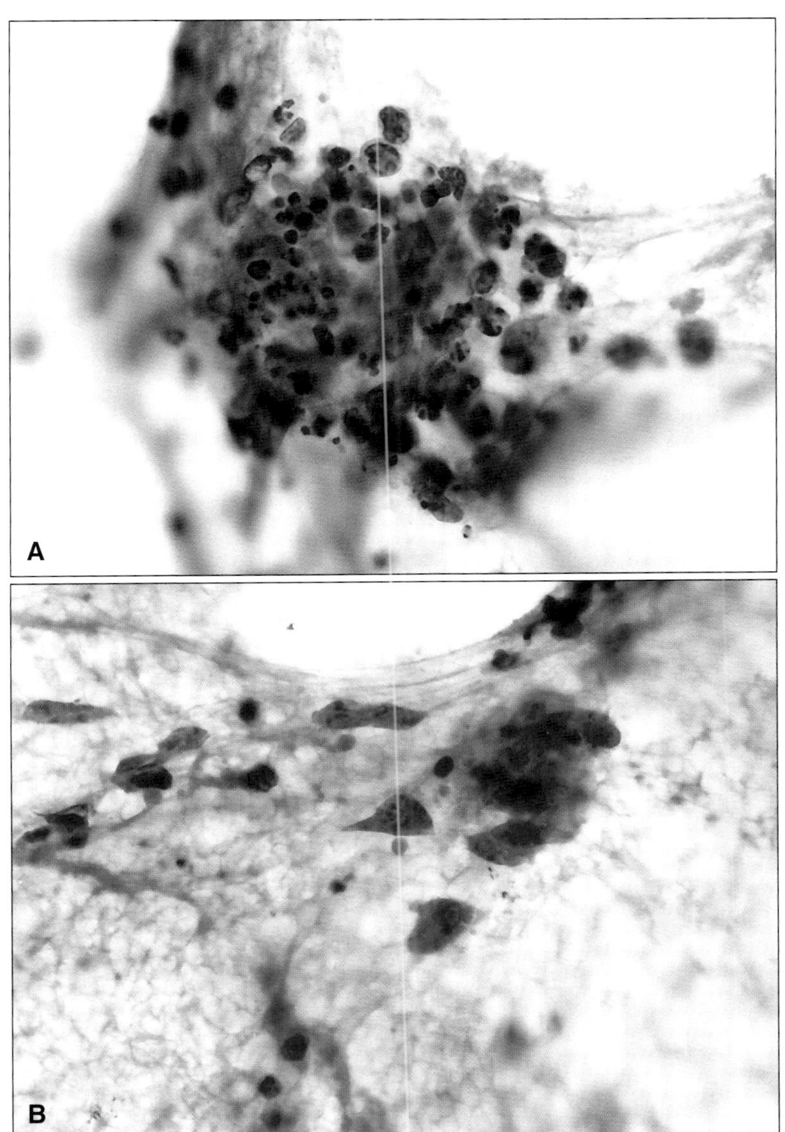

Fig. 7.20 (A,B) Fine-needle aspiration of large cell lymphoma yields a monotonous population of dyscohesive single cells with a high nuclear:cytoplasmic ratio and prominent nucleoli. There is inconspicuous, scant, basophilic cytoplasm. Lymphoglandular bodies (shreds of cytoplasm) are apparent in the background.

mous carcinoma is very rare in the renal pelvis. Malignant squamous cells and glandular cells are seen.

OTHER RENAL TUMORS

Lymphoma

Malignant lymphoma typically presents as an unencapsulated, infiltrative, solitary mass in the kidney. Except in the renal transplant population, primary extranodal renal lymphoma is rare; commonly, renal lymphoma occurs in association with nodal involvement or generalized disease. Renal intravascular lymphomatosis has been rarely reported. Post-transplant lymphomas are commonly present at extranodal sites, including the kidney, and so are an exception to this rule. The most frequent subtype of lymphoma in kidney is diffuse large cell B lymphoma (DLCL). However, other low-grade B cell lymphomas such as mucosa-associated lymphoid tissue (MALT) lymphoma of kidney may occur.

DLCL is frequently misdiagnosed as chromophobe RCC, as both entities may present with 'bare' nuclei, which in the case of chromophobe RCC represents stripping of cytoplasm due to its fragility or smearing technique. High-grade RCC, metastatic poorly differentiated carcinoma, and Wilms' tumor (WT) are other common pitfalls regarding differential diagnosis. Establishing monoclonality with immunohistochemical stains, as well as flow cytometry, aid in the diagnosis.[3] EMA and CK7 will similarly be positive if RCC is present and will be negative in lymphoma. (Fig. 7.20)

Renal sarcoma

Primary sarcoma of the kidney is extremely rare. Leiomyosarcoma is the most common type, followed by malignant fibrous histiocytoma, hemangiopericytoma, fibrosarcoma, and unclassified sarcomas. Prognosis is poor, with a mean survival of 23 months. Cytology is identical to that of sarcomas elsewhere.

Metastatic malignancy of the kidney

Metastasis is two to three times as common as RCC. The most common primary sources are breast, lung, intestine, opposite kidney, and stomach. Metastatic tumors of the kidney are often bilateral and multifocal. The history of a previous primary lesion and an immunohistochemical panel aid in the diagnosis. (Fig. 7.21)

PEDIATRIC RENAL TUMORS

Wilms' tumor (nephroblastoma)

Nephroblastoma (WT) is the most common renal malignancy of childhood. It accounts for 6% of all pediatric cancers. Most cases occur in patients younger than 3 years, and only 3% of cases occur in children older than 10 years. Boys and girls are affected equally.

Clinical presentation is typically as a unilateral mass, possibly accompanied by hematuria. Occasional cases present with acute abdomen secondary to intratumoral bleeding or, rarely, metastasis. Survival rate is 85%. Unfavorable prognostic factors include diffuse anaplasia (about 5% of cases), higher stage, and older age.

A genetic predisposition with an autosomal dominant inheritance pattern or a chromosomal abnormality involving the short arm of chromosome 11 can be found in some cases. The classic genetic abnormality is alteration of *WT1* at 11p13; however, WT is a genetically heterogeneous entity with loss of heterozygosity described at 11p, 16q, 1p, and 9q.[24]

FNA of nephroblastoma is rarely performed, as the clinicoradiologic presentation is usually sufficient for presumptive diagnosis, and preoperative biopsy may upstage an organ-confined tumor. Differential diagnosis includes the usual pediatric 'round blue cell' tumors: embryonal rhabdomyosarcoma, neuroblastoma, lymphoma, and possibly primitive neuroectodermal tumor. (Figs 7.22 & 7.23)

Cystic nephroma

This benign neoplasm may be seen in both adults and children. It presents as a sharply demarcated, multicystic mass. The pediatric tumors are considered analogs of nephroblastoma exhibiting complete differentiation. This interpretation is supported by the observation that the similar pediatric tumor, cystic partially differentiated nephroblastoma, although also clinically benign, contains microscopic, non-expansile nests of blastema in some septa. Cystic nephroma in adults likely has a different histogenesis from the pediatric form, but is also clinically benign. In a child, the diagnosis includes cystic nephroblastoma. In an adult, the differential diagnosis includes cystic RCC. (Fig. 7.24)

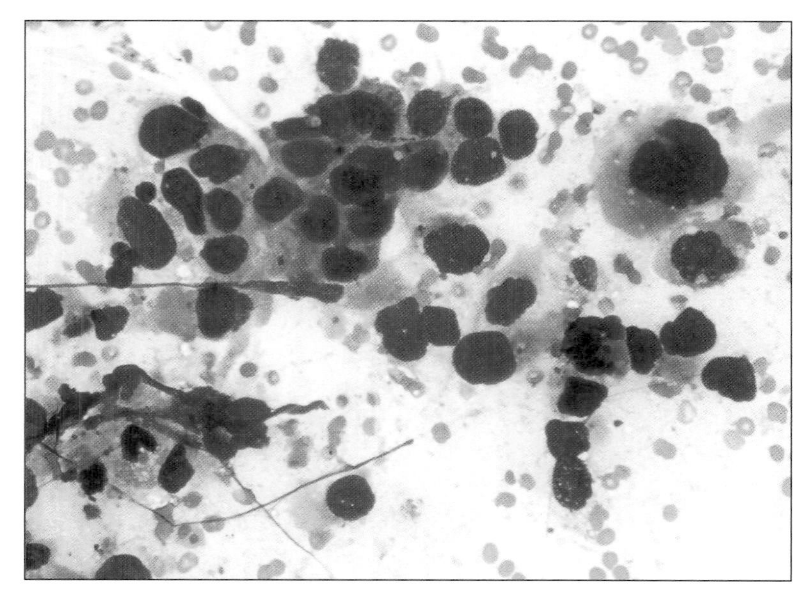

Fig. 7.21 Bronchogenic adenocarcinoma metastatic to kidney from a fine-needle aspiration biopsy shows clusters of epithelioid cells that, on immunohistochemical staining, are positive for cytokeratin 7, negative for cytokeratin 20, and positive for thyroid transcription factor-1.

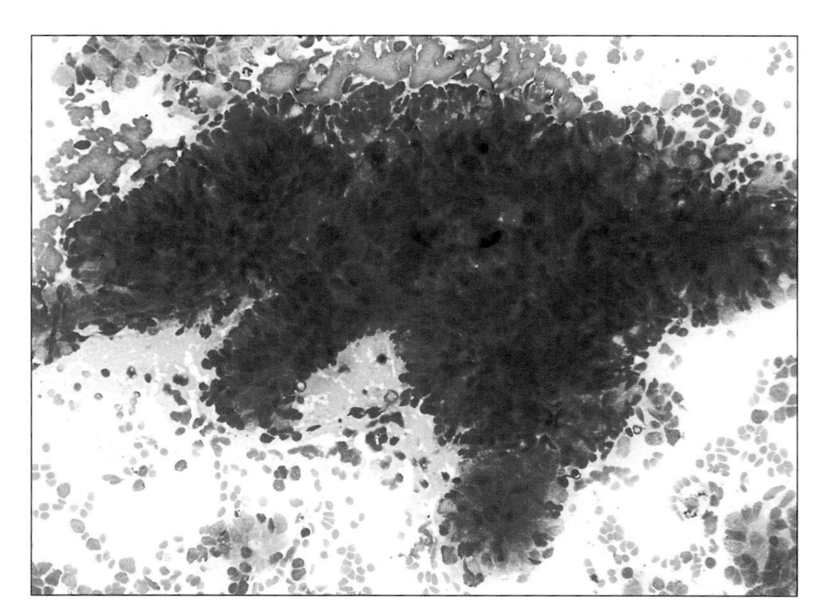

Fig. 7.22 Nephroblastoma has three components: epithelium, stroma, and blastema. Any or all of these components can be identified on cytology. Blastemal cells are small round blue cells with scant cytoplasm, dark blue nuclei, fine granular chromatin, and inconspicuous nucleoli. These cells are usually distributed haphazardly, but dense groups with variable nuclear molding and occasional rosetting may be seen.

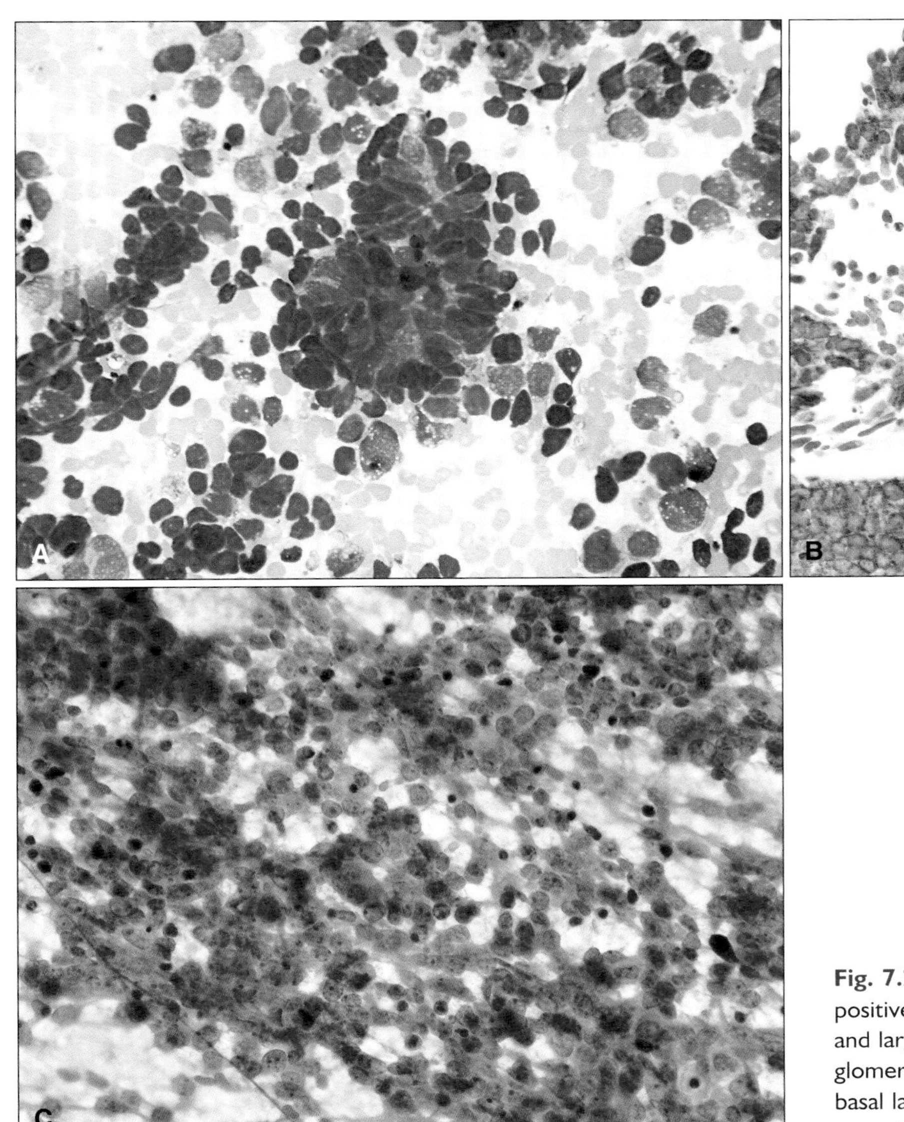

Fig. 7.23 (A–C) In nephroblastoma, epithelial cells are cytokeratin positive and slightly larger than blastemal cells, with abundant cytoplasm and larger nuclei. They can form nests and primitive tubular and glomeruloid structures. The cellular clusters are bounded by a cyanophilic basal lamina. Stromal cells are spindle cells arranged in loose sheets in a metachromatic myxoid stroma.

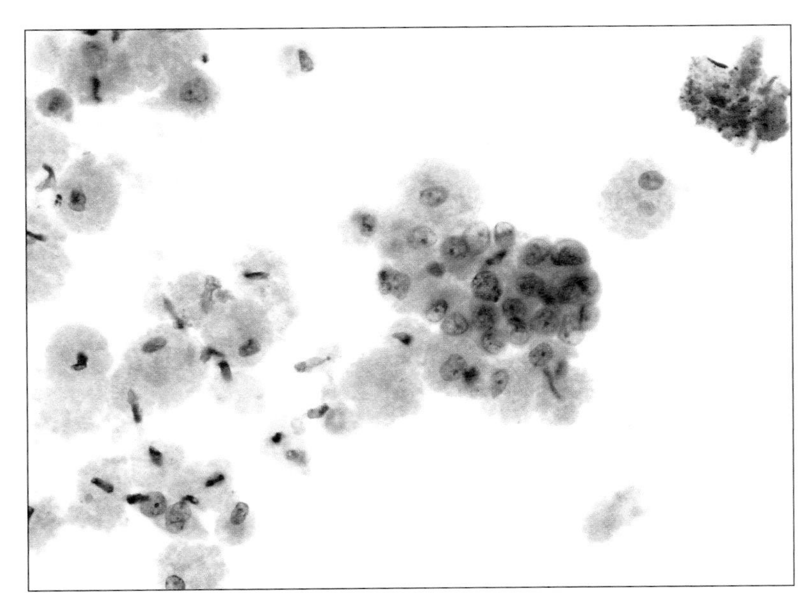

Fig. 7.24 In cystic nephroma, small flat sheets of epithelial cells with well-defined borders, single larger epithelial cells with eccentric hyperchromatic nuclei, and densely packed mesenchymal cells are seen in a background of histiocytes.

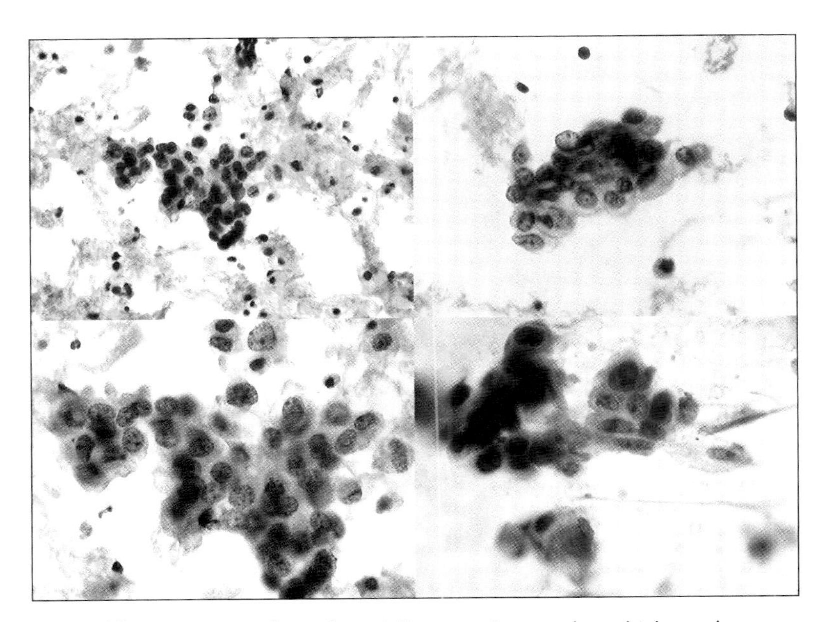

Fig. 7.25 Aspirates of renal medullary carcinoma show high-grade epithelial malignancy with gland-like, cribriform, and strand-like growth patterns. Tumor diathesis is present.

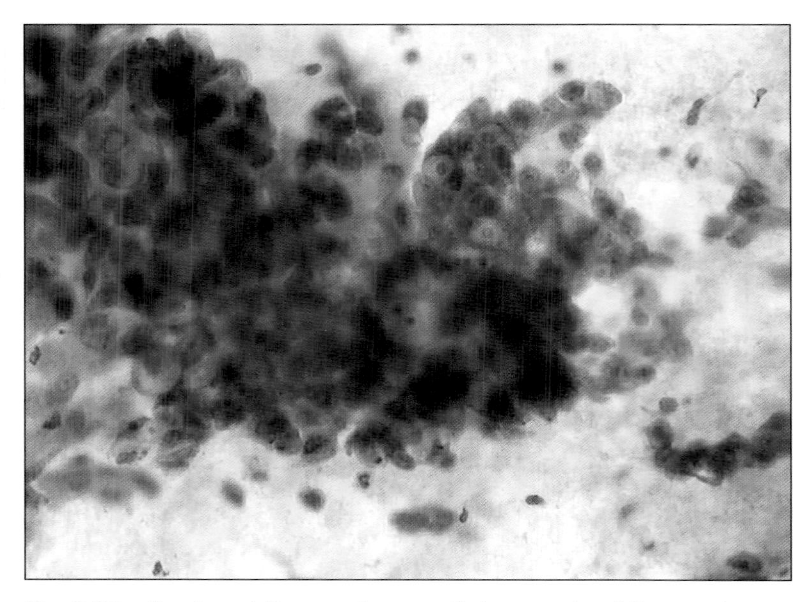

Fig. 7.26 Renal medullary carcinoma cells have eosinophilic cytoplasm. Many cells have eosinophilic cytoplasmic inclusions resembling those of rhabdoid tumor.

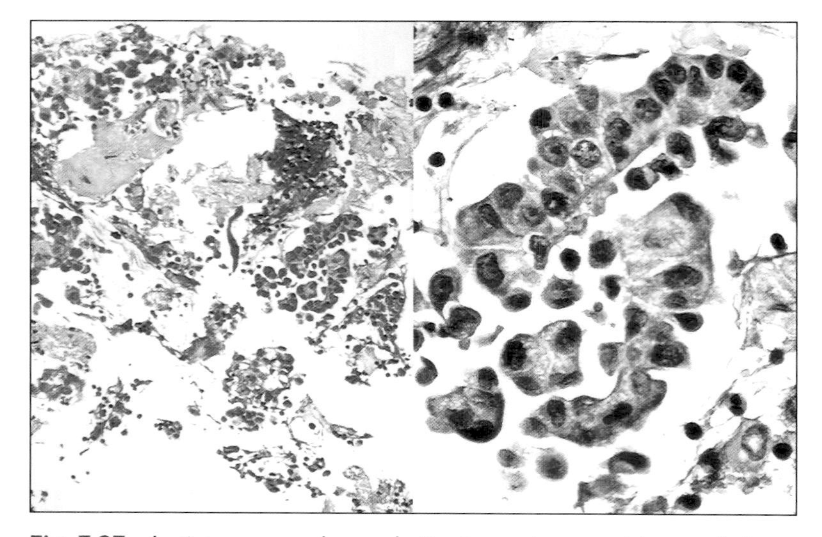

Fig. 7.27 In tissue cores, desmoplastic stroma is present in association with high-grade carcinoma.

Renal medullary carcinoma

RMC is a rare high-grade malignancy associated with sickle-cell trait that occurs primarily in children and young adults.[21,25] It arises in the renal medulla. It is a clinically aggressive tumor, with a mean survival of only 4 months. (Figs 7.25–7.27)

REFERENCES

1. Katz RL. Kidneys, adrenals and retroperitoneum. In: Bibbo M, ed. Comprehensive cytopathology. 2nd edn. Philadelphia: WB Saunders; 1997:781–821.
2. Renshaw AA, Granter SR, Cibas E. Fine-needle aspiration of the adult kidney. Cancer 1997;81:71–88.
3. Truong LD, Todd TD, Dhurandhar B, et al. Fine-needle aspirations of renal masses in adults. Analysis of results and diagnostic problems in 108 cases. Diagn Cytopathol 1999;20:339–349.
4. Gibbons RP, Bush WH Jr, Burnett LL. Needle tract seeding following aspiration of renal cell carcinoma. J Urol 1977;118:865–867.
5. Kiser GC, Totonchy M, Barry JM. Needle tract seeding after percutaneous renal adenocarcinoma aspiration. J Urol 1986;136:1292–1293.
6. Silverman JF, Gurley AM, Harris JP, et al. Fine needle aspiration cytology of renal infarcts. Cytomorphologic findings and potential diagnostic pitfalls in two cases. Acta Cytol 1991;35:736–741.
7. Grignon DJ, Eble JN. Papillary and metanephric adenomas of the kidney. Semin Diagn Pathol 1998;15:41–53.
8. Liu J, Fanning CV. Can renal oncocytomas be distinguished from renal cell carcinoma on fine-needle aspiration specimens? A study of conventional smears in conjunction with ancillary studies. Cancer 2001;93:390–397.
9. Baiyee D. CD3: good marker for oncocytoma (Abstract). Annual Meeting of the United States and Canadian Academy of Pathology, Chicago, Illinois, 2002.
10. Avery AK, Beckstead J, Renshaw AA, et al. Use of antibodies to RCC and CD10 in the differential diagnosis of renal neoplasms. Am J Surg Pathol 2000;24:203–210.
11. Kim MK, Kim S. Immunohistochemical profile of common epithelial neoplasms arising in the kidney. Appl Immunohistochem Mol Morphol 2002;10:332–338.
12. Al Nazer M, Mourad WA. Successful grading of renal-cell carcinoma in fine-needle aspirates. Diagn Cytopathol 2000;22:223–226.
13. Cajulis RS, Katz RL, Dekmezian R, et al. Fine needle aspiration biopsy of renal cell carcinoma. Cytologic parameters and their concordance with histology and flow cytometric data. Acta Cytol 1993;37:367–372.
14. Bostwick DG, Murphy GP. Diagnosis and prognosis of renal cell carcinoma: highlights from an international consensus workshop. Semin Urol Oncol 1998;16:46–52.
15. Mejean A, Hopirtean V, Bazin JP, et al. Prognostic factors for the survival of patients with papillary renal cell carcinoma: meaning of histological typing and multifocality. J Urol 2003;170:764–767.
16. Gattuso P, Ramzy I, Truong LD, et al. Utilization of fine-needle aspiration in the diagnosis of metastatic tumors to the kidney. Diagn Cytopathol 1999;21:35–38.
17. Tretiakova MS, Sahoo S, Takahashi M, et al. Expression of alpha-methylacyl-CoA racemase in papillary renal cell carcinoma. Am J Surg Pathol 2004;28:69–76.
18. Ro JY, Ayala AG, Sella A, et al. Sarcomatoid renal cell carcinoma: clinicopathologic. A study of 42 cases. Cancer 1987;59:516–526.
19. Auger M, Katz RL, Sella A, et al. Fine-needle aspiration cytology of sarcomatoid renal cell carcinoma: a morphologic and immunocytochemical study of 15 cases. Diagn Cytopathol 1993;9:46–51.
20. Layfield LJ. Fine-needle aspiration biopsy of renal collecting duct carcinoma. Diagn Cytopathol 1994;11:74–78.
21. Assad L, Resetkova E, Oliveira VL, et al. Cytologic features of renal medullary carcinoma. Cancer 2005;1051:28–34.
22. Caraway NP, Wojcik EM, Katz RL, et al. Cytologic findings of collecting duct carcinoma of the kidney. Diagn Cytopathol 1995;13:304–309.
23. Ono K, Nishino E, Nakamine H. Renal collecting duct carcinoma. Report of a case with cytologic findings on fine needle aspiration. Acta Cytol 2000;44:380–384.
24. Ruteshouser EC, Hendrickson BW, Colella S, et al. Genome-wide loss of heterozygosity analysis of WT1-wild-type and WT1-mutant Wilms tumors. Genes Chromosomes Cancer 2005;43:172–180.
25. Swartz MA, Karth J, Schneider DT, et al. Renal medullary carcinoma: clinical, pathologic, immunohistochemical, and genetic analysis with pathogenetic implications. Urology 2002;60:1083–1089.

8

TUMORS AND TUMOR-LIKE CONDITIONS OF THE KIDNEY

Satish K. Tickoo and Mahul B. Amin

BENIGN EPITHELIAL NEOPLASMS

RENAL ONCOCYTOMA

Renal oncocytoma is the most common benign renal tumor for which planned nephrectomy is performed, and comprises about 3–7% of all primary renal neoplasms.[1–5] It shows a wide age distribution at presentation, with a peak incidence in the seventh decade of life. Males are affected nearly twice as often as females. The majority of cases are asymptomatic; most are discovered during the work-up of unrelated conditions. A minority present with hematuria, flank pain, or a palpable mass.

Cytogenetics

The most frequently reported genetic changes are the loss of chromosomes 1 and Y (Table 8.1). Less commonly, translocations t(9;11)(p23;q13) and t(5;11)(q35;q13) have been reported.[6–10] Few familial cases have been described, some of which are now considered to be examples of Birt–Hogg–Dubé syndrome (see below).

Immunohistochemistry

Oncocytomas are usually positive for cytokeratin, epithelial membrane antigen (EMA), antimitochondrial antibody, and parvalbumin, but are negative for vimentin. Stains for CD10 and renal cell carcinoma (RCC) antibody are also usually negative (Table 8.2).

Ultrastructure

By ultrastructural examination, renal oncocytoma is characterized by cells containing numerous mitochondria with lamellar cristae. Other cytoplasmic organelles are sparse and unremarkable.[11,12]

Differential diagnosis

The differential diagnosis of oncocytoma includes any renal neoplasm with granular eosinophilic cytoplasm, including the eosinophilic variant of chromophobe RCC, eosinophilic variant of clear cell (conventional) RCC, papillary renal cell carcinoma (PRCC) with abundant granular cytoplasm, rare cases of (oncocytoma-like) angiomyolipoma, and rare (oncocytoma-like) RCCs, unclassified (Table 8.3). Careful attention to the architectural and cytologic features allows for the correct classification on routine hematoxylin–eosin (H&E)-stained sections in the vast majority of cases.

While renal oncocytoma has uniform, round nuclei with evenly dispersed chromatin and usually with central

Table 8.1 Diagnostic cytogenetic/molecular features of common renal tumors

Tumor	Features
Clear cell RCC	Loss of 3p Mutations/hypermethylations of *VHL* gene
Papillary RCC	Trisomies 7 and 17; loss of chromosome Y *MET* mutations in familial and some sporadic cases Additional aberrations including gains of 3q, 8p, 12q, 16q, and 20q
Chromophobe RCC	Hypodiploidy, losses of chromosomes 1, Y, 6, 10, 13, 17, 21
Renal oncocytoma	Losses of chromosomes 1 and Y t(9;11)(p23;q13), t(5;11)(q35;q13)
Collecting duct carcinoma	Monosomies 1, 6, 14, 15, 22; loss of heterozygosity 1q; minimal deletion at 1q32.1–32.2
Carcinoma with Xp11 chromosomal aberrations	t(X;1)(p11.2;q21) or t(X;17)(p11.2;q25)
Mucinous tubular and spindle cell carcinoma	Losses at chromosomes 1, 4q, 6, 8p, 11q, 13, 14, 15; gains at chromosomes 11q, 16q, 17, 20q
Angiomyolipoma	*TSC1* and *TSC2* gene inactivation, frequent in cases with tuberous sclerosis, but also in some sporadic angiomyolipomas
Wilms' tumor	Deletions of *WT1* in WAGR syndrome and point mutations *WT1* in Denys–Drash syndrome; *WT2* gene involvement in Beckwith–Wiedemann syndrome; no consistent abnormalities in sporadic cases; *p53* mutations in Wilms' tumor with anaplasia
Mesoblastic nephroma	t(12;15)(p13;q25) and *ETV6–NTRK3* gene fusion – only in cellular variant
Rhabdoid tumor of the kidney	Inactivation of *hSNF5/INI1* gene on chromosome 22
Metanephric adenoma	2p losses (? trisomies 7 and 17; ? losses of sex chromosomes)

RCC, renal cell carcinoma; WAGR, Wilms' tumor, aniridia, genitourinary abnormalities, and mental retardation.

Table 8.2 Immunohistochemical staining in the differential diagnosis of renal tumors

Antibody	*Clear cell RCC*	*Papillary RCC*	*Chromophobe RCC*	*Collecting duct carcinoma*	*Renal oncocytoma*	*AML*
CD10	+ (membranous)	+ (membranous)	+/– (cytoplasmic, if positive)	–/+	+/– (cytoplasmic, if positive)	ND
RCC	+ (membranous)	+ (membranous)	+/– (membranous)	–	weak cytoplasmic, if positive	ND
Vimentin	+	+	–	ND	–	+
Antimitochondrial	+ (eosinophilic variants), diffuse, coarse	+ (eosinophilic variants), diffuse, coarse	+ coarse with peripheral accentuation	ND	+ diffuse, fine	ND
CK7	–	+	+	+/–	–	–
Parvalbumin	–/+	–/+	+	ND	+/–	ND
FHIT	–/+	+	+	ND	+	ND
HMWCK	–	–	–	+	–	–
Ulex europaeus/PNA/SBA	–	–	–	+	–	–

RCC, renal cell carcinoma; AML, angiomyolipoma; CK7, cytokeratin 7; FHIT, fragile histidine triad; HMWCK, high molecular weight cytokeratin (CK903/34βE12); PNA, peanut lectin agglutinin; SBA, soybean lectin agglutinin; ND, not done/tested.

Table 8.3 Differential diagnosis of renal oncocytoma

	Renal oncocytoma	*Chromophobe RCC (eosinophilic variant)*	*Clear cell RCC (eosinophilic variant)*	*Papillary RCC (eosinophilic variant)*	*Angiomyolipoma (oncocytoma-like)*
Gross features	Mahogany-brown, brown, or pale-tan cut surface	Usually brown cut surface	Usually brown cut surface	Usually brown cut surface Gross hemorrhage and necrosis frequent	Usually brown cut surface Yellow foci of fat, and large vessels may be identifiable
Microscopic features	Solid acinar, sheet-like, tubular, cystic architecture Cells filled with finely granular eosinophilic cytoplasm Round, uniform nuclei with frequent, uniform nucleoli	Solid sheets separated by incomplete fibrous septa, acinar, tubular architecture Hyperchromatic, raisinoid nuclei, at least focally Frequent perinuclear halos Accentuated cell borders	Solid or acinar architecture, with at least focal, intricate, arborizing, fine vasculature Granular, eosinophilic cytoplasm with large, pleomorphic (usually at least grade 3) nuclei Large, pleomorphic nucleoli	Papillary architecture Rarely areas with prominent tubular or solid acinar features, but papillary areas predominate Stromal foamy macrophages Granular, eosinophilic cytoplasm with large, pleomorphic (usually at least grade 3) nuclei	Solid or solid alveolar architecture Foci of fat and abnormal vessels may or may not be present Cells filled with finely to irregularly granular eosinophilic cytoplasm Nucleoli usually large and irregular
Antimitochondrial antibody	Positive; diffuse, finely granular	Positive; diffuse, coarsely granular with peripheral accentuation	Positive, irregularly distributed cytoplasmic	Positive, irregularly distributed cytoplasm	ND
Parvalbumin	Positive, usually focal	Positive, diffuse and strong	Negative	Usually negative but may be positive	ND
Vimentin	Negative	Negative	Positive	Positive	ND
CD10	Negative	Positive	Positive	Positive	Negative
RCC	Negative	Positive	Positive	Positive	ND
HMB45	Negative	Negative	Negative	Negative	Positive
Melan-A	Negative	Negative	Negative	Negative	Positive
CK7	Negative	Positive	Negative	Positive	Negative
Colloidal iron stain	Negative to focally (usually luminal) positive	Diffusely positive	Negative to focal droplet-like positive	Negative to focal droplet-like positive	Negative
Ultrastructure	Numerous mitochondria, most with lamellar cristae	Microvesicles, usually abundant Numerous mitochondria, with predominant tubulo-vesicular cristae	Prominent mitochondria, usually swollen and pleomorphic, with short attenuated cristae Lipid and glycogen prominent	Prominent mitochondria with variable cristae, usually lamellar Usually many phagolysosomes	ND
Genetics	–1, –Y, t(5;11), t(9;11)	Multiple monosomies	–3p, *VHL* alterations	Trisomy 7/17, –Y, in some cases Additional aberrations	ND

RCC, renal cell carcinoma; CK7, cytokeratin 7; ND, not done/tested.

nucleoli, chromophobe RCC shows, at least focally, hyperchromatic, wrinkled nuclei, many surrounded by a perinuclear halo. Rare cases may require ancillary studies (Tables 8.1–8.3). Hale's colloidal iron stain may help in distinguishing oncocytoma from chromophobe RCC, but it is a fastidious stain and requires strict adherence to proper technique.

Eosinophilic variant of clear cell (conventional) RCC usually has a high nuclear grade with prominent nucleoli, and shows more nuclear pleomorphism, as well as the intricate vasculature characteristic of clear cell RCC.

Eosinophilic variant of PRCC has a prominent papillary architecture that is not a feature of renal oncocytoma. Presence of foamy macrophages also favor PRCC.

In contrast to renal oncocytoma, the vast majority of angiomyolipomas are immunoreactive for HMB-45, smooth muscle actin, microphthalmia transcription factor, and Melan-A (A103).

Tumors with cytoarchitectural features of renal oncocytoma but showing atypical features like diffuse nuclear irregularities, easily identifiable mitotic figures, or very prominent and irregular nucleoli, should not be considered as renal oncocytoma or 'atypical oncocytoma', and must be designated as RCC, unclassified.

When the above-described diagnostic criteria are strictly adhered to, renal oncocytomas are benign neoplasms. Early reports of metastatic or 'malignant' oncocytomas include tumors that would now be classified as chromophobe or other RCCs with eosinophilic features. (Figs 8.1–8.12)

RENAL ONCOCYTOSIS

Oncocytosis is an unusual condition in which the kidney contains numerous oncocytic tumors, often together with oncocytic changes in intact cortical tubules.[13] (Figs 8.13–8.15) Birt-Hogg-Dubé syndrome (see below) is a consideration in the differential diagnosis.

PAPILLARY/TUBULOPAPILLARY (CHROMOPHIL) ADENOMA

These microscopic lesions are common findings in surgical and autopsy specimens of the kidney, and greater than 25% incidence has been reported in well-sampled specimens at autopsy. The tumor is always an incidental finding, found in kidneys removed for other clinically apparent tumors/lesions, or in kidneys examined at autopsy.

Cytogenetics

Like most PRCCs, adenomas also show trisomies of chromosomes 7 and 17, and loss of chromosome Y (in males).

Differential diagnosis

All agree that the diagnosis of adenoma is appropriate only for small tumors, but the maximum size has been controversial. As proposed in the Heidelberg and WHO/AJCC

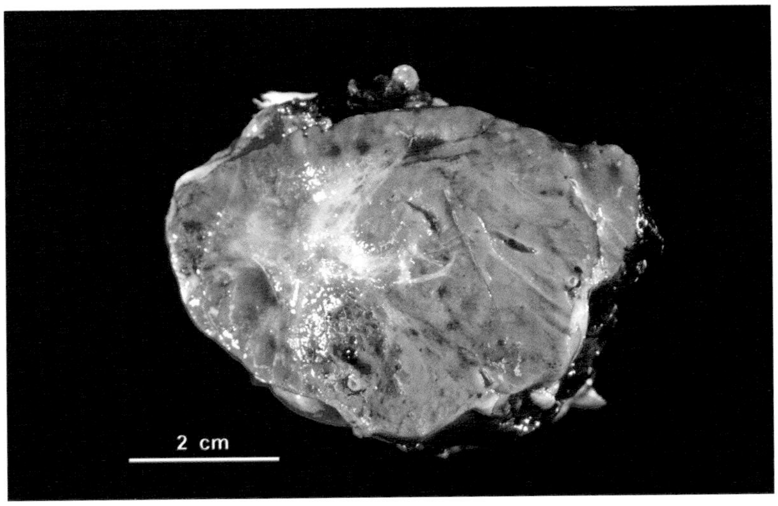

2 cm

Fig. 8.1 Oncocytoma is a well-circumscribed, non-encapsulated neoplasm, classically with a mahogany-brown cut surface. Less frequently, it may be tan to pale yellow in color. Focal hemorrhage may be present, but gross necrosis is rare. Cysts and gross extension into perinephric adipose tissue may be seen, but are unusual.

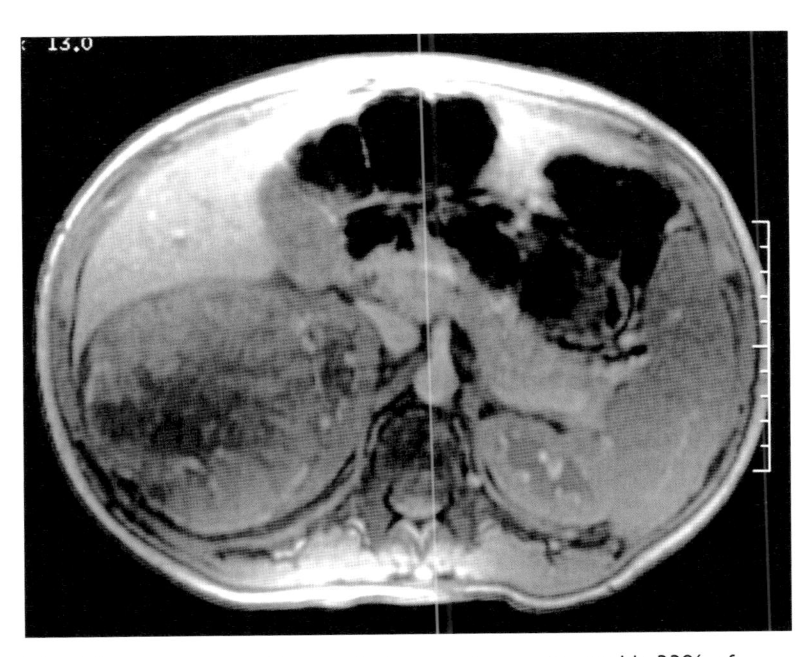

Fig. 8.2 A central, stellate, radiating scar is seen in roughly 33% of renal oncocytomas. The scar is generally present in tumors of large size. However, similar scars may also be seen in other low-grade tumors, such as low-grade clear cell (conventional) renal cell carcinoma and chromophobe renal cell carcinoma. Tumors are multifocal in up to 15% of the cases and bilateral in 4%.[1–5]

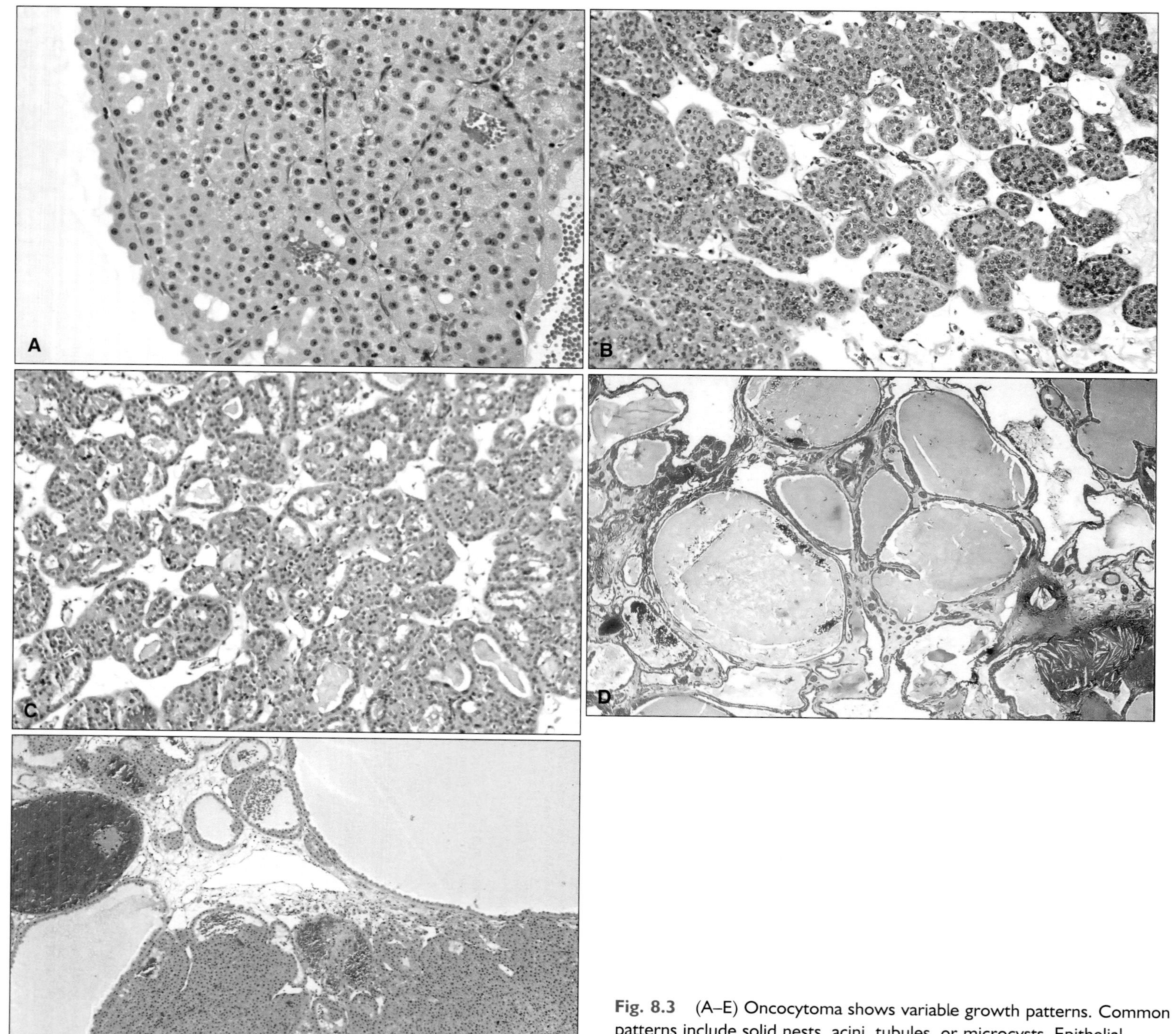

Fig. 8.3 (A–E) Oncocytoma shows variable growth patterns. Common patterns include solid nests, acini, tubules, or microcysts. Epithelial elements are embedded within a hypocellular hyalinized or myxoid stroma. Most tumors contain a variety of architectural patterns.

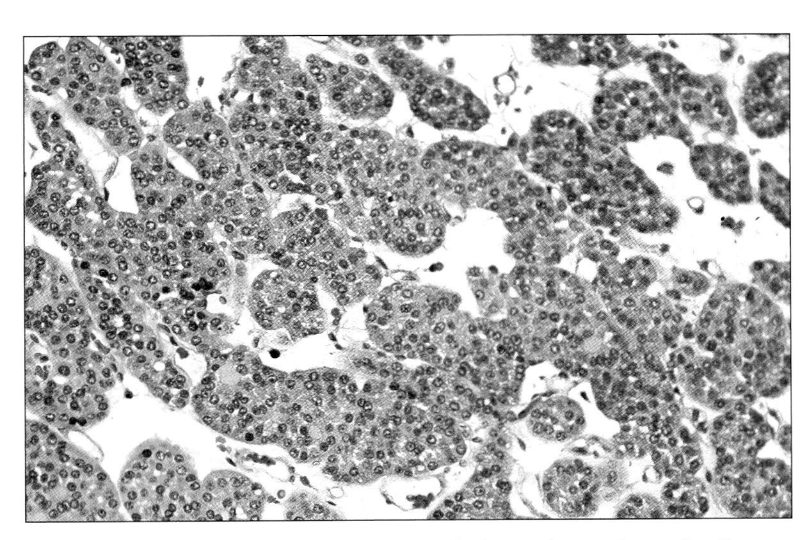

Fig. 8.4 Renal oncocytoma is composed of round to polygonal cells with finely granular eosinophilic cytoplasm. Nuclei are central, round, and uniform, with evenly dispersed chromatin, and often a central nucleolus.

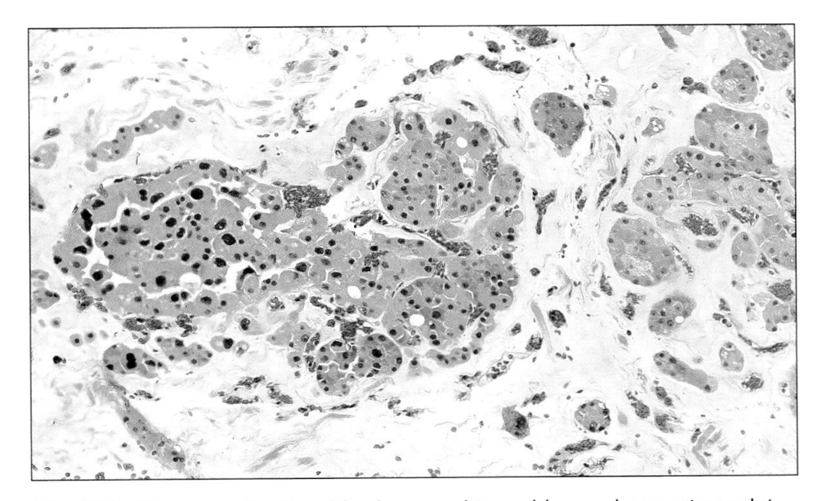

Fig. 8.5 Clusters of cells with pleomorphic and hyperchromatic nuclei are seen in many renal oncocytomas, and usually represent degenerative changes. Such cells do not show mitotic activity, and are almost always negative for immunohistochemical proliferation markers, such as MIB-1.

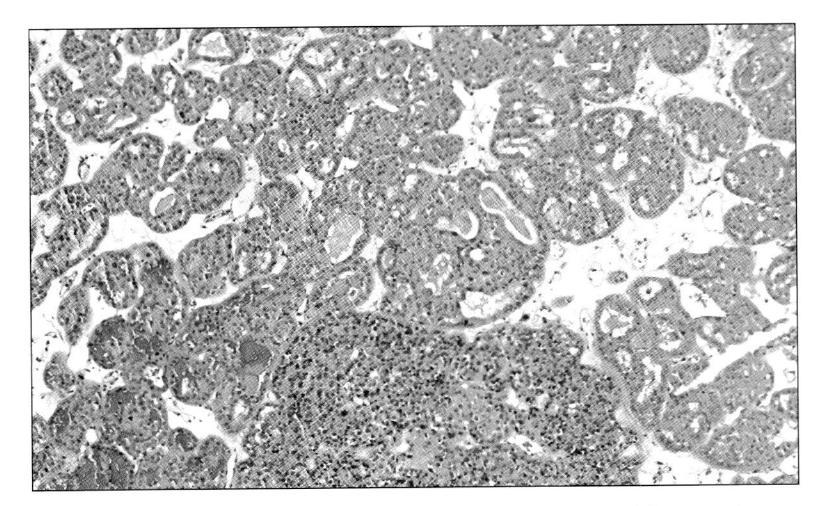

Fig. 8.6 A smaller population of cells with scant eosinophilic cytoplasm, a high nuclear:cytoplasmic ratio, and resultant darker appearance (so-called oncoblasts) are also common in oncocytomas. Mitotic activity is rare; if easily identifiable mitoses are observed, other diagnoses should be considered. Atypical mitotic figures are not seen; necrosis is uncommon.

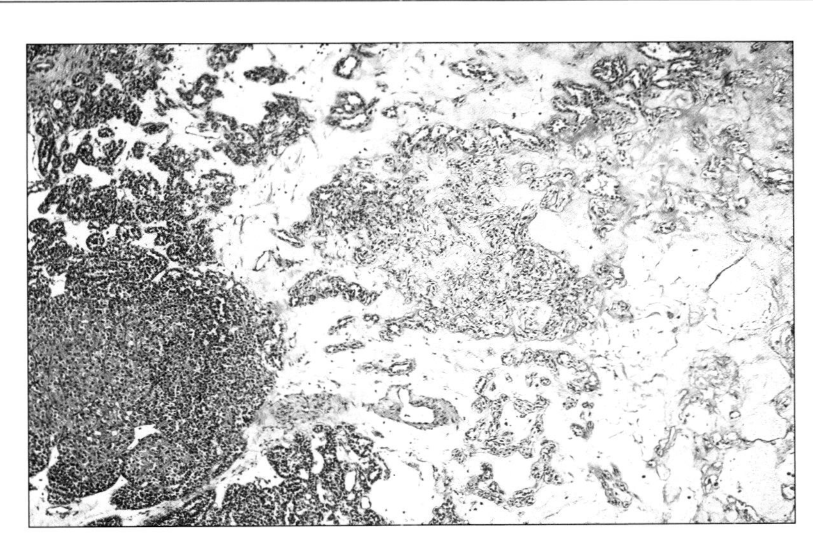

Fig. 8.7 Focal clear cell change may be present in renal oncocytoma, usually in areas of stromal hyalinization.

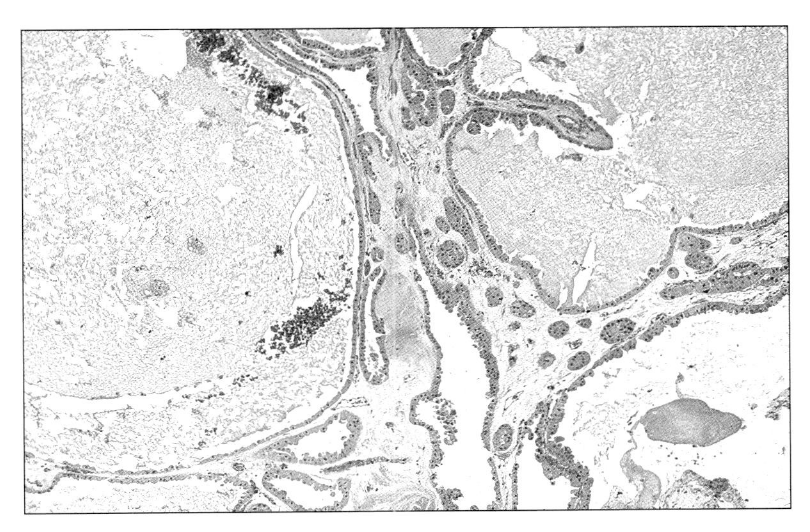

Fig. 8.8 Focal intratubular epithelial tufts or small papillations may be present, but extensive papillary architecture is not a feature of renal oncocytoma.

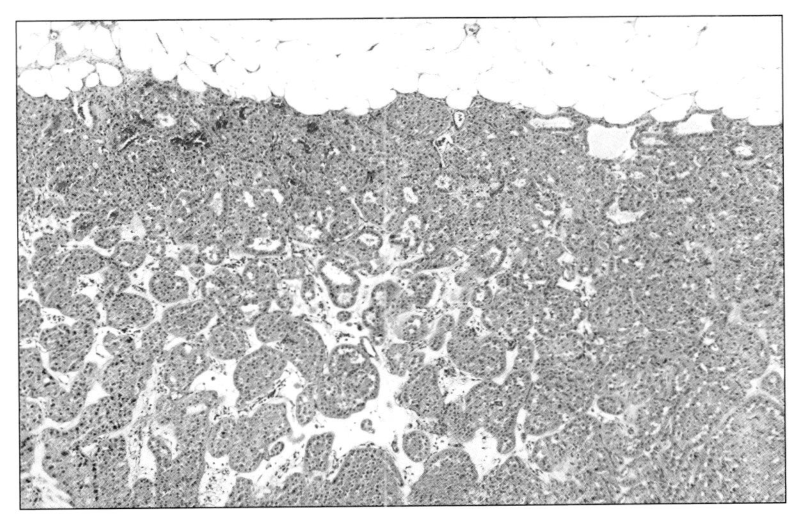

Fig. 8.9 Extension into perinephric adipose tissue is seen in up to 20% of renal oncocytomas. Generally, no desmoplastic or fibrous response is present around such foci.

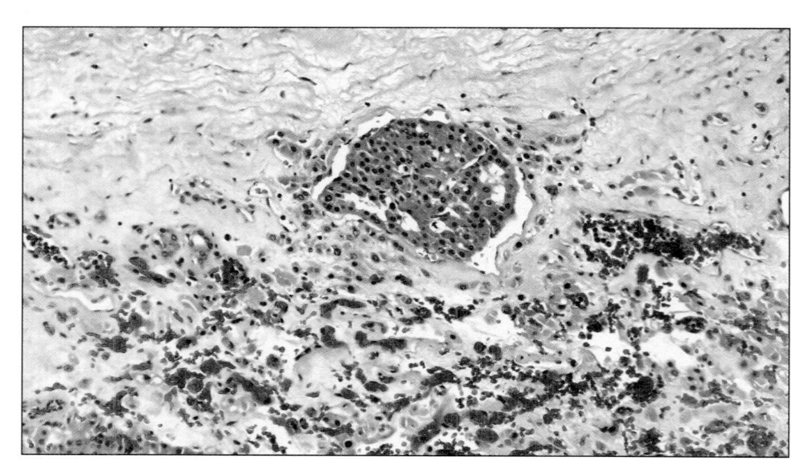

Fig. 8.10 Small vessel invasion may be occasionally seen in renal oncocytoma; invasion into larger vascular channels is extremely uncommon. In the presence of other classical features, perinephric tumor extension and vascular invasion are acceptable as rare features of renal oncocytoma. Nuclear grading and tumor staging in renal oncocytoma is of no clinical use, as these are benign tumors.

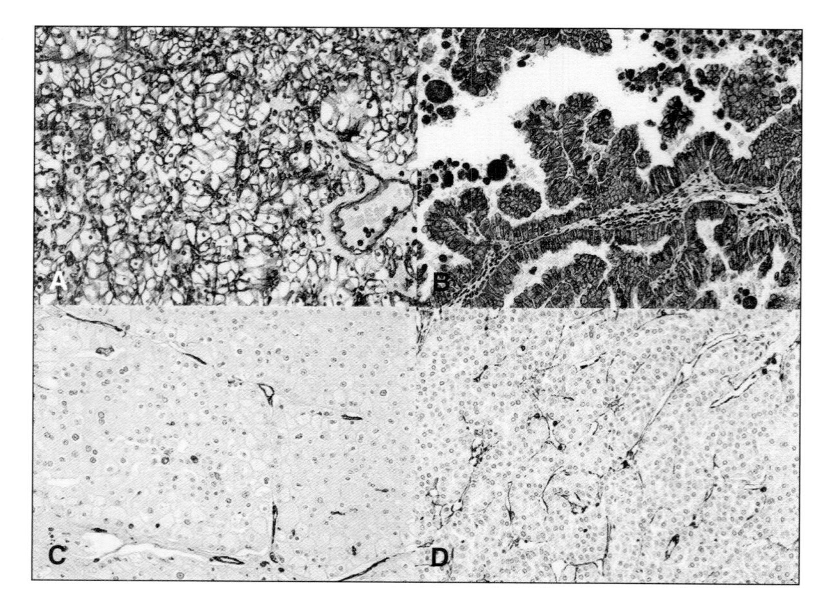

Fig. 8.11 Immunostaining for vimentin in common renal epithelial neoplasms: (A) clear cell (conventional) renal cell carcinoma (RCC), (B) papillary RCC, (C) chromophobe RCC, and (D) renal oncocytoma.

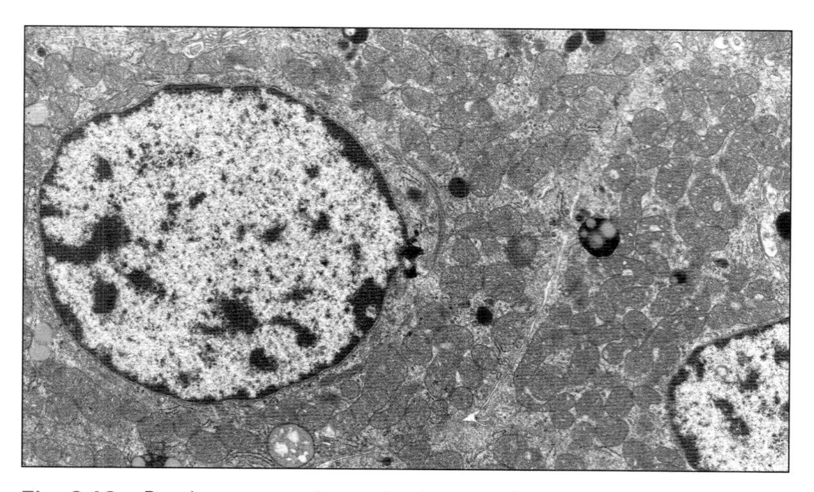

Fig. 8.12 By ultrastructural examination, renal oncocytoma is characterized by cells containing numerous mitochondria with lamellar cristae. Other cytoplasmic organelles are sparse and unremarkable.[11,12]

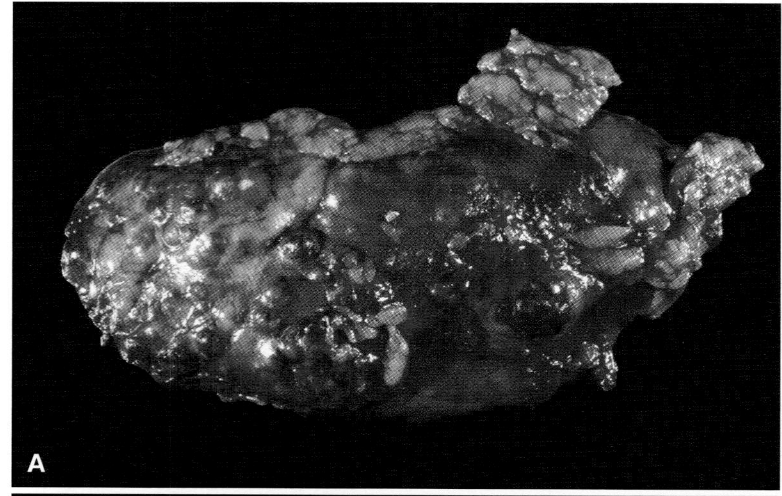

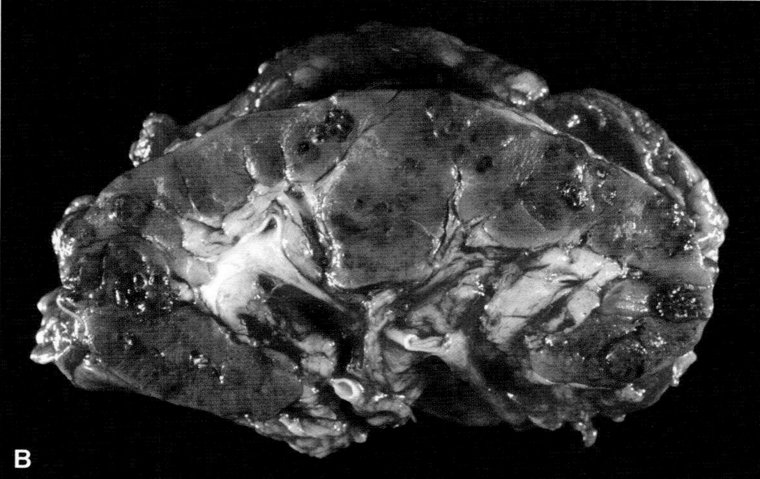

Fig. 8.13 The external (A) and cut (B) surface of a kidney affected by oncocytosis is studded with numerous tumor nodules that have gross features similar to those of renal oncocytoma.

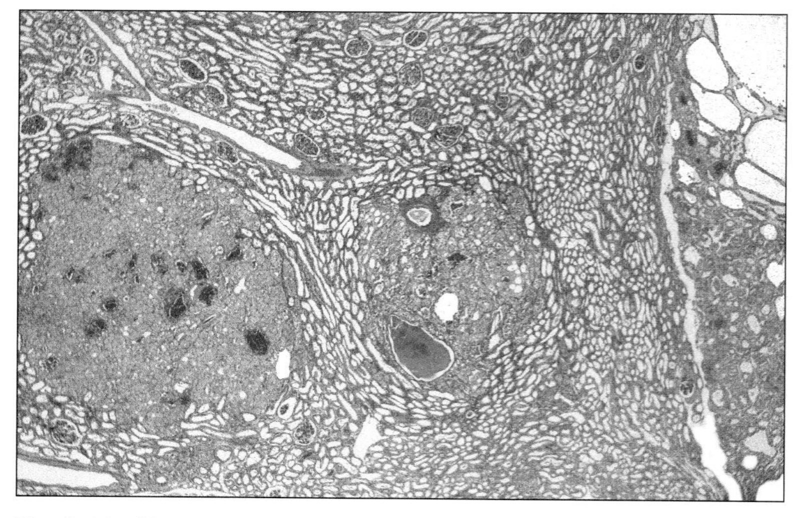

Fig. 8.14 Microscopic features of renal oncocytosis include extreme multifocality, oncocytic change in benign tubules, microcysts lined by oncocytic cells, and neoplastic oncocytes infiltrating between benign tubules.[13] In this image, three microscopic oncocytic nodules are present in this single field.

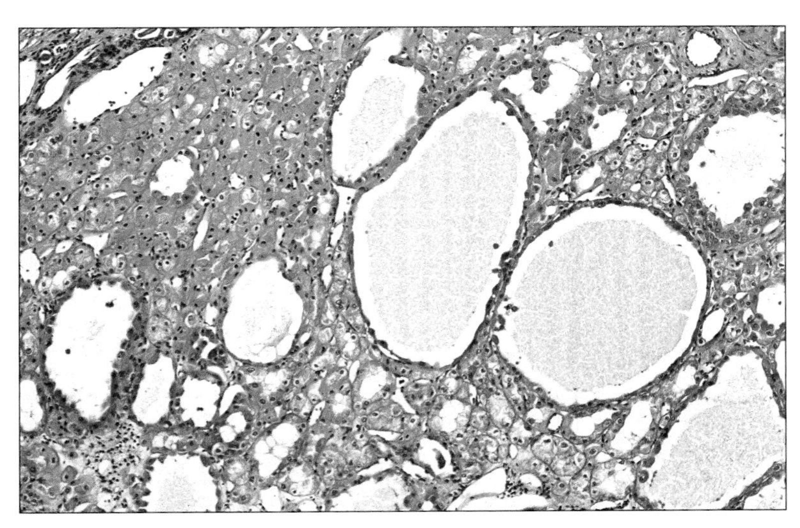

Fig. 8.15 While most of the nodules in renal oncocytosis resemble typical renal oncocytoma on microscopic evaluation, some have hybrid features of renal oncocytoma (lower left), with round, uniform nuclei, and chromophobe renal cell carcinoma (right), with nuclear irregularities and perinuclear halos. Until the clinical behavior of such hybrid tumors has been better defined, it is best to regard them as low-grade malignant neoplasms like pure chromophobe renal cell carcinoma.

consensus classifications, most pathologists now accept 5 mm as the upper limit for the size.[14,15] By definition, the presence of any clear cell carcinoma features, even in a lesion smaller than 5 mm, excludes it from the category of adenoma, although no studies indicate malignant behavior in such small clear cell tumors. (Fig. 8.16)

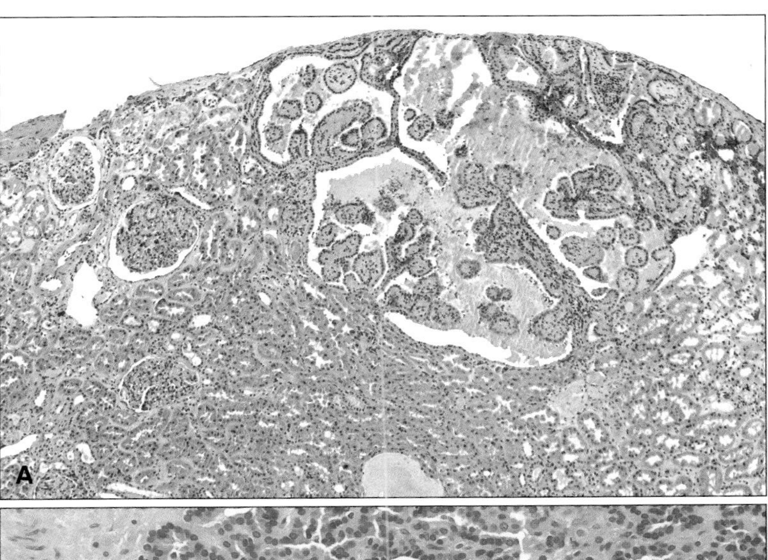

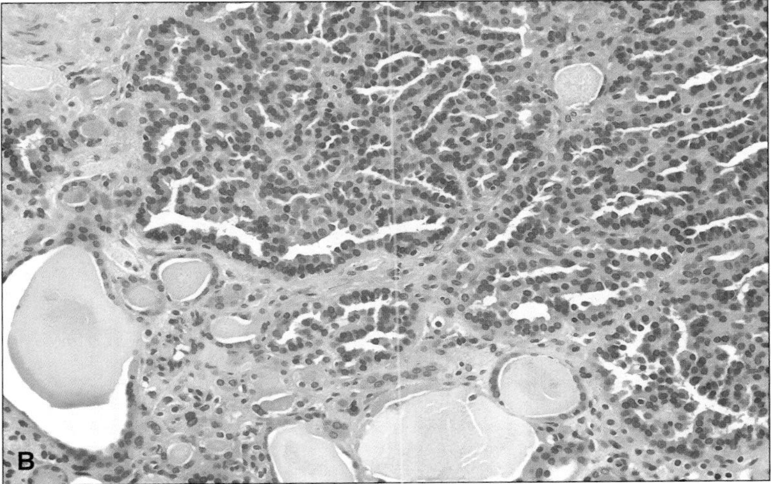

Fig. 8.16 Tubulopapillary adenoma, usually an incidental, small (less than 5 mm) lesion, may show either (A) papillary or (B) tubulopapillary architecture and low nuclear grade. Presence of clear cell features excludes a lesion from this category.

METANEPHRIC ADENOMA, METANEPHRIC ADENOFIBROMA, AND METANEPHRIC STROMAL TUMOR

Metanephric adenoma, and the closely related metanephric adenofibroma and metanephric stromal tumor, are recently characterized benign renal cortical neoplasms.[16–21] Affected patients are in the first through ninth decades of life, with a female-to-male ratio of 2 : 1. Presenting signs and symptoms are similar to those of other renal mass lesions; but polycythemia has been reported in approximately 12% of the patients.

Cytogenetics

Cytogenetic studies have shown variable results, including normal karyotypes, trisomies of chromosomes 7 and 17 and loss of sex chromosomes, and more recently 2p losses.[19,22–25]

Immunohistochemistry

The epithelial components of metanephric adenoma and adenofibroma are positive for pan-cytokeratin. Positive reactions with EMA are uncommon and usually confined to papillary/cystic areas. The stromal component in each is positive for vimentin, and is CD34-positive in metanephric stromal tumor.

Ultrastructure

Electron microscopy shows variable numbers of microvilli and few cytoplasmic organelles consisting mainly of free ribosomes and mitochondria in the epithelial components.

Differential diagnosis

Wilms' tumor and papillary renal carcinoma are important considerations in the differential diagnosis. In contrast to Wilms' tumor, metanephric adenoma shows minimal mitotic activity, and is composed of bland cells with small nuclei. No blastemal elements or nephrogenic rests are present. Distinguishing some cases of PRCC from metanephric adenoma may pose a more difficult diagnostic challenge. Unlike metanephric adenoma, PRCC frequently contains numerous foamy histiocytes, and is multifocal in up to half of cases. Nuclear atypia, prominent nucleoli, and a well-formed capsule are not the features of metanephric adenoma. Metanephric stromal tumor may be confused with clear cell sarcoma, but the characteristic vascular pattern of the latter, and the typical morphologic features of the former, should help in this differentiation. (Figs 8.17–8.21)

RENAL CELL CARCINOMA

The majority of renal tumors are of epithelial origin and most are malignant. Until about a decade ago, renal carcinomas were broadly classified as clear cell, granular cell, and sarcomatoid carcinoma. Recent studies have resulted in a better understanding of the clinicopathologic spectrum of these tumors. The resultant current classification of renal tumors (Table 8.4) is clinically highly relevant. This classification also is further validated by numerous cytogenetic and molecular studies.[26–32] As a result of our newly found knowledge about these tumors and their more accurate classification, much of the old literature on 'renal carcinomas' has become obsolete, especially that which deals with clear cell, granular cell, or sarcomatoid tumors. All of these groups, as we understand now, include a mixture of entities with diverse natural histories.

RCC accounts for approximately 2% of all cancers.[33] Its incidence varies among countries, with the highest rates in North America and Scandinavia.[34] It occurs twice

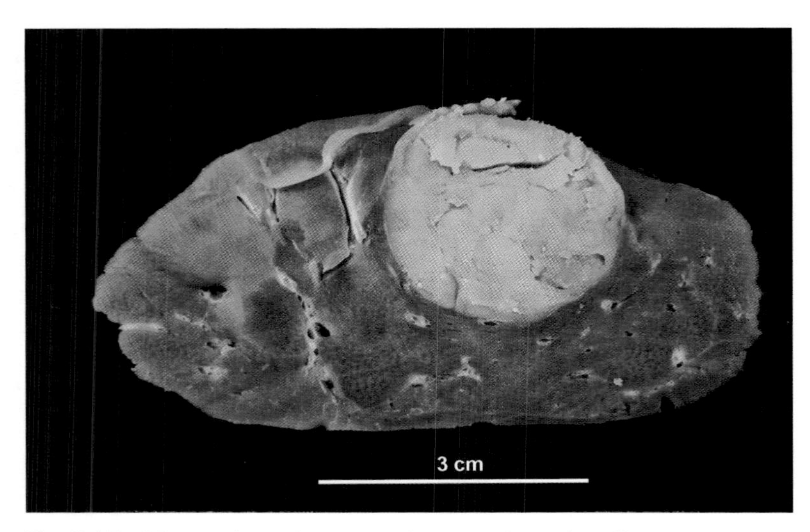

Fig. 8.17 Metanephric adenoma and metanephric adenofibroma are well-circumscribed cortical neoplasms, usually unencapsulated but sharply demarcated from the surrounding renal parenchyma. They are solid, range from tan to yellow, and often show areas of necrosis, hemorrhage, hyalinization, and cystic degeneration. Calcifications may be apparent grossly. Multifocal tumors are rare and bilateral tumors have not been reported.

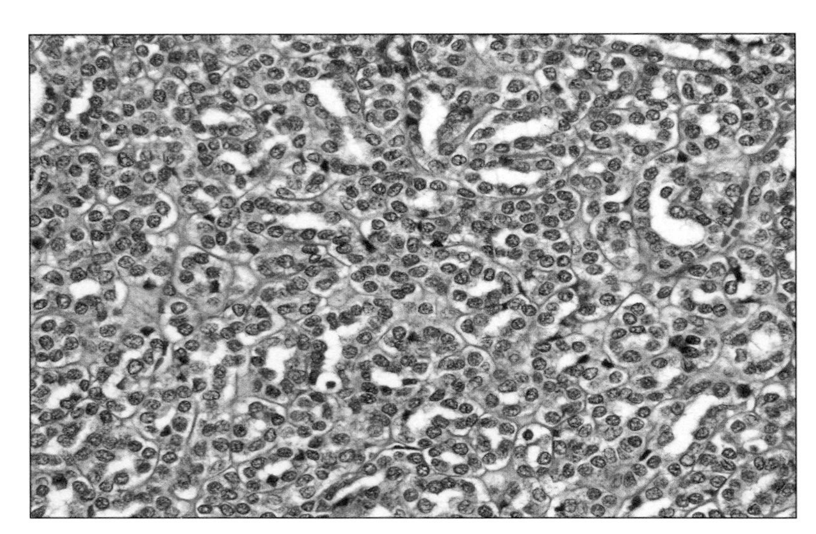

Fig. 8.19 Metanephric adenoma is characterized by tightly packed small tubules separated by a modest amount of stroma. Cytoplasm is scant. Nuclei are small, round to ovoid, and often overlap. Nucleoli are typically inconspicuous, and mitotic figures are rare.

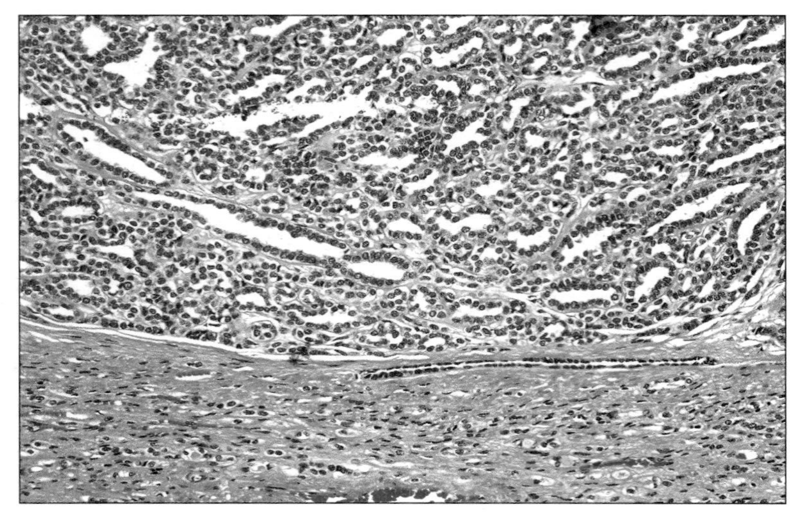

Fig. 8.18 Metanephric adenoma shows clear demarcation from the surrounding renal parenchyma, without a distinct capsule.

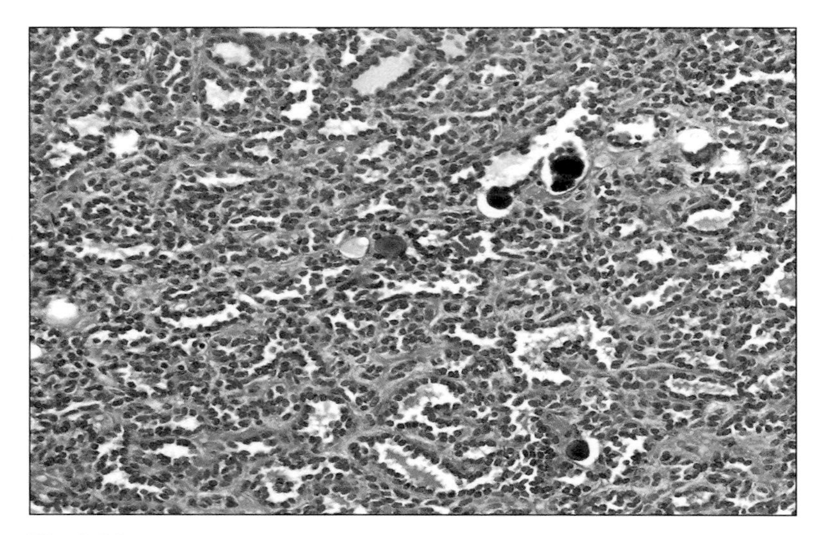

Fig. 8.20 Papillary or glomeruloid components are seen in roughly half of metanephric adenomas and are often associated with microcalcifications, including psammoma bodies.

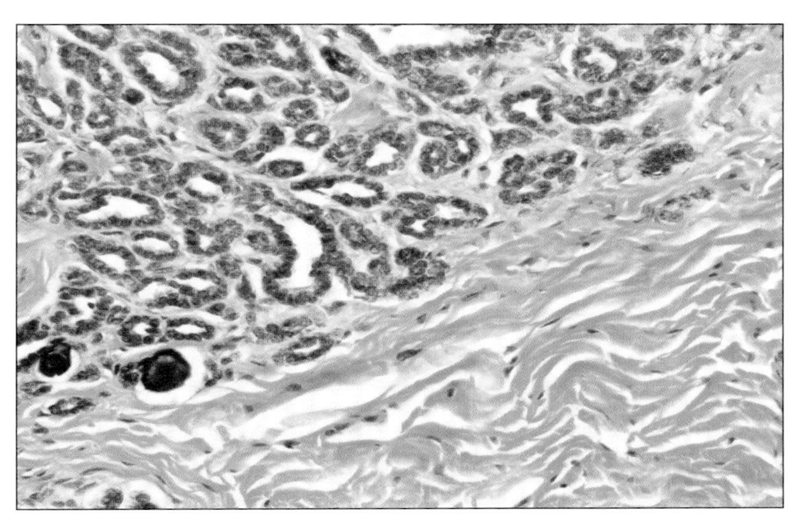

Fig. 8.21 Metanephric adenofibroma is a biphasic neoplasm with an epithelial component identical to metanephric adenoma and a mesenchymal component of bland fibroblast-like cells in interlacing fascicles with focal hyalinization and myxoid change.[22] Metanephric stromal tumor is histologically identical to the stromal component of metanephric adenofibroma. It is an unencapsulated spindle cell lesion with alternating high and low cellularity, onion-skin cuffing around entrapped renal tubules, heterologous differentiation (glial or cartilaginous), and vascular alterations (including angiodysplasia).[16]

as frequently in men as in women. In 2002, approximately 32 000 new cases of kidney cancer were diagnosed in the USA, with close to 12 000 deaths reported. The disease resulted in more than 91 000 deaths worldwide in the year 2000.[35] RCC may occur at any age, with peak incidence in the sixth and seventh decades of life. The incidence has increased substantially over the last two decades, undoubtedly at least in part due to improved diagnostic techniques.

Fuhrman's nuclear grading system remains the most popular and clinically useful grading system for renal carcinoma, although many grading schemes have been proposed.[36,37] Tumors are graded from grade 1 to 4, according to nuclear size and shape, and nucleolar prominence. Tumor is classified according to the highest nuclear grade present, even when focal.

For practical purposes, if nucleoli are not apparent at low magnification (×100), the tumor is either grade 1 or 2; easily identifiable nucleoli at this magnification correspond to grade 3 or 4 tumors. If nucleoli are easily identified at high magnification (×400), it is a grade 2 tumor, and if not, the tumor is best classified as a grade 1 tumor. Marked nuclear pleomorphism separates grade 4 from grade 3 tumors (see Figs 8.26–8.28).

Although nuclear grading of chromophobe and papillary RCCs has been used by some authors,[38,39] in our experience it is of limited or no use in chromophobe RCC, and its clinical utility in PRCC, at best, remains controversial. Grading is most useful in clear cell (conventional) and the other subtypes of RCC.

The tumor, nodes, metastases (TNM) staging proposed by Union Internationale Contre le Cancer/American Joint Committee on Cancer (UICC/AJCC) (most recently modified in 2002)[40] is widely used for staging of renal cancers

Table 8.4 Classification of renal neoplasms (non-urothelial) and tumor-like conditions

Renal epithelial tumors
Benign
Renal oncocytoma
Papillary/tubulopapillary adenoma
Metanephric adenoma
Metanephric adenofibroma
Malignant
Clear cell (conventional) renal cell carcinoma
Papillary renal cell carcinoma
Chromophobe renal cell carcinoma
Collecting duct carcinoma
Medullary carcinoma
Mucinous tubular and spindle cell carcinoma
Carcinomas associated with Xp11 chromosomal aberrations
Renal cell carcinoma, unclassified
Tumor of undetermined malignant potential
Multilocular cystic renal cell carcinoma
Non-epithelial tumors
Benign
Angiomyolipoma
Renomedullary interstitial cell tumor (medullary fibroma)
Juxtaglomerular cell tumor
Metanephric stromal tumor
Solitary fibrous tumor
Leiomyoma
Hemangioma
Lymphangioma
Lipoma
Malignant
Leiomyosarcoma
Rhabdosarcoma
Synovial sarcoma
Liposarcoma
Others
Mixed epithelial and stromal tumors
Mixed epithelial and stromal tumor
Cystic nephroma
Miscellaneous tumors
Carcinoid tumor
Primitive neuroectodermal tumor
Small cell carcinoma
Metastatic tumors
Hematopoeitic tumors
Pediatric tumors
Wilms' tumor (nephroblastoma)
Nephrogenic rests and nephroblastomatosis
Cystic partially differentiated nephroblastoma
Cystic nephroma
Mesoblastic nephroma
Clear cell sarcoma
Rhabdoid tumor
Ossifying renal tumor
Tumor-like conditions
Xanthogranulomatous pyelonephritis
Tuberculosis
Malakoplakia
Renal abscess

Table 8.5 TNM staging of renal tumors

Primary tumor (T)	
T1a:	4 cm or less, organ-confined
T1b:	>4 to 7 cm, organ-confined
T2:	more than 7 cm, organ-confined
T3a:	direct invasion into perinephric fat, including renal sinus fat, or adrenal gland, but confined within Gerota's fascia
T3b:	gross tumor in renal vein(s), its segmental (muscle-containing) branches, or vena cava below diaphragm
T3c:	gross tumor in vena cava above diaphragm, or invading the wall of vena cava
T4:	tumor beyond Gerota's fascia
Regional lymph nodes (N)	
NX:	regional nodes cannot be assessed
N0:	no regional node metastasis
N1:	metastasis in a single node
N2:	metastasis in more than one regional node
Comments:	Laterality does not affect N classification.
	If a lymph node dissection is performed, there should be at least eight nodes for pathologic evaluation
Distant metastasis (M)	
MX:	distant metastasis cannot be assessed
M0:	no distant metastasis
M1:	distant metastasis

(Table 8.5). The changes in the current compared with the previous staging are:

- pT1 tumors are divided into pT1a (up to 4 cm in size) and pT1b (>4 to 7 cm in size);
- stage pT3a includes tumors invading into renal sinus fat;
- stage pT3b includes tumors with gross involvement of segmental (muscle-containing) 'branches' of renal vein;
- stage pT3c includes tumors invading the wall of vena cava.

CLEAR CELL (CONVENTIONAL) RENAL CELL CARCINOMA

Clear cell (conventional) RCC comprises approximately 60–65% of renal epithelial neoplasms.[5,41] Males are affected more commonly than females, in a ratio of 1.7–2.0 to 1. Age at presentation ranges from 34 to 90 years, with a mean of 61 years. Only occasional cases are reported in children and young adults.[41] In sporadic disease, both kidneys are affected equally and most tumors are solitary. Bilateral disease is seen in 3.5% of cases, and multifocality in approximately 11%.[5,41] Hereditary clear cell RCC tends to arise at an earlier age, and is more likely to be bilateral and multifocal.

The most common symptoms at the time of presentation are hematuria, abdominal pain, and a palpable mass, although the combination of all three features ('classic triad') occurs in less than 10% of cases. Other nonspecific signs and symptoms include fever, night sweats, general malaise, and weight loss. Currently, 50% or more of cases are asymptomatic, incidental findings, detected using modern imaging techniques (see Fig. 8.25).[42–45]

Disease-free and overall survival correlates with grade and stage. The overall 5- and 10-year disease-specific survival rates are approximately 76% and 70% respectively.[5,41] Survival in cases presenting with metastatic disease is dismal. Effective systemic therapy remains elusive, making surgical resection the best chance for cure.

Cytogenetics and molecular biology

Clearcell RCC is characterized by the loss of genetic material from the short arm of chromosome 3 (3p) and mutations in the *VHL* gene. In patients with von Hippel–Lindau disease, such losses and mutations are described in virtually all cases.[26–32,46–49] Somatic mutations/hypermethylations in the same region can be found in 75–80% of the more common sporadic tumors, too (see Table 8.1).[50]

Immunohistochemistry

Clear cell RCCs, particularly of lower grade, usually show strong membrane-predominant immunoreactivity with antibodies to cytokeratin, EMA, CD10 (see Fig. 8.40), RCC antigen, and vimentin (Table 8.2). Stains for parvalbumin are usually negative.

Ultrastucture

Tumor cells with clear cytology contain abundant glycogen and lipid, with few mitochondria and sparse endoplasmic reticulum. Eosinophilic cells tend to have relatively less glycogen and lipid but numerous mitochondria, prominent Golgi apparatus, and prominent endoplasmic reticulum. The mitochondria are pleomorphic, generally swollen, and with short attenuated cristae. Both types of cell show pinocytotic vesicles at the cell membranes and numerous luminal microvilli.

Differential diagnosis

Adequate sampling and understanding of the morphologic diversity in clear cell (conventional) RCC should minimize errors in classification. Some tumors may be confused with papillary or chromophobe RCCs, although thorough microscopic examination should reveal areas with classic histologic features.

In most cases of clear cell (conventional) RCC with papillary growth, this pattern is, at the most, focal. Histiocytes are unlikely to be present within the fibrovascular 'stalk' in these papillary/pseudopapillary areas, and intracellular hemosiderin deposition is absent. Rare cases of PRCC may have prominent clear cell cytology. However, the predominant papillary architecture and fibrous encapsulation are usually keys to the correct diagnosis. Immunohistochemical staining for cytokeratin 7 (CK7) may also help, as papillary carcinomas usually express CK7 whereas conventional tumors do not.

Chromophobe RCC has characteristic nuclear and cytoplasmic features that are rarely (and only focally) seen in clear cell tumors. Rarely, clear cell RCC may have very prominent cell borders, raising the differential diagnostic possibility of a chromophobe RCC. Areas with classic clear cell features, including clear and not bubbly cytoplasm and the intricate, arborizing vasculature, are the key to the diagnosis. Diffuse cytoplasmic positivity for Hale's colloidal iron is a hallmark of chromophobe tumors. Electron microscopy is a more reliable means to resolve the differential diagnosis. Cytogenetics and molecular genetics, if available, can resolve the difficulties of classification in the more problematic cases.

Epithelioid variants of angiomyolipomas can be readily mistaken for a clear cell (conventional) RCC. Unlike clear cell carcinomas, such tumors are not usually organized in nests, but in sheets, and may show focal presence of fat. Close attention to morphologic features, immunohistochemistry, electron microscopy, and even cytogenetic properties can help in correct diagnosis. Clear cell (conventional) RCC is usually immunoreactive for cytokeratin CAM 5.2, as well as EMA, whereas angiomyolipoma is not. Also, angiomyolipoma stains for HMB-45, Melan-A (A103), and smooth muscle actin.

Some poorly differentiated clear cell RCCs may raise the suspicion of metastatic tumors. Knowledge of the patient's prior medical history will help.

Adrenocortical carcinoma enter the differential diagnosis, particularly in tumors of the upper pole. Adrenocortical tumors are not immunoreactive for EMA and are rarely positive for cytokeratins; they also express inhibin and Melan-A (A103). (Figs 8.22–8.41)

MULTILOCULAR CYSTIC RENAL CELL CARCINOMA

Multilocular cystic RCC is a rare variant of clear cell (conventional) renal carcinoma, constituting between 3% and 6% of clear cell RCCs. The mean age at presentation is 51 years. None of the reported cases has progressed.[51–55]

Differential diagnosis

The differential diagnosis includes cystic nephroma and extensively cystic clear cell (conventional) RCC.

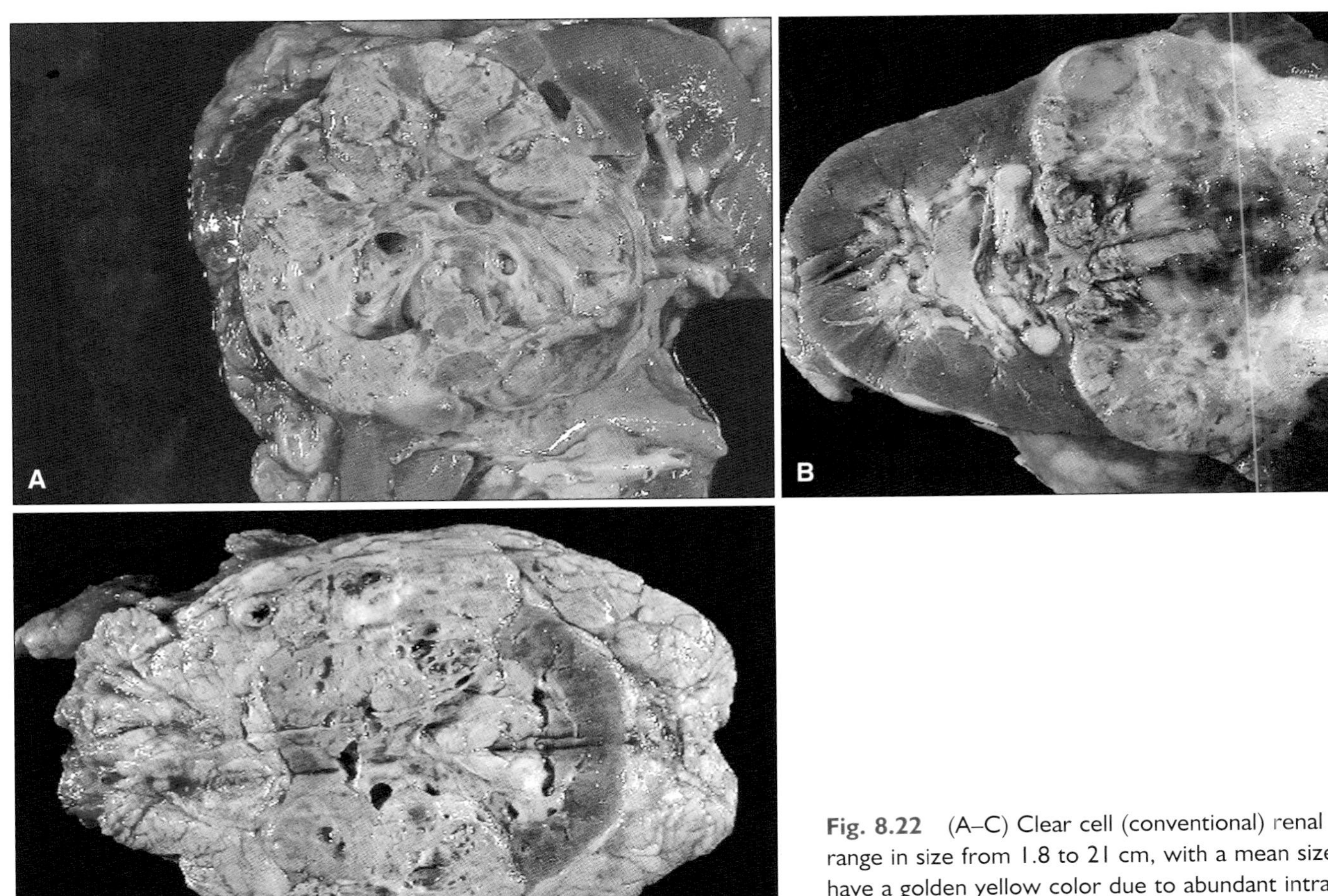

Fig. 8.22 (A–C) Clear cell (conventional) renal cell carcinoma. Tumors range in size from 1.8 to 21 cm, with a mean size of 7.1 cm. Classic cases have a golden yellow color due to abundant intracytoplasmic lipid. Higher grade tumors contain less lipid and have a more varied appearance. (Courtesy of Dr Victor E. Reuter, Memorial Sloan-Kettering Cancer Center, New York.)

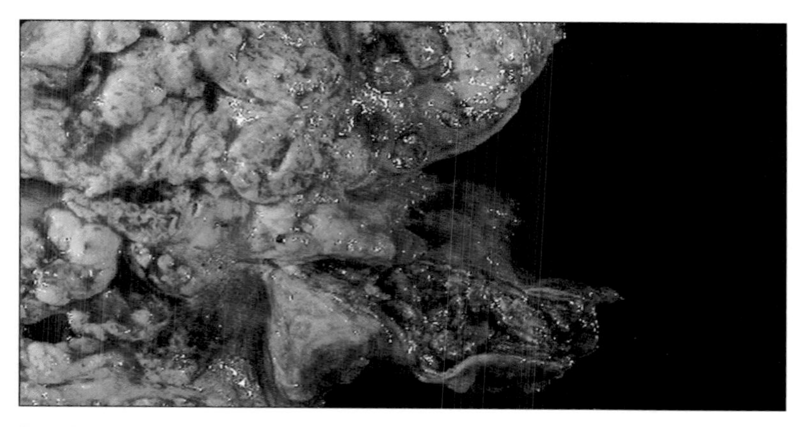

Fig. 8.23 Gross renal vein invasion is identified in approximately 30% of clear cell (conventional) renal cell carcinomas. Approximately half of the cases present with disease extending outside the kidney (pT3 or higher). However, modern imaging techniques and early detection have brought about a significant stage migration in the past few years.[42–45] (Courtesy of Dr Victor E. Reuter, Memorial Sloan-Kettering Cancer Center, New York.)

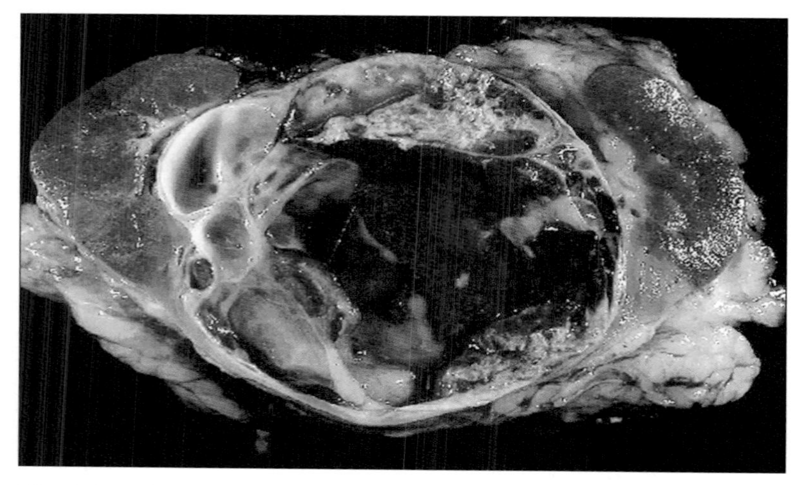

Fig. 8.24 Cystic change and necrosis are frequent, and some tumors may be extensively cystic. (Courtesy of Dr Victor E. Reuter, Memorial Sloan-Kettering Cancer Center, New York.)

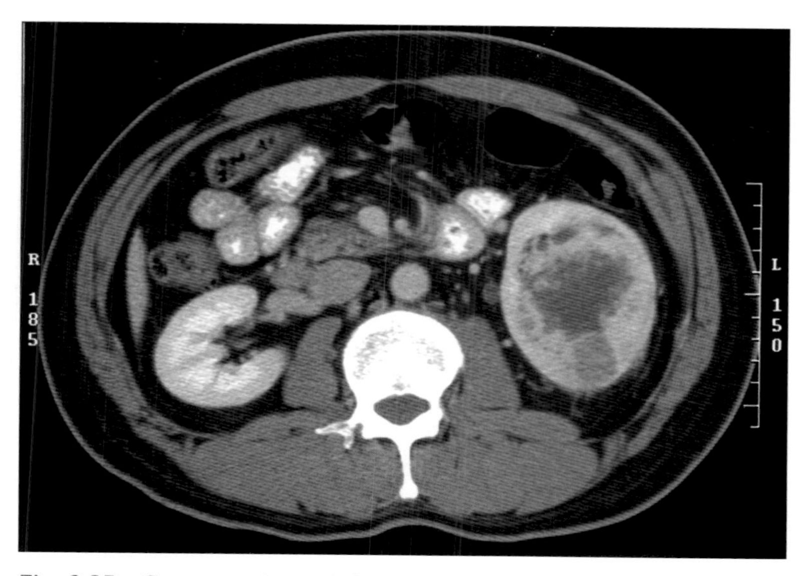

Fig. 8.25 Contrast-enhanced CT scan of a clear cell (conventional) renal cell carcinoma. The decreased attenuation in the central part of the tumor indicates hemorrhage or necrosis. Irregular extensions on the posterior aspect of the tumor suggest extrarenal soft tissue extensions.

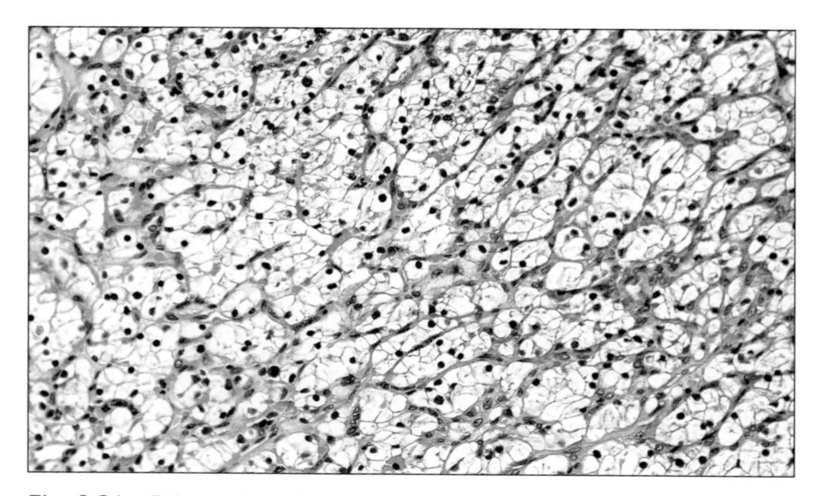

Fig. 8.26 Fuhrman's nuclear grading system correlates with tumor stage and reliably stratifies patients into prognostic groups. Mitotic activity is not a prominent feature of these tumors, with very few cases exhibiting more than five mitoses per ten high-power fields. This figure is of a Fuhrman's nuclear grade I tumor showing a classic solid acinar growth pattern, separated by delicate, arborizing fibrovascular septa.

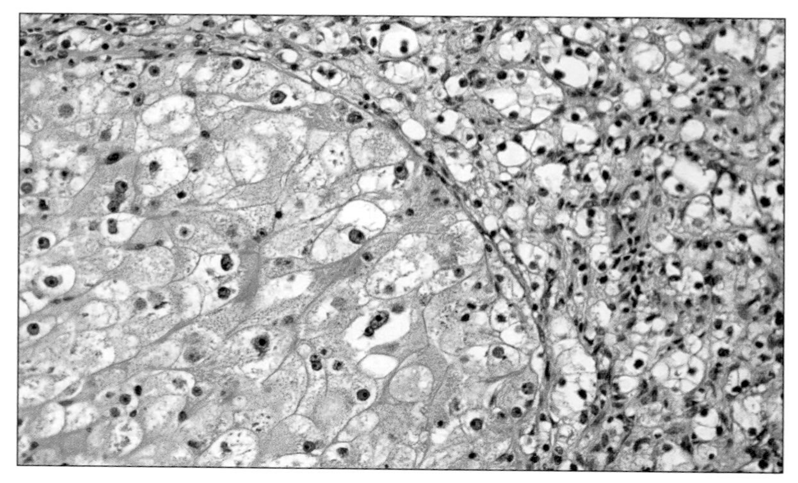

Fig. 8.27 Clear cell (conventional) renal cell carcinoma, Fuhrman's nuclear grade 3. The tumors are graded according to the highest nuclear grade present, even if focal. This example shows grade 2 nuclei on the right side; however, the focal presence of grade 3 areas (left) upgrades it to a nuclear grade 3 carcinoma.

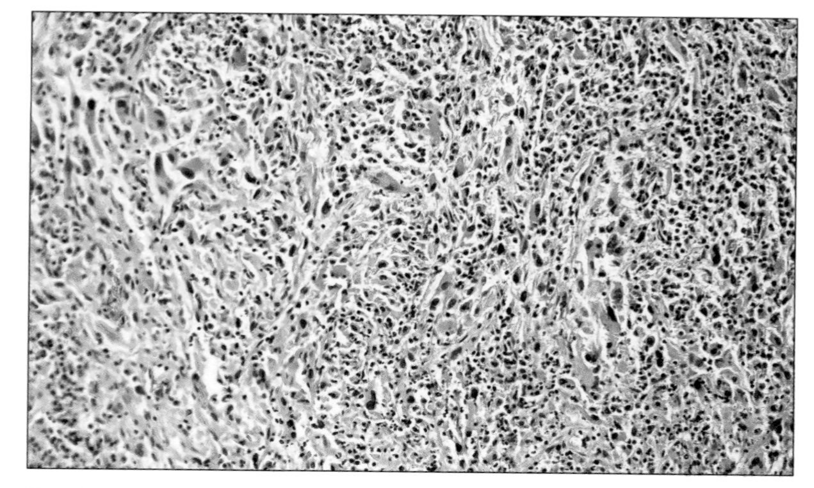

Fig. 8.28 Clear cell (conventional) renal cell carcinoma, Fuhrman's nuclear grade 4 lesions contain bizarre, pleomorphic cells. The nuclei show marked pleomorphism and focal multilobulation.

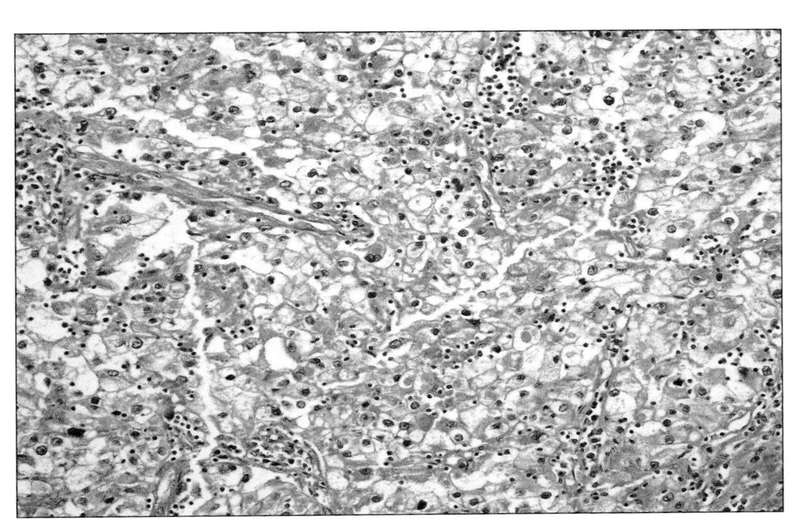

Fig. 8.29 Clear cell (conventional) renal cell carcinoma with solid sheet-like architecture. The thin, arborizing fibrovascular septa are easily discernible. In other cases, the acinar pattern may not be as prominent and the tumor may show solid sheet-like, cystic, papillary/pseudopapillary, tubular and sarcomatoid growth patterns.

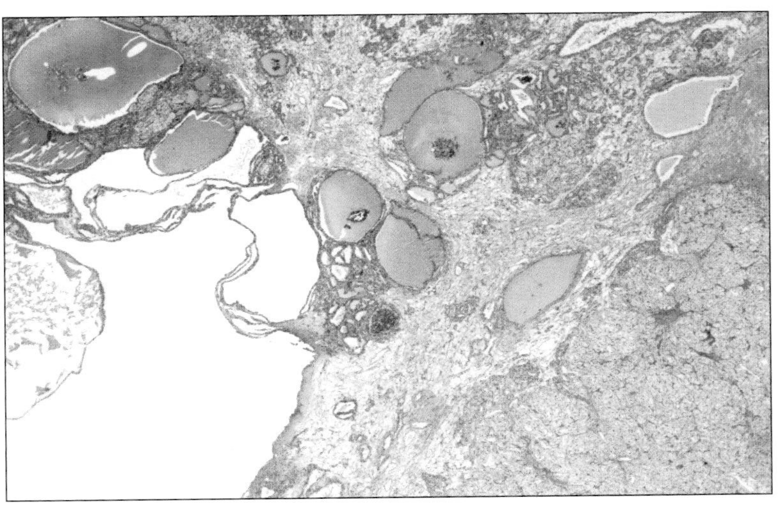

Fig. 8.30 Clear cell (conventional) renal cell carcinoma with multiple cyst formation.

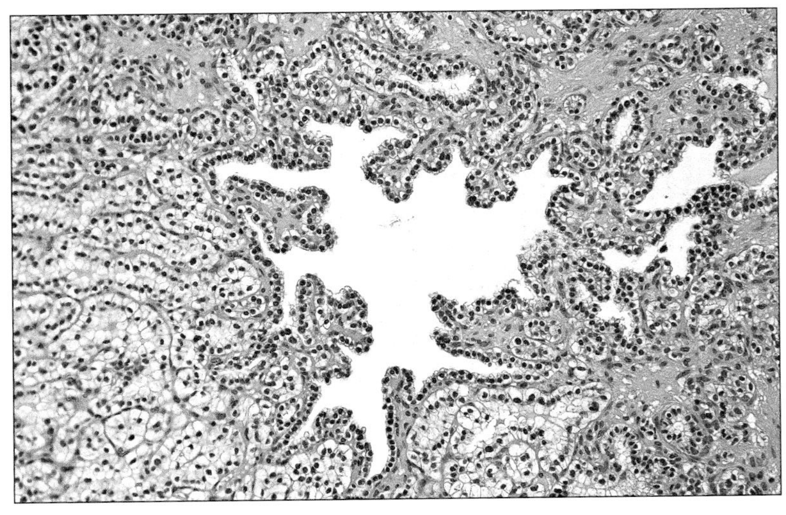

Fig. 8.31 Focal papillary infoldings in a cyst. Such focal changes are not infrequent in clear cell (conventional) renal cell carcinoma, but a prominent papillary architecture is not a feature of this tumor.

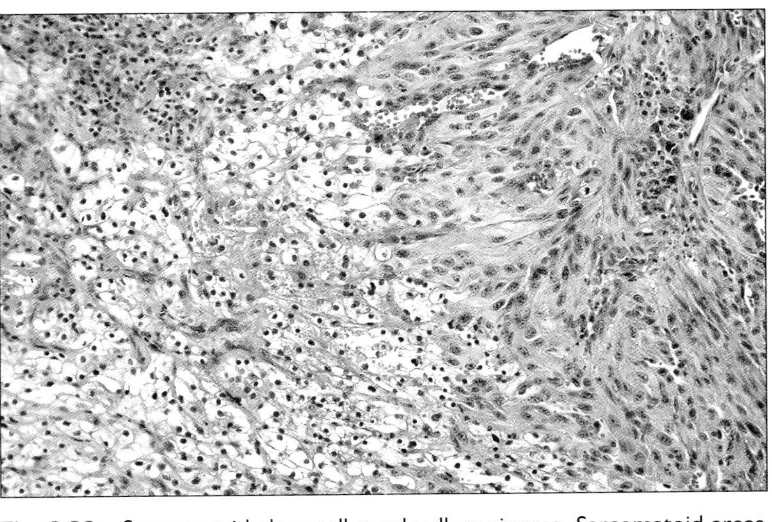

Fig. 8.32 Sarcomatoid clear cell renal cell carcinoma. Sarcomatoid areas are indicative of a high-grade tumor. A rich capillary vascular network is prominent in all architectural patterns of clear cell renal cell carcinoma except the sarcomatoid areas.

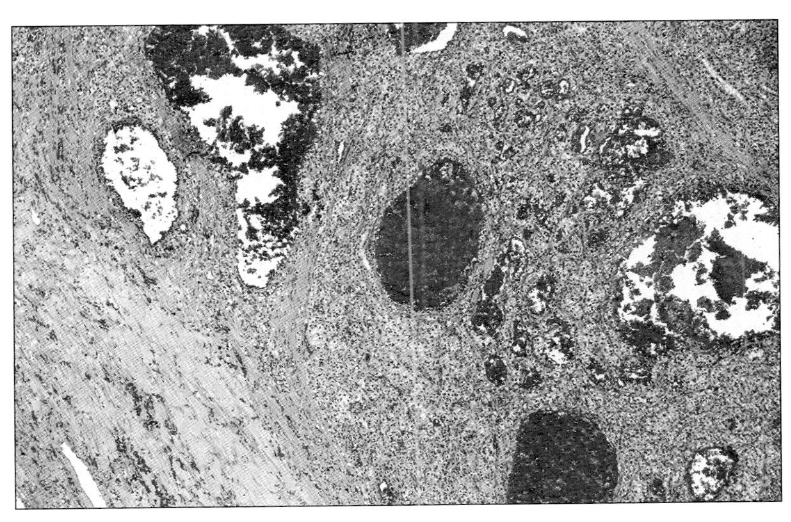

Fig. 8.33 The presence of fresh blood in the acini is a common finding in clear cell (conventional) renal cell carcinoma, and may help narrow the differential diagnostic possibilities in a metastasis of unknown origin.

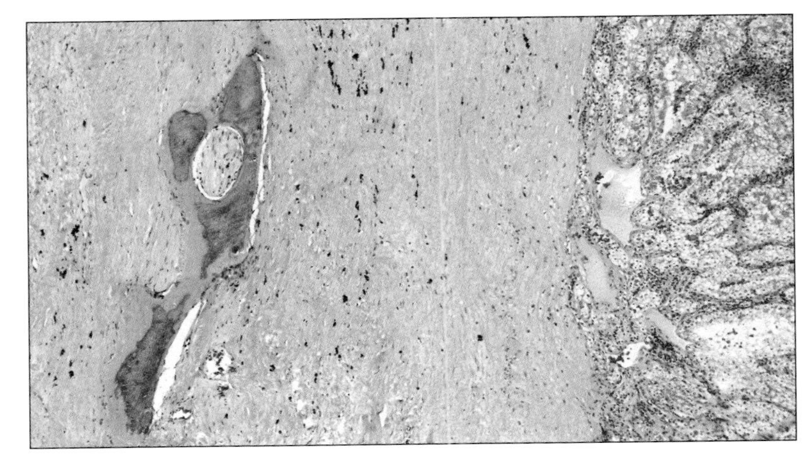

Fig. 8.34 Focal fibrosis or hyalinization is common in clear cell (conventional) renal cell carcinomas, but true desmoplasia is absent or minimal. Geographic necrosis and focal hemorrhage are frequent. Calcifications and osseous metaplasia (shown here) are seen in up to 10% and 4% of cases, respectively.[41]

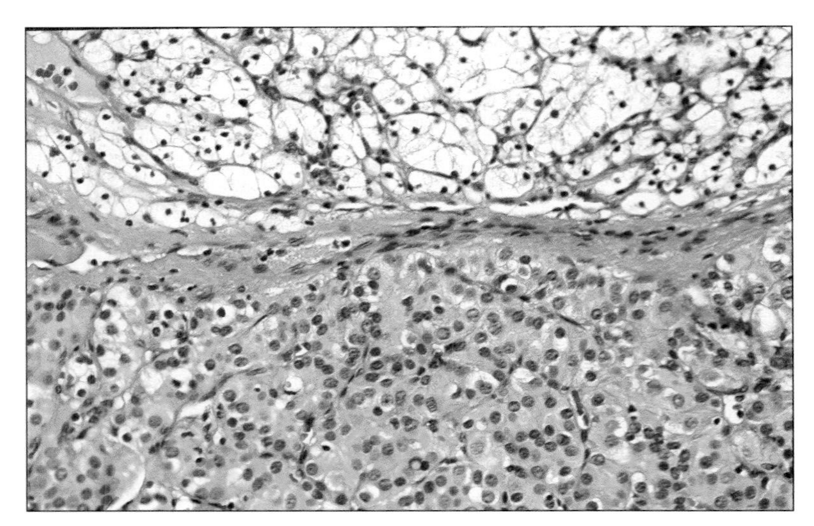

Fig. 8.35 The majority of clear cell (conventional) renal cell carcinomas show a mixture of cells with clear or granular–eosinophilic cytoplasm. The cytoplasmic features generally correlate with tumor grade. Grade I lesions invariably contain clear cytoplasm, whereas the cytoplasm of higher-grade lesions is more likely to be variably eosinophilic.

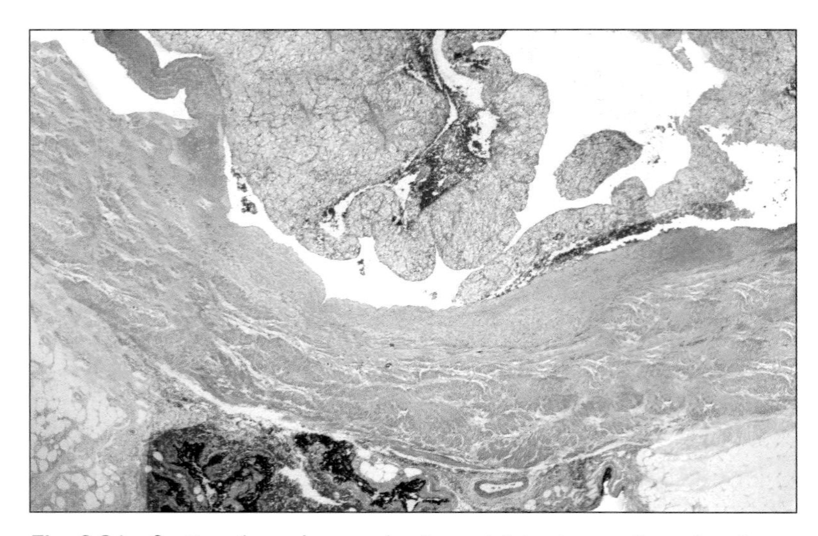

Fig. 8.36 Section through a renal vein containing tumor thrombus from a clear cell (conventional) renal cell carcinoma.

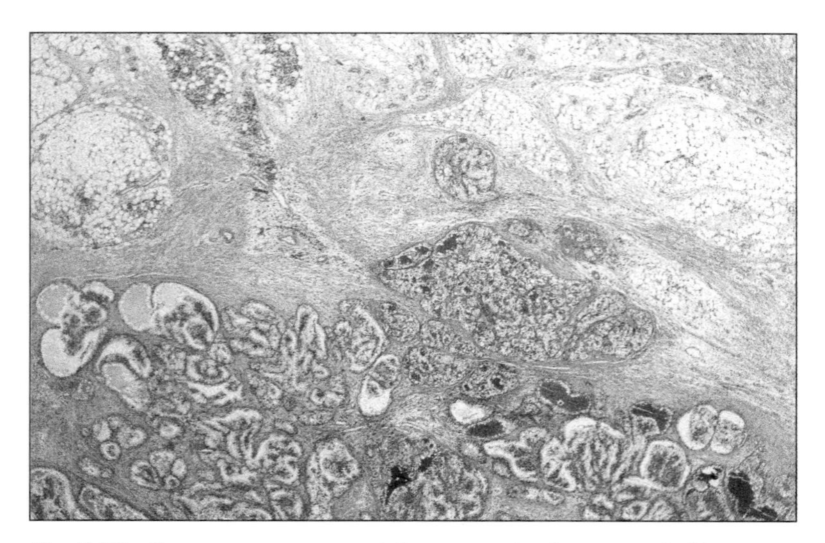

Fig. 8.37 Some tumors are partially or completely surrounded by a fibrous capsule, whereas most are non-encapsulated. This figure shows a clear cell (conventional) renal cell carcinoma with perinephric fat invasion.

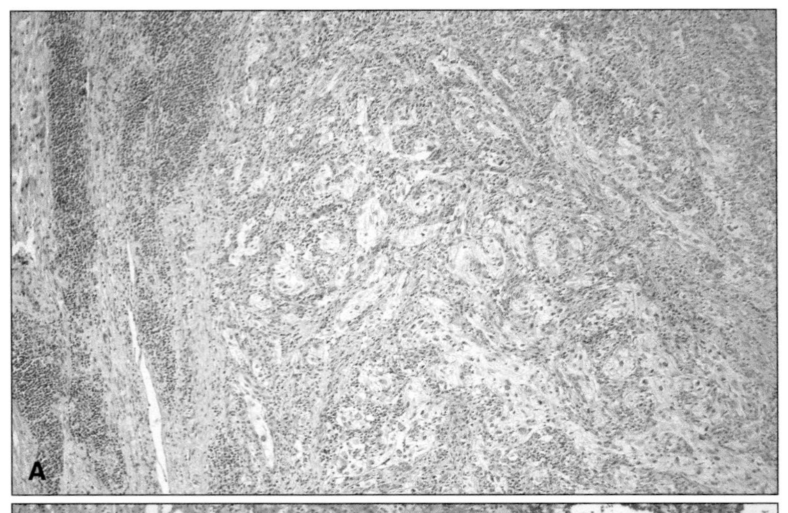

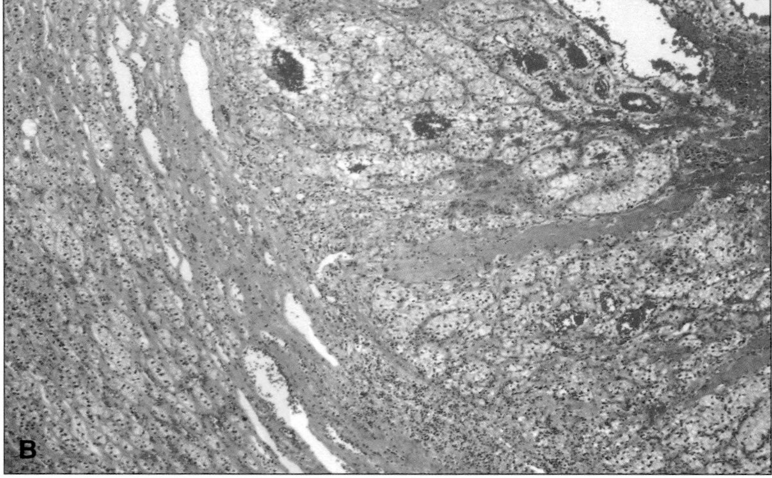

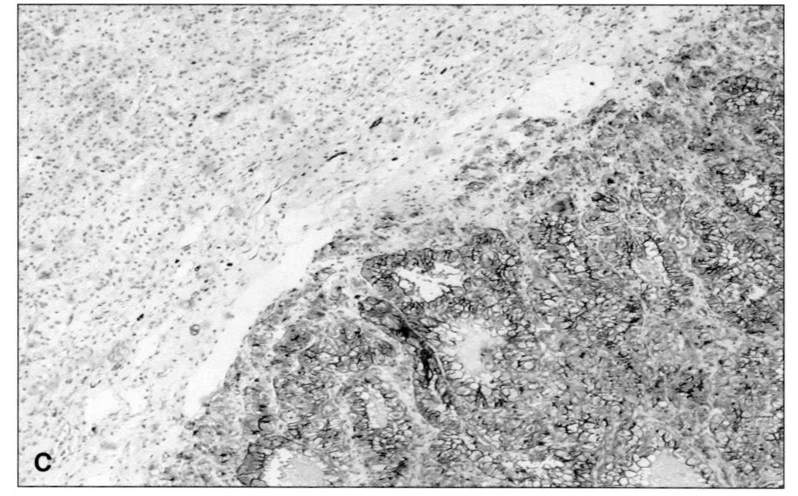

Fig. 8.38 Regional lymph node (A) and adrenal gland (B) metastasis from a clear cell renal cell carcinoma. Metastasis from a clear cell renal cell carcinoma is confirmed by the immunostain for CD10 (C).

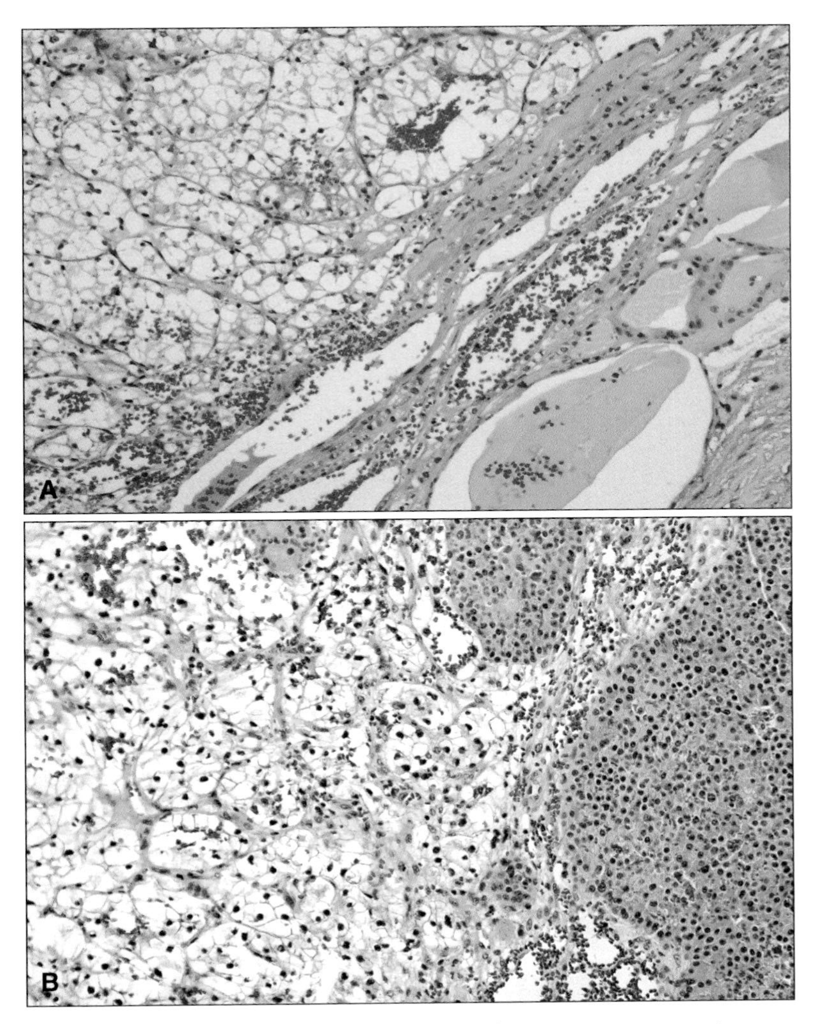

Fig. 8.39 Clear cell (conventional) renal cell carcinoma, metastatic to unusual sites: thyroid (A), and a pancreatic endocrine tumor (B).

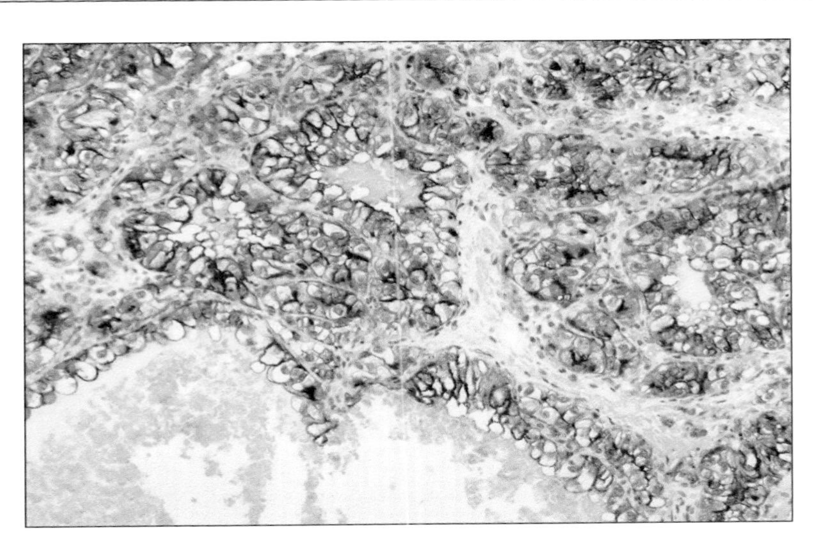

Fig. 8.40 Clear cell (conventional) renal cell carcinoma showing diffuse and strong membrane-predominant immunoreactivity with the antibody CD10.

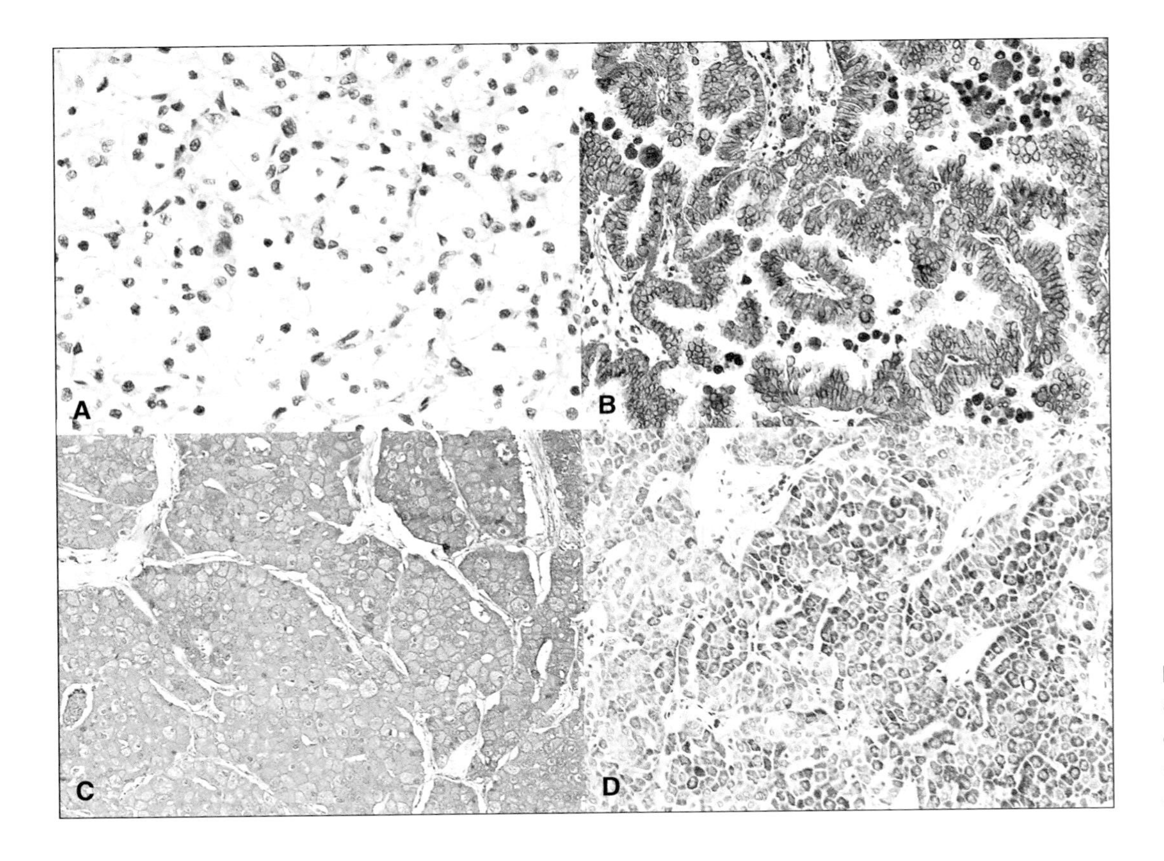

Fig. 8.41 Parvalbumin immunostain: (A) clear cell (conventional) renal cell carcinoma, (B) papillary renal cell carcinoma, (C) chromophobe renal cell carcinoma, and (D) renal oncocytoma.

Cystic nephromas are usually lined by a single layer of flattened or hobnail epithelium. The fibrous stroma may be more cellular, resembling ovarian stroma. The septa may contain small tubules lined by bland epithelial cells, reminiscent of renal tubules. In the presence of any expansile or solid tumor masses in the septa (particularly if the solid areas constitute more than 10% of the tumor), the diagnosis of clear cell (conventional) RCC is more appropriate. (Figs 8.42–8.44)

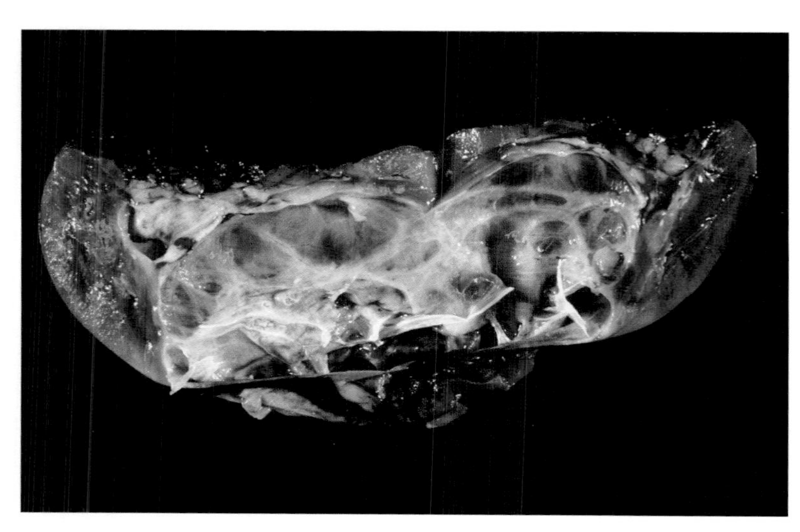

Fig. 8.42 Grossly, multilocular cystic renal cell carcinoma is a well-circumscribed, multicystic mass that is separated from the adjacent renal parenchyma by a fibrous pseudocapsule. Size is quite variable, but may reach up to 13 cm. The cysts are variable in size, separated by thin fibrous septa, and may contain serous or bloody fluid or clots. No solid or expansile masses of tumor are present.

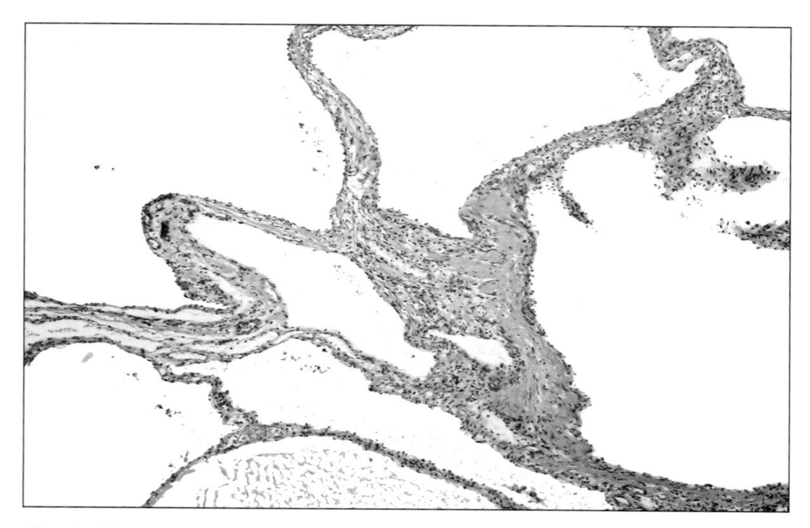

Fig. 8.43 Microscopically, in multilocular cystic renal cell carcinoma, the thin fibrous septa are lined by one or more layers of neoplastic epithelial cells with clear cytoplasm and Fuhrman nuclear grade I or 2. Focally, and, in some cases, in most of the tumor, the epithelial lining may be absent. Foamy macrophages may also line the cyst wall. Small collections of tumor cells are almost always present within the fibrous septa or in the tumor capsule, but no expansile or solid masses of tumor are evident. Occasionally the tumor cells exhibit papillary tufting into the cyst lumen.

PAPILLARY (CHROMOPHIL) RENAL CELL CARCINOMA

PRCC is the second most common RCC, comprising approximately 7–15% of renal cell neoplasms.[5,39,56–60]

Patients present in the third to eighth decades of life. An increasing number of tumors are discovered as incidental masses during work-up for unrelated conditions. The male-to-female ratio ranges from 2:1 to 3.9:1. While the majority are unilateral, PRCC is the most common multifocal or bilateral renal tumor (see Fig. 8.46)

PRCC has a more favorable prognosis than clear cell carcinoma, and a less favorable one than chromophobe RCC. The reported 5-year disease-free survival rate varies from 79% to 92%.[5] Grading remains controversial. While some investigators report it as a strong predictor of survival, others have not found any significant association with prognosis.

Some authors have proposed subtyping PRCC into type 1 and type 2 lesions, based on architectural and cytologic features.[39,61] Some genetic differences have also been reported between the type 1 and type 2 tumors,[62,63] and subsequently differences in survival between the two groups.[61] However, the utility of subtyping of PRCC is still controversial, and remains to be clinically proven.

Cytogenetics and molecular biology

PRCCs are characterized by trisomy of chromosomes 7 and 17, as well as loss of chromosome Y (see Fig. 8.45). Some investigators have suggested that tumors exhibiting only trisomy 7 and 17 are likely to be benign, and require additional genetic abnormalities to acquire more aggressive behavior.[59,60,64,65]

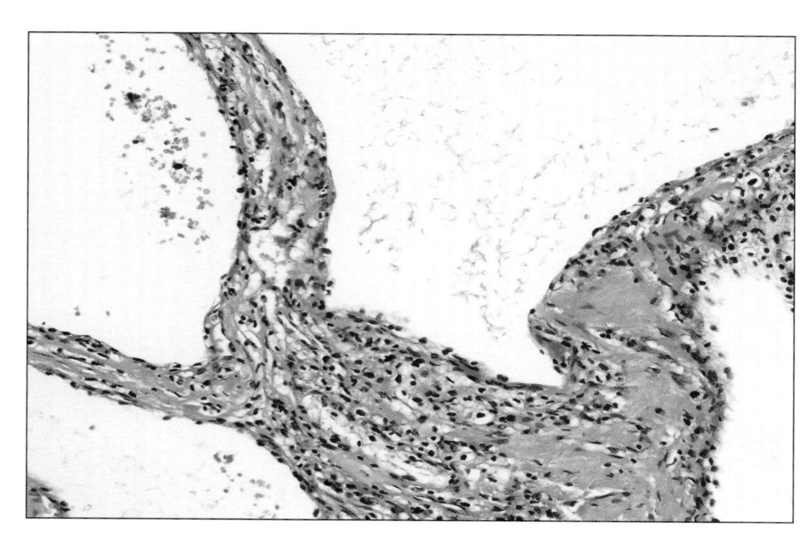

Fig. 8.44 At higher magnification, multilocular cystic renal cell carcinoma shows cysts lined by clear cells with low nuclear grade. Small clusters of clear cells are also present in the septa, but no expansile tumor masses are seen.

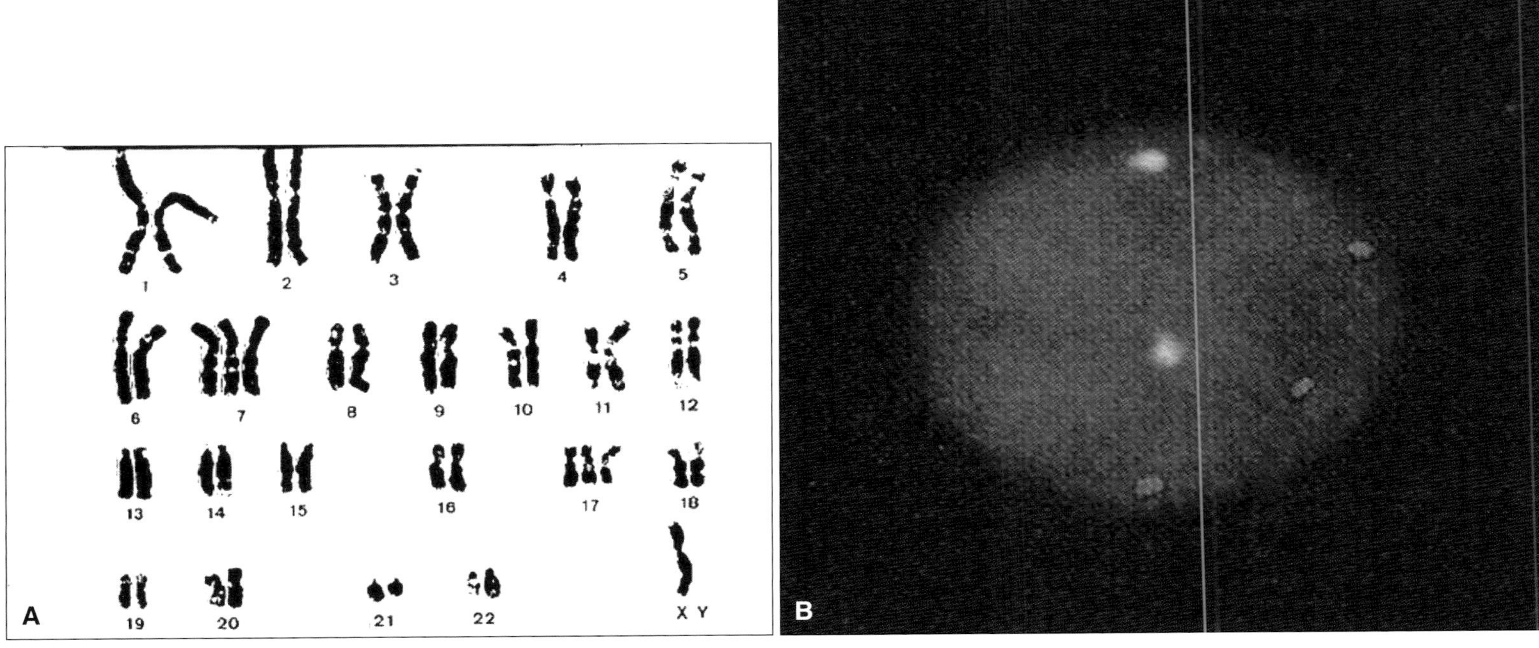

Fig. 8.45 The characteristic karyotype of a papillary renal cell carcinoma, showing trisomy 7 and 17 (A), and trisomy 7 by fluorescence in situ hybridization (FISH) analysis in another case (B).

Recently, some RCCs with nested to papillary architecture, prominent clear cell cytology, and a predilection to occur in children or young adults have been shown to bear a translocation involving the *TFE3* gene at chromosome Xp11.2 [t(X;1)(p11.2;q21) and t(X;17)(p11.2;q25)].[66–68] These tumors are now redesignated as Xp11 translocation carcinomas.

Differential diagnosis

PRCCs may be confused principally with clear cell carcinomas exhibiting a papillary or pseudopapillary growth, and with collecting duct carcinomas (CDCs).

PRCCs may contain tumor cells with clear cytoplasm focally, especially in areas with a solid growth pattern. PRCCs with predominantly clear cell cytology are exquisitely uncommon.[69] Clear cell RCC may be focally papillary, although this is usually due to cell drop-off in areas away from feeding vessels, creating a pseudopapillary appearance. Adequate sampling should clarify the issue. Psammoma, bodies, hemosiderin deposition within tumor cells, and fibrovascular cores containing foamy macrophages are more likely to be seen in PRCC. CK7 immunoreactivity is present at least focally in many PRCCs, whereas it is negative in most conventional RCCs (see differential diagnosis, clear cell RCC). If needed, molecular genetics can be used to solve difficult cases.[69]

Tumors with papillary architecture and prominent clear cell cytology, particularly in young patients, may represent Xp11.2 tumors. Immunostaining with TFE3 antibody, and molecular studies if frozen tissue is available, will clarify the issue.

CDCs may have a papillary growth pattern and resemble PRCC. CDCs are centered in the medulla, are virtually always high grade, invariably invade into adjacent renal parenchyma, and are associated with a desmoplastic stroma. Intracytoplasmic and luminal mucin is a common feature, as are reactivity for carcinoembryonic antigen (CEA), the lectins peanut and soybean agglutinin, and *Ulex europaeus*, and high molecular weight cytokeratin. CK7 may be expressed in both tumors. Cytogenetic studies may be used to solve difficult diagnostic problems. (Figs 8.45–8.58)

CHROMOPHOBE RENAL CELL CARCINOMA

Chromophobe RCCs comprise 6–11% of renal epithelial tumors.[5,71–74] The age and sex distribution is similar to that seen in clear cell RCC; the mean age at presentation is 59 years. While some patients present with a palpable mass or hematuria, the majority are asymptomatic. Most cases are unilateral and approximately 11% are bilateral. Radiographic examination may reveal a central scar, similar to that seen in oncocytomas and large, low-grade clear cell (conventional) RCCs, and most tumors appear hypovascular on angiographic evaluation.

Stage for stage, chromophobe RCC has a significantly better prognosis than clear cell (conventional) RCC.[73–75] The 5- and 10-year disease-specific survival rates are close to 95% and 90%, respectively.[5] Since its morphologic features may overlap with those of other tumors that have entirely different biologic behavior, the identification and proper diagnosis of chromophobe RCC is essential.

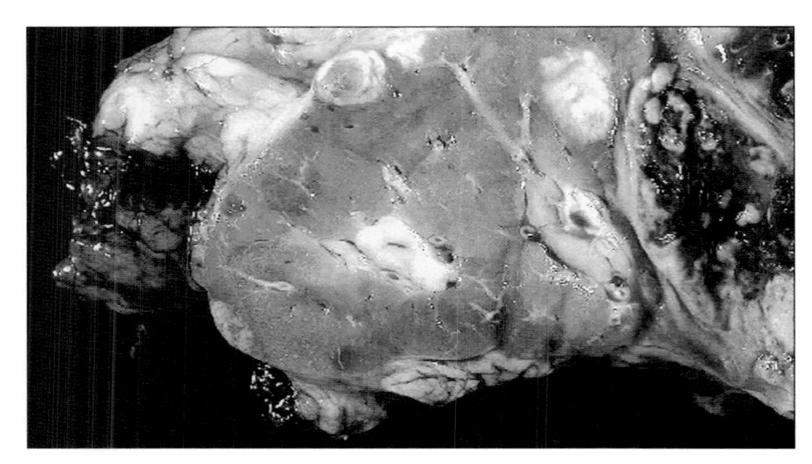

Fig. 8.46 Papillary renal cell carcinomas can range from 1.0 to 18.0 cm in maximum diameter (mean, 6.3 cm). The tumor is commonly multifocal. (Courtesy of Dr Victor E. Reuter, Memorial Sloan-Kettering Cancer Center, New York.)

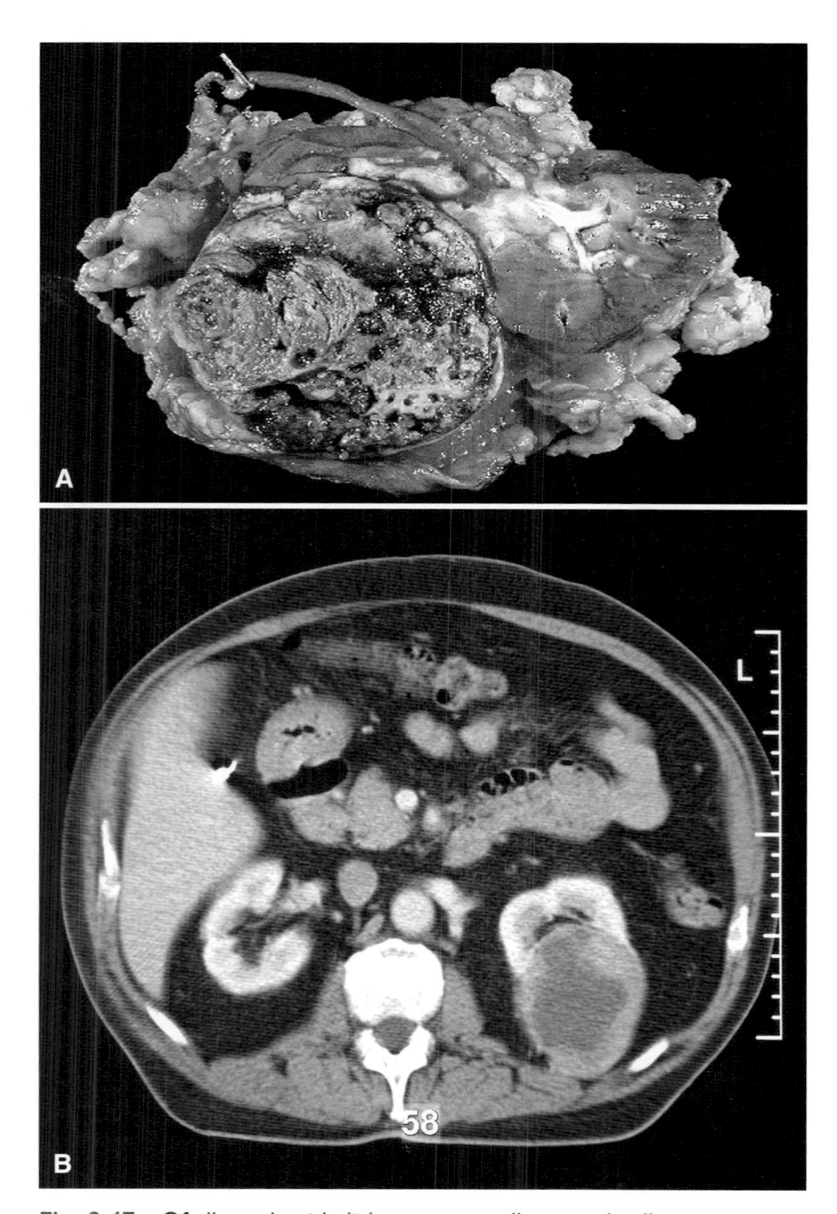

Fig. 8.47 Of all renal epithelial tumors, papillary renal cell carcinomas are the most likely to be surrounded by a fibrous capsule. Gross necrosis and hemorrhage are common, as are the areas of gross cystic change (A). Necrosis and cystic change are also evident in this enhanced computed tomographic scan of the tumor (B).

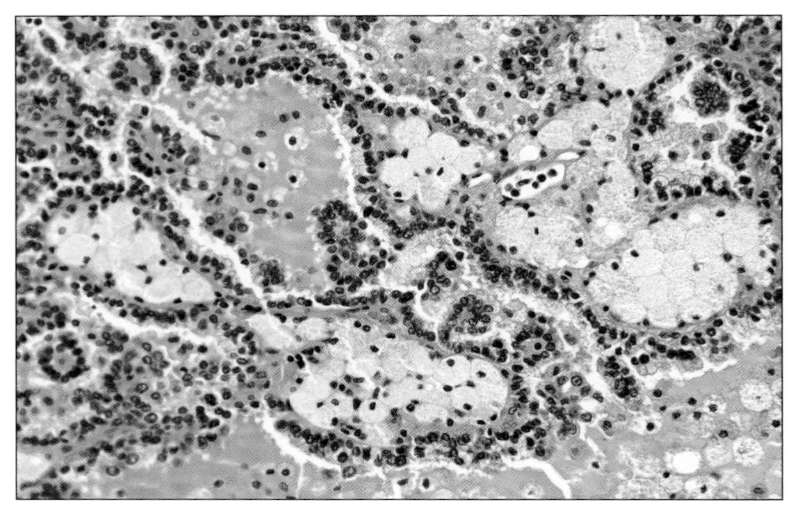

Fig. 8.48 Most papillary renal cell carcinomas exhibit a variegated appearance. Tumors containing abundant foamy macrophages are tan to yellow, whereas those with intratumoral hemorrhage are dark tan to brown. Tumors with lower-grade cytology tend to be more solid; higher-grade tumors more often show hemorrhage and cystic change.

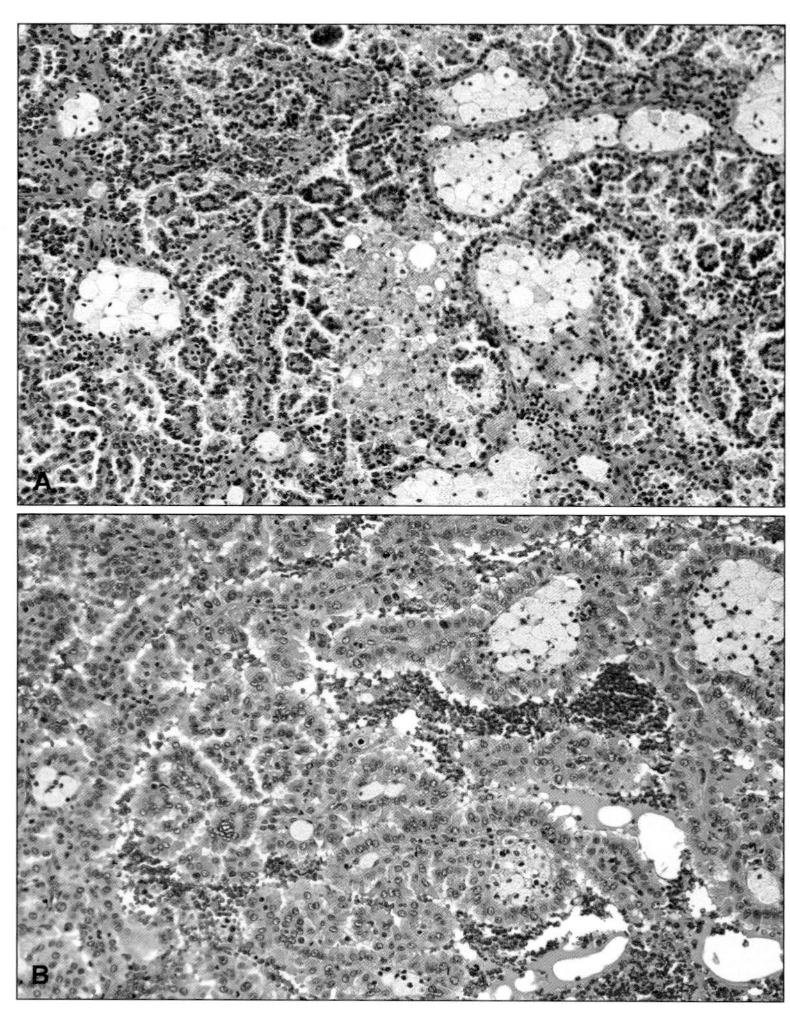

Fig. 8.49 Papillary renal cell carcinoma exhibits a broad morphologic spectrum. The classic papillary pattern is characterized by discrete papillary fronds lined by neoplastic epithelial cells and containing a central fibrovascular core. Two cytologic variants occur: (A) basophilic/type 1 cells, with scant cytoplasm, relatively high nuclear:cytoplasmic ratio; (B) eosinophilic/type 2 cells, with abundant eosinophilic cytoplasm and higher-grade nuclei.

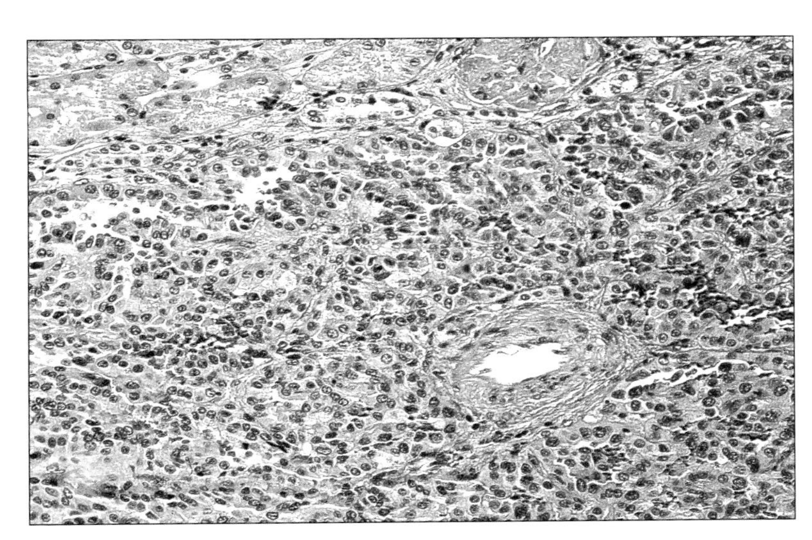

Fig. 8.50 Other architectural patterns may be seen in papillary renal cell carcinoma (PRCC). Some tumors contain trabecular and solid areas in which the papillae are closely packed, masking their true growth pattern. Areas of true solid growth are usually small, and are present adjacent to areas of more conventional PRCC.

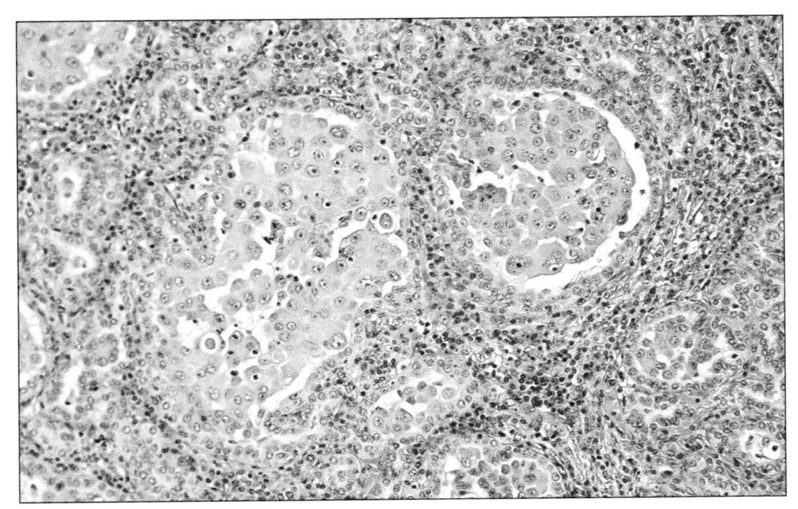

Fig. 8.51 The tubular growth pattern in papillary renal cell carcinoma is characterized by small to medium-sized tubules lined by cuboidal or columnar-shaped tumor cells, usually with sparse intervening stroma. The glomeruloid pattern (shown here) consists of closely juxtaposed small tubule-like structures with intraluminal tufting of tumor cells. The cells lining the tubule-like structures are smaller and contain scant to moderate amounts of mostly amphophilic cytoplasm, whereas the cells tufting into the lumen are larger and contain more abundant, often eosinophilic, cytoplasm and are of higher nuclear grade. In rare cases, the glomeruloid growth pattern may predominate or may comprise the entire tumor.

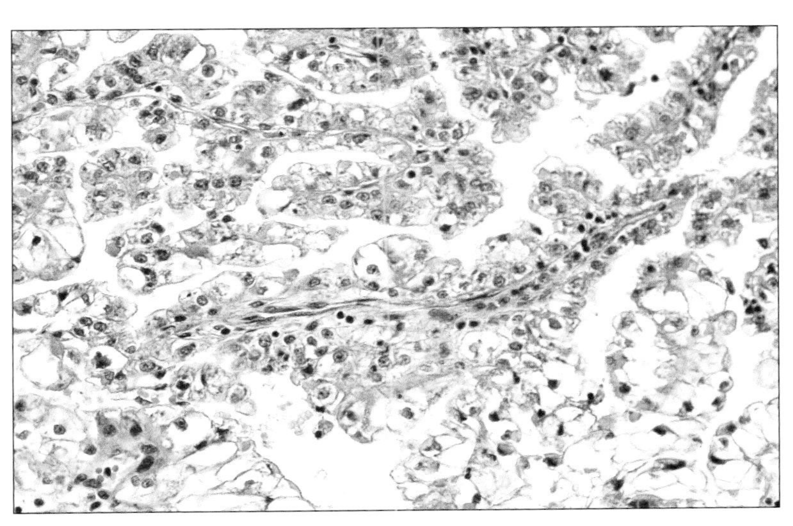

Fig. 8.52 Xp11.2 renal carcinomas feature nested to papillary architecture, and are characterized by polygonal cells with clear to eosinophilic, granular cytoplasm. Foam cells and psammoma bodies are often present. The combination of tumor cells with clear cytoplasm and papillary architecture is uncommon in other renal carcinomas. The renal carcinomas bearing the t(X;17) and resulting *ASPL–TFE3* gene fusion usually have more voluminous cytoplasm, more loosely packed cells, and more prominent psammoma bodies, compared with those in t(X;1) carcinomas. Both of these tumors show strong and diffuse nuclear immunoreactivity with TFE3 antibody.[70]

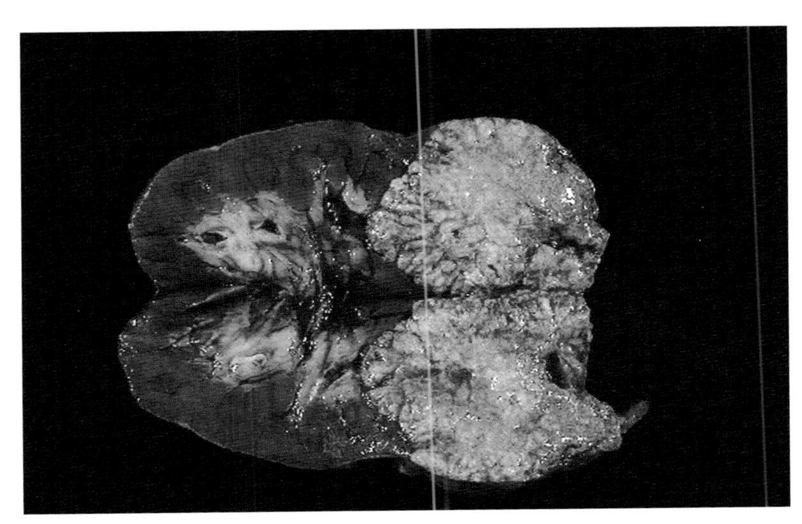

Fig. 8.53 While a papillary growth pattern predominates in the majority of papillary renal cell carcinomas (PRCCs), some cases exhibit a less prominent component of papillary architecture. Therefore, the percentage of papillary architecture alone should not be used to determine whether a tumor is a PRCC or not. Sarcomatoid features (as seen in this gross figure) are a sign of aggressive disease.

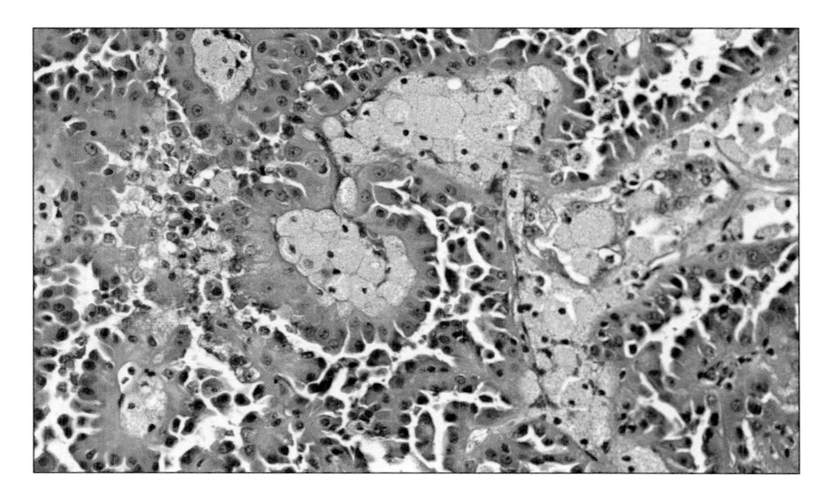

Fig. 8.54 Nuclear features can be quite variable in papillary renal cell carcinoma. Small, round nuclei with inconspicuous nucleoli generally occur in basophilic areas. Large, moderately irregular nuclei containing coarse chromatin and prominent nucleoli are generally seen in eosinophilic areas. Prominent foamy macrophages are seen within the fibrovascular cores.

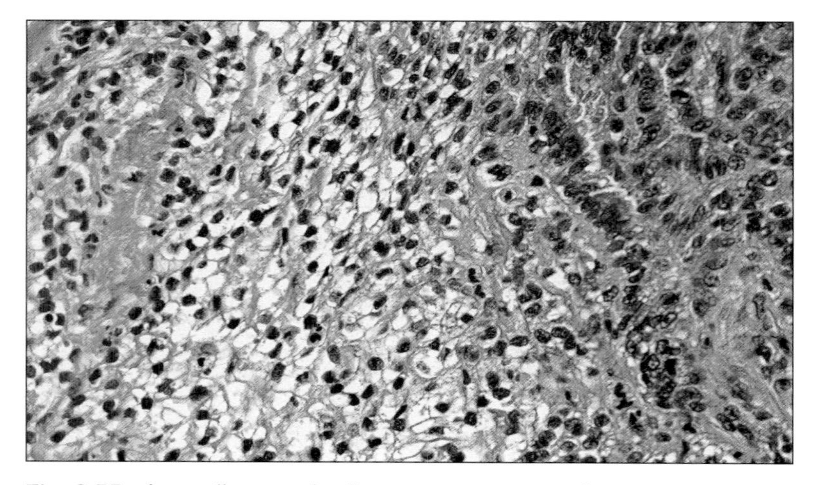

Fig. 8.55 In papillary renal cell carcinoma, tumor cells with clear cytoplasm are almost always a focal finding. They are seen predominantly in association with a solid growth pattern or in areas in close association with necrosis and degenerative changes.

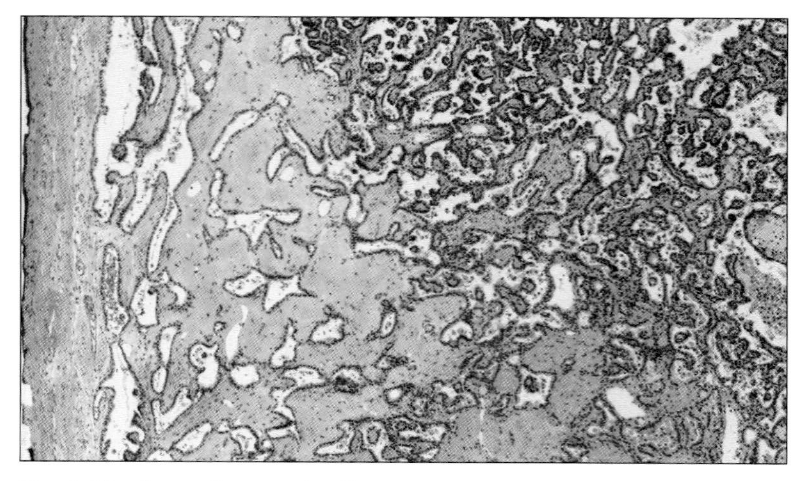

Fig. 8.56 In papillary renal cell carcinoma, psammoma bodies and foamy macrophages are typical within the fibrovascular stalk. Necrosis with secondary cystic change is common. The stalk may be hyalinized or fibrotic (shown here), masking the papillary nature of the lesion.

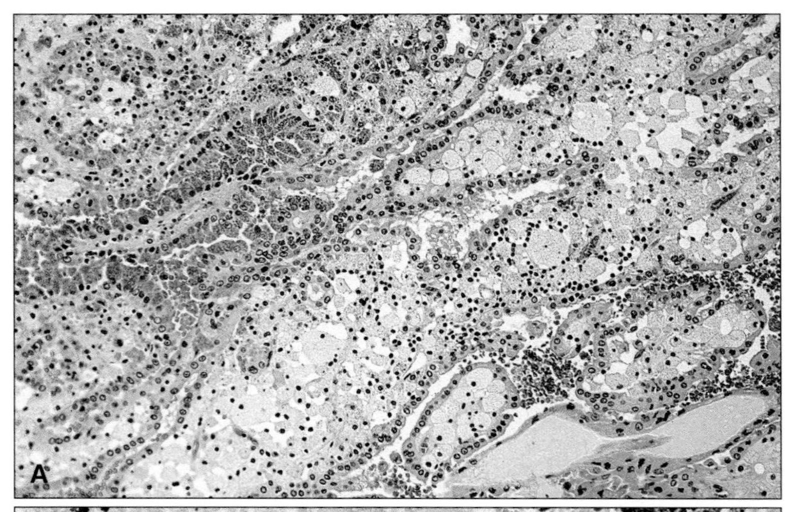

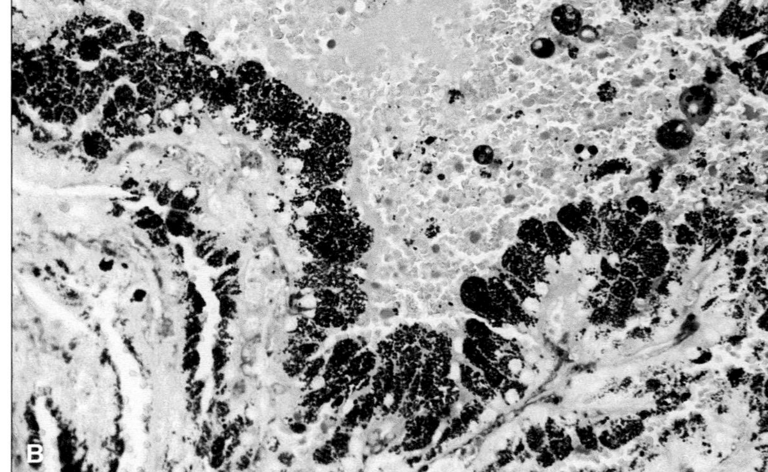

Fig. 8.57 Papillary renal cell carcinoma. Hemosiderin pigment may be present in the cytoplasm of the tumor cells in a patchy distribution, and is more often seen in eosinophilic tumors. (A) Marked hemosiderin deposition within both the epithelial cells and the foamy macrophages. (B) Prussian-blue stain highlighting the presence of iron pigment in the cells.

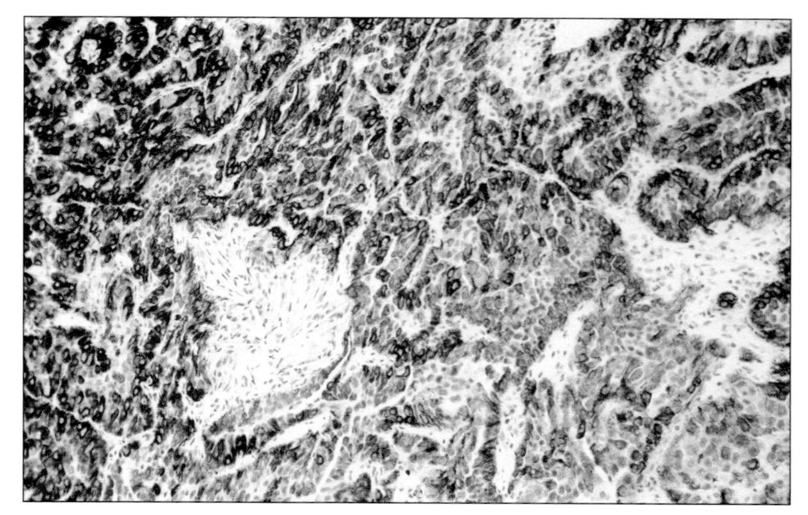

Fig. 8.58 By immunohistochemical staining, most papillary renal cell carcinomas are positive for cytokeratin 7 (CK7). However, some high-grade tumors (particularly the eosinophilic variants) may not be positive for CK7. Like clear cell (conventional) renal cell carcinoma, papillary renal cell carcinoma is usually positive for epithelial membrane antigen, CD10, and vimentin.

While rare classic chromophobe RCC may metastasize, those with a sarcomatoid component are the most likely to behave in an aggressive fashion.[76] Some studies have shown increased predilection for sarcomatoid change in these tumors.[77]

The recognition of chromophobe RCCs in humans in 1985 led to a reassessment of the morphologic classification of renal tumors and has served as the foundation for the current classification of renal tumors.[71-74]

Chromophobe RCCs are thought to arise from intercalated cells of the renal cortex, similar to oncocytomas. Several investigators have recently drawn attention to the possible link between chromophobe RCC and renal oncocytoma, indicating that 'hybrid' tumors may exist.

Cytogenetics

Chromophobe RCCs are characterized genetically by losses of multiple chromosomes, including chromosome 1, Y, 6, 10, 13, 17, and 21.[78-82] Loss of multiple chromosomes leads to hypodiploid tumor cells, a unique feature seen in many chromophobe RCCs.

Immunohistochemistry

Tumor cells show immunoreactivity for EMA, as well as low molecular weight cytokeratins such as CAM 5.2 and AE1/AE3. Parvalbumin is usually strongly positive (see Table 8.2). Vimentin is positive only in the sarcomatoid areas. High molecular weight cytokeratin 34βE12 is generally negative. While these tumors have been reported to show a characteristic staining pattern with antimitochondrial antibody (113-1),[83] the staining patterns of oncocytomas and the eosinophilic variant of chromophobe RCC may show some overlap.

Differential diagnosis

Given the differing clinical behavior, it is essential to differentiate chromophobe RCC from other renal tumors with eosinophilic cytoplasm, like clear cell RCC or renal oncocytoma. The distinction between them can be performed easily in most cases by adequate sampling and paying close attention to the morphologic characteristics of the tumor (see Table 8.3). Electron microscopy as well as cytogenetics may be useful in difficult cases. (Figs 8.59–8.70)

RENAL TUMORS OF BIRT–HOGG–DUBÉ SYNDROME

Renal tumors in the rare, autosomal dominant Birt–Hogg–Dubé syndrome are usually multifocal and bilateral. Most tumors have oncocytic features, and are either chromophobe RCC, renal oncocytoma, or tumors with hybrid features of both.[88-90] Rare clear cell (conventional) RCCs have also been described in this setting. Additionally, many kidneys contain microscopic oncocytic nodules, somewhat similar to those described in renal oncocytosis.

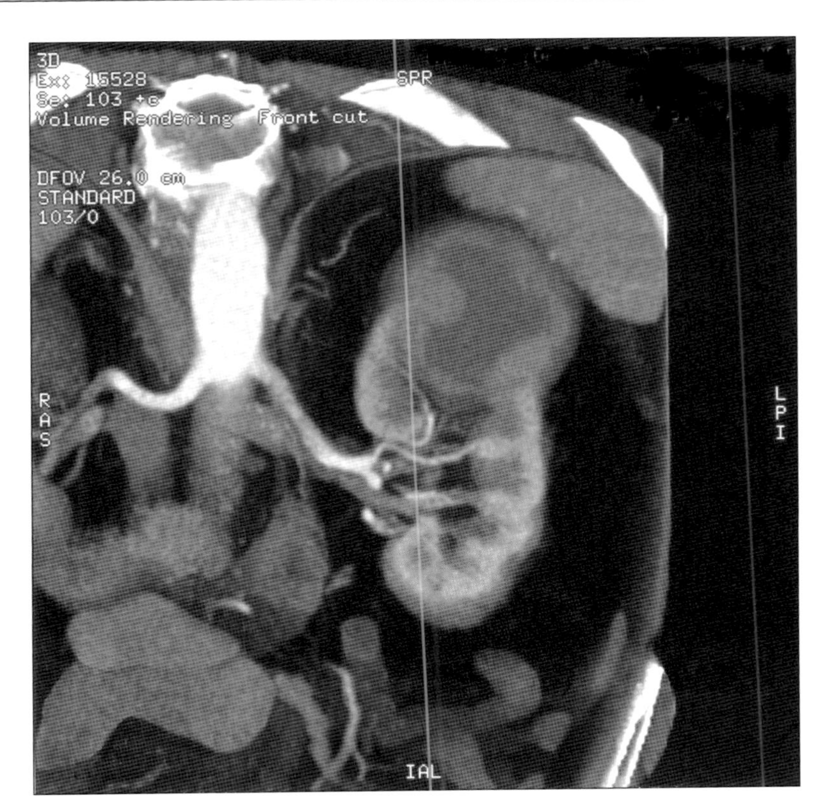

Fig. 8.59 Chromophobe renal cell carcinoma has the largest mean size among all epithelial renal tumors; tumors may range in size from 2.0 to 23.0 cm, with a mean size of 8.4 cm. Tumors commonly have a lobulated appearance and roughly one-fourth to one-third of cases exhibit gross hemorrhage or necrosis. Gross involvement of the renal vein may be seen in a small number of cases, while up to a third may exhibit disease invading perirenal adipose tissue. On arteriography the tumors are often hypovascular, unlike other renal cell carcinomas.

COLLECTING DUCT CARCINOMA

CDC, also known as Bellini duct carcinoma, is rare, comprising less than 1% of renal epithelial tumors.[91-96] While many of the aggressive tumors have distinctive morphologic features, the true morphologic spectrum of CDC remains to be defined. CDC may occur at any age; the age at presentation ranges from 13 to 83 years. However, in general, cases tend to present in younger patients. Hematuria is the most common symptom at presentation, followed by pain, weight loss, and the presence of a palpable mass. Classic cases are characterized by aggressive behavior. Over 50% of patients present with metastatic disease and most die within 24 months of presentation. Nodal, osseous, and visceral metastases are common, and the metastases to bone are usually osteoblastic.

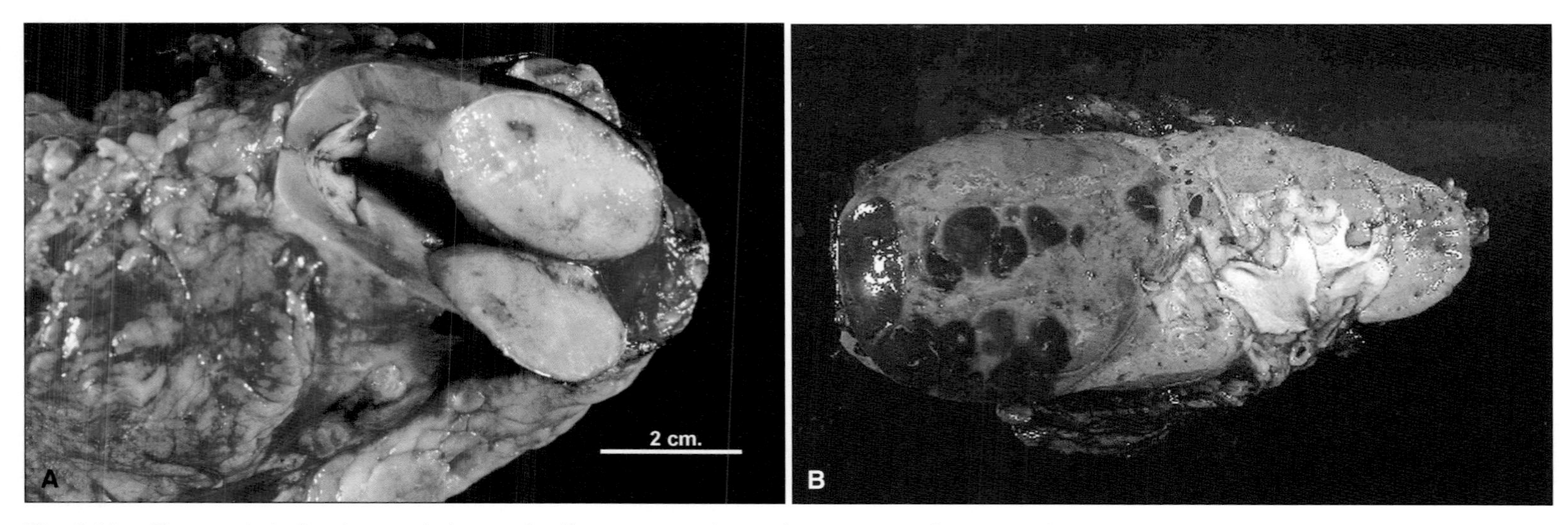

Fig. 8.60 Characteristically, chromophobe renal cell carcinomas show a homogeneous beige or pale-tan cut surface (A). They usually lack a distinct capsule. A central scar is present in 7–15% of cases.[5,41] Some tumors may have a dark brown and mahogany color (B), and such tumors are predominantly composed of eosinophilic cells (eosinophilic variant). Tumors commonly have a lobulated appearance and roughly one-fourth to one-third of cases exhibit gross hemorrhage or necrosis. Gross cystic areas are quite rare.

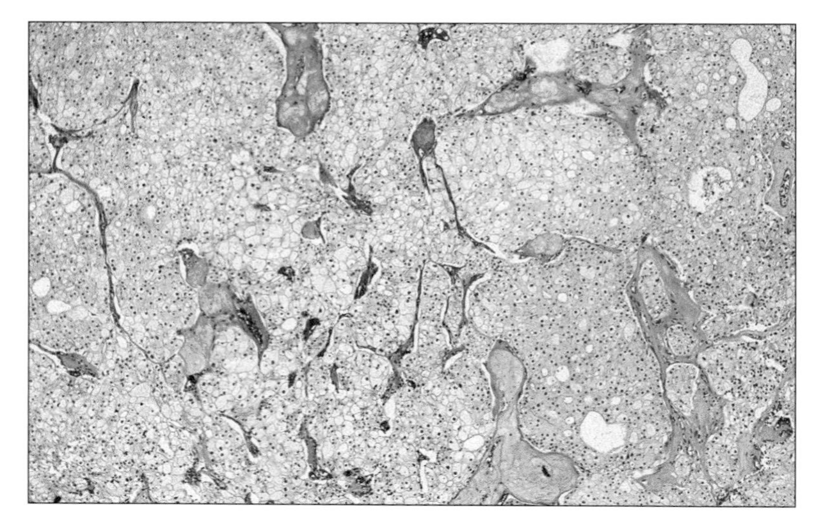

Fig. 8.61 Microscopically, the pattern of growth in chromophobe renal cell carcinoma is predominantly solid, often with incomplete, thin, fibrous septations. Necrosis and calcification are frequently seen.

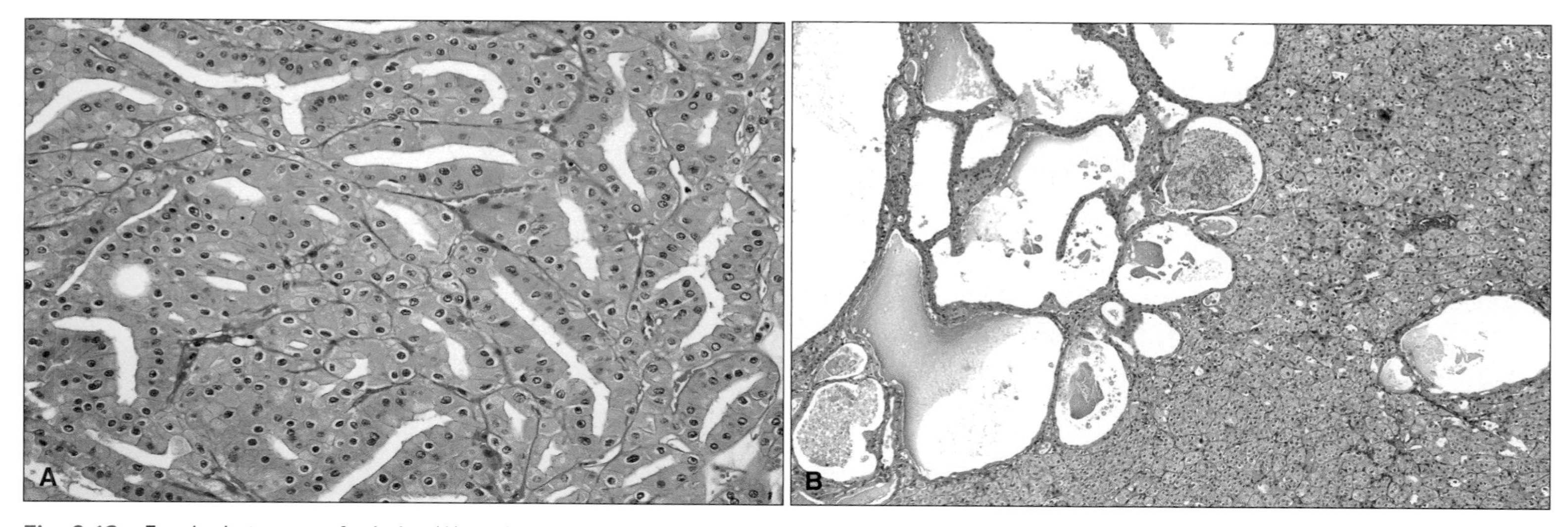

Fig. 8.62 Focal admixtures of tubular (A), trabecular, and cystic (B) patterns may occur in chromophobe renal cell carcinoma.

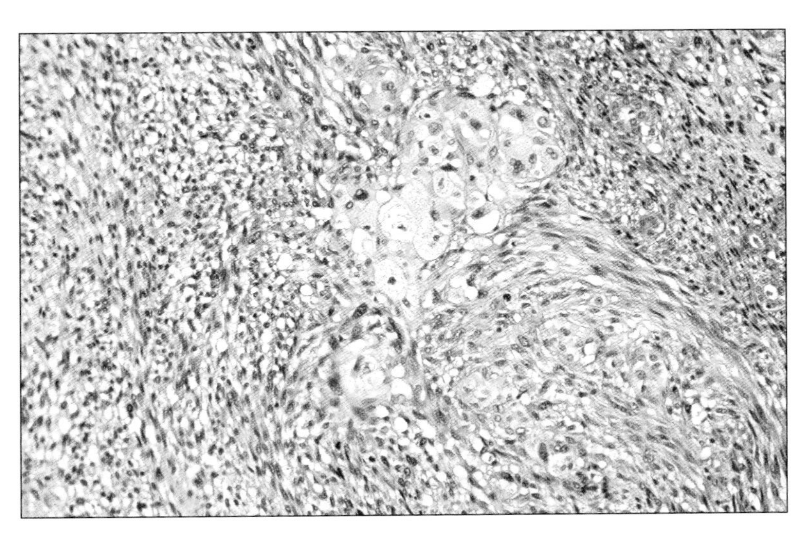

Fig. 8.63 A small percentage of chromophobe renal cell carcinomas exhibit a sarcomatoid pattern of growth.

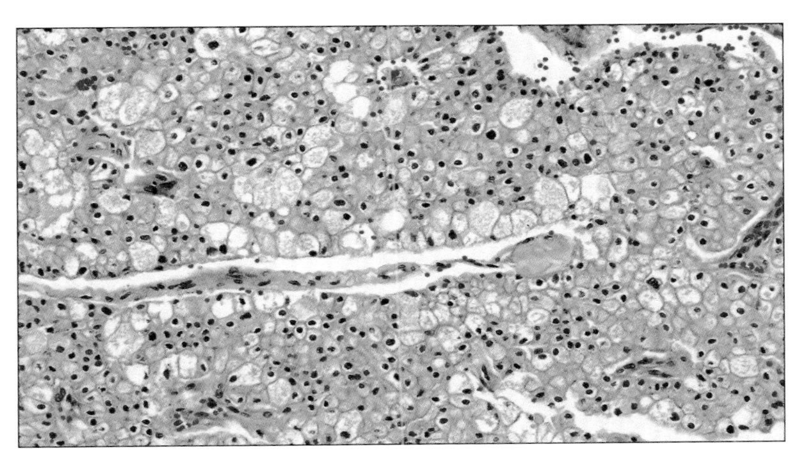

Fig. 8.66 A combination of pale and eosinophilic cells in variable proportions is seen in virtually all chromophobe renal cell carcinomas. Perinuclear halos are invariably seen. In many areas, the cell membranes appear accentuated as a result of cytoplasmic organelles being pushed to the periphery of the cytoplasm.

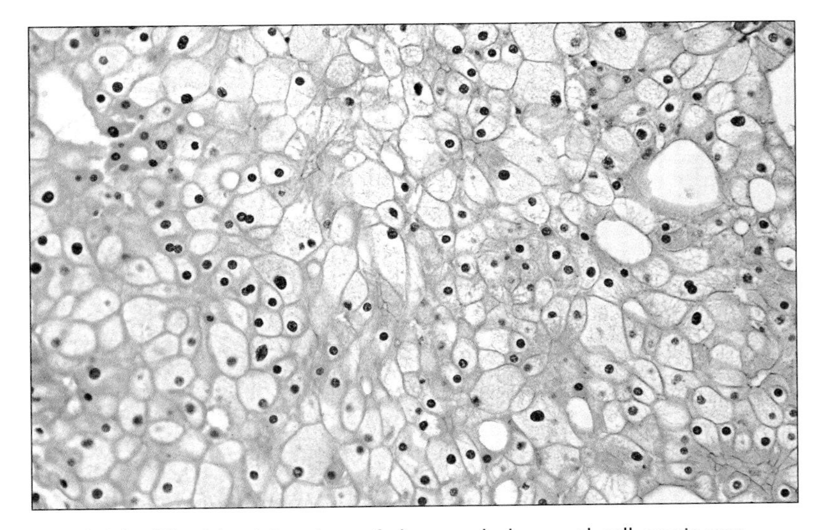

Fig. 8.64 The 'classic' variant of chromophobe renal cell carcinoma consists of predominantly large, round to polygonal cells with well-defined cell borders and pale cytoplasm. The cytoplasm, in fact, is not totally clear but translucent and finely reticulated. Many cases contain larger cells with abundant clear to foamy ('hydropic') cytoplasm.

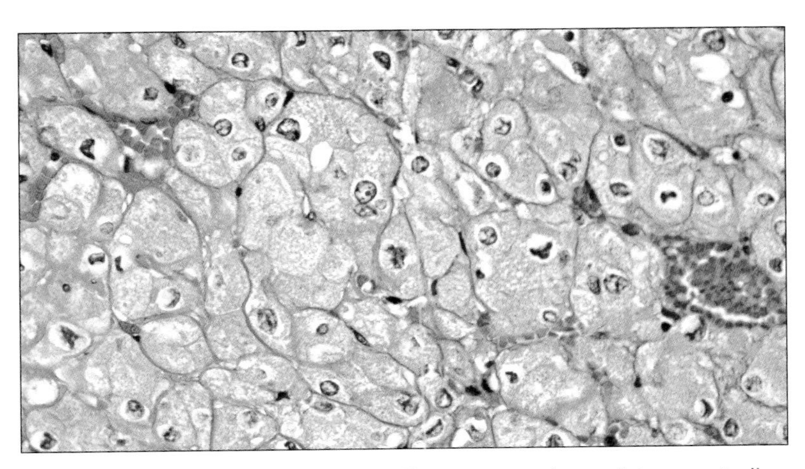

Fig. 8.67 In chromophobe renal cell carcinoma, the nuclei are typically hyperchromatic, with an irregular nuclear membrane.[84] Binucleate cells are present in all cases. Focal cytologic atypia with bizarre nuclei is seen in half the cases, but is a prominent feature in only a small minority of tumors. Round nuclei with only focally wrinkled contours may be present in rare tumors. Mitotic activity is very low, except in sarcomatoid areas.

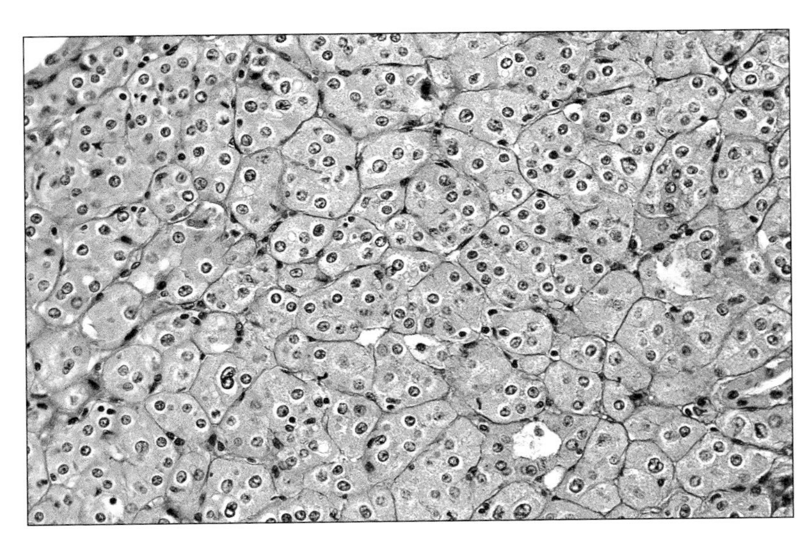

Fig. 8.65 A predominance of tumor cells with more dense eosinophilic cytoplasm is seen in 30% of cases, and these constitute the 'eosinophilic variants' of chromophobe renal cell carcinoma.

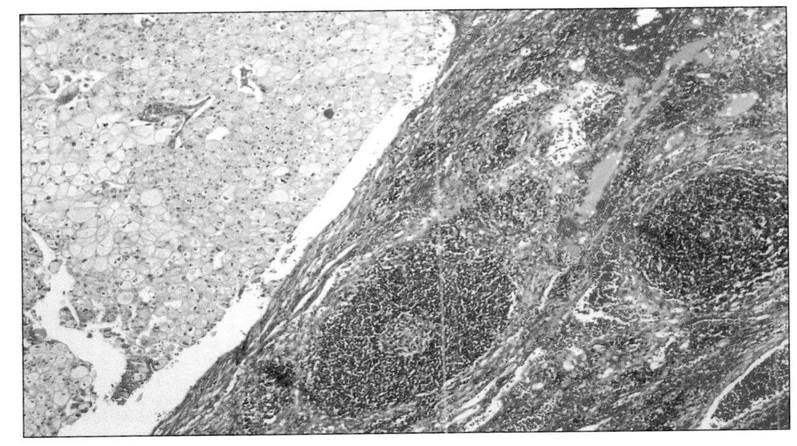

Fig. 8.68 Although a few tumors show extrarenal soft tissue extension (pT3), metastatic disease (metastasis to regional lymph node shown here) at presentation is uncommon.

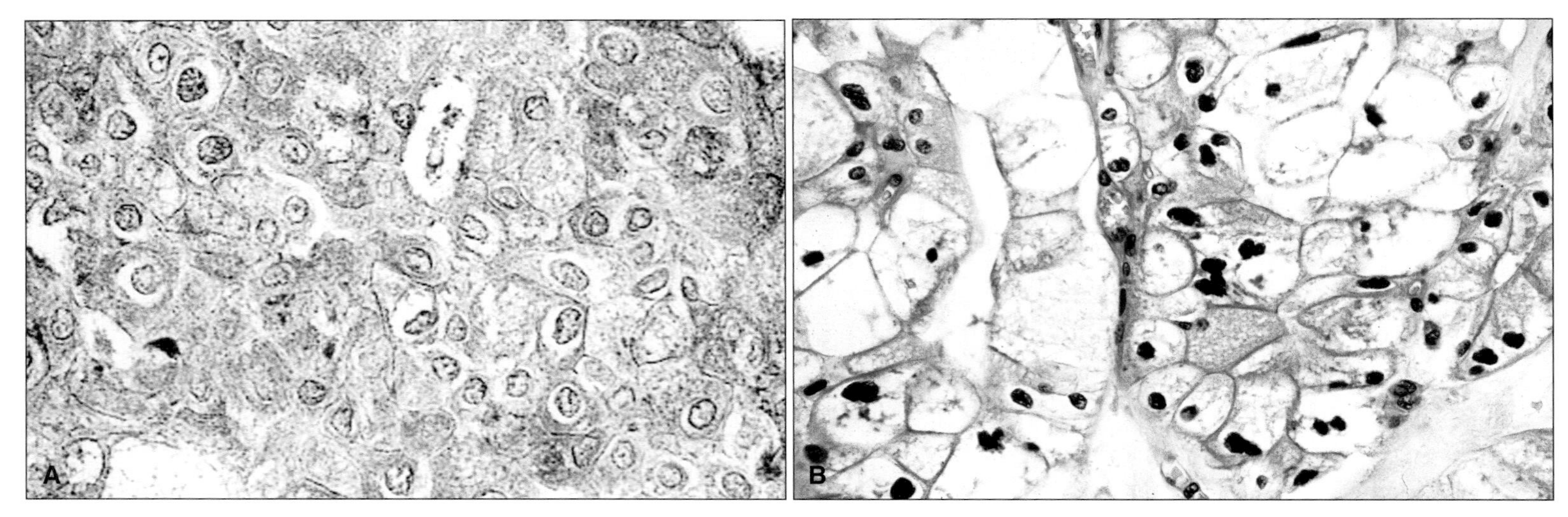

Fig. 8.69 (A,B) Variable granular or reticular and diffuse cytoplasmic staining with Hale's colloidal iron is reported in the majority of cases. Diffuse, reticular positivity with Hale's colloidal iron stain, when present, is highly characteristic of chromophobe renal cell carcinoma.[85,86] However, the stain is highly fastidious and procedure-dependent. Weak Hale's colloidal iron positivity has been demonstrated in other renal tumors, including a focal droplet-like staining in clear cell (conventional) and papillary renal cell carcinoma, and focal, or sometimes diffuse, but chiefly luminal, staining in renal oncocytoma.

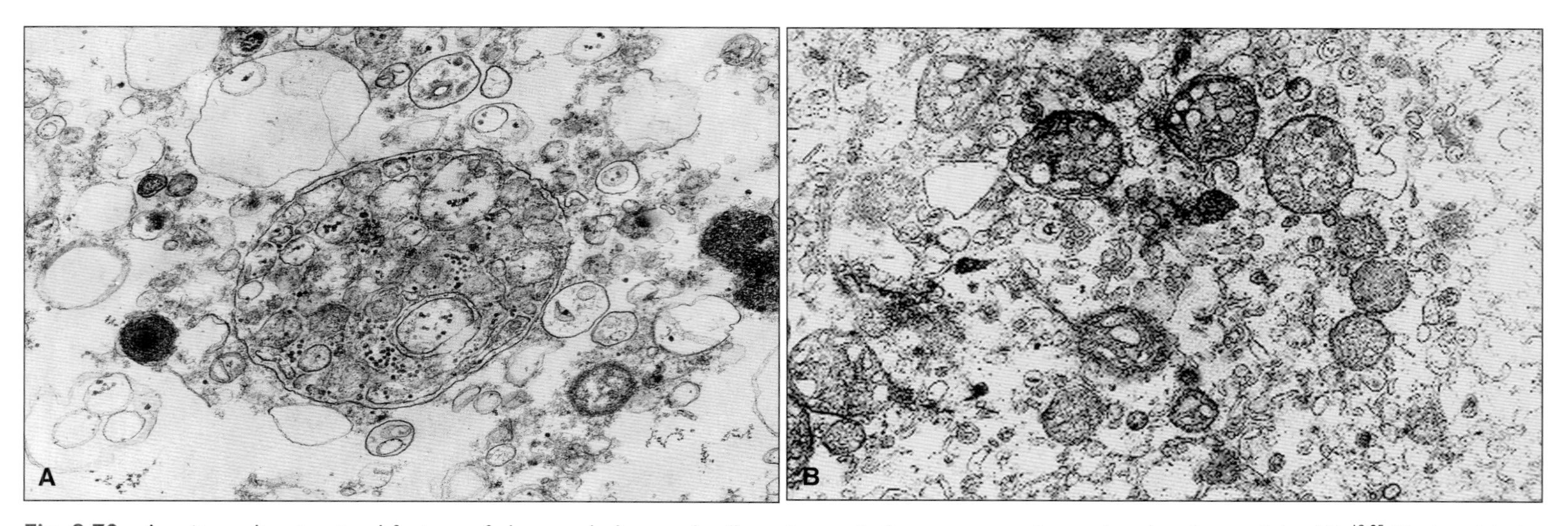

Fig. 8.70 A unique ultrastructural feature of chromophobe renal cell carcinoma is the presence of cytoplasmic microvesicles (A).[12,85] Their origin is believed to be related to defective mitochondriogenesis. Tissue processing for paraffin embedding results in disruption of these vesicles and cannot be employed for the ultrastructural confirmation of a histologic diagnosis of chromophobe renal cell carcinoma.[87] The mitochondria often show tubulocystic cristae (B).

Cytogenetics

The genetic and molecular genetic findings have not been studied well. The reported findings include monosomy of chromosomes 1, 6, 14, 15, and 22, loss of heterozygosity of chromosomal arm 1q, and minimal area of deletion at 1q32.1–32.2.[97–101] Importantly, of all the tumors studied, none has shown trisomy 7 or 17 or losses of chromosome 3.

Immunohistochemistry

The tumors show immunoreactivity for CEA, peanut agglutinin, soybean agglutinin, and *Ulex europaeus* agglutinin (see Table 8.2).[93,94,96] Cytokeratin 34βE12 and CK7 may be positive as well. While this immunophenotype may help distinguish CDC from PRCC, it is not specific, as a similar staining profile may be seen in urothelial tumors, including those arising in the renal pelvis.

Differential diagnosis

Classic tumors are morphologically distinct. In other cases, the differential diagnosis may include PRCC, medullary carcinoma, and, more commonly, urothelial carcinoma of the pelvicalyceal system invading the renal parenchyma. PRCCs are rarely associated with desmoplastic stroma and the papillae are more likely to contain foamy macrophages. Histochemical, immunohistochemical, and genetic features can also aid in classifying these tumors.

Distinguishing between high-grade urothelial carcinoma and CDC may present a more difficult problem since both may be associated with an inflamed, fibrotic, or desmoplastic stroma and may contain neoplastic cells within adjacent renal tubules. In addition, both may have a tubular or tubulopapillary pattern of growth and a similar immunophenotype. Intracytoplasmic mucin may be seen in urothelial tumors as well. Although the presence of squamous differentiation and a more solid nested architectural pattern favors urothelial carcinoma, the best way to resolve this differential diagnosis is by looking for in situ urothelial carcinoma. Molecular studies may also be of diagnostic utility. (Figs 8.71–8.75)

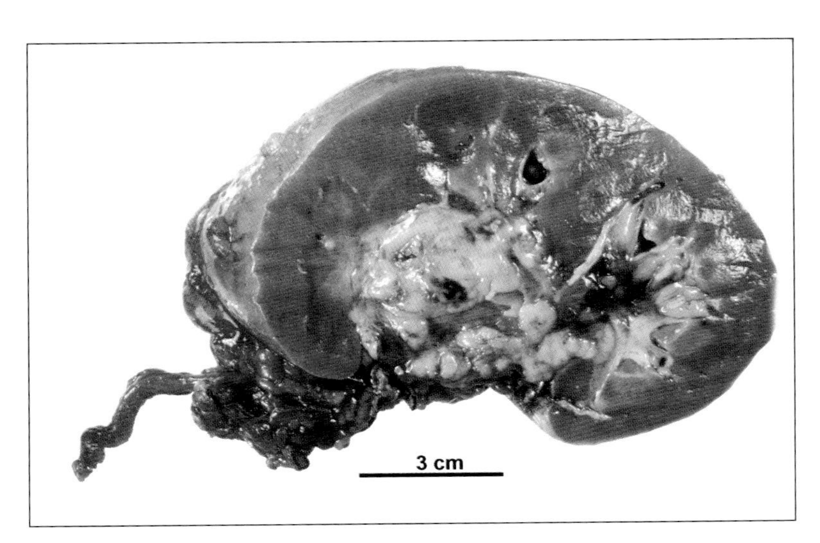

Fig. 8.71 Collecting duct carcinomas are centered in the medulla, although large tumors may occupy the cortex as well. They are usually poorly circumscribed, and often extend into the renal sinus and hilar fat. The cut surface is solid, tan–white, and firm, but may show cysts as well as gross evidence of hemorrhage and necrosis.

MEDULLARY CARCINOMA

This unique group of highly aggressive tumors predominantly affects young patients of African-American descent.[104–109] Patients present at a mean age of 22 years (range, 11–39 years), although rare cases in older patients have been described. Males predominate, especially in patients below the age of 25. Almost all patients have sickle cell trait except for rare cases that have sickle cell disease or hemoglobin SC disease.[104–110] Most cases reported had metastatic disease at the time of presentation, and mean survival is approximately 4 months.[110]

These tumors are believed to arise from the distal collecting ducts. Morphologically, they share features with high-grade CDC, and many have considered them to be a variant of CDC. Recently, however, many differences between the two entities have been reported.[110]

Differential diagnosis

Differential diagnosis includes collecting duct and high-grade urothelial carcinoma. Careful sampling and attention to the clinical features of the case may be needed to accurately classify the tumor. The immunohistochemical features of the three tumor types overlap significantly. However, the authors of a recent study did not find the presence of high molecular weight cytokeratin (34βE12) in any of their medullary carcinoma cases, although most patients with CDC and urothelial carcinoma are positive for this antibody.[110] (Figs 8.76–8.78)

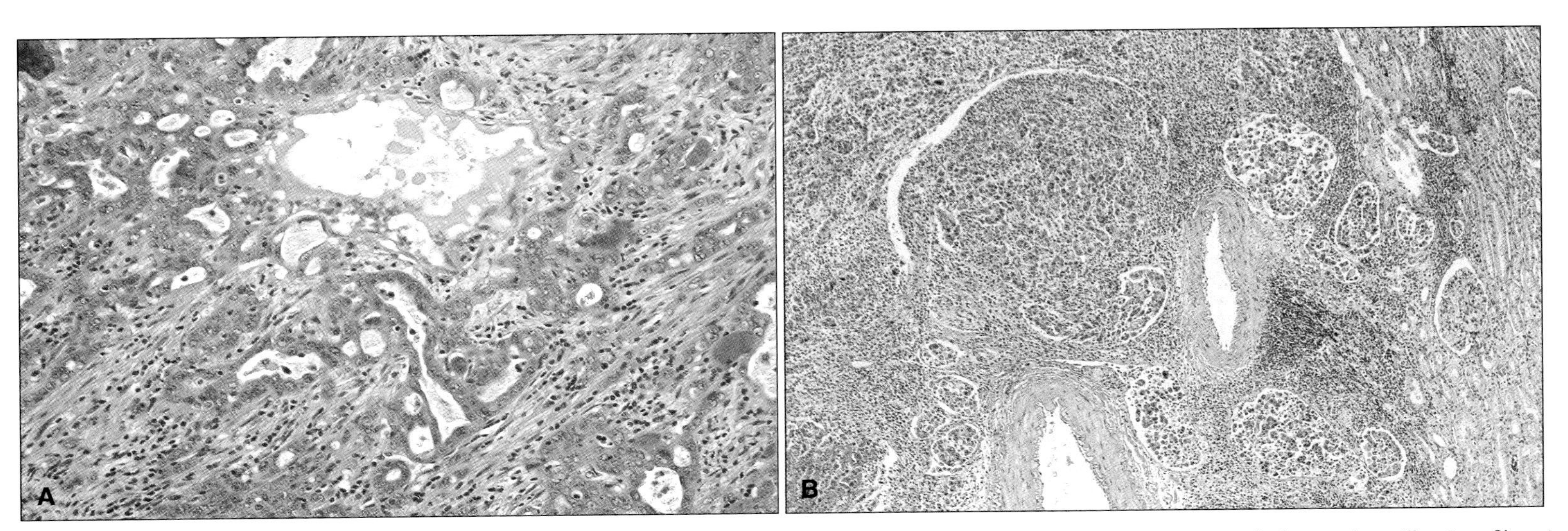

Fig. 8.72 (A,B) The histologic features of classic collecting duct carcinomas are multinodularity, and neoplastic ducts, tubules, and papillae in a fibrotic or desmoplastic stroma. The tumor cells have eosinophilic, basophilic, or amphophilic cytoplasm, high-grade nuclei, and prominent nucleoli. Some cases may be focally or predominantly sarcomatoid.[102] Cytoplasmic and luminal mucin is frequently present.

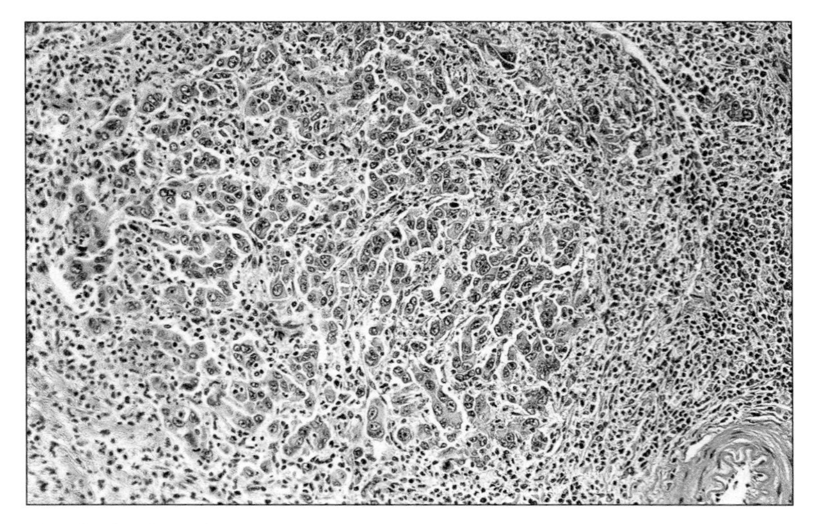

Fig. 8.73 In collecting duct carcinoma, the papillae rarely, if ever, contain foamy macrophages. Acute or chronic inflammatory cells are usually abundant within the surrounding stroma (shown here). Psammoma bodies are rare.

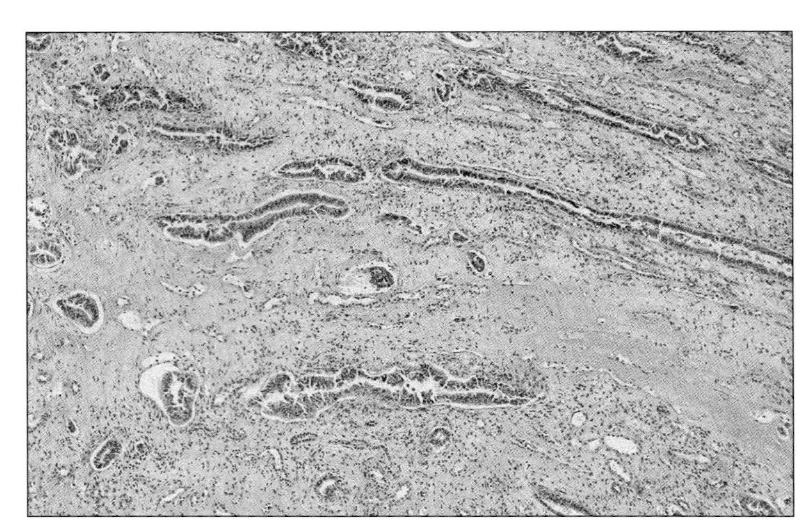

Fig. 8.74 Characteristically, in collecting duct carcinoma, adjacent renal tubules are lined by dysplastic cells.

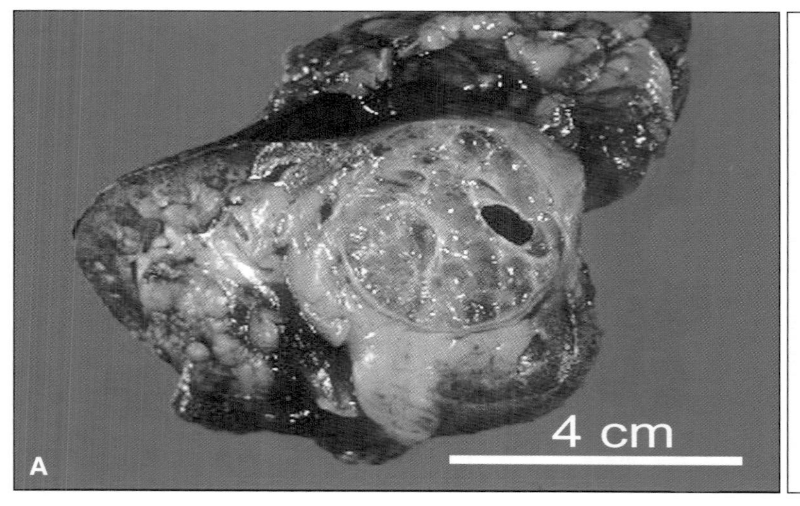

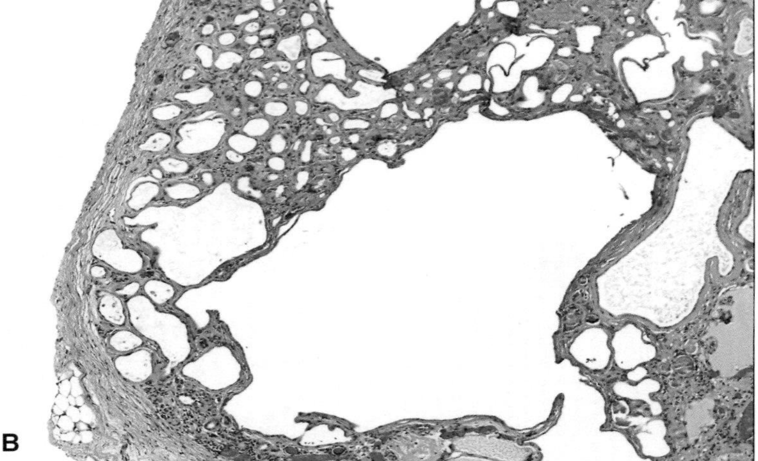

Fig. 8.75 The morphologic spectrum of collecting duct carcinoma (CDC) has been expanded recently to include not only sarcomatoid lesions but also 'low-grade' tumors. These are characterized by multilocular cystic gross appearance (A) and tubulocystic pattern of growth, tumor cells with low-grade nuclei, hobnailed cytoplasm, and mucin production on microscopic evaluation (B).[103] No molecular studies are available for this subtype of CDC.

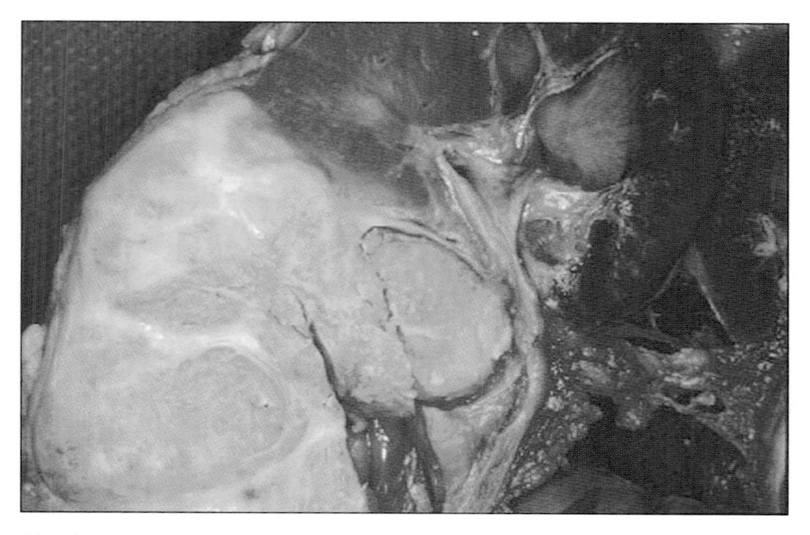

Fig. 8.76 Medullary carcinomas tend to be centered in the medulla of the kidney. Mean tumor size is 7.0 cm (range, 4.0–12.0 cm).

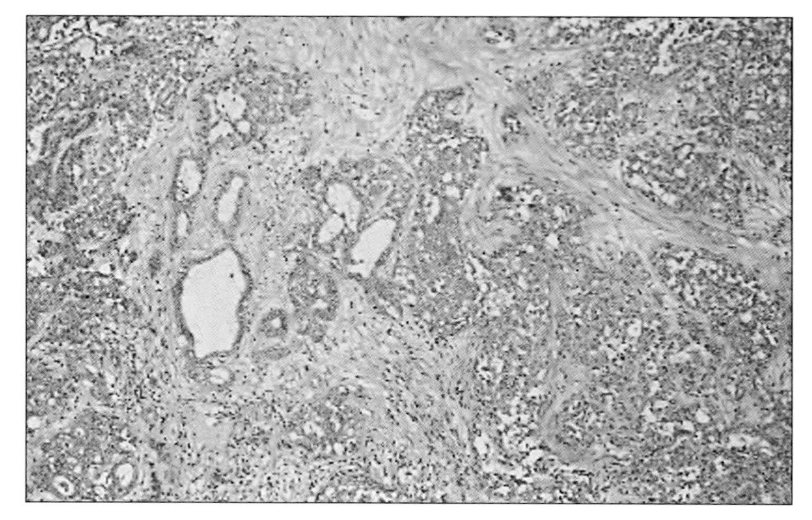

Fig. 8.77 Medullary carcinomas are composed of cells with high-grade nuclei and prominent nucleoli arranged in solid nests or irregular tubules. Microcystic or reticular growth like that seen in yolk sac tumors is common. Areas resembling adenoid cystic carcinoma have also been described.

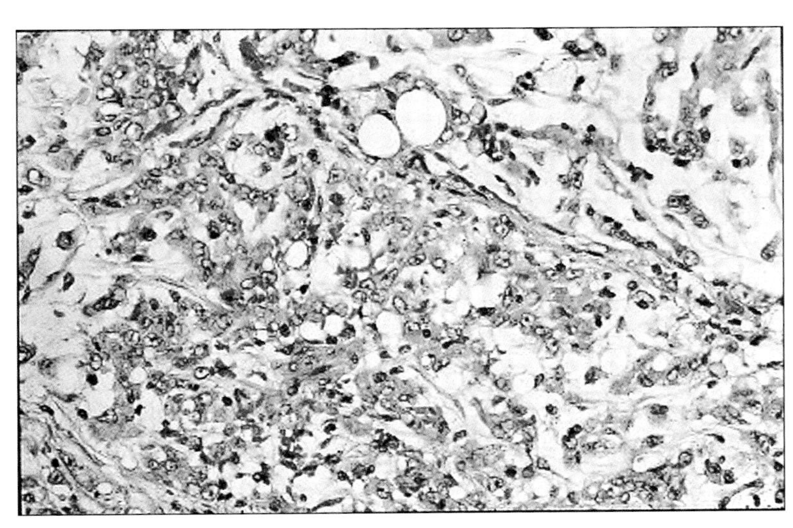

Fig. 8.78 In medullary carcinoma, the surrounding stroma is usually fibrotic or desmoplastic. Stroma is infiltrated by abundant inflammatory cells, mostly polymorphonuclear cells. Many blood vessels in the tissue sections contain irregular or sickled red blood cells.

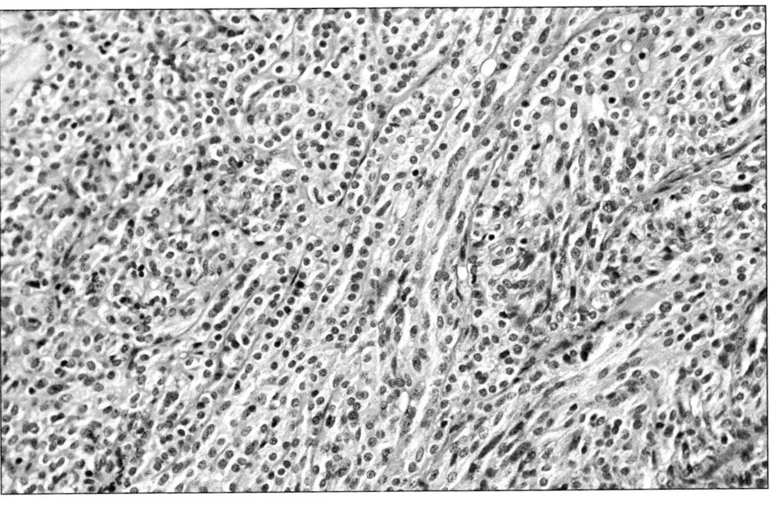

Fig. 8.79 Microscopically, mucinous tubular and spindle cell carcinoma is composed of elongated, interconnected tubules, many appearing straight and with slit-like lumina, solid compressed cord-like structures, and prominent low-grade spindle cell areas. The cells, other than those in the spindled areas, are low cuboidal with small amounts of eosinophilic cytoplasm, and with low-grade bland-appearing nuclei. Papillary areas and cysts are not identified.

MUCINOUS TUBULAR AND SPINDLE CELL CARCINOMA (LOW-GRADE BIPHASIC RENAL CELL CARCINOMA OF POSSIBLE COLLECTING DUCT OR LOOP OF HENLE ORIGIN)

This recently described tumor is unique among renal epithelial neoplasms in being a tumor with a less aggressive biologic behavior in spite of containing a spindle cell component that morphologically mimics a low-grade sarcoma. Most have been reported in females, with age ranges of 17 to 78 years (average, 53 years).[111–114]

Ultrastructure

Ultrastructural evaluation done on a few cases shows close resemblance to the normal loop of Henle. Comparative genomic hybridization (CGH) data available on a few cases show frequent losses at chromosomes 1, 4q, 6, 8p, 11q, 13, 14, and 15, with gains at 11q, 16q, 17, and 20q. No evidence of *VHL* deletions was found by FISH analysis.[114]

Gross appearance

Grossly, it is a well-circumscribed tumor with a tan–white cut surface that sometimes shows areas of hemorrhage and necrosis. The epicenter is usually located in the renal medulla. (Figs 8.79 & 8.80)

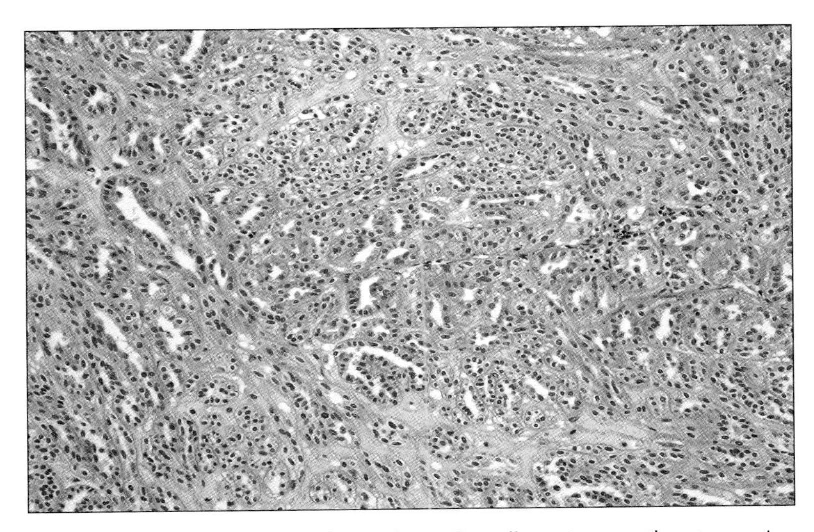

Fig. 8.80 In mucinous tubular and spindle cell carcinoma, the stroma is characteristically, and at least focally, myxoid, and usually contains some inflammatory cell infiltrates.

RENAL CELL CARCINOMA, UNCLASSIFIED

This diagnostic category includes the renal carcinomas that do not fit into any of the above-described categories, even after genetic analysis. Thus, tumors of unrecognizable cell or architectural type, or those with apparent composites of the recognized types, are all included in this category.[14,15] These form up to 6% of all renal epithelial tumors.[5]

While many of the tumors from this category are of high cytoarchitectural grade and behave in an aggressive manner, by definition, it is not a pure entity limited to only such aggressive tumors. Many other less aggressive tumors also belong to this group of renal neoplasms.

MIXED EPITHELIAL AND STROMAL NEOPLASMS

MIXED EPITHELIAL AND STROMAL TUMOR

This entity has various synonyms, including adult mesoblastic nephroma, cystic hamartoma of renal pelvis, leiomyomatous renal hamartoma, solid and cystic biphasic tumor, etc.[115–120] The tumor appears biphasic, composed of mesenchymal (stromal) and epithelial components. Some authors consider the latter entrapped renal tubules, while others believe they represent neoplastic elements. The tumor differs from the congenital form of mesoblastic nephroma in many ways, and even lacks the genetic alterations typical of cellular congenital mesoblastic nephroma.[121] Therefore the term mesoblastic nephroma is not appropriate in this setting.

Patients range in age from 19 to 78 years, and most reported cases have been females (male-to-female ratio, 1 : 10). Presenting signs and symptoms most commonly include a palpable abdominal or flank mass, flank pain, or hematuria. However, in a recent study, most were incidental findings.[120] All reported cases of adult mixed epithelial and stromal tumors have behaved in a benign manner following surgical excision, though one recurred locally 21 years after resection.[116]

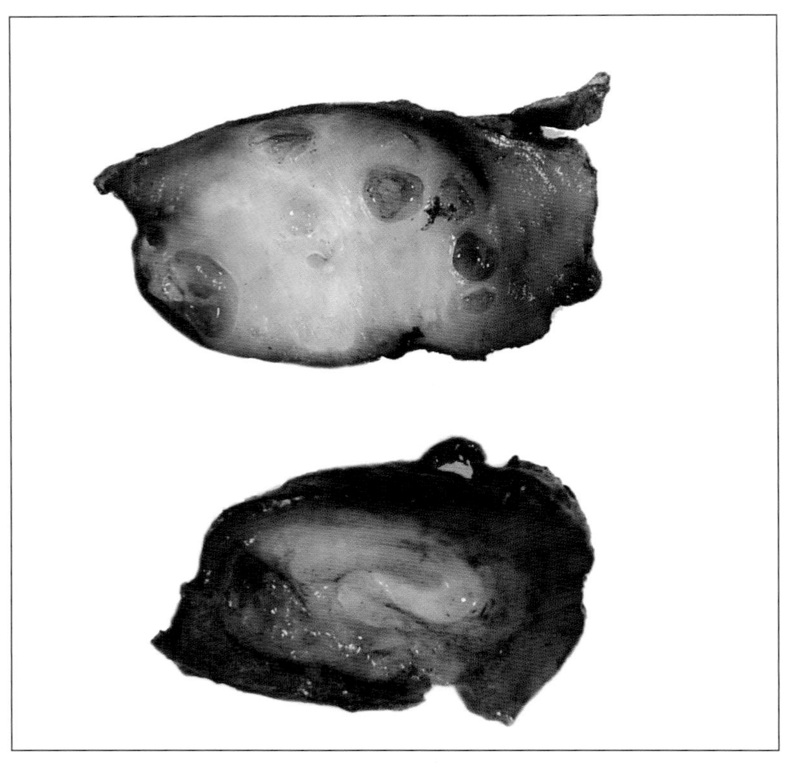

Fig. 8.81 Mixed epithelial and stromal tumors are solid or solid and cystic, tan to yellow, and well circumscribed and encapsulated, and range in size from 2 to 24 cm. In some cases, a cystic component predominates and is associated with a solid mural nodule. In other cases, the appearance may mimic multilocular cystic renal cell carcinoma.

Immunohistochemistry

The immunohistochemical profile of the mesenchymal component reflects the degree of smooth muscle differentiation seen on routine H&E-stained sections. The epithelial components are positive for both low and high molecular weight cytokeratins and *Ulex europaeus* lectin. Positive reactions with antibodies to estrogen and progesterone receptors (ER and PR) have recently been described.[120] (Figs 8.81–8.83)

Table 8.6 Features differentiating adult and pediatric cystic nephroma

Cystic nephroma of childhood	*Cystic nephroma of adults*
Age at presentation usually less than 4 years	Age at presentation usually more than 30 years
Male:female ratio 2:1	Male:female ratio 1:8
Pathogenesis related to Wilms' tumor, considered to be fully differentiated CPDN	Not related to Wilms' tumor
Stroma consists of myxoid to collagenous fibrous tissue	Stroma may resemble ovarian stroma, which may be ER/PR positive

CPDN, cystic partially differentiated nephroblastoma; ER, estrogen receptor; PR, progesterone receptor.

CYSTIC NEPHROMA

Adult cystic nephroma (CN) predominantly affects females.[54,122] (See Table 8.6 for differences from childhood CN.) Most tumors are asymptomatic or present as a palpable abdominal mass. There is some overlap between adult CN and adult mixed epithelial and stromal tumors, although the exact relationship between the two tumors remains undefined. We reserve the term cystic nephroma for the lesions that are grossly multicystic without any solid nodules, and adult mixed epithelial and stromal tumor for the tumors with variable solid and cystic appearance.

Gross appearance

Grossly, CN is well circumscribed, and is composed of multiple, non-communicating cysts that vary in size and contain clear fluid. No communication with the pelvicalyceal system is present. No solid expansile nodules, hemorrhage, or necrosis is identified. (Figs 8.84 & 8.85)

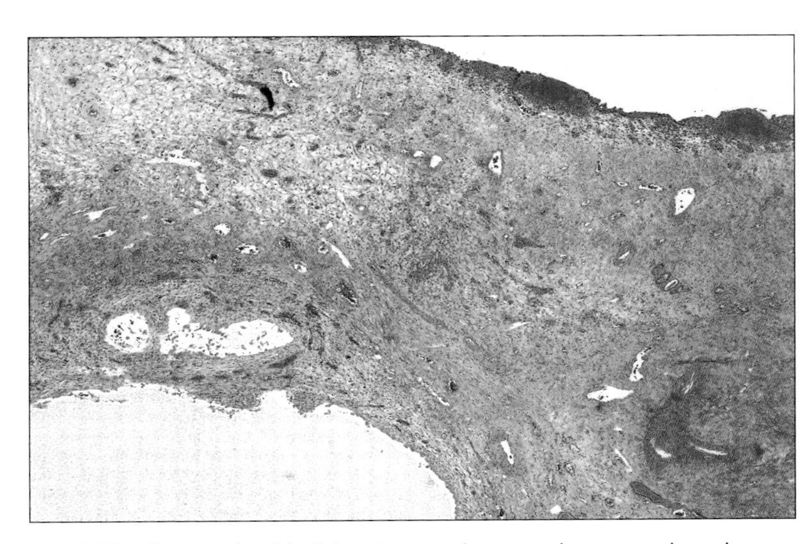

Fig. 8.82 In mixed epithelial and stromal tumor, the mesenchymal component is characterized by fascicles and sheets of spindle cells showing variable degrees of smooth muscle, fibroblastic, or myofibroblastic differentiation with interspersed collagen. In some cases, the mesenchymal component resembles ovarian stroma (see also Fig. 8.84). Mitotic figures, hemorrhage, and necrosis are uncommon.

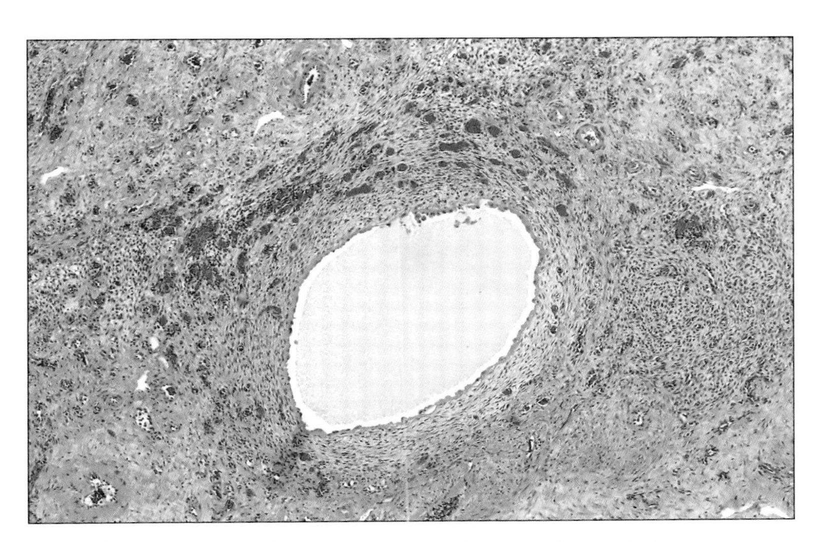

Fig. 8.83 In mixed epithelial and stromal tumor, the epithelial components vary from round and regular tubules to more complex structures that show papillations and cystic dilatation. They are lined by cuboidal to flattened epithelium that may show clear cell change or have a hobnail appearance. Unlike mesoblastic nephroma, the epithelial components may be found interspersed throughout the mesenchymal components and not merely restricted to the periphery of the tumor nodules.

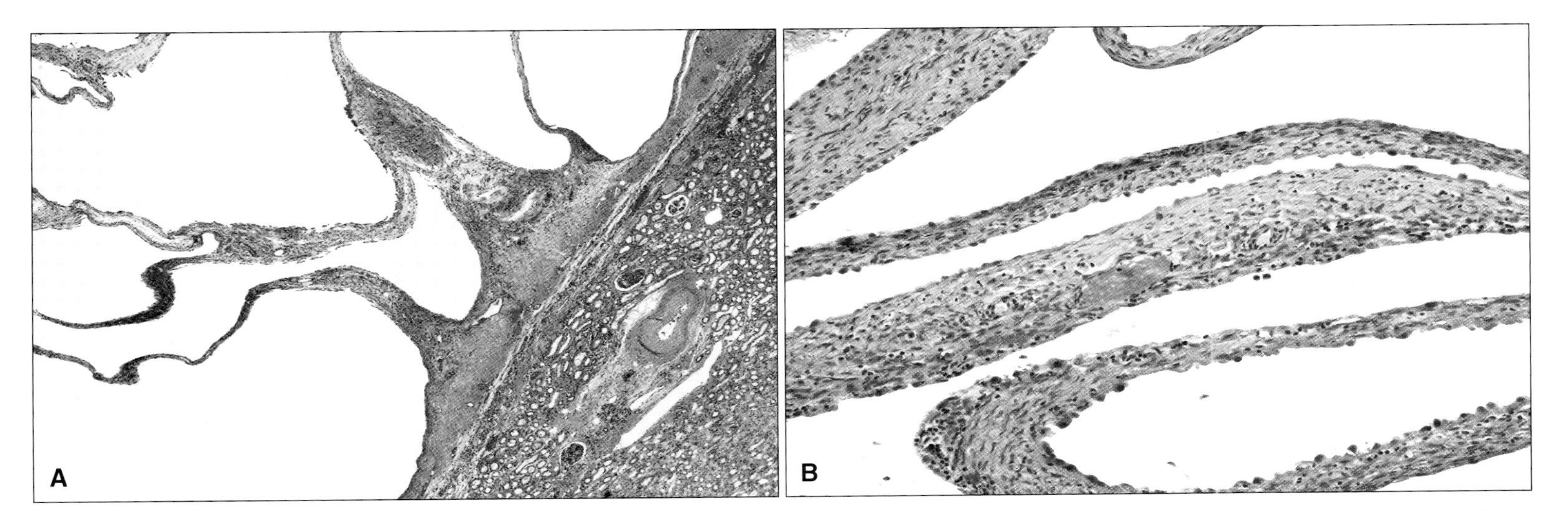

Fig. 8.84 (A,B) Microscopically, in cystic nephroma, the cysts are lined by flattened, cuboidal, or hobnail cells and the septa are composed of fibrous tissue of variable cellularity, at times having the appearance of ovarian-type stroma. The ovarian-type stroma frequently shows positive immunohistochemical reaction for estrogen and progesterone receptors. The fibrous septa may contain microscopic cysts lined by bland cuboidal cells reminiscent of renal tubules.

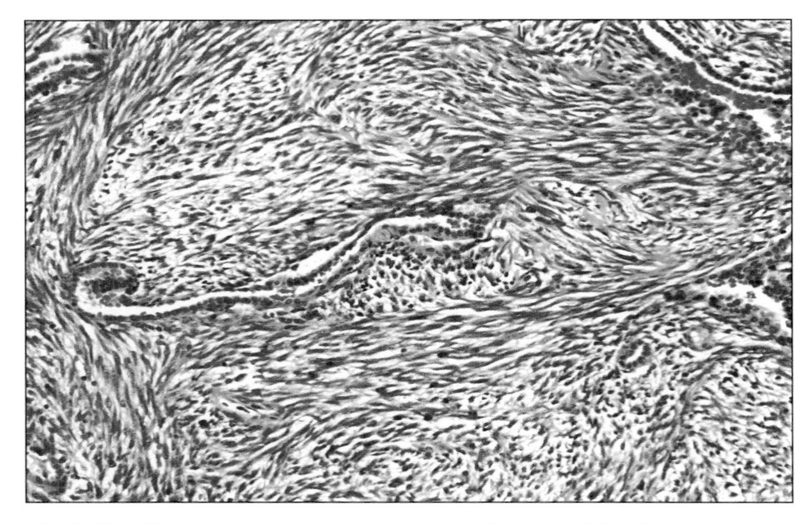

Fig. 8.85 Sarcomas have rarely been described as arising from cystic nephromas.[123,124] Most are undifferentiated embryonal-type tumors. Recently, some embryonal sarcomas arising in the background of cystic nephroma were found to have the *SYT–SSX* gene fusion resulting from the translocation t(X;18), a characteristic of synovial sarcoma.[124] These tumors have been redesignated as 'primary renal synovial sarcomas'.

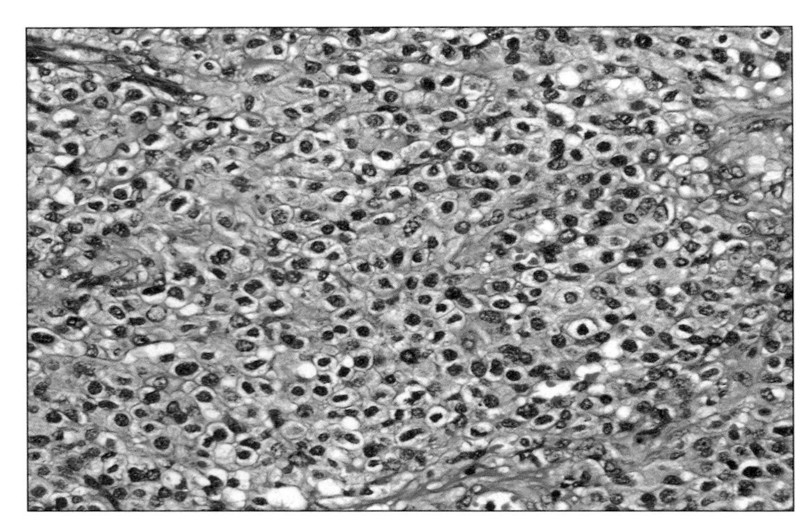

Fig. 8.86 The histologic appearance of juxtaglomerular cell tumors is variable. Classic examples have a glomus tumor-like appearance and are composed of sheets of homogeneous round to polygonal cells with clear to slightly eosinophilic cytoplasm and distinct cell borders. Others consist of sheets or irregular cords of polygonal to spindle cells with indistinct cell borders. Some tumors contain well-developed tubules. A papillary pattern has been described in which the neoplastic cells form papillary fronds lined by cuboidal cells.[128]

MISCELLANEOUS TUMORS

JUXTAGLOMERULAR CELL TUMOR

Juxtaglomerular cell tumor is an extremely uncommon renal tumor of young adults in the second and third decades of life; a few cases have been described in the sixth and seventh decades.[125–127] Signs and symptoms of hyper-reninism are the hallmark of juxtaglomerular cell tumor and include hypertension, hyperaldosteronism, and hypokalemia. Females outnumber males by a roughly 1.5 : 1 margin. Juxtaglomerular cell tumors are benign neoplasms. Surgical resection of the affected kidney cures systemic hypertension in most patients.

Immunohistochemistry

Immunohistochemistry shows diffuse positive staining with antibodies to renin and vimentin. A variable number of common muscle actin (HHF-35), smooth muscle actin, and CD34-positive cells may be found, while neuroendocrine markers are negative. Cytokeratin stains label the cuboidal epithelium of the tubules but not the polygonal or spindle cells.

Ultrastructure

Electron microscopy shows distinctive membrane-bound rhomboid and polygonal granules that are immunoreactive with antibodies to renin.

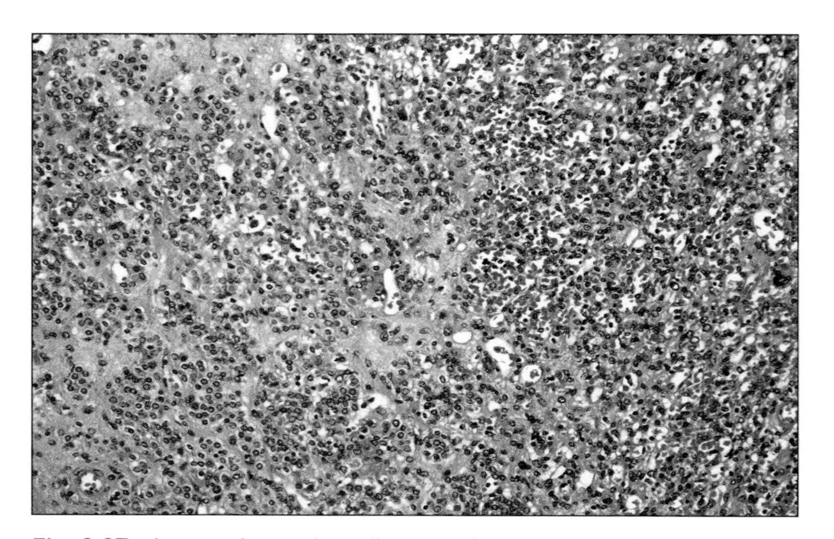

Fig. 8.87 In juxtaglomerular cell tumor, the stroma may be scanty or consist of large areas of hyalinized or myxoid fibrous tissue and often contains a scattered lymphoplasmacytic infiltrate. Numerous capillaries and branching blood vessels and sinusoids similar to those of hemangiopericytoma are typically found. Pleomorphism and mitotic activity are uncommon. Periodic acid–Schiff (PAS) stain reveals cytoplasmic granules in a subset of cells.

Gross appearance

Juxtaglomerular cell tumors are well-encapsulated, light tan to yellow, unilateral and solitary tumors. Most are solid, though small cysts may be present. The majority of the tumors are relatively small, ranging in diameter from 2 to 3 cm. (Figs 8.86 & 8.87)

CARCINOID TUMOR

Carcinoid tumor of the kidney is very rare and less than 50 cases have been described in the literature.[129–132] Before accepting a tumor as primary carcinoid tumor of the kidney, it is imperative to exclude the possibility of a metastasis. In a case of renal carcinoid tumor with vascular invasion, the latter is more likely, and the primary source may become apparent only after prolonged follow-up.

Most patients with carcinoid of the kidney present in the fifth to seventh decades of life. Males and females are affected equally. Most cases are discovered incidentally following radiologic investigation for other diseases; overt endocrine disturbances, including the carcinoid syndrome, are uncommon.[133–136] Few present with nonspecific signs and symptoms including flank pain, vague abdominal discomfort, or hematuria.

Approximately one-third of patients show metastases to sites including regional lymph nodes, liver, lung, and bone, and many deaths due to disease have been reported. Like carcinoids found elsewhere, histologic features do not predict outcome. However, in one study, mitotic activity and pleomorphism were shown to be associated with an aggressive behavior.[131]

Immunohistochemistry

By immunohistochemistry, renal carcinoids show positive reactions to neuron-specific enolase (NSE), chromogranin, synaptophysin, serotonin, somatostatin, pancreatic polypeptide, and glucagon. Like hindgut carcinoids, positive reactions to prostatic acid phosphatase have been reported.[137] Electron microscopy confirms the presence of dense core granules.

Rare cases have been described as components of cystic teratoma of the kidney.[138] (Figs 8.88 & 8.89)

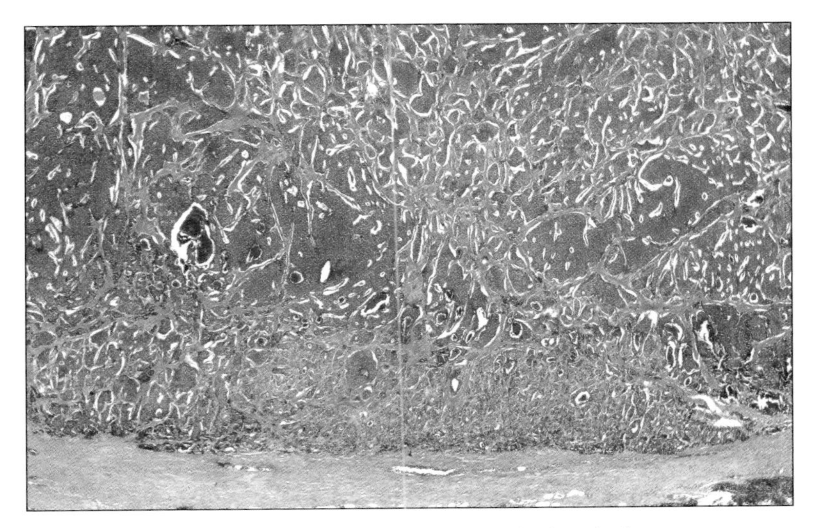

Fig. 8.88 Renal carcinoids are well-circumscribed and often encapsulated, tan to yellow, solid and fleshy tumors that frequently show areas of hemorrhage and necrosis or cystic degeneration. Reported tumors have ranged in size from 2 to 30 cm in greatest dimension (mean, 9 cm). Diffuse infiltration of renal parenchyma is not a feature of renal carcinoid, though invasion of perinephric adipose tissue and renal vein have been described. Some examples have been described in horseshoe kidneys.[139]

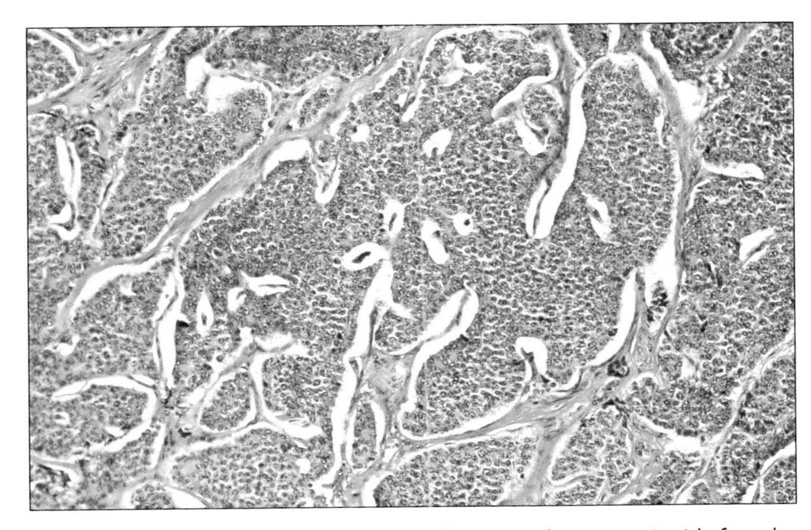

Fig. 8.89 Histologically, renal carcinoids are similar to carcinoids found at other sites, with nested or trabecular architecture supported by a well-vascularized stroma. They possess the characteristic 'salt and pepper' appearance of generally uniform, round nuclei. Though focal pleomorphism may be seen, mitotic figures and vascular invasion are uncommon.

OTHER NEUROENDOCRINE NEOPLASMS

Primary renal small cell carcinoma, pheochromocytoma, and neuroblastoma have been described. Small cell carcinomas are large, locally invasive neoplasms that often present with regional or distant metastases. Before accepting a tumor as primary small cell carcinoma of the kidney, the possibility of metastasis must be excluded.

PRIMITIVE NEUROECTODERMAL TUMOR

Primary primitive neuroectodermal tumors (PNETs) of the kidney are quite rare,[140–143] but recently two studies with large numbers of cases were published, including 79 cases from the files of the National Wilms' Tumor Study Group.[144,145] Patients range in age from 4 to 61 years, with the majority in the second and third decades of life. Presenting signs and symptoms are nonspecific.

Cytogenetics

Similar to the PNET/Ewing's sarcomas at other sites, most renal PNETs show the translocation t(11;22)(q24;q12), which results in most cases of fusion of the *ews* gene on chromosome 22 to the *Fli-1* gene on chromosome 11.[142–146]

Demonstration of the characteristic t(11;22), or, less frequently, t(21;22), may help to confirm the diagnosis of renal PNET.

Immunohistochemistry

Expression of the *MIC2* gene product by immunohistochemistry using the O13 or HBA71 antibody is characteristic, and approximately two-thirds of the tumors show Fli-1 nuclear positivity.[145] The majority of PNETs are positive with antibodies to vimentin and NSE, while a minority are positive with S-100 protein and cytokeratin.

Ultrastructure

Electron microscopy demonstrates primitive cells with interdigitating cell processes and containing occasional dense core granules and microtubules.

Gross appearance

Renal PNETs tend to be large at presentation and may entirely replace the underlying renal parenchyma. Reported size has ranged from 4 to 24 cm (mean, 16 cm). Grossly, PNETs are tan–white to gray and contain areas of hemorrhage, necrosis, and cystic degeneration. Invasion into adjacent tissues, including perinephric adipose tissue, renal vein, or inferior vena cava, may be seen. (Fig. 8.90)

ANGIOMYOLIPOMA

Angiomyolipomas are distinctive neoplasms composed of variable combinations of smooth muscle, adipose tissue, and blood vessels. Though most commonly found within the kidneys,[147,148] they may occur at extrarenal sites including liver, lungs, lymph nodes, and retroperitoneal soft tissues. While less than half of all cases occur in patients with tuberous sclerosis, approximately 80% of patients with tuberous sclerosis develop an angiomyolipoma.[149–151]

The overwhelming majority of angiomyolipomas behave in a benign fashion. The primary complication is retroperitoneal hemorrhage, which can rarely be fatal.[152] Size greater than 4 cm is considered to be an important factor for hemorrhage. Renal failure may complicate massive bilateral disease, particularly in patients with tuberous sclerosis.[153] Epithelioid tumors with pleomorphic monotypic features mimicking high-grade or sarcomatous RCC tend to behave in a more aggressive fashion.[154,155] Rare examples of 'sarcomatous transformation' to high-grade sarcomas with subsequent distant metastases have been reported.[156–158]

Angiomyolipomas are believed to arise from a putative precursor 'perivascular epithelioid cell', and appear to be related to a family of mesenchymal tumors that includes lymphangioleiomyomatosis, clear cell 'sugar' tumors of the lung, pancreas and uterus, and cardiac rhabdomyomas.

Immunohistochemistry

All are immunoreactive with the antibody HMB-45.[148,159,160]

Ultrastructure

Ultrastructural examination reveals spherical structures with internal lamellations, consistent with aberrant melanosomes, in a subset of cases. Rare type-2 premelanosomes and rhomboid crystals may also be seen. (Figs 8.91–8.99)

LIPOMA AND LIPOSARCOMA

Intrarenal lipoma is a rare neoplasm with a predilection for middle-aged females.[165] None has been reported in patients

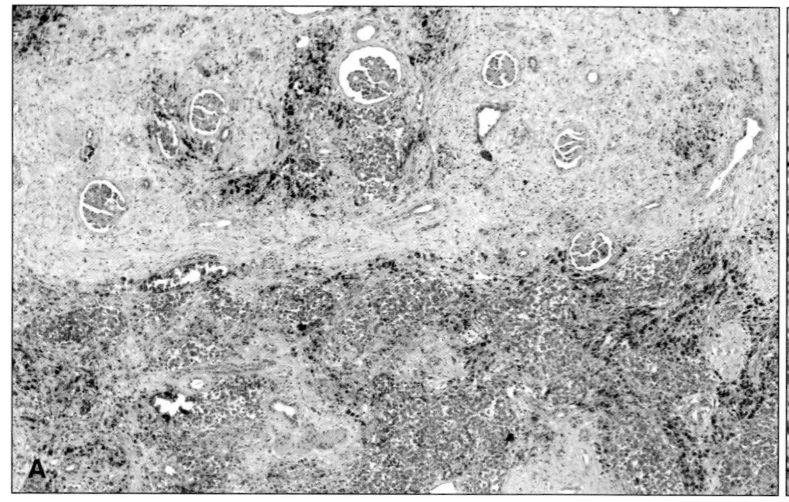

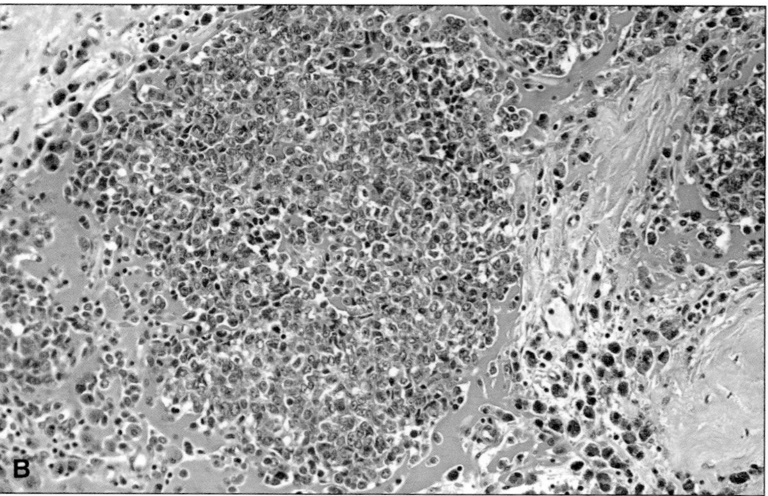

Fig. 8.90 (A,B) Microscopically, primitive neuroectodermal tumors (PNETs) of the kidney resemble PNETs found elsewhere and consist of sheets of monotonous cells with scant cytoplasm traversed by thin fibrous bands. Perivascular pseudorosettes may be seen, but true rosettes are uncommon.

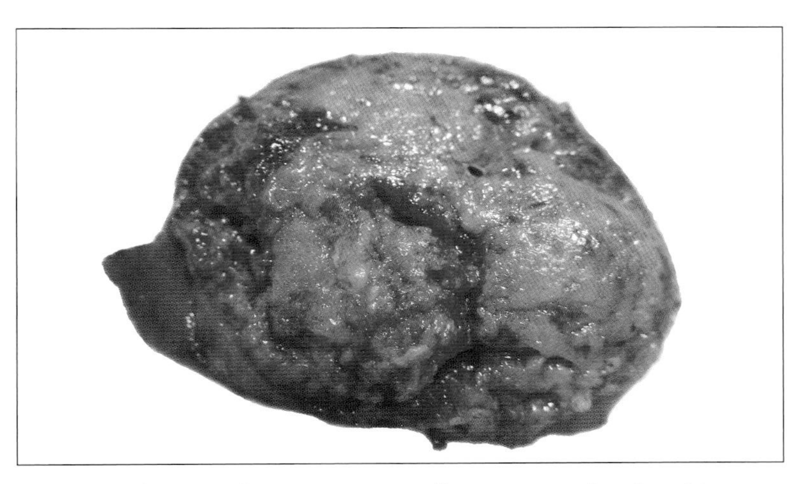

Fig. 8.91 Angiomyolipomas are generally not encapsulated, and have pushing rather than infiltrative borders. Size can range from 0.5 to 25 cm. The color and consistency are variable and reflect the relative proportion of adipose tissue and smooth muscle in a neoplasm. Classic examples contain soft yellow regions admixed with more firm tan regions.

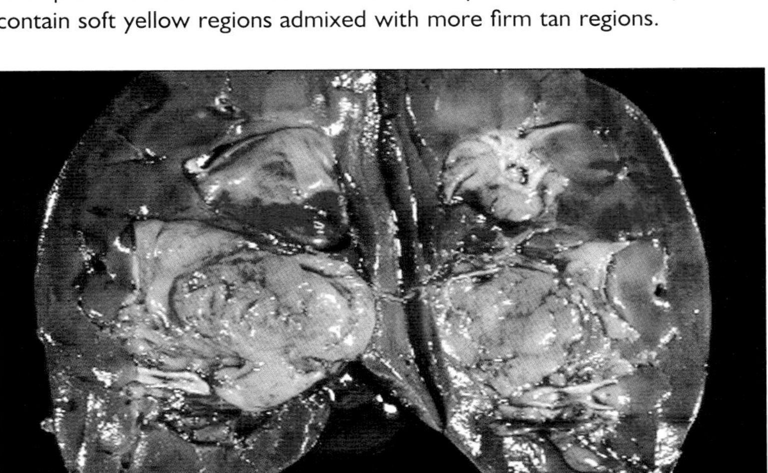

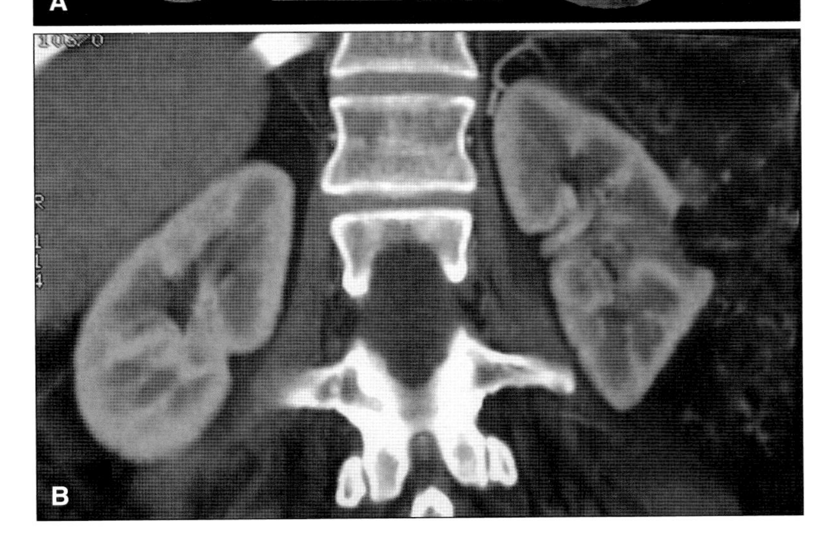

Fig. 8.92 (A,B) The majority of angiomyolipomas are unilateral and unifocal. The presence of bilateral or multifocal tumors, or tumors with epithelioid histology, strongly suggests the diagnosis of tuberous sclerosis. Small foci of hemorrhage are common, but extensive intratumoral hemorrhage is rare. Tumors with abundant intratumoral fat are easily diagnosed on radiologic evaluation. Tumors composed predominantly of adipose tissue may be confused with well-differentiated liposarcoma,[161] while others composed predominantly of smooth muscle may be confused with leiomyoma, leiomyosarcoma, or sarcomatoid renal cell carcinoma.

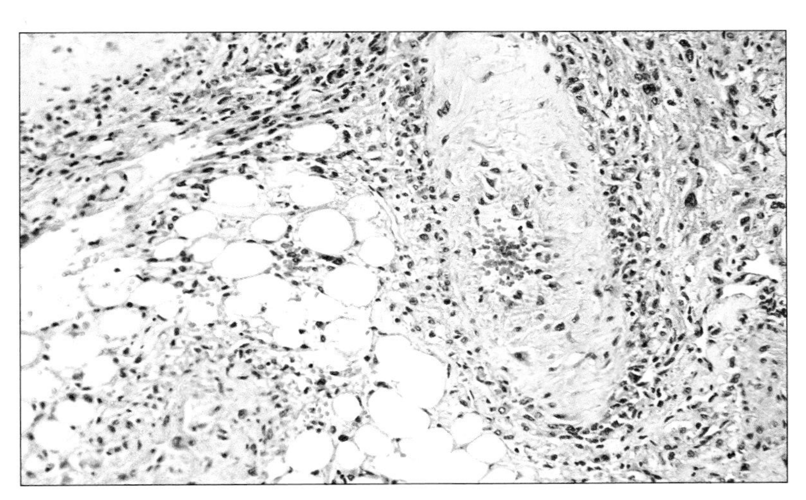

Fig. 8.93 Angiomyolipomas are composed of adipose tissue, smooth muscle, and vasculature in variable proportions. Over 90% of tumors contain at least focal areas of mature adipose tissue.

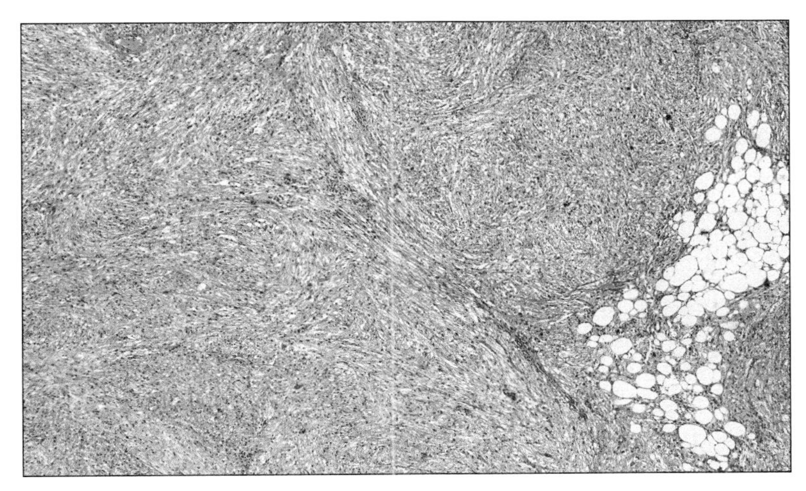

Fig. 8.94 The smooth muscle component of angiomyolipoma ranges from fascicles of elongated spindle cells to sheets of epithelioid cells with abundant eosinophilic granular cytoplasm. The smooth muscle cells often appear to originate and radiate from vessel walls.

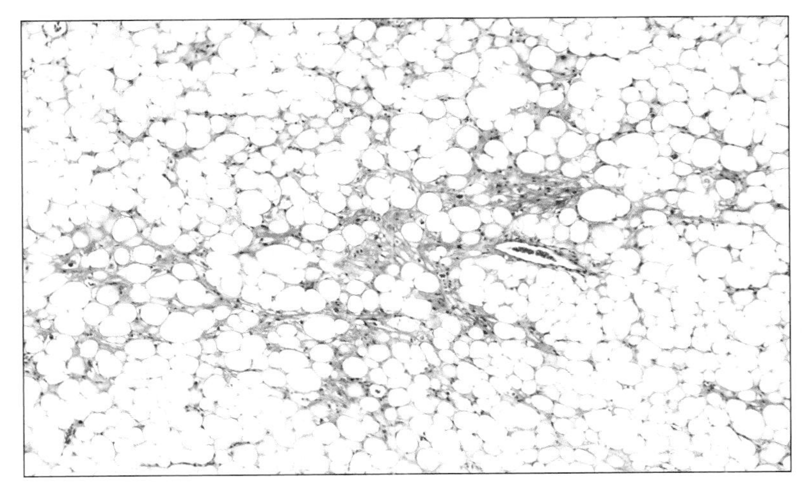

Fig. 8.95 The morphology of the vascular component of angiomyolipoma is variable, and thickened and hyalinized vessels with eccentric lumina are seen in most cases. Plump epithelioid cells often surround vascular structures and may provide an important clue to the diagnosis, particularly in tumors composed predominantly of adipose tissue. Mitotic activity is rare.

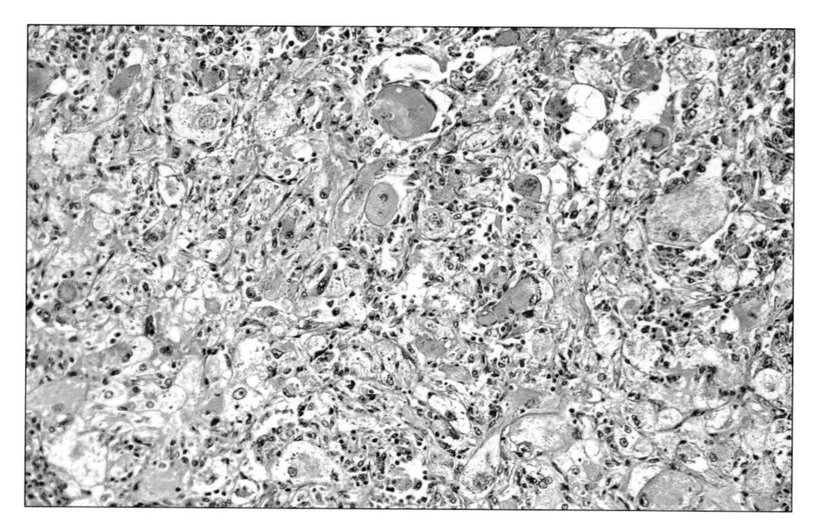

Fig. 8.96 The recently described epithelioid variant of angiomyolipoma (renal epithelioid oxyphilic neoplasm [REON]/perivascular epithelioid cell tumor [PECOMA]) is composed either exclusively or predominantly of polygonal cells with densely eosinophilic cytoplasm.[154] A variable degree of nuclear atypia is seen, including cells with multilobulated nuclei and multinucleation.

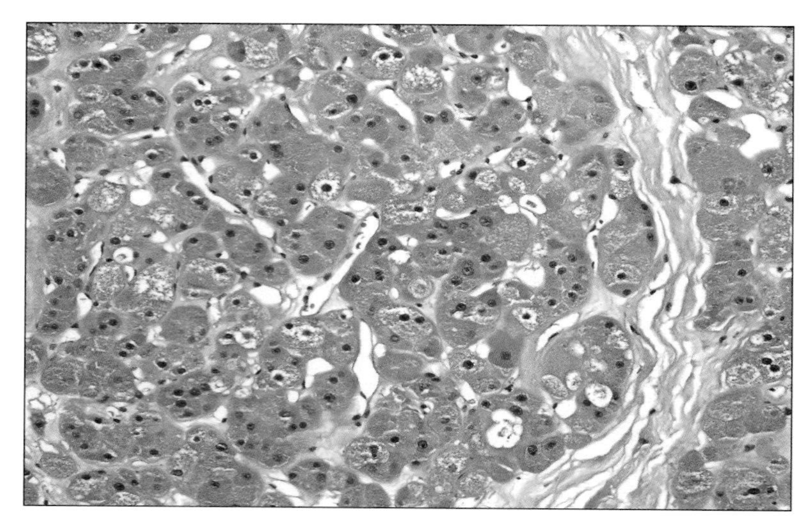

Fig. 8.97 Variable, usually focal, cytoplasmic clearing may be present in angiomyolipoma. Extensive intratumoral hemorrhage and necrosis are common in the epithelioid variant. Rare examples of angiomyolipoma composed predominantly of epithelioid cells with densely eosinophilic cytoplasm reminiscent of oncocytoma have been described recently ('oncocytoma-like angiomyolipoma').[155]

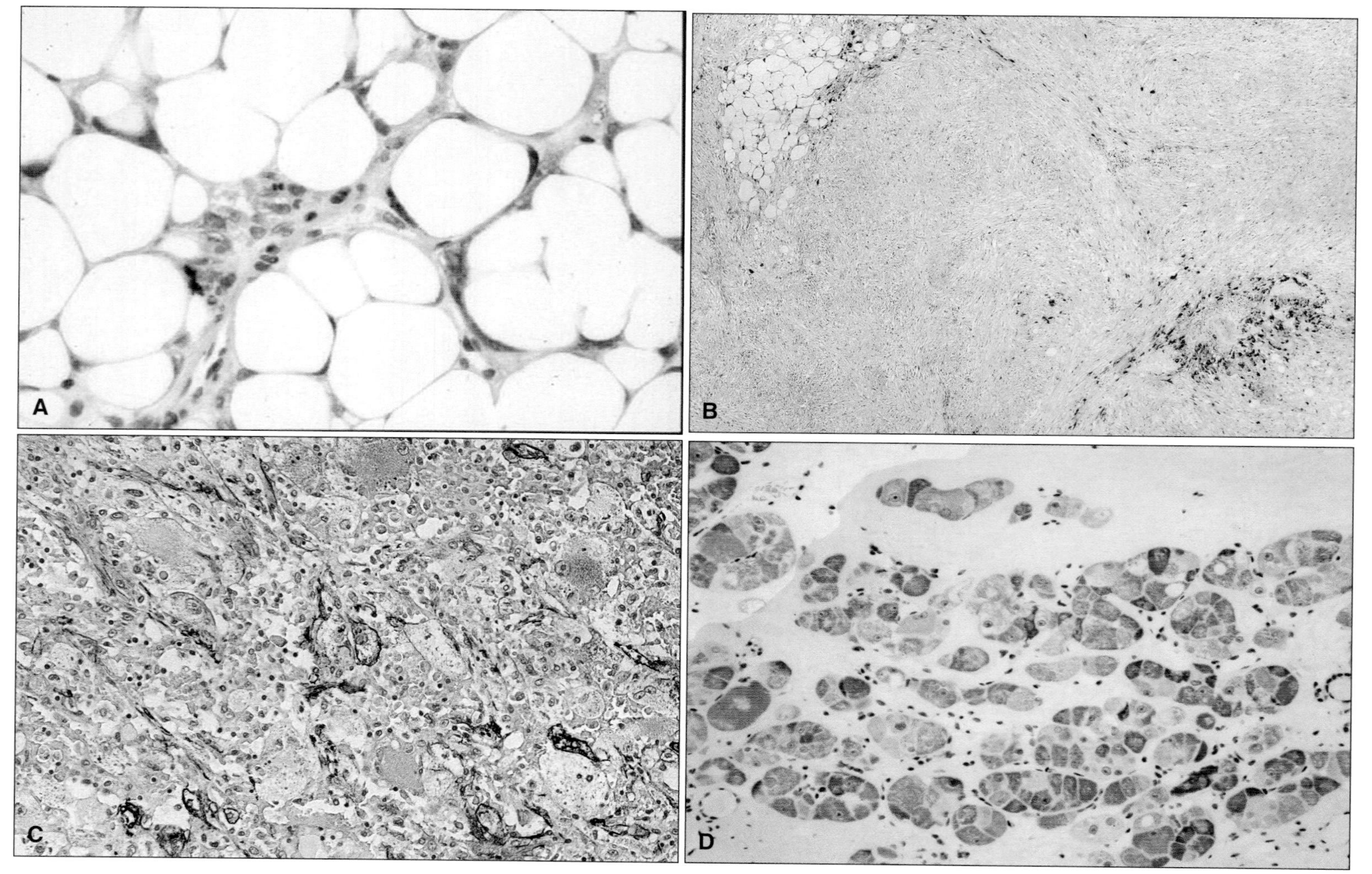

Fig. 8.98 Antibodies to several melanoma-related antigens, including HMB-45, tyrosinase, microphthalmia transcription factor, and A103 (Melan-A/MART-1), are at least focally positive in the majority of angiomyolipomas.[148,154,155,162–164] The epithelioid smooth muscle cell components are most often positive with these antibodies, though the spindled smooth muscle and adipose tissue components may also be positive. HMB-45 positivity is shown here in predominantly lipomatous (A), leiomyomatous (B), pleomorphic epithelioid (C), and 'oncocytoma-like' (D) angiomyolipomas.

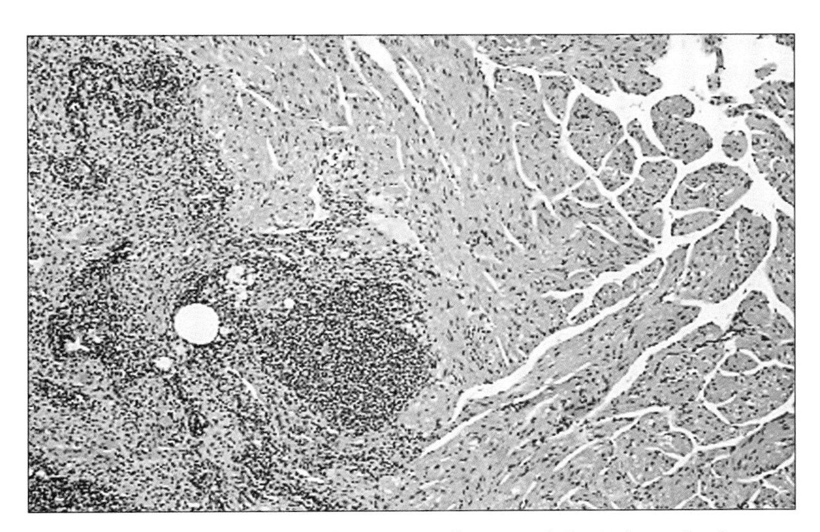

Fig. 8.99 Some patients with angiomyolipoma of the kidney also have angiomyolipomas involving non-contiguous sites, particularly regional lymph nodes. Sometimes the tumor may extend into the renal vein or inferior vena cava. The former are considered to represent multifocal rather than metastatic disease, since no such patient has died from disease progression.

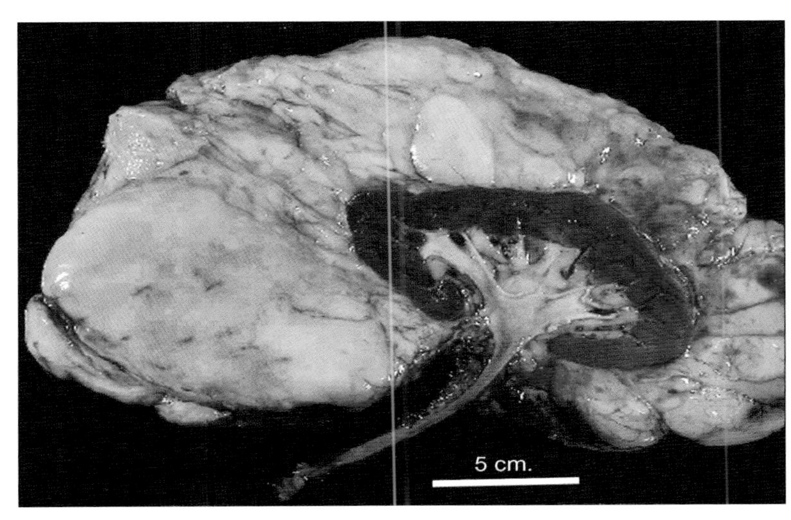

Fig. 8.100 Liposarcomas involving the kidneys or perirenal tissues are most often primary in the retroperitoneum. Careful examination of the gross specimen is helpful in distinguishing primary versus secondary renal liposarcoma, though in some cases a definitive separation may be impossible. This distinction is of little clinical significance, since therapy is surgical resection regardless of primary site and even intrarenal tumors may recur and show dedifferentiation following primary resection.

with tuberous sclerosis. The gross and microscopic features are similar to those of lipomas found at other sites. Careful examination of multiple tissue sections and immunohistochemistry with antibodies to HMB-45 may be necessary to rule out the diagnosis of angiomyolipoma.

Differential diagnosis

Primary liposarcoma of the kidney is rare. All reported renal liposarcomas have been of the well-differentiated or myxoid type. Of more importance is the distinction of predominantly lipomatous angiomyolipoma from well-differentiated liposarcoma. Adequate sampling of the tumor and immunohistochemistry using antibodies to HMB-45 are helpful in this differential. (Fig. 8.100)

SMOOTH MUSCLE TUMORS OF THE KIDNEY

Smooth muscle tumors of the kidney can be either leiomyomas that resemble uterine fibroids, or other smooth muscle tumors that are immunoreactive with HMB-45, Melan-A (A103), and other related antibodies. The latter most likely represent leiomyomatous angiomyolipomas.[122] Unlike the uterine leiomyoma-like tumors, the leiomyomatous angiomyolipomas usually arise in the renal capsule, and have been included among the renal 'capsulomas'.[122]

Acceptable examples of renal leiomyoma are rare. Tumors range from incidental, microscopic lesions found at autopsy to symptomatic masses as large as 37 kg.[166,167] Other than leiomyomatous angiomyolipoma, the differential diagnosis for leiomyomas includes mesoblastic nephroma.

Primary renal sarcomas comprise roughly 1% of all renal neoplasms and the majority of these are leiomyosarcomas.[168–170] Many tumors arise from within the kidney or hilar blood vessels; a few appear to arise from the renal capsule. Extension into perirenal adipose tissue and adjacent organs is common.

Gross appearance

The majority of cases have been at least 10 cm in greatest dimension. Grossly, they are firm, white to tan, and multinodular or lobulated. Hemorrhage and necrosis are uncommon. Like smooth muscle tumors found elsewhere, mitotic activity, nuclear atypia, necrosis, and large size are indicative of malignancy. Prognosis is poor, though rare long-term survivors have been reported. The differential diagnoses include sarcomatoid RCC and angiomyolipoma. (Fig. 8.101)

MEDULLARY FIBROMA (RENOMEDULLARY INTERSTITIAL CELL TUMOR)

Medullary fibroma (renomedullary interstitial cell tumor) is most often an unsuspected finding uncovered at the time of autopsy or in kidneys removed for other reasons.[171] An association between multiple medullary fibromas and systemic hypertension has been reported.[172] (Fig. 8.102)

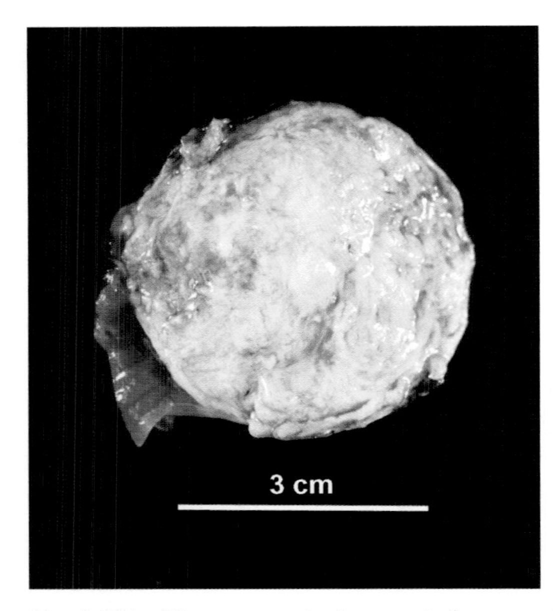

Fig. 8.101 The gross and microscopic features of renal leiomyomas (shown here) are similar to those of uterine leiomyomas. As is the case with smooth muscle neoplasms arising in the retroperitoneum, mitotic activity, nuclear atypia, necrosis, and, to some extent, large size favor the diagnosis of leiomyosarcoma.

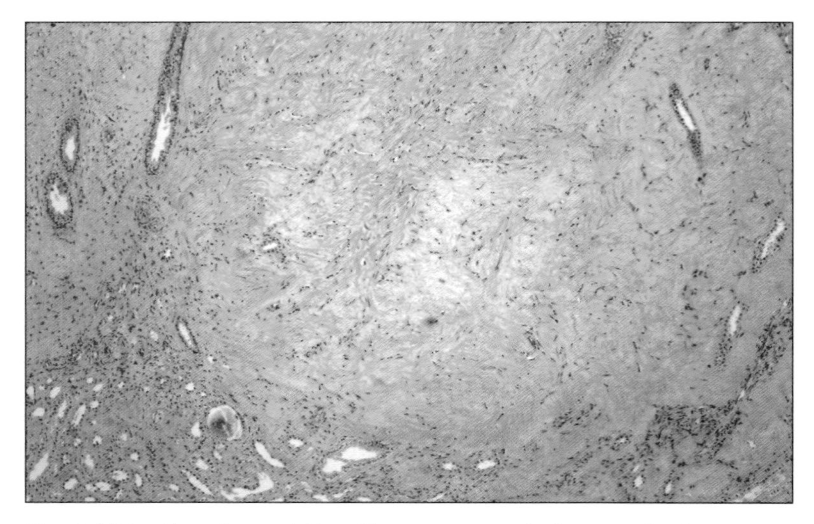

Fig. 8.102 Grossly, medullary fibromas are well circumscribed, tan to white, and found within the renal medulla. Most measure less than 5 mm in greatest dimension, although rare lesions large enough to be detected by imaging studies have been reported.[173] Microscopically, they consist of bland stellate cells set within a loose to densely sclerotic collagenous background. Entrapped tubules may be seen at the periphery of the nodules.

OTHER MESENCHYMAL NEOPLASMS

A wide variety of other mesenchymal neoplasms occur rarely in the adult kidney and benign tumors include solitary (localized) fibrous tumor, schwannoma, neurofibroma, myxoma, hemangioma, and lymphangioma.[122,174–181]

Renal rhabdomyosarcomas in the adult are most often of the pleomorphic type and are highly aggressive.[182] Wilms' tumor is an important consideration in the differential diagnosis. Malignant fibrous histiocytoma, fibrosarcoma, osteosarcoma, chondrosarcoma, mesenchymal chondrosarcoma, malignant mesenchymoma, and angiosarcoma have also been described.[168,183–189] Consideration should be given to sarcomatoid RCC before making the diagnosis of any primary renal sarcoma, necessitating a liberal sampling of such tumors.

HEMATOLOGIC MALIGNANCIES

These are described in detail in Chapter 14.

PEDIATRIC RENAL TUMORS

Pediatric renal tumors are extremely uncommon, and only approximately 500 such tumors are diagnosed annually in the United States. Proper diagnosis and staging are extremely important, as both the management and prognosis are highly dependent on these factors.

Stage is the major determinant of therapy and prognosis in pediatric renal tumors. Previously, violation of the hilar plane, an arbitrary plane connecting the medial borders of the upper and lower poles, was the major basis for distinguishing between stage I and II tumors. Because of poor reliability and total dependence on the interpretation of this plane by the grossing pathologist, hilar plane has now been discarded as the basis for this distinction. The currently accepted staging system by the National Wilms' Tumor Study Group (NWTS-5) is tabulated (Table 8.7).[190,191]

WILMS' TUMOR (NEPHROBLASTOMA)

Wilms' tumor (WT) is the most common pediatric renal neoplasm, except during the first 3 months of life.[191,192] Most

Table 8.7	Staging of pediatric renal tumors (NWTS-5)
Stage I	Tumor limited to the kidney and completely resected No capsular penetration by the tumor No tumor invasion of the veins or lymphatics of renal sinus No nodal or hematogenous spread
Stage II	Tumor extending beyond the kidney but completely resected Tumor penetrates renal capsule, but with margins clear Tumor in lymphatics or veins of renal sinus Tumor in renal vein with margin not involved Biopsy (except FNA) or local intraoperative spillage confined to flank No nodal or hematogenous metastases
Stage III	Residual tumor or nonhematogenous metastases confined to abdomen Involvement of abdominal nodes Peritoneal contamination or tumor implant/s Gross residual tumor in abdomen Resection margins involved by tumor
Stage IV	Hematogenous metastases or spread beyond abdomen
Stage V	Bilateral renal tumors When possible, a substage designation should be provided, according to stage of the most advanced individual tumor (e.g. stage V, substage I)

cases are diagnosed between the ages of 2 and 5 years; 90% are diagnosed by the age of 6 years.[191-193] Cases in adults are very rare. The most common sites of metastasis are regional lymph nodes, lungs, and liver. Spread to other organs is rare.

Cytogenetics and molecular biology

No single consistent cytogenetic or molecular abnormality has been found in WT.[194] In the genetic settings, the *WT1* gene, located on chromosome 11p13, is consistently deleted in the WT associated with aniridia and genital anomalies (WAGR syndrome), and point mutations in the gene are seen in Denys–Drash syndrome (pseudohermaphroditism, severe glomerulopathy, and WT). However, this gene is normal in more than 50% of sporadic WT specimens. Another gene, *WT2*, located on 11p15, is involved in WT associated with Beckwith–Wiedemann syndrome (organomegaly, hemihypertrophy, renal cysts, WT, adrenal or hepatic tumors).

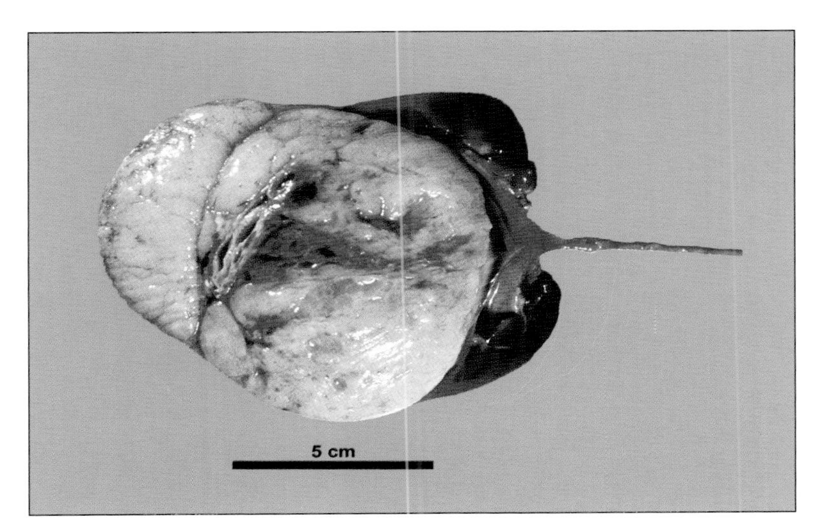

Fig. 8.103 Wilms' tumor (WT) typically presents as a sharply demarcated solitary spherical mass, but approximately 10% are multicentric, and 5–6% are bilateral at presentation. The cut surface of WT is usually pale gray and uniform, soft and friable. Focal hemorrhage, necrosis, and cysts are commonly encountered. Abundant stroma in the tumor may lead to a firm consistency or a nodular appearance. Polypoid masses protruding into the pelvicalyceal system may also occur.

Immunohistochemistry

The diversity of cell lines and degrees of differentiation imparts a correspondingly varied profile of immunohistochemical results.[195] Immunoreactivity for WT-1 protein is typically limited to the blastema and epithelial components of WT; the stroma is usually negative.[196] While WT-1 immunoreactivity may help distinguish WT from PNET, the reactivity is not specific for WT. Positive results may be observed in desmoplastic small round cell tumor.

Ultrastructure

Ultrastructural analysis may occasionally be needed to distinguish this lesion from other undifferentiated round cell neoplasms; otherwise, it is rarely required to establish the diagnosis of WT. (Figs 8.103–8.109)

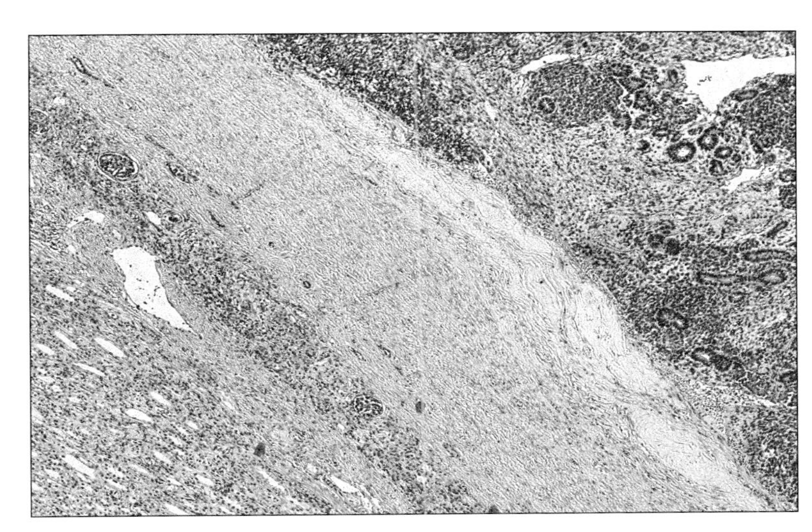

Fig. 8.104 Wilms' tumor. A thick reactive capsule is present.

Wilms' tumor with anaplasia

Approximately 5% of WTs show anaplastic features.[198-200] Anaplastic nuclear change is the only criterion of 'unfavorable histology' in WT, and all WTs lacking this feature are designated as having 'favorable histology'. Furthermore, anaplasia may be focal or diffuse,[200] but only tumors with diffuse anaplasia are of 'unfavorable histology'. Tumors with focal anaplasia behave like those without anaplasia.

Anaplasia is an indicator of increased resistance to adjuvant therapy, and is not a marker of increased tumor aggressiveness. Enlarged nuclei in differentiated skeletal muscle cells of a WT do not signify anaplasia, unless accompanied by multipolar mitotic figures. Anaplasia usually correlates with the presence of *p53* gene mutations.[201] (Fig. 8.110)

Cystic variants of Wilms' tumor

Scattered cysts are commonly encountered in conventional WT, but rarely the tumor is composed entirely of cystic spaces and delicate septa, without an expansile solid component. Tumors composed entirely of multilocular cysts are designated as cystic nephroma (CN). If the septa contain embryonal cell types, the designation of cystic partially differentiated nephroblastoma (CPDN) is used.[202]

The epithelial cells lining the cysts of CN and CPDN range from flattened to columnar, and are often of the

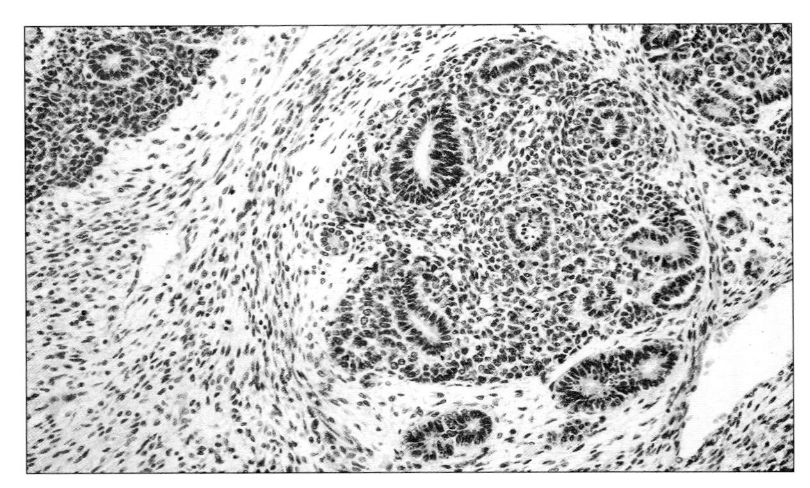

Fig. 8.105 Most Wilms' tumors exhibit a triphasic appearance, with cells of blastemal, stromal, and epithelial lineage in variable proportions. However, many tumors consist of any one or two of these cell lineages.

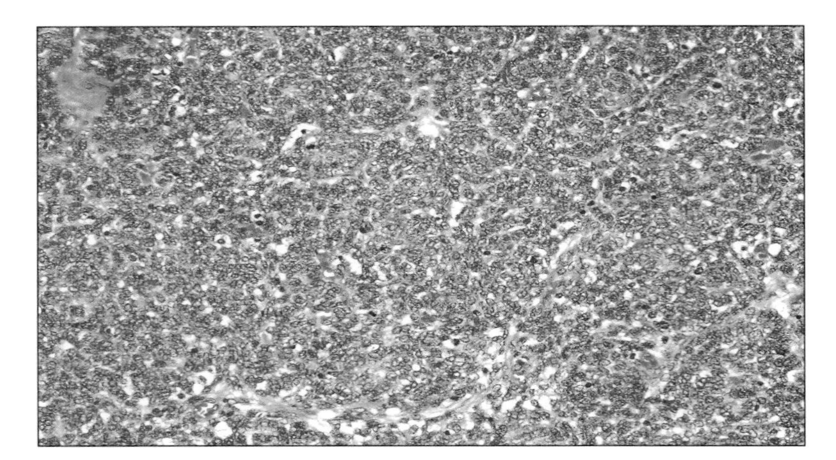

Fig. 8.106 The blastemal component of Wilms' tumor comprises small, closely packed cells with a high nuclear:cytoplasmic ratio, and round or oval nuclei with moderately coarse chromatin, occasional nuclear molding, and inconspicuous nucleoli. Predominantly blastemal tumors consist of sheets of cells, usually with invasive margins (diffuse blastemal pattern). This pattern frequently presents with stage III or IV disease.[197]

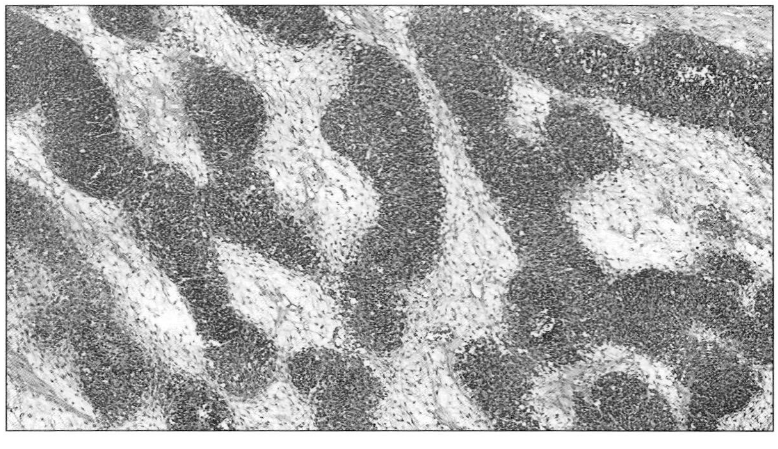

Fig. 8.107 Alternatively, in Wilms' tumor, the blastemal cells may form serpiginous, anastomosing cords in a loose, stellate, or spindled stroma (serpentine blastema), or rounded blastemal nests (nodular blastema), or may be outlined by a layer of cuboidal or columnar cells, reminiscent of basal cell carcinoma (basaloid blastema). These patterns usually lack the invasive margins seen with the diffuse blastemal pattern.

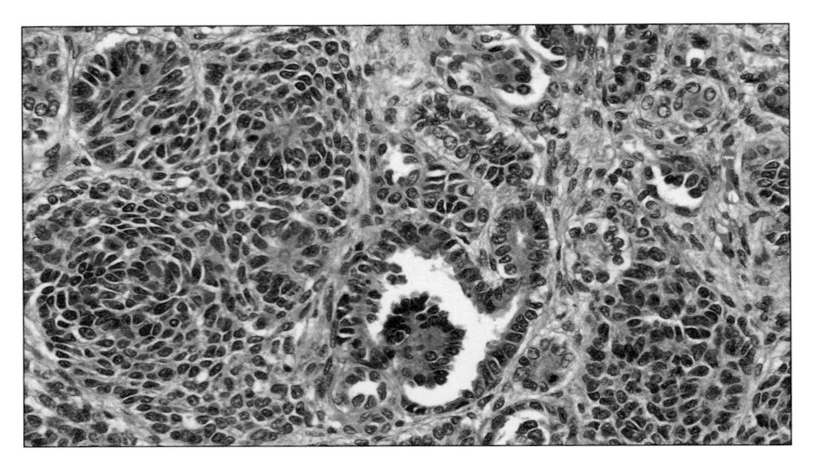

Fig. 8.108 Epithelial differentiation in Wilms' tumor may produce ill-formed to well-defined tubular differentiation. Glomerular differentiation may be present as simple papillary formations barely suggesting glomerulogenesis to mature tumor glomeruli resembling those of normal kidneys. Rarely, heterologous epithelial cell types including mucinous and squamous cells, or even neurons and neuroendocrine cells, may be seen.

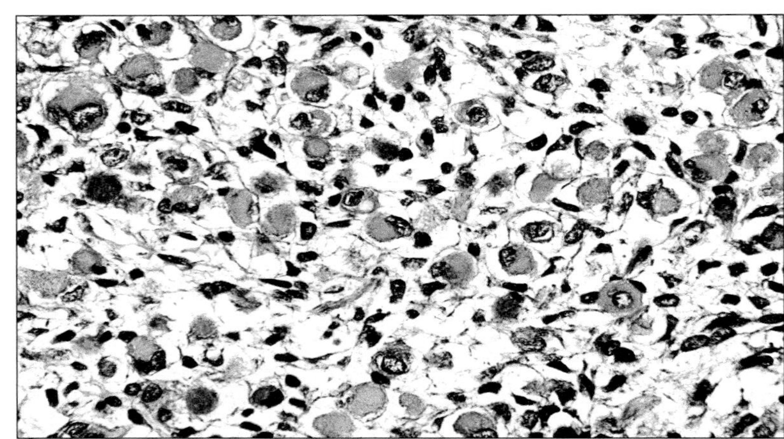

Fig. 8.109 The stromal component in Wilms' tumor may be in the form of immature myxoid and spindled mesenchyme, or heterologous cell types like skeletal muscle (shown here), fibroblastic/myofibroblastic, smooth muscle, adipose cells, cartilage, osteoid or bone, or neuroglial cells.

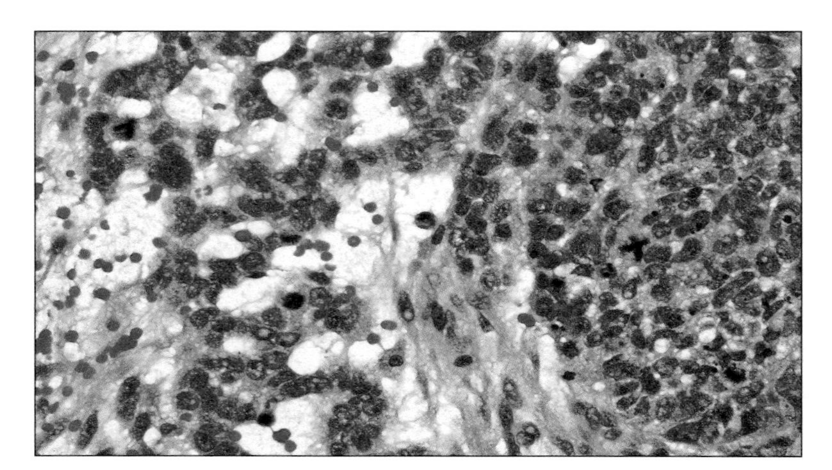

Fig. 8.110 Anaplastic nuclear change in Wilms' tumor is easily apparent under low magnification. The features of anaplasia as defined by the National Wilms' Tumor Study Group include (a) markedly enlarged tumor cell nuclei with increased chromatin content, and (b) multipolar or obviously polyploid mitotic figures.

'hobnail' type, with prominent eosinophilic cytoplasm. The cyst walls are composed of variably cellular fibrous tissue (also see CN in adults, page 8–28 and Table 8.6). The distinction of CN from CPDN has little or no clinical importance when the lesion is completely resected, as both lesions are curable by resection alone.

Differential diagnosis

Triphasic tumors rarely present a problem in diagnosis. However, in small biopsies from large retroperitoneal masses of uncertain origin or from metastatic sites, other small round cell tumors, including immature teratoma, hepatoblastoma, pancreatoblastoma, and desmoplastic small round cell tumor, may enter in the differential diagnosis. The presence of nuclear molding or the focal presence of tubular differentiation will often make the diagnosis clear. Ancillary studies such as immunohistochemistry, electron microscopy, and molecular studies may be required to distinguish some of these lesions from WT.

Epithelial-predominant WT can rarely be difficult to differentiate from PRCC with a predominant tubular or solid component, or metanephric adenoma, particularly when the tumor is from an adolescent or adult. Unequivocal glomerular differentiation, characteristic blastemal aggregation patterns, or the presence of heterologous cell types can confirm the diagnosis of WT. Diffuse positive staining for CK7 may be a useful marker for PRCC, although focal positive staining may be present in many WTs. Nuclear labeling for *WT1* may also help. More difficult cases will require molecular or cytogenetic studies.

Nephrogenic rests and nephroblastomatosis

Nephrogenic rests (NRs) are the persistent embryonal tissue representing precursor lesions of WT, and are identified in more than 30% of kidneys resected for WT.[191,203,204] The presence of multiple or diffusely distributed NRs is termed nephroblastomatosis.

Based on their relation to the renal lobe, two categories of NR are recognized: perilobar nephrogenic rests (PLNRs) and intralobar nephrogenic rests (ILNRs). ILNRs may occur anywhere in the renal lobe. They may also occur within the renal sinus, including the walls of the pelvicalyceal system. ILNRs are characterized by poor circumscription and irregular extensions between nephrons, and contain blastema, tubules, and cysts in a predominant background of stromal elements. PLNRs usually are discrete structures that are clearly demarcated from adjacent nephrons. Unlike ILNRs, they are usually numerous, are not admixed with nephrons, and contain minimal or sclerotic stroma.

Hyperplastic changes in the NRs may produce large masses with numerous mitotic figures. A section from the interior of a hyperplastic NR may be indistinguishable from WT. An important feature distinguishing hyperplastic NRs from WT is the usual absence of a pseudocapsule at the interface between hyperplastic NRs and renal parenchyma.

The presence of NRs in a kidney removed for WT correlates with an increased risk of subsequent tumor formation in the remaining kidney. Children with WT who also have NRs, particularly of the perilobar type, have a markedly increased risk of developing contralateral disease.[203,205] (Fig. 8.111)

MESOBLASTIC NEPHROMA

Mesoblastic nephroma (MN) comprises only 2–3% of pediatric renal tumors, but it is the most common renal neoplasm in the first 3 months of life. Approximately two-thirds of the cases are diagnosed in the first 3 months of life, and 90% are diagnosed in the first year.[206,207] This diagnosis should be considered suspect in any patient beyond the second year of life (see mixed epithelial and stromal tumor, page 8–28).[191]

MN is generally associated with good outcome, and most cases are treated by nephrectomy alone. However, recurrences and/or metastases do occur in about 5% of cases.

The cells of MN show immunostaining features consistent with those of myofibroblasts (positive for vimentin, muscle-specific actin, and occasionally desmin), and ultrastructural studies confirm the fibroblastic or myofibroblastic nature of the tumor cells.

In spite of the highly cellular and mitotically active appearance of many tumors, the vast majority of MNs are cured by nephrectomy alone if the lesion is completely resected. The critical prognostic issue is whether the lesion was completely resected.

Most relapsed cases recur within 1 year of nephrectomy. MNs of older infants and children are somewhat more likely to behave aggressively than those in neonates.

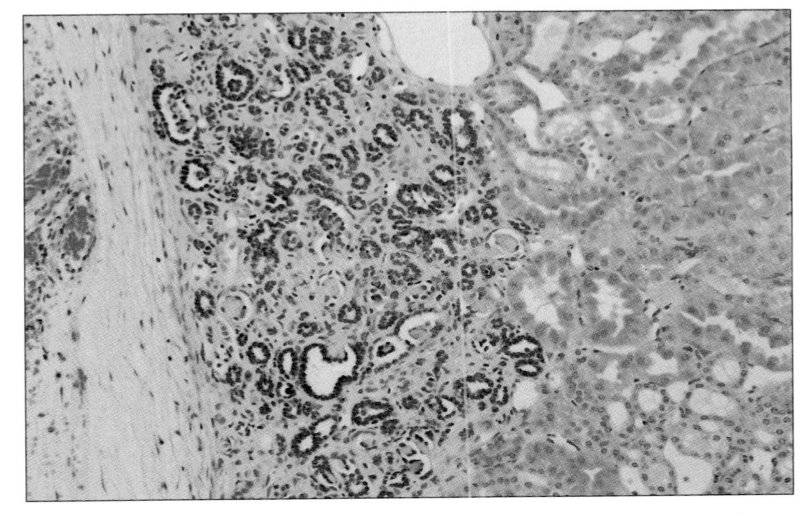

Fig. 8.111 A perilobar nephrogenic rest is a discete structure clearly demarcated from adjacent nephrons.

Recurrent MN is usually limited to the retroperitoneum. Rare cases may metastasize, and the lung is the most common metastatic site; a few cases of brain metastasis have been reported.[208,209] Relapses may respond to adjuvant therapy. However, some relapsed tumors are highly resistant, and complete surgical removal of recurrent disease is advisable whenever possible.

Cytogenetics

Cellular MN shares many histopathologic features with infantile fibrosarcoma. In addition, the t(12;15)(p13;q25) chromosome translocation and the resultant *ETV6–NTRK3* gene fusion are also found in both entities.[210,211] Classic MN does not demonstrate this gene fusion. In tumors with mixed morphology, the gene fusion is found in the cellular areas, but not in classic areas.

Differential diagnosis

The neoplasms most likely to be confused with MN in the infantile kidney are WT, clear cell sarcoma, and rhabdoid tumor (see below). Because of markedly different biologic behaviors, the establishment of a correct diagnosis is extremely important.

Untreated WT composed predominantly of stromal cells is uncommon, but rare examples do occur. In most such cases, the presence of immature or mature skeletal muscle readily excludes the diagnosis of MN. WT removed after chemotherapy may show only a residual stromal component, because treatment often ablates the embryonal, proliferating elements of a WT but tends to spare stromal cells. A diagnosis of MN should be considered suspect in a patient who has received prior therapy, unless the clinical and other features are characteristic. Bilaterality or the presence of NRs strongly favors WT. (Figs 8.112 & 8.113)

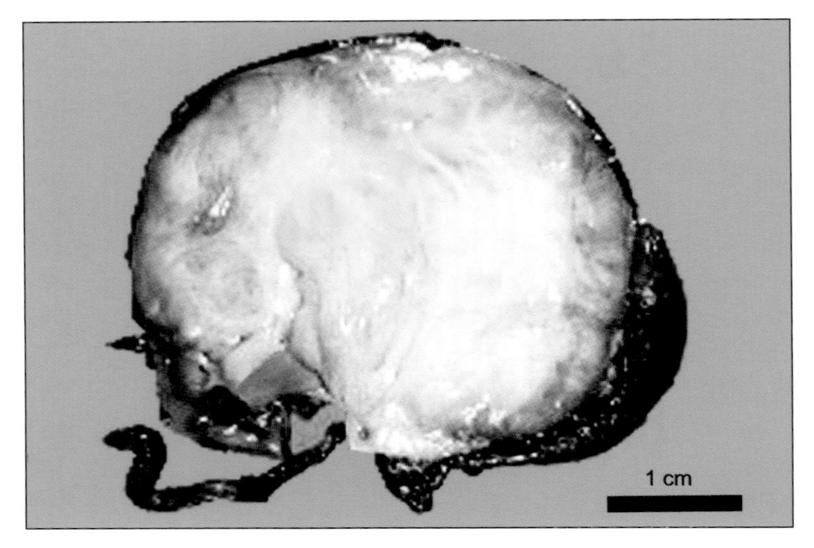

Fig. 8.112 Mesoblastic nephromas usually arise near the renal sinus, and the sinus and adjacent structures on the medial side of the kidney are major sites of extrarenal spread. The appearance of the cut surface is variable. Some tumors have a firm, whorled appearance resembling leiomyoma, but a soft and friable cut surface is more frequent. Hemorrhage, necrosis, and cyst formation are not uncommon.

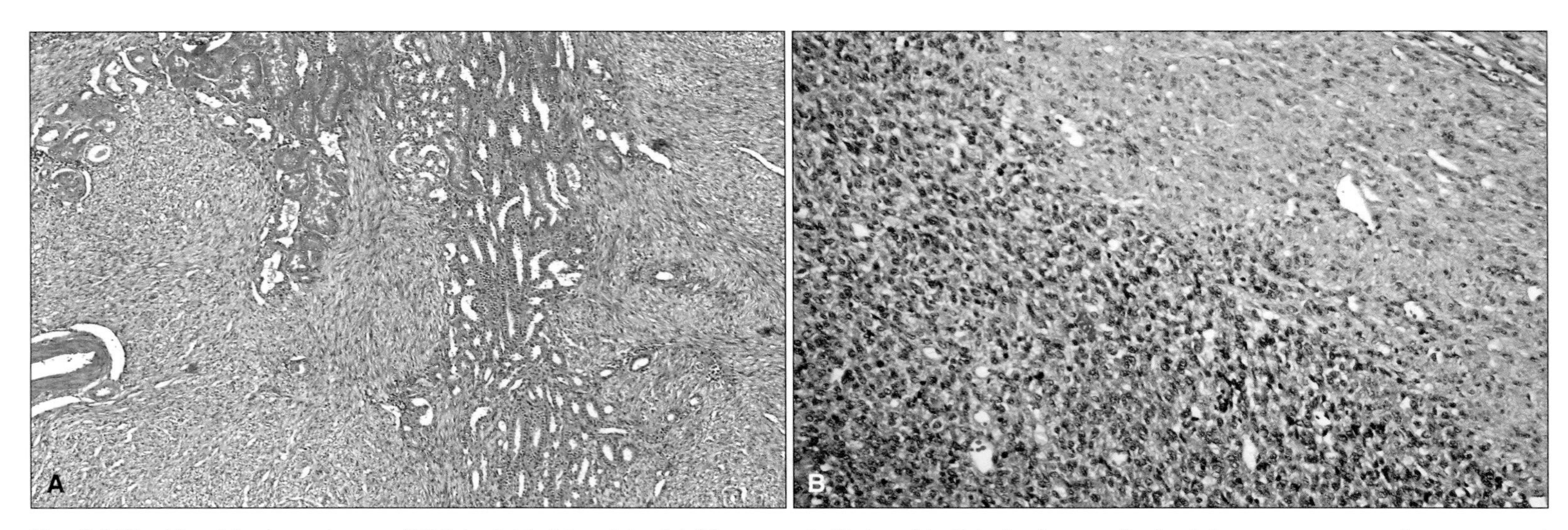

Fig. 8.113 Mesoblastic nephroma (MN) is divided into 'classic' (fibromatosis-like) and 'cellular' subtypes. Both of these patterns may be seen together, as the cellular pattern usually arises in a background of the classic pattern. (A) Classic MN is characterized by relatively low cellularity, low to moderate mitotic index, and long tongues of tumor extending irregularly into adjacent kidney and soft tissue. Only about one-fourth of MNs are of the pure classic pattern. In addition to involving the renal sinus and adjacent soft tissues, classic MN may also extend into perirenal fat. Cartilage or other dysplastic changes may be found in the renal parenchyma adjacent to tumor, sometimes becoming surrounded by tumor. Tumors of the pure classic pattern are usually small. Cellular MN is characterized by densely packed spindle cells with a high mitotic rate. This is the predominant or exclusive pattern in approximately two-thirds of MNs. Composite specimens, composed of both cellular and classic patterns, are not uncommon (B). Many cellular MNs, particularly in tumors of large size, may have a pushing border, instead of the interdigitating pattern seen in the classic subtype. Cellular MN may attain a very large size, with nephrectomy specimens sometimes exceeding 1 kg.

CLEAR CELL SARCOMA OF THE KIDNEY

Clear cell sarcoma of the kidney (CCSK), previously also known as 'bone metastasizing renal tumor of childhood', constitutes about 3% of childhood renal tumors.[191] This neoplasm has a propensity for widespread metastases and for recurrence after therapy. Metastases may occur in a variety of sites, including sites that are unusual for WT, such as bone, brain, and soft tissues.[212] Approximately 5% of cases present with hematogenous metastases.

CCSK is rare in the first 6 months of life, but the incidence increases rapidly thereafter, peaking in the second and third years. Very occasional cases are reported in adolescents and young adults.[213] The male-to-female ratio is 2:1. No bilateral cases are known.[212]

Patients with stage I disease have close to a 100% survival even without adjuvant therapy. For patients with stage II or III disease, actuarial 6-year survival has risen from the previous 30% to the current 75% with the addition of doxorubicin (Adriamycin) to chemotherapeutic regimens.[191,212–216] Recurrences may occur many years (i.e. greater than a decade) after the initial diagnosis; therefore close follow-up is required for longer periods than is needed for most WTs.

Most CCSKs have a typical, classic appearance, but variations from this classic pattern produce many problems in the differential diagnosis. At low-power examination, CCSK usually has a thick pseudocapsule; however, at higher-magnification evaluation, the capsule shows infiltration by single cells and cell clusters that extend a short distance into the surrounding renal parenchyma, sometimes with entrapment of renal tubules. Dilatation of these entrapped tubules produces intratumoral cysts that may mimic CN.

The classic pattern of CCSK predominates in most specimens and is present at least focally in over 90% of tumors. Variant morphologies include epithelioid, spindle cell (resulting from either proliferation of septal cells or spindling of the epithelial cells), myxoid and sclerosing, palisading (Verocay body-like), and monstrocellular (anaplastic) patterns.[191]

Immunohistochemistry

Immunohistochemistry shows staining for vimentin and sometimes bcl-2. Stains for cytokeratins, EMA, S-100 protein, chromogranin, synaptophysin, CD34, CD117 (c-kit), and CD99 (MIC2) are consistently negative.

Ultrastructure

Ultrastructural studies show the tumor cells with elongated irregular processes surrounding abundant intercellular matrix, which is responsible for the vacuoles seen on light microscopy. True desmosomes are not seen, but primitive cell junctions may be numerous. The cytoplasm tends to be poor in organelles.

Differential diagnosis

The differential diagnostic considerations include WT, MN, and rhabdoid tumor of the kidney (RTK). Closely packed cells showing overlapping nuclei and nuclear molding favor the diagnosis of WT over CCSK. Heterologous tissues such as skeletal muscle are never seen in CCSK. Sclerotic, hyalinized stroma in an untreated tumor favors CCSK over WT. Cellular MN sometimes has considerable resemblance to spindled variants of CCSK, and the age ranges of these two entities overlap. Small foci resembling CCSK may occur in MN, but MN lacks the diversity of morphologic patterns that typifies CCSK. In some difficult cases, molecular studies may be essential. Differentiation from RTK is discussed below. (Figs 8.114–8.116)

RHABDOID TUMOR OF THE KIDNEY

RTK is a rare, clinically aggressive, renal neoplasm of young children, comprising approximately 2% of pediatric renal tumors.[191,217,218] Most cases are at an advanced stage when diagnosed, even in the newborns. Median age at diagnosis for RTK is 13 months; the diagnosis is considerably less likely in any patient older than 3 years and extremely suspect beyond 5 years. Most extrarenal rhabdoid tumor (RT) and RT-like neoplasms in adults are probably other entities that show only some morphologic resemblance to RTK.

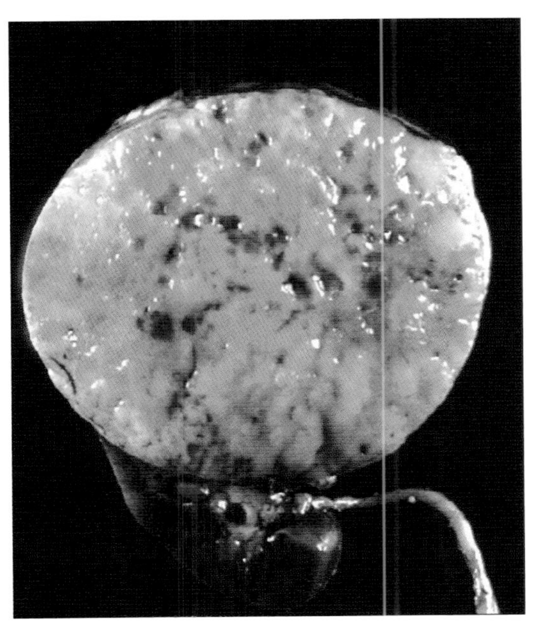

Fig. 8.114 Clear cell sarcomas of the kidney are usually relatively large, with a mean diameter of more than 11 cm. The tumor is often irregular in shape, but with a distinct tumor–kidney junction. The color is variable, but a glistening, gelatinous surface is often seen. Cysts are almost always present and may be very prominent. Multicentricity is not a feature.

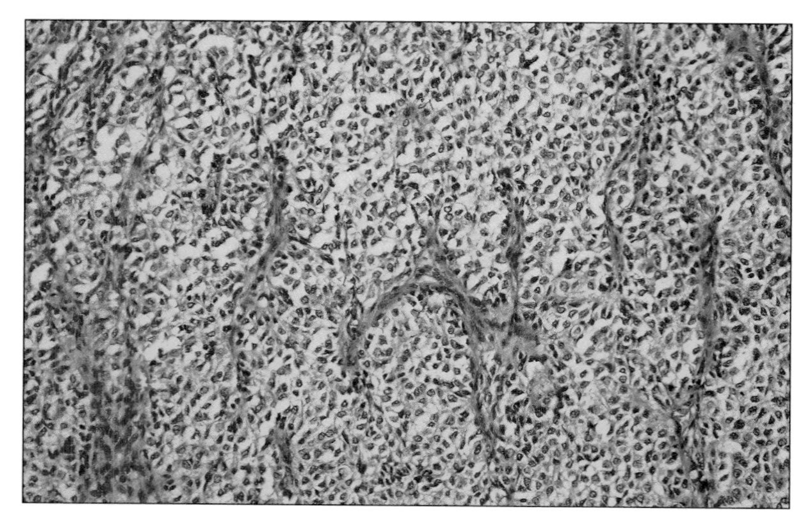

Fig. 8.115 The hallmark of classic-pattern clear cell sarcoma of the kidney is an evenly distributed network of vascular septa, connected at frequent intervals by transverse arcades. These fibrovascular septa subdivide the tumor into a classic pattern of cords six to ten cells thick, and nests.

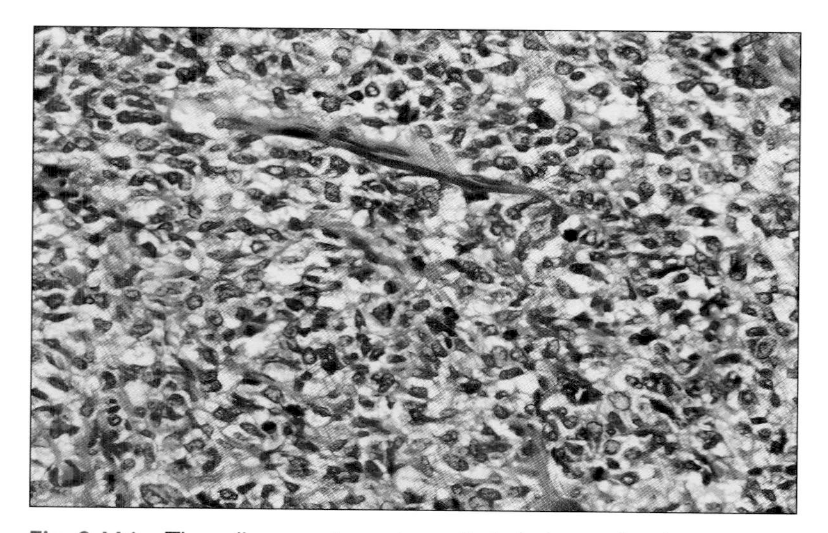

Fig. 8.116 The cells are polygonal, usually lack distinct borders, and enclose vacuoles of extracellular mucopolysaccharides, which are a distinctive and prominent feature of most clear cell sarcomas of the kidney (CCSKs) and contribute to their usually pale appearance on stained slides. These vacuoles may appear empty or contain blue-stained granular material. Some CCSKs contain cells with eosinophilic, sharply demarcated cytoplasm. These cells can be present either focally or diffusely. Nuclear chromatin is usually finely granular, with inconspicuous nucleoli. Mitotic figures are variable in number but are usually less numerous than those in Wilms' tumor.

RTK is among the most malignant neoplasms of childhood and, despite the intensified therapeutic regimens used now, the prognosis remains poor. Most patients either present with or develop metastases to bone, brain, and other sites, and death usually occurs within 1 year of diagnosis in more than 75% of patients.

Molecular biology

The molecular hallmark of RTK is the inactivation of the *hSNF5/INI1* gene on chromosome 22. This inactivation has also been demonstrated in morphologically similar aggressive tumors of the brain and soft tissue in infants.[219-222] Approximately 15% of RTK cases are associated with PNET of the posterior cranial fossa. Most, but not all, of these central nervous system (CNS) tumors resemble medulloblastoma. Genetic studies support the view that these CNS tumors are independent primaries arising in a background of an underlying genetic predisposition.[223]

Immunohistochemistry

Polyphenotypic immunohistochemical results are commonly observed in RTK, which limits the value of immunostains in establishing this diagnosis. Vimentin is almost always expressed in RTK, and coexpression of cytokeratin and EMA is frequently observed. Stains for muscle markers may be positive in some cases, but are limited to the cytoplasmic inclusions.[217]

Ultrastructure

The most distinctive ultrastructural feature of RTK consists of whorled arrays of intermediate filaments that are responsible for the cytoplasmic inclusions seen on light microscopy. Myofilaments are not observed. The most important role of the ultrastructural study of RT is in excluding alternative diagnoses, such as rhabdomyosarcoma or neuroendocrine neoplasms.

Differential diagnosis

Both blastemal and myogenic elements of WT may contain cytoplasmic inclusions resembling those of RTK. The presence of blastemal aggregation patterns or of embryonal and better-differentiated tubules, or heterologous cells such as differentiated skeletal muscle, will facilitate the correct diagnosis in most instances. The huge nucleoli, characteristic of RTK, are not seen in WT, with the exception of some anaplastic specimens.

The cellular subtype of MN occasionally may have vesicular nuclei with prominent nucleoli, and a rare MN contains foci with hyaline cytoplasmic inclusions. The far less invasive tumor periphery will favor the diagnosis of cellular MN, and the immunohistochemical presence of cytokeratin and EMA will support RTK. However, cytogenetic and/or molecular analysis may be needed for this distinction in more difficult cases.

The rare occurrence of prominent nucleoli focally in CCSK can rarely lead to difficulty in distinguishing these entities. The presence of classic histologic and cytologic features of CCSK elsewhere is a major clue to the correct diagnosis in such instances. Additionally, CCSK lacks the extreme invasiveness of RTK.

Gross appearance

RTKs typically present as a bulky mass, frequently replacing the kidney. Tumor diameter ranges from 3 to 17 cm (mean, 9.6 cm). Hemorrhage and necrosis are commonly seen, and satellite nodules in the renal parenchyma or capsular invasion are frequent. The medial portion of the kidney is consistently involved. The tumor–kidney junction is usually poorly defined; invasion into adjacent soft tissues and angiolymphatic spaces is frequently observed. This aggressive appearance is an important clue to the diagnosis, and, in specimens lacking this feature, alternative diagnoses must be seriously considered.[191] (Fig. 8.117)

OSSIFYING RENAL TUMOR OF INFANCY

This rare infantile neoplasm is usually seen clinically as a calcified mass located predominantly within the pelvicalyceal system. It is often thought to represent a staghorn calculus on imaging studies, but surgical exploration reveals dense adherence to the renal parenchyma, usually in the region of a medullary papilla.[224] Microscopically, the lesion consists of a spindle cell stroma similar to that of MN, with variably large regions of osteoid material. This lesion is clinically benign.

NON-NEOPLASTIC TUMOR-LIKE CONDITIONS

XANTHOGRANULOMATOUS PYELONEPHRITIS

Xanthogranulomatous pyelonephritis may mimic RCC on clinical, radiologic, and even gross evaluation.[225]

It is usually a disease of older females, although cases may be seen in children, as well as in adult males.[226] A history of urinary tract infection is frequent, and urine cultures may reveal *E. coli*, *Proteus* species, or other Gram-negative organisms.[227]

Distinction from clear cell (conventional) RCC is usually straightforward on the basis of histologic features. Numerous lymphocytes and plasma cells admixed with, and between, aggregates of clear cells should raise the caution of xanthogranulomatous pyelonephritis in a lesion being considered a clear cell RCC. In rare instances, immunostaining for cytokeratin and histiocytic markers (CD68) may be required for this differentiation. (Figs 8.118 & 8.119)

MALAKOPLAKIA

Kidney is the second most common site of genitourinary malakoplakia, after bladder. The lesion bears considerable gross and microscopic resemblance to xanthogranulomatous pyelonephritis,[228] and clinically and grossly may also mimic a renal neoplasm.[229] (Figs 8.120 & 8.121)

TUBERCULOSIS

In spite of the recent decline in cases of tuberculosis, the incidence of genitourinary tuberculosis has not shown a concomitant decline.[230] The kidney remains the most common site of genitourinary tuberculosis.[231]

Renal tuberculosis may be of the miliary type, which is characterized grossly by numerous tiny, white bilateral nodules (millet seed-like), and well-developed tubercles with no to minimal necrosis on microscopy. It is most

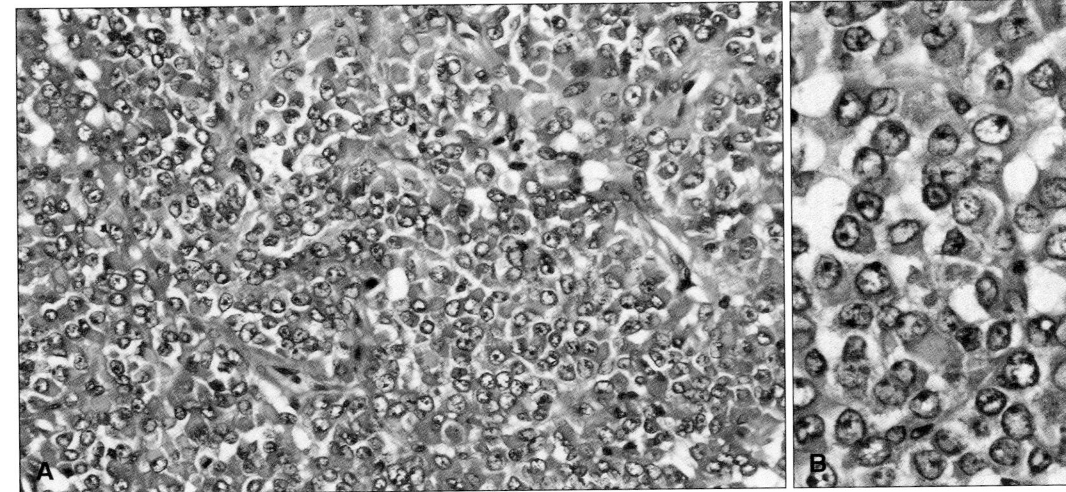

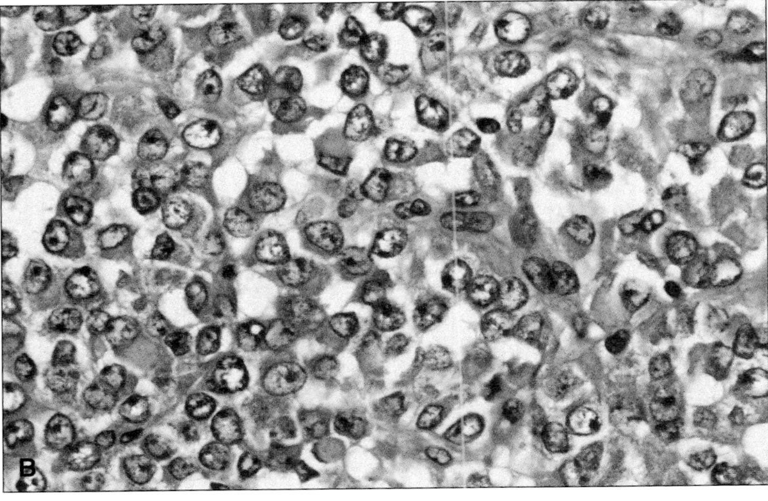

Fig. 8.117 (A,B) The cells of rhabdoid tumor of the kidney (RTK) are relatively large and usually round or polygonal, with abundant eosinophilic or amphophilic cytoplasm. Nuclei are relatively large and vesicular, with very prominent nucleoli. Eosinophilic and homogeneous to finely filamentous cytoplasmic inclusions are a characteristic feature of RTK. These inclusions are variably prominent in a given tumor, and may be focal, requiring extensive search. They are often most readily found near foci of necrosis.

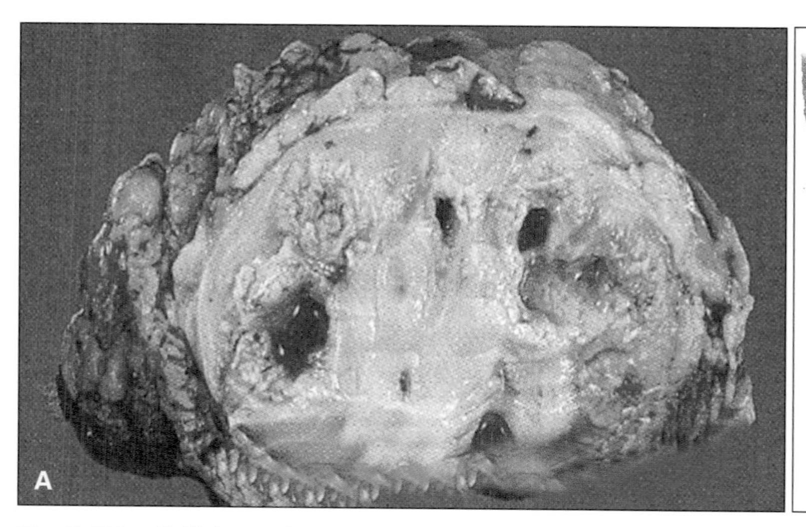

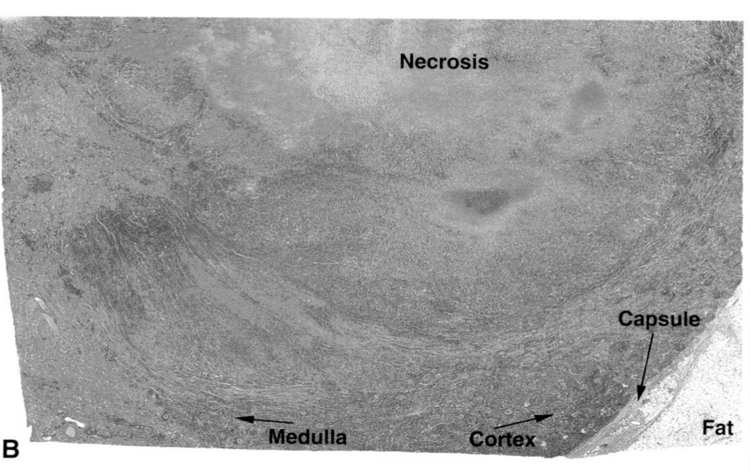

Fig. 8.118 (A,B) In xanthogranulomatous pyelonephritis, grossly, the renal cut surface shows a single or multiple confluent yellow nodular areas, usually with central necrosis. The lesions often surround the pelvicalyceal system, but may be present in the renal parenchyma away from the renal pelvis. Abundant admixed or surrounding gray–white fibrous areas are frequent. Extensions beyond the renal capsule may be present, and this feature, along with the yellow cut surface, is reminiscent of renal cell carcinoma.

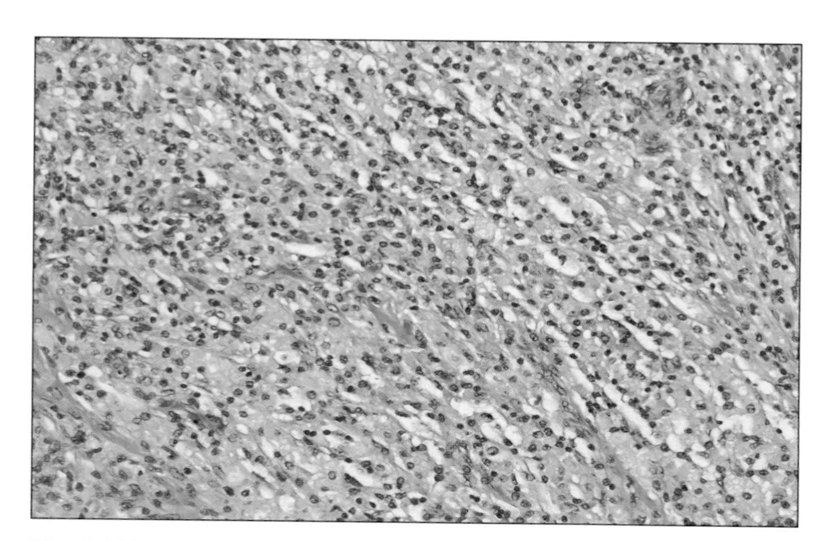

Fig. 8.119 Microscopically, xanthogranulomatous pyelonephritis is characterized by large numbers of foamy histiocytes, usually admixed with variable proportions of plasma cells, lymphocytes, and neutrophils. Cholesterol clefts with associated foreign body-type giant cells are common within the infiltrates.

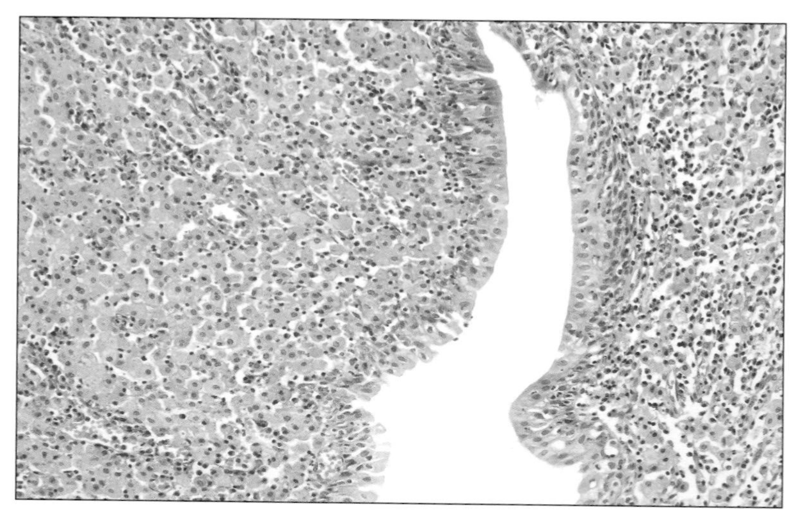

Fig. 8.120 In renal malakoplakia, sectioning shows patchy, nodular or diffuse parenchymal replacement by usually yellow, or, less commonly, tan or brown tissue. Microscopically, the renal parenchyma is replaced by abscesses, and large histiocytes by granular eosinophilic to foamy cytoplasm (von Hansemann cells) usually admixed with a mixed inflammatory infiltrate.

common in children, and is part of a generalized disease. The other more common form is of the ulceronecrotic type. (Figs 8.122 & 8.123)

PERINEPHRIC AND RENAL ABSCESSES

Perinephric and renal abscesses are not common. They form less than 1% of all intra-abdominal abscesses.[232]

In the pre-antibiotic era, most renal and perinephric abscesses were hematogenous, and *Staphylococcus aureus* was the commonest causative organism. Now, the most common route is ascending infection from the bladder to the kidney, with pyelonephritis occurring first. The organisms most frequently encountered in perinephric and renal abscesses are *E. coli*, and *Proteus* and *Klebsiella* species, although, in rare instances, other unusual pathogens (e.g. actinomycetes) may be isolated.[232,233]

The most important risk factor is the presence of nephrolithiasis producing local obstruction to urinary flow. Of patients with perinephric abscess, 20–60% have renal stones. (Fig. 8.124)

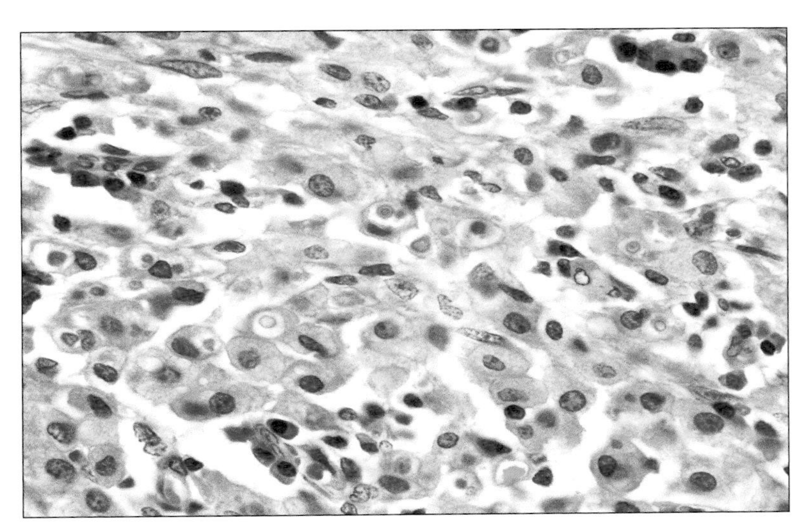

Fig. 8.121 Some of the histiocytes in malakoplakia contain the characteristic targetoid, calcific, basophilic inclusions (Michaelis–Guttman bodies). Ultrastructurally, these bodies are phagolysosomes that contain the breakdown products of bacteria, usually *E. coli*.

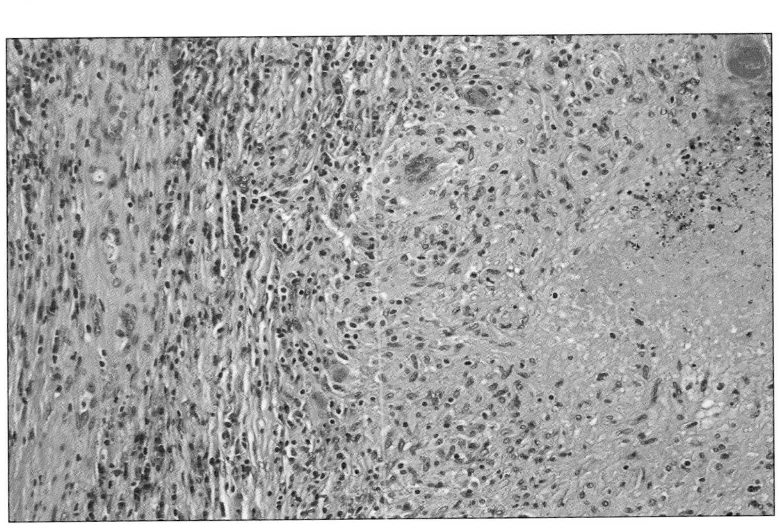

Fig. 8.123 On microscopy, the typical necrotizing epithelioid granulomas, usually with multiple Langhans-type and other giant cells, are easily identified in the ulceronecrotic form of renal tuberculosis.

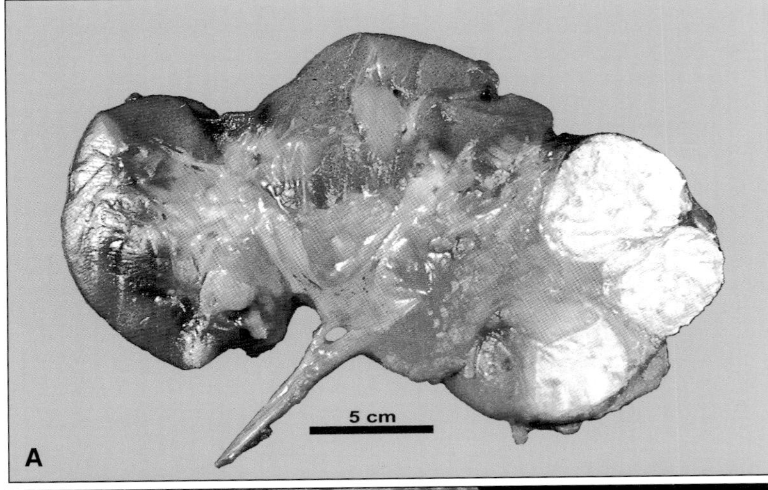

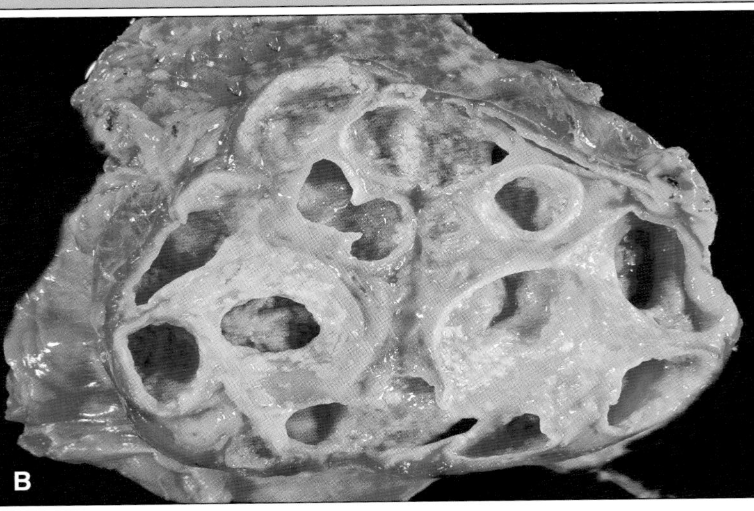

Fig. 8.122 The ulceronecrotic form of renal tuberculosis is more common in adults, and is accompanied by active pulmonary disease in only a very small proportion of cases. Grossly, the kidney may show multiple, variably sized areas of caseation necrosis, and necrotic material may fill the pelvicalyceal system as well. Extensive fibrosis in and around the lesions may result in one or multiple masses that can superficially resemble tumors (A). Ureteral involvement may lead to obstruction to outflow, and resultant pyonephrosis (B).

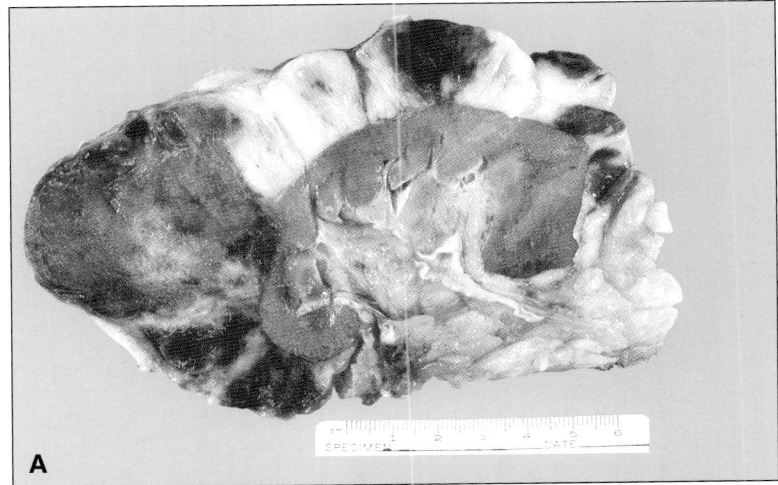

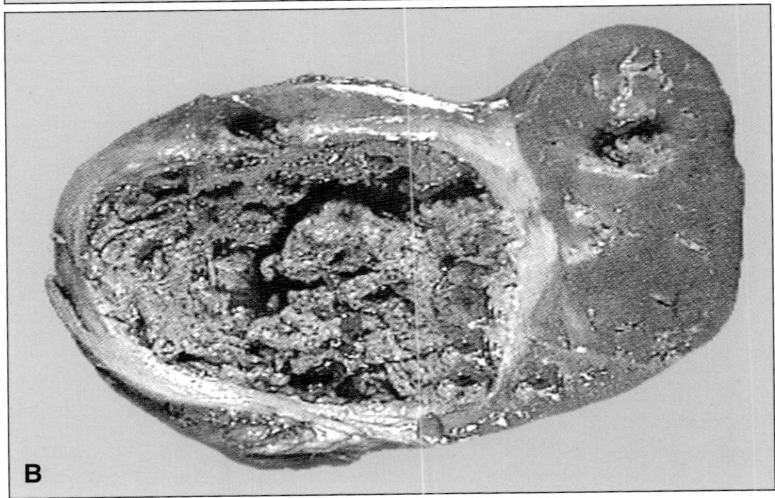

Fig. 8.124 (A,B) Renal and perirenal abscesses may occasionally be associated with a renal neoplasm, or rarely may even simulate a renal neoplasm.[232,234,235]

REFERENCES

1. Davis CJ, Mostofi FK, Sesterhenn I, Ho CK. Renal oncocytoma. Clinicopathological study of 166 patients. J Urogen Pathol 1991;1:41–52.
2. Lieber MM, Tomera KM, Farrow GM. Renal oncocytoma. J Urol 1981;125: 481–485.
3. Amin MB, Crotty TB, Tickoo SK, Farrow GM. Renal oncocytoma: a reappraisal of morphologic features with clinicopathologic findings in 80 cases. Am J Surg Pathol 1997;21:1–12.
4. Perez-Ordonez B, Hamed G, Campbell S, et al. Renal oncocytoma: a clinicopathologic study of 70 cases. Am J Surg Pathol 1997;21:871–883.
5. Amin MB, Tamboli P, Javidan J, et al. Prognostic impact of histologic subtyping of adult renal epithelial neoplasms: an experience of 405 cases. Am J Surg Pathol 2002;26:281–291.
6. Walter TA, Pennington RD, Decker HJ, Sandberg AA. Translocation t(9;11)(p23;q12): a primary chromosomal change in renal oncocytoma. J Urol 1989;142:117–119.
7. Crotty TB, Lawrence KM, Moertel CA, et al. Cytogenetic analysis of six renal oncocytomas and a chromophobe cell renal carcinoma. Evidence that –Y, –1 may be a characteristic anomaly in renal oncocytomas. Cancer Genet Cytogenet 1992;61:61–66.
8. Fuzesi L, Gunawan B, Braun S, Boeckmann W. Renal oncocytoma with a translocation t(9;11)(p23;q13). J Urol 1994;152:471–472.
9. van den Berg E, Dijkhuizen T, Storkel S, et al. Chromosomal changes in renal oncocytomas. Evidence that t(5;11)(q35;q13) may characterize a second subgroup of oncocytomas. Cancer Genet Cytogenet 1995;79: 164–168.
10. Neuhaus C, Dijkhuizen T, van den Berg E, et al. Involvement of the chromosomal region 11q13 in renal oncocytoma: case report and literature review. Cancer Genet Cytogenet 1997;94:95–98.
11. Tickoo SK, Lee MW, Eble JN, et al. Ultrastructural observations on mitochondria and microvesicles in renal oncocytoma, chromophobe renal cell carcinoma, and eosinophilic variant of conventional (clear cell) renal cell carcinoma. Am J Surg Pathol 2000;24:1247–1256.
12. Erlandson RA, Shek TW, Reuter VE. Diagnostic significance of mitochondria in four types of renal epithelial neoplasms: an ultrastructural study of 60 tumors. Ultrastruct Pathol 1997;21:409–417.
13. Tickoo SK, Reuter VE, Amin MB, et al. Renal oncocytosis: a morphologic study of fourteen cases. Am J Surg Pathol 1999;23:1094–1101.
14. Kovacs G, Akhtar M, Beckwith BJ, et al. The Heidelberg classification of renal cell tumours. J Pathol 1997;183:131–133.
15. Storkel S, Eble JN, Adlakha K, et al. Classification of renal cell carcinoma: Workgroup No. 1. Union Internationale Contre le Cancer (UICC) and the American Joint Committee on Cancer (AJCC). Cancer 1997;80: 987–989.
16. Argani P, Beckwith JB. Metanephric stromal tumor: report of 31 cases of a distinctive pediatric renal neoplasm. Am J Surg Pathol 2000;24: 917–926.
17. Davis CJ, Barton JH, Sesterhenn IA, Mostofi FK. Metanephric adenoma. Clinicopathological study of fifty patients. Am J Surg Pathol 1995;19:1101–1114.
18. Jones EC, Pins M, Dickersin GR, Young RH. Metanephric adenoma of the kidney. A clinicopathological, immunohistochemical, flow cytometric, cytogenetic, and electron microscopic study of seven cases. Am J Surg Pathol 1995;19:615–626.
19. Gatalica Z, Grujic S, Kovatich A, Petersen RO. Metanephric adenoma: histology, immunophenotype, cytogenetics, ultrastructure. Mod Pathol 1996;9:329–333.
20. Bouzourene H, Blaser A, Francke ML, Chaubert P, Bouzourene N. Metanephric adenoma of the kidney: a rare benign tumour of the kidney. Histopathology 1997;31:485–486.
21. Kuroda N, Tol M, Hiroi M, Enzan H. Review of metanephric adenoma of the kidney with focus on clinical and pathobiological aspects. Histol Histopathol 2003;18:253–257.
22. Hennigar RA, Beckwith JB. Nephrogenic adenofibroma. A novel kidney tumor of young people. Am J Surg Pathol 1992;16:325–334.
23. Granter SR, Fletcher JA, Renshaw AA. Cytologic and cytogenetic analysis of metanephric adenoma of the kidney: a report of two cases. Am J Clin Pathol 1997;108:544–549.
24. Brown JA, Anderl KL, Borell TJ, Qian J, Bostwick DG, Jenkins RB. Simultaneous chromosome 7 and 17 gain and sex chromosome loss provide evidence that renal metanephric adenoma is related to papillary renal cell carcinoma. J Urol 1997;158:370–374.
25. Stumm M, Koch A, Wieacker PF, et al. Partial monosomy 2p as the single chromosomal anomaly in a case of renal metanephric adenoma. Cancer Genet Cytogenet 1999;115:82–85.
26. Presti JC Jr, Rao PH, Chen Q, et al. Histopathological, cytogenetic, and molecular characterization of renal cortical tumors. Cancer Res 1991;51:1544–1552.
27. Fleming S. The impact of genetics on the classification of renal carcinoma. Histopathology 1993;22:89–92.
28. Kovacs G. Molecular differential pathology of renal cell tumours. Histopathology 1993;22:1–8.
29. Bugert P, Kovacs G. Molecular differential diagnosis of renal cell carcinomas by microsatellite analysis. Am J Pathol 1996;149:2081–2088.
30. Steiner G, Sidransky D. Molecular differential diagnosis of renal carcinoma: from microscopes to microsatellites. Am J Pathol 1996;149: 1791–1795.
31. Wagner JR, Linehan WM. Molecular genetics of renal cell carcinoma. Semin Urol Oncol 1996;14:244–249.
32. Bodmer D, van den Hurk W, van Groningen JJ, et al. Understanding familial and non-familial renal cell cancer. Hum Mol Genet 2002;11: 2489–2498.
33. Kosary C, McLaughlin J. Kidney and renal pelvis. NIH Publication No. 93-2789. Bethesda, MD: National Cancer Institute; 1993.
34. Parkin DM, Pisani P, Ferlay J. Estimates of the worldwide incidence of eighteen major cancers in 1985. Int J Cancer 1993;54:594–606.
35. Anonymous. Cancer incidence, mortality and prevalence worldwide. Vol. 5. 1.0 edn. Lyon: IARC Press; 2001.
36. Fuhrman SA, Lasky LC, Limas C. Prognostic significance of morphologic parameters in renal cell carcinoma. Am J Surg Pathol 1982;6:655–663.
37. Medeiros LJ, Jones EC, Aizawa S, et al. Grading of renal cell carcinoma: Workgroup No. 2. Union Internationale Contre le Cancer and the American Joint Committee on Cancer (AJCC). Cancer 1997;80:990–991.
38. Lohse CM, Blute ML, Zincke H, Weaver AL, Cheville JC. Comparison of standardized and nonstandardized nuclear grade of renal cell carcinoma to predict outcome among 2,042 patients. Am J Clin Pathol 2002;118: 877–886.
39. Delahunt B, Eble JN. Papillary renal cell carcinoma: a clinicopathologic and immunohistochemical study of 105 tumors. Mod Pathol 1997;10: 537–544.
40. Green F, Page D, Fleming I, et al. AJCC cancer staging manual. 6th edn. New York: Springer; 2002.
41. Reuter VE, Tickoo SK. Adult renal tumors. In: Mills SE, ed. Sternberg's Diagnostic surgical pathology. 4th edn. Philadelphia: Lippincott Williams & Wilkins; 2004:1955–1999.
42. Ritchie AW, Chisholm GD. The natural history of renal carcinoma. Semin Oncol 1983;10:390–400.
43. Porena M, Vespasiani G, Rosi P, et al. Incidentally detected renal cell carcinoma: role of ultrasonography. J Clin Ultrasound 1992;20:395–400.
44. Konnak JW, Grossman HB. Renal cell carcinoma as an incidental finding. J Urol 1985;134:1094–1096.
45. Thompson IM, Peek M. Improvement in survival of patients with renal cell carcinoma – the role of the serendipitously detected tumor. J Urol 1988;140:487–490.
46. Linehan WM, Lerman MI, Zbar B. Identification of the von Hippel–Lindau (*VHL*) gene. Its role in renal cancer. JAMA 1995;273:564–570.
47. Poston CD, Jaffe GS, Lubensky IA, et al. Characterization of the renal pathology of a familial form of renal cell carcinoma associated with von Hippel–Lindau disease: clinical and molecular genetic implications. J Urol 1995;153:22–26.
48. Richards FM, Payne SJ, Zbar B, Affara NA, Ferguson-Smith MA, Maher ER. Molecular analysis of de novo germline mutations in the von Hippel–Lindau disease gene. Hum Mol Genet 1995;4:2139–2143.
49. Suzuki H, Ueda T, Komiya A, et al. Mutational state of von Hippel–Lindau and adenomatous polyposis coli genes in renal tumors. Oncology 1997;54:252–257.
50. Zbar B. Von Hippel–Lindau disease and sporadic renal cell carcinoma. Cancer Surv 1995;25:219–232.
51. Taxy JB, Marshall FF. Multilocular renal cysts in adults. Possible relationship to renal adenocarcinoma. Arch Pathol Lab Med 1983;107: 633–637.
52. Tamura Y, Okamura K, Ogura H, et al. [Multilocular cystic renal cell carcinoma: a report of 2 cases.] Hinyokika Kiyo 1990;36:437–441.
53. Murad T, Komaiko W, Oyasu R, Bauer K. Multilocular cystic renal cell carcinoma. Am J Clin Pathol 1991;95:633–637.
54. Eble JN, Bonsib SM. Extensively cystic renal neoplasms: cystic nephroma, cystic partially differentiated nephroblastoma, multilocular cystic renal cell

carcinoma, and cystic hamartoma of renal pelvis. Semin Diagn Pathol 1998;15:2–20.
55. Nassir A, Jollimore J, Gupta R, Bell D, Norman R. Multilocular cystic renal cell carcinoma: a series of 12 cases and review of the literature. Urology 2002;60:421–427.
56. Amin MB, Corless CL, Renshaw AA, Tickoo SK, Kubus J, Schultz DS. Papillary (chromophil) renal cell carcinoma: histomorphologic characteristics and evaluation of conventional pathologic prognostic parameters in 62 cases. Am J Surg Pathol 1997;21:621–635.
57. Weiss LM, Gelb AB, Medeiros LJ. Adult renal epithelial neoplasms. Am J Clin Pathol 1995;103:624–635.
58. Renshaw AA, Corless CL. Papillary renal cell carcinoma. Histology and immunohistochemistry. Am J Surg Pathol 1995;19:842–849.
59. Lager DJ, Huston BJ, Timmerman TG, Bonsib SM. Papillary renal tumors. Cancer. 1995;76:669–673.
60. Henn W, Zwergel T, Wullich B, Thonnes M, Zang KD, Seitz G. Bilateral multicentric papillary renal tumors with heteroclonal origin based on tissue-specific karyotype instability. Cancer 1993;72:1315–1318.
61. Delahunt B, Eble JN, McCredie MR, Bethwaite PB, Stewart JH, Bilous AM. Morphologic typing of papillary renal cell carcinoma: comparison of growth kinetics and patient survival in 66 cases. Hum Pathol 2001;32: 590–595.
62. Jiang F, Richter J, Schraml P, et al. Chromosomal imbalances in papillary renal cell carcinoma: genetic differences between histological subtypes. Am J Pathol 1998;153:1467–1473.
63. Sanders ME, Mick R, Tomaszewski JE, Barr FG. Unique patterns of allelic imbalance distinguish type 1 from type 2 sporadic papillary renal cell carcinoma. Am J Pathol 2002;161:997–1005.
64. Kovacs G. Papillary renal cell carcinoma. A morphologic and cytogenetic study of 11 cases. Am J Pathol 1989;134:27–34.
65. Lager DJ, Huston BJ, Timmerman TG, Bonsib SM. Papillary renal tumors. Morphologic, cytochemical, and genotypic features. Cancer 1995;76: 669–673.
66. Sidhar SK, Clark J, Gill S, et al. The t(X;1)(p11.2;q21.2) translocation in papillary renal cell carcinoma fuses a novel gene *PRCC* to the *TFE3* transcription factor gene. Hum Mol Genet 1996;5:1333–1338.
67. Ladanyi M, Lui MY, Antonescu CR, et al. The der(17)t(X;17)(p11;q25) of human alveolar soft part sarcoma fuses the *TFE3* transcription factor gene to *ASPL*, a novel gene at 17q25. Oncogene 2001;20:48–57.
68. Argani P, Antonescu CR, Illei PB, et al. Primary renal neoplasms with the *ASPL–TFE3* gene fusion of alveolar soft part sarcoma: a distinctive tumor entity previously included among renal cell carcinomas of children and adolescents. Am J Pathol 2001;159:179–192.
69. Fuzesi L, Gunawan B, Bergmann F, Tack S, Braun S, Jakse G. Papillary renal cell carcinoma with clear cell cytomorphology and chromosomal loss of 3p. Histopathology 1999;35:157–161.
70. Argani P, Antonescu CR, Couturier J, et al. *PRCC–TFE3* renal carcinomas: morphologic, immunohistochemical, ultrastructural, and molecular analysis of an entity associated with the t(X;1)(p11.2;q21). Am J Surg Pathol 2002;26:1553–1566.
71. Thoenes W, Storkel S, Rumpelt HJ. Human chromophobe cell renal carcinoma. Virchows Arch B Cell Pathol Incl Mol Pathol 1985;48:207–217.
72. Thoenes W, Storkel S, Rumpelt HJ, Moll R, Baum HP, Werner S. Chromophobe cell renal carcinoma and its variants – a report on 32 cases. J Pathol 1988;155:277–287.
73. Akhtar M, Kardar H, Linjawi T, McClintock J, Ali MA. Chromophobe cell carcinoma of the kidney. A clinicopathologic study of 21 cases. Am J Surg Pathol 1995;19:1245–1256.
74. Crotty TB, Farrow GM, Lieber MM. Chromophobe cell renal carcinoma: clinicopathological features of 50 cases. J Urol 1995;154:964–967.
75. Cochand-Priollet B, Molinie V, Bougaran J, et al. Renal chromophobe cell carcinoma and oncocytoma. A comparative morphologic, histochemical, and immunohistochemical study of 124 cases. Arch Pathol Lab Med 1997; 121:1081–1086.
76. de Peralta-Venturina M, Moch H, Amin M, et al. Sarcomatoid differentiation in renal cell carcinoma: a study of 101 cases. Am J Surg Pathol 2001;25:275–284.
77. Akhtar M, Tulbah A, Kardar AH, Ali MA. Sarcomatoid renal cell carcinoma: the chromophobe connection. Am J Surg Pathol 1997;21: 1188–1195.
78. Bugert P, Gaul C, Weber K, et al. Specific genetic changes of diagnostic importance in chromophobe renal cell carcinomas. Lab Invest 1997;76:203–208.
79. Schwerdtle RF, Storkel S, Neuhaus C, et al. Allelic losses at chromosomes 1p, 2p, 6p, 10p, 13q, 17p, and 21q significantly correlate with the chromophobe subtype of renal cell carcinoma. Cancer Res 1996;56: 2927–2930.
80. Kovacs A, Kovacs G. Low chromosome number in chromophobe renal cell carcinomas. Genes Chromosomes Cancer 1992;4:267–268.
81. Akhtar M, Al-Sohaibani MO, Haleem A, et al. Flow cytometric DNA analysis of chromophobe cell carcinoma of the kidney. J Urol Pathol 1996; 4:15–23.
82. Kovacs A, Storkel S, Thoenes W, Kovacs G. Mitochondrial and chromosomal DNA alterations in human chromophobe renal cell carcinomas. J Pathol 1992;167:273–277.
83. Tickoo SK, Amin MB, Linden MD, Lee MW, Zarbo RJ. Antimitochondrial antibody (113-1) in the differential diagnosis of granular renal cell tumors. Am J Surg Pathol 1997;21:922–930.
84. Tickoo SK, Amin MB. Discriminant nuclear features of renal oncocytoma and chromophobe renal cell carcinoma. Analysis of their potential utility in the differential diagnosis. Am J Clin Pathol 1998;110: 782–787.
85. Tickoo SK, Amin MB, Zarbo RJ. Colloidal iron staining in renal epithelial neoplasms, including chromophobe renal cell carcinoma: emphasis on technique and patterns of staining. Am J Surg Pathol 1998;22: 419–424.
86. DeLong WH, Sakr W, Grignon DG. Chromophobe renal cell carcinoma. A comparative histochemical and immunohistochemical study. J Urol Pathol 1996;4:1–8.
87. Bonsib SM, Bray C, Timmerman TG. Renal chromophobe cell carcinoma: limitations of paraffin-embedded tissue. Ultrastruct Pathol 1993;17: 529–536.
88. Zbar B, Alvord WG, Glenn G, et al. Risk of renal and colonic neoplasms and spontaneous pneumothorax in the Birt–Hogg–Dubé syndrome. Cancer Epidemiol Biomarkers Prev 2002;11:393–400.
89. Khoo SK, Giraud S, Kahnoski K, et al. Clinical and genetic studies of Birt–Hogg–Dubé syndrome. J Med Genet 2002;39:906–912.
90. Pavlovich CP, Walther MM, Eyler RA, et al. Renal tumors in the Birt–Hogg–Dubé syndrome. Am J Surg Pathol 2002;26:1542–1552.
91. Fleming S, Lewi HJ. Collecting duct carcinoma of the kidney. Histopathology 1986;10:1131–1141.
92. Kennedy SM, Merino MJ, Linehan WM, Roberts JR, Robertson CN, Neumann RD. Collecting duct carcinoma of the kidney. Hum Pathol 1990;21:449–456.
93. Amin MB, Varma MD, Tickoo SK, et al. Collecting duct carcinoma of the kidney. Adv Anat Pathol 1997;4:85–94.
94. Srigley JR, Eble JN. Collecting duct carcinoma of kidney. Semin Diagn Pathol 1998;15:54–67.
95. Rumpelt HJ, Storkel S, Moll R, Scharfe T, Thoenes W. Bellini duct carcinoma: further evidence for this rare variant of renal cell carcinoma. Histopathology 1991;18:115–122.
96. Dimopoulos MA, Logothetis CJ, Markowitz A, Sella A, Amato R, Ro J. Collecting duct carcinoma of the kidney. Br J Urol 1993;71:388–391.
97. Polascik TJ, Cairns P, Epstein JI, et al. Distal nephron renal tumors: microsatellite allelotype. Cancer Res 1996;56:1892–1895.
98. Schoenberg M, Cairns P, Brooks JD, et al. Frequent loss of chromosome arms 8p and 13q in collecting duct carcinoma (CDC) of the kidney. Genes Chromosomes Cancer 1995;12:76–80.
99. Steiner G, Cairns P, Polascik TJ, et al. High-density mapping of chromosomal arm 1q in renal collecting duct carcinoma: region of minimal deletion at 1q32.1-32.2. Cancer Res 1996;56:5044–5046.
100. Gregori-Romero MA, Morell-Quadreny L, Llombart-Bosch A. Cytogenetic analysis of three primary Bellini duct carcinomas. Genes Chromosomes Cancer 1996;15:170–172.
101. Fuzesi L, Cober M, Mittermayer C. Collecting duct carcinoma: cytogenetic characterization. Histopathology 1992;21:155–160.
102. Baer SC, Ro JY, Ordonez NG, et al. Sarcomatoid collecting duct carcinoma: a clinicopathologic and immunohistochemical study of five cases. Hum Pathol 1993;24:1017–1022.
103. MacLennan GT, Farrow GM, Bostwick DG. Low-grade collecting duct carcinoma of the kidney: report of 13 cases of low-grade mucinous tubulocystic renal carcinoma of possible collecting duct origin. Urology 1997;50:679–684.
104. Davis CJ Jr, Mostofi FK, Sesterhenn IA. Renal medullary carcinoma. The seventh sickle cell nephropathy. Am J Surg Pathol 1995;19:1–11.
105. Figenshau RS, Basler JW, Ritter JH, Siegel CL, Simon JA, Dierks SM. Renal medullary carcinoma. J Urol 1998;159:711–713.
106. Avery RA, Harris JE, Davis CJ Jr, Borgaonkar DS, Byrd JC, Weiss RB. Renal medullary carcinoma: clinical and therapeutic aspects of a newly described tumor. Cancer 1996;78:128–132.

107. Rodriquez-Jurado R, Gonzalez-Crussi F. Renal medullary carcinoma. Immunohistochemical and ultrastructural observations. J Urol Pathol 1996; 4:191–203.
108. Friedrichs P, Lassen P, Canby E, Graham C. Renal medullary carcinoma and sickle cell trait. J Urol 1997;157:1349.
109. Herring JC, Schmetz MA, Digan AB, Young ST, Kalloo NB. Renal medullary carcinoma: a recently described highly aggressive renal tumor in young black patients. J Urol 1997;157:2246–2247.
110. Swartz MA, Karth J, Schneider DT, Rodriguez R, Beckwith JB, Perlman EJ. Renal medullary carcinoma: clinical, pathologic, immunohistochemical, and genetic analysis with pathogenetic implications. Urology 2002;60: 1083–1089.
111. Otani M, Shimizu T, Serizawa H, Ebihara Y, Nagashima Y. Low-grade renal cell carcinoma arising from the lower nephron: a case report with immunohistochemical, histochemical and ultrastructural studies. Pathol Int 2001;51:954–960.
112. Parwani AV, Husain AN, Epstein JI, Beckwith JB, Argani P. Low-grade myxoid renal epithelial neoplasms with distal nephron differentiation. Hum Pathol 2001;32:506–512.
113. Srigley J, Eble JN, Grignon DHR. Unusual renal cell carcinoma with prominent spindle cell change possibly related to the loop of Henle. Mod Pathol 1999;12:107A.
114. Srigley JR, Kapusta L, Reuter V, et al. Phenotypic, molecular and ultrastructural studies of a novel low grade renal epithelial neoplasm possibly related to the loop of Henle. Mod Pathol 2002;12:182A.
115. Durham JR, Bostwick DG, Farrow GM, Ohorodnik JM. Mesoblastic nephroma of adulthood. Report of three cases. Am J Surg Pathol 1993;17: 1029–1038.
116. Levin NP, Damjanov I, Depillis VJ. Mesoblastic nephroma in an adult patient: recurrence 21 years after removal of the primary lesion. Cancer 1982;49:573–577.
117. Pawade J, Soosay GN, Delprado W, Parkinson MC, Rode J. Cystic hamartoma of the renal pelvis. Am J Surg Pathol 1993;17:1169–1175.
118. Prats Lopez J, Palou Redorta J, Morote Robles J, Martinez Perez E, Ruiz Marcellan C. Leiomyomatous renal hamartoma in an adult. Eur Urol 1988;14:80–82.
119. Trillo AA. Adult variant of congenital mesoblastic nephroma. Arch Pathol Lab Med 1990;114:533–535.
120. Adsay NV, Eble JN, Srigley JR, Jones EC, Grignon DJ. Mixed epithelial and stromal tumor of the kidney. Am J Surg Pathol 2000;24:958–970.
121. Pierson CR, Schober MS, Wallis T, et al. Mixed epithelial and stromal tumor of the kidney lacks the genetic alterations of cellular congenital mesoblastic nephroma. Hum Pathol 2001;32:513–520.
122. Tamboli P, Ro JY, Amin MB, Ligato S, Ayala AG. Benign tumors and tumor-like lesions of the adult kidney. Part II: Benign mesenchymal and mixed neoplasms, and tumor-like lesions. Adv Anat Pathol 2000;7:47–66.
123. Antonescu CR, Bisceglia M, Reuter V. Sarcomatous transformation of cystic nephroma in adults. Mod Pathol 1997;10:69A.
124. Argani P, Faria PA, Epstein JI, et al. Primary renal synovial sarcoma: molecular and morphologic delineation of an entity previously included among embryonal sarcomas of the kidney. Am J Surg Pathol 2000;24: 1087–1096.
125. Kodet R, Taylor M, Vachalova H, Pycha K. Juxtaglomerular cell tumor. An immunohistochemical, electron-microscopic, and in situ hybridization study. Am J Surg Pathol 1994;18:837–842.
126. Squires JP, Ulbright TM, DeSchryver-Kecskemeti K, Engleman W. Juxtaglomerular cell tumor of the kidney. Cancer 1984;53:516–523.
127. Tanaka T, Okumura A, Mori H. Juxtaglomerular cell tumor. Arch Pathol Lab Med 1993;117:1161–1164.
128. Tetu B, Vaillancourt L, Camilleri JP, Bruneval P, Bernier L, Tourigny R. Juxtaglomerular cell tumor of the kidney: report of two cases with a papillary pattern. Hum Pathol 1993;24:1168–1174.
129. McDonald EC, Mukai K, Burke BA, Sibley RK. Primary carcinoid tumor of the kidney: a light and electron microscopic, and immunohistochemical study. J Urol 1983;130:333–335.
130. Goldblum JR, Lloyd RV. Primary renal carcinoid. Case report and literature review. Arch Pathol Lab Med 1993;117:855–858.
131. Raslan WF, Ro JY, Ordonez NG, et al. Primary carcinoid of the kidney. Immunohistochemical and ultrastructural studies of five patients. Cancer 1993;72:2660–2666.
132. Takeshima Y, Inai K, Yoneda K. Primary carcinoid tumor of the kidney with special reference to its histogenesis. Pathol Int 1996;46:894–900.
133. Hannah J, Lippe B, Lai-Goldman M, Bhuta S. Oncocytic carcinoid of the kidney associated with periodic Cushing's syndrome. Cancer 1988;61: 2136–2140.
134. Gleeson MH, Bloom SR, Polak JM, Henry K, Dowling RH. Endocrine tumour in kidney affecting small bowel structure, motility, and absorptive function. Gut 1971;12:773–782.
135. Hamilton I, Reis L, Bilimoria S, Long RG. A renal vipoma. Br Med J 1980; 281:1323–1324.
136. Resnick ME, Unterberger H, McLoughlin PT. Renal carcinoid producing the carcinoid syndrome. Med Times 1966;94:895–896.
137. Azumi N, Traweek ST, Battifora H. Prostatic acid phosphatase in carcinoid tumors. Immunohistochemical and immunoblot studies. Am J Surg Pathol 1991;15:785–790.
138. Kojiro M, Ohishi H, Isobe H. Carcinoid tumor occurring in cystic teratoma of the kidney: a case report. Cancer 1976;38:1636–1640.
139. van den Berg E, Gouw AS, Oosterhuis JW, et al. Carcinoid in a horseshoe kidney. Morphology, immunohistochemistry, and cytogenetics. Cancer Genet Cytogenet 1995;84:95–98.
140. Gupta NP, Singh BP, Raina V, Gupta SD. Primitive neuroectodermal kidney tumor: 2 case reports and review of the literature. J Urol 1995;153: 1890–1892.
141. Takeuchi T, Iwasaki H, Ohjimi Y, et al. Renal primitive neuroectodermal tumor: an immunohistochemical and cytogenetic analysis. Pathol Int 1996;46:292–297.
142. Marley EF, Liapis H, Humphrey PA, et al. Primitive neuroectodermal tumor of the kidney – another enigma: a pathologic, immunohistochemical, and molecular diagnostic study. Am J Surg Pathol 1997;21:354–359.
143. Sheaff M, McManus A, Scheimberg I, Paris A, Shipley J, Baithun S. Primitive neuroectodermal tumor of the kidney confirmed by fluorescence in situ hybridization. Am J Surg Pathol 1997;21:461–468.
144. Parham DM, Roloson GJ, Feely M, Green DM, Bridge JA, Beckwith JB. Primary malignant neuroepithelial tumors of the kidney: a clinicopathologic analysis of 146 adult and pediatric cases from the National Wilms' Tumor Study Group Pathology Center. Am J Surg Pathol 2001;25:133–146.
145. Jimenez RE, Folpe AL, Lapham RL, et al. Primary Ewing's sarcoma/primitive neuroectodermal tumor of the kidney: a clinicopathologic and immunohistochemical analysis of 11 cases. Am J Surg Pathol 2002;26:320–327.
146. Quezado M, Benjamin DR, Tsokos M. EWS/FLI-1 fusion transcripts in three peripheral primitive neuroectodermal tumors of the kidney. Hum Pathol 1997;28:767–771.
147. Farrow GM, Harrison EG Jr, Utz DC, Jones DR. Renal angiomyolipoma. A clinicopathologic study of 32 cases. Cancer 1968;22:564–570.
148. Stone CH, Lee MW, Amin MB, et al. Renal angiomyolipoma: further immunophenotypic characterization of an expanding morphologic spectrum. Arch Pathol Lab Med 2001;125:751–758.
149. Bernstein J, Robbins TO. Renal involvement in tuberous sclerosis. Ann N Y Acad Sci 1991;615:36–49.
150. Stillwell TJ, Gomez MR, Kelalis PP. Renal lesions in tuberous sclerosis. J Urol 1987;138:477–481.
151. van Baal JG, Fleury P, Brummelkamp WH. Tuberous sclerosis and the relation with renal angiomyolipoma. A genetic study on the clinical aspects. Clin Genet 1989;35:167–173.
152. Beh WP, Barnhouse DH, Johnson SH 3rd, Marshall M, Price SE Jr. A renal cause for massive retroperitoneal hemorrhage – renal angiomyolipoma. J Urol 1976;116:372–374.
153. Kalra OP, Verma PP, Kochhar S, Jha V, Sakhuja V. Bilateral renal angiomyolipomatosis in tuberous sclerosis presenting with chronic renal failure: case report and review of the literature. Nephron 1994;68: 256–258.
154. Eble JN, Amin MB, Young RH. Epithelioid angiomyolipoma of the kidney: a report of five cases with a prominent and diagnostically confusing epithelioid smooth muscle component. Am J Surg Pathol 1997;21:1123–1130.
155. Martignoni G, Pea M, Bonetti F, Brunelli M, Eble JN. Oncocytoma-like angiomyolipoma. A clinicopathologic and immunohistochemical study of 2 cases. Arch Pathol Lab Med 2002;126:610–612.
156. Ferry JA, Malt RA, Young RH. Renal angiomyolipoma with sarcomatous transformation and pulmonary metastases. Am J Surg Pathol 1991;15: 1083–1088.
157. Lowe BA, Brewer J, Houghton DC, Jacobson E, Pitre T. Malignant transformation of angiomyolipoma. J Urol 1992;147:1356–1358.
158. Cibas ES, Goss GA, Kulke MH, Demetri GD, Fletcher CD. Malignant epithelioid angiomyolipoma ('sarcoma ex angiomyolipoma') of the kidney: a case report and review of the literature. Am J Surg Pathol 2001;25: 121–126.

159. Bonetti F, Pea M, Martignoni G, et al. Clear cell (sugar) tumor of the lung is a lesion strictly related to angiomyolipoma – the concept of a family of lesions characterized by the presence of the perivascular epithelioid cells (PEC). Pathology 1994;26:230–254.
160. Chan JK, Tsang WY, Pau MY, Tang MC, Pang SW, Fletcher CD. Lymphangiomyomatosis and angiomyolipoma: closely related entities characterized by hamartomatous proliferation of HMB-45-positive smooth muscle. Histopathology 1993;22:445–455.
161. Hruban RH, Bhagavan BS, Epstein JI. Massive retroperitoneal angiomyolipoma. A lesion that may be confused with well-differentiated liposarcoma. Am J Clin Pathol 1989;92:805–808.
162. Zavala-Pompa A, Folpe AL, Jimenez RE, et al. Immunohistochemical study of microphthalmia transcription factor and tyrosinase in angiomyolipoma of the kidney, renal cell carcinoma, and renal and retroperitoneal sarcomas: comparative evaluation with traditional diagnostic markers. Am J Surg Pathol 2001;25:65–70.
163. Pea M, Bonetti F, Zamboni G, et al. Melanocyte-marker-HMB-45 is regularly expressed in angiomyolipoma of the kidney. Pathology 1991;23: 185–188.
164. Jungbluth AA, Busam KJ, Gerald WL, et al. A103: an anti-melan-a monoclonal antibody for the detection of malignant melanoma in paraffin-embedded tissues. Am J Surg Pathol 1998;22:595–602.
165. Dineen MK, Venable DD, Misra RP. Pure intrarenal lipoma – report of a case and review of the literature. J Urol 1984;132:104–107.
166. Clinton-Thomas CL. A giant leiomyoma of the kidney. Br J Urol 1956;43: 497–501.
167. Fisher KS, van Blerk PJ. Childhood leiomyoma of kidney. Urology 1983;21: 74–75.
168. Farrow GM, Harrison EG, Utz DC Jr, ReMine WH. Sarcomas and sarcomatoid and mixed malignant tumors of the kidney in adults. I. Cancer 1968;22:545–550.
169. Srinivas V, Sogani PC, Hajdu SI, Whitmore WF Jr. Sarcomas of the kidney. J Urol 1984;132:13–16.
170. Ng WD, Chan KW, Chan YT. Primary leiomyosarcoma of renal capsule. J Urol 1985;133:834–835.
171. Lerman RJ, Pitcock JA, Stephenson P, Muirhead EE. Renomedullary interstitial cell tumor (formerly fibroma of renal medulla). Hum Pathol 1972;3:559–568.
172. Mullick T, Hutchins GM. Multiple medullary fibromas of the kidney are associated with systemic hypertension. Mod Pathol 1998;8:80A.
173. Mai KT. Giant renomedullary interstitial cell tumor. J Urol 1994;151:986–988.
174. Alvarado-Cabrero I, Folpe AL, Srigley JR, et al. Intrarenal schwannoma: a report of four cases including three cellular variants. Mod Pathol 2000;13:851–863.
175. Fain JS, Eble JN, Nascimento AG, Farrow GM, Bostwick DG. Solitary fibrous tumor of the kidney. J Urol Pathol 1996;4:227–238.
176. Gelb AB, Simmons ML, Weidner N. Solitary fibrous tumor involving the renal capsule. Am J Surg Pathol 1996;20:1288–1295.
177. Melamed J, Reuter VE, Erlandson RA, Rosai J. Renal myxoma. A report of two cases and review of the literature. Am J Surg Pathol 1994;18:187–194.
178. Wang T, Palazzo JP, Mitchell D, Petersen RO. Renal capsular hemangioma. J Urol 1993;149:1122–1123.
179. Anderson C, Knibbs DR, Ludwig ME, Ely MG 3rd. Lymphangioma of the kidney: a pathologic entity distinct from solitary multilocular cyst. Hum Pathol 1992;23:465–468.
180. Ordonez NG, Bracken RB, Stroehlein KB. Hemangiopericytoma of kidney. Urology 1982;20:191–195.
181. Ligato S, Ro JY, Tamboli P, Amin MB, Ayala AG. Benign tumors and tumor-like lesions of the adult kidney. Part I: Benign renal epithelial neoplasms. Adv Anat Pathol 1999;6:1–11.
182. Grignon DJ, McIsaac GP, Armstrong RF, Wyatt JK. Primary rhabdomyosarcoma of the kidney. A light microscopic, immunohistochemical, and electron microscopic study. Cancer 1988;62: 2027–2032.
183. Joseph TJ, Becker DI, Turton AF. Renal malignant fibrous histiocytoma. Urology 1991;37:483–489.
184. O'Malley FP, Grignon DJ, Shepherd RR, Harker LA. Primary osteosarcoma of the kidney. Report of a case studied by immunohistochemistry, electron microscopy, and DNA flow cytometry. Arch Pathol Lab Med 1991;115: 1262–1265.
185. Nativ O, Horowitz A, Lindner A, Many M. Primary chondrosarcoma of the kidney. J Urol 1985;134:120–121.
186. Malhotra CM, Doolittle CH, Rodil JV, Vezeridis MP. Mesenchymal chondrosarcoma of the kidney. Cancer 1984;54:2495–2499.
187. Mead JH, Herrera GA, Kaufman MF, Herz JH. Case report of a primary cystic sarcoma of the kidney, demonstrating fibrohistiocytic, osteoid, and cartilaginous components (malignant mesenchymoma). Cancer 1982;50: 2211–2214.
188. Tsuda N, Chowdhury PR, Hayashi T, et al. Primary renal angiosarcoma: a case report and review of the literature. Pathol Int 1997;47:778–783.
189. Farrow GM, Harrison EG, Utz DC Jr. Sarcomas and sarcomatoid and mixed malignant tumors of the kidney in adults. II. Cancer 1968;22: 551–555.
190. Beckwith JB. National Wilms Tumor Study: an update for pathologists. Pediatr Dev Pathol 1998;1:79–84.
191. Beckwith JB. Renal neoplasms of childhood. In: Sternberg SS, ed. Diagnostic surgical pathology. Philadelphia: Lippincott Williams & Wilkins; 1999:1825–1852.
192. Breslow NG, Beckwith JB, Ciol M, Sharples K. Age distribution of Wilms' tumor: report from the National Wilms' Tumor Study. Cancer Res 1988;48:1653–1657.
193. Breslow N, Olshan A, Beckwith JB, Green DM. Epidemiology of Wilms tumor. Med Pediatr Oncol 1993;21:172–181.
194. Coppes MJ, Campbell CE, Williams BRG. Wilms tumor: clinical and molecular characterization. Austin, TX: RG Landes; 1995.
195. Wick MR, Cherwitz DL, Manivel C, Sibley R. Immunohistochemical findings in tumors of the kidney. In: Eble JN, ed. Tumors and tumor-like conditions of the kidneys and ureters. New York: Churchill Livingstone; 1990:207–247.
196. Grubb GR, Yun K, Williams BR, Eccles MR, Reeve AE. Expression of WT1 protein in fetal kidneys and Wilms tumors. Lab Invest 1994;71: 472–479.
197. Beckwith JB, Zuppan CE, Browning NG, Moksness J, Breslow NE. Histological analysis of aggressiveness versus responsiveness in Wilms' tumor. Med Pediatr Oncol 1996;27:422–428.
198. Beckwith JB, Palmer NF. Histopathology and prognosis of Wilms' tumor: results from the First National Wilms' Tumor Study. Cancer 1978;41: 1937–1948.
199. Zuppan CW, Beckwith JB, Luckey DW. Anaplasia in unilateral Wilms' tumor: a report from the National Wilms' Tumor Study Pathology Center. Hum Pathol 1988;19:1199–1209.
200. Faria P, Beckwith JB, Mishra K, et al. Focal versus diffuse anaplasia in Wilms tumor: new definitions with prognostic significance: a report from the National Wilms Tumor Study Group. Am J Surg Pathol 1996;20: 909–920.
201. Bardeesy N, Falkoff D, Petruzzi MJ, et al. Anaplastic Wilms' tumor, a subtype displaying poor prognosis, harbours *p53* gene mutations. Nat Genet 1994;7:91–97.
202. Joshi VV, Beckwith JB. Multilocular cyst of the kidney (cystic nephroma) and cystic, partially differentiated nephroblastoma: terminology and criteria for diagnosis. Cancer 1989;64:466–479.
203. Beckwith JB, Kiviat NB, Bonadio JF. Nephrogenic rests, nephroblastomatosis, and the pathogenesis of Wilms' tumor. Pediatr Pathol 1990;10:1036.
204. Beckwith JB. Precursor lesions of Wilms tumor: clinical and biological implications. Med Pediatr Oncol 1993;21:158–168.
205. Coppes MJ, Arnold M, Beckwith JB, et al. Factors affecting the risk of contralateral Wilms tumor development. Cancer 1999;85:1616–1625.
206. Bolande RP. Congenital mesoblastic nephroma of infancy. Perspect Pediatr Pathol 1973;1:227–250.
207. Pettinato G, Manivel JC, Wick MR, Dehner LP. Classical and cellular (atypical) congenital mesoblastic nephroma: a clinicopathologic, ultrastructural, immunohistochemical, and flow cytometric study. Hum Pathol 1989;20:682–690.
208. Heidelberger KP, Ritchey ML, Dauser RC, McKeever PE, Beckwith JB. Congenital mesoblastic nephroma metastatic to the brain. Cancer 1993;72: 2499–2502.
209. Schlesinger AE, Rosenfield NS, Castle VP, Jasty R. Congenital mesoblastic nephroma metastatic to the brain: a report of two cases. Pediatr Radiol 1995;25:S73–S75.
210. Knezevich SR, Garnett MJ, Pysher TJ, Beckwith JB, Grundy PE, Sorensen PH. *ETV6-NTRK3* gene fusions and trisomy 11 establish a histogenetic link between mesoblastic nephroma and congenital fibrosarcoma. Cancer Res 1998;58:5046–5048.
211. Rubin BP, Chen CJ, Morgan TW, et al. Congenital mesoblastic nephroma t(12;15) is associated with *ETV6-NTRK3* gene fusion: cytogenetic and molecular relationship to congenital (infantile) fibrosarcoma. Am J Pathol 1998;153:1451–1458.

212. Argani P, Perlman EJ, Breslow NE, et al. Clear cell sarcoma of the kidney: a review of 351 cases from the National Wilms Tumor Study Group Pathology Center. Am J Surg Pathol 2000;24:4–18.
213. Amin MB, de Peralta-Venturina MN, Ro JY, et al. Clear cell sarcoma of kidney in an adolescent and in young adults: a report of four cases with ultrastructural, immunohistochemical, and DNA flow cytometric analysis. Am J Surg Pathol 1999;23:1455–1463.
214. Haas JE, Bonadio JF, Beckwith JB. Clear cell sarcoma of the kidney with emphasis on ultrastructural studies. Cancer 1984;54:2978–2987.
215. Marsden HB, Lawler W. Bone metastasizing renal tumor of childhood: histopathological and clinical review of 38 cases. Virchows Arch A Pathol Anat Histopathol 1980;387:341–351.
216. Green DM, Breslow ME, Beckwith JB, Moksness J, Finklestein JZ, D'Angio GJ. Treatment of children with clear-cell sarcoma of the kidney: a report from the National Wilms Tumor Study Group. J Clin Oncol 1994;12: 2132–2137.
217. Weeks DA, Beckwith JB, Mierau GW, Luckey DW. Rhabdoid tumor of kidney: a report of 111 cases from the National Wilms' Tumor Study Pathology Center. Am J Surg Pathol 1989;13:439–458.
218. Wick M, Ritter JH, Dehner LP. Malignant rhabdoid tumors: a clinicopathologic review and conceptual discussion. Semin Diagn Pathol 1995;12:233–248.
219. Versteege I, Sevenet N, Lange J, et al. Truncating mutations of *hSNF5/INI1* in aggressive paediatric cancer. Nature 1998;394:203–206.
220. Biegel JA, Zhou JY, Rorke LB, et al. Germ-line and acquired mutations of *INI1* in atypical teratoid and rhabdoid tumors. Cancer Res 1999;59: 74–79.
221. Savla J, Chen TT, Schneider NR, Timmons CF, Delattre O, Tomlinson GE. Mutations of the *hSNF5/INI1* gene in renal rhabdoid tumors with secondary brain tumors. J Natl Cancer Inst 2000;92:648–650.
222. Sevenet N, Sheridan E, Amram D, Schneider P, Handgretinger R, Delattre O. Constitutional mutations of the *hSNF5/INI1* gene predispose to a variety of cancers. Am J Hum Genet 1999;65:1342–1348.
223. Lee HY, Yoon CS, Sevenet N, Rajalingam V, Delattre O, Walford NQ. Rhabdoid tumor of the kidney is a component of the rhabdoid predisposition syndrome. Pediatr Devel Pathol 2002;5: 395–399.
224. Sotelo-Avila C, Beckwith JB, Johnson JE. Ossifying renal tumor of infancy: a clinicopathologic study of nine cases. Pediatr Pathol Lab Med 1995;15: 745–762.
225. Tolia BM, Iloreta A, Freed SZ, Fruchtman B, Bennett B, Newman HR. Xanthogranulomatous pyelonephritis: detailed analysis of 29 cases and a brief discussion of atypical presentations. J Urol 1981;126: 437–442.
226. Malek RS, Elder JS. Xanthogranulomatous pyelonephritis: a critical analysis of 26 cases and of the literature. J Urol 1978;119:589.
227. Moller JC, Kristensen IB. Xanthogranulomatous pyelonephritis. A clinico-pathological study with special reference to pathogenesis. Acta Pathol Microbiol Scand [A] 1980;88:89–96.
228. Esparza AR, McKay DB, Cronan JJ, Chazan JA. Renal parenchymal malakoplakia. Histologic spectrum and its relationship to megalocytic interstitial nephritis and xanthogranulomatous pyelonephritis. Am J Surg Pathol 1989;13:225–236.
229. Trillo A, Lorentz WB, Whitley NO. Malakoplakia of kidney simulating renal neoplasm. Urology 1977;10:472.
230. Petersen L, Mommsen S, Pallisgaard G. Male genitourinary tuberculosis. Report of 12 cases and review of the literature. Scand J Urol Nephrol 1993; 27:425–428.
231. Wise GJ, Marella VK. Genitourinary manifestations of tuberculosis. Urol Clin North Am 2003;30:111–121.
232. Fowler JE Jr, Perkins T. Presentation, diagnosis and treatment of renal abscesses: 1972–1988. J Urol 1994;151:847–851.
233. Leach TD, Sadek SA, Mason JC. An unusual abdominal mass in a renal transplant recipient. Transpl Infect Dis 2002;4:218–222.
234. Gillitzer R, Melchior SW, Hampel C, Pfitzenmaier J, Thuroff JW. Transitional cell carcinoma of the renal pelvis presenting as a renal abscess. Urology 2002;60:165.
235. Angel C, Shu T, Green J, Orihuela E, Rodriquez G, Hendrick E. Renal and peri-renal abscesses in children: proposed physio-pathologic mechanisms and treatment algorithm. Pediatr Surg Int 2003;19:35–39.

CYTOLOGY OF THE URINARY TRACT

Ricardo H. Bardales and Klaus Schreiber

SAMPLE CONSIDERATIONS

The sampling method and the site both influence the cell composition of urine specimens. Ureteral and renal pelvis specimens are usually the most cellular. Umbrella and squamous cells predominate in urethral specimens. In contrast, few or no squamous cells are present in bladder, renal pelvis, and ureteral samples.

VOIDED URINE

Voided urine is simply and noninvasively obtained. The second morning mid-stream urine specimen is most satisfactory, as the first morning urine specimen has many degenerated cellular elements. Collection on three consecutive days provides a high diagnostic yield for urothelial carcinoma, particularly if high grade.[1,2] Voided urine cytology is accurate in predicting bladder cancer recurrence. (Fig. 9.1)

URINE OBTAINED BY INSTRUMENTATION

Instrumented urine specimens are highly cellular and preserve optimal cytologic detail. Bladder catheterization may be used to obtain urine or to perform bladder wash/barbotage. Because of the high cellular yield, bladder washes are valuable for detecting recurrences in patients with bladder cancer and for obtaining cells for ancillary testing. The ureter, renal pelvis, and calyces can be accessed with a flexible ureteropyeloscope under anesthesia. The value of cytologic examination of ureteral or renal pelvis washes is enhanced by bilateral specimen collections; comparison of the cell morphology from both sides allows the detection of subtle cytologic abnormalities. Brush cytology is sensitive and specific for high-grade urothelial carcinoma of the upper urinary tract, but is technically difficult. Brushes yield fewer umbrella cells and more basal and intermediate cell clusters than do washes. (Figs 9.2–9.4)

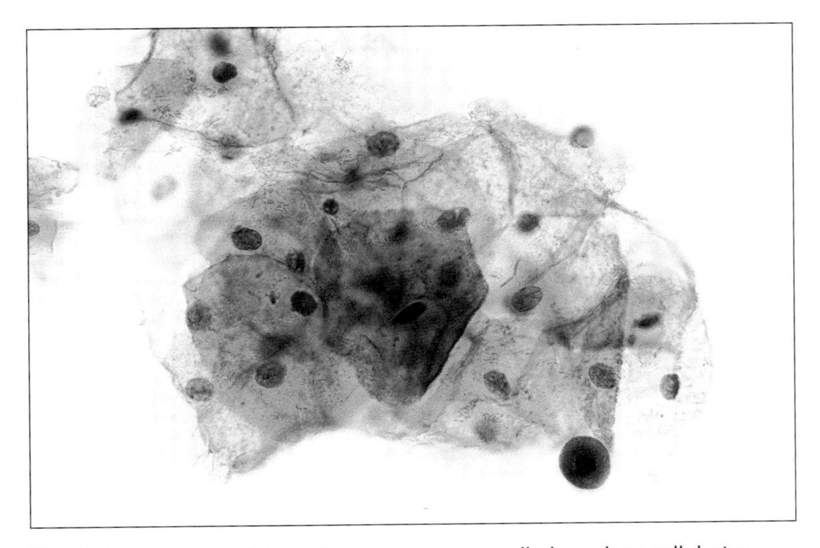

Fig. 9.1 Normal voided urine specimens usually have low cellularity. The urothelial cells come from the superficial urothelial 'field of umbrellas'. Squamous cells may be contamination from the external genitalia, or may represent squamous metaplasia of the bladder trigone.[1] Rare red blood cells, segmented leukocytes, lymphocytes, and degenerated renal tubular cells may be present.

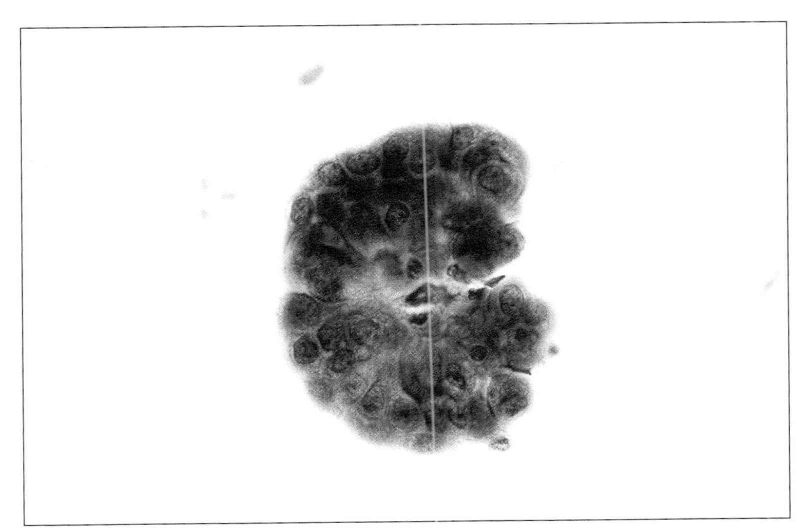

Fig. 9.2 Bladder wash preparations show cohesive cell aggregates forming balls or pseudopapillary clusters. The clusters show smooth and even borders and may have a densely stained cytoplasmic collar.[3] Small clusters, triplets, pairs, or single cells in smaller numbers may be seen. Variable numbers of squamous and red blood cells are present.

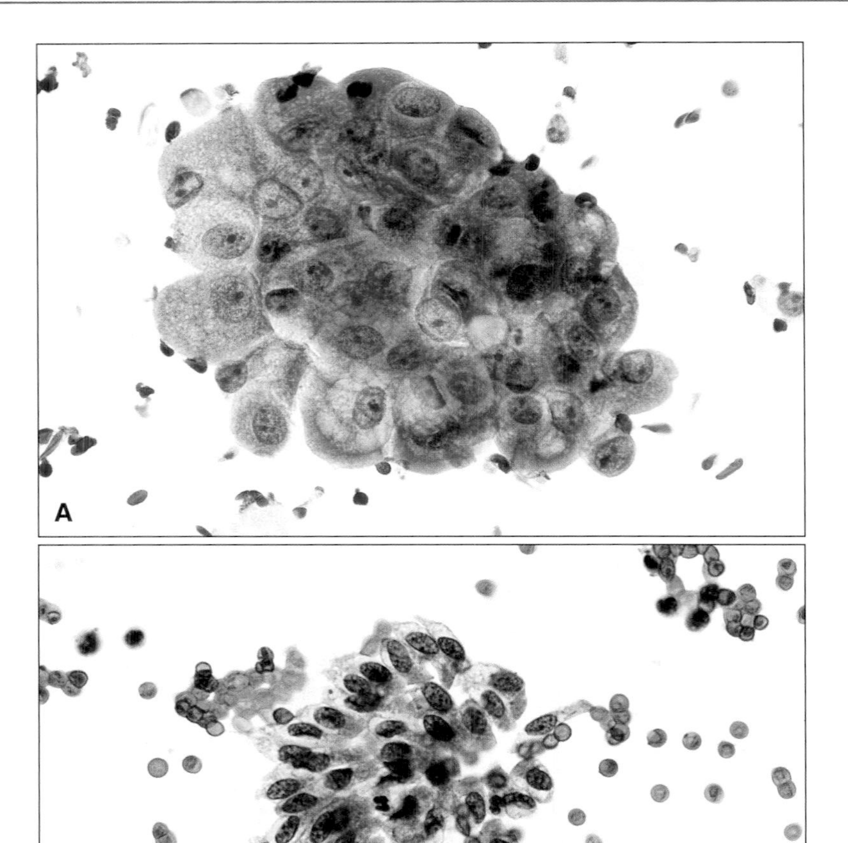

Fig. 9.3 (A,B) Ureteral wash/brush preparations show a mixture of umbrella cells and cuboidal and columnar intermediate/basal cells. Renal tubular cells may be identified. Inflammatory cells are variably present. More intact red blood cells are present in brushings than in washings.

PREPARATIVE PROCEDURES

Urine should be transported promptly to the laboratory for processing. If delay is anticipated, the specimen must be refrigerated. Alternatively, the sample may be fixed with an equal volume of 50–70% ethyl alcohol with 2% Carbowax. For brush cytology, immediate immersion of the brush in a cytology fixative is recommended, particularly for thin-layer preparations.

Conventional or cytospin smears should be prepared immediately after the specimen is received. Monolayer technologies (e.g. Cytyc®, Marlborough, MA; Surepath®, Burlington, NC) may reduce the number of inadequate samples and yield better cell morphology, but experience in the cytologic interpretation of these preparations is limited.[4]

NORMAL URINARY TRACT CYTOLOGY

Normal urine contains three types of epithelial cells. *Umbrella cells* are always benign, although they may coexist with urothelial neoplasms. Umbrella cells need to be distinguished from parabasal squamous cells, which are round and lack a biconvex shape, and from uni- or multinucleated macrophages or histiocytes, which are round and have reniform nuclei. Cuboidal or columnar *intermediate* or *basal urothelial cells* are smaller than umbrella cells. In voided urine specimens, they may be present singly and in small numbers, but a rare cluster of such cells may be identified. These cells are numerous in instrumented urine specimens. (Figs 9.5 & 9.6)

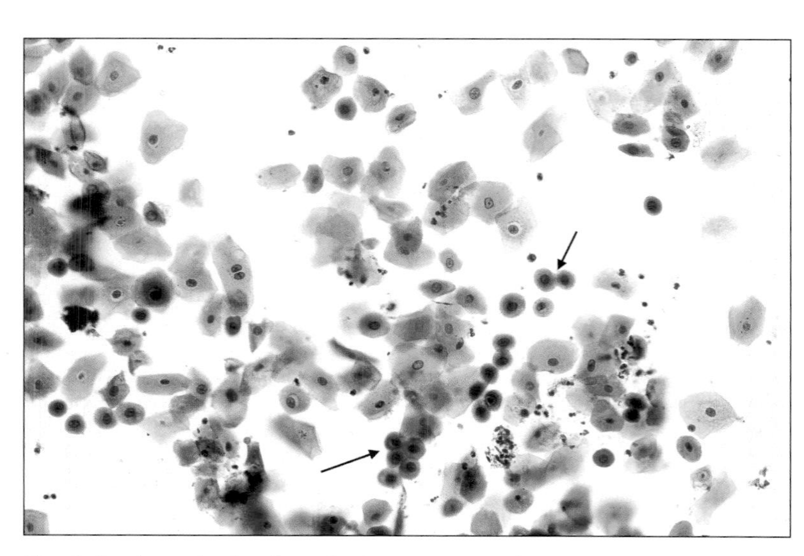

Fig. 9.4 A urethral catheterization specimen shows numerous squamous cells and fewer umbrella cells (arrows).

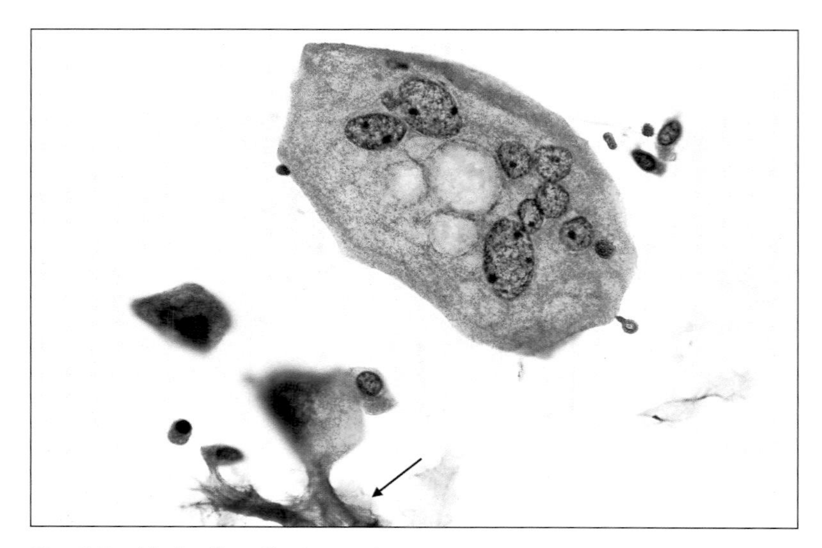

Fig. 9.5 Umbrella cells show a biconvex cytoplasmic outline, one border flatter than the other. The round central nucleus has powdery, regular chromatin and small chromocenters. Cytoplasm may be dense, thin, or vacuolated, with well-defined, smooth borders. Rare multinucleated umbrella cells with anisonucleosis may be seen. Smaller basal/intermediate cells are also seen. Lubricant (arrow) suggests instrumentation.

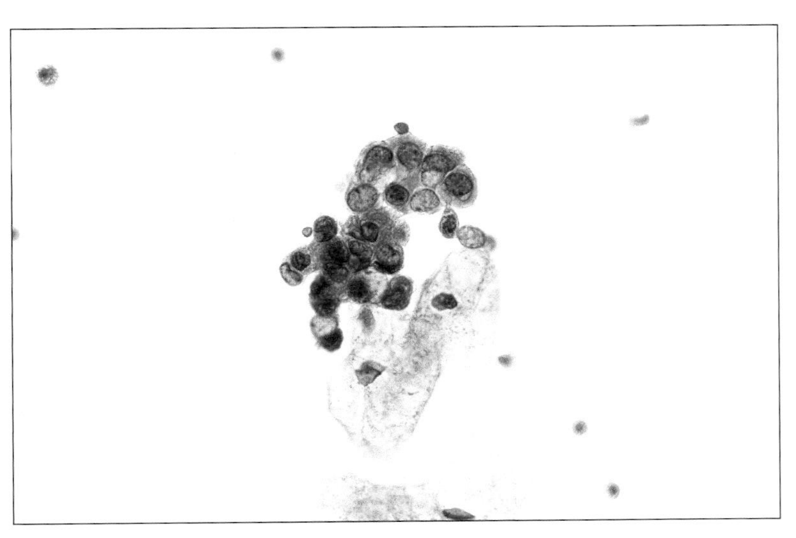

Fig. 9.6 Intermediate and basal cells have thin cytoplasm and a low nuclear:cytoplasmic ratio. The nucleus is round and smooth. Chromatin is powdery and regular. Careful examination of cells at the edge of a cluster will display characteristics similar to those of single cells. Odd cell shapes suggest urothelial pathology. Mitotic figures are rare without urothelial pathology.

SURGICALLY ALTERED URINARY TRACT

Urine obtained through a stent

The double-J ureteral stent is used in ureteral obstruction caused by urolithiasis or trauma. Urine cytology specimens obtained through a stent are similar to those obtained by other instrumentation methods. Low-grade urothelial carcinoma may be difficult to distinguish from stent effect. The rubbing effect of the tip on the renal pelvis causes marked squamous metaplasia, which may mimic changes seen in high-grade urothelial or squamous carcinoma. The finding of cell clusters and crystals in a background of tissue damage, and absence of high-grade tumor cells should dissuade from a diagnosis of malignancy. (Figs 9.7 & 9.8)

Enterostomy urine

The ileal conduit is the most common urinary diversion following total cystectomy. Colonic urinary diversions (colon conduit, cecal reservoir, ureterosigmoidostomy) are less usual. The ileal mucosa shows progressive shortening, loss of microvilli, and goblet cell hyperplasia during the first 3 years after surgery. Later, the epithelium becomes largely flat, avillous, and without mucin secretion.

Complications of enteric urinary diversion include stricture, pyelonephritis, and lithiasis. Development of urothelial carcinoma in an ileal loop is exceedingly rare, and no cases of adenocarcinoma of the ileum have been reported. By contrast, colonic urinary diversions have a high incidence of intestinal and, less commonly, urothelial carcinoma.

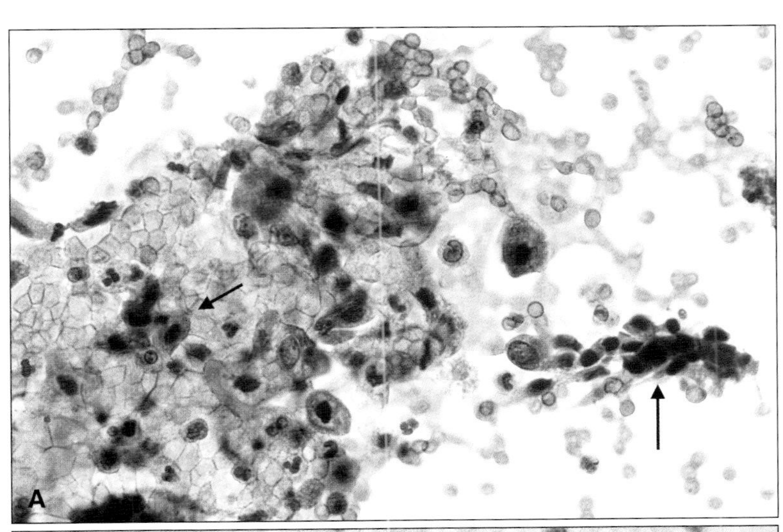

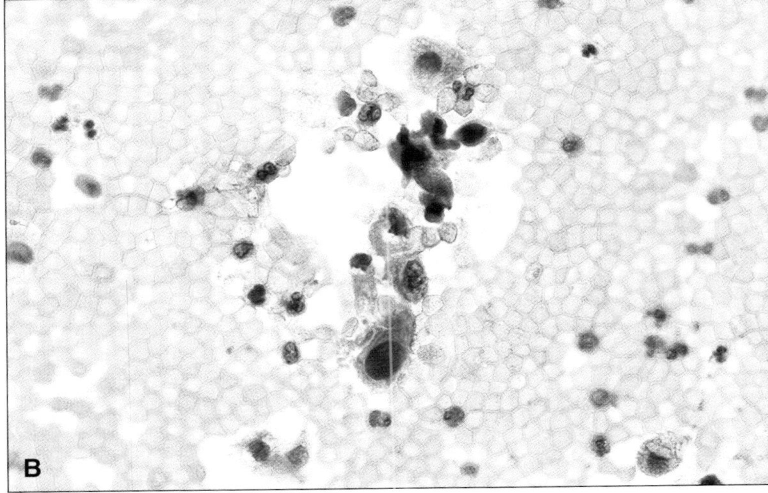

Fig. 9.7 (A,B) With stent urine, smears show reactive urothelial cells and cellular or non-cellular elements associated with the underlying obstructive process. Crystals are usually seen with urolithiasis. The background shows evidence of tissue damage, including debris and variable numbers of inflammatory cells. Squamous metaplastic cells with marked nuclear atypia may predominate (arrows).

Urine cytology is accurate and can reveal recurrent urothelial carcinoma even before it is clinically evident.[5] Well-preserved, high-grade tumor cells with a distinct cytoplasmic border, anaplastic nuclei, and tumor diathesis indicate recurrent urothelial carcinoma. However, chemotherapy and radiation effect should be considered. (Figs 9.9–9.11)

INFECTIONS AND INFESTATIONS OF THE URINARY TRACT

KIDNEY, RENAL PELVIS, AND URETERS

Acute pyelonephritis

Acute pyelonephritis is commonly bacterial. It is usually an ascending infection from the lower urinary tract, but hematogenous seeding may occur in sepsis. The most

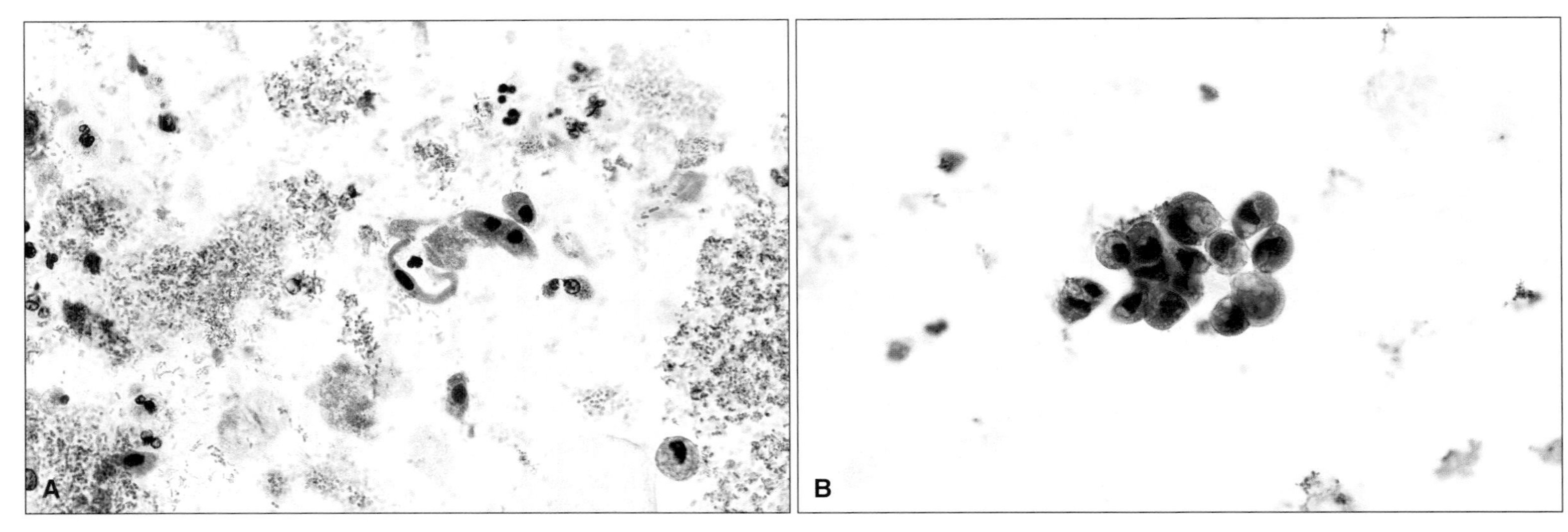

Fig. 9.8 (A,B) Similar, but less striking, cell changes may be identified in urine samples from patients with a neurogenic bladder and a permanent urinary bladder catheter. Columnar cells with vacuolated cytoplasm, dark degenerated nuclei, bacterial overgrowth, and paucity of inflammatory cells are common in urine specimens obtained from these patients. Degenerated nuclei resembling low-grade papillary urothelial carcinoma may be seen.

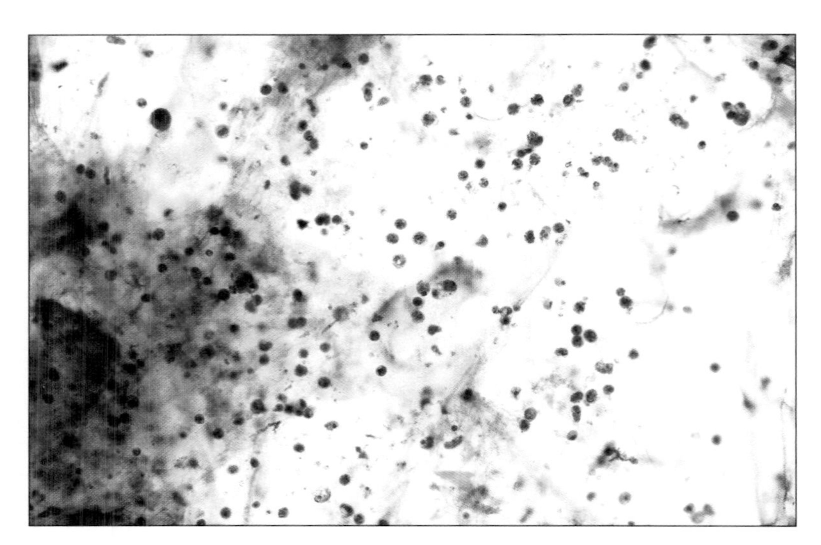

Fig. 9.9 The smear pattern of ileal-conduit urine is characteristic. Smears are markedly cellular. Discohesive, degenerated cells are present on a granular background without inflammation or blood. The cells are small, round or cuboidal, with indistinct cell borders, granular cytoplasm, and pyknotic, eccentric nuclei.

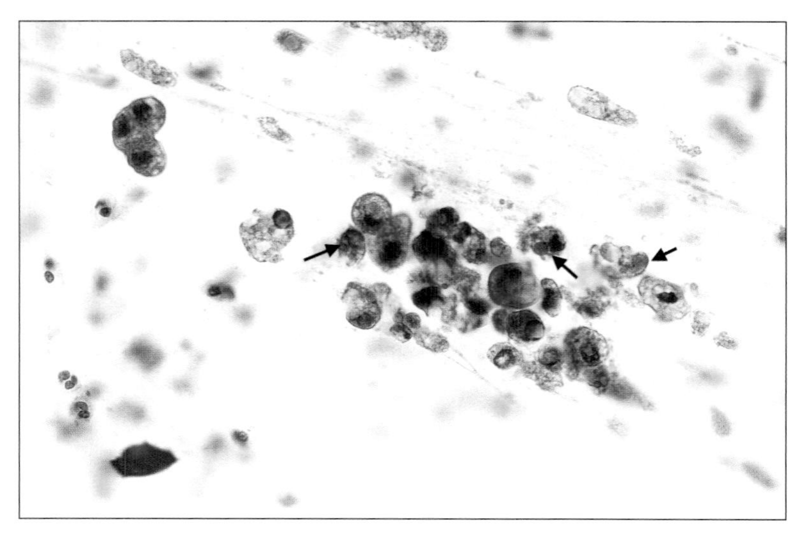

Fig. 9.10 Round eosinophilic cytoplasmic inclusions (arrows) are common in enterostomy urine. Nuclei are often pyknotic.

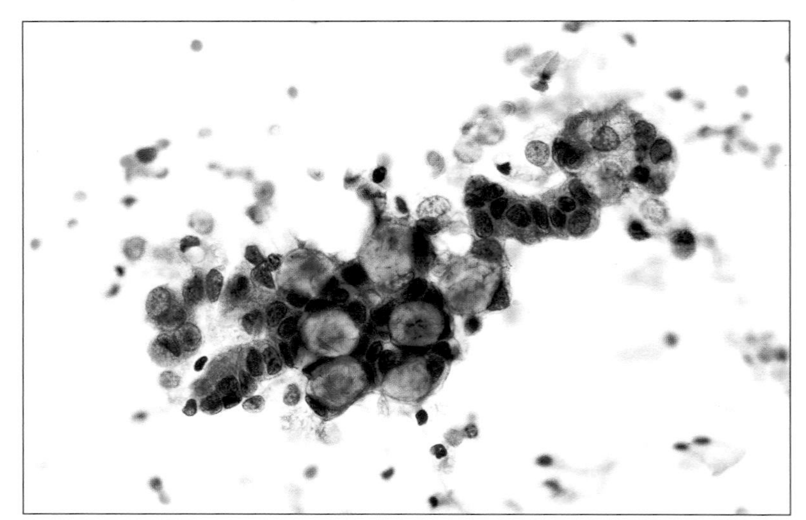

Fig. 9.11 Enterostomy urine cytology. Well-preserved, cohesive clusters of round or cuboidal cells with sharp cytoplasmic borders, dense cytoplasm, and subtle nuclear abnormalities may suggest a low-grade urothelial neoplasm. Less degenerated, loosely cohesive clusters of intestinal cells show ample vacuolated cytoplasm and a round, hyperchromatic nucleus. A honeycomb appearance or basally located uniform round nuclei help one to recognize the intestinal origin of the cells. These cell clusters are most obvious in the first 3 years after surgery.

frequent pathogens are coliform bacteria such as *Escherichia coli*, *Proteus*, *Enterobacter*, and *Klebsiella*. Predisposing factors include urinary obstruction, instrumentation, vesicoureteral reflux, diabetes mellitus, and immunosuppression.

Fungal acute pyelonephritis and acute interstitial nephritis due to cytomegalovirus (CMV), herpesvirus, and the BK polyomavirus are seen in immunocompromised patients. No specific therapy is at present available for BK virus nephropathy.[6] White blood cell casts in urine samples are characteristic of acute bacterial pyelonephritis. Reactive

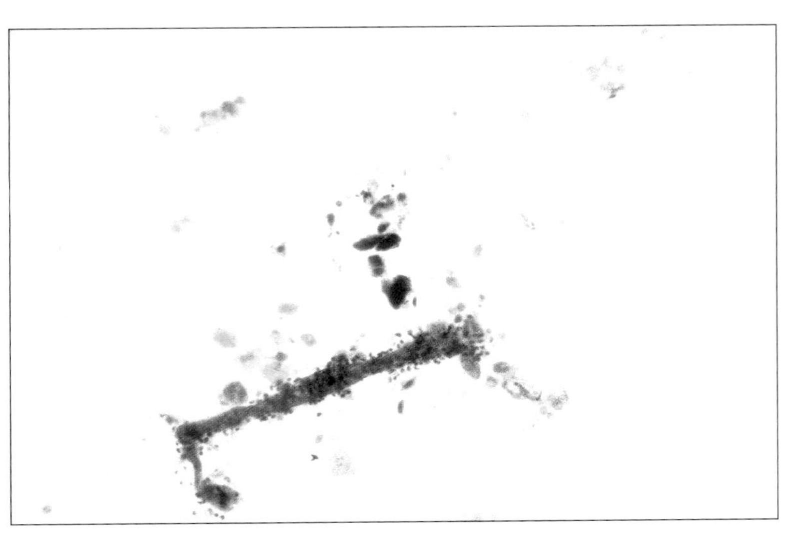

Fig. 9.12 Fungal elements are occasionally identified in urine cytology samples from patients with renal candidiasis, mucormycosis, or coccidioidomycosis.[7] Broad hyphae surrounded by bacteria and debris are seen in a silver stain of a voided urine sample from a diabetic with renal zygomyosis. Proof of renal involvement may require direct ureteral or renal pelvis catheterization.

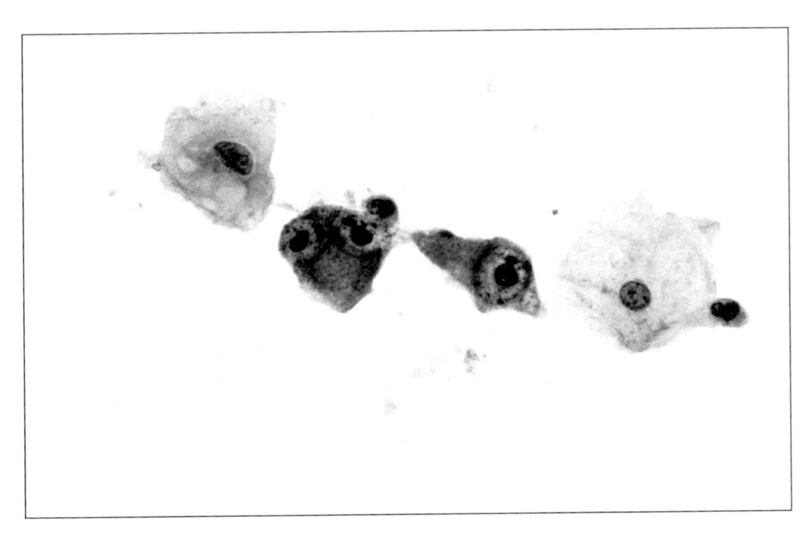

Fig. 9.13 Intranuclear inclusions are seen in the renal tubular cells in cytomegalovirus (CMV), polyomavirus, and adenovirus infections. In this urine smear from a patient with systemic CMV infection, large cells of renal tubular origin show eosinophilic nuclear inclusions with perinuclear clearing.

urothelial cells are also identified, and are more numerous if cystitis or urethritis coexists. Red blood cells may be present in severe bacterial infections. Without acute inflammation, bacteria or yeast in a urine smear usually represent overgrowth and not active infection. (Figs 9.12 & 9.13)

Papillary necrosis

(Fig. 9.14)

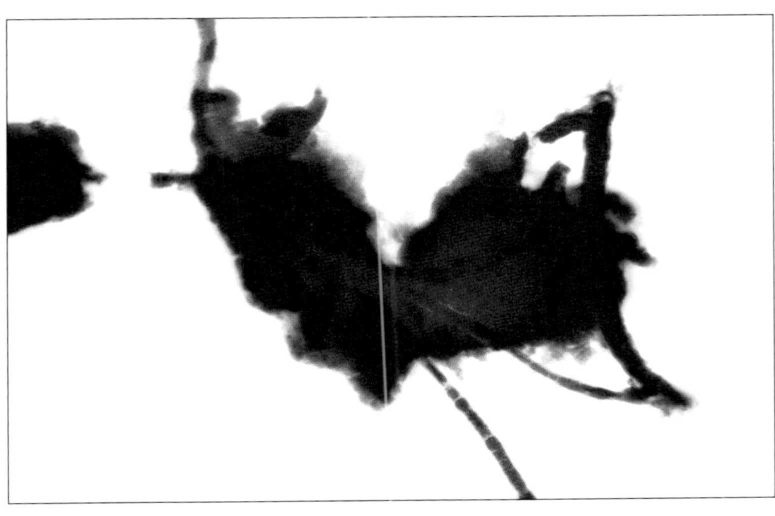

Fig. 9.14 In papillary necrosis, a complication of acute pyelonephritis seen in diabetics, coagulative necrosis of the papillary tips occurs, with only a limited acute inflammatory response. The clinical picture varies from an acute disease to a more chronic process with renal failure and polyuria caused by an inability to concentrate urine. Small fragments of degenerated tissue with capillaries may be identified with debris and red blood cells.

Chronic pyelonephritis

Chronic pyelonephritis occurs in 10–20% of patients in transplant or dialysis units. Chronic nonobstructive (reflux) nephropathy, a congenital disorder that occurs early in childhood, is the most common form of chronic pyelonephritis. Histologic findings include tubular atrophy and dilatation, interstitial fibrosis, and chronic inflammation. The characteristic 'thyroidization' of the tubules results from dilatation and accumulation of eosinophilic casts within the lumen. (Fig. 9.15)

Xanthogranulomatous pyelonephritis

Xanthogranulomatous pyelonephritis (XGP) is an uncommon form of chronic pyelonephritis that presents as a mass. The presence of a tumor elicits a clinical differential diagnosis that includes renal cell carcinoma,[8] but <5% of patients with XGP develop urologic neoplasms. XGP is often associated with staghorn calculi. Histologically, sheets of foamy histiocytes containing fragments of phagocytosed bacteria form ill-defined granulomas with occasional plasma cells and lymphocytes. *E. coli* (67%) and *Proteus mirabilis* (26%) are commonly isolated.

Cytologic examination of serial voided urine and ureteral washings yields a diagnostic accuracy rate of 80%. The differential diagnosis of XGP in urine includes tuberculosis and malakoplakia.[9] The abundant reactive histiocytes on a hemorrhagic, inflammatory background in urine may mimic well-differentiated renal cell carcinoma. Urine shows scattered histiocytes with abundant foamy cytoplasm and an eccentric nucleus. The histiocytes may have basophilic

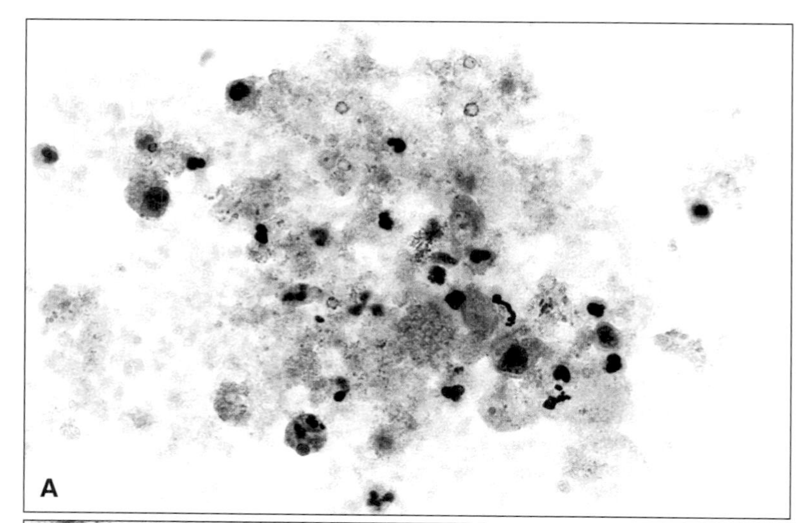

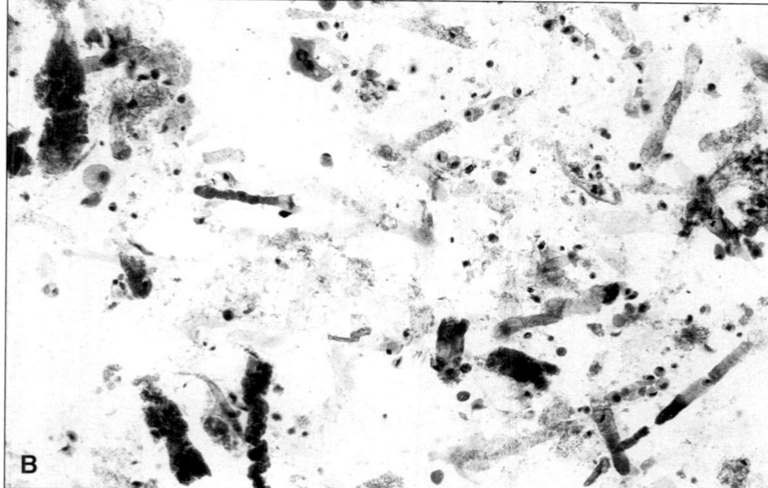

Fig. 9.15 (A,B) Urine cytology findings in chronic pyelonephritis are nonspecific. Mononuclear cell inflammation is usually sparse. Neutrophils predominate in bouts of acute infection, and occasional white blood cell casts may be found. The background is granular, with broad waxy casts and occasional hyaline or fine granular casts. Coarse granular casts may be present when there is proteinuria.

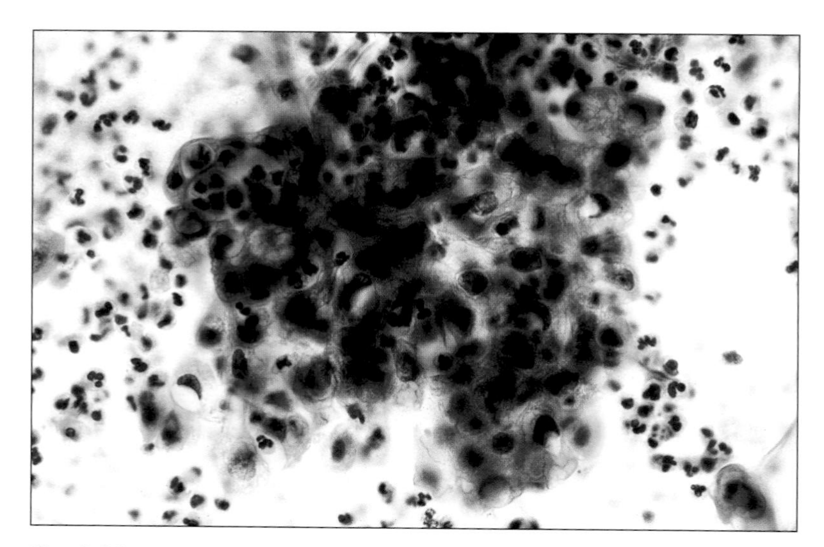

Fig. 9.16 Voided urine smears of bacterial cystitis show variable numbers of segmented leukocytes and intact red blood cells in a non-necrotic background. Reactive urothelial cells exhibit vacuolated cytoplasm, round nuclei, and prominent nucleoli. Nuclei may be hyperchromatic, but the chromatin distribution is uniform and the nuclear contours are smooth. The nuclear:cytoplasmic ratio is normal or slightly increased.

intracytoplasmic periodic acid–Schiff (PAS)-negative inclusions.[9] Multinucleated histiocytes may be identified. In the background are squamous metaplastic cells and intense inflammation along with lymphocytes and plasma cells.

Renal tuberculosis

Renal tuberculosis is uncommon. Most patients lack evident pulmonary disease when renal involvement is diagnosed. It is a granulomatous, cavitary process with an epicenter in the cortex, which subsequently expands to produce papillary necrosis with consequent seeding of the ureters and bladder. The differential diagnosis includes renal cell carcinoma, malakoplakia, and bacille Calmette-Guérin (BCG) infection in patients who have been treated for bladder neoplasia. Epithelioid histiocytes, granulomas, multinucleated Langhans'-type giant cells, and amorphous debris in urine cytology support the diagnosis of tuberculosis. Metaplastic squamous cells from the renal pelvis may be found in inactive renal tuberculosis.

URINARY BLADDER AND URETHRA

Acute inflammation may be a part of the necrotic background seen in invasive urothelial carcinoma. The presence of white blood cell casts indicates acute pyelonephritis, commonly associated with bacterial cystitis.

Bacterial cystourethritis

Bacterial cystitis affects predominantly women of reproductive age, and results from ascending bacterial infection from the introitus and distal urethra. The most common pathogenic organisms are Gram-negative enteric bacteria (*E. coli*, followed by *Proteus*, *Enterobacter*, and *Klebsiella*). Mycobacterial or actinomycotic cystitis is rare. (Figs 9.16–9.18)

Fungal cystitis

Predisposing factors for fungal cystitis include immunosuppression (including steroid therapy), diabetes, bladder outlet obstruction, and the presence of an indwelling catheter. Pyuria and microhematuria are seen in the urinalysis. *Candida albicans* is the most common etiologic agent in diabetics and has been associated with formation of a 'fungus ball' leading to obstructive uropathy. However, candiduria may represent noninvasive colonization, low-grade infection, or extensive urinary tract infection. Less

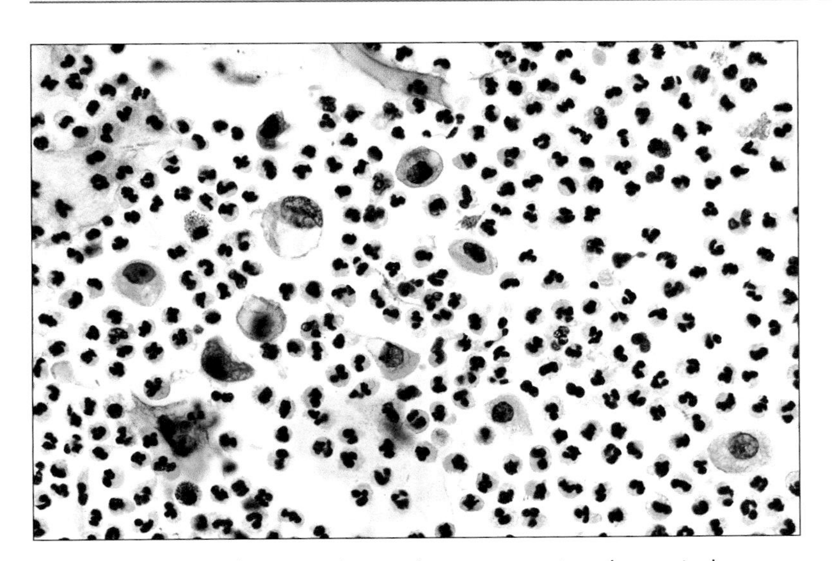

Fig. 9.17 Bacterial cystitis. A monolayer preparation shows single reactive cells and marked acute inflammation. The cytoplasm may be vacuolated and contain neutrophils.

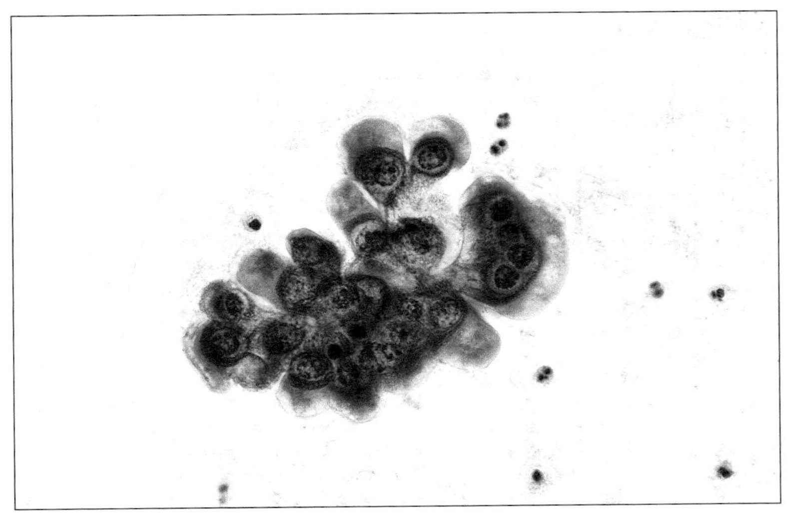

Fig. 9.18 Degenerated cells, debris, and eosinophils may be present in subacute or chronic cystitis. Subacute cystitis may yield highly reactive, small umbrella cells with a perinuclear halo, reminiscent of those seen in cervicovaginal smears.

common causes of fungal cystitis are *Aspergillus*, *Mucor*, *Blastomyces*, *Histoplasma*, *Cryptococcus*, and *Coccidioides*, particularly in immunosuppressed hosts. (Figs 9.19–9.22)

Viral cystitis

Viral cystitis is rare. However, polyomavirus, papillomavirus, and adenovirus type II have been detected in urine specimens from healthy people. Herpes simplex virus (HSV) type 2, CMV, and polyomavirus are the DNA viruses that most often affect the urinary tract. No RNA viruses or oncogenic RNA viruses (Retroviridae) have been detected.

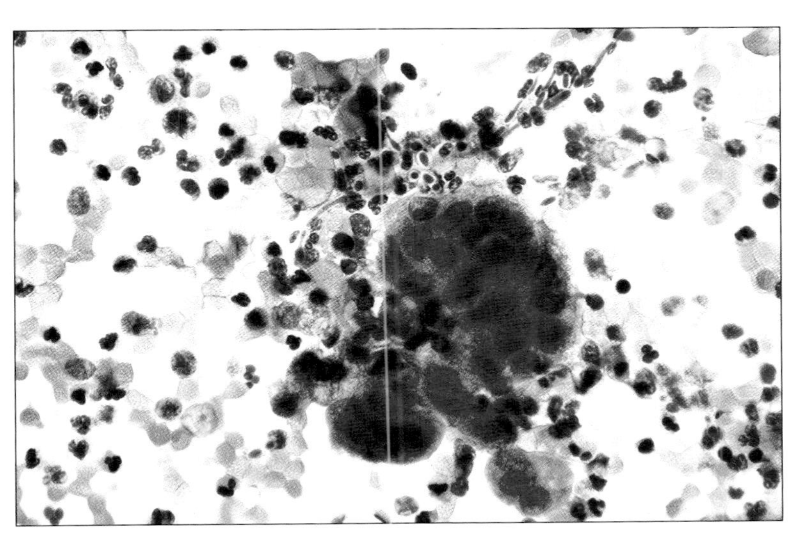

Fig. 9.19 Pseudohyphae and budding yeast are characteristic of *Candida* species. *Candida* organisms in the urine should be noted in the cytology report, but the diagnosis of urinary tract candidiasis is suggested only when acute inflammation, tissue damage, and reactive cellular changes are present.

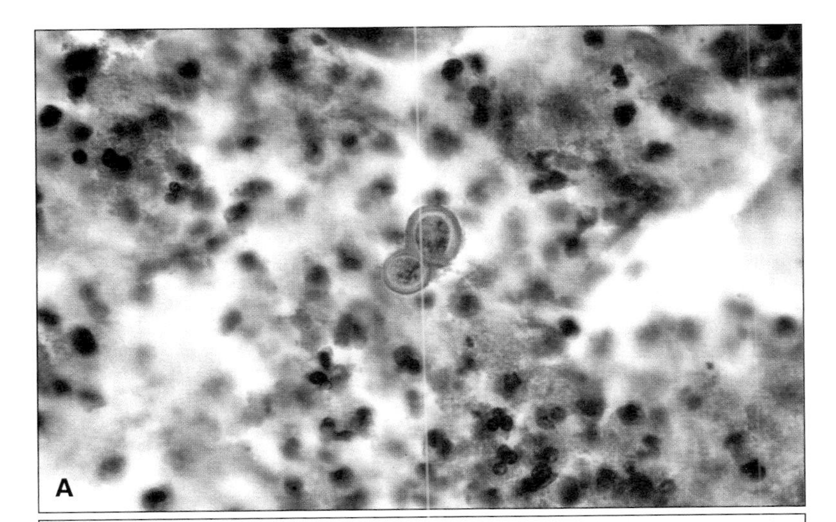

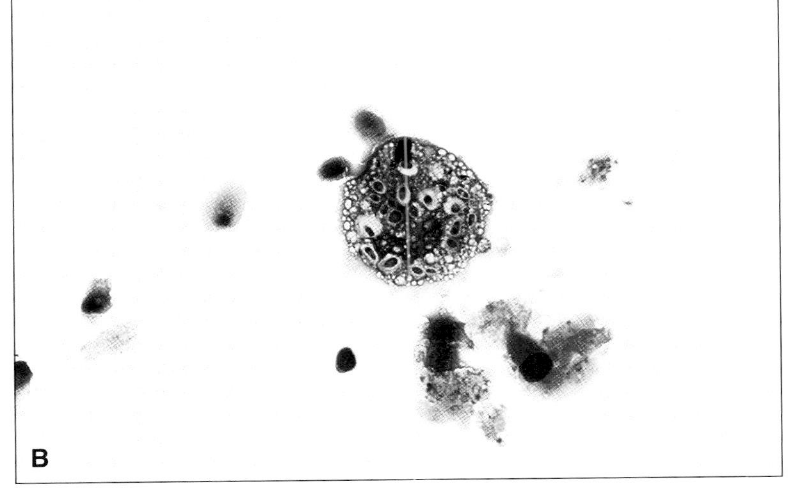

Fig. 9.20 Dimorphic fungi occasionally cause urinary tract infection. Blastomycosis commonly involves the prostate or testis, less often the urinary tract. Broad-based budding yeasts are diagnostic of blastomycosis (A). Small, intracellular yeasts are characteristic of histoplasmosis. The intracellular organisms are best seen with the use of periodic acid–Schiff or silver stain (B). Such infections are vanishingly rare.

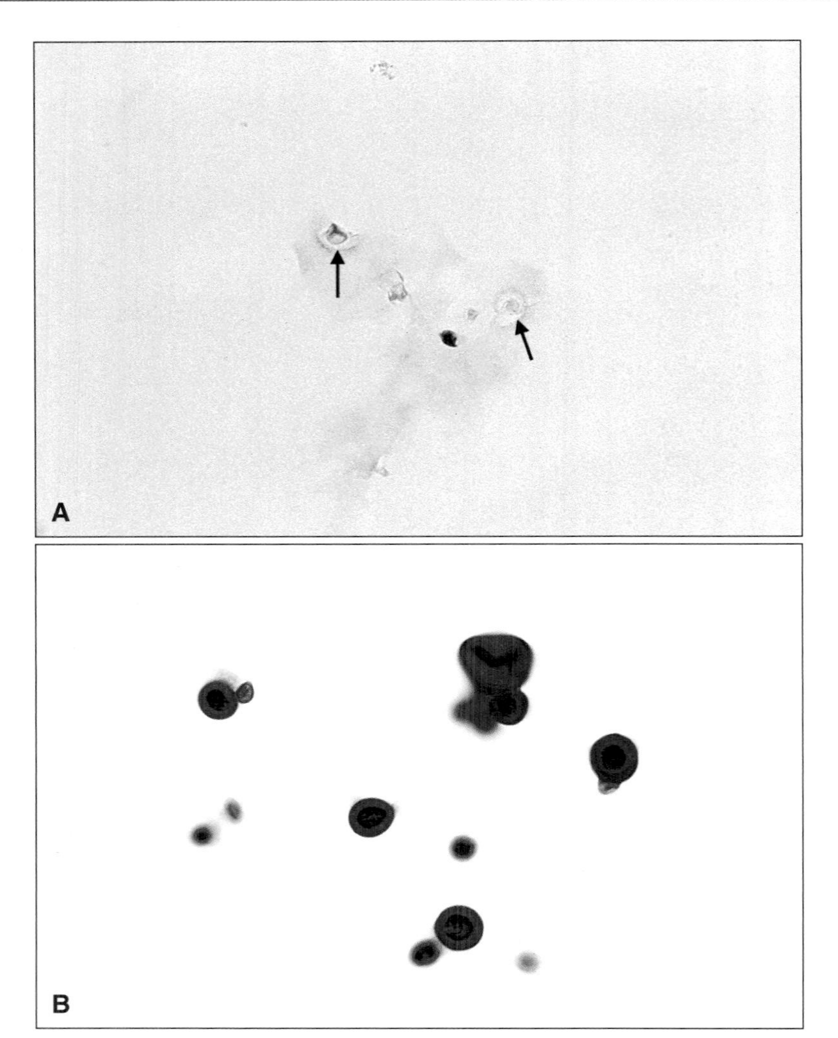

Fig. 9.21 (A,B) Large, clear capsules (arrows) surrounding yeast forms are present in *Cryptococcus*. The organisms are best seen with the use of mucicarmine stain or India ink preparations.

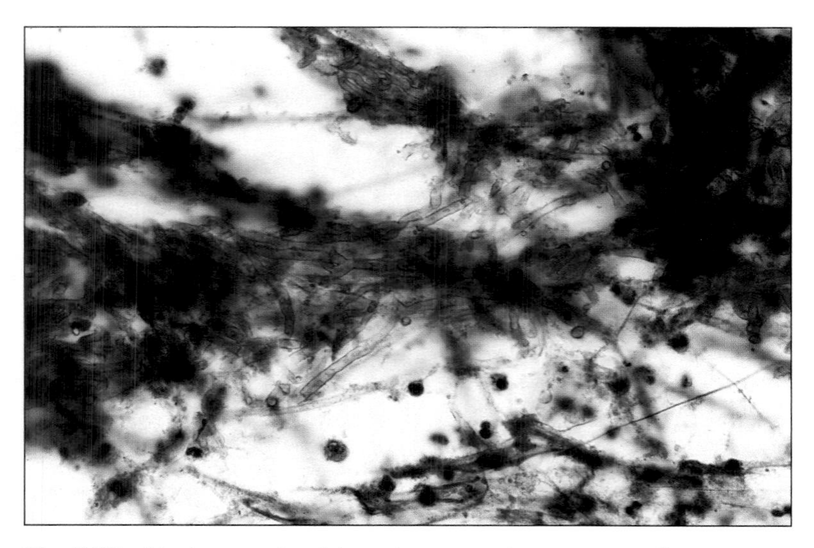

Fig. 9.22 Hyphomycosis of the urinary tract is uncommon. Septate hyphal forms are seen in *Aspergillus* species (shown here), and *Pseudallescheria* and *Fusarium* species. *Rhizopus* species have wide hyphae with irregular contours and rare septa. However, tissue degeneration may preclude the precise evaluation of these features.

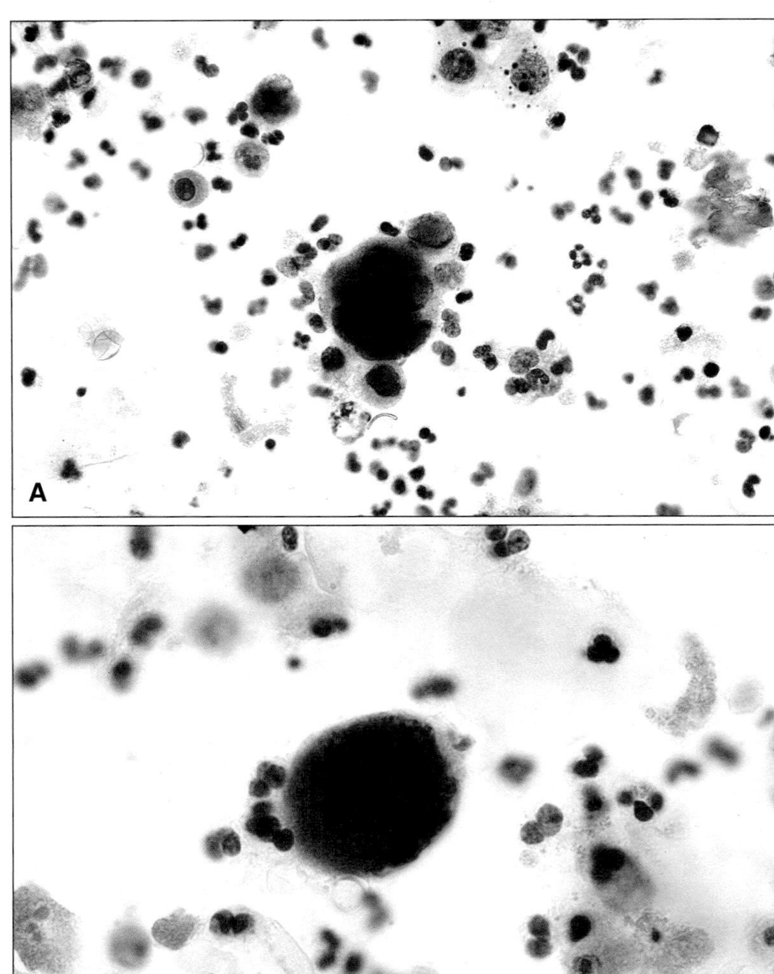

Fig. 9.23 (A,B) Hemorrhagic herpes simplex virus cystitis can occur with genital herpetic lesions, occasionally even in immunocompetent hosts. This figure is from a renal transplant patient. Cell enlargement, multinucleation, nuclear molding, and ground-glass nuclei are present in a background of acute inflammation. Cowdry A eosinophilic irregular nuclear inclusions may be present.

Herpes simplex virus (Fig. 9.23)

Cytomegalovirus CMV hemorrhagic cystitis can occur on a background of chemotherapy for bone marrow transplantation, AIDS, or other immunosuppression. Urine culture is insensitive for the diagnosis of CMV in these patients. Infected renal tubular cells or stromal cells show enlargement and a single eosinophilic nuclear inclusion surrounded by a clear halo. Occasionally, intracytoplasmic inclusions are also seen. Scattered lymphocytes and red blood cells are common in the background.

BK polyomavirus Most persons acquire polyomavirus early in life, but clinically evident disease occurs only with immunosuppression and presents with hematuria and/or cystitis. Urine cytology is inexpensive, rapid, and accurate for detecting polyomavirus, and cytopathic effect may persist for several months after symptoms subside.[10] Polyomavirus also causes tubulointerstitial disease in renal allograft recipients. Preliminary data suggest that urine cytology is sensitive for this diagnosis.[11] (Figs 9.24 & 9.25)

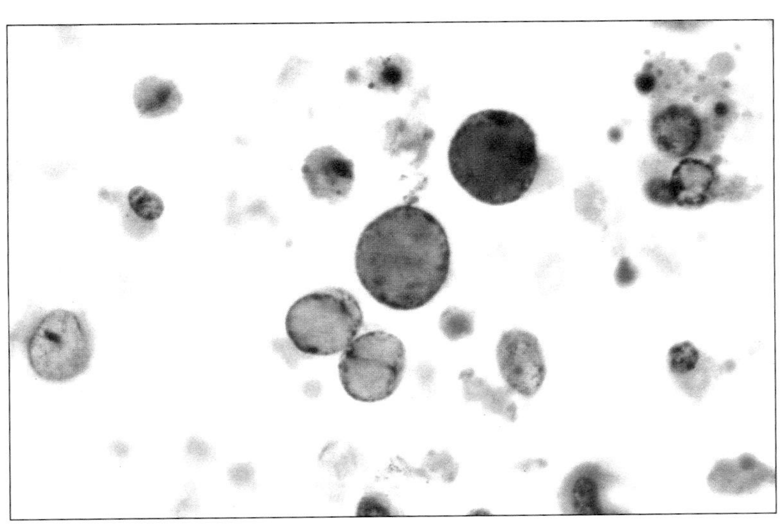

Fig. 9.24 Polyomavirus infection. Urine cytology shows many cells with classical large, homogeneous, and basophilic intranuclear inclusions. Degenerated intranuclear inclusion-bearing cells with coarse chromatin can be seen, particularly in adults. The nuclei of polyomavirus-infected cells may resemble those of urothelial carcinoma in situ when the inclusion is degenerated and coarse.

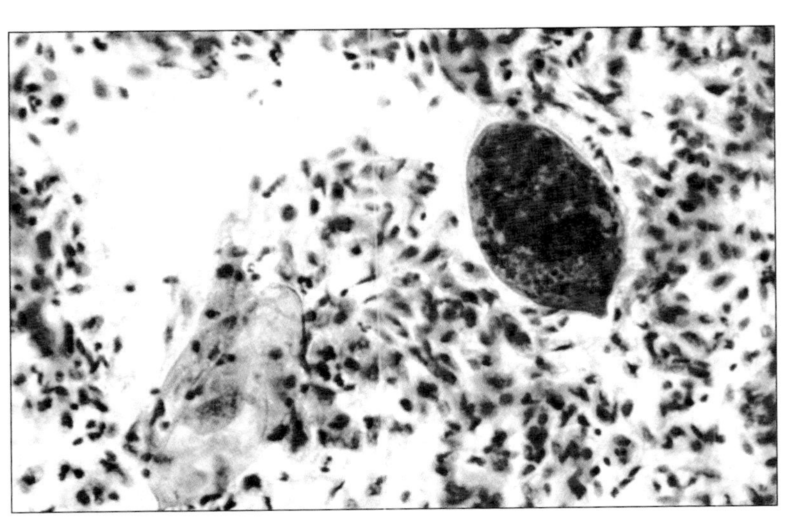

Fig. 9.26 Urinary schistosomiasis causes eosinophiluria, proteinuria, and hematuria. *Schistosoma haematobium* eggs (shown here) are oval, 100–150 μm, and have a small, terminal spine. *Schistosoma mansoni* eggs, rarely found in the urine, have a lateral spine. Viable or calcified eggs, and empty shells can be identified in the smears. Urothelial cells show squamous metaplasia with varying degrees of keratinization and nuclear atypia.

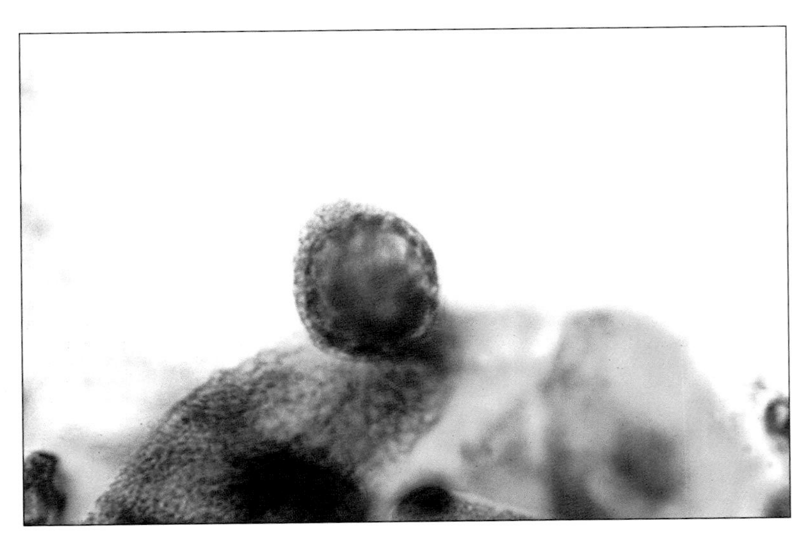

Fig. 9.25 Polyomavirus infection. Distinction from the cytopathic effect of herpes infection is based on the nuclear characteristics and multinucleation. Adenovirus has a large homogeneous intranuclear basophilic inclusion resembling that of polyomavirus. The coexistence of multiple small and irregular intranuclear inclusions and nuclear clearing in the same urine sample favors the diagnosis of adenovirus.

Human papillomavirus

Bladder condyloma is more common in women. It often results from anogenital condylomas extending into the urethra and bladder. Human papillomavirus (HPV) types 6 and 11 have been found in bladder condylomas. The pathogenetic role of HPV infection in the development of urothelial carcinoma is controversial, although it is conceivable that the various types of HPV can act as oncogenic agents, particularly in immunosuppressed patients. Koilocytes, characterized by a wrinkled and hyperchromatic nucleus, a perinuclear cavity with thick outlines, and dense cytoplasm, may be detected in urine samples. As in urethral condylomas, the yield of urine cytology is low in comparison with brush cytology. Before a urine cytology diagnosis of bladder condyloma is made, condyloma of the urethra and external genitalia should be excluded.

Parasitic infections

Schistosomiasis *Schistosoma haematobium*, endemic in Africa and Mediterranean Asia, inhabits the pelvic veins and sheds its eggs into the urinary bladder, causing hematuria or chronic cystitis. Urinary egg excretion has diurnal periodicity, with more pronounced egg shedding at midday. Bladder biopsy shows urothelial squamous and intestinal metaplasia and mural granulomas, fibrosis, and calcified eggs. The association between bladder schistosomiasis and urothelial squamous cell carcinoma is well documented. Occasionally, *Schistosoma mansoni* eggs, typically shed in the stool, may be found in the urine. (Fig. 9.26)

Trichomoniasis Trichomoniasis of the urinary tract is rare, presents as urethritis and/or cystitis, and is often associated with genital trichomoniasis. Cytologic findings in urine are similar to those of cervicovaginal trichomoniasis. (Fig. 9.27)

NONINFECTIOUS INFLAMMATORY CONDITIONS

MALAKOPLAKIA

Malakoplakia is an uncommon granulomatous disease that affects primarily the urinary tract, frequently the urinary

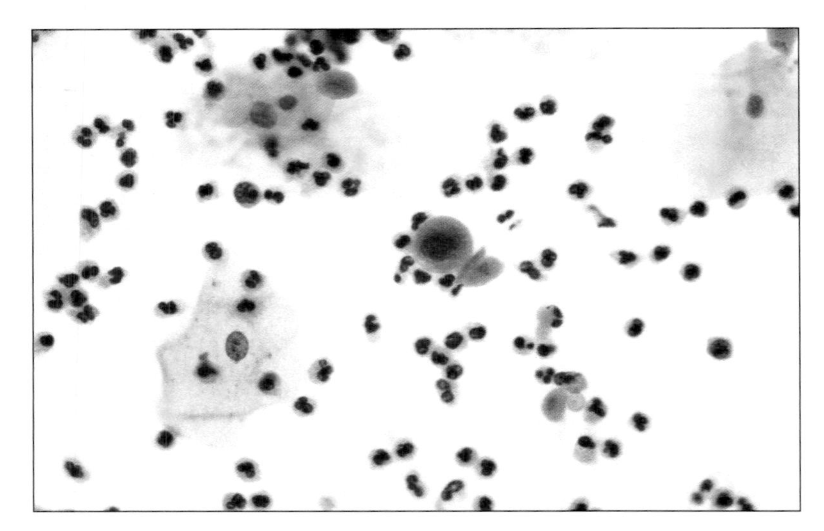

Fig. 9.27 Trichomoniasis. Smears show marked acute inflammation with aggregates of neutrophils, squamous metaplasia, few urothelial cells, and red blood cells. The organism is a light-gray, 15–50-μm pear-shaped protozoon with a small, dark, slit-like, eccentric nucleus and cytoplasmic eosinophilic granules. The flagellum is not obvious. Trichomonads may resemble superficial urothelial cells or renal tubular cells.

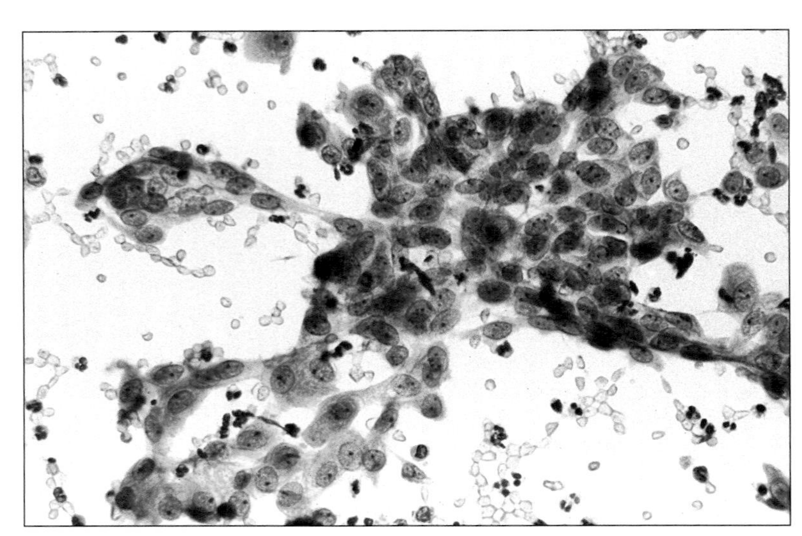

Fig. 9.29 Malakoplakia. The smear background is granular, with necrotic debris and a few plasma cells. Sheets of reactive, reparative urothelial cells and acute inflammation are present.

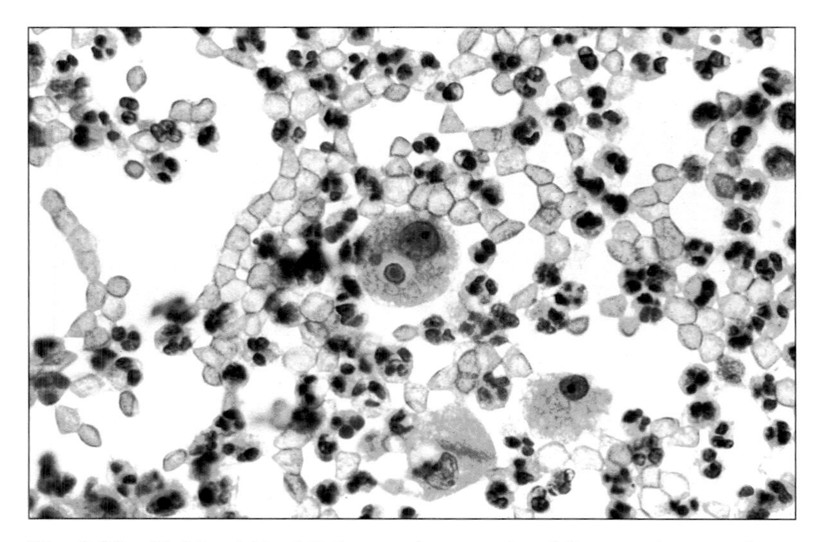

Fig. 9.28 Malakoplakia. Histiocytes have eosinophilic granular cytoplasm with one or more basophilic, 5–10-μm bodies with concentric laminations (Michaelis–Gutmann bodies). The differential diagnosis includes xanthogranulomatous pyelonephritis.

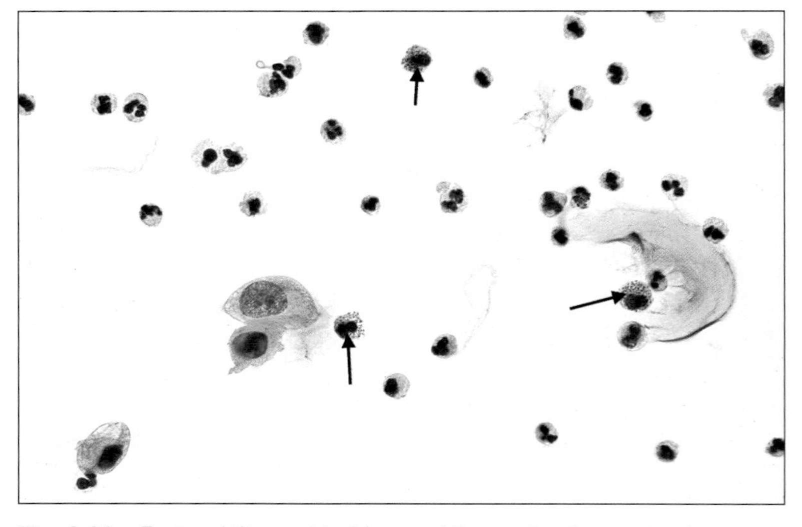

Fig. 9.30 Eosinophilic cystitis. Neutrophils may be the predominant inflammatory cell population, with only small numbers of eosinophils (arrows). Thus, it is not possible to diagnose eosinophilic cystitis by urine cytology alone.

bladder and ureters, of middle-aged women. Bladder malakoplakia manifests as urinary tract infection and gross hematuria; urine culture frequently isolates *E. coli*. Histologically, submucosal aggregates of large histiocytes (von Hansemann cells) contain cytoplasmic Michaelis–Gutmann bodies that may represent mineralized fragments of bacteria. (Figs 9.28 & 9.29)

EOSINOPHILIC CYSTITIS

Eosinophilic cystitis[12] is rare and may be associated with allergic diseases, hypereosinophilic syndrome, and bladder trauma, including bladder surgery. Pyuria and microhematuria are commonly present. Histologically, there is edema of the lamina propria with mixed inflammation and eosinophils. (Fig. 9.30)

FOLLICULAR CYSTITIS

Lymphoid follicles in the lamina propria of the bladder, resembling Peyer's patches in the intestine, characterize follicular cystitis. It occurs with urinary tract infection, particularly in prepubertal girls and in patients with bladder cancer. (Fig. 9.31)

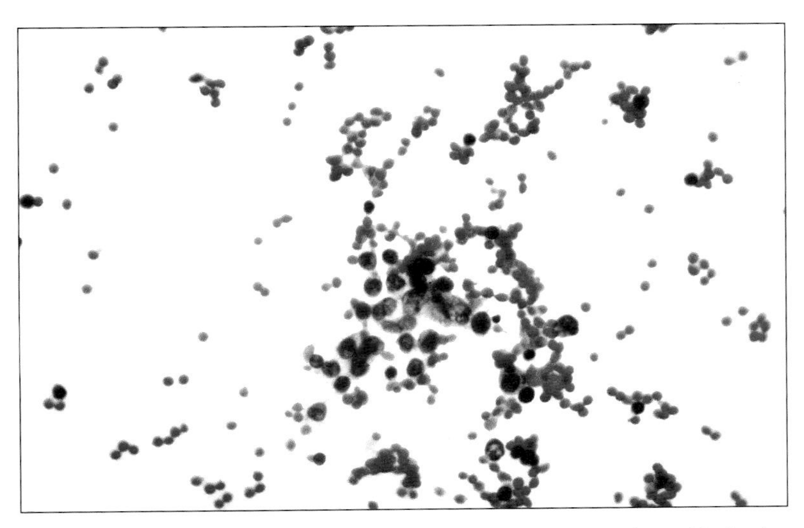

Fig. 9.31 A polymorphous population of lymphocytes and tingible-body macrophages in the urine smear is characteristic of follicular cystitis. This appearance is similar to that in follicular cervicitis, in which the lesion is associated with *Chlamydia* infection. No such connection is known in the bladder.

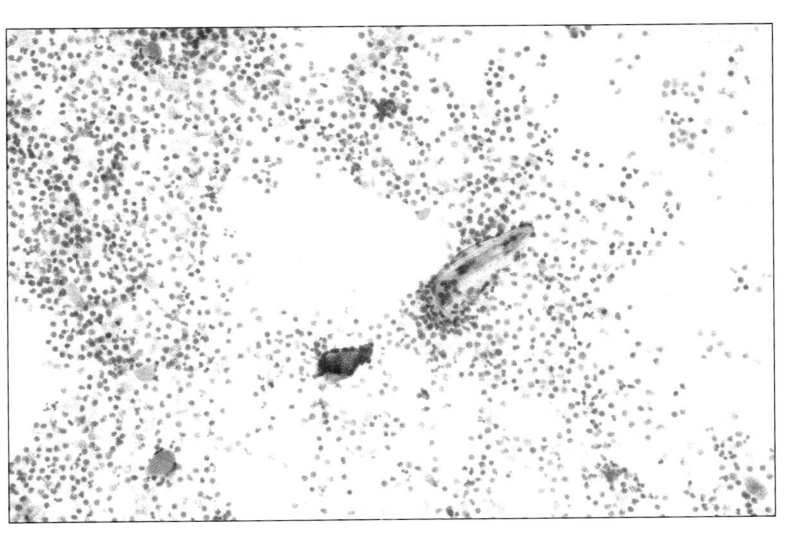

Fig. 9.32 Vegetable cells, fibers, amorphous debris, and numerous bacilli identify fecal matter in urine. A few reactive urothelial cells may be present.

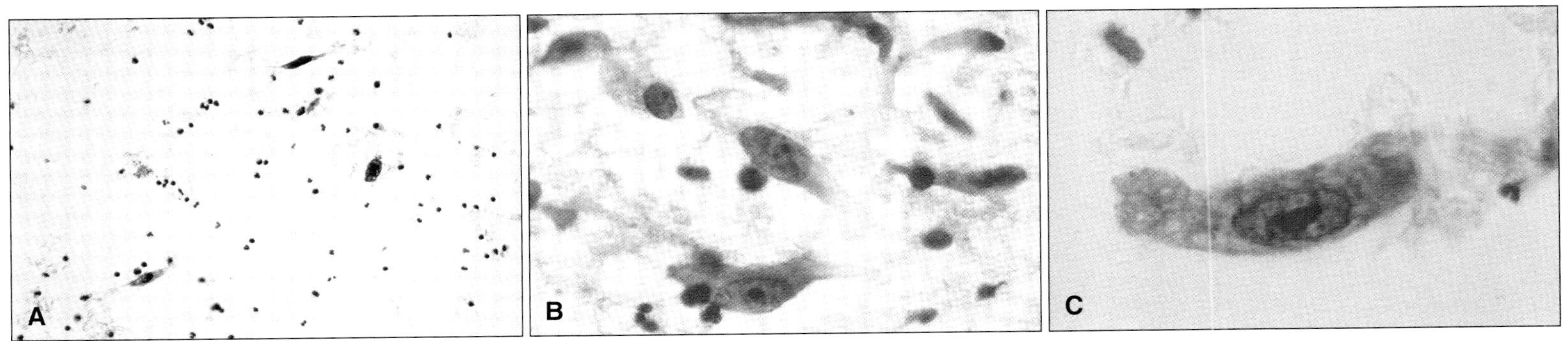

Fig. 9.33 (A–C) Inflammatory pseudotumor. Atypical spindle cells, resembling those of sarcoma, may be present in urine samples. The spindle cells lack mitosis and nuclear anaplasia, and no diathesis is seen. Eosinophilic cytoplasm may be seen in some spindle cells. Myofibroblasts may be positive for keratin and epithelial membrane antigen, erroneously suggesting carcinosarcoma. (Reproduced with permission from Acta Cytol 1999;43:259.)

VESICOENTERIC FISTULA

Vesical fistulas are more common in men and occur as complications of diverticulitis, colon cancer, inflammatory bowel disease, radiation, surgery, or infection. Fecaluria and pneumaturia are uncommon. (Fig. 9.32)

INFLAMMATORY PSEUDOTUMOR

Inflammatory pseudotumor[13] (inflammatory myofibroblastic tumor) is a rare lesion, unrelated to bladder trauma. It occurs typically in young adult women, who commonly have gross hematuria. It presents as a polypoid intravesical mass ranging from 1.5 cm to 13 cm. Microscopically, the lesions show spindle myofibroblasts, myxoid stroma, and variable numbers of lymphocytes, plasma cells, and red blood cells. (Fig. 9.33)

CYSTITIS GLANDULARIS AND CYSTITIS CYSTICA

Cystitis glandularis and cystitis cystica are present in over 60% of normal bladders, commonly in the trigone. The frequency increases with age. Similar lesions occur in the ureter and renal pelvis. In cystitis glandularis, microsocopic glands with columnar or cuboidal epithelium including variable numbers of goblet cells are located in the lamina propria. In cystitis cystica, cystoscopically visible cysts lined with urothelial cells contain proteinaceous fluid with a few inflammatory cells.[14] (Fig. 9.34)

SQUAMOUS METAPLASIA

Nonkeratinized squamous cells without atypia are common in urine smears obtained from women of childbearing age

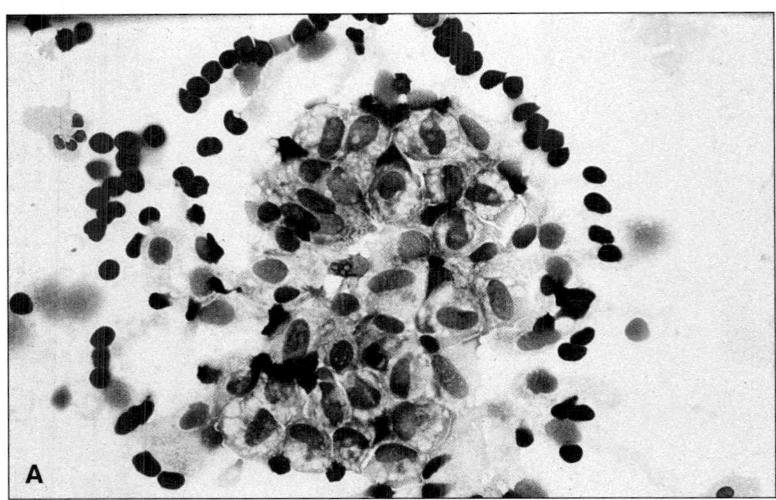

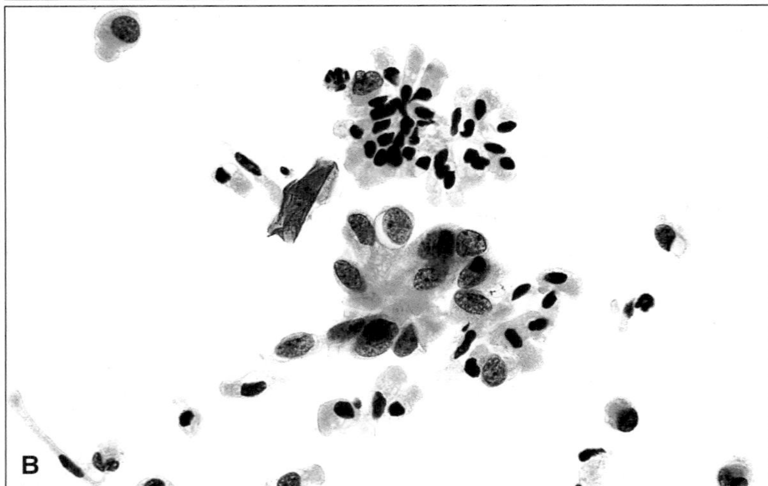

Fig. 9.34 (A,B) Cystitis glandularis. Smears have low cellularity, and cohesive groups of columnar cells with bland nuclei. Admixed goblet cells are variably present. The smear background is clean. Benign adenomatous polyps of the prostatic urethra may show similar cytologic characteristics.[15] Low-grade bladder adenocarcinoma of intestinal type is distinguished by its necrotic background, high cellularity, and nuclear anaplasia.

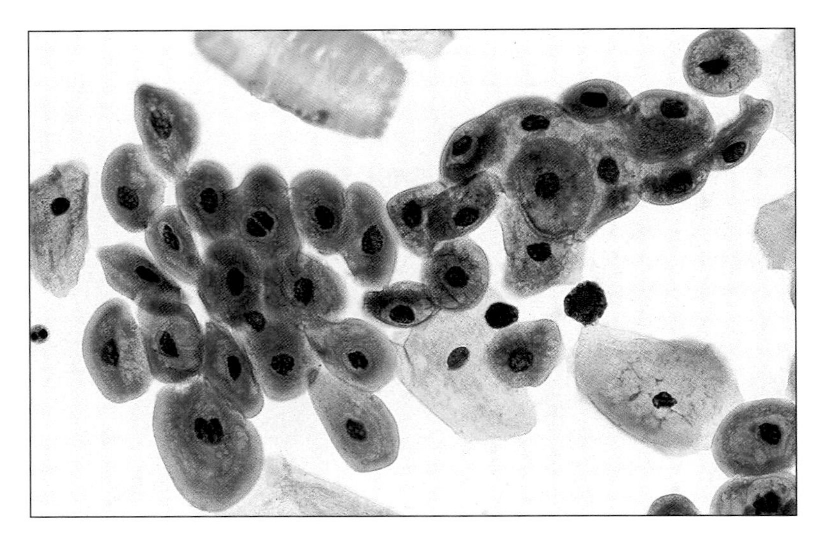

Fig. 9.35 In this case of nonkeratinizing squamous metaplasia, umbrella cells retain their general shape. However, the cells tend to mold and aggregate. This change carries no pre-neoplastic implications.

and in patients receiving hormonal therapy for prostatic adenocarcinoma, and their presence does not connote neoplasia. Keratinizing squamous metaplasia or leukoplakia occurs more often in the bladder than in the renal pelvis, ureter, and urethra, and is associated with inflammation, chronic infection, or squamous carcinoma. Squamous metaplastic cells with varying degrees of keratinization and atypia have been found in patients with chronic indwelling urinary catheters and schistosomiasis, who have elevated risk for squamous cell carcinoma. (Fig. 9.35)

NEPHROGENIC ADENOMA

Nephrogenic adenoma (nephrogenic metaplasia) is associated with urothelial chronic inflammation or trauma. The bladder is the most common site, but the lesion has been described in the urethra, ureters, and renal pelvis.[14] It is most common in adult males, and may accompany urothelial carcinoma treated with intravesical BCG or chemotherapy, or renal transplantation.[16] It may cause hematuria or urinary frequency, or it may be asymptomatic and diagnosed incidentally.

Nephrogenic adenomas are papillary or polypoid, usually <1 cm, and mimic urothelial carcinoma cystoscopically. Microscopically, various architectural patterns are seen, but cuboidal to low-columnar hobnail cells with rare mitotic figures and fine chromatin are characteristic.[14] The differential diagnosis includes clear cell adenocarcinoma, prostate adenocarcinoma, renal cell carcinoma, and low-grade papillary urothelial carcinoma. (Fig. 9.36)

BCG EFFECT

Adjuvant intravesical immunotherapy with BCG is effective treatment for noninvasive bladder cancer, presumably stimulating immune destruction of tumor cells. BCG produces an intense cystitis with dysuria, frequency, and hematuria. Microscopic changes include urothelial degeneration and denudation, eosinophilic cystitis, and noncaseating granulomatous inflammation. Voided urine cytologic examination has been used for monitoring response to therapy and in follow-up.[17] (Figs 9.37 & 9.38)

INTRAVESICAL CHEMOTHERAPY

Intravesical chemotherapy with mitomycin C, thiotepa, or doxorubicin does not produce the marked cellular atypia seen after cyclophosphamide therapy. Urothelial cell changes are more evident in the non-neoplastic superficial cell layer than in the basal–intermediate cell layer and tend to subside after removal of the drug. These forms of therapy

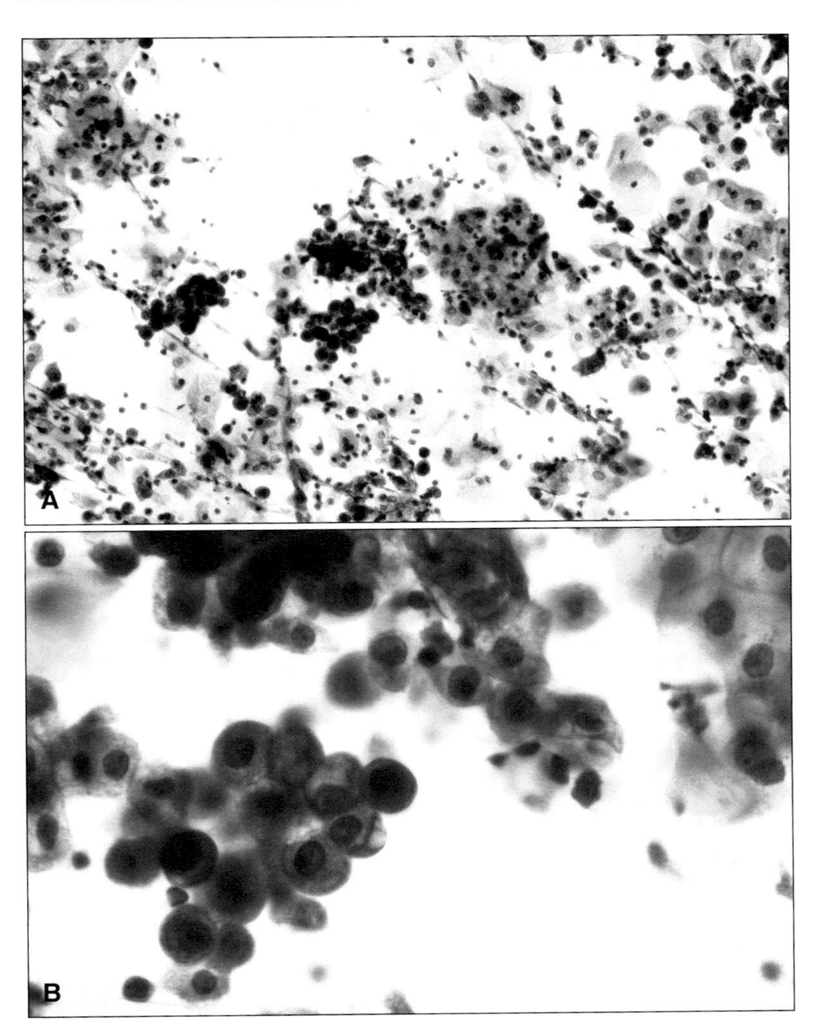

Fig. 9.36 (A,B) Nephrogenic adenoma. Cuboidal cells with fine cytoplasmic vacuolization occur in variously cohesive aggregates. Columnar cells and glands may be seen. The nucleus is round to oval and central, with fine chromatin. Mild nuclear atypia may be present. Background shows acute inflammation. The most common initial cytologic diagnosis is negative or atypical.

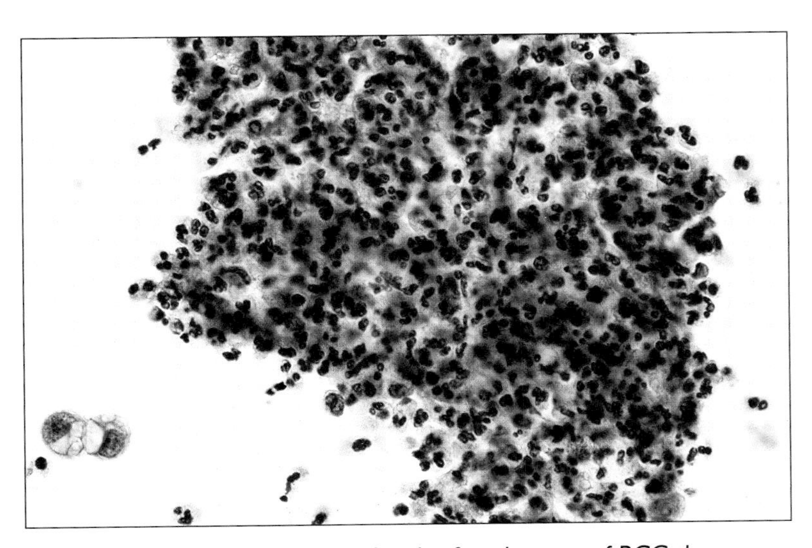

Fig. 9.37 Leukocyturia is seen shortly after the start of BCG therapy, and seems to correlate with the efficacy of therapy.[18] Urothelial cells may show enlarged, hyperchromatic nuclei with prominent nucleoli, anisonucleosis, vacuolated cytoplasm, and a high nuclear:cytoplasmic ratio.[19,20] Cytologic changes persist in urine specimens for months after termination of BCG therapy.

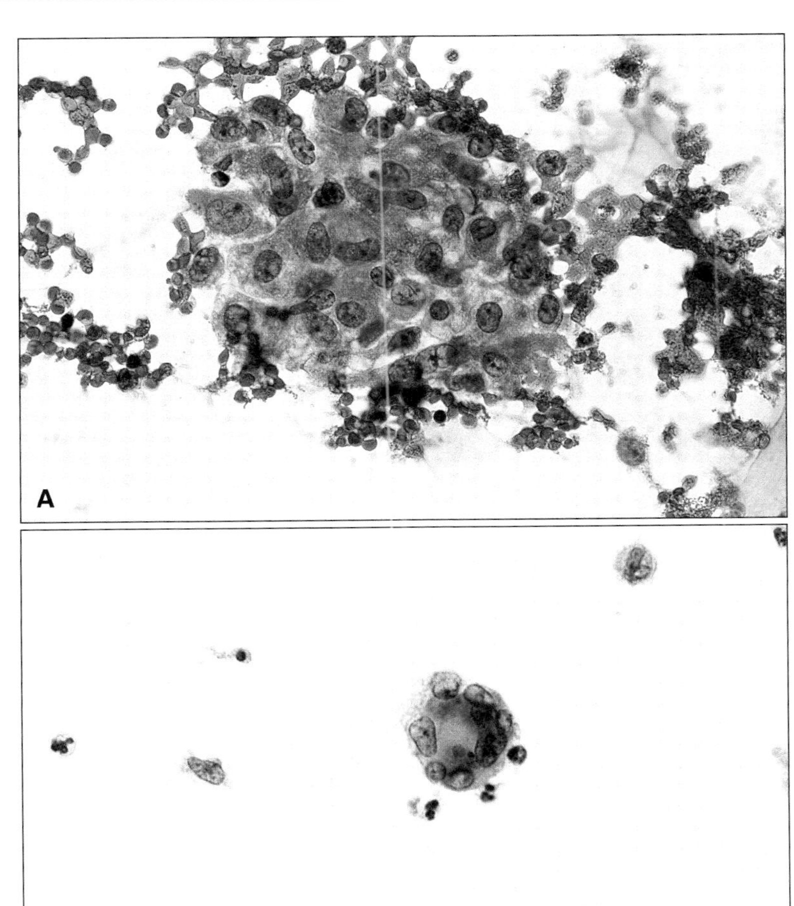

Fig. 9.38 (A,B) BCG effect. Granulomas are present in between 1.3% and 76% of urine cytology specimens. In urine specimens obtained by instrumentation, granulomas are rare. The cytologic characteristics are indistinguishable from those seen in tuberculous cystitis.

do not alter the cytomorphology of low- or high-grade carcinoma. (Fig. 9.39)

UROLITHIASIS

Urolithiasis is commonly diagnosed in men in the third to fifth decade of life. Patients with a neurogenic bladder are predisposed to urolithiasis. Calculi may form anywhere in the urinary tract, but are most frequent in the urinary bladder and renal pelvis. They may be clinically silent or cause hematuria, or abdominal or lumbar pain.

Calcium oxalate stones are associated with hypercalcemia, intestinal disease or surgery, chronic renal failure, and diet. Triple phosphate calculi are more frequent in women, usually in association with bacterial and xanthogranulomatous pyelonephritis. Uric acid stones are associated with gout, dehydration, and malignancy with rapid cell turnover. Rarely, calculi may form as a result of foreign bodies, infections, or other unknown factors.

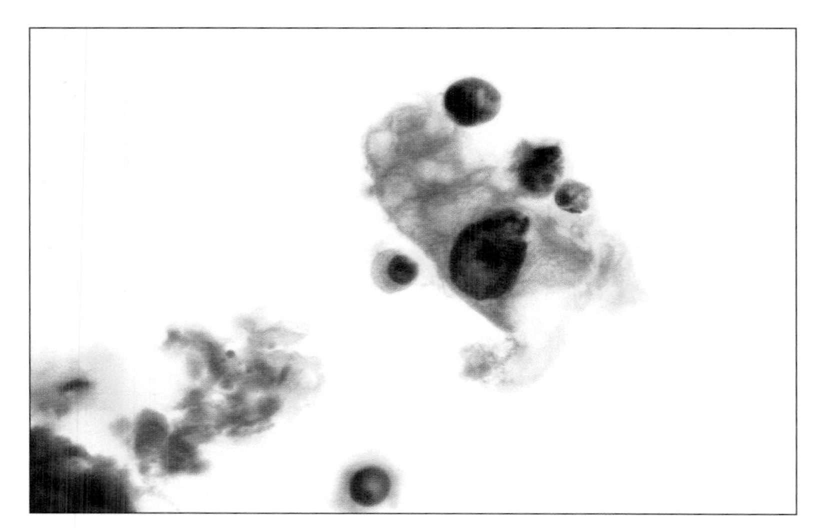

Fig. 9.39 Urine specimens from patients receiving intravesical chemotherapy are of high cellularity and contain acute inflammatory cells. As shown here, mitomycin C therapy produces nuclear and cytoplasmic enlargement, nucleoli, and anisokaryosis. Multinucleated cells may be present. Cytologic changes are first observed 4 months after therapy begins, and persist for at least 18 months after completion. Thiotepa causes similar but less pronounced changes. Cytologic criteria of malignancy, such as coarse chromatin and an elevated nuclear:cytoplasmic ratio, are uncommon in relapse-free mitomycin C-treated patients.

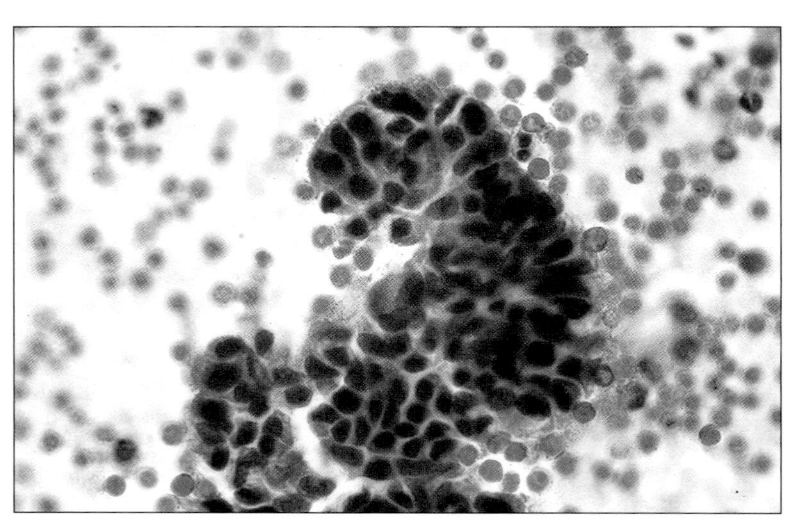

Fig. 9.40 Most cases of urolithiasis show clusters of umbrella cells with smooth, round borders, a normal to slightly increased nuclear:cytoplasmic ratio, abundant vacuolated cytoplasm, a round nucleus with uniform contours and powdery chromatin, and round, conspicuous nucleoli. Basal and intermediate cell clusters are usually round with smooth borders, but frayed edges and cells with irregular nuclear contours and hyperchromasia are present occasionally. All urothelial cell changes revert to normal once the calculi are removed.

Urinary crystals and cytologic changes may not be detected in all patients with urolithiasis, and crystals may be identified in the absence of calculi.

Low-grade urothelial carcinoma and instrumentation effect have cytomorphology almost identical to that of urolithiasis. Atypical squamous metaplastic cells on a background of lysed blood and acute inflammation can mimic invasive carcinoma. However, the severe nuclear anaplasia seen in high-grade urothelial carcinoma is absent in urolithiasis. Lysed blood, extensive cellular degeneration, and variable numbers of squamous metaplastic and multinucleated giant cells may be present, particularly in patients with staghorn stones in the renal pelvis and in those with large bladder stones. Bladder calculi usually induce less shedding and often little cytologic abnormality. These features are indistinguishable from those of low-grade urothelial carcinoma (transitional cell carcinoma [TCC] grades 1 and 2). (Fig. 9.40)

Table 9.1 Histologic grading and classification of urothelial neoplasms

WHO 1973	*WHO/ISUP 1998*	*WHO 1999*	*Cheng 2000*	*Ancona 2001*
		Papillary		
Papilloma	Papilloma	Papilloma	Papilloma	Papilloma
Grade 1	PUNLMP	Grade 1	Grade 1	Grade 1
Grade 2	Low grade	Grade 2	Grade 2	Grade 2
Grade 3	High grade	Grade 3	Grade 3	Grade 3
		Flat		
	Reactive atypia		Reactive atypia	Reactive atypia
	Atypia of unknown significance			Metaplasia
	Dysplasia		Dysplasia	Dysplasia
	CIS/severe dysplasia		CIS/severe dysplasia	CIS

WHO, World Health Organization; ISUP, International Society of Urological Pathology; PUNLMP, papillary urothelial neoplasm of low malignant potential; CIS, carcinoma in situ.
Modified from Bardales.[21]

URINARY TRACT NEOPLASIA

Urothelial neoplasms comprise 80–90% of urinary tract neoplasms. Squamous cell carcinomas account for <5%; mixed carcinomas, ~5%; adenocarcinomas, <2%; and mesenchymal and miscellaneous tumors, ~5%.

Urothelial neoplasms are of two types, papillary and flat. Papillary neoplasms are usually of low grade. Flat carcinoma in situ (CIS) is more aggressive than papillary carcinoma and frequently accompanies invasive urothelial carcinoma.

Urine cytology is recommended for monitoring patients with established urothelial neoplasia and as a screening tool for patients at risk for urothelial carcinoma. Grading systems for urothelial carcinoma are reviewed in Table 9.1.

Table 9.2 Suggested cytology report format for diagnosis of urinary tract neoplasms

Cytologic category	*Corresponding cytologic diagnosis**
'Negative for malignancy'	Normal urothelial cells Reactive urothelial cells
'Atypical urothelial cells'†	Descriptive diagnosis
'Positive for malignant cells'	Low-grade papillary urothelial carcinoma High-grade papillary urothelial carcinoma Carcinoma in situ Invasive urothelial carcinoma Adenocarcinoma (if deemed; see text) Squamous carcinoma (if deemed; see text) Small cell carcinoma Other malignancies

*Description of additional cellular and noncellular elements, i.e. inflammation, blood, crystals, casts, etc., should be included.
†This category includes the following histologic diagnoses: papillary urothelial neoplasm of low malignant potential (grade I TCC, WHO 1973), some low-grade papillary urothelial carcinomas (grade 2 TCC, WHO 1973), and dysplastic flat urothelial lesions (WHO/ISUP 1998; Ancona 2001).
Modified from Bardales.[21]

Table 9.3 Corresponding histologic and cytologic diagnoses of urothelial neoplasms

Histology (various terminologies)	*Cytology*
Papillary neoplasms	
Papilloma	Normal urothelial cells
PUNLMP*	Reactive urothelial cells Atypical urothelial cells
Grade 1 TCC†	Reactive urothelial cells Atypical urothelial cells
Grade 2 TCC†	Low-grade urothelial carcinoma Atypical urothelial cells
Low-grade urothelial carcinoma*	Low-grade urothelial carcinoma Atypical urothelial cells
Grade 3 TCC†	High-grade urothelial carcinoma
High-grade urothelial carcinoma*	High-grade urothelial carcinoma
Flat lesions	
Reactive atypia*	Reactive urothelial cells
Urothelial hyperplasia‡	Normal/reactive urothelial cells
Dysplasia	Atypical urothelial cells
Carcinoma in situ	Carcinoma in situ

PUNLMP, papillary urothelial neoplasm of low malignant potential; TCC, transitional cell carcinoma.
*World Health Organization/International Society of Urological Pathology (WHO/ISUP) 1998.
†WHO 1973 and 1999.
‡Ancona 2001.
Modified from Bardales.[21]

CYTOLOGIC CLASSIFICATION OF UROTHELIAL NEOPLASIA

The diagnostic accuracy of urine cytology for low-grade papillary neoplasms (TCC grades 1 and 2) is low and variable. However, for high-grade tumors, including invasive carcinoma and CIS, urine cytology is highly accurate. A tentative classification of urine cytology diagnoses of neoplasms of the urinary tract and their histologic counterparts are in Tables 9.2 and 9.3.

Nuclear characteristics distinguish between a reactive atypia and high-grade urothelial carcinoma. The high cellularity and cell clusters so characteristic of instrumented urine specimens make the diagnosis of low-grade urothelial neoplasms (grades 1 and 2) difficult. Sometimes, washings or brushings allow the diagnosis of grade 2 carcinomas, particularly those with markedly discohesive cells and recognizable nuclear abnormalities. Because low-grade urothelial neoplasms may display an overlying umbrella cell layer, the presence of umbrella cells in the cell clusters of brushings or washings lacks diagnostic significance.

The abrasive effect of lithiasis on the urothelium induces exfoliation of urothelial cell clusters that are indistinguishable from the cell clusters seen in washings and brushings of low-grade urothelial neoplasms. Therefore, the distinction between instrumentation effect, urolithiasis, and low-grade urothelial neoplasms is always difficult, and often impossible.

PAPILLARY UROTHELIAL NEOPLASIA

Urothelial papilloma

Cytology: 'Negative for malignancy. Normal urothelial cells'

Urothelial papilloma is composed of a delicate fibrovascular core surrounded by architecturally and cytologically normal urothelium. Urothelial papilloma represents less than 3% of papillary urothelial neoplasms. Patients with urothelial papilloma have little risk of developing urothelial carcinoma.[22]

The diagnosis of urothelial papilloma is made strictly histologically. Urine cytology specimens show an increased number of exfoliated cells, rare cells with minimal atypia, and a small number of red blood cells.

Urothelial atypia

The diagnosis of 'atypia' implies cellular changes that fall short of those seen in malignancy, but beyond those of reactive processes. The term is highly subjective. Ideally, cases should correspond to almost all papillary urothelial neoplasms of low malignant potential (PUNLMPs, grade 1 TCC), some low-grade papillary urothelial carcinomas (grade 2 TCC), and dysplastic flat lesions. Therefore, the cytologic diagnosis of atypia has clinical implications and should trigger the investigation of a significant urothelial lesion. (Figs 9.41 & 9.42)

Papillary urothelial neoplasm of low malignant potential (grade I TCC)

Cytology: 'Reactive urothelial cells' or 'Atypical urothelial cells'

PUNLMP or grade 1 TCC is defined as a 'papillary urothelial lesion with more than seven layers of orderly arranged cells within papillae with minimal architectural abnormalities and mild nuclear atypia'.[24] Patients are at risk of local recurrence (30%), progression (3%), and death from bladder cancer (3–4%) after 10 years.[25] Urine cytologic examination has low sensitivity for this neoplasm because of the similarity of the cells to normal or reactive urothelial cells.

Cytologic features of PUNLMP are summarized in Table 9.4, but are nonspecific. Features favoring reactive process include vacuolated cytoplasm, smooth nuclear borders, lack of anisonucleosis, and a prominent round nucleolus in a background of inflammation, crystals, and/or red blood cells.

The value of papillary clusters as a diagnostic criterion for PUNLMP is controversial. Cell clusters are common in urine of patients with benign conditions such as urolithiasis.[26] The presence of a fibrovascular core is the only diagnostic feature of papillary urothelial carcinoma, best seen in cell block preparations.

A densely staining cytoplasmic collar of instrumentation effect might be helpful to distinguish reactive from neoplastic clusters, but its accuracy remains untested.[27] (Figs 9.43 & 9.44)

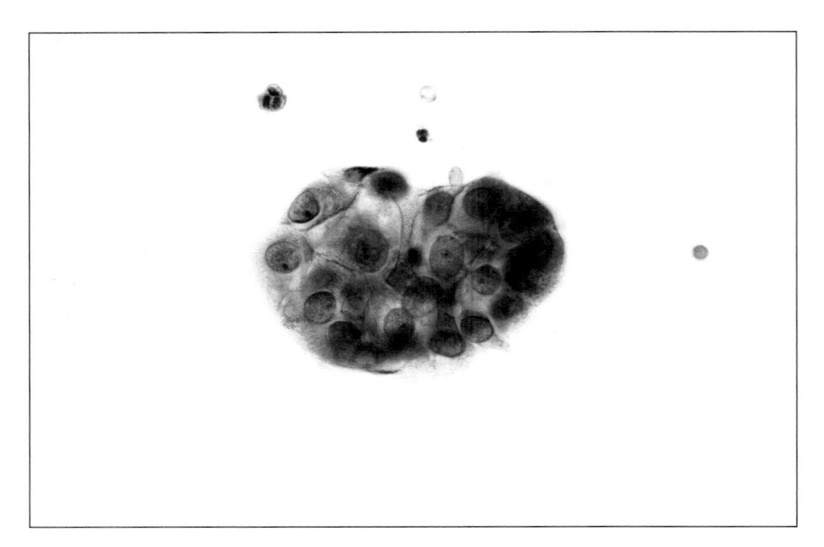

Fig. 9.41 'Atypia' encompasses combinations of some possibly reactive features (cytoplasmic vacuolation, prominent round nucleoli) and others concerning for low-grade neoplasia (cell clusters in instrumented urine, cells with a high nuclear:cytoplasmic ratio and round nucleus).[23] This figure shows minimal, nondiagnostic cytologic changes in a patient with grade I papillary urothelial carcinoma.

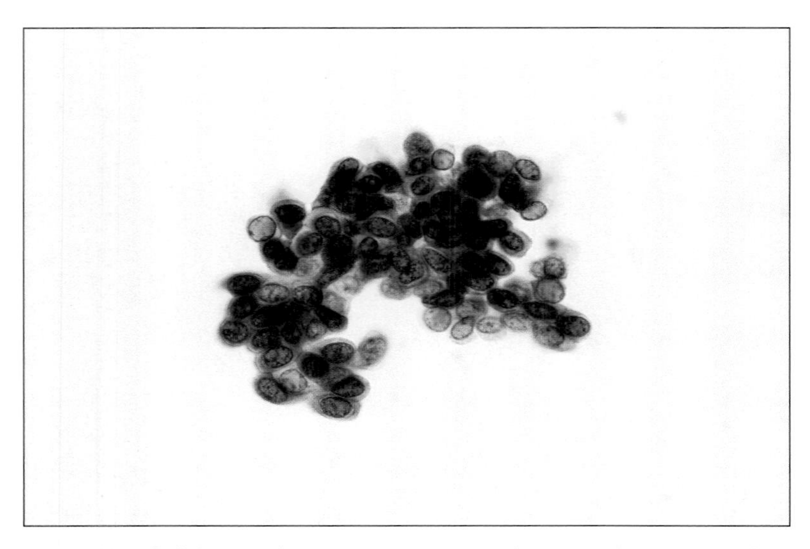

Fig. 9.42 Cellular overlapping, some anisonucleosis, and an increased nuclear:cytoplasmic ratio are 'atypical' features. This figure shows another case of grade I papillary urothelial carcinoma, originally interpreted as reactive.

Low-grade papillary urothelial carcinoma (grade 2 TCC)

Cytology: 'Positive for malignancy. Low-grade papillary urothelial carcinoma'

Most of these tumors yield abnormal cells in urine and are thus diagnosable by cytology, although inconspicuous clusters of malignant cells may be missed on low-power examination. In practice, the cytologic diagnosis ranges from

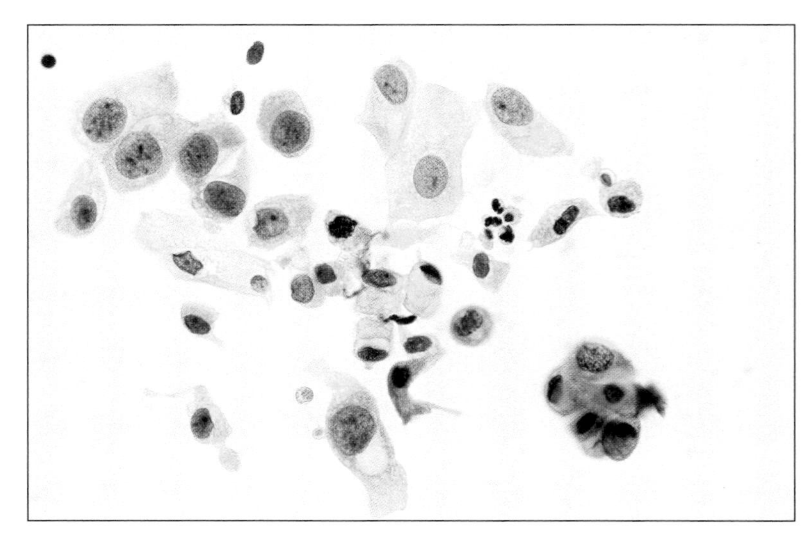

Fig. 9.43 Homogeneous cytoplasm, irregular nuclear membrane, and an increased nuclear:cytoplasmic ratio are the most useful features separating low-grade urothelial carcinoma from benign processes. Secondary criteria include nuclear hyperchromasia and eccentrically placed nuclei. In this example of grade I transitional cell carcinoma, cytologic abnormalities are minimal; this case would be difficult to diagnose definitively as carcinoma.

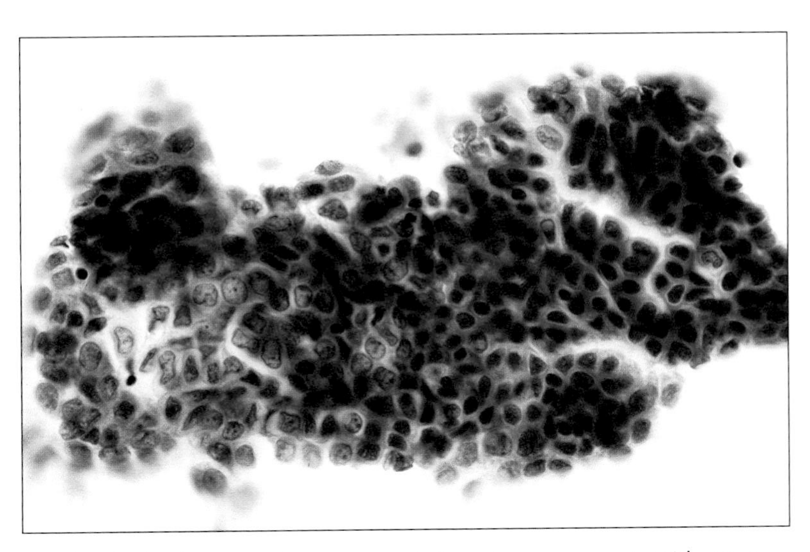

Fig. 9.44 In this example, a range of alterations is present, with some groups showing evident anisonucleosis and irregularities of nuclear contour. The diagnosis in this case was 'atypical urothelial cells, favor low-grade urothelial carcinoma'.

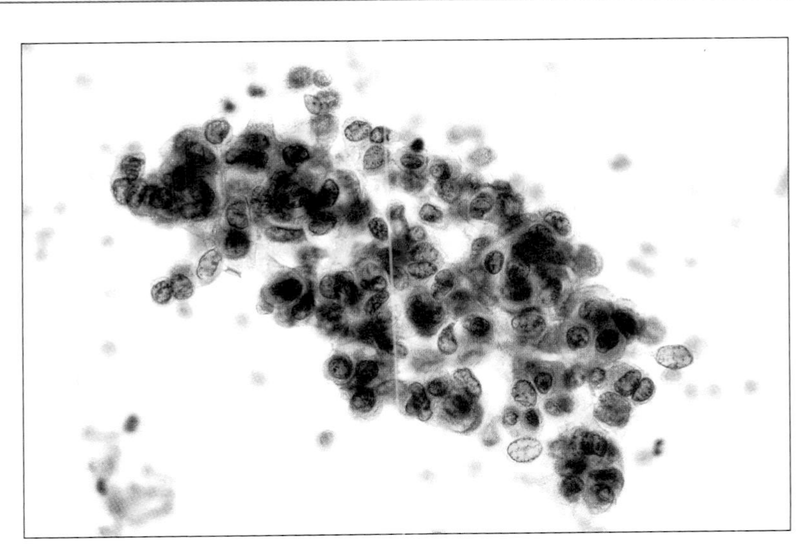

Fig. 9.45 Low-grade papillary urothelial carcinoma. Cellular changes are evident and include cellular disarray, anisonucleosis, irregular nuclear contours, an increased nuclear:cytoplasmic ratio, and thin cytoplasm.

Table 9.4 Cytology of papillary urothelial neoplasms

	Reactive	*PUNLMP**	*LG-PUC*†
Single cells	Rare	Rare	Variable
Cell arrangement	Papillary	Papillary	Papillary and loose
Cell size	Increased and uniform	Increased and uniform	Increased and variable
Cytoplasm	**Vacuolated**	**Usually homogeneous**	**Homogeneous**
NCR	**Preserved**	**Slightly increased**	**Increased**
Nuclear			
Position	**Central/eccentric**	**Eccentric**	**Eccentric**
Size variation	Absent/slight	Slight	Moderate
Shape	Oval	Oval/round	Round and variable
Shape variation	Absent (uniform)	Slight	Moderate
Contours	**Smooth**	**Smooth**	**Few notches**
Pleomorphism	Absent	Absent	Mild to moderate
Hyperchromasia	**Absent**	**Absent/mild**	**Mild/moderate**
Nucleolus	Large, round	Inconspicuous	Variable

NCR, nuclear:cytoplasmic ratio; PUNLMP, papillary urothelial neoplasm of low malignant potential; LG-PUC, low-grade papillary urothelial carcinoma.
*Includes grade 1 TCC (WHO 1973).
†Includes low-grade papillary urothelial carcinomas (WHO/ISUP 1998) or grade 2 TCC (WHO 1973).
Bold type indicates the most salient features.
Modified from Bardales.[21]

'atypia' in few cases to 'low-grade papillary urothelial carcinoma'. Cytologic features in instrumented urine specimens are summarized in Table 9.4.

Instrumentation, urolithiasis, and polypoid cystitis exfoliate atypical urothelial fragments with a high nuclear:cytoplasmic ratio. Smooth nuclear contours, uniform nuclei, and vacuolated cytoplasm favor a benign diagnosis. (Figs 9.45 & 9.46)

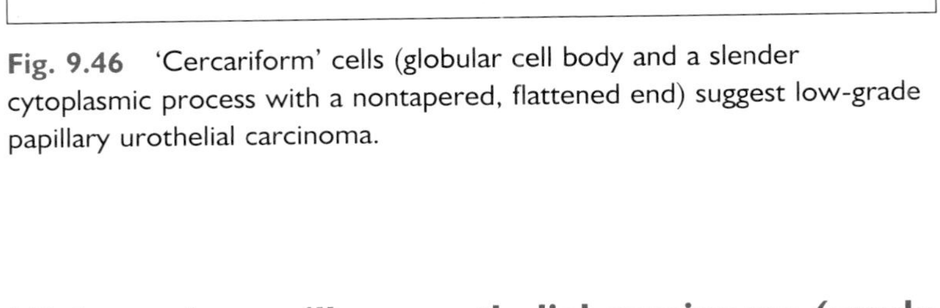

Fig. 9.46 'Cercariform' cells (globular cell body and a slender cytoplasmic process with a nontapered, flattened end) suggest low-grade papillary urothelial carcinoma.

High-grade papillary urothelial carcinoma (grade 3 TCC)

Cytology: 'Positive for malignancy. High-grade urothelial carcinoma'

High-grade papillary urothelial carcinoma shows marked cellular abnormalities, and urine cytology is accurate for screening and surveillance. Instrumented urine specimens usually exhibit high cellularity and numerous high-grade tumor cells, and are preferred for diagnosis; tumor cells may be absent in some voided urines. Cytologic features of high-grade papillary urothelial carcinoma are summarized in Table 9.5. (Figs 9.47–9.51)

Table 9.5 Cytology of high-grade papillary urothelial carcinoma and invasive urothelial carcinoma

	*HG-PUC**	*Invasive UC*
Single cells	Numerous	Numerous
Cell arrangement	**Tight and loose clusters**	**Loose clusters**
Cell size	Large, pleomorphic	Large, pleomorphic
Cytoplasm	Homogeneous/vacuolated	Homogeneous/vacuolated
NCR	Variable	Variable
Nuclear		
Enlargement	Marked	Marked
Size variation	Marked	Marked
Pleomorphism	Moderate/marked	Moderate/marked
Contours	Irregular, notches	Irregular, notches
Shape	Marked variation	Marked variation
Chromatin	Irregular, coarse	Irregular, coarse
Nucleolus	Variable/large, irregular	Variable/large, irregular
Necrosis	**Absent**	**Present**

NCR, nuclear:cytoplasmic ratio; HG-PUC, high-grade papillary urothelial carcinoma; UC, urothelial carcinoma.
*Includes grade 3 papillary urothelial carcinoma (WHO/ISUP 1998) or grade 3 TCC (WHO 1973).
Bold type indicates the most salient features.
Modified from Bardales.[21]

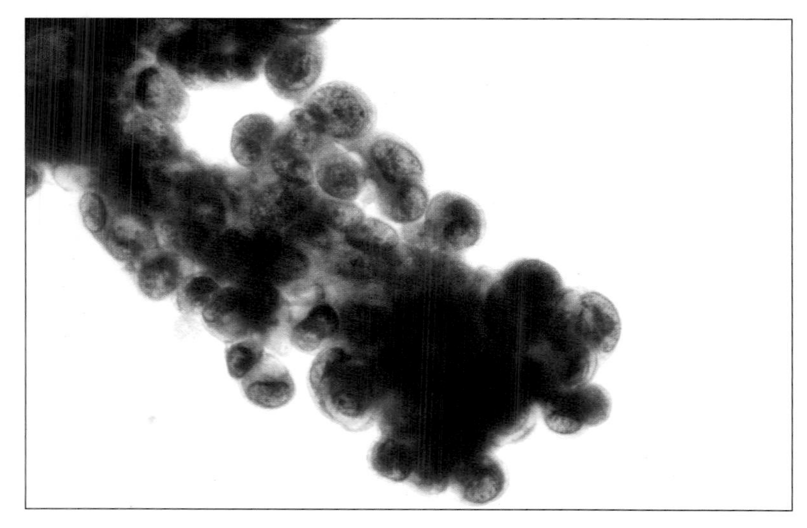

Fig. 9.47 A papillary cell cluster shows a high nuclear:cytoplasmic ratio and frankly anaplastic nuclei. High-grade papillary urothelial carcinoma yields large, pleomorphic cells, whereas the cells of flat carcinoma in situ (see Fig. 9.54) are relatively uniform.

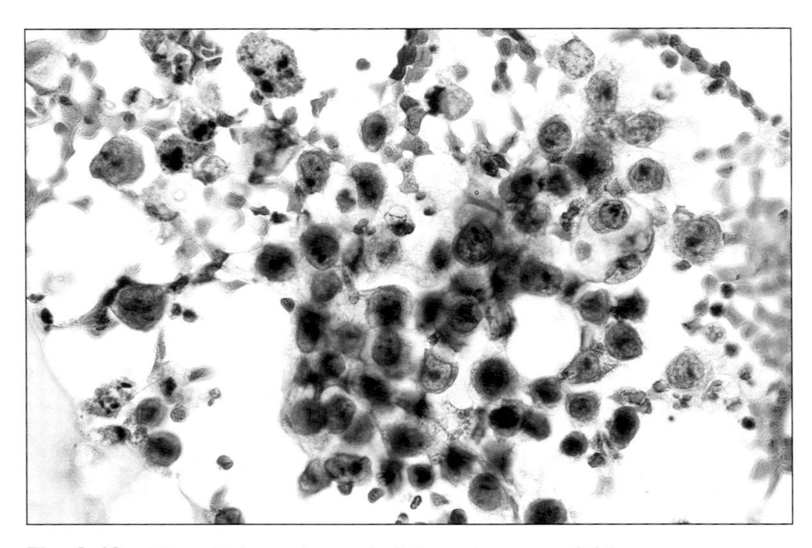

Fig. 9.48 Many high-grade urothelial carcinomas exhibit squamous (20% of tumors) or glandular (60% of tumors) metaplasia. Keratinized squamous cells and mucin-producing cells are not therefore evidence of squamous cell carcinoma or adenocarcinoma.

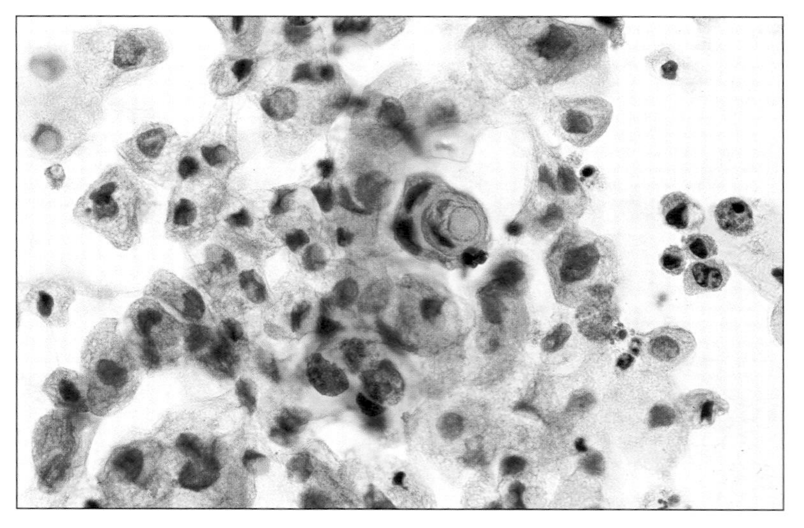

Fig. 9.49 Cytophagocytosis or 'cannibalism' appears to indicate high-grade, invasive urothelial carcinoma. The background is clean, suggesting noninvasive tumor.

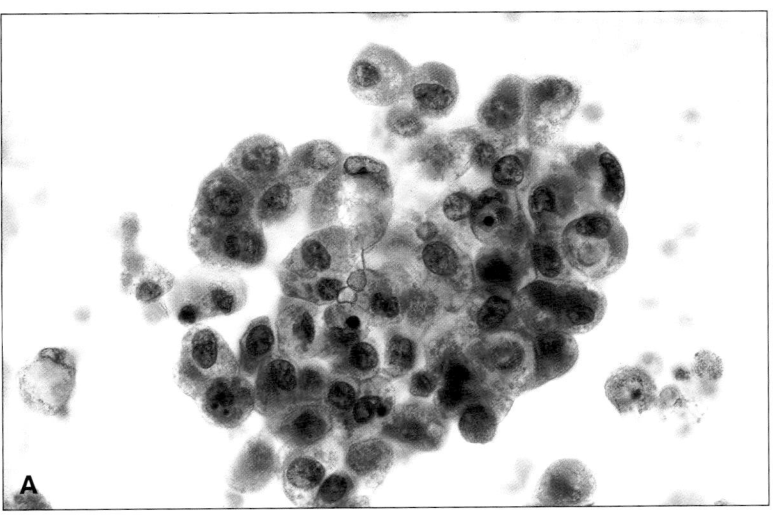

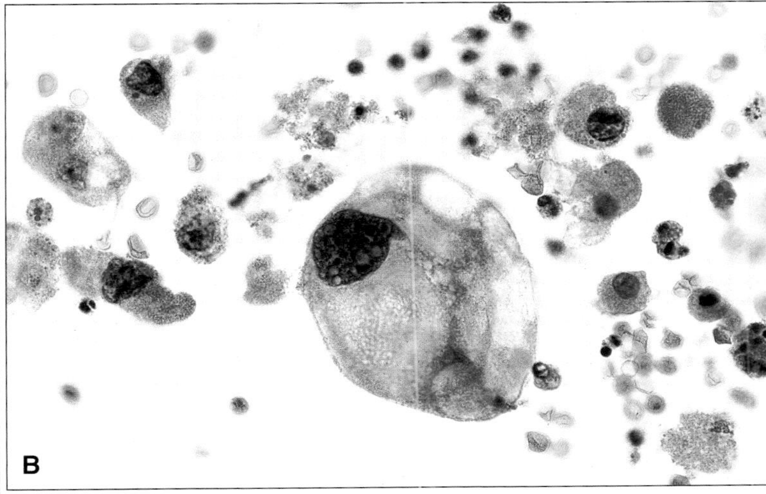

Fig. 9.50 High-grade papillary urothelial carcinoma. (A) Vacuolated cytoplasm and prominent nucleoli may suggest a reactive process, but the anaplastic nuclear and nucleolar characteristics distinguish carcinoma. (B) A single enlarged cell with vacuolated cytoplasm mimics chemotherapy effect. However, the surrounding smaller malignant cells share similar nuclear features.

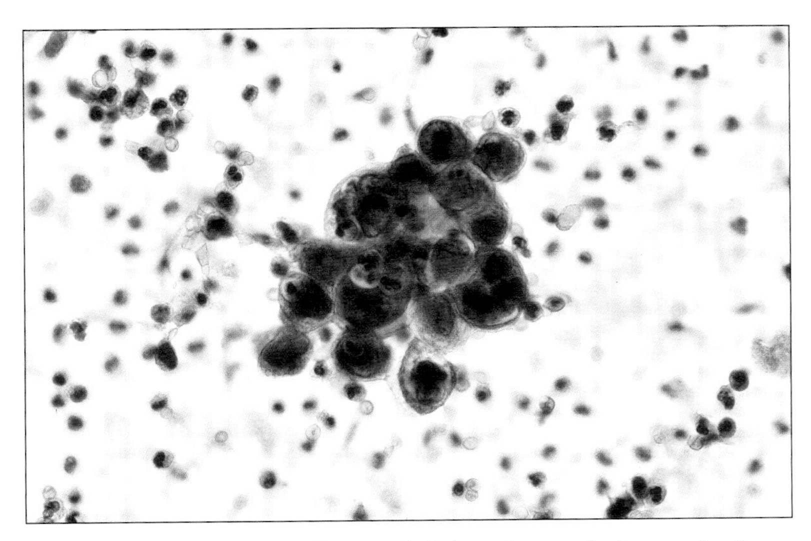

Fig. 9.51 High-grade papillary urothelial carcinoma. A cluster of cells with phagocytosis of neutrophils resembles acute cystitis. Despite the inflammatory background, nuclear anaplasia is evident.

FLAT UROTHELIAL NEOPLASIA

'Reactive atypia'

Cytology: 'Negative for malignant cells. Reactive urothelial cells'

Patients with this histologic lesion do not have adverse clinical outcomes. By contrast, patients with urothelial dysplasia are at increased risk for developing carcinoma.[28] Therefore, the term 'reactive urothelial cell changes', which has no neoplastic connotation, might be preferable. Unfortunately, in practice, these lesions may be difficult to reliably separate from urothelial dysplasia. The cytologic features are those of 'reactive urothelial cells' described previously.

'Urothelial dysplasia'

Cytology: 'Atypical urothelial cells'

Urothelial dysplasia is the precursor of in situ and invasive urothelial carcinoma.[29] Dysplasia is defined as architectural and cytologic changes short of carcinoma, but beyond those of a reactive process.[28] Until accurate cytologic criteria for dysplasia are established, use of the term 'urothelial dysplasia' should be avoided in urine cytology, and the term 'urothelial cell atypia' should be used instead. The cytologic diagnosis of 'atypia' as used here implies the presence of a significant flat lesion, which should be followed up by cystoscopic investigation and biopsy. Cytologic features of 'atypia' seen in instrumented urine specimens are summarized in Table 9.6. (Figs 9.52 & 9.53)

Urothelial carcinoma in situ

Cytology: 'Positive for malignancy. Carcinoma in situ'

CIS, a flat urothelial neoplasm, is a precursor of invasive cancer. It is usually multifocal and may appear granular, velvety, and erythematous on cystoscopic examination. Considerable nuclear anaplasia is present. Urothelial thickness varies from monolayered to hyperplastic; in contrast to papillary neoplasms, cytologic abnormalities predominate over architectural ones. Cytologically, just as histologically, in some cases, small, fairly uniform cells predominate (small cell CIS); in other cases, large, pleomorphic, obviously malignant cells are present (large cell CIS).

The cytologic features of CIS are summarized in Table 9.6. Absence of necrosis favors CIS over invasive carcinoma (see below), but does not absolutely exclude invasion.

Table 9.6 Cytology of flat urothelial lesions

	*Reactive**	*Dysplasia*	*CIS*
Single cells	Rare	Scattered	Numerous
Cell arrangement	**Papillary, loose**	**Loose clusters**	**Loose**
Cell size	Increased, uniform	Increased, uniform	Increased, variable
Cytoplasm	**Vacuolated**	**Clear/ homogeneous**	**Homogeneous**
NCR	**Preserved**	**Slightly increased**	**Markedly increased**
Nuclear			
Enlargement	Slight	Slight	Moderate/marked
Size variation	Absent	Slight	Moderate/marked
Shape	Oval	Oval/round	Variable
Shape variation	Absent (uniform)	Slight	Moderate/marked
Contours	**Regular, smooth**	**Irregular, notches**	**Pleomorphic**
Pleomorphism†	Absent	Mild	Moderate/severe
Hyperchromasia	Absent	Mild	Moderate/marked
Chromatin	**Fine, regular**	**Granular, irregular**	**Coarse, irregular**
Nucleolus	Large, round	Absent or small	Variable, large

CIS, carcinoma in situ; NCR, nuclear:cytoplasmic ratio.
*Includes 'reactive atypia' (WHO/ISUP 1998).
†Refers to uniform nuclear enlargement in all cells.
Bold type indicates the most salient features.
Modified from Bardales.[21]

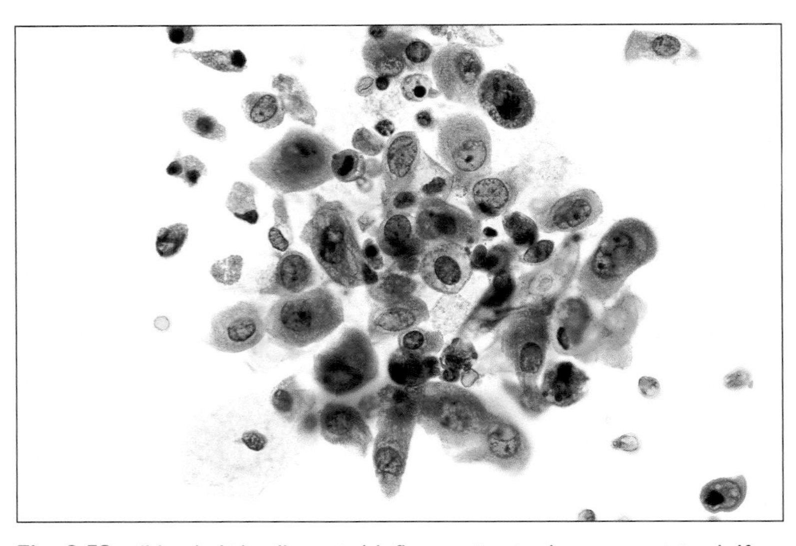

Fig. 9.53 'Urothelial cell atypia.' Inflammation is absent or minimal. If inflammation is present, these patients need to be re-evaluated once the inflammation subsides. Necrosis is absent. It may be difficult to differentiate 'atypia' from reactive urothelial cell changes associated with instrumentation, inflammation, lithiasis, infections, or intravesical or systemic chemotherapy.

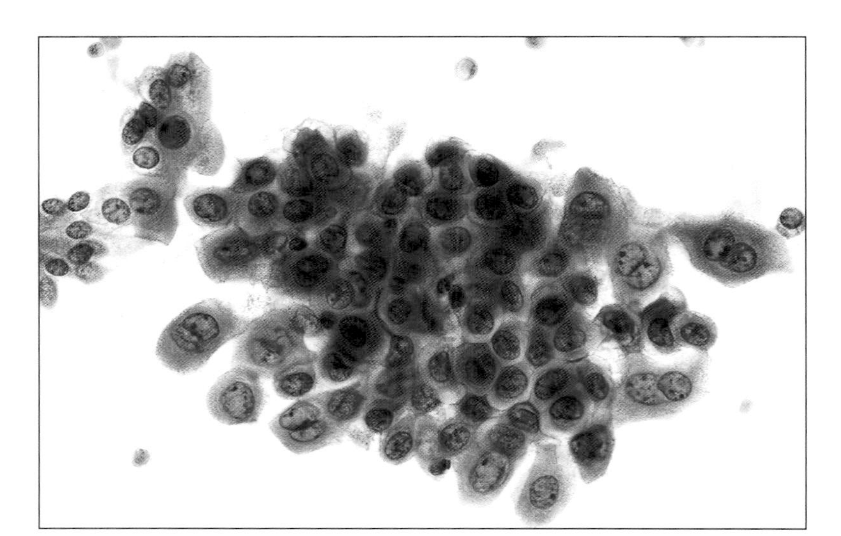

Fig. 9.52 Loose cellular arrangement, clear cytoplasm, slight nuclear enlargement, irregular nuclear contours with few notches, mild hyperchromasia, irregular chromatin distribution without clumping, and mild pleomorphism characterize cells dervied from dysplastic urothelium. The cytologic diagnosis is 'atypical urothelial cells', followed by a description of the findings and diagnostic considerations. The degree of cell disaggregation favors the diagnosis of urothelial dysplasia over a low-grade papillary lesion.

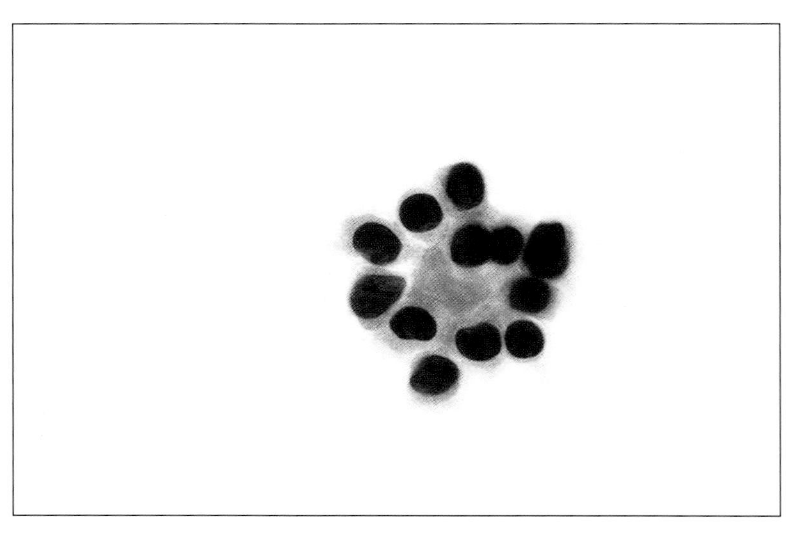

Fig. 9.54 Carcinoma in situ (CIS). Smears are of variable cellularity and show small clusters and single cells. Malignant cells are usually uniform with dense or vacuolated cytoplasm, a variable nuclear:cytoplasmic (N:C) ratio, and anaplastic nuclei. Red blood cells may be identified, but necrosis is absent. Small cell CIS (shown here) has small, uniform cells with a high N:C ratio, hyperchromatic, irregular nuclei, coarse chromatin, and inconspicuous nucleoli.

Intravesical chemotherapy and photodynamic therapy effect can mimic large cell CIS. Systemic cyclophosphamide therapy causes changes cytologically indistinguishable from CIS. Polyomavirus cytopathic effect (see above) may also mimic CIS. (Figs 9.54 & 9.55)

INVASIVE UROTHELIAL CARCINOMA

Cytology: 'Positive for malignancy. High-grade urothelial carcinoma'

Invasive urothelial carcinoma is typically of high cytologic grade. Admixed squamous, glandular, or small cell (neuroendocrine) differentiation is an unfavorable prognostic factor and may alter management.

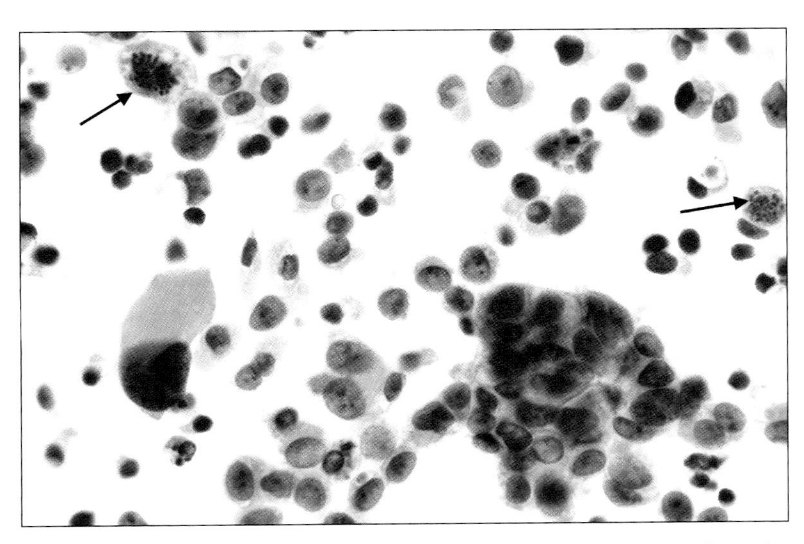

Fig. 9.55 Large cell carcinoma in situ has larger, pleomorphic cells with abundant cytoplasm, a variable nuclear:cytoplasmic ratio, and large nuclei with irregular nuclear contours, coarse chromatin, and large, irregular nucleoli. Abnormal mitotic figures are present (arrows).

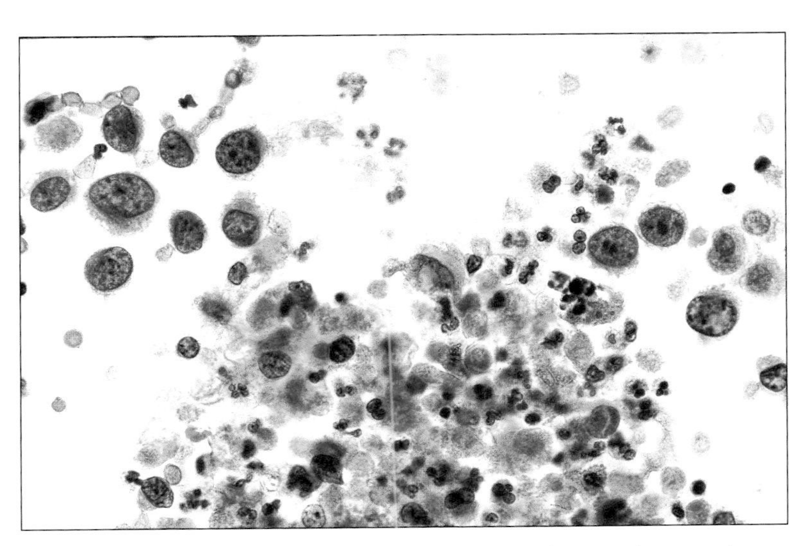

Fig. 9.57 When the triad of high cellularity, cell pleomorphism, and necrosis is present, the cytologic diagnosis of invasive urothelial carcinoma can be made with certainty. This bladder washing shows the classic smear pattern of necrosis and numerous single high-grade malignant cells.

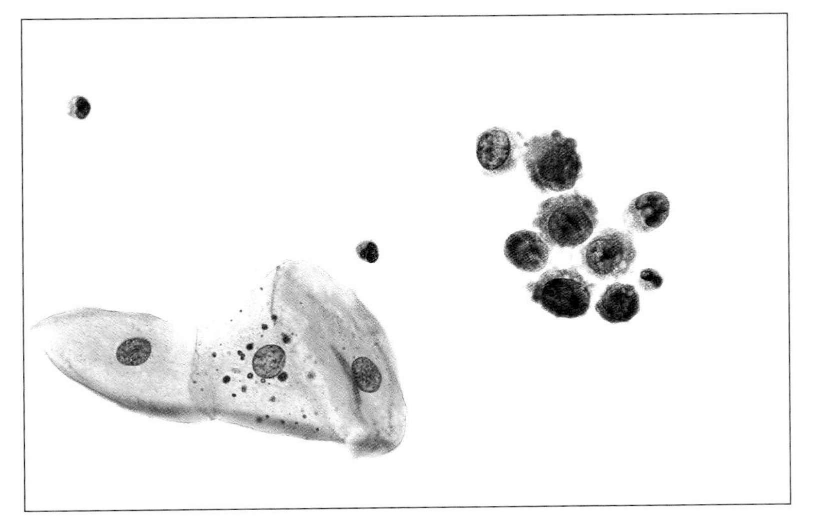

Fig. 9.56 Invasive urothelial carcinoma. Voided and instrumented urine smears show irregular, three-dimensional cell groups and numerous discohesive cells. Malignant cells are large and show abundant dense or vacuolated cytoplasm, enlarged pleomorphic nuclei, coarse and irregular chromatin, and a single large nucleolus or multiple small nucleoli. Abnormal mitotic figures may be present. In this voided urine specimen, necrosis is absent, yet the patient had a stage IV carcinoma.

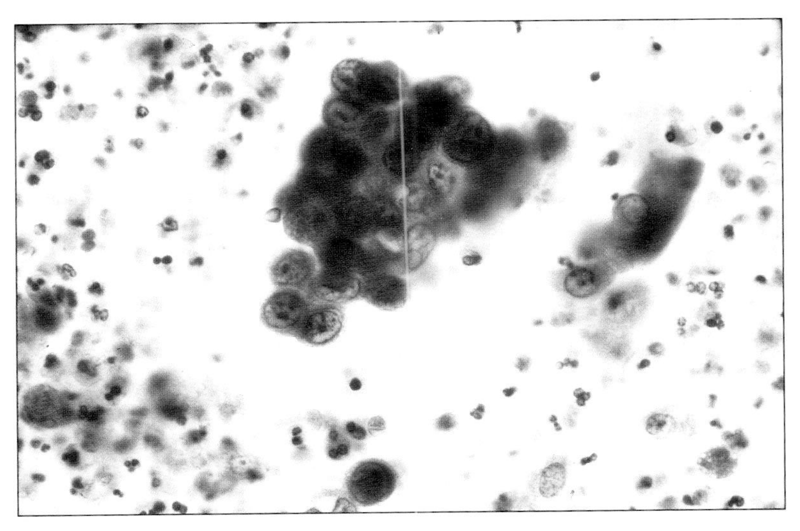

Fig. 9.58 Invasive urothelial carcinoma. The precursor lesion may have been either a flat in-situ or a preinvasive papillary lesion. However, residual papillary architecture is discernible in only a minority of cases. In this case, papillary clusters composed of malignant cells and necrosis are seen in bladder washings, indicating that the precursor was a papillary carcinoma.

The background may show necrosis with lysed blood, granular debris, and inflammatory cells, but absence of a diathesis does not exclude invasion.

Urine obtained shortly after a biopsy may show markedly abnormal cells that mimic malignancy, but even though acute inflammation is present, necrosis is absent. Tissue damage and atypical squamous metaplastic cells are seen with large bladder calculi, but high-grade cancer cells are absent. (Figs 9.56–9.60)

CARCINOMA OF THE UPPER URINARY TRACT

Less than 10% of urinary tract cancers occur in the ureter and renal pelvis. A cytologic diagnosis is commonly made by transurethral selective catheterization, ideally with brushings and washings. Endoscopic renal pelvis brush cytology of grade 1 and 2 urothelial carcinoma has >90% diagnostic accuracy. Larger lesions can be sampled by fine-needle aspiration biopsy or percutaneous translumbar brush cytology.[30] Voided urine specimens are

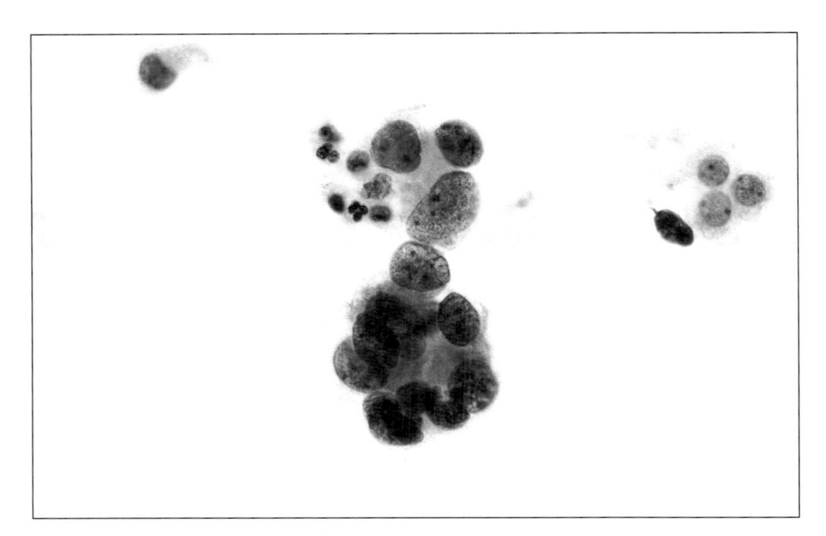

Fig. 9.59 Admixed malignant mucin-secreting cells are more common in invasive than in noninvasive tumors. Their presence does not change the classification of the tumor as urothelial, nor should it be diagnosed as a 'mixed' carcinoma. The example shown here should be diagnosed as 'invasive urothelial carcinoma with glandular differentiation'.

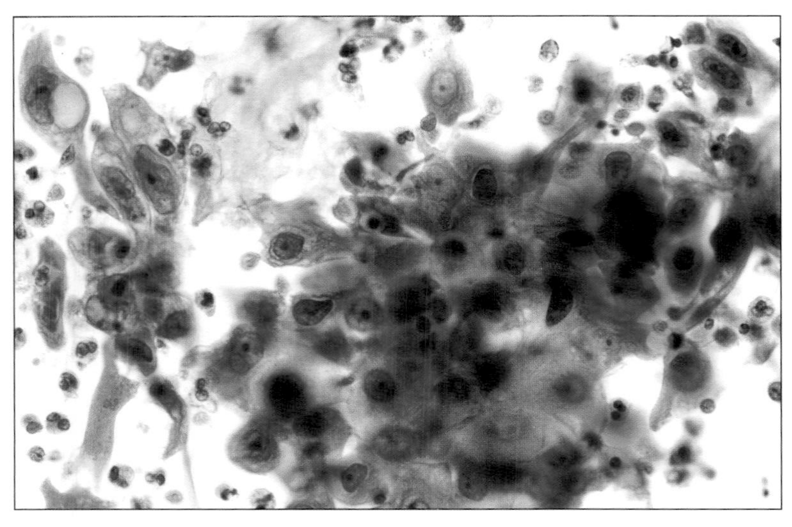

Fig. 9.60 Squamous differentiation is relatively common in invasive urothelial carcinomas. Urothelial carcinomas with a prominent squamous component may be relatively radioresistant. This bladder washing shows highly anaplastic malignant cells with abundant cytoplasm, well-defined cytoplasmic borders, and focal keratinization.

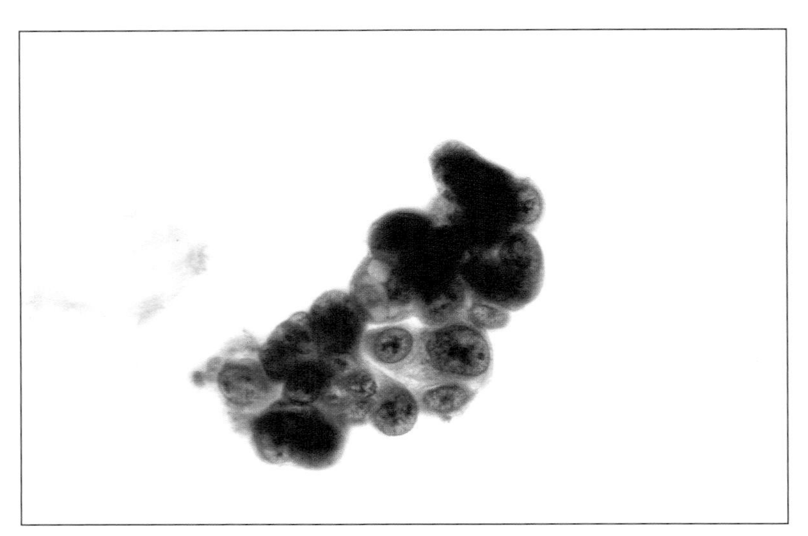

Fig. 9.61 Carcinomas of the upper urinary tract are most commonly papillary in type. Urine smears show true papillary fragments with a fibrovascular core. In this voided urine sample, a papillary cluster together with some discohesive high-grade malignant cells is seen. Subsequent nephrectomy showed a high-grade papillary carcinoma of the renal pelvis.

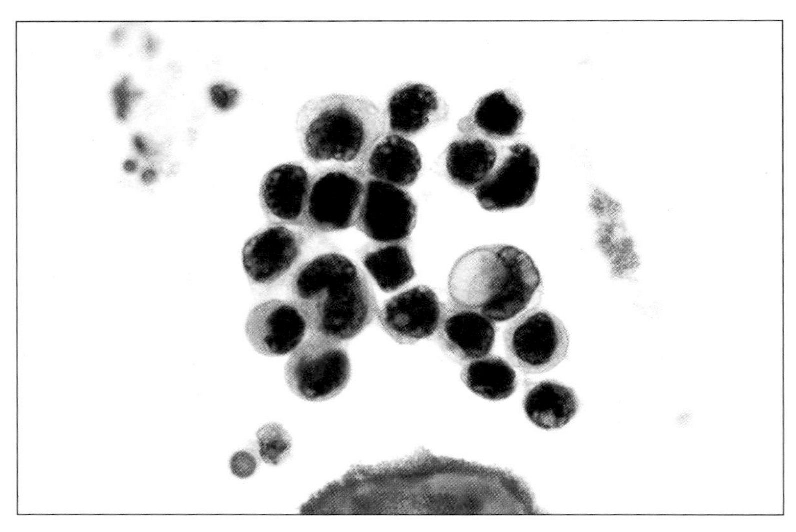

Fig. 9.62 Another case of papillary carcinoma of the renal pelvis detected in voided urine. Note that the cytomorphology is identical to that of urinary bladder papillary carcinoma. Brush specimens of low-grade carcinomas of the renal pelvis typically contain columnar urothelial cells and monomorphic single cells with irregular nuclear membranes.

suboptimal for evaluating the upper urinary tract. (Figs 9.61–9.70)

SQUAMOUS CELL CARCINOMA

Cytology: 'Positive for malignancy. High-grade carcinoma with squamous component'

To qualify as squamous cell carcinoma, a tumor should lack any urothelial component and the surrounding urothelium should exhibit keratinizing squamous metaplasia. Predisposing factors for squamous cell carcinoma include schistosomiasis, severe chronic inflammation, longstanding lithiasis, nonfunctioning bladder, indwelling catheter, and renal transplant.[32] Squamous cell carcinoma invading the bladder from the uterine cervix or vagina appears identical. (Figs 9.71–9.74)

ADENOCARCINOMA

Cytology: 'Positive for malignancy. Adenocarcinoma or poorly differentiated carcinoma'

Adenocarcinoma accounts for less than 2% of bladder carcinomas and can arise with similar morphology in the

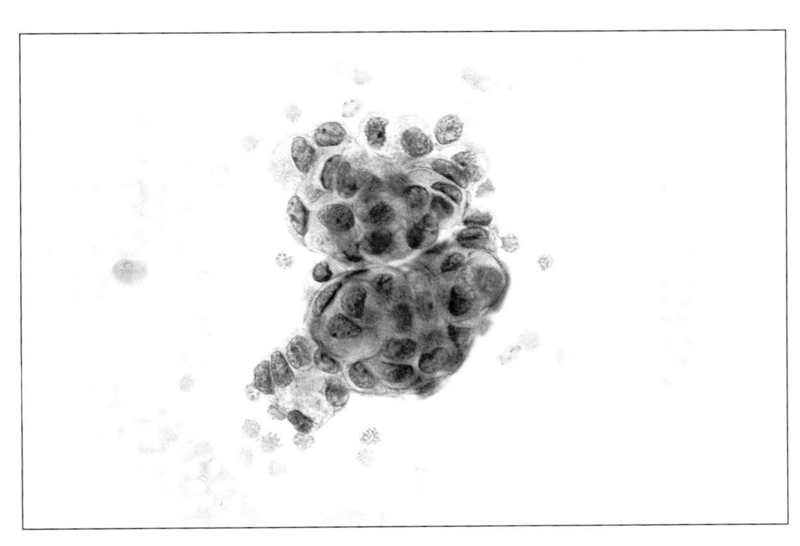

Fig. 9.63 The deceptively atypical appearance of the benign upper urinary tract cells can complicate the cytologic evaluation of upper urinary tract carcinoma.[31] Bilateral ureteral collections are therefore helpful as a cytologic control, particularly for low-grade tumors. This ureteral washing shows forcefully exfoliated umbrella cells, some with large, irregular nuclei; these cells are benign.

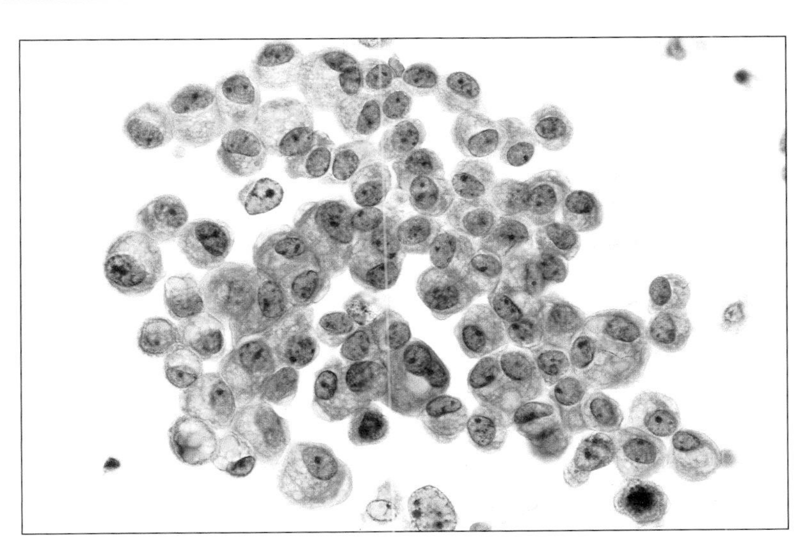

Fig. 9.65 Grading criteria for carcinomas of the urinary bladder apply equally to the upper urinary tract. This grade I urothelial carcinoma of the ureter shows minimal cytologic abnormalities, except for occasional cells with large nuclei and prominent nucleoli.

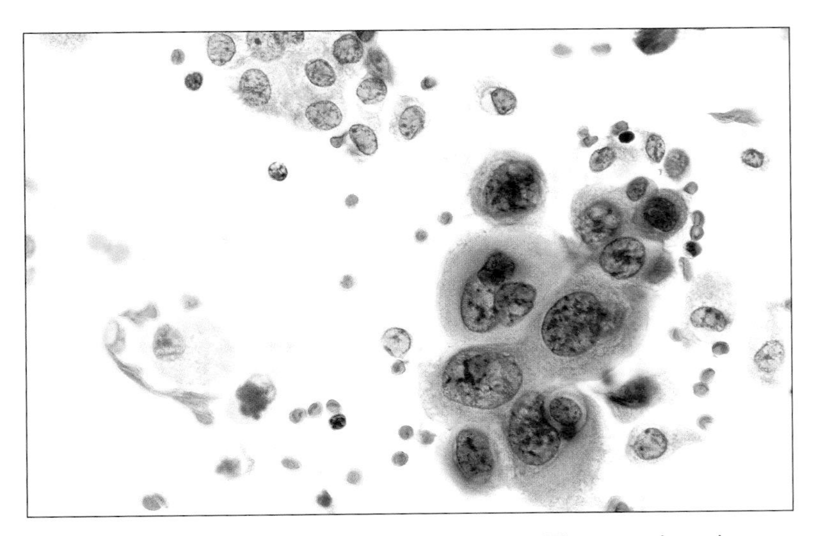

Fig. 9.64 Carcinoma of the upper urinary tract. The contralateral ureteral washing shows large cells with enlarged nuclei and clear features of malignancy. Comparison of this with Fig. 9.63 illustrates the utility of bilateral specimens in achieving diagnostic certainty.

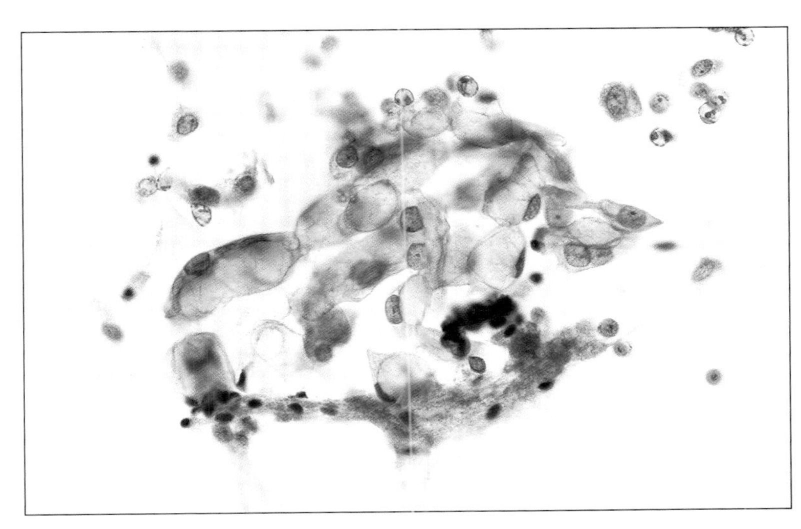

Fig. 9.66 Large cells with abnormal shapes, abundant vacuolated cytoplasm, and bland nuclear features are seen in a ureteral washing from a patient with grade I carcinoma.

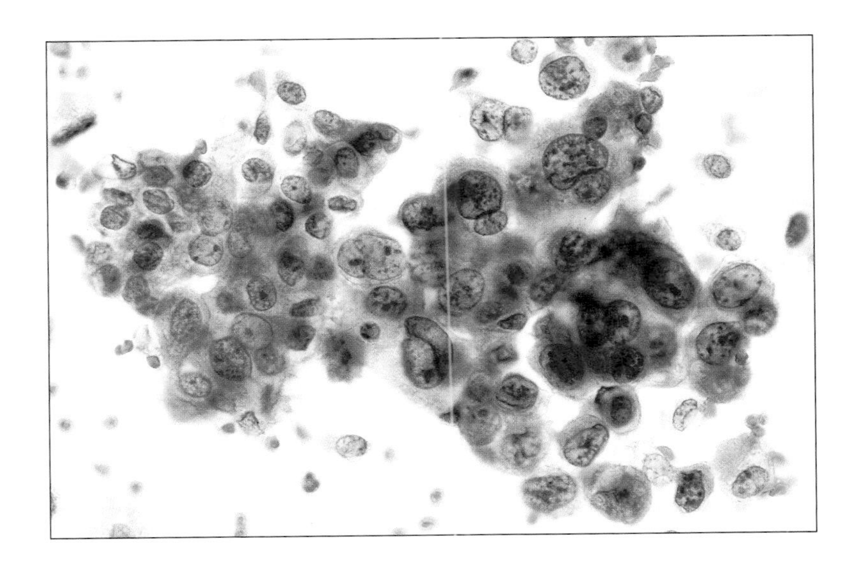

Fig. 9.67 Grade 2 urothelial carcinoma of the ureter exhibits greater nuclear pleomorphism, coarsened chromatin, and nucleoli.

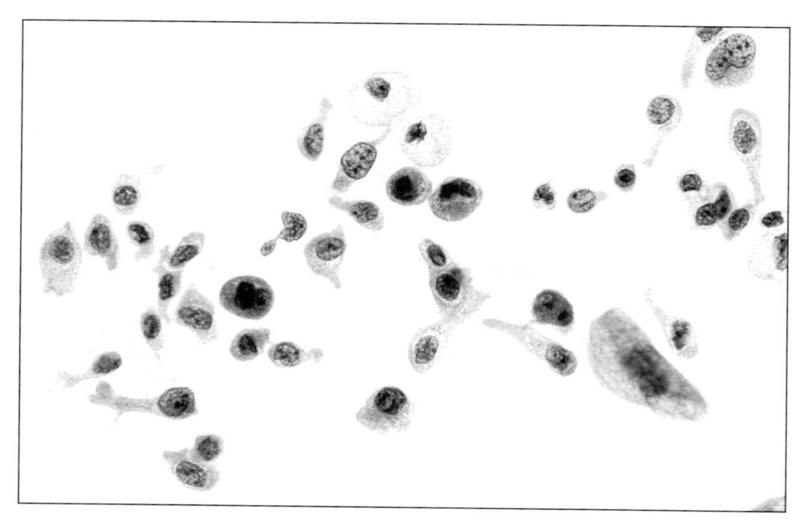

Fig. 9.68 In this ureteral washing of grade 2 carcinoma, moderately pleomorphic cells are accompanied by scattered cercariform cells.

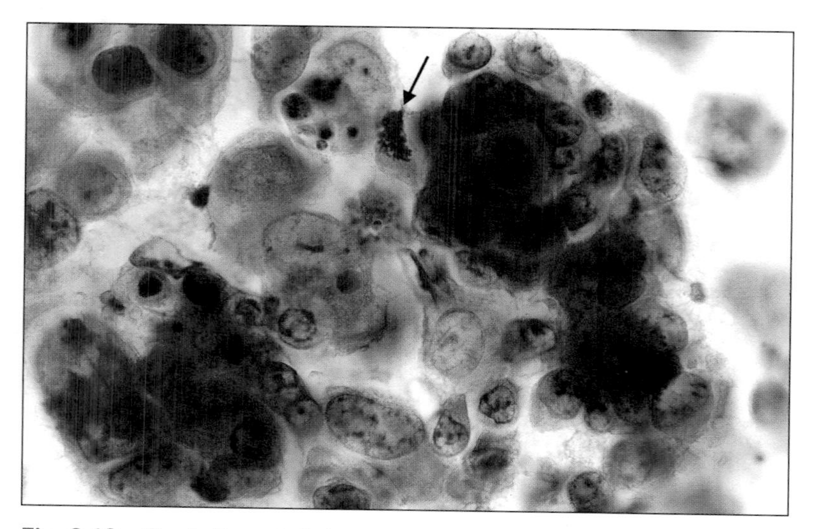

Fig. 9.69 Grade 3 urothelial carcinoma of the upper urinary tract shows marked anisocytosis and anisonucleosis, irregular nuclear contours, and occasional atypical mitoses (arrow). Invasive urothelial carcinomas often show vacuolated cytoplasm, hyperchromasia, prominent nucleoli, and necrosis, features that may resemble those present in lithiasis of the renal pelvis. Numerous anaplastic cells and necrosis indicate invasive carcinoma.

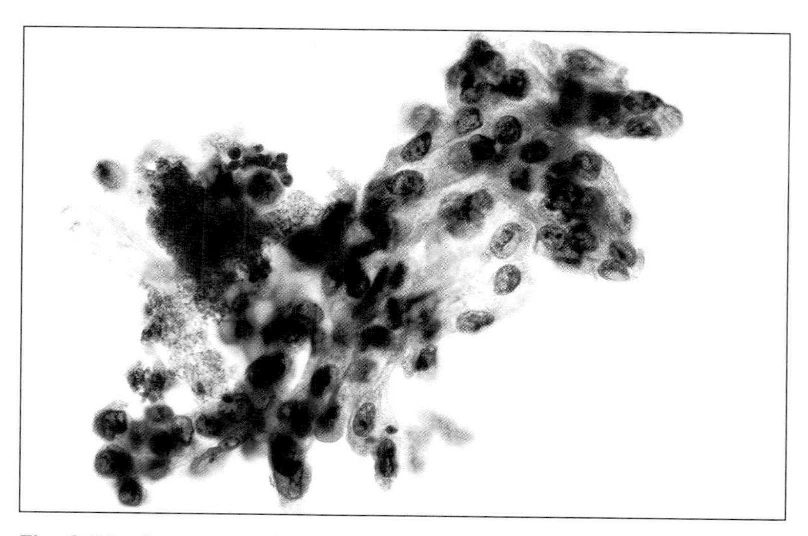

Fig. 9.70 Reactive urothelial cell changes associated with instrumentation effect, urolithiasis, or inflammatory disorders should be carefully considered in upper tract specimens. This sheet of benign reactive and elongated reparative urothelial cells from a ureteral washing might be overinterpreted as atypia or malignancy. Papillary clusters with nuclear crowding, a high nuclear:cytoplasmic ratio, anisonucleosis, and peripheral cell palisading favor a neoplasm over an instrumentation effect.

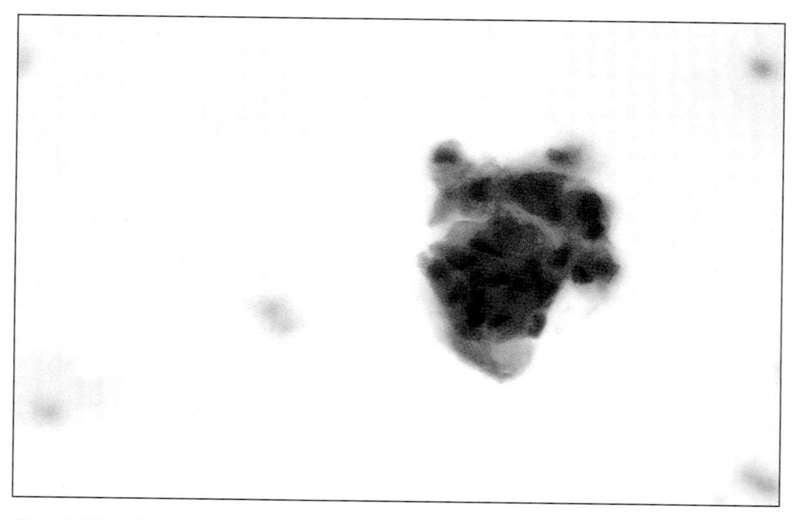

Fig. 9.71 With squamous cell carcinoma, keratin fragments and necrosis are commonly present in the smear background. This voided urine specimen shows scant cellularity, cellular degeneration, and rare, small fragments of keratinized cells with hyperchromatic nuclei.

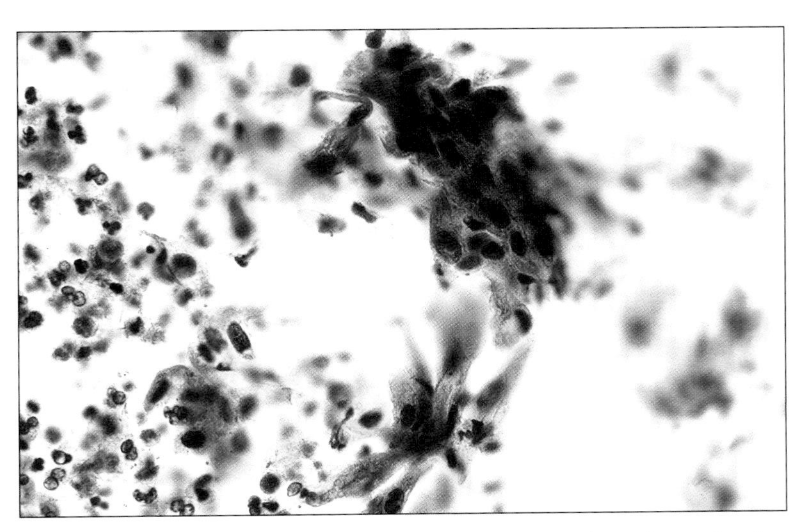

Fig. 9.72 Squamous cell carcinoma. This bladder washing shows focally keratinized, spindled cells with hyperchromatic, irregular nuclei and dense cytoplasm. Distinction from high-grade urothelial carcinoma with squamous differentiation is not possible by cytology alone, and it is preferable simply to describe 'high-grade neoplasm with a squamous component'.

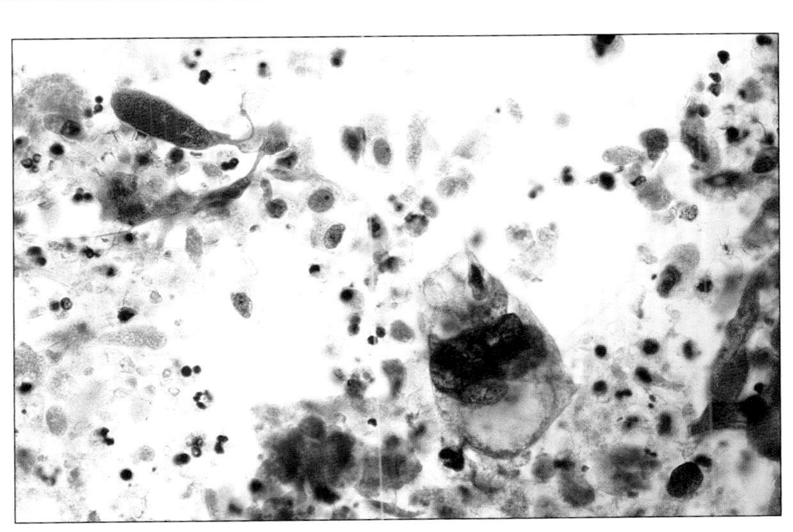

Fig. 9.74 Bladder calculus causes marked squamous metaplasia, keratinization, occasional multinucleated cells, and necrosis. Despite the atypical appearance, the findings are entirely benign. Lack of nuclear anaplasia permits distinction.

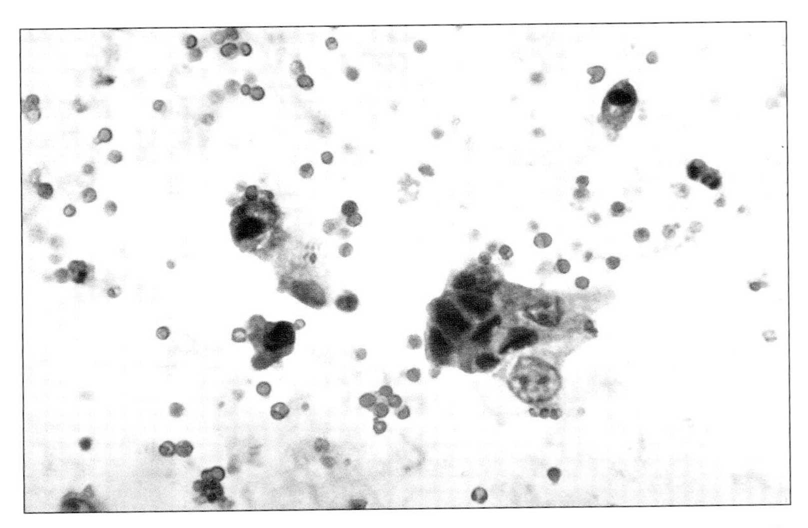

Fig. 9.73 Another voided urine specimen showing poorly differentiated squamous cell carcinoma presents with extensive cell necrosis and degeneration.

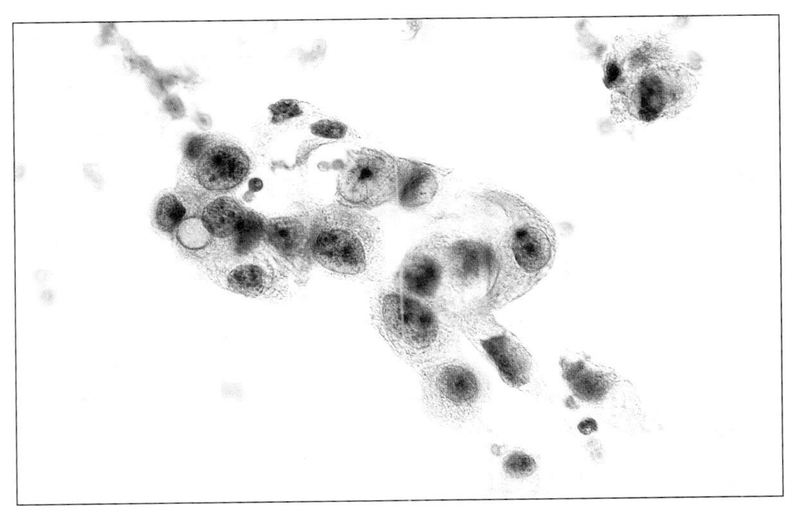

Fig. 9.75 Glandular structures and single cells with thin or finely vacuolated cytoplasm, vesicular chromatin, and prominent nucleoli are seen in adenocarcinoma. This bladder washing comes from a patient with well-differentiated adenocarcinoma.

urinary bladder itself or in the urachus. Predisposing factors include schistosomiasis, bladder augmentation, protracted chronic cystitis, and neurogenic bladder. Histologically, the intestinal type is the most common and is indistinguishable from colorectal adenocarcinoma. Other types include mucinous (colloid), signet ring cell, and clear cell types.[33] Mucinous adenocarcinoma of the renal pelvis appears similar, showing round clusters of cells in a mucinous background.[34]

The differential diagnosis includes metastatic adenocarcinoma, papillary clear cell adenocarcinoma of the urethra, urothelial carcinoma with glandular differentiation, cystitis glandularis, benign adenomatous polyp of the prostatic urethra,[15] nephrogenic adenoma, and endometriosis/endocervicosis of the bladder. (Figs 9.75–9.79)

SMALL CELL CARCINOMA

Cytology: 'Small cell carcinoma'

Small cell neuroendocrine carcinoma of the urinary tract[35] is highly aggressive and accounts for less than 1% of

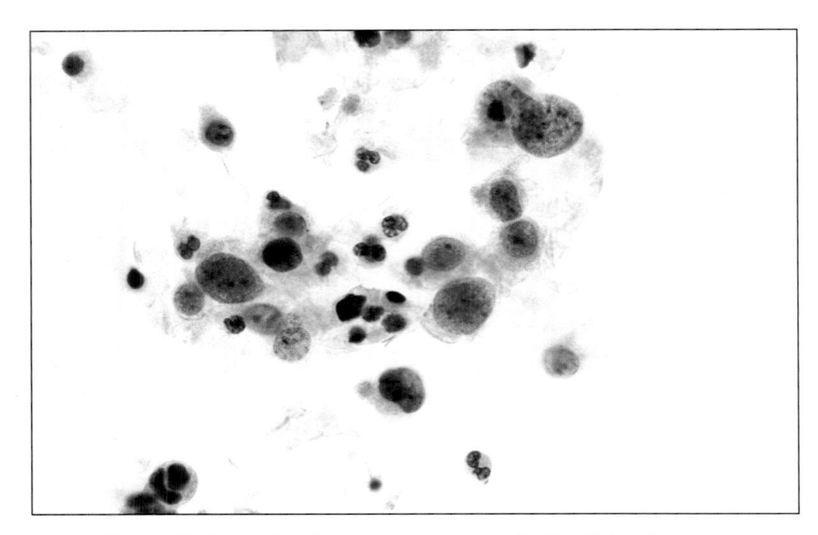

Fig. 9.76 In high-grade adenocarcinoma, marked cellular degeneration, necrosis, and low cellularity are usually seen, as in this bladder washing. The specific diagnosis of adenocarcinoma by means of urine cytology can be made in approximately two-thirds of cases; the remainder – as seen here – are indistinguishable from poorly differentiated urothelial carcinomas.

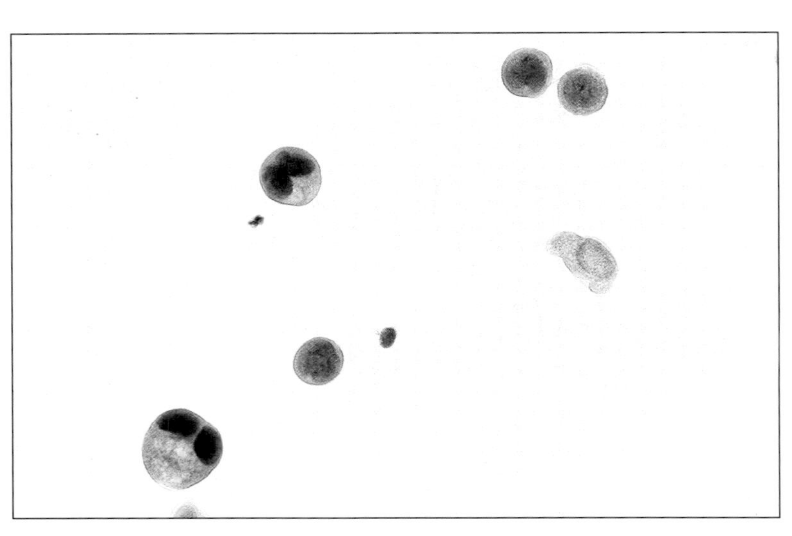

Fig. 9.77 Round cells with a large cytoplasmic vacuole and a hyperchromatic nucleus are seen in signet ring cell adenocarcinoma (voided urine specimen). The signet ring cell type has a particularly poor prognosis; otherwise, subtyping has little prognostic significance.

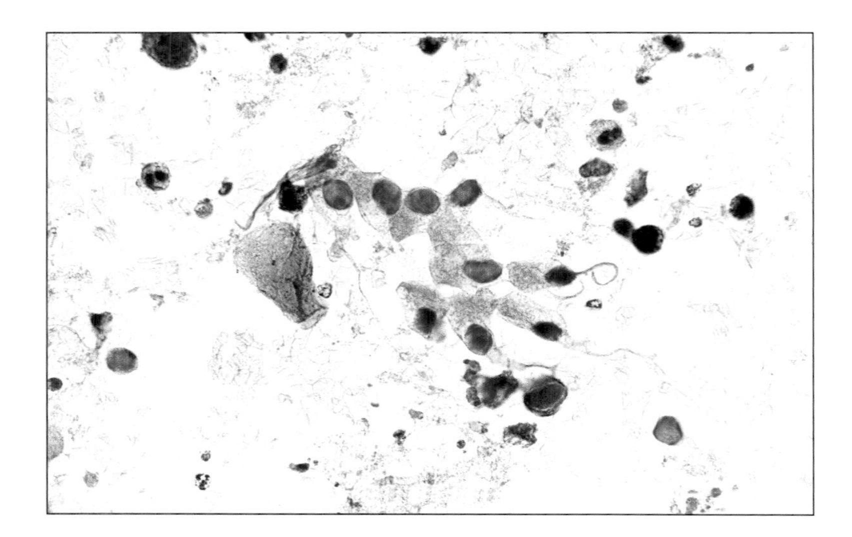

Fig. 9.78 Urine specimens from patients with intestinal-type adenocarcinoma show single and clustered degenerated columnar and pleomorphic cells in a mucinous and necrotic background. Voided urine smears (seen here) show similar findings, but have lower cellularity.

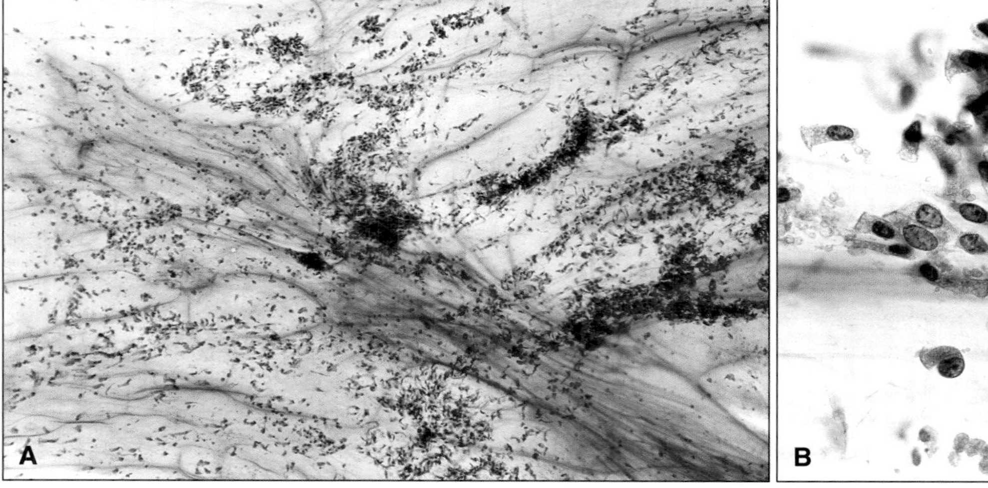

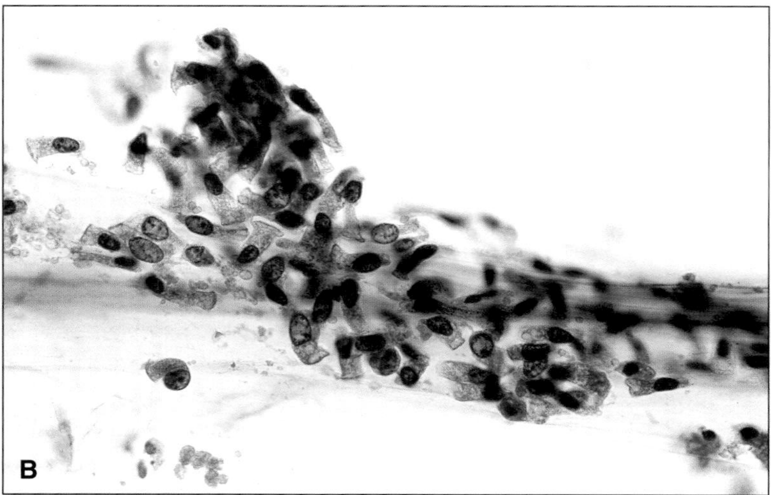

Fig. 9.79 Urachal carcinoma has a variety of types, but is often well-differentiated adenocarcinoma. (A) Low-power image shows single cells and clusters in a background of mucus. (B) Numerous deceptively bland columnar cells with oval nuclei and abundant extracellular mucin may be found in urine specimens from patients with urachal adenocarcinoma.

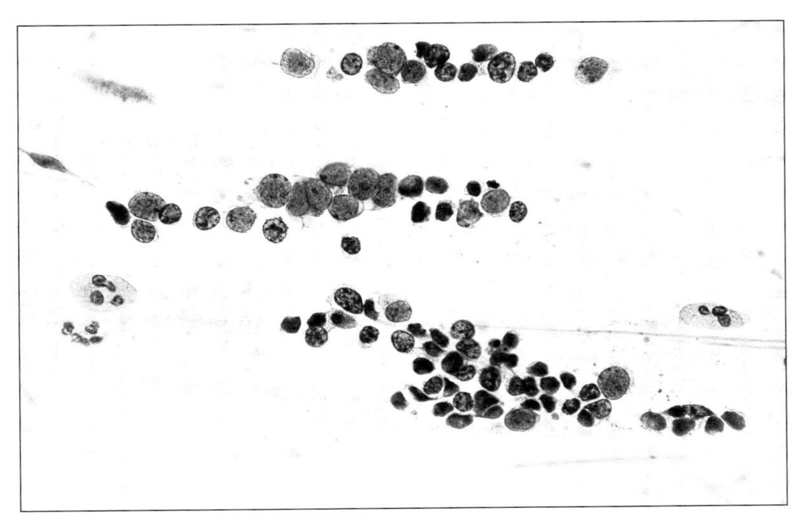

Fig. 9.80 Smears of small cell carcinoma have high cellularity, numerous naked and karyorrhectic nuclei, and necrosis. The 'intermediate' cell type shows nuclear pleomorphism, hyperchromasia, and small nucleoli; the 'oat' cell type shows minimal pleomorphism and less hyperchromasia. Cells are round to oval, with scant cytoplasm, arranged often singly or in variably cohesive clusters. Cytophagocytosis, nuclear molding, and rare abnormal mitotic figures may be seen. Immunohistochemical stains for neuroendocrine markers are helpful.

Table 9.7 Secondary neoplasms commonly involving the urinary tract
Direct extension from a primary tumor of:
Kidney
Prostate
Colon
Female genital tract
Male genital tract
Retroperitoneum
Metastasis from a distant primary tumor
Carcinomas
Hematolymphoid malignancies
Melanoma
Sarcomas
Germ cell tumors
Modified from: Bardales.[37]

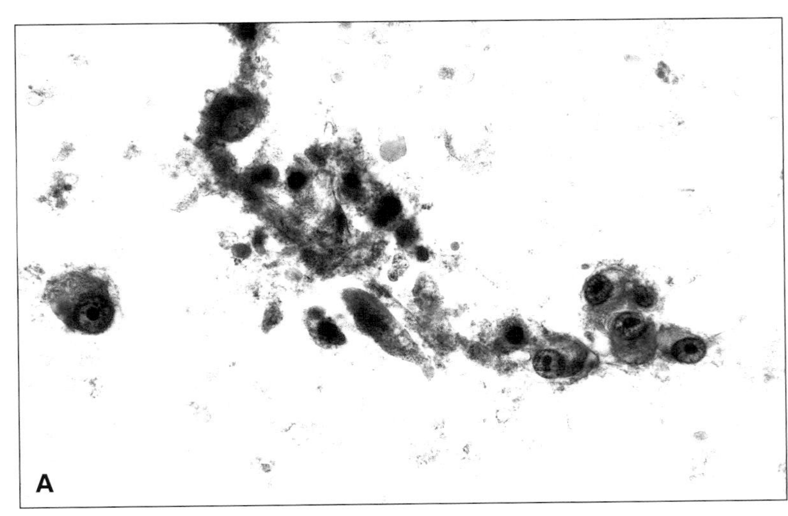

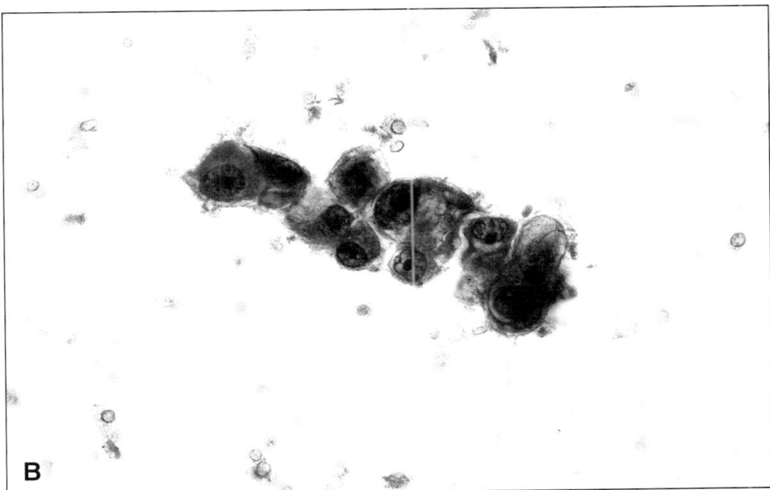

Fig. 9.81 (A,B) Renal cell clear cell carcinoma exfoliates large cells with thin, clear or vacuolated cytoplasm, an eccentric round nucleus, irregular vesicular chromatin, and a large round eosinophilic nucleolus. Granular and dense cytoplasm may be present in some cells. Multinucleated cells with anaplastic nuclei and occasionally benign-appearing multinucleated cells can be identified. Necrosis and blood are usually present.

bladder malignancies. Most cases occur in combination with urothelial carcinoma and, because of its ominous significance, any component of small cell carcinoma should be reported.

Metastatic neuroendocrine carcinoma, extension from small cell carcinoma of the prostate, and the small cell subtype of urothelial CIS should be excluded. The rare primary carcinoid tumor of the urinary tract has less anaplasia and lacks background necrosis.[36] (Fig. 9.80)

SECONDARY NEOPLASMS OF THE URINARY TRACT

Contiguous spread of a malignancy in an adjacent organ is more common than metastasis from a distant primary (Table 9.7). In adults, the most common distant primary sites include the stomach, breast, and lung. In children, leukemias, neuroblastoma, and Wilms' tumor have been detected in urine specimens. (Figs 9.81–9.89)

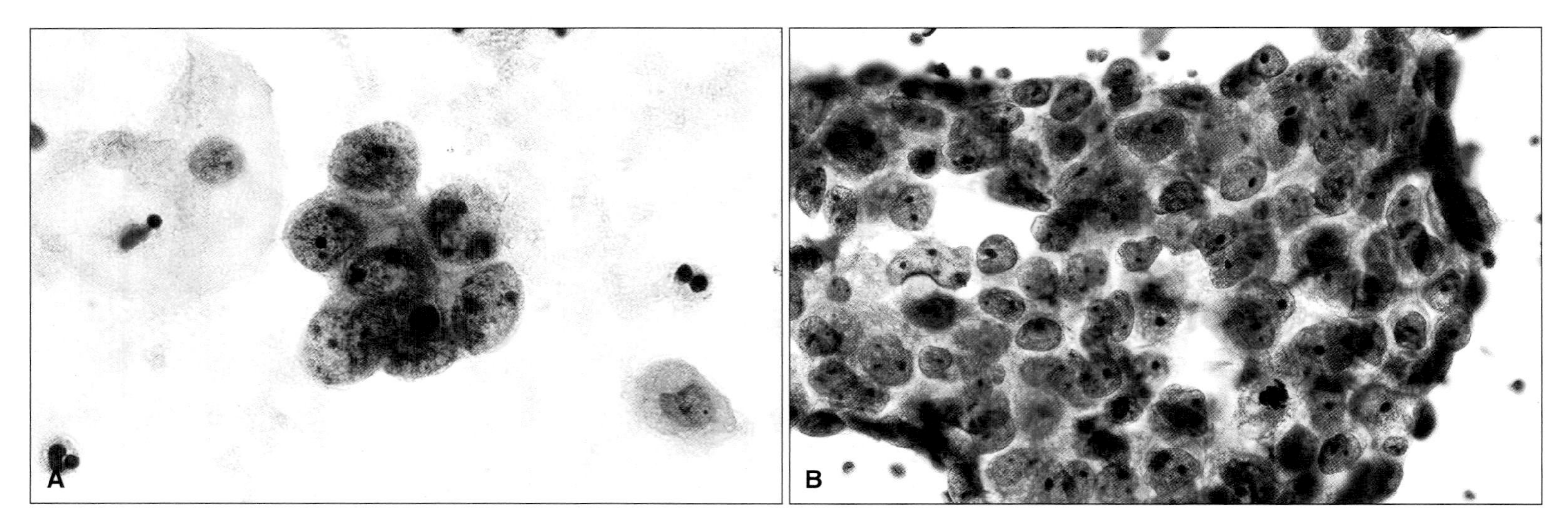

Fig. 9.82 Prostatic adenocarcinoma, of acinar or ductal origin, can involve the bladder neck or prostatic urethra, or metastasize to the urinary bladder wall and yield malignant cells in urine specimens. Urine specimens are of variable cellularity, the lowest being found in voided urine (A). Necrosis and acute inflammation are evident when there is mucosal ulceration. Bladder washing (B) shows a larger cluster of highly anaplastic cells.

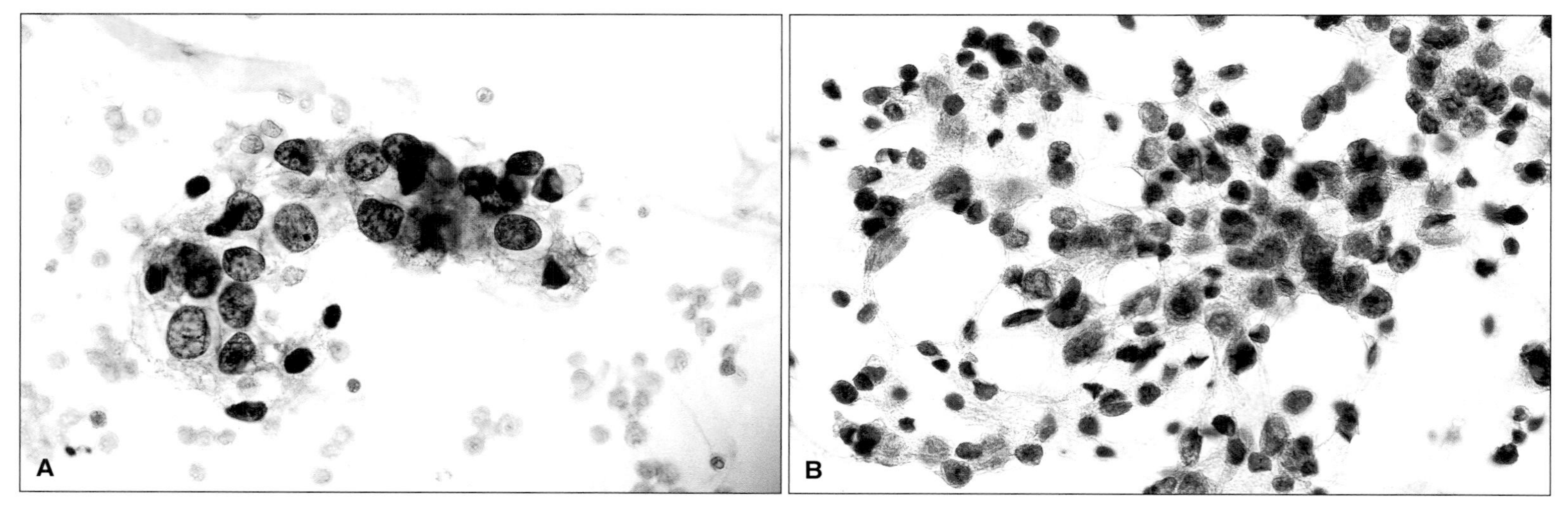

Fig. 9.83 (A,B) Malignant cells of acinar-type prostatic adenocarcinoma in voided urine specimens are commonly seen in small aggregates, with only few cells found singly or in pairs. Cells have very scant vacuolated or thin cytoplasm, ill-defined cytoplasmic borders, a high nuclear:cytoplasmic ratio, round or oval nuclear borders, and large, often multiple, nucleoli. These two bladder wash specimens illustrate typical findings.

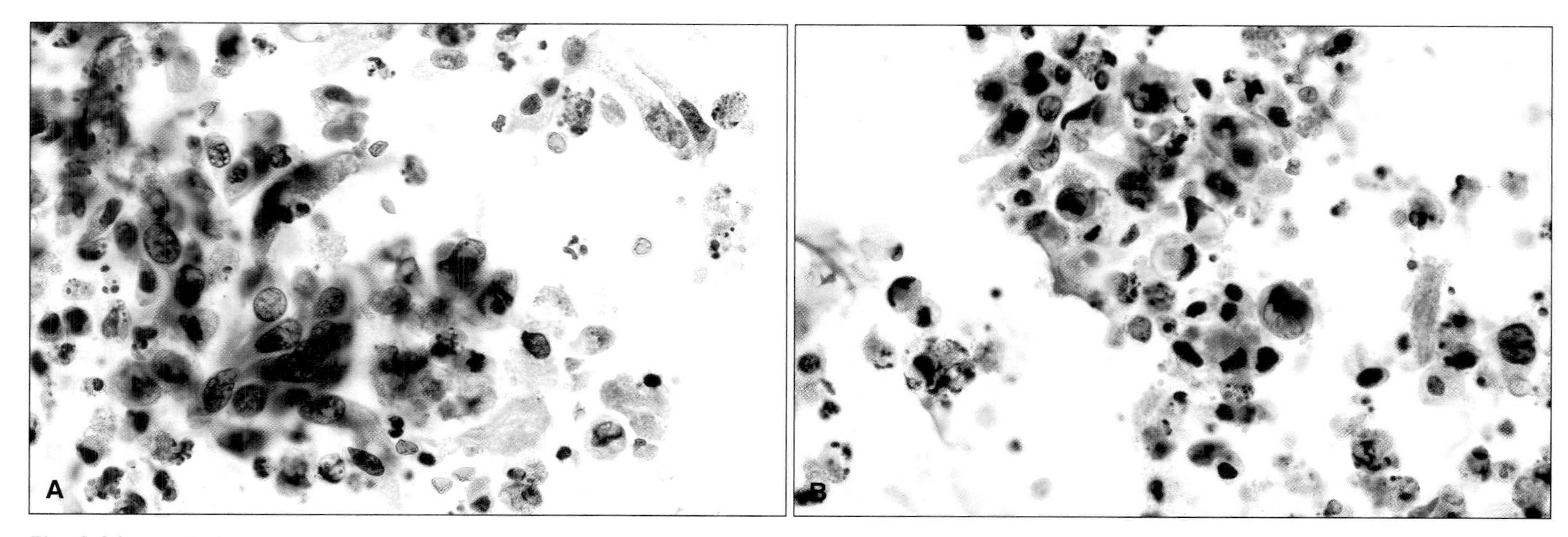

Fig. 9.84 (A,B) Colon carcinoma involving the bladder by direct extension yields highly cellular urine smears with a necrotic background. Columnar cells and gland formation are helpful features. Cells with vacuolated cytoplasm are found. Primary intestinal-type urinary bladder adenocarcinoma shows cytomorphology identical to that of colonic adenocarcinoma.

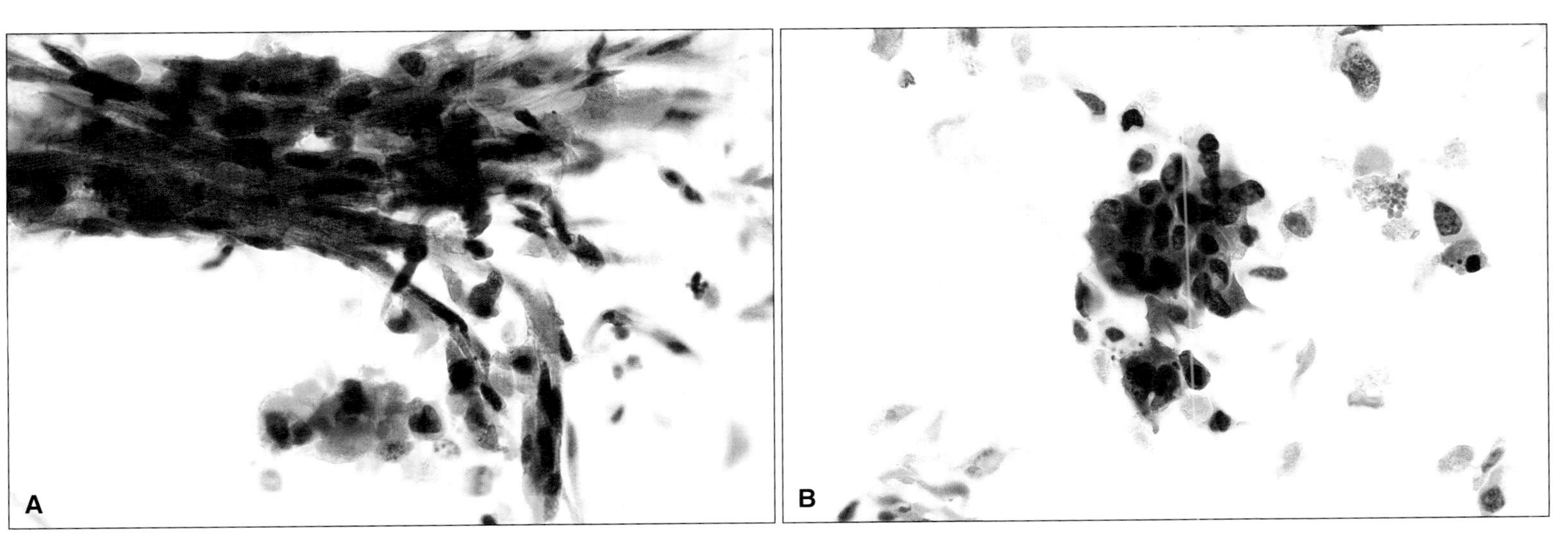

Fig. 9.85 (A,B) Squamous cell carcinoma of the cervix/vagina and primary squamous carcinoma of the urinary bladder appear identical in urine of bladder washes.

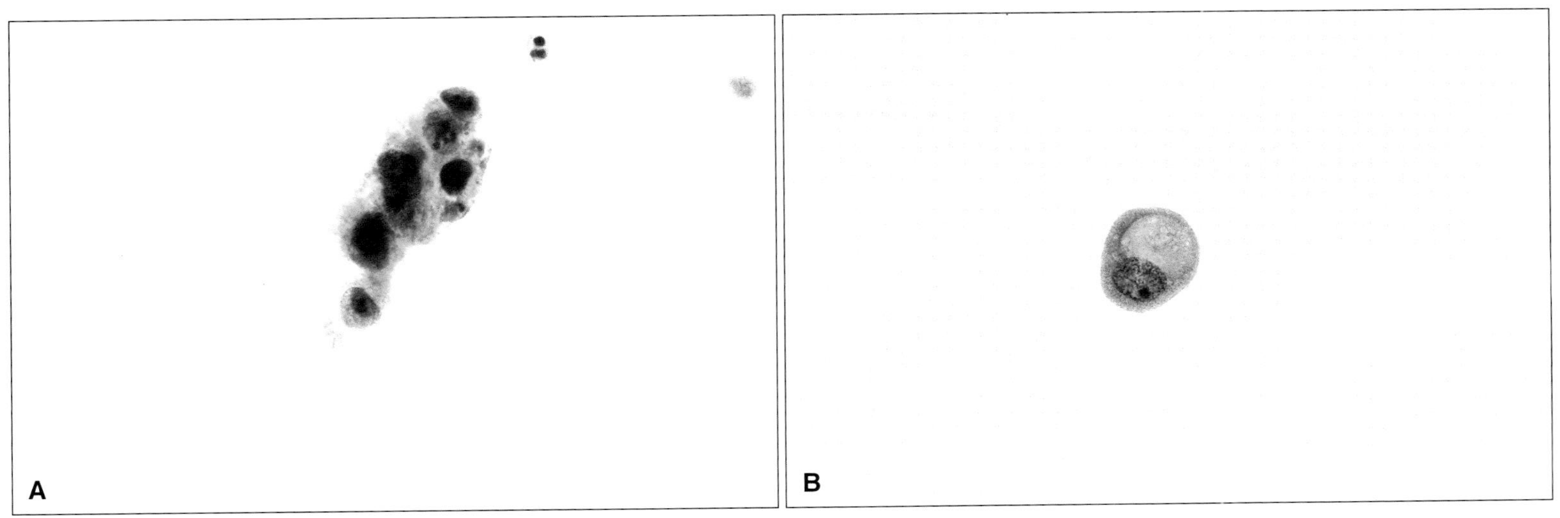

Fig. 9.86 (A,B) Large cells with a large nucleus, prominent nucleoli, and vacuolated cytoplasm are seen in endometrial or endocervical adenocarcinoma. Here, a voided urine sample from a patient with clear cell adenocarcinoma of the endometrium shows degenerated cells and a single large malignant cell with a cytoplasmic vacuole. Urine cytologic findings of metastatic adenocarcinomas appear similar to those of primary adenocarcinoma or metastases from other sources.

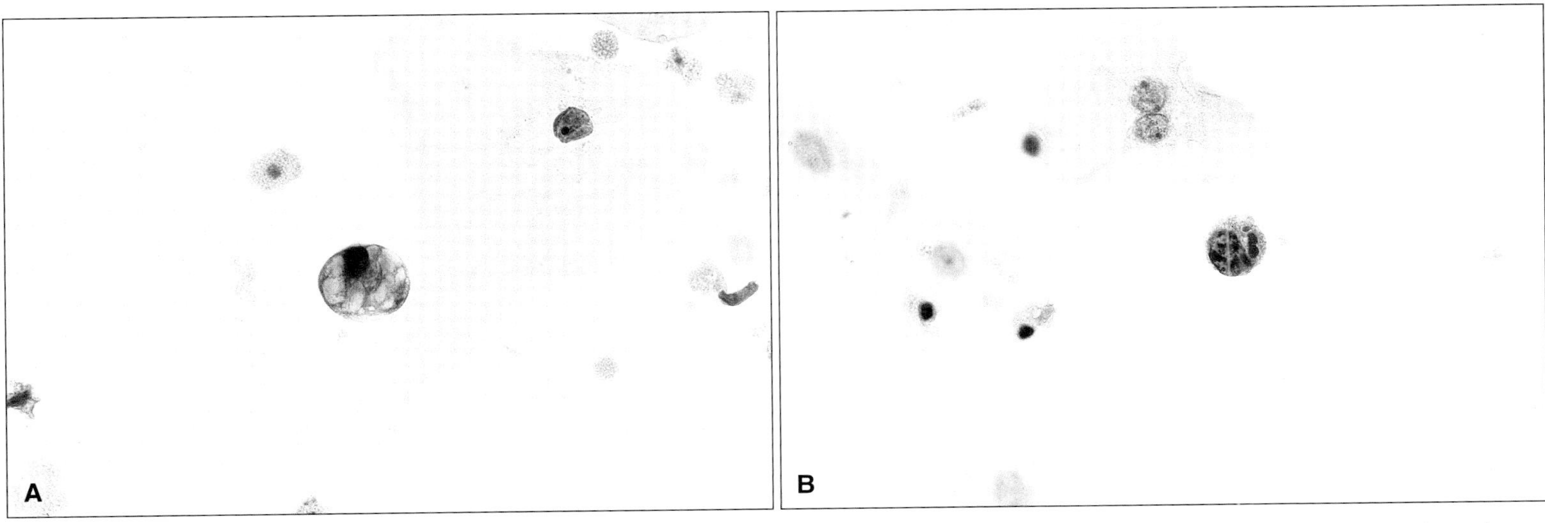

Fig. 9.87 (A,B) Voided urine specimens from breast carcinoma metastatic to the urinary tract show large, round cells with ample cytoplasm, large vacuole(s), an eccentric nucleus, and often a prominent nucleolus. The cellularity is scant, and the background may be clean. Voided urine specimens from metastatic lobular breast carcinoma show smaller cells arranged singly or in a short linear arrangement or clusters. Cells have scant cytoplasm and hyperchromatic nuclei. Metastatic breast carcinomas in the ureter may present as a collection of urine (urinoma) that may be aspirated for diagnostic purposes.

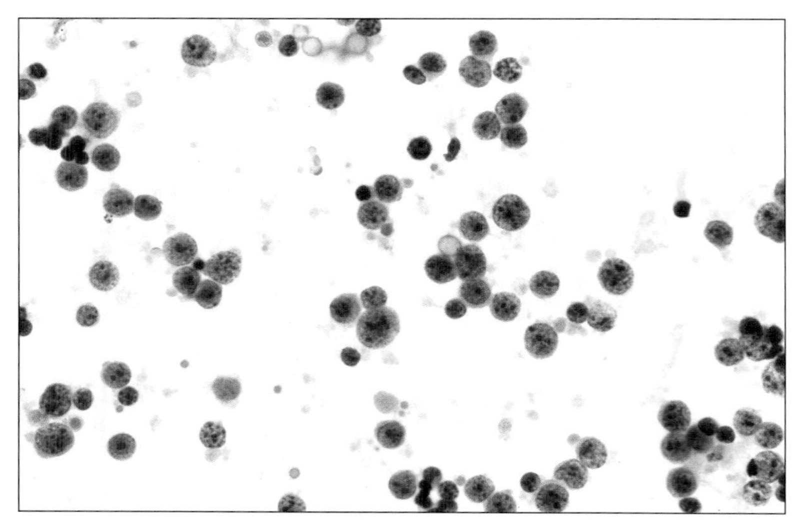

Fig. 9.88 Genitourinary tract involvement by malignant lymphoma in autopsies is >50%. The kidney is most commonly involved. Most cases are of the diffuse large cell type. Smears are variably cellular, with single monomorphic mononuclear cells with nuclear folds and coarse chromatin. Cell degeneration is present, along with necrosis and inflammation. With renal involvement, malignant cells are present, along with pathologic casts, damaged renal tubular cells, or fragments of necrotic parenchyma. Their absence suggests lower urinary tract and not renal involvement, as in this bladder washing.

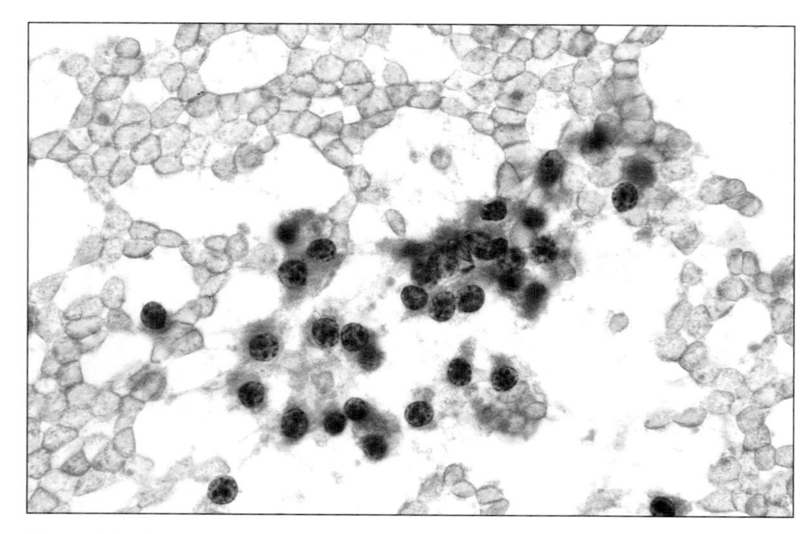

Fig. 9.89 Involvement of the urinary tract by primary or metastatic plasma cell myeloma is rare. Voided urine smears show rare degenerated abnormal plasma cells with dense cytoplasm with focal paranuclear clearing, eccentric nuclei, coarse and clumped chromatin, and variable nucleoli.

REFERENCES

1. Bardales R. Constituents of urinary tract specimens in the absence of disease. In: Bardales R, ed. Practical urologic cytopathology. New York: Oxford University Press; 2002:38–52.
2. Koss L, Deitch D, Ramanathan R, et al. Diagnostic value of cytology of voided urine. Acta Cytol 1985;29:810–816.
3. Kannan V, Bose S. Low grade transitional cell carcinoma and instrument artifact: a challenge in urinary cytology. Acta Cytol 1993;37:899–902.
4. Luthra U, Dey P, George J, et al. Comparison of ThinPrep and conventional preparations: urine cytology evaluation [letter]. Diagn Cytopathol 1999;21:364–366.
5. Anagnostopoulou I, Rammou-Kinia R, Likourinas M. Urine cytology evaluation in cases of uretero-ileal cutaneous diversion. Cytopathology 1995;6:268–272.
6. Boubenider S, Hiesse C, Marchand S, et al. Post-transplantation polyomavirus infections. J Nephrol 1999;12:24–29.
7. Bardales R. Infections and infestations of the urinary tract. In: Bardales R, ed. Practical urologic cytopathology. New York: Oxford University Press; 2002:53–87.
8. Gregg C, Rogers T, Munford R. Xanthogranulomatous pyelonephritis. Curr Clin Top Infect Dis 1999;19:287–304.
9. Bosch-Princep R, Salvado-Usach M, Martinez-Gonzalez S, et al. Xanthogranulomatous pyelonephritis: urinary and fine needle aspiration cytology [letter]. Acta Cytol 1998;42:1062–1064.
10. Masuda K, Akutagawa K, Yutani C, et al. Persistent infection with human polyomavirus revealed by urinary cytology in a patient with heart transplantation: a case report. Acta Cytol 1998;42:803–806.
11. Drachenberg C, Beskow C, Cangro C, et al. Human polyoma virus in renal allograft biopsies: morphological findings and correlation with urine cytology. Hum Pathol 1999;30:970–977.
12. Itano N, Malek R. Eosinophilic cystitis in adults. J Urol 2001;165:805–807.
13. Iczkowski K, Shanks J, Gadaleanu V, et al. Inflammatory pseudotumor and sarcoma of urinary bladder: differential diagnosis and outcome in thirty-eight spindle cell neoplasms. Mod Pathol 2001;14:1043–1051.
14. Young R. Pseudoneoplastic lesions of the urinary bladder and urethra: a selective review with emphasis on recent information. Semin Diagn Pathol 1997;14:133–146.
15. Schnadig V, Adesokan A, Neal D, et al. Urinary cytologic findings in patients with benign and malignant adenomatous polyps of the prostatic urethra. Arch Pathol Lab Med 2000;124:1047–1052.
16. Tse V, Khadra M, Eisinger D, et al. Nephrogenic adenoma of the bladder in renal transplant and non-renal transplant patients: a review of 22 cases. Urology 1997;50:690–696.
17. Skemp N, Fernandes E. Routine bladder biopsy after bacille Calmette-Guerin treatment: is it necessary? Urology 2002;59:224–226.
18. Saint F, Patard J, Irani J, et al. Leukocyturia as a predictor of tolerance and efficacy of intravesical BCG maintenance therapy for superficial bladder cancer. Urology 2001;57:617–621; discussion 621–622.
19. Mack D, Frick J. Diagnostic problems of urine cytology on initial follow-up after intravesical immunotherapy with Calmette-Guerin bacillus for superficial bladder cancer. Urol Int 1994;52:204–207.
20. Takashi M, Schenck U, Koshikawa T, et al. Cytological changes induced by intravesical bacillus Calmette-Guerin therapy for superficial bladder cancer. Urol Int 2000;64:74–81.
21. Bardales R. Primary tumors of the urinary tract. In: Bardales R, ed. Practical urologic cytopathology. New York: Oxford University Press; 2002:122–202.
22. Cheng L, Darson M, Cheville J, et al. Urothelial papilloma of the bladder: clinical and biologic implications. Cancer 1999;86:2098–2101.
23. Renshaw A. Subclassifying atypical urinary cytology specimens. Cancer 2000;90:222–229.
24. Epstein J, Amin M, Reuter V, et al. The World Health Organization/International Society of Urological Pathology consensus classification of urothelial (transitional cell) neoplasms of the urinary bladder. Bladder Consensus Conference Committee [see comments]. Am J Surg Pathol 1998;22:1435–1448.
25. Cheng L, Neumann R, Bostwick D. Papillary urothelial neoplasms of low malignant potential: clinical and biologic implications [see comments]. Cancer 1999;86:2102–2108.
26. Goldstein M, Whitman T, Renshaw A. Significance of cell groups in voided urine. Acta Cytol 1998;42:290–294.
27. Renshaw A, Nappi D, Weinberg D. Cytology of grade 1 papillary transitional cell carcinoma: a comparison of cytologic/architectural and morphometric criteria in cystoscopically obtained urine. Acta Cytol 1996;40:676–682.
28. Cheng L, Cheville JC, Neumann RM, et al. Natural history of urothelial dysplasia of the bladder. Am J Surg Pathol 1999;23:443–447.
29. Amin MB, Young RH. Intraepithelial lesions of the urinary bladder with a discussion of the histogenesis of urothelial neoplasia. Semin Diagn Pathol 1997;14:84–97.
30. Dodd LG, Johnston WW, Robertson CN, et al. Endoscopic brush cytology of the upper urinary tract: evaluation of its efficacy and potential limitations in diagnosis. Acta Cytol 1997;41:377–384.

31. Potts SA, Thomas PA, Cohen MB, et al. Diagnostic accuracy and key cytologic features of high-grade transitional cell carcinoma in the upper urinary tract. Mod Pathol 1997;10:657–662.
32. Eble JN, Young RH. Carcinoma of the urinary bladder: a review of its diverse morphology. Semin Diagn Pathol 1997;14:98–108.
33. Grignon DJ, Ro JY, Ayala AG, et al. Primary adenocarcinoma of the urinary bladder: a clinicopathologic analysis of 72 cases. Cancer 1991;67:2165–2172.
34. Yonekawa M, Hoshida Y, Hanai J, et al. Catheterized urine cytology of mucinous carcinoma arising in the renal pelvis: a case report. Acta Cytol 2000;44:442–444.
35. Ali SZ, Reuter VE, Zakowski MF. Small cell neuroendocrine carcinoma of the urinary bladder: a clinicopathologic study with emphasis on cytologic features. Cancer 1997;79:356–361.
36. Rudrick B, Nguyen GK, Lakey WH. Carcinoid tumor of the renal pelvis: report of a case with positive urine cytology. Diagn Cytopathol 1995;12: 360–363.
37. Bardales R. Secondary neoplasms of the urinary tract. In: Bardales R, ed. Practical urologic cytopathology. New York: Oxford University Press; 2002: 203–233.

10

RENAL PELVIS AND URETER

Maria M. Shevchuk and Myron Tannenbaum

NORMAL ANATOMY AND HISTOLOGY

Epithelium

The renal calyces, renal pelvis, and ureter are lined by urothelium, with surface umbrella cells similar to those of the bladder.

The lining, particularly of the pelvis, is frequently thrown into folds and deep crypt-like indentations. (Fig. 10.1)

A thin layer of loose connective tissue is present between urothelium and muscularis propria.[1]

Muscle

The pelvis and ureters are surrounded by a continuous muscle layer. It begins as small fascicles near the minor calyces and becomes a single layer with spiral architecture around the pelvis and ureter. Distally, the ureter acquires an external muscle coat from the bladder muscularis propria.[1] No muscle is present over the renal papilla, where urothelium is juxtaposed with renal medulla.

Outside the muscle, there are varying amounts of peripelvic and periureteral adipose tissue.

CONGENITAL MALFORMATIONS

CONGENITAL URETERAL ANOMALIES

The double ureter is the most common anomaly, seen in approximately 0.8% of autopsies. It is frequently associated with a double renal pelvis. Distally, the ureters may join to form a single vesicle orifice, or have two orifices into the bladder. Occasionally, one ureter, usually from the upper pole, implants extravesically.[2] (Figs 10.2 & 10.3)

Ureteral agenesis may be localized or associated with ipsilateral renal and hemitrigone agenesis.[2]

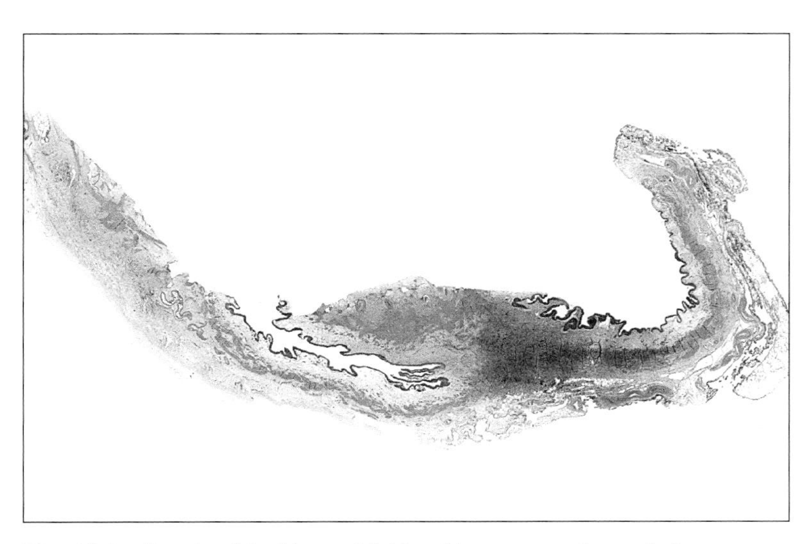

Fig. 10.1 Renal pelvis. Mucosal folds with attenuated muscle layers beneath the folds.

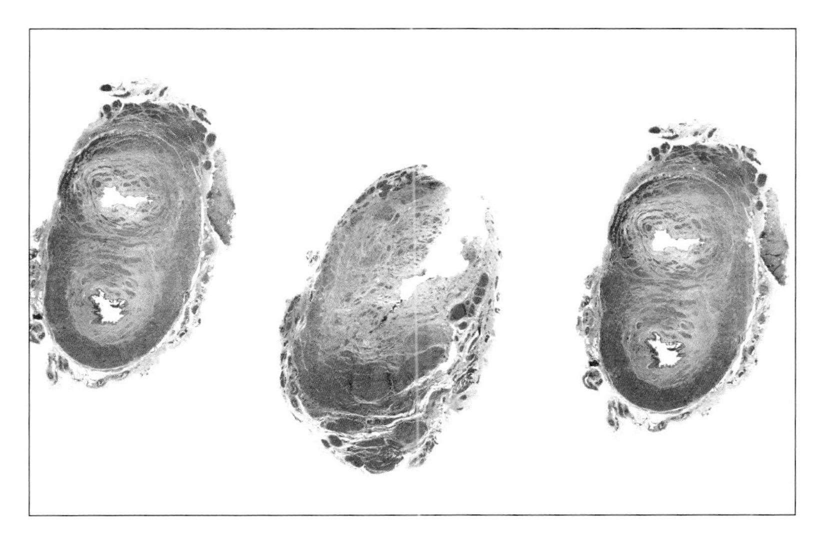

Fig. 10.2 Double ureter. There are complete muscle layers around each ureteral lumen.

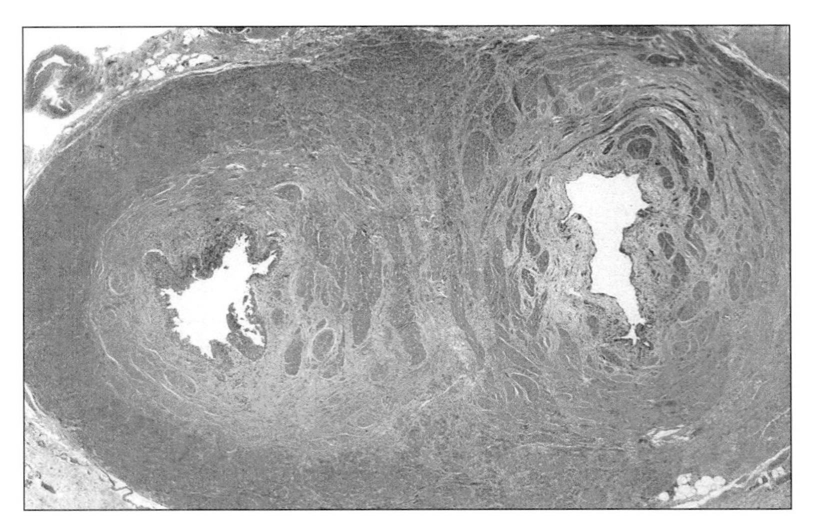

Fig. 10.3 Photomicrograph from a section of ureteral lumina from a double ureter. There are complete muscle layers around each ureteral lumen.

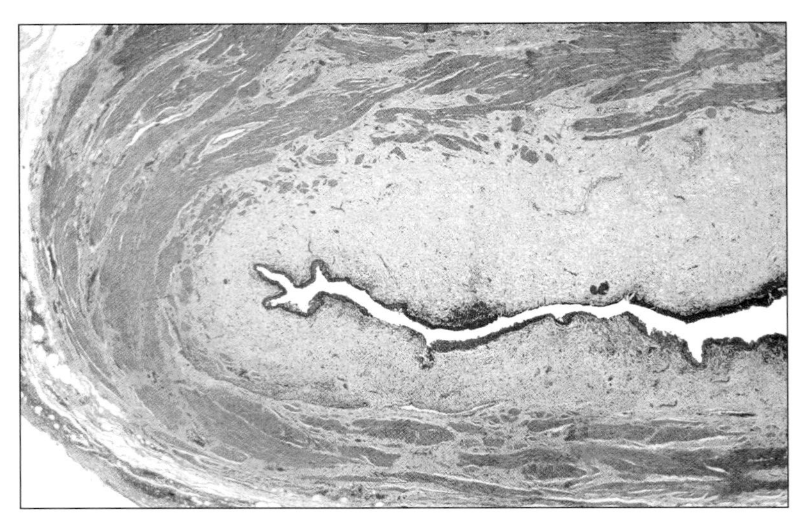

Fig. 10.4 Submucosal fibrosis surrounding the ureteral lumen, with intact urothelium and submucosal urothelial nests.

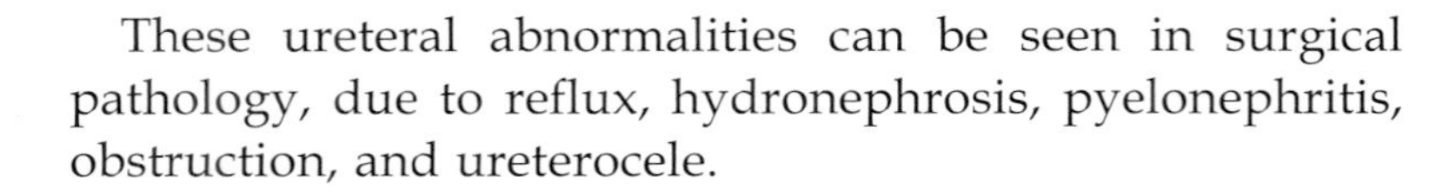

These ureteral abnormalities can be seen in surgical pathology, due to reflux, hydronephrosis, pyelonephritis, obstruction, and ureterocele.

MEGALOURETER

Refluxing megaloureter

Clinical This lesion is present in children with reflux and recurrent infections. The female to male ratio is 5:1.

Pathology There is a deficiency of longitudinal muscle fibers in the distal intramural segment of the ureter. This segment should be resected.[3]

Histology There is an absence or a thinning of the longitudinal muscle fibers, best seen in longitudinal section (especially with trichrome stain) of distal ureter. However, histologic diagnosis is difficult.

Primary megaloureter

Clinical This is a non-refluxing lesion.

Gross The distal ureter is narrow/normal with marked dilatation of the remaining proximal ureter.

Histology The distal segment is abnormal in most cases, and should be resected. There is either a preponderance of circular muscle, or a fibrosis of muscle and adventitia.[4,5] (Fig. 10.4)

URETERAL DYSPLASIA

Clinical These ureters may be atretic or dilated (primary megaloureter). In 50–70% of cases, they are associated with renal dysplasia.

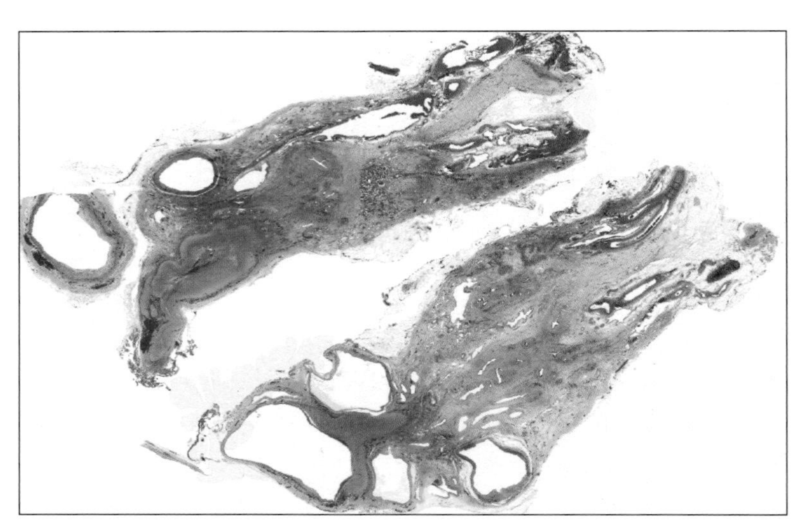

Fig. 10.5 Renal dysplasia. Abnormal renal pelvis and ureter with parenchymal fibrosis.

Pathology In most cases, the muscle is markedly thinned or lacking in the affected ureters.[5] (Figs 10.5–10.7)

URETEROCELE

A ureterocele is a congenital dilatation of the distal and intramural portion of the ureter, frequently deforming the trigone and sometimes resulting in obstruction or reflux.[6]

Histology There is usually atrophic or absent muscularis propria in the distal ureter, which may be associated with an adjacent segment of muscular hyperplasia.

OBSTRUCTION

Non-neoplastic ureteral obstruction can be intrinsic or extrinsic.

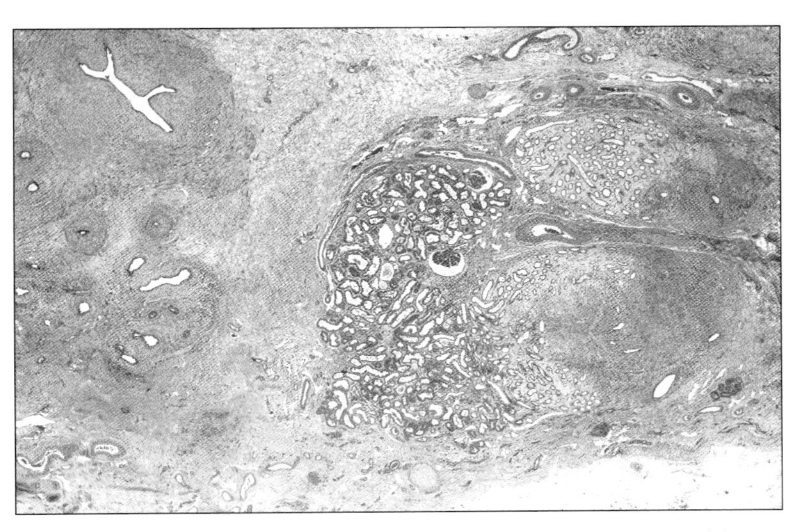

Fig. 10.6 Section of dysgenetic kidney with renal pelvis separated from renal parenchyma and with disconnected collecting system, fibrosis, and occasional foci of cartilage.

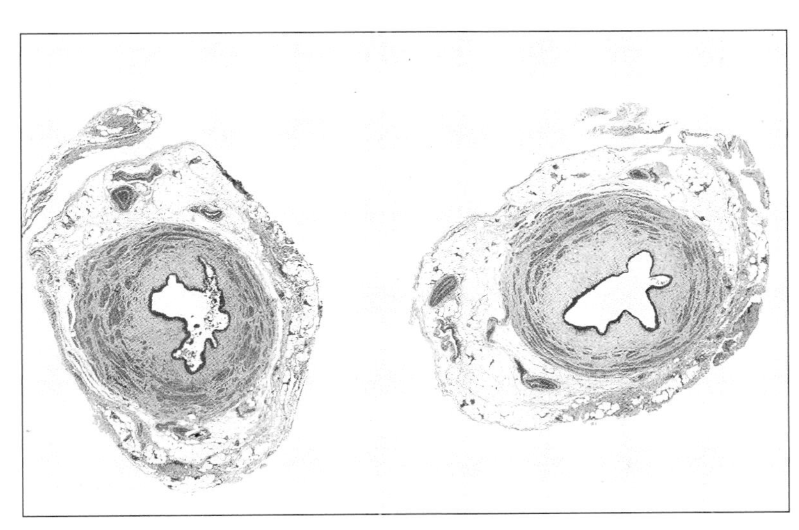

Fig. 10.8 Endoureteral fibrosis surrounds ureteral lumina.

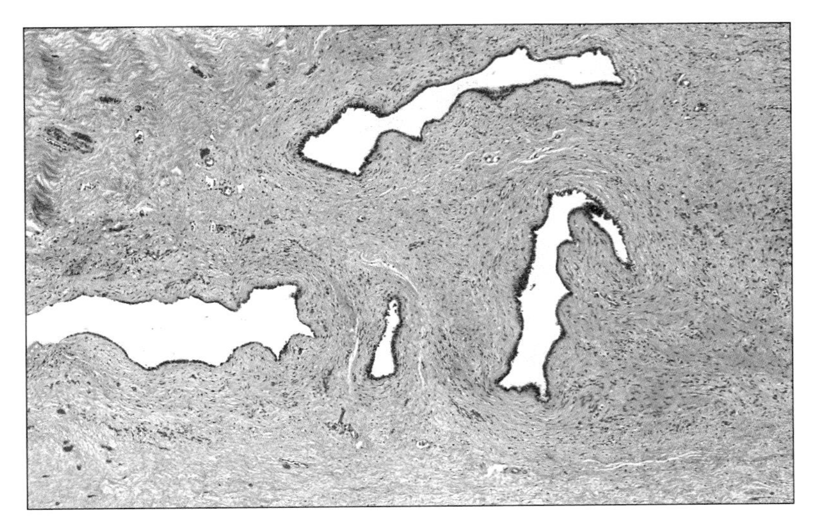

Fig. 10.7 Section of dysgenetic kidney with renal pelvis separated from renal parenchyma with fibrosis and scant muscle around calyceal system.

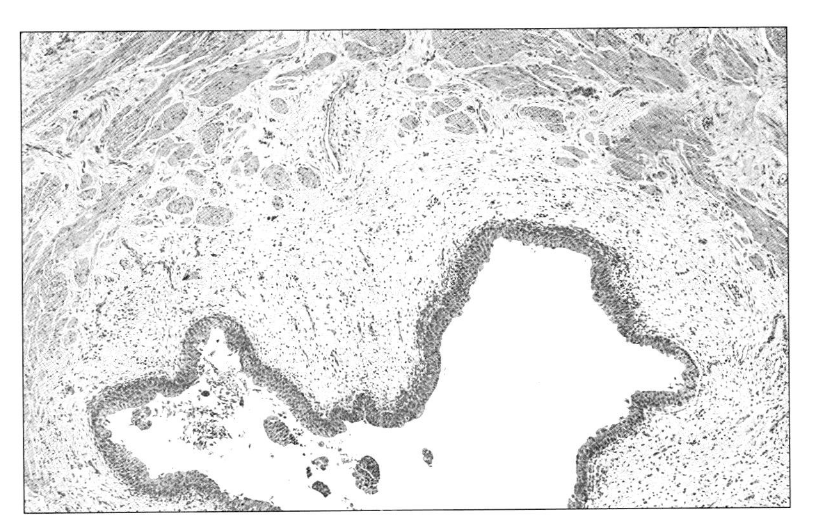

Fig. 10.9 Endoureteral fibrosis surrounds ureteral lumen. Portion of smooth muscle wall is above endoureteral fibrosis and ureteral lumen.

INTRINSIC OBSTRUCTION

The most common site of ureteral obstruction is the ureteropelvic junction.

Clinical Childhood ureteropelvic junction obstruction is frequently bilateral, or, if unilateral, more common on the left, and more common in boys. In adulthood, the lesion is more common in women and unilateral.[7]

Gross The ureteropelvic junction frequently contains a thickened area of stenosis with a funnel-like configuration proximally.

Histology The involved segment of ureter may have:

- smooth muscle thinning (usually with loss of the longitudinal fibers);
- focal loss of smooth muscle;
- mucosal valve or fold;[8]
- lamina propria and muscular fibrosis.

(Figs 10.8–10.14)

EXTRINSIC OBSTRUCTION

- Extrinsic causes of obstruction include: compression by vessels, usually abnormally located polar vessels in a nonrotated kidney.[9]
- Retroperitoneal fibrosis:[10,11]
  either idiopathic with/without Gartner's syndrome or secondary to retroperitoneal involvement by infections or tumors.[12] (Fig. 10.11)

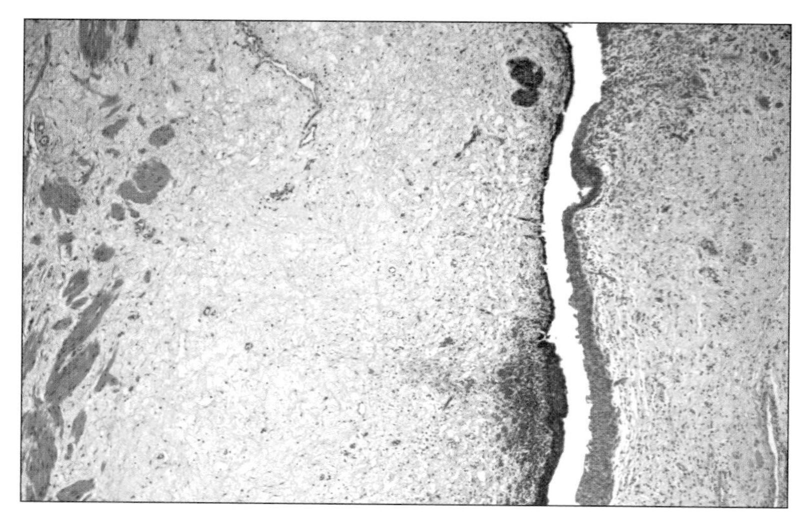

Fig. 10.10 Submucosal fibrosis with a submucosal urothelial nest in the fibrosis to the left of the ureteral lumen.

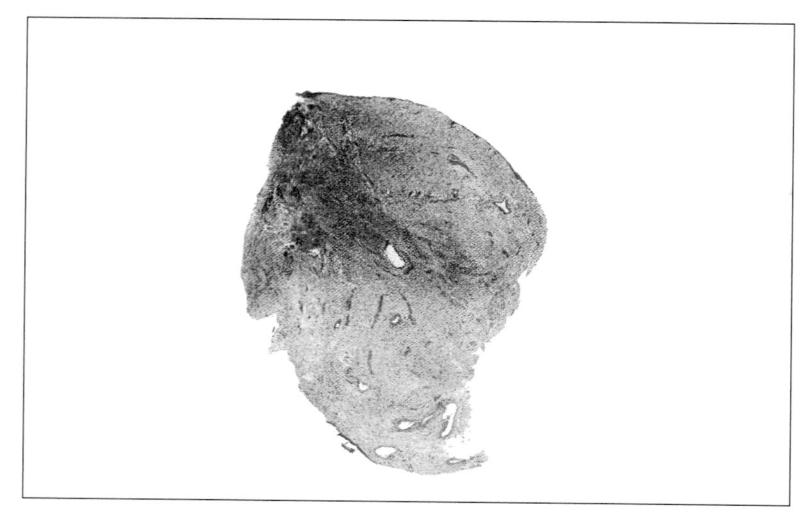

Fig. 10.11 Ureteral obstruction can be associated with infection, stones, as well as tumors. This ureter shows marked fibrosis of its wall and involvement by tumor.

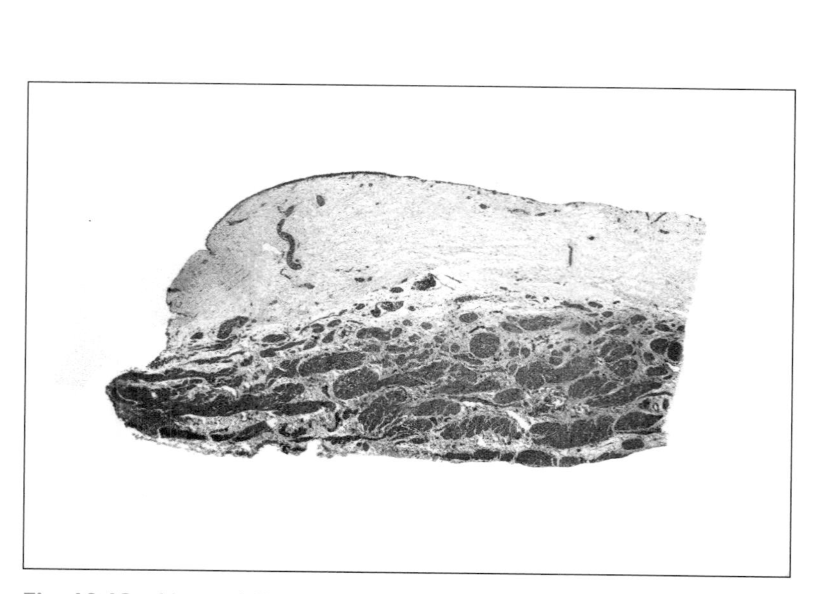

Fig. 10.12 Ureteral fibrosis at the ureteropelvic junction can cause obstruction. There are also submucosal fibrosis and von Brunn's nests in the submucosal connective tissue.

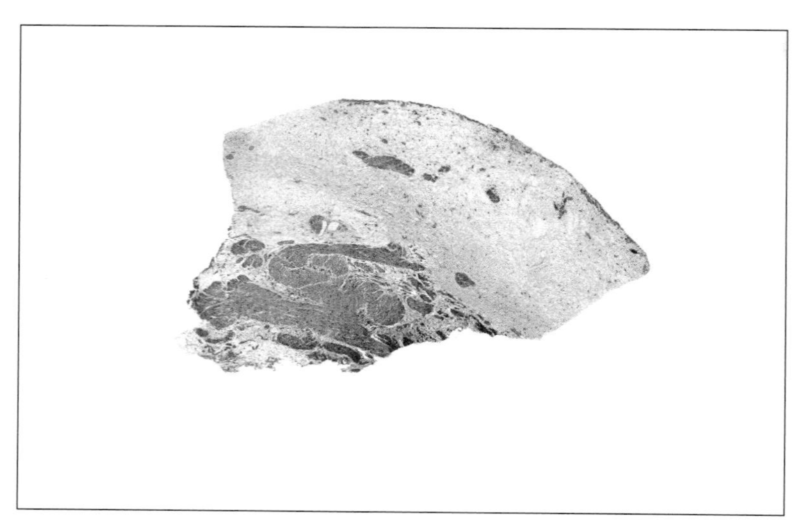

Fig. 10.13 Ureteral fibrosis at the ureteropelvic junction can cause obstruction. There are also submucosal fibrosis and von Brunn's nests.

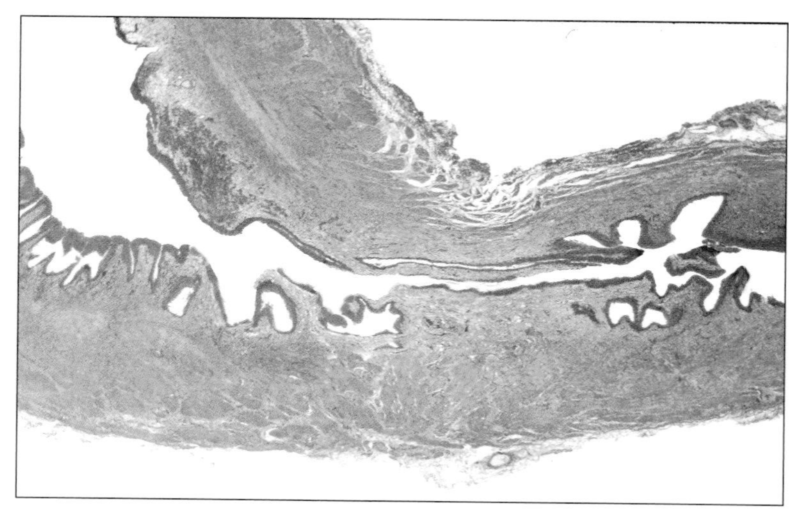

Fig. 10.14 Ureteropelvic junction proximal to the ureteral stenosis. Note the pyelitis cystica and the complex invaginations of urothelium.

Idiopathic retroperitoneal fibrosis

Gross Frequently, there is medial deviation of the ureter on radiologic examination. The ureter and vessels are encased in firm fibrotic tissue.

Histology There are varying amounts of fibrosis with collagen deposition. In areas, the lesion shows a chronic inflammatory infiltrate, consisting predominantly of lymphocytes and plasma cells with occasional lymphoid nodule formation. Stromal edema can also be seen.

INFLAMMATORY LESIONS

MALAKOPLAKIA

Clinical Malakoplakia is associated with recurrent infections. It is less common in the pelvis and ureter than in the kidney.

Histology Malakoplakia is a granulomatous inflammation with large eosinophilic histiocytes (von Hansemann cells) containing intracytoplasmic Michaelis–Gutmann bodies, which are positive for periodic acid–Schiff (PAS), iron, and calcium.[13,14]

NEPHROLITHIASIS

Clinical Nephrolithiasis is associated with many conditions, including metabolic diseases, obstruction, and infections.[15]

Stone types
- Calcium-containing (most common).
- Struvite (most often seen in staghorn calculi).
- Uric acid.
- Cystine.
- Matrix stone.

STONE GRANULOMA

Clinical Stone granuloma usually follows ureteroscopy and stone fragmentation.

Histology Stone fragments are imbedded in the ureteral wall, with histiocytes and foreign body giant cells.[16]

PROLIFERATIVE AND TUMOR-LIKE LESIONS

VON BRUNN'S NESTS

These nest-like invaginations of the urothelium are common in the renal pelvis and ureter. Although often considered normal, they tend to be more numerous in patients with renal and ureteral pathology, and are probably a reactive change.

Histology Von Brunn's nests in the upper tracts can differ from those of the bladder. They are frequently smaller and more irregular in shape. (See Figs 10.10, 10.15, 10.16 & 10.18)

Practical point Since von Brunn's nests in the upper tracts can be smaller and more irregular, it is harder to distinguish them from invasive urothelial carcinoma, when both are present in the same tissue. Von Brunn's nests can be distinguished from nests of invasive carcinoma mainly by their benign cytology and by comparing them to other similar von Brunn's nests in the specimen. (Figs 10.17 & 10.18)

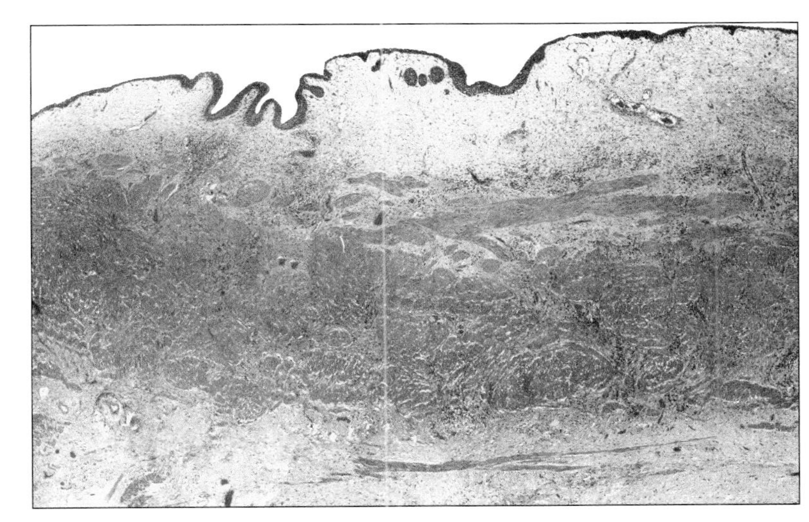

Fig. 10.15 Von Brunn's urothelial nests can be seen in submucosal tissue in the upper middle portions of this low-power photomicrograph.

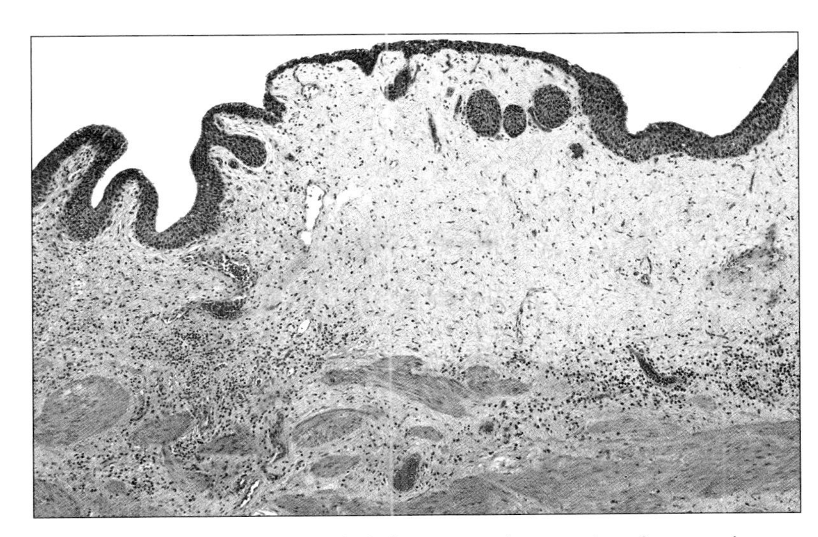

Fig. 10.16 Von Brunn's urothelial nests can be seen in submucosal tissue in the upper middle portions of this medium-power photomicrograph.

PYELITIS AND URETERITIS CYSTICA

Von Brunn's nests can develop a central lumen, and the lining cells can undergo metaplasia to glandular cells.[17,18]

The diagnosis of pyelitis and ureteritis cystica covers the whole spectrum of change, and the term glandularis is not necessary, although it can be added to emphasize extensive glandular metaplasia.

Gross In the renal pelvis and ureter, pyelitis or ureteritis cystica can present as nodules (similar to those in the

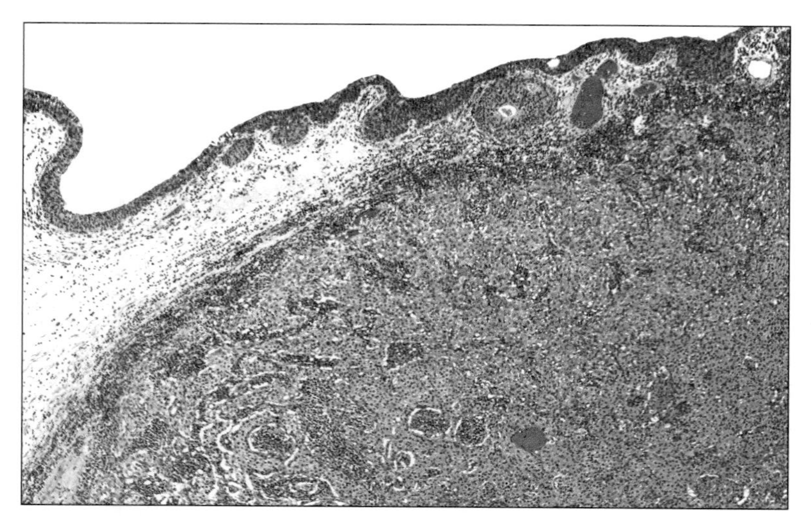

Fig. 10.17 In this specimen, urothelial carcinoma in situ involves von Brunn's nests. There is adjacent invasive carcinoma.

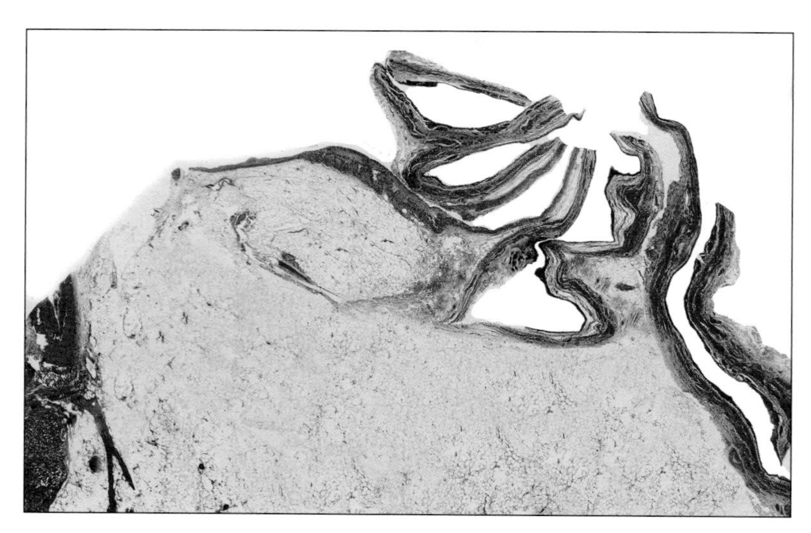

Fig. 10.19 Complex pyelitis cystica.

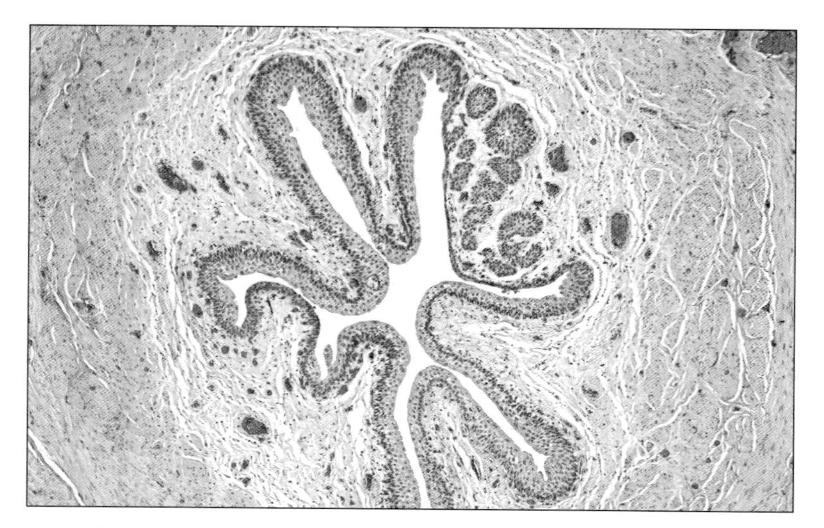

Fig. 10.18 Von Brunn's nests can be seen in submucosal tissue in the upper right-hand corner of this low-power photomicrograph. Note the irregular shapes and sizes of these benign urothelial nests.

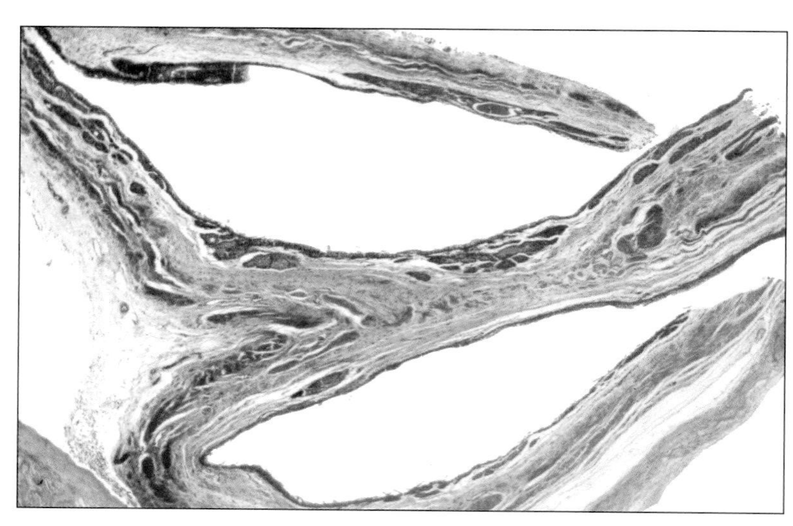

Fig. 10.20 Complex pyelitis cystica. There are submucosal urothelial nests and branching.

bladder), but in the upper tracts a characteristic gross appearance of these lesions is that of blister-like, clear fluid-filled subepithelial cysts.

Histology The lesions of pyelitis and ureteritis cystica range from small cysts lined by multilayered urothelial cells, through urothelial-lined cysts with luminal cells showing glandular metaplasia, to cysts lined exclusively by glandular cells, sometimes of intestinal type.

The large cysts of pyelitis and ureteritis cystica are usually lined by a few layers of urothelial cells with pressure atrophy of the luminal cell layer. (Figs 10.14, 10.19–10.21)

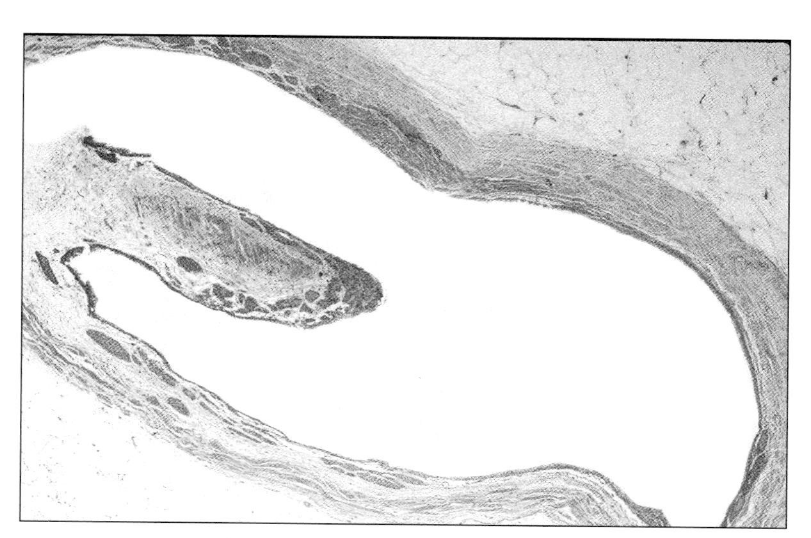

Fig. 10.21 Complex pyelitis cystica. There are submucosal urothelial nests and branching.

UROTHELIAL HYPERPLASIA

Urothelial hyperplasia is an increased number of cells, and is usually a reactive change.

METAPLASIA

Squamous metaplasia

Clinical Squamous metaplasia is associated with long-standing infections, and particularly with stone disease.

- *Nonkeratinizing* squamous metaplasia is reactive and is not known to pose a significant risk of carcinoma.
- *Keratinizing* squamous metaplasia is more common, and is associated with an increased risk of squamous cell carcinoma of the renal pelvis and ureter.
- *Leukoplakia* is squamous metaplasia with a thick layer of keratin (hyperkeratosis), which appears as a thick white plaque.[19,20]
- *Cholesteatoma* is a localized collection of keratin from keratinizing squamous metaplasia.[20]

Practical point If keratinizing squamous metaplasia is diagnosed, the rest of the specimen should be examined carefully to exclude carcinoma, and the patient needs to be followed.

Glandular metaplasia

Glandular metaplasia is usually of the intestinal type. It is rather uncommon in the pelvis and even more so in the ureter. However, it is seen adjacent to adenocarcinoma of these organs.[18,21]

BENIGN NEOPLASMS

FIBROEPITHELIAL POLYP

Clinical Fibroepithelial polyps are benign lesions, probably acquired, which may present as pelvic/calyceal masses or as ureteral obstruction.

Histology Fibroepithelial polyps are urothelial-lined fibrous proliferations. The fibrous component can consist of loose connective tissues, be variably collagenized, and contain varying amounts of smooth muscle and blood vessels.

Occasionally, instead of a single polyp, there are multiple polypoid projections of the mucosa, known as *polypoid ureteritis* and *pyelitis*.[22,23] (Figs 10.22–10.26)

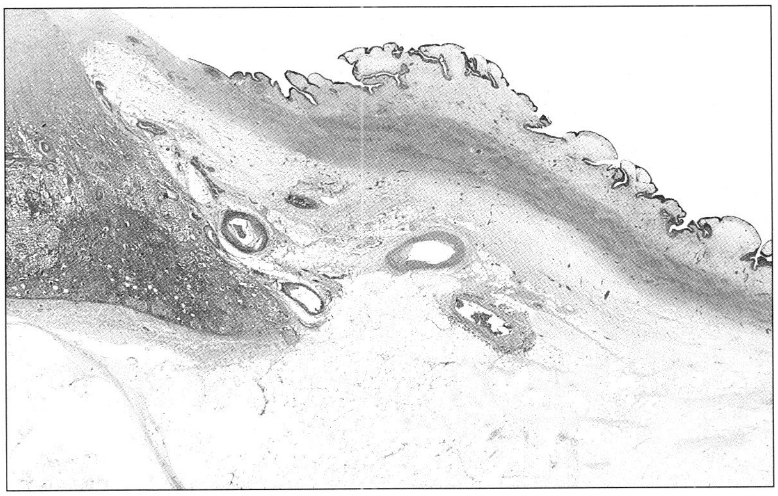

Fig. 10.22 Low-power photomicrograph of luminal surface with multiple small fibroepithelial polyps (upper half). Tumor is present in the renal pelvis at the left. In the same slide, at higher magnification (Fig. 10.23), there is papillary hyperplasia with mild urothelial atypia. The gross appearance is similar to that found in polypoid cystitis.

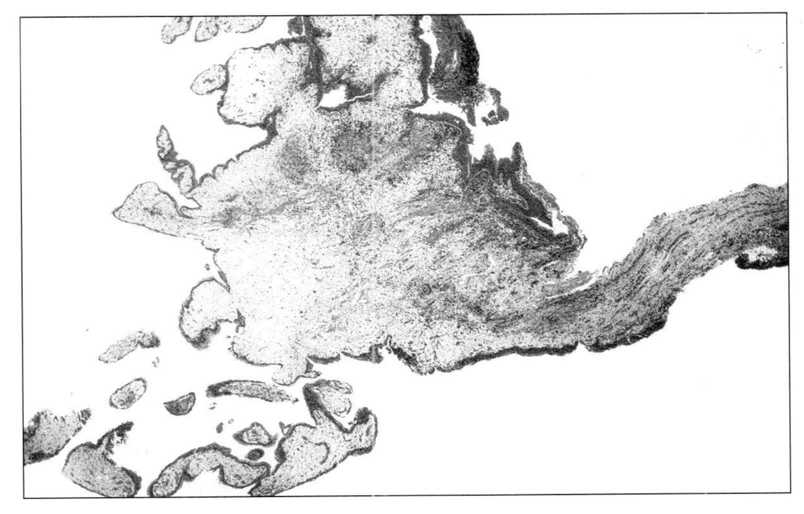

Fig. 10.23 Fibroepithelial polyp with inflammation.

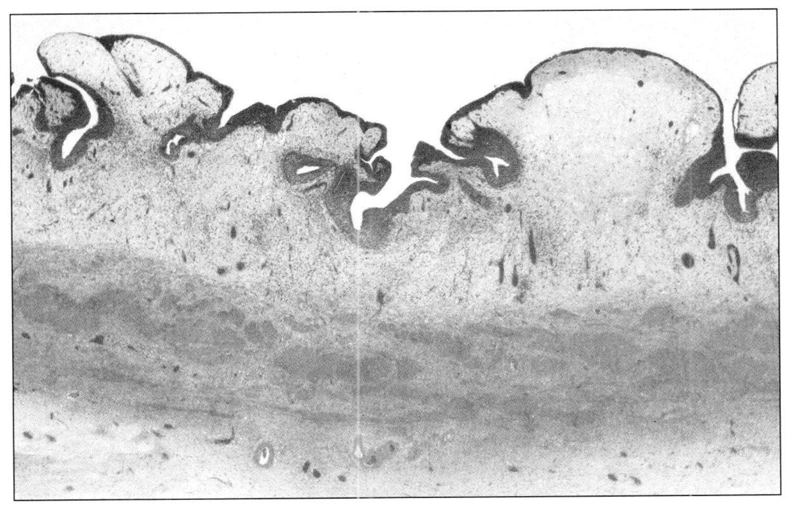

Fig. 10.24 Polypoid lesions with mild urothelial atypia. The appearance is similar to that found in polypoid cystitis.

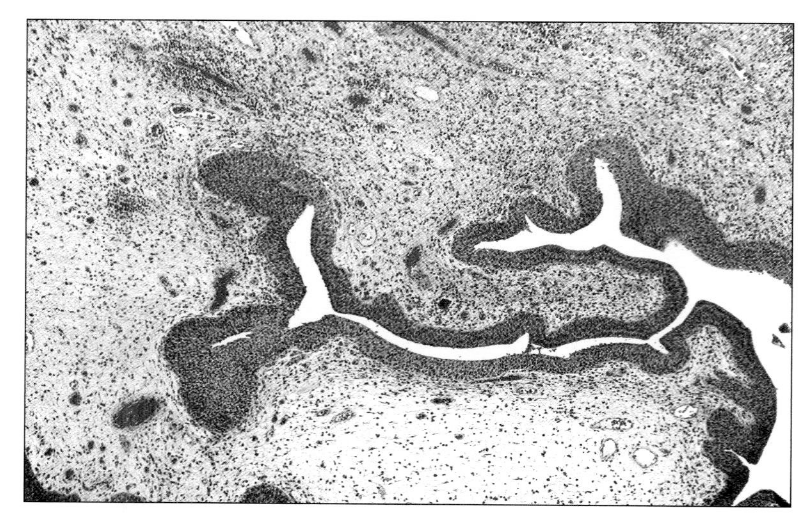

Fig. 10.25 Polypoid lesions with mild urothelial atypia. The appearance is similar to that seen in polypoid cystitis.

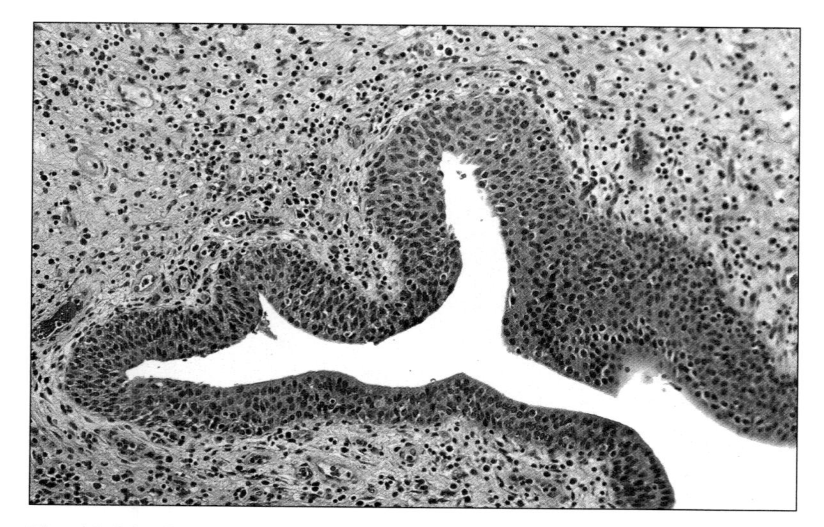

Fig. 10.26 Polypoid lesions with mild urothelial atypia. The appearance is similar to that seen in polypoid cystitis.

NEPHROGENIC ADENOMA

Clinical Nephrogenic adenoma is much less common in the upper urinary tract than in the bladder.

Gross This lesion frequently appears as an exophytic lesion.

Histology Nephrogenic adenoma consists of benign cuboidal or hobnail cells in a papillary or tubular configuration.[24–26]

CYSTIC HAMARTOMA

Cystic hamartoma is a multicystic lesion of the renal pelvis and calyces.[27]

Histology Cystic hamartoma is a benign biphasic lesion with the following components:

- the epithelial component consists of cuboidal or columnar cells forming tubules and cysts;
- the stromal component is predominantly fibroblastic, but may contain smooth muscle.

UROTHELIAL PAPILLOMA

Clinical Papilloma is a rare small benign lesion.

Histology Urothelial papilloma consists of a fibrovascular core lined by a layer of benign urothelial cells that is of normal thickness.[28] (Fig. 10.31)

Practical point Just as in the bladder, urothelial papilloma of the pelvis or ureter is rare, and care must be taken not to misdiagnose a low-grade papillary carcinoma as papilloma.

INVERTED PAPILLOMA

Clinical Inverted papilloma is a benign tumor that is less common in the ureter than in the bladder, and less common still in the pelvis. The lesion is more often seen in men, with a mean age in the sixties. Patients can present with hematuria.

Gross Inverted papilloma grossly resembles a carcinoma and can be multifocal.

Histology The tumor consists of interconnecting trabeculae of benign-appearing urothelial cells extending into the lamina propria. Glandular change can be focally present.[29–31]

Inverted papilloma can be associated with a urothelial carcinoma in adjacent structures, or rarely it can evolve into a carcinoma, especially in the ureter.[32,33]

RARE BENIGN LESIONS

- *Pelvic lipomatosis* consists of excessive proliferation of peripelvic adipose tissue.[34]
- *Amyloid tumor* is a nodular collection of amyloid, present in the ureteral wall.[35]
- *Hemangioma*, *leiomyoma*, *neurofibroma*, and *myofibroblastic tumor* can be seen in the renal pelvis and ureter.[36,37]

MALIGNANT NEOPLASMS

Urothelial dysplasia and *carcinoma in situ* of the renal pelvis and ureter are similar to these lesions in the bladder. However, in the upper tracts, they are usually in specimens with a urothelial carcinoma. They are concentrated in areas adjacent to the invasive carcinoma, but can also represent separate satellite lesions. In such cases, there is an increased risk of tumors elsewhere in the urothelial tract.[38,39]

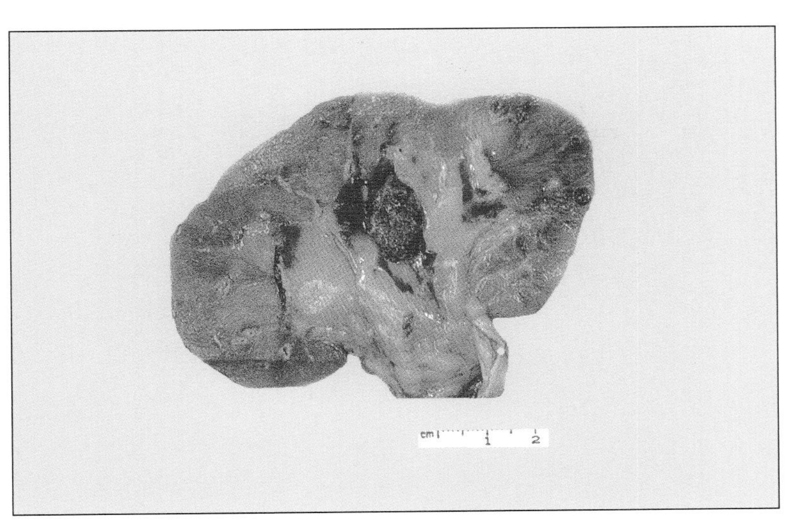

Fig. 10.27 Papillary urothelial carcinoma. This appearance is similar to that seen in papillary urothelial carcinoma of the urinary bladder.

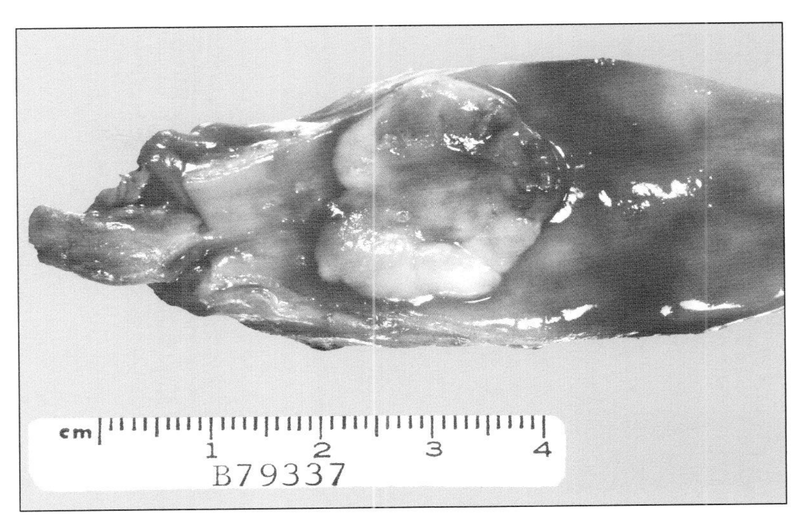

Fig. 10.29 Papillary urothelial carcinoma in the lower third of the ureter, near the bladder cuff. This appearance is similar to that seen in papillary urothelial carcinomas of the urinary bladder.

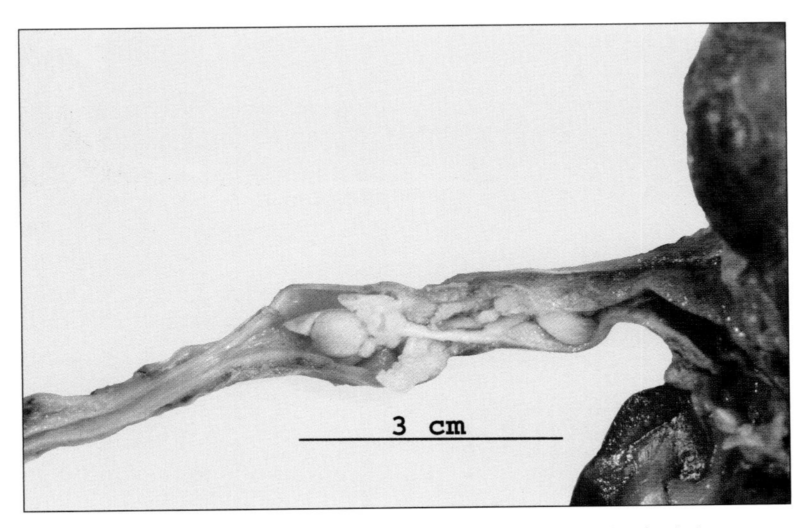

Fig. 10.28 Papillary urothelial carcinoma in the upper third of the ureter. This appearance is similar to that seen in papillary urothelial carcinoma of the urinary bladder.

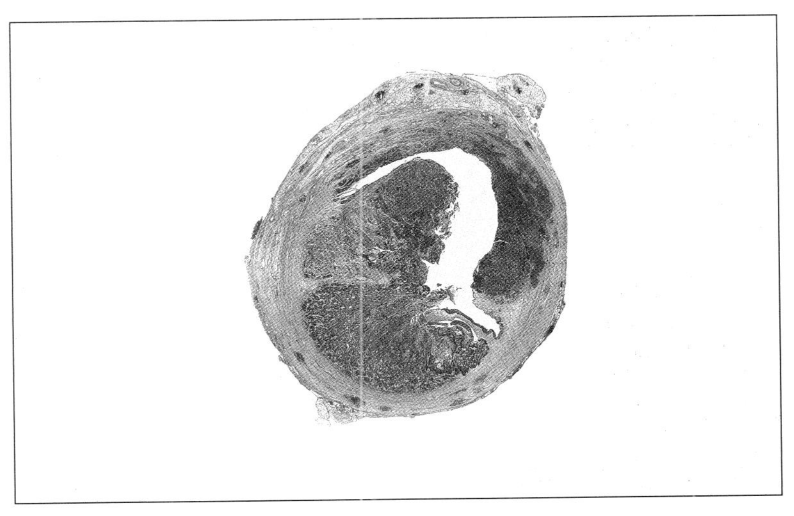

Fig. 10.30 Cross-section of papillary urothelial carcinoma in the upper third of the ureter. It is invasive into the wall of the ureter, causing obstruction.

Because of the multifocal nature of the urothelial neoplasia, representative sections should be taken from the entire urothelial tract, including grossly uninvolved areas of the renal pelvis/calyces and ureter.

UROTHELIAL CARCINOMA

Epidemiology Some risk factors for urothelial carcinoma of the upper urinary tracts are similar to those for bladder: smoking, chemical carcinogens, and cyclophosphamide. Other factors are more specific for the upper tract: analagesic abuse, Thorotrast radiologic contrast material, and Balkan nephropathy.[40–42]

Clinical Fifty percent of patients with renal pelvic or ureteral urothelial carcinomas also have other lesions in the urinary tract at some time. For this reason, a nephroureterectomy should include the bladder cuff with the intramural portion of the ureter.[43]

Symptoms include hematuria and flank pain.

Gross Ureteral tumors are usually exophytic and obstructive lesions, resulting in hydronephrosis. Renal pelvic or calyceal tumors can cause segmental obstruction with hydronephrosis, or grow in an endophytic fashion into the renal parenchyma. (Figs 10.27–10.30)

Histology Renal pelvic and ureteral tumors are graded like bladder tumors.[28,44] The microscopic spectrum includes all the variants of urothelial carcinoma, and there may be focal *squamous, glandular, sarcomatoid, small cell, micropapillary, osteoclastic, rhabdoid,* and *trophoblastic change.*[44] Urothelial dysplasia and carcinoma in situ adjacent to the invasive tumor helps to identify it as urothelial in difficult cases.

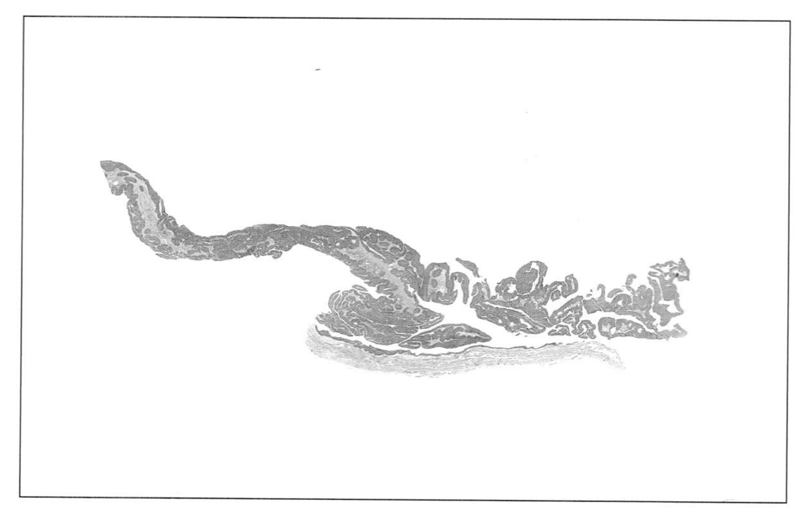

Fig. 10.31 Ureteral papillary tumor: papilloma. There is a stalk in the left of the photomicrograph and submucosal urothelial nests and extensions in the wall of the ureter (bottom of photomicrograph). The whole section must be observed under higher magnification in order to rule out a higher grade of urothelial neoplasia.

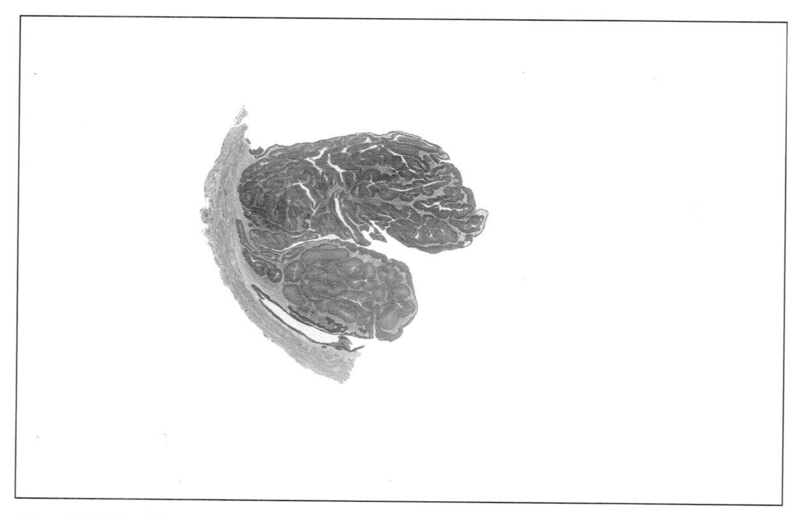

Fig. 10.32 Ureteral papillary tumor: low-grade carcinoma. There is fusion of the papillary tumor stalks. In the left of the photomicrograph, there is the wall of the ureter. There is no invasion of the wall.

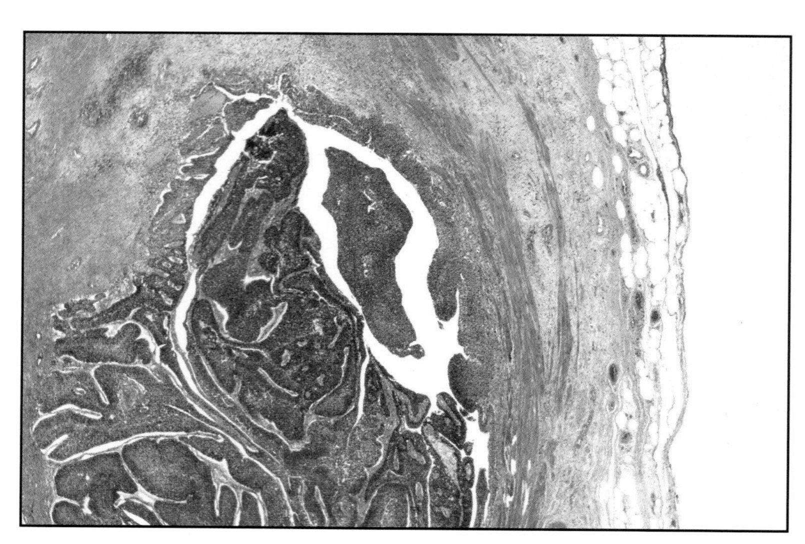

Fig. 10.33 Ureteral papillary tumor: low-grade carcinoma. There is fusion of the papillary tumor stalks, and invasion into the wall of the ureter. Almost complete luminal obstruction was noted on pyelography. Low-power photomicrograph.

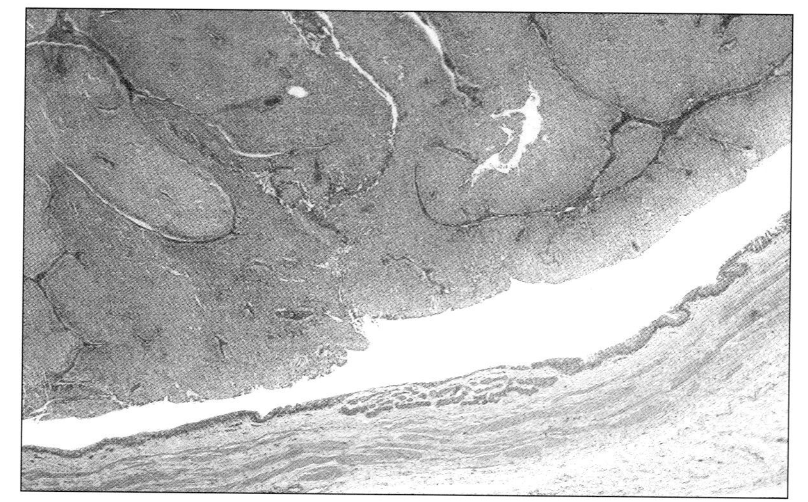

Fig. 10.34 Ureteral papillary tumor: low-grade carcinoma. There is fusion of the papillary tumor stalks (upper two-thirds of photomicrograph), and the urothelial lining of the ureteral lumen has von Brunn's nests and urothelial extensions (lower third). Almost complete blockage of the ureteral lumen was noted on pyelography.

Urothelial carcinoma of the renal pelvis frequently extends into the collecting ducts in an in-situ fashion. (Figs 10.32–10.59)

Immunohistochemistry can be helpful in identifying tumors as urothelial. Recent studies indicate that uroplakin III is a specific marker for urothelial tumors, but it is present in only about 50% of cases. Thrombomodulin, CK903 (34βE12), CK7, and CK20 are not specific for urothelial carcinoma, but are useful because they are present in 69%, 80%, 100%, and 48% of cases, respectively. A panel incorporating some or all of these markers may be supportive of urothelial origin.[45]

Practical point The prognosis of renal pelvic and ureteral carcinomas is strongly correlated with stage, especially with invasion of muscularis. This is more difficult to diagnose in the upper tracts than in the bladder, because of their anatomy. The muscular layer is much thinner in the upper tract and can more easily be replaced by a desmoplastic fibrotic response. Further difficulties arise from the irregular folded contour of the pelvic and ureteral surfaces. One should not mistake a papillary, noninvasive tumor within a tissue fold as invasive carcinoma. Another pitfall is the presence of numerous irregular von Brunn's nests, which are frequently present underneath in situ carcinoma. These must be distinguished from nests of invasive

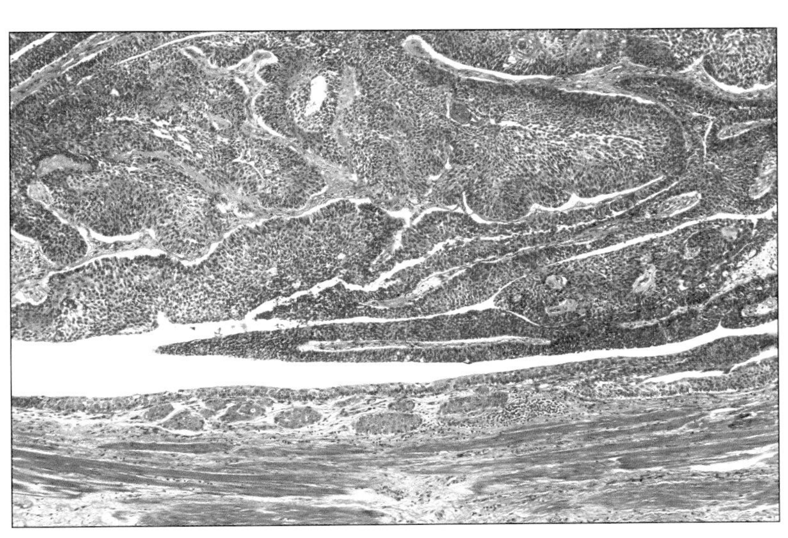

Fig. 10.35 Ureteral papillary tumor: high-grade carcinoma. There is fusion of the papillary tumor stalks (upper two-thirds of photomicrograph), and the urothelial lining (lower third) is dysplastic, with von Brunn's nest involvement by urothelial dysplasia.

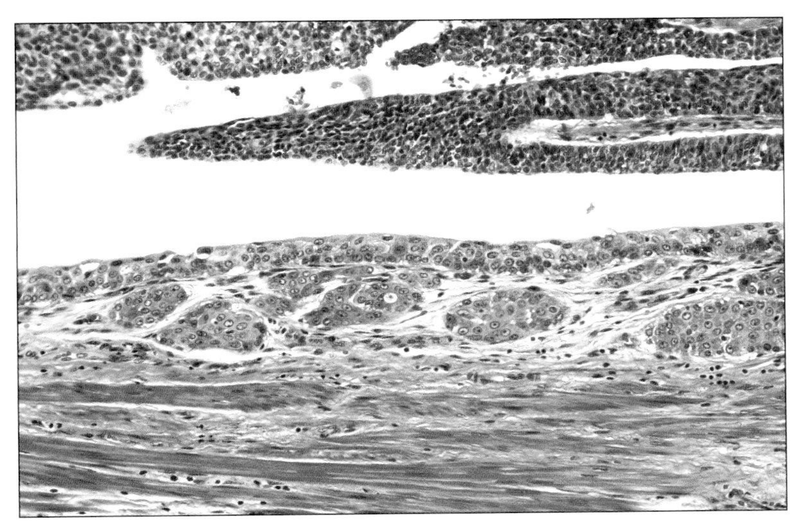

Fig. 10.36 Higher magnification of Fig. 10.35.

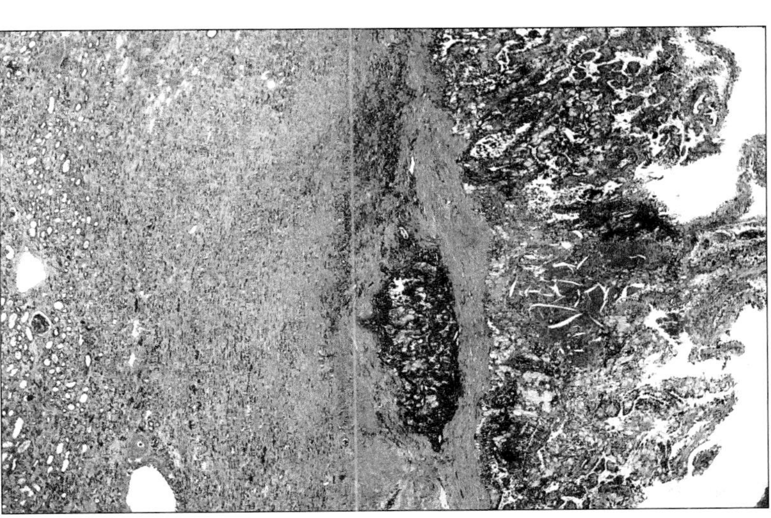

Fig. 10.37 Papillary urothelial carcinoma, low grade (right side of photomicrograph) with parenchymal invasion (mid photomicrograph). This appearance is similar to that seen in papillary urothelial carcinoma of the urinary bladder.

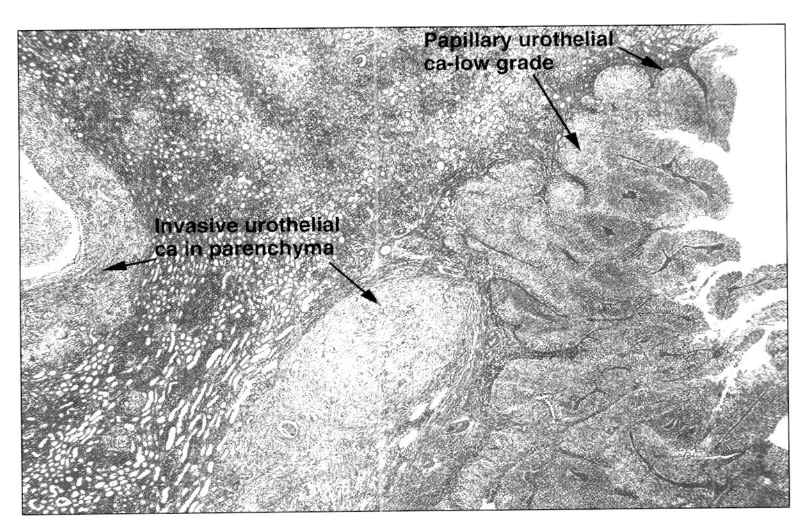

Fig. 10.38 Papillary urothelial carcinoma, low grade (arrows, right side) with parenchymal invasion (arrows, mid photomicrograph) of tubules and lymphatics.

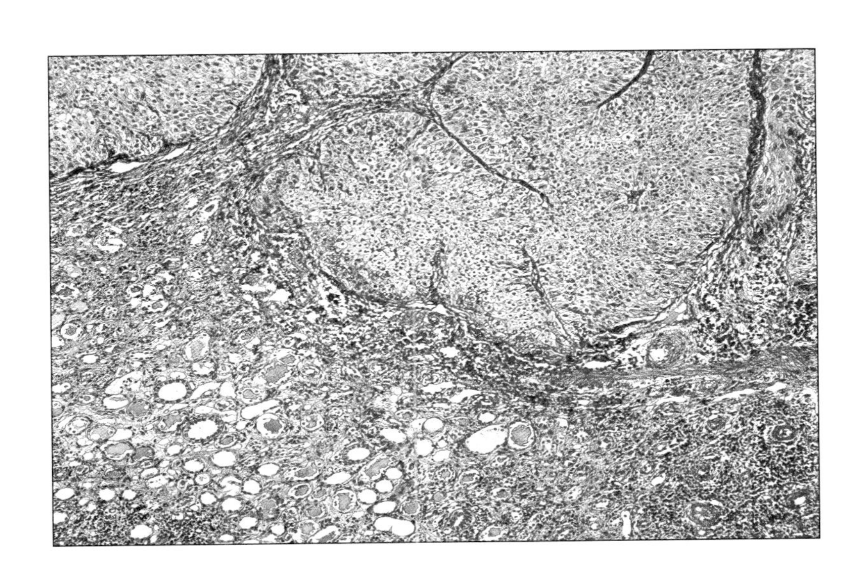

Fig. 10.39 Papillary urothelial carcinoma, high grade (upper half of photomicrograph) with chronic pyelonephritis (lower half).

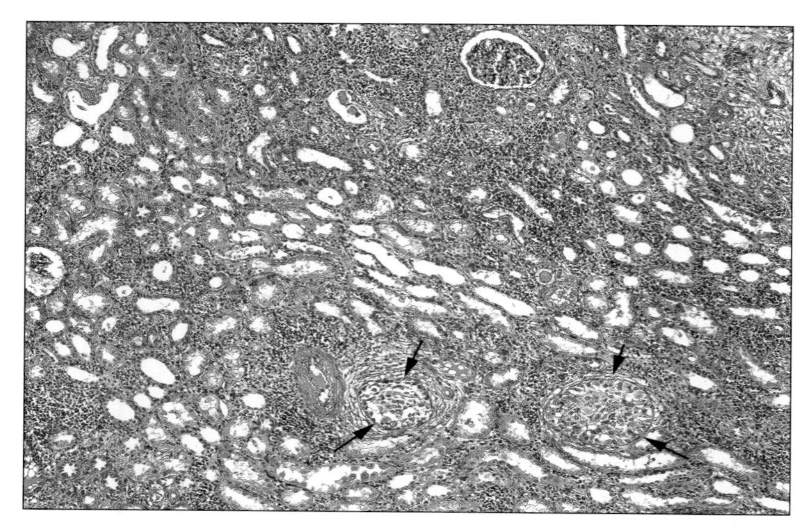

Fig. 10.40 Parenchymal invasion by urothelial cancer (arrows) of renal tubules and lymphatics.

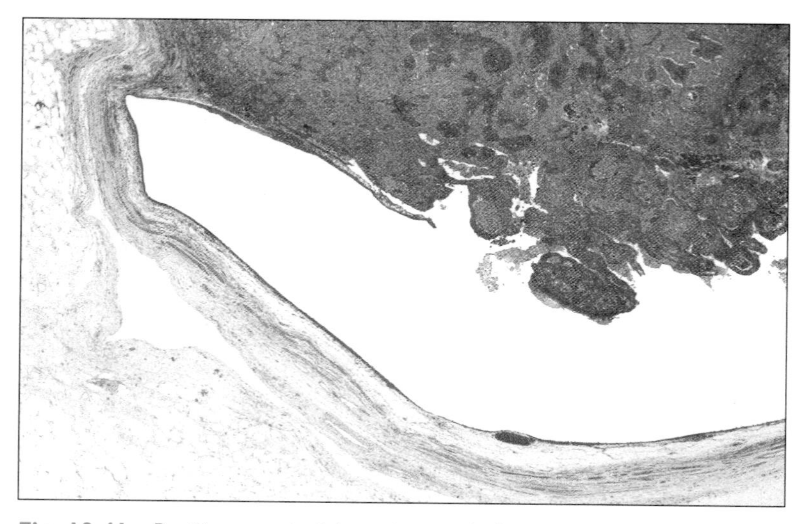

Fig. 10.41 Papillary urothelial carcinoma, high grade, with an endophytic growth pattern (upper half of photomicrograph). There are fused neoplastic urothelial nests beneath the urothelial mucosa of the renal pelvis.

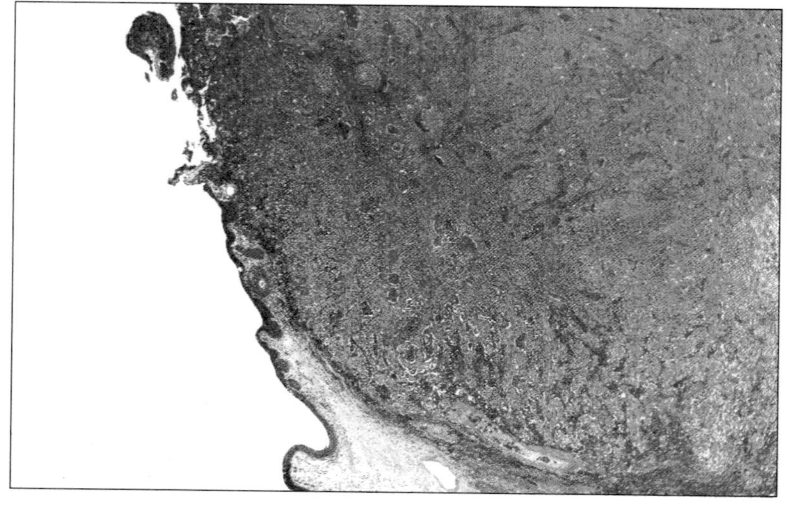

Fig. 10.42 Papillary urothelial carcinoma, high grade, with an exophytic and endophytic growth pattern (right two-thirds of photomicrograph). There are neoplastic urothelial nests beneath the urothelial mucosa of the renal pelvis (left third).

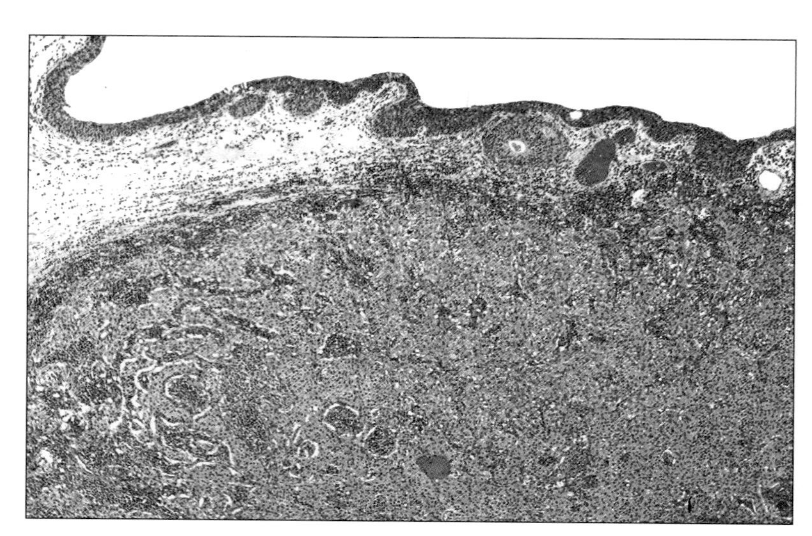

Fig. 10.43 Higher magnification of urothelial carcinoma, high grade, with an endophytic growth pattern (lower two-thirds of photomicrograph). There is urothelial carcinoma in situ of renal pelvis mucosa with involvement of underlying von Brunn's nests (upper third).

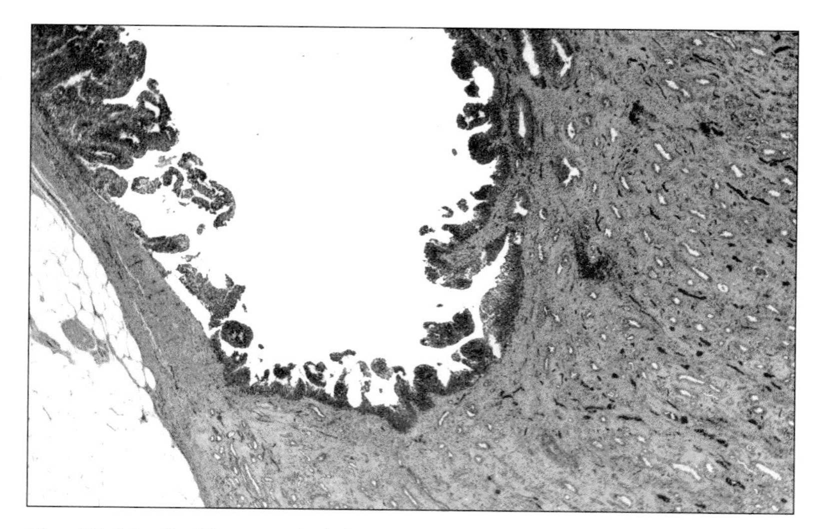

Fig. 10.44 Papillary urothelial carcinoma, low grade, with an exophytic growth pattern (left two-thirds); renal parenchyma (right) with focal intraepithelial involvement of collecting ducts.

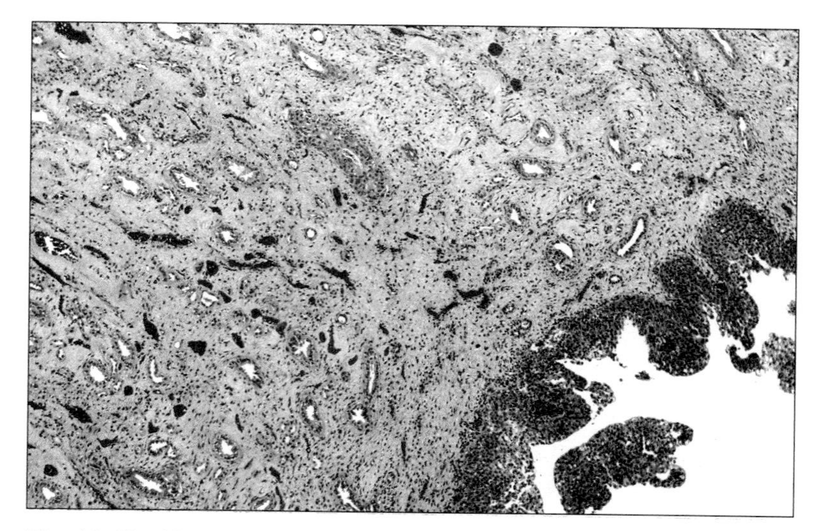

Fig. 10.45 Higher magnification of papillary urothelial carcinoma, low grade, with an exophytic growth pattern (right third of photomicrograph); renal parenchyma (left) with focal intramucosal collecting duct involvement.

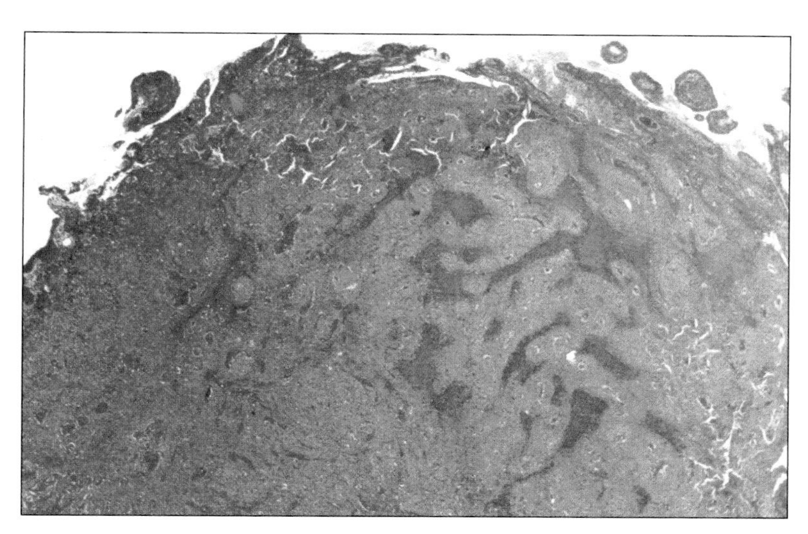

Fig. 10.46 Papillary urothelial carcinoma, high grade, with an exophytic (upper third of photomicrograph) and endophytic (lower two-thirds) growth pattern.

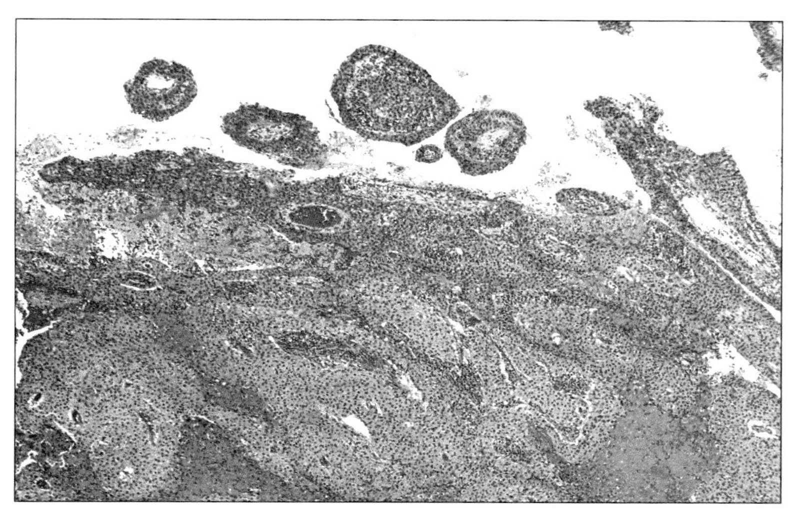

Fig. 10.47 Papillary urothelial carcinoma, high grade, with an exophytic (upper third of photomicrograph) and endophytic (lower two-thirds) growth pattern.

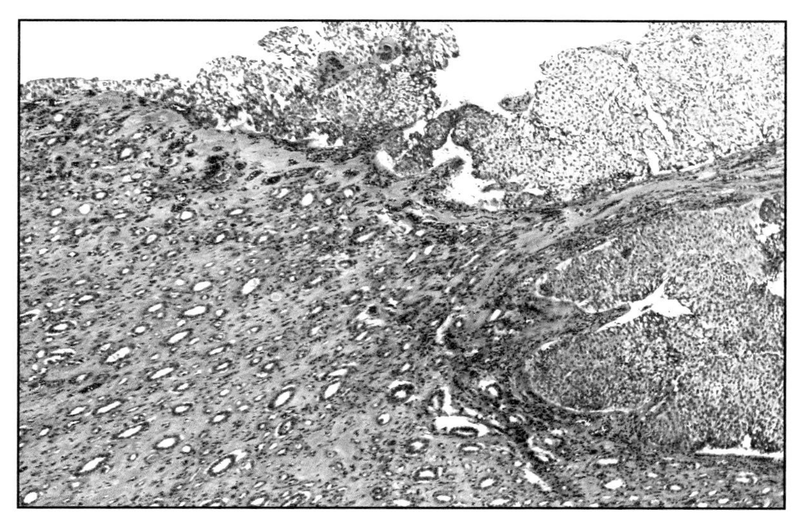

Fig. 10.48 Papillary urothelial carcinoma, low grade, with an exophytic growth pattern (right half of photomicrograph); renal parenchyma (left) with no tubular involvement.

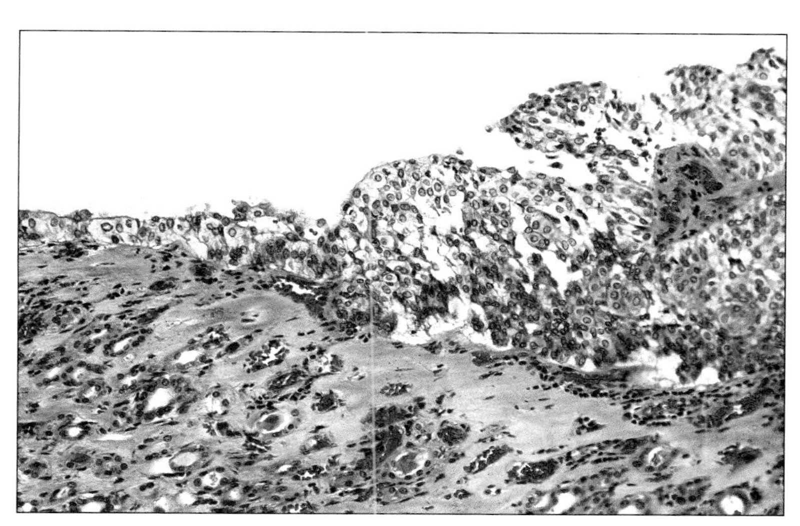

Fig. 10.49 Higher magnification of Fig. 10.48, showing a papillary urothelial carcinoma, low grade, with an exophytic growth pattern (right half of photomicrograph). There is renal parenchyma in the lower half, with no tubular involvement by tumor.

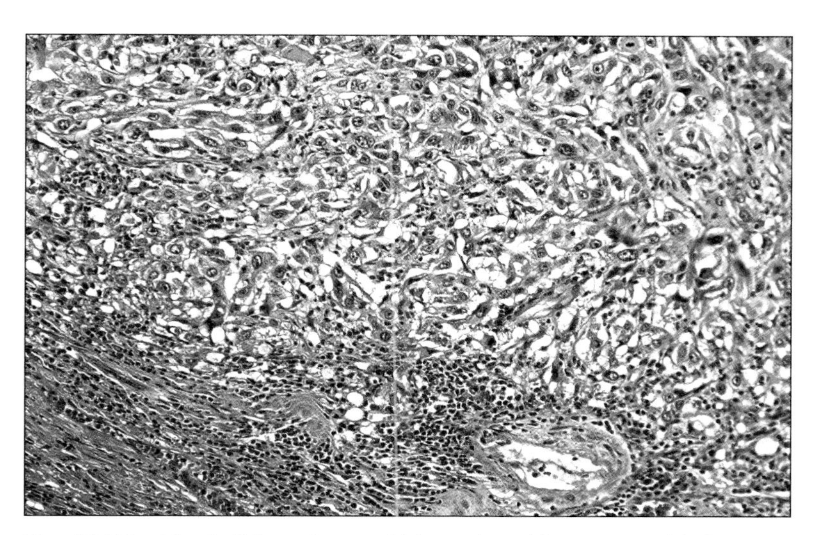

Fig. 10.50 Urothelial carcinoma, high grade, with sarcomatoid change and an endophytic growth pattern (upper two-thirds of photomicrograph), with chronically inflamed renal parenchyma (lower left third).

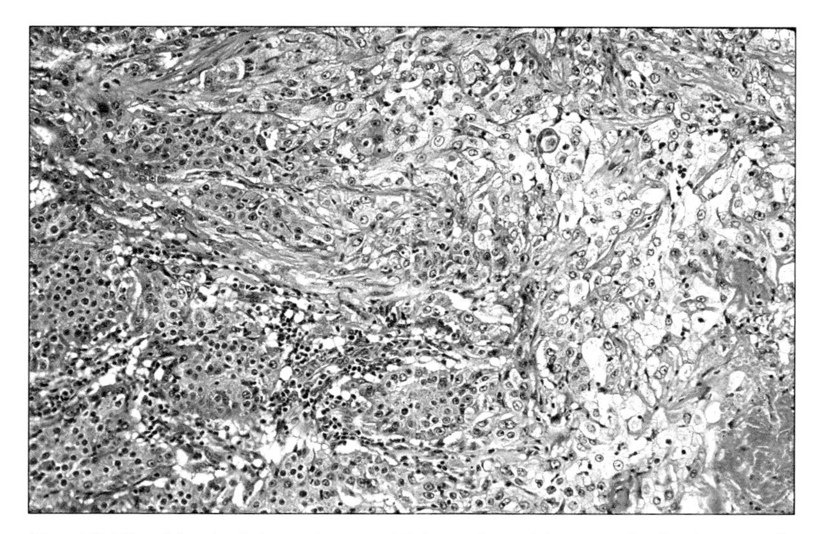

Fig. 10.51 Urothelial carcinoma, high grade, with an endophytic growth pattern.

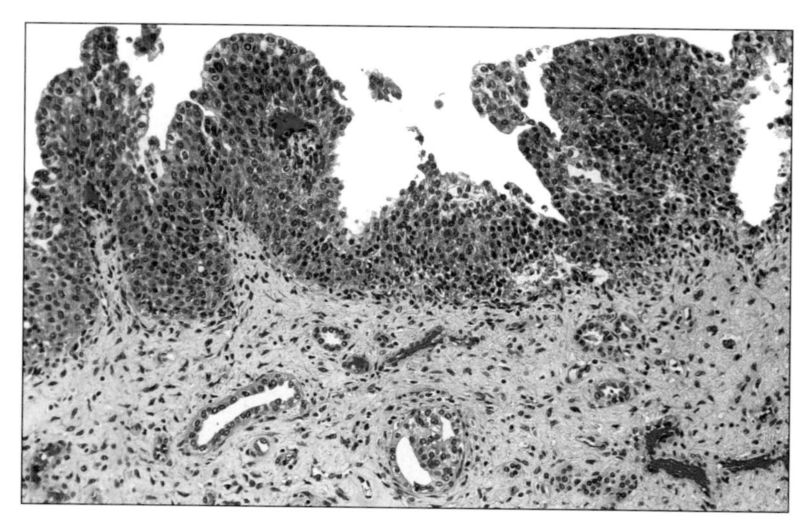

Fig. 10.52 Papillary urothelial carcinoma, low grade, with an exophytic growth pattern (upper half of photomicrograph); renal parenchyma (lower half) with no tubular involvement.

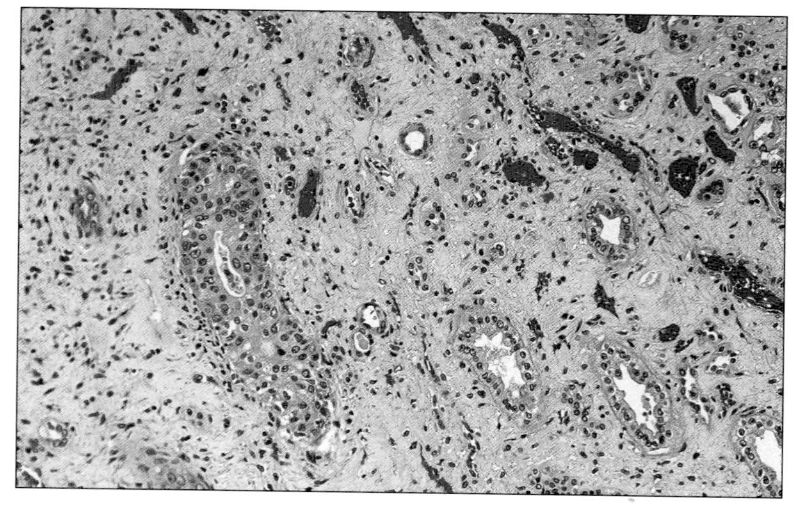

Fig. 10.53 Papillary urothelial carcinoma, low grade, with focal collecting duct involvement.

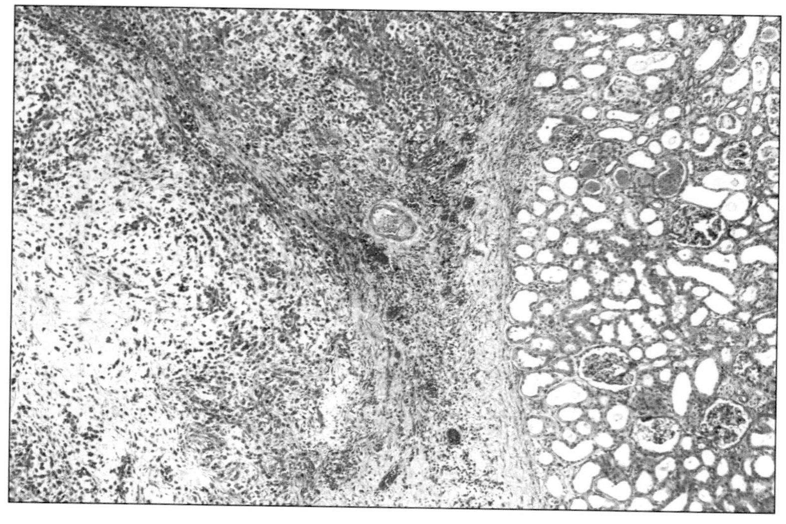

Fig. 10.54 Papillary urothelial carcinoma, high grade, with a spindle cell change (sarcomatoid change). The endophytic growth pattern is seen in the middle upper third of the photomicrograph. The sarcomatoid change is seen in the left third of the photomicrograph.

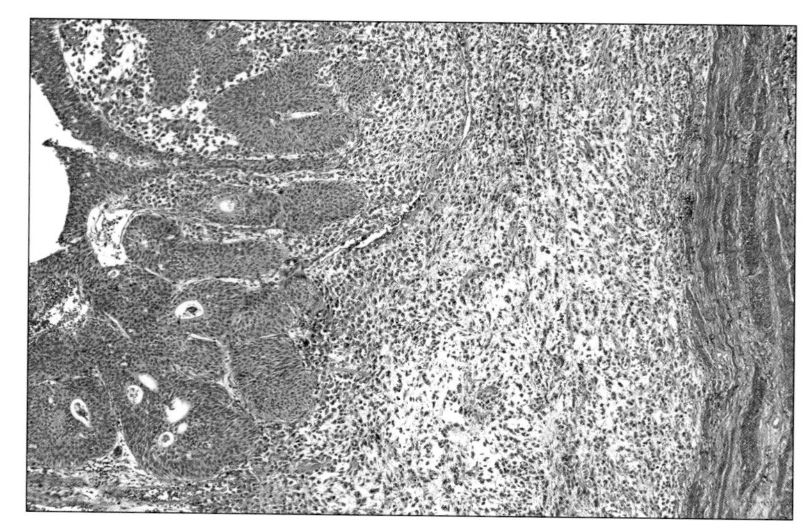

Fig. 10.55 Urothelial carcinoma, high grade, with a spindle cell change (sarcomatoid change). There is urothelial carcinoma in situ with neoplastic involvement of the urothelial nests below the flat surface of the urothelial tumor. The sarcomatoid change (middle third of photomicrograph) is adjacent to the urothelial cancer on the left of the photomicrograph.

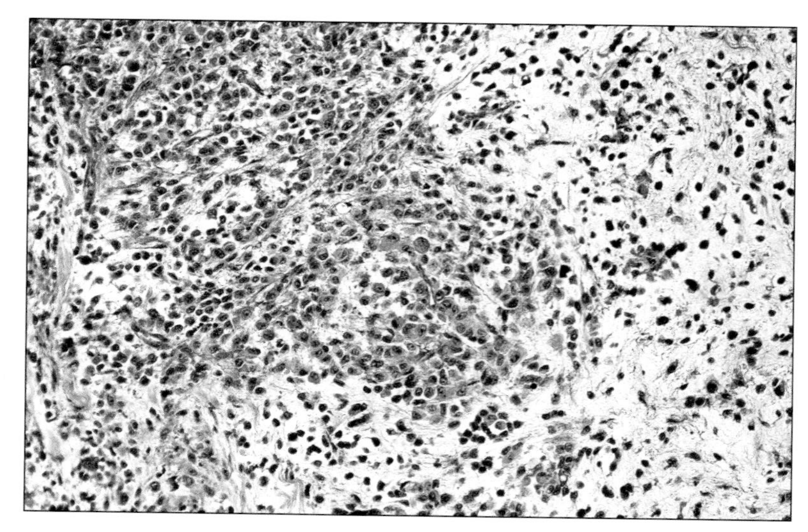

Fig. 10.56 Urothelial carcinoma, high grade, mixed with a spindle cell change (sarcomatoid change).

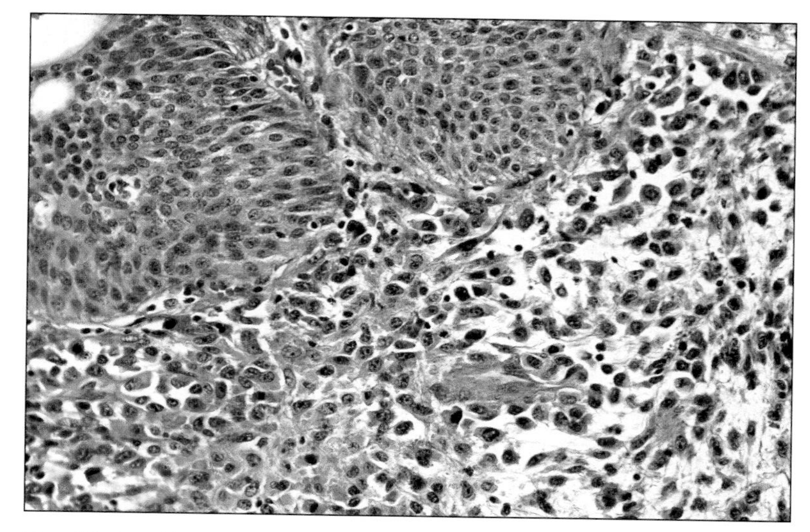

Fig. 10.57 Urothelial carcinoma, high grade, mixed with a spindle cell variant change (sarcomatoid change).

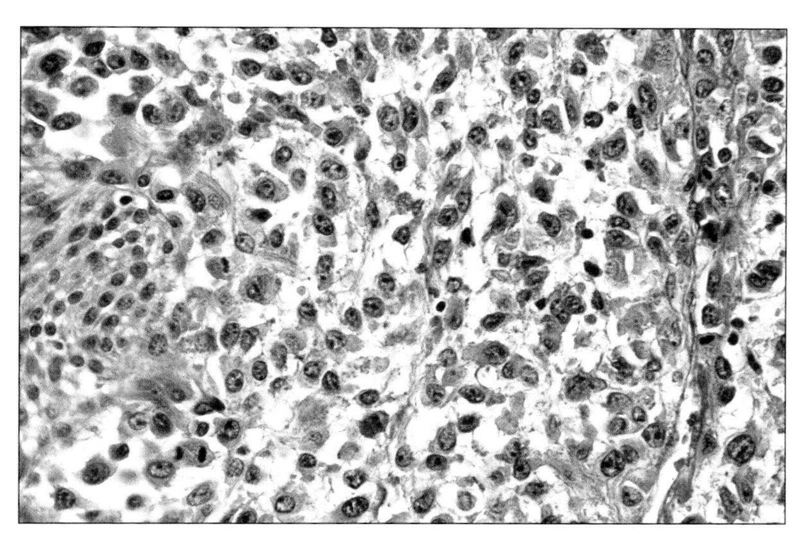

Fig. 10.58 Urothelial carcinoma, high grade, mixed with a spindle cell variant change (sarcomatoid change). It has a rhabdoid appearance in some areas.

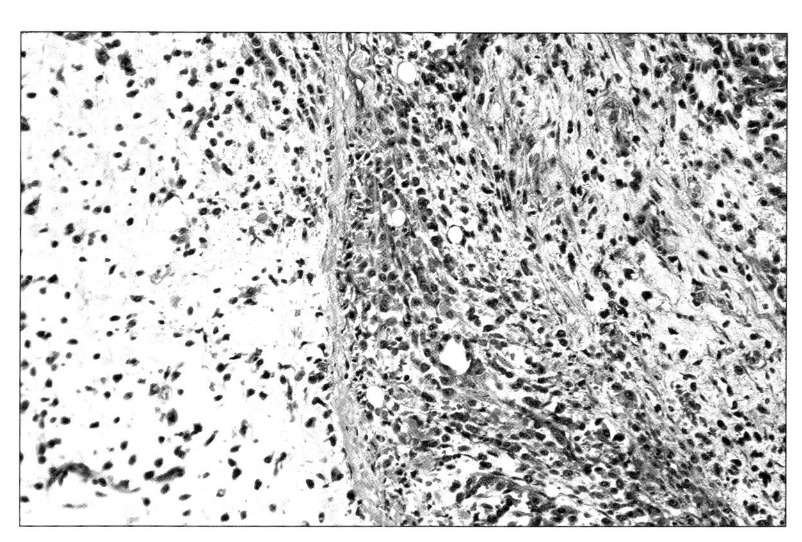

Fig. 10.60 Urothelial carcinoma, high grade (right half of photomicrograph), adjacent to spindle cell change (sarcomatoid change) area (left half).

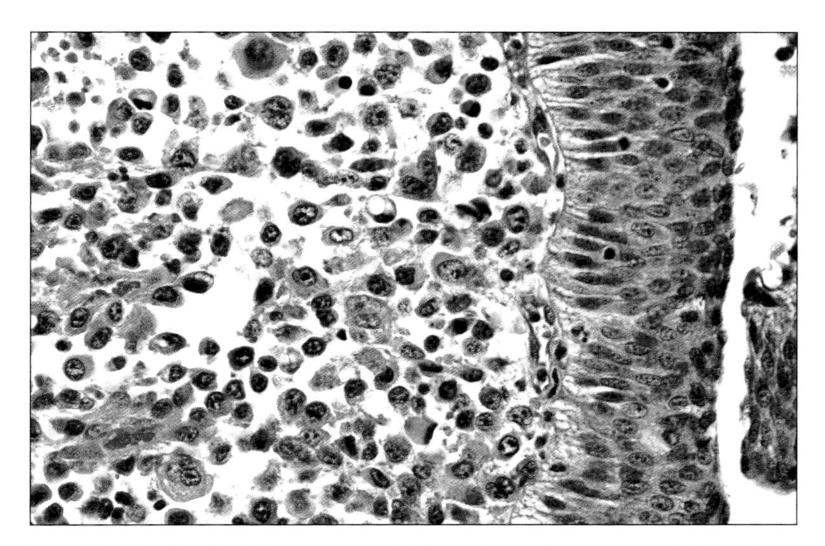

Fig. 10.59 Urothelial carcinoma, high grade, with sarcomatoid (focally rhabdoid) change. The sarcomatoid or spindle cell change is in the left two-thirds of the photomicrograph. The atypical urothelium is on the right side.

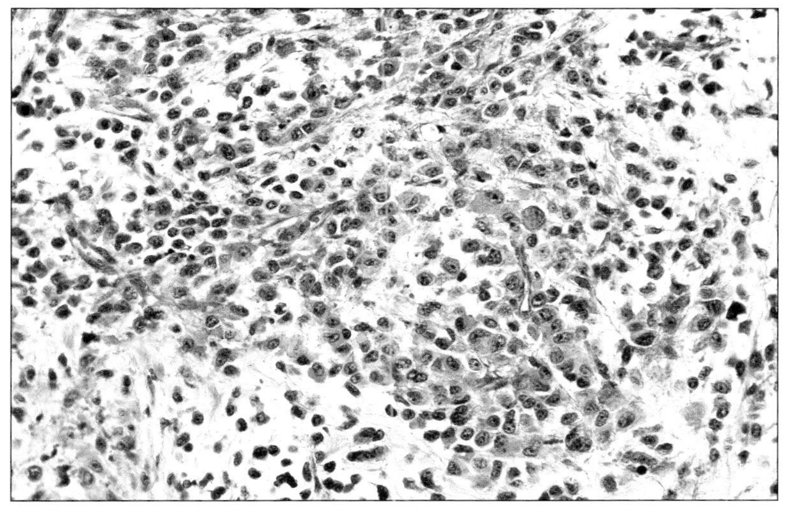

Fig. 10.61 Urothelial carcinoma, high grade (right half of photomicrograph), mixed with spindle cell change (sarcomatoid change).

carcinoma (see above in 'von Brunn's nests' and Figs 10.34–10.36).

SQUAMOUS CELL CARCINOMA AND ADENOCARCINOMA

Clinical Pure squamous cell carcinoma of the renal pelvis comprises approximately 10% of renal pelvic tumors and a much smaller percentage of ureteral tumors.[46,47]

Pure adenocarcinoma of the renal pelvis and ureters is rare and must be distinguished from focal glandular change of urothelial carcinoma, which is common and does not entail a worse prognosis.[48–50]

Pure squamous cell carcinoma and adenocarcinoma have a much worse prognosis than urothelial carcinoma with squamous or glandular change. These tumors are often associated with stones (staghorn calculi) and chronic infections.

Gross Squamous cell carcinoma and adenocarcinoma of the renal pelvis and ureter can present as exophytic masses. Often, however, these tumors form firm, plaque-like areas in the renal pelvis, with desmoplastic invasion into the renal parenchyma, sometimes extending into the perinephric adipose tissues.

Histology Most squamous cell carcinomas are high grade and resemble squamous cell carcinoma elsewhere. Leukoplakia is frequently found adjacent to tumor.

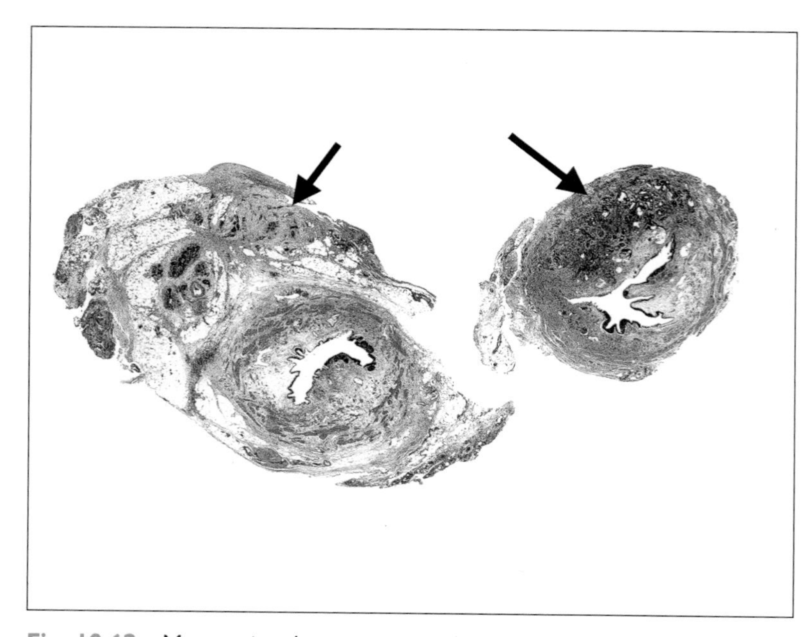

Fig. 10.62 Metastatic adenocarcinoma from the pancreas to the left periureteral tissue (arrows). Pancreatic carcinoma metastasizes more often to the left ureter than to the right. Primary adenocarcinomas of the ureters are very rare. Other primary sites should first be considered, as from the colon, prostate, etc.

Adenocarcinoma has several histologic appearances. Some resemble colonic adenocarcinoma, colloid (mucinous) carcinoma or signet ring cell carcinoma, and there is a single hepatoid case.[50] It is important to recognize the existence of these variants of adenocarcinoma, in order to identify these rare tumors as primary tumors of the renal pelvis or ureter and properly distinguish them from gastrointestinal metastases. (Fig. 10.62)

Practical point Since both squamous cell carcinoma and adenocarcinoma of the renal pelvis frequently present as fibrotic areas in renal pelves damaged by stones and infections, they can easily be mistaken for scarring. Therefore, thick scars in the pelves or ureters removed for longstanding stone disease or infection should be adequately examined microscopically, so that a malignant tumor is not missed.

NON-EPITHELIAL MALIGNANT TUMORS

- Sarcomas of the renal pelvis and ureter are distinctly uncommon lesions. *Leiomyosarcoma*,[51] *malignant schwannoma*, and *osteogenic sarcoma* have been reported.
- Rarely, a *malignant melanoma* can arise from the pelvic mucosa.
- *Lymphoma* usually involves the renal pelvis and ureter by extension from disseminated disease.[52]

REFERENCES

1. Matsuno T, Tokunaka S, Koyanagi T. Muscular development in the urinary tract. J Urol 1984;132:148–152.
2. Mackie GG. Abnormalities of the ureteral bud. Urol Clin North Am 1978;5: 161–174.
3. Tanagho EA, Guthrie TH, Lyon RP. The intravesical ureter in primary reflux. J Urol 1969;101:824–832.
4. Belman AB. Megaureter, classification, etiology, and management. Urol Clin North Am 1974;1:497–513.
5. Tokunaka S, Koyanagi T. Morphologic study of primary nonreflux megaureters with particular emphasis on the role of ureteral sheath and ureteral dysplasia. J Urol 1982;128:399–402.
6. Tokunda S, Gotoh T, Kayanagi T, et al. Morphological study of the ureterocele: a possible clue to its embryogenesis as evidenced by a locally arrested myogenesis. J Urol 1981;126:726–729.
7. Johnston JH, Evans JP, Glassberg KI, et al. Pelvic hydronephrosis in children: a review of 219 personal cases. J Urol 1977;117:97–101.
8. Maizels M, Stephens FD. Valves of the ureter as a cause of primary obstruction of the ureter: anatomic, embryologic and clinical aspects. J Urol 1980;123:742–747.
9. Stephens FD. Ureterovascular hydronephrosis and the "aberrant" renal vessels. J Urol 1982;128:984–987.
10. Lepor H, Walsh PC. Idiopathic retroperitoneal fibrosis. J Urol 1979;122:1–6.
11. Mitchinson MJ. Retroperitoneal fibrosis revisited. Arch Pathol Lab Med 1986;110:784–786.
12. Recloux P, Weiser M, Piccart M, Sculier J-P. Ureteral obstruction in patients with breast cancer. Cancer 1988;61:1904–1907.
13. Matthews PN, Greenswood RN, Hendry WF, Cattell WR. Extensive pelvis malacoplakia. Observations on management. J Urol 1986;135:132–134.
14. Rudd EG, Matthews MD. Malacoplakia: an unusual etiology of ureteral obstruction. Obstet Gynecol 1982;60:134–136.
15. Pac CYC. Etiology and treatment of urolithiasis. Am J Kidney Dis 1991;18: 624–637.
16. Dretler SP, Young RH. Stone granuloma. A cause of ureteral stricture. J Urol 1993;150:1800–1802.
17. Morse HD. The etiology and pathology of pyelitis cystica, ureteritis cystica and cystitis cystica. Am J Pathol 1928;4:33–49.
18. Bullock PS, Thoni DE, Murphy WM. The significance of colonic mucosa (intestinal metaplasia) involving the urinary tract. Cancer 1987;59: 2086–2090.
19. Reece RW, Koontz WW Jr. Leukoplakia of the urinary tract: a review. J Urol 1975;114:165–171.
20. Hertle L, Androulakakis P. Keratinizing desquamative squamous metaplasia of the upper urinary tract: leukoplakia-cholesteatoma. J Urol 1982;127:631–635.
21. Krag DO, Alcott DL. Glandular metaplasia of the renal pelvis, report of a case. Am J Clin Pathol 1957;27:672–680.
22. Edelman R, Kim ES, Bard RH. Benign fibroepithelial polyp of the renal pelvis. Br J Urol 1982;54:321–322.
23. Macksood MJ, Roth DR, Chang C-H, Perlmutter AD. Benign fibroepithelial polyps as a cause of intermittent ureteropelvic junction obstruction in a child. A case report and review of the literature. J Pathol 1985;134:951–952.
24. Fernandez PL, Nogales FF, Zuluaga A. Nephrogenic adenoma of the ureter. Br J Urol 1991;68:104–105.
25. Kunze E, Fischer G, Dembowski J. Tubulo-papillary adenoma (so-called nephrogenic adenoma) arising in the renal pelvis. Report of a case with a critical consideration of histogenesis and terminology. Pathol Res Pract 1993;189:217–225.
26. Martinez-Pineiro L, Hidalgo L, Picazo ML, Cozar JM, Martinez-Pineiro JA. Nephrogenic adenoma of the renal pelvis. Br J Urol 1991;67:101.
27. Pawade J, Soosay GN, Delprado W, Parkinson MC, Rode J. Cystic hammartoma of the renal pelvis. Am J Surg Pathol 1993;17:1169–1175.
28. Epstein JL, Amin MB, Reuter VR, et al. The World Health Organization/International Society of Urological Pathology consensus classification of urothelial (transitional cell) neoplasms of the urinary bladder: Bladder Consensus Conference Committee. Am J Surg Pathol 1998;22:1435–1448.
29. Fromowitz FB, Steinbook ML, Lautin EM, et al. Inverted papilloma of the ureter. J Urol 1981;126:113–116.
30. Kyriakos M, Royce RK. Multiple simultaneous inverted papillomas of the upper urinary tract. A case report with a review of ureteral and renal pelvis inverted papillomas. Cancer 1989;63:368–380.

31. Kunze E, Schauer A, Schnitt M. Histology and histogenesis of two different types of inverted urothelial papillomas. Cancer 1983;51:348–358.
32. Kimura G, Tsuboi N, Nakajima H, et al. Inverted papilloma of the ureter with malignant transformation: a case report and review of the literature. Urol Int 1987;42:30–36.
33. Grainger R, Gikas PW, Grossman HB. Urothelial carcinoma occurring within an inverted papilloma of the ureter. J Urol 1990;143:802–804.
34. Hurwitz RS, Benjamin JA, Cooper JF. Excessive proliferation of peripelvic fat of the kidney. Urology 1978;11:448–456.
35. Farrands PA, Tribe CR, Slade N. Localized amyloid of the ureter. Case report and review of the literature. Histopathology 1983;7:613–622.
36. Edward HG, Deweerd JH, Woolner LB. Renal hemangiomas. Proc Staff Meetings Mayo Clin 1962;37:545–551.
37. Uchida M, Watanabe H, Mishina T, Shemada N. Leiomyoma of the renal pelvis. J Urol 1981;125:572–574.
38. McCarton JP Jr, Chasko SB, Gray GF Jr. Systematic mapping of nephroureterectomy specimens removed for urothelial cancer: pathological findings and clinical correlation. J Urol 1982;128:243–246.
39. Heney NM, Nocks BN, Daly JJ, et al. Prognostic factors in carcinoma of ureter. J Urol 1981;125:632–636.
40. McLaughlin JK, Blot WJ, Mandel JS, et al. Etiology of cancer of the renal pelvis. J Natl Cancer Inst 1983;71:287–291.
41. Palvio DHB, Andersen JC, Falk E. Transitional cell tumors of the renal pelvis and ureter associated with capillarosclerosis indicating analgesic abuse. Cancer 1987;59:972–976.
42. Christensen P, Rorbaek Madsen M, Myhre Jensen O. Latency of Thorotrast-induced renal tumors. Scand J Urol Nephrol 1983;17:127–130.
43. Bonsib SM. Pathology of the renal pelvis and ureter. In: Eble JN, ed. Tumors and tumor-like conditions of the kidneys and ureters. New York: Churchill Livingstone; 1990.
44. Bonsib SM, Eble JN. Renal pelvis and ureter. In: Bostwick DG, Eble JN, eds. Urological surgical pathology. St Louis: Mosby; 1997.
45. Parker DC, Folpe AL, Bell J, et al. Potential utility of uroplakin III, thrombomodulin, high molecular weight cytokeratin, and cytokeratin 20 in noninvasive, invasive and metastatic urothelial (transitional cell) carcinomas. Am J Surg Pathol 2003;27:1–10.
46. Vyas MCR, Joshi KR, Mathur DR, et al. Primary squamous cell carcinoma of the renal pelvis, a report of four cases with review of literature. J Pathol Microbiol 1982;25:151–155.
47. Blacher EJ, Johnson DE, Abdul-Karim FW, et al. Squamous cell carcinoma of renal pelvis. Urology 1985;25:124–125.
48. Stein A, Sova Y, Lurie M, et al. Adenocarcinoma of the renal pelvis, report of two cases, one with simultaneous transitional cell carcinoma of the bladder. Urol Int 1988;43:299–301.
49. Aufderheide AC, Streitz JM. Mucinous adenocarcinoma of the renal pelvis. Report of two cases. Cancer 1974;33:167–173.
50. Ishikura H, Ishiguro T, Enatsu C, et al. Hepatoid adenocarcinoma of the renal pelvis producing alpha-fetoprotein of hepatic type and bile pigment. Cancer 1991;67:3051–3056.
51. Werner JR, Klingersmith W, Denko JV. Leiomyosarcoma of the ureter. Case report and review of literature. J Urol 1959;82:68–71.
52. Scharifker D, Chalasani A. Ureteral involvement by malignant lymphoma. Ten years experience. Arch Pathol Lab Med 1978;102:541–542.

PATHOLOGY OF UROTHELIAL BLADDER CANCER

Myron Tannenbaum, John F. Madden, and Maria M. Schevchuk

11

INTRODUCTION

The barnyard pen metaphor, which is frequently used to describe the pathobiology of prostate cancer, can also be applied to the variants of urothelial cancer. Urothelial bladder cancer can be likened to a barnyard pen in which there are animals going nowhere (incidental non-lethal cancers, e.g. papillary urothelial neoplasm of low malignant potential), rabbits ready to hop out at any time (potentially lethal cancers that might benefit from treatment, e.g. carcinoma in situ (CIS), low-grade papillary urothelial carcinoma), and birds (T2 and T3 lesions: urothelial cancers that may be beyond cure at the time of diagnosis).[1] In this chapter, we will try to shed some light on each 'animal' in this barnyard pen.

In the early 1970s, investigators from the National Bladder Research Program defined the nature of some of the challenges in urothelial cancer. Researchers from different medical specialties and from many countries participated in the program. Since that time, epidemiologists, pathologists, chemotherapists, radiotherapists, and urologists have been gathering knowledge that could clarify the processes involved in the initiation and progression of urothelial cancer (Fig. 11.1).

In taking the lives of so many individuals, including a candidate for the US presidency, urothelial cancer has altered the course of human history. In the USA, more than 51 000 new cases of bladder cancer are diagnosed annually; 10 500 people are dying from the disease. Many of these patients (80%) are first seen with 'superficial' disease. However, 20% and 5% present with invasive and metastatic disease, respectively. Carcinoma of the bladder affects men more than women in a ratio of 3–4:1; this may be due to differences in smoking habits and occupational exposures. The incidence of bladder cancer in the USA varies across different states and counties. Furthermore, different incidences are observed between adjacent urban and rural areas, implying that social, occupational, environmental, or dietary factors may promote the development of bladder cancer.[2]

HISTOLOGY OF UROTHELIUM

Light histology and ultrastructure of normal and then neoplastic urothelium will be considered first. We then focus on bladder biopsy, which is important in the pathologic determination of staging and cytologic grading of the urothelial neoplasm. Urothelial dysplasia and carcinoma in situ, a term coined almost 50 years ago by the pathology and urology departments of Columbia-Presbyterian Medical School, will also be discussed. Before a final decision is made with regard to the treatment of the patient, another variable of paramount importance is the multicentricity of carcinoma in the urothelial system; this factor will be examined in great detail. We have elected to exclude a review of urinary cytology, which has been comprehensively elaborated in a previous chapter. We have also opted not to write about the new molecular pathology, for to do so would serve only to make this chapter more voluminous. However, in omitting these elements, we do not intend to detract from the major importance that each of these tools has in the clinical management and understanding of the pathobiology of urothelial cancer.

Transitional epithelium or urothelium of the urinary bladder exhibits a large variety of histologic patterns that can easily be demonstrated on conventional light histology. It lines the urinary conduit 'waterway' from the renal calyceal system, ureters, urinary bladder, periurethral ducts, and urethra to the outside of the body. The classification of the histopathology of the urinary bladder carcinomas has been extensively documented by numerous authors.[3–5] Even though a large amount of information and atlases on the pathology of these neoplasms are available, much remains an enigma to those healthcare providers who are in the daily position of evaluating the pathobiology of these tumors. There is a need for the urologic pathologist to communicate the histopathology to the chemotherapist, the radiologist, and now the environmentalist, as well as lastly, but yet most importantly, the urologic surgeon. It is the purpose of this chapter to bring into focus, from the point of view of the urologic

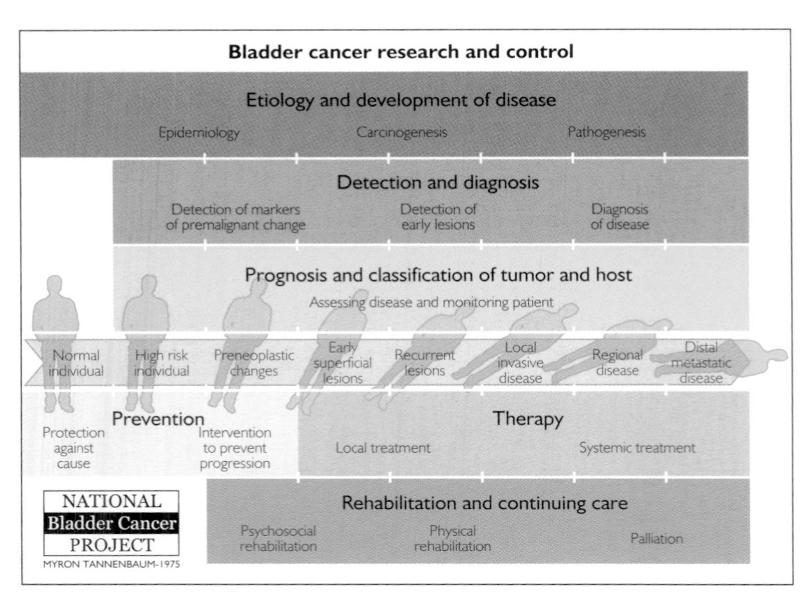

Fig. 11.1 The National Bladder Cancer Project. The falling person shows the progression of bladder cancer as it relates to detection and prevention.

pathologist, what might be some of the points of confusion regarding the biology of the urothelial system. For CIS, the cytologic grade and stage of single and/or multicentric papillary tumors need to be critically determined, and the evaluation of such tumors communicated to those in the various medical disciplines who clinically treat these patients. There may also be correlation of urinary cytology with the grading of these multiple bladder biopsies. We will deal with these topics, but it will be more propitious to first discuss the architecture and structure of normal urothelium.

HISTOLOGY OF NON-NEOPLASTIC UROTHELIUM (TRANSITIONAL EPITHELIUM)

Urothelium, or transitional epithelium, lines the urinary bladder, ureters, and renal pelvis. It was originally called transitional epithelium because its histologic appearance was transitional between non-keratinizing squamous and pseudostratified columnar epithelium. In the past several years, many histologists and pathologists have used urothelium as a more appropriate term.

Light histologic tissue sections reveal that the cellular thickness of the urothelium depends not only on the degree of distension in the urinary bladder but also on the plane through which the tissue is cut. If the knife cut is tangential to the basement membrane, a histologic picture is generated where there appears to be an artificially thickened urothelial mucosa. Therefore urothelial cellular thickness is of marginal help in assessing urothelial neoplasms.

The thickness of the normal urothelium varies according to the degree of distension and anatomic location. The

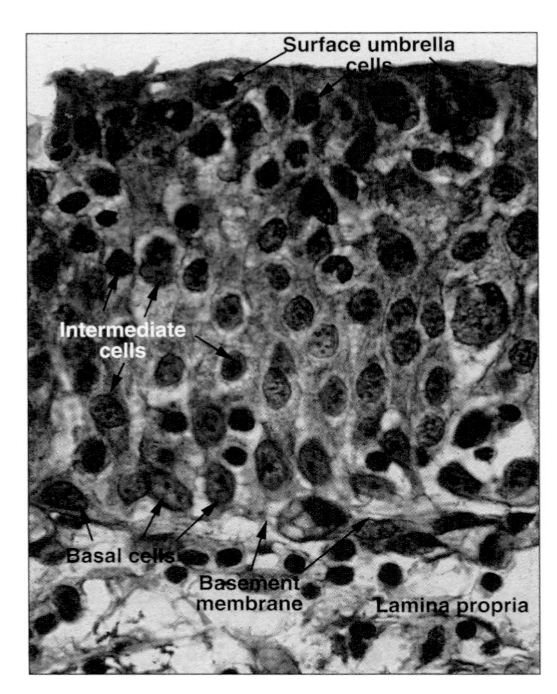

Fig. 11.2 Light histology of normal urothelium with a few chronic inflammatory cells and some urothelial atypia. Surface, intermediate, and basal cells are present. Some of the urothelial atypia is due to the anaplasia of repair.

urothelium is usually six or seven cells in thickness, and in the ureter three to five cells in thickness; however, it may be only two or three cell layers thick along the minor calyces of the kidney. In the urothelium of the urinary bladder, three different cellular regions can be identified (Figs 11.2 and 11.3). The superficial cells, or umbrella cells, are in contact with the urinary space. Beneath these cells, there are the intermediate cells and then the basal cells, which lie on a basement membrane.[6] In the distended bladder, the urothelium may be only two or three cells in thickness and flattened. The long axis of these flattened cells is horizontal to the basement membrane. Superficial cells are large elliptical cells that may appear umbrella-like over the smaller intermediate cells. The superficial cells may be binucleated and have abundant eosinophilic cytoplasm. When the urinary bladder is distended with urine, these cells become flattened and are barely visible on histologic sectioning. The presence of these cells is taken as a sign of normal differentiation within the architecture of the urothelium. Conversely, it is also possible to see these umbrella cells overlying frank carcinoma. In summary, the presence or absence of superficial cells cannot always be used as a determining factor of malignancy.

The intermediate cell layer may vary from one to five cells in thickness in the contracted bladder, where they are oriented with the long axis perpendicular to the basement membrane. The nuclei are oval and have finely stippled chromatin with absent or minute nucleoli. There is ample cytoplasm, which may be vacuolated. The cytoplasmic

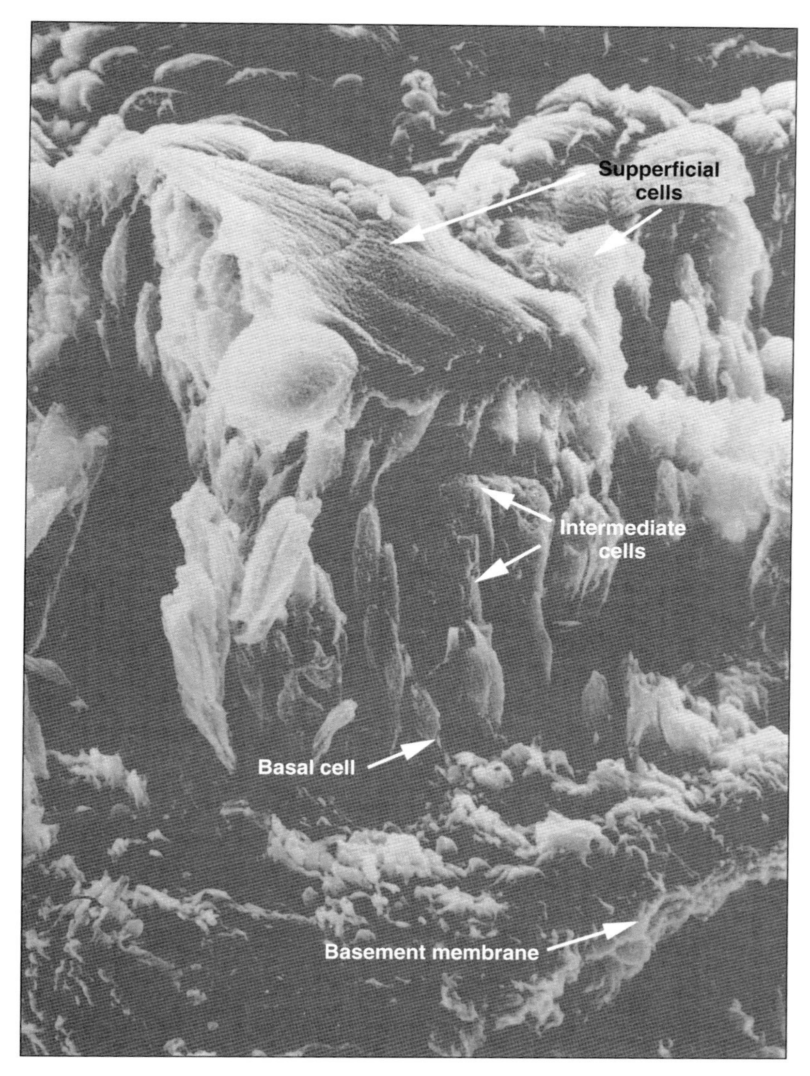

Fig. 11.3 Scanning electron microscopy of normal urothelium, demonstrating a three-dimensional view of the surface, intermediate, and basal cells sitting on the basement membrane.

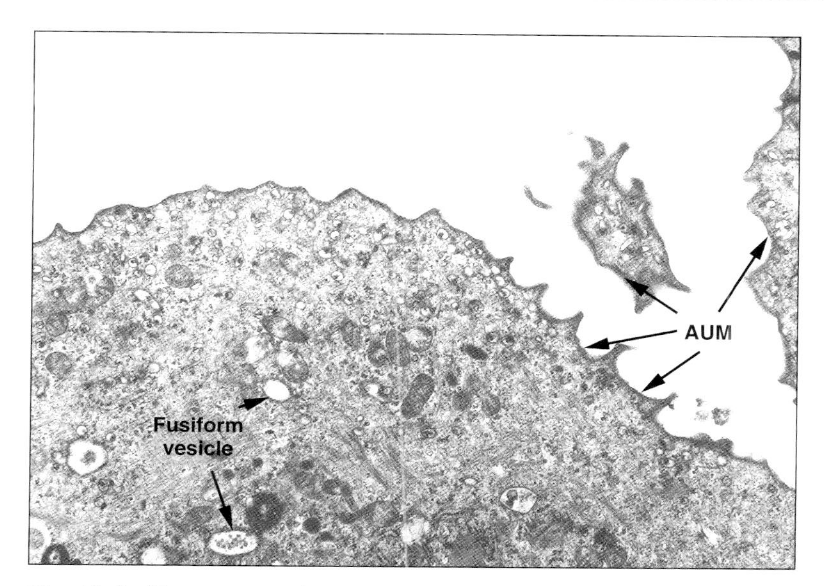

Fig. 11.4 Transmission electron microscopy of the surface cells, showing the asymmetric unit membrane (AUM) on the luminal surface of the urothelial cell.

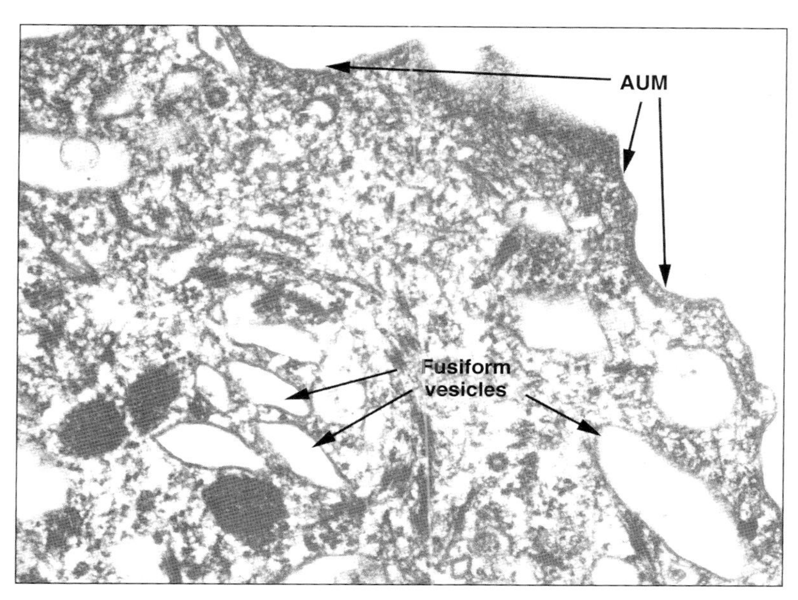

Fig. 11.5 Transmission electron microscopy of the surface cells, showing the asymmetric unit membrane (AUM) on the luminal surface of the urothelial cell and the fusiform vesicles that form the AUM by fusing to it.

membranes are distinct. The intermediate cells are attached to each other by desmosomes. In the distended state, this layer may be inconspicuous or only one cell thick and flattened.

The basal cell layer comprises cuboidal cells that are evident only in the contracted bladder, and in non-malignant urothelium are attached by hemidesmosomes to a thin but continuous basement membrane composed of a lamina lucida, lamina densa, and anchoring fibrils.[6]

By means of transmission and scanning electron microscopy, ultrastructural studies have shown that the urothelium and especially the superficial urothelial cells have a unique membrane surface that is lined by a cytoplasmic membrane three layers thick (Figs 11.4–11.9). There are two electron-dense layers and a central lucent layer. The two dense layers are of unequal thickness. The cytoplasmic surface membrane is known as the asymmetric unit membrane (AUM).[6] In reality, although the trilaminar arrangement of the cytoplasmic membrane can readily be observed, it is difficult to see the asymmetry of the dense layers. The membrane contains frequent invaginations, giving it a scalloped appearance. The cytoplasm of the superficial cells, and sometimes the upper intermediate cells, has cytoplasm, which contains fusiform vesicles that are also lined by the AUM. It is believed that during the process of urinary bladder distension, these invaginations and fusiform vesicles are incorporated into the surface membrane. This is a mechanism for increasing the surface area of the cells and maintaining the structural integrity of the urothelium.

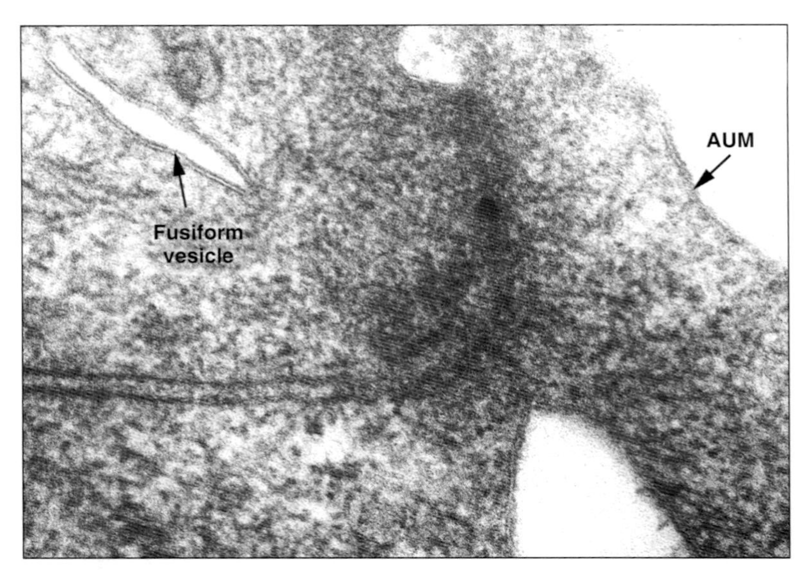

Fig. 11.6 Asymmetric unit membrane (AUM) and fusiform vesicles at higher magnification.

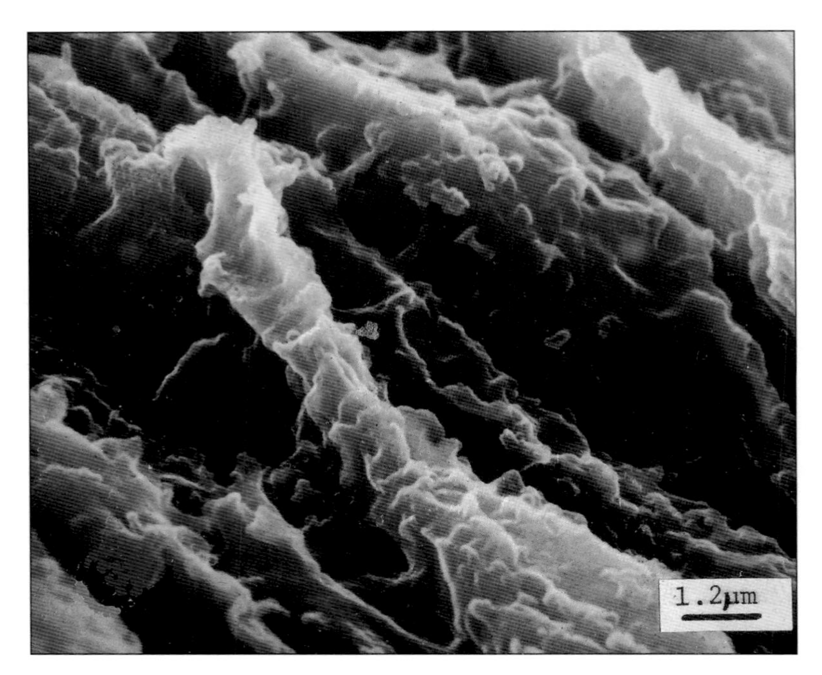

Fig. 11.8 Scanning electron microscopy of the spindle-shaped intermediate cells, demonstrating the absence of the asymmetric unit membrane on their surface.

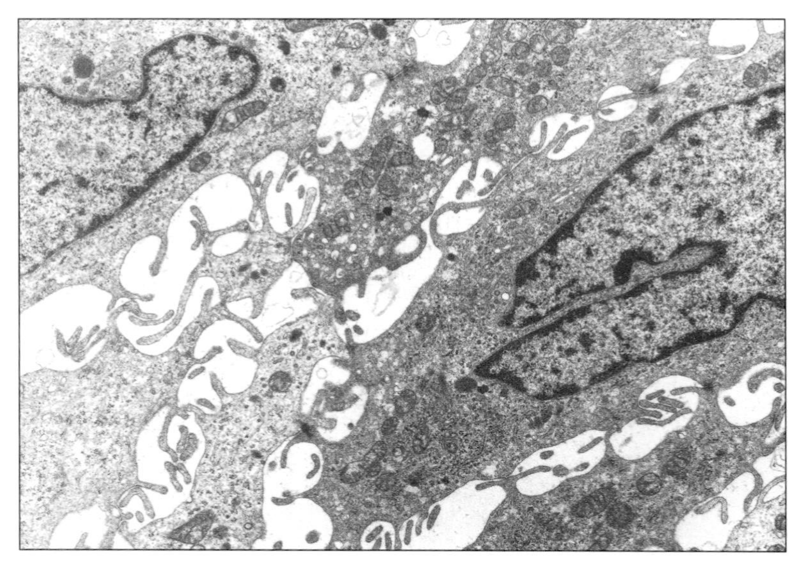

Fig. 11.7 Transmission electron microscopy of the intermediate cells, demonstrating the absence of the asymmetric unit membrane on their surface. Fusiform vesicles are present but no tripartite junctional complexes.

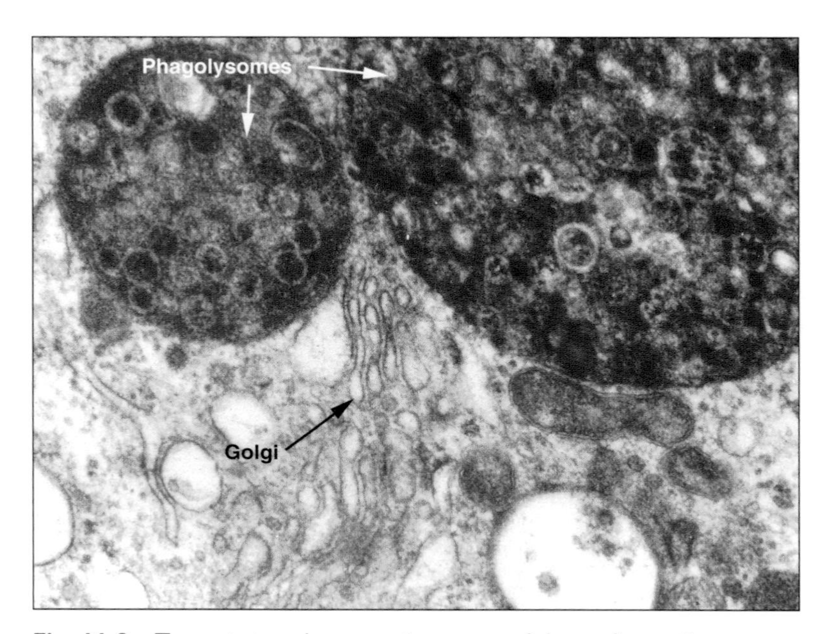

Fig. 11.9 Transmission electron microscopy of the surface cells, demonstrating the presence of phagolysosomes. These structures help digest bacteria that have been phagocytosed, and increase in number in the surface and intermediate cells when there is bacterial infection.

BLADDER BIOPSIES

To evaluate the progression of neoplasia of the urothelium, it is important to understand the interplay between the urologist and the surgical pathologist. Biopsies are taken to confirm the urinary cytologic, clinical, and cystoscopic findings (Figs 11.10–11.12). In obtaining the cystoscopic biopsies of the bladder mucosa, the urothelium may become detached during manipulation or processing of the surgical material. In most instances, however, this does not occur. Table 11.1 summarizes the cytologic and cystoscopic findings.

One urologic pathology textbook recommends that tissue taken by means of a 'cold cup' cutting forceps from endoscopically visible lesions or apparently normal mucosa at adjacent, random, or preselected sites be placed immediately in the proper fixatives. The author notes that the biopsy tends to 'ball up' in the fixative so that the mucosa covers most of the underlying tissue, and in

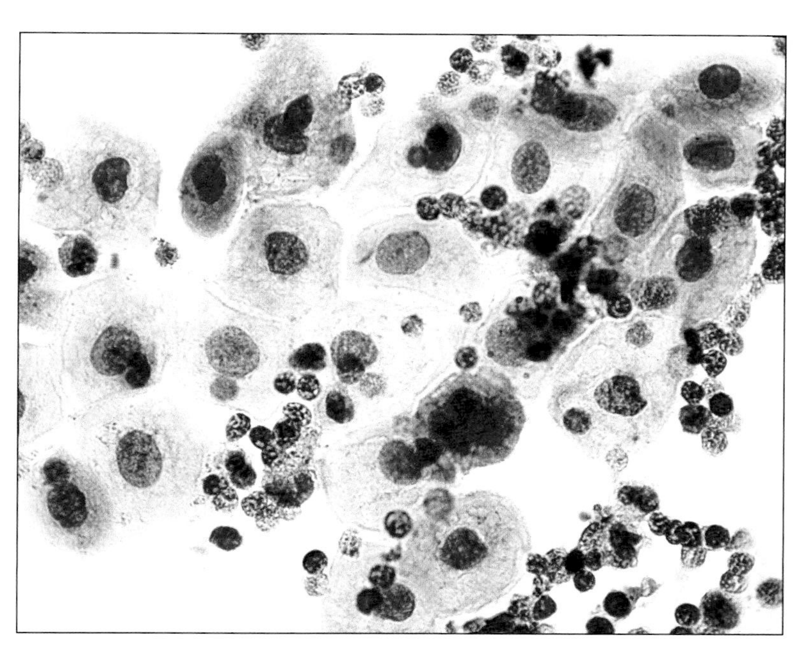

Fig. 11.10 Urine cytology: benign urinary cells mixed with red blood cells and inflammatory cells.

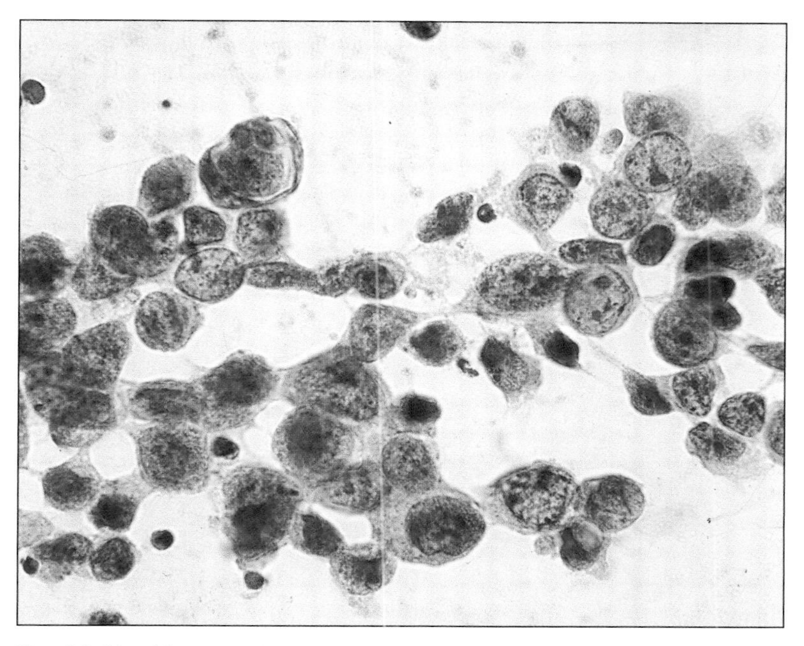

Fig. 11.11 Urine cytology: malignant urinary cells (high grade).

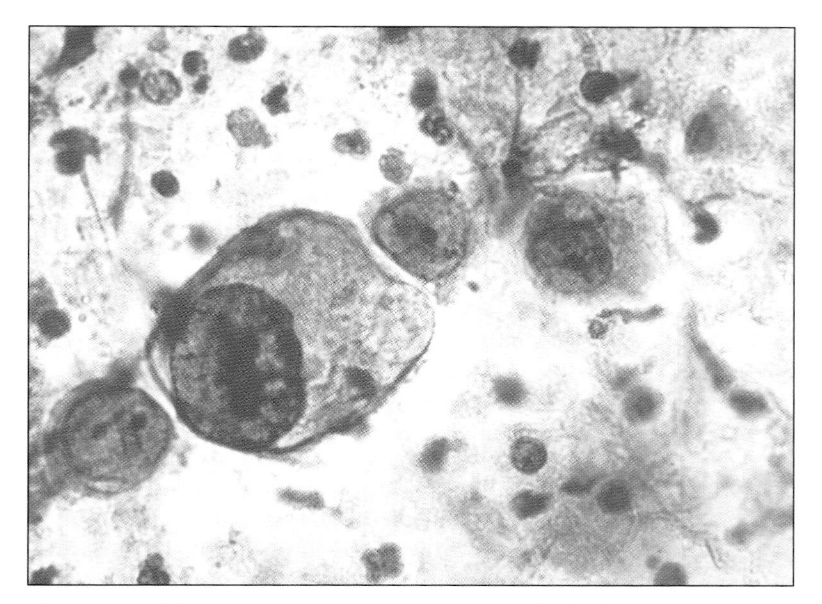

Fig. 11.12 Urine cytology: malignant urinary cells (high grade) that are of adenocarcinomatous origin.

Table 11.1 Cytologic and cystoscopic findings in urothelial bladder cancer

Cytology	*Cystoscopy*	*Interpretation*
Negative	Visible papillary lesion(s)	Papillary lesion of low grade No significant epithelial atypia
Marked atypia (suspicious)	Visible papillary lesion(s)	Papillary lesion of moderate grade, peripheral epithelial atypia, or both
Positive (cancer cells present)	Visible papillary lesion(s)	Papillary lesion of low grade with peripheral carcinoma in situ Papillary lesion of high grade with or without carcinoma in situ
	Visible nonpapillary lesion	Invasive carcinoma with or without carcinoma in situ
	Nonvisible lesions	Carcinoma in situ (common) Metastatic carcinoma (rare) Carcinoma in diverticulum (very rare)

(After Koss 1972,[7] with permission of JB Lippincott.)

most cases orientation is not of great concern. Gross examination of bladder biopsies is generally unrevealing, and emphasis should be given to recording the number and size of the tissues in each specimen container. The weight of a bladder biopsy is unimportant. The entire specimen should be embedded. Depending on the size, bisection might be beneficial. The exact number of sections necessary to reveal all significant pathologic processes in a cold cup biopsy has not been established, but most laboratories prepare multiple sections from each specimen. Tissue sectioning at the periphery of the tissue ball can create a tangential appearance, producing artifacts that may augment small remnants of 'muscularis mucosae'. These are muscle fibers that often exist in a syncytial pattern in the lamina propria.

It is of paramount importance that accurate staging and cytologic grading of these urothelial cancers be critically evaluated so that effective treatment can be instituted.

RULES FOR THE CLINICAL AND PATHOLOGIC STAGING OF UROTHELIAL TUMORS[8]

Primary tumor assessment involves bimanual examination under anesthesia before and after endoscopic surgery (biopsy or transurethral resection), and histologic verification of the presence or absence of tumor. The results of bimanual examination following endoscopic surgery indicate clinical stage. The finding of bladder wall thickening, a mobile mass, or a fixed mass suggests the presence of T3a, T3b, and T4b disease, respectively. We indicate 'm' for multiple tumors and insert 'is' to any T to note an associated CIS. Appropriate imaging techniques for lymph node evaluation should be used, and evaluation for distant metastases should include imaging of the chest, biochemical studies, and isotopic studies for the detection of common metastatic sites. Computed tomography or other modalities may be used to supply additional information concerning minimal requirements for staging. The primary tumor may be superficial or invasive, and can be partially or totally resected with sufficient tissue from the tumor base for evaluation of the full depth of tumor invasion. Visually adjacent cystoscopically normal–appearing mucosa should be considered for biopsy. Urinary cytology and pyelography are also important.

Pathologic staging also involves microscopic examination and confirmation of the extent of the neoplasia in the urothelium. Total cystectomy and lymph node dissection are generally the only final answer for the staging.

The biopsy of the primary tumor (T) may be classified as follows.

- TX, primary tumor cannot be assessed.
- T0, no evidence of primary tumor.
- Ta, noninvasive papillary carcinoma (stage 0).
- Tis, CIS or 'flat tumor'.
- T1, tumor invades subepithelial connective tissue (stage A).
- T2, tumor invades muscle (muscularis propria) (stage B).
  T2a, tumor invades superficial muscle of muscularis propria (inner half) (stage B1).
  T2b, tumor invades deep muscle of muscularis propria (outer half) (stage B2).
- T3, tumor invades perivesical tissue (stage C):
  T3a, microscopically;
  T3b, macroscopically (extravesical mass).
- T4, tumor invades any of prostate, uterus, vagina, pelvic wall, or abdominal wall:
  T4a, tumor invades prostate, uterus, or vagina;
  T4b, tumor invades pelvic wall or abdominal wall.

In addition, different surgical pathologists have attempted to further stratify the stage T1 urothelial cell carcinoma into substages (see Table 11.2).

These results are helpful in clarifying the early pathobiology of these tumors, but they are not always that easily obtainable because of sampling and cautery artifacts.

HISTOPATHOLOGY OF NEOPLASTIC UROTHELIAL (TRANSITIONAL) TUMORS

When the tumor is detected cytologically and cystoscopically, a biopsy specimen is obtained and several variegated patterns of tumor spread can be revealed. The possible life cycle of untreated tumors of the urinary bladder has been postulated by researchers at Columbia-Presbyterian Medical Center.[12] Many of these tumors, both in the flat as well as in the exophytic papillary form, must have cell extension beyond the basement membrane of the urothelium in order to invade. Once this occurs, there is invasion through the lamina propria and then, with the course of time (which is ill defined), invasion of both the muscle and/or the lymphatics. Frequently, tumors that are of the solid nonpapillary type can spread laterally. At the same time, they may perforate the submucosa and spread as finger-like projections into the muscularis propria of the bladder (see Fig. 11.13). At first, the papillary tumors are exophytic into the bladder lumen, and consequently they are readily seen cystoscopically. In both forms, the flat in

Table 11.2 Substages of stage T1 urothelial cell carcinoma

	Subclassification	*Level of invasion*	*Results*
Younes et al. (1990)[9]	T1a	Connective tissue superficial to muscularis mucosae	75% 5-year survival
	T1b	To muscularis mucosae	75% 5-year survival
	T1c	Through muscularis mucosae but superficial to muscularis propria	11% 5-year survival
Hasui et al. (1994)[10]	T1a	Superficial to muscularis mucosae	0.7% progression
	T1b	Deep to muscularis mucosae	53.5% progression
Angulo et al. (1995)[11]	T1a	Invading lamina propria but not muscularis mucosae	86% 5-year survival
	T1b	Invading submucosa	52% 5-year survival

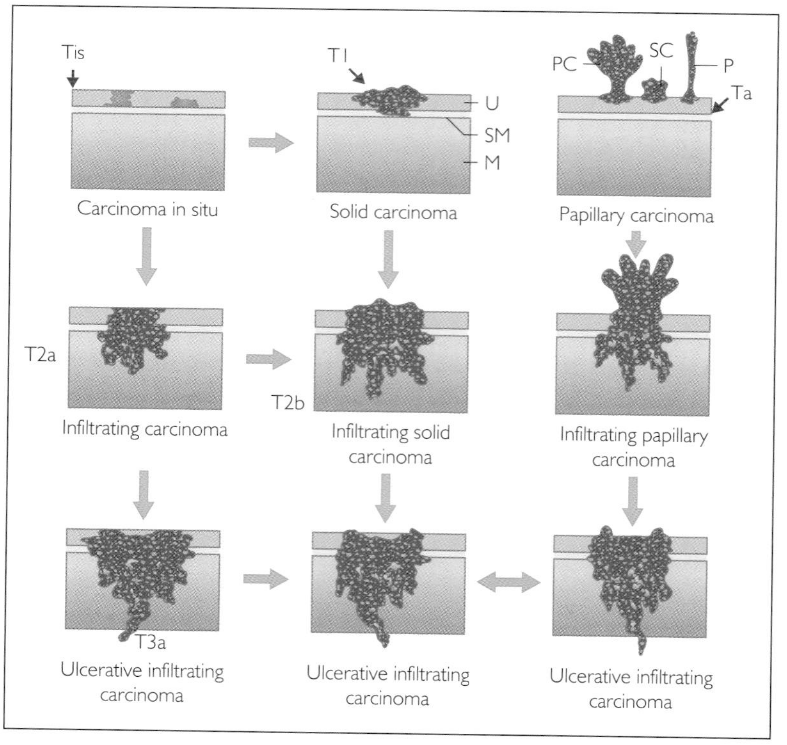

Fig. 11.13 The natural history of urinary bladder cancers. (After Melicow 1974[12] and Tannenbaum 1984,[13] with permission.) U, urothelium; SM, submucosa; M, mucosa; PC, papillary carcinoma; SC, solid carcinoma; P, papilloma.

situ cancer and the papillary exophytic type tend to shower off cells into the lumen of the bladder. Depending on the grade of the tumor, they can be readily detected by urinary cytology. The higher the grade, the easier it is to detect the cancer cytologically. Many of the papillary tumors will also bleed, because the tumor has delicate fibrovascular stalks that contain blood vessels without smooth muscle. If these tumors twist, branches of the tumor break off into the urine, and blood will also pulsate out from the vessels in the tumor branches. The papillary tumors also break through the basement membrane that envelops their base, and they then invade the lamina propria or submucosa, and perhaps, in some instances, the muscularis propria. All types eventually become ulcerated and infected. At this time, it becomes difficult to determine whether the tumors are originally of the solid or papillary form. If urinary cytology is used with increased frequency, many of these tumors can be detected at very early stages, i.e. before they reach stage T2a or T2b, as represented in the upper third of Fig. 11.13. At all times, it is extremely difficult for any pathologist to critically separate advanced-stage T2b from early T2a lesions. This difficulty is compounded when the specimens are cauterized, and especially when there is no specific orientation of the specimens for histologic sectioning.

The topographic distribution and cell types of bladder tumors are seen in Fig. 11.14. The majority of bladder tumors (70%) are located on the posterior and lateral walls near the ureteral orifices. Most of the tumors in these sites are papillary, as they have fibrovascular stalks. The remaining 20% are in a solid invasive form and have no fibrovascular formation. They also commonly extend through the basement membrane that surrounds the nests of von Brunn. There is also a varying amount of CIS (see Figs 11.15–11.21) associated with these bladder neoplasms in about 3% of these cases.[12] However, it is our impression that this percentage is a variable one. It is greatly dependent on whether the pathologist, in cooperation with the urologist, spends a considerable amount of time looking for this lesion in the associated biopsy specimens. These biopsies should be taken at least within a 1-cm distance from the exophytic tumors. If this is done, the incidence of CIS is considerably greater than 3%. These figures vary at each institution

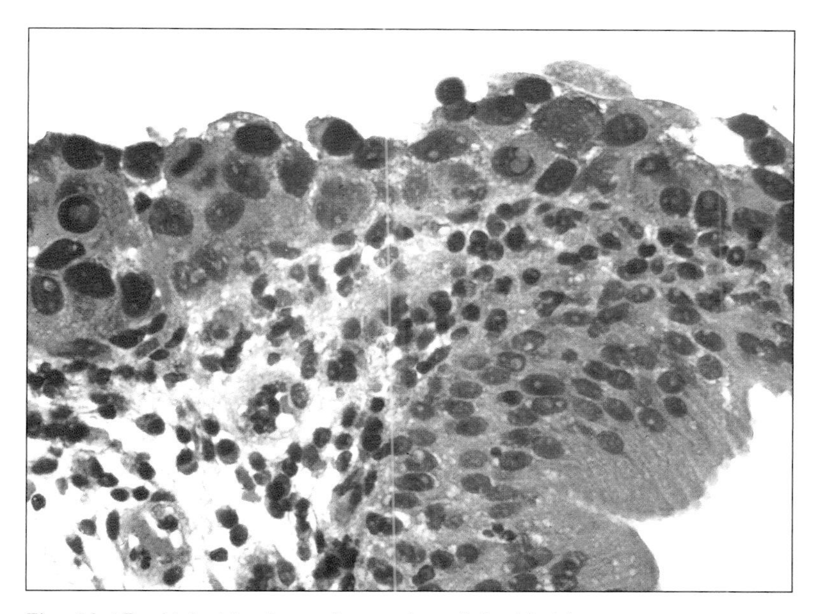

Fig. 11.15 Light histology of a portion of the bladder mucosa, demonstrating carcinoma in situ (CIS) in the upper third of the photomicrograph. The tumor covers the opening of a von Brunn nest, which is lined by non-neoplastic urothelium. Note the markedly enlarged nuclei in the CIS and the normal-sized nuclei in the epithelium of the von Brunn nest.

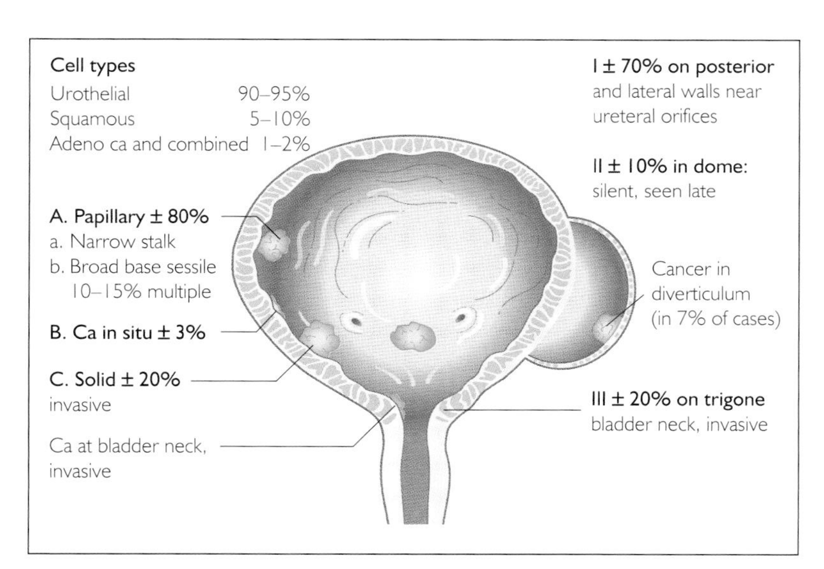

Fig. 11.14 The distribution and cell types of urothelial neoplasms of the urinary bladder. (After Melicow 1974[12] and Tannenbaum 1984,[13] with permission.)

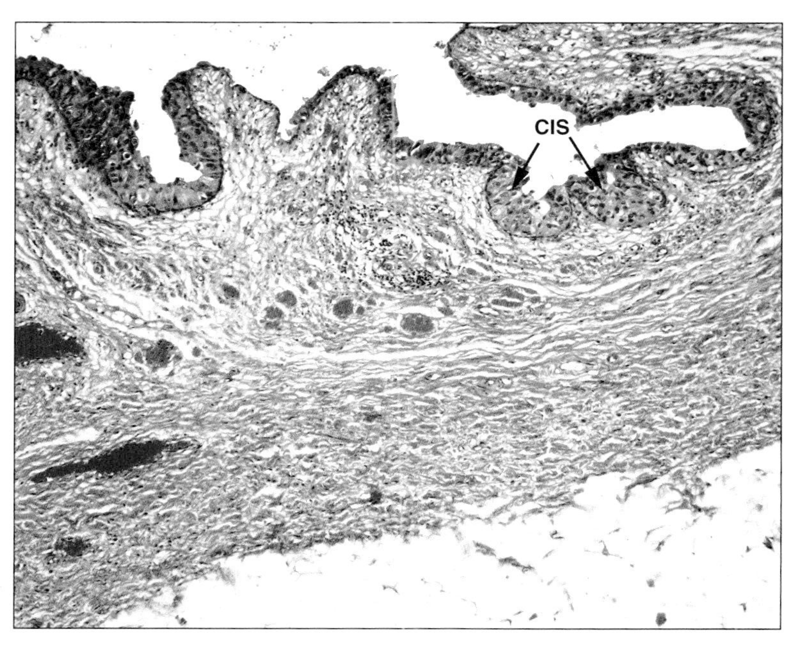

Fig. 11.16 Urothelial carcinoma in situ (CIS) in the mouth of a diverticulum of the urinary bladder. There is dysplasia in other areas of the urothelium.

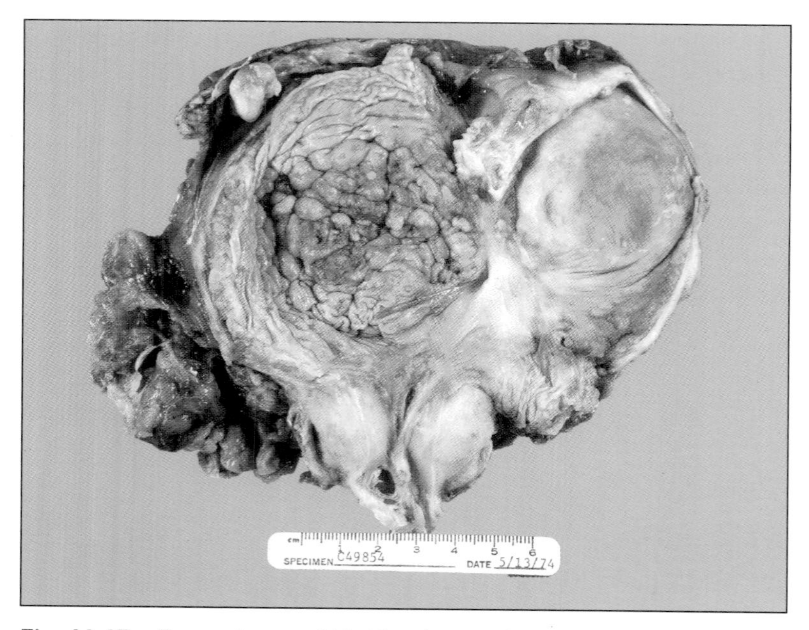

Fig. 11.17 Gross picture of bladder diverticulum on the right, with urothelial carcinoma in situ in the mouth of a diverticulum of the urinary bladder. There was dysplasia in other areas of the urothelium of the diverticulum and urinary bladder.

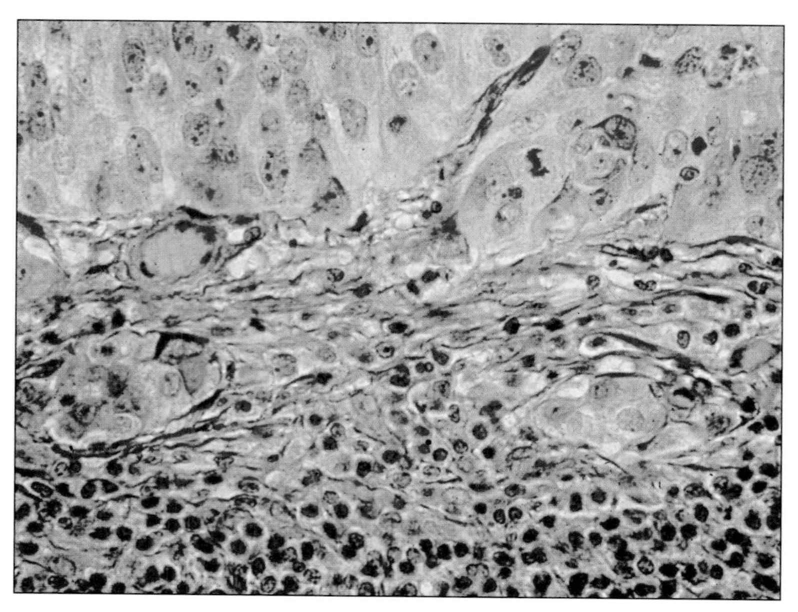

Fig. 11.19 A higher magnification of another portion of the bladder mucosa with carcinoma in situ overlying an invasive focus of carcinomatous urothelium (stage T1 or stage A).

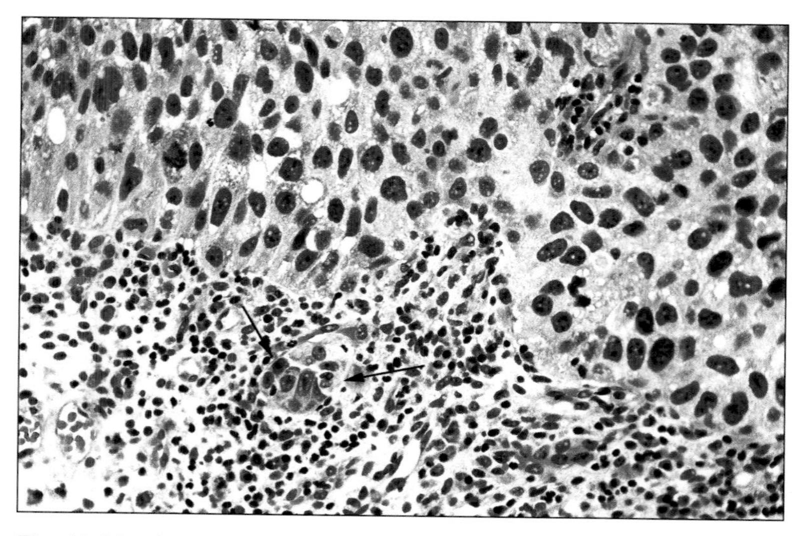

Fig. 11.18 Another portion of the bladder mucosa with carcinoma in situ, but it is overlying an invasive focus of carcinomatous urothelium (arrows) (stage T1 or stage A).

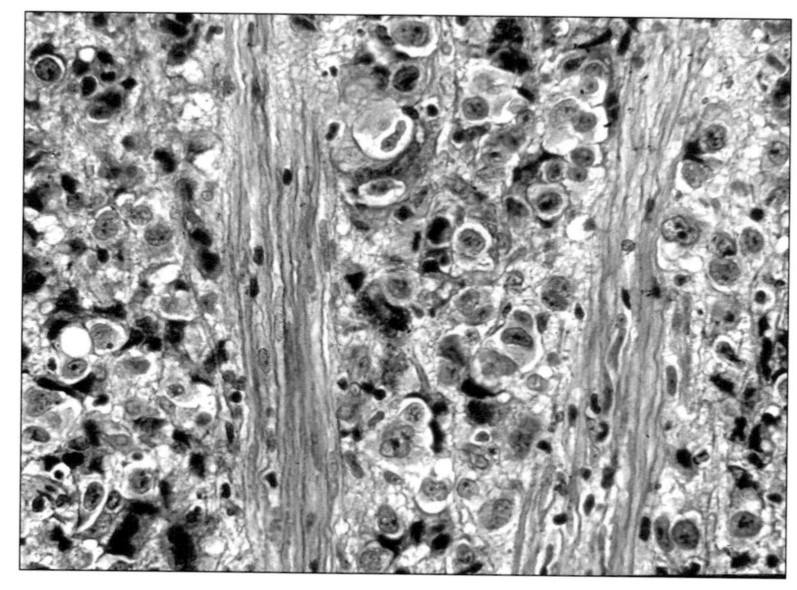

Fig. 11.20 Light histology photomicrograph of another area of the bladder tumor from Figs 11.18 and 11.19. Here there is a high-grade (grade 3) urothelial carcinoma invading the muscularis propria, which is being split apart.

depending on many factors, i.e. the tissue fixatives, the methods of handling the specimen, and whether the pathologist has spent the time looking for these lesions.

As can be seen from Fig. 11.14, a small proportion of urothelial tumors are found in the dome of the bladder (10%). However, a significant percentage of these urothelial tumors occur in the region of the bladder neck (20%). The majority of these bladder neck tumors are 90–95% urothelial; about 5% demonstrate a squamous cell component and approximately 1% are adenocarcinoma in cell type. It is a common occurrence, in that there can be varying percentages of each of these cell types associated with the other. However, it is rare that all three types are found simultaneously.

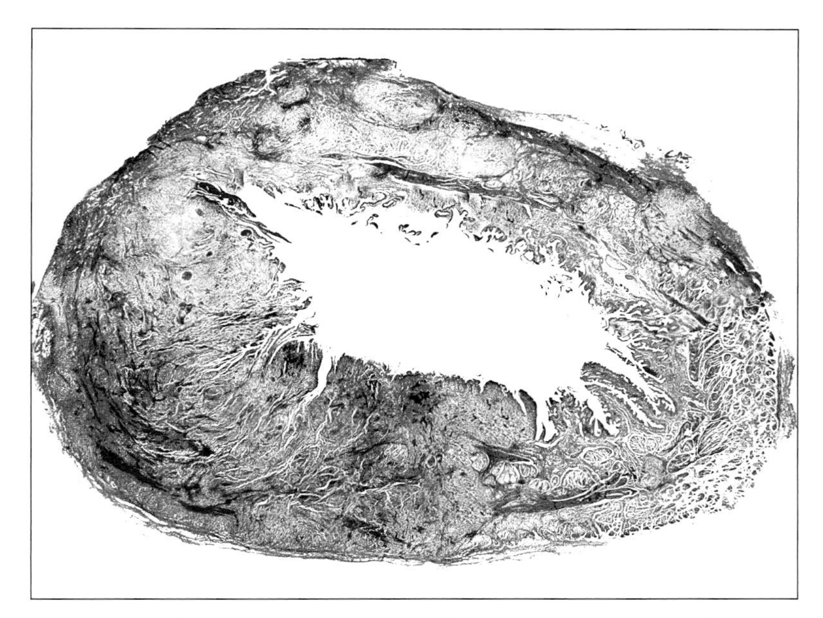

Fig. 11.21 Giant microtome section of a whole cross-section of a bladder with numerous high-grade urothelial tumors that invade through the muscularis propria into the perivesical connective tissue.

When 840 primary vesical tumors were studied over a period of 10 years, there was a varying distribution of the grades, incidence, age, group, and sex. It was noted that 97% of the tumors developed after the patient was 40 years old. In the series studied by Melicow,[12] the greatest incidence occurred between the ages of 50 and 79. The male-to-female ratio was approximately 3:1. The extremely well-differentiated grade 1 and grade 2 tumors reached a peak incidence within the sixth to seventh decade of life and then showed a relative decrease within the next decade. The high-grade tumors were fewer in number but continued to be relatively prominent from the seventh decade on.

GRADING OF UROTHELIAL TUMORS

Similar to the stage, the grade of the urothelial tumor has prognostic significance. On different occasions, the reproducibility of the grading of the same urothelial tumor by the same pathologist and between different pathologists was studied.[14,15] Ooms and colleagues performed an analysis of the performance of pathologists in the grading of bladder tumors. Using the World Health Organization (WHO) grading system, 57 transurethrally resected bladder tumors were analyzed to determine whether different pathologists graded the same bladder tumor differently (interindividual consistency) and whether the same pathologist graded a bladder tumor differently at different times (intraindividual consistency). Disturbingly, high interindividual and intraindividual inconsistencies in the grading of bladder tumors were found. All pathologists showed essentially the same degree of intraindividual inconsistency. In almost 50% of the cases, the same pathologist graded the tumor differently at different times. In clinical decision making, these inconsistencies might invalidate the usefulness of bladder tumor grading.

Ooms and coworkers also described the results of grading of bladder tumors using morphometry and then compared these with the results of histologic grading of the same tumor by different pathologists.[15] The nuclear sizes of cells obtained from the superficial and deep cell layers of each carcinoma and from giant cells were measured in 27 cases in which the histologic grading by different pathologists was unequivocal. In cells from all three areas, the nuclear area increased with higher grades of tumor. However, significant differences in size of only the large cells were seen in tumors of grade 1 and 2. It can be seen from this study that morphometry is a valuable tool in the objective grading of bladder tumors, with the exception of CIS lining the bladder lumen.

Recently, the grading of papillary tumors has taken on even more significance in our cost-effective society. This fact is brought into focus by an article evaluating recurrence and progression in low-grade papillary urothelial tumors. Holmäng and colleagues reported on long-term follow-up data on patients from western Sweden.[16] They specifically studied the WHO group of grade 1 bladder tumors, and determined whether further histopathologic subgrouping of these papillary neoplasms into groups of low malignant potential and low-grade papillary carcinoma was of clinical value (see Figs 11.22–11.36). Six hundred and eighty patients in western Sweden were first diagnosed with bladder carcinoma from 1987 to 1988 and were registered and followed for at least 5 years. Of the tumors in these patients, 255 (37.5%) were stage Ta, WHO grade 1. Tumors were further classified as papillary neoplasm of low malignant potential in 95 patients and low-grade papillary carcinoma in 160 according to the WHO and the International Society of Urological Pathology consensus classification of urothelial (transitional cell) neoplasms of the bladder.[17] It was demonstrated that the mean age of patients first diagnosed with low-grade papillary carcinoma was 69 years, which was 4.6 years higher than those with papillary neoplasm of low malignant potential ($P < 0.005$). During a mean observation time of 60 months, the researchers' 255 patients underwent 577 operations for recurrences and had 1858 negative cystoscopies. The risk of recurrence was significantly lower in patients with papillary neoplasm of low malignant potential as compared with those with low-grade papillary carcinoma (35% versus 71%, $P < 0.001$). The risk of recurrence was higher in patients first diagnosed

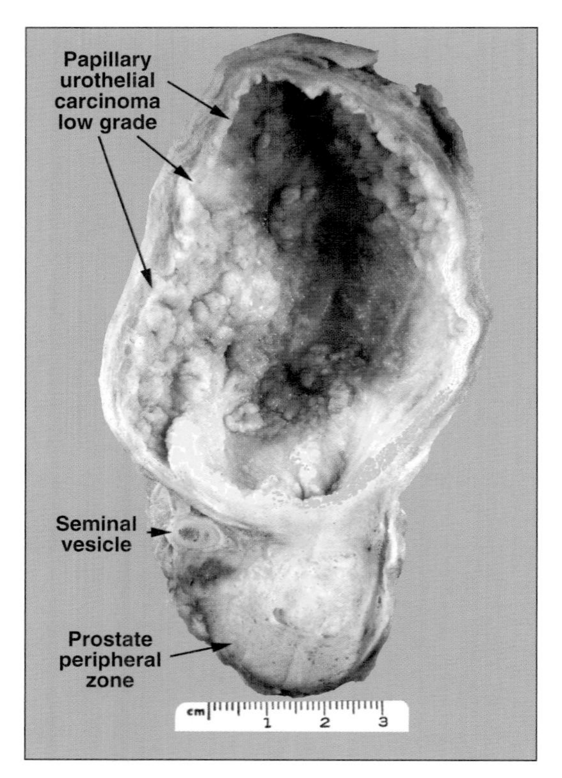

Fig. 11.22 Gross specimen of a radical cystoprostatectomy in which the entire urothelial surface has multiple papillary urothelial tumors as well as invasive urothelial cancer in some foci (pT2 lesions).

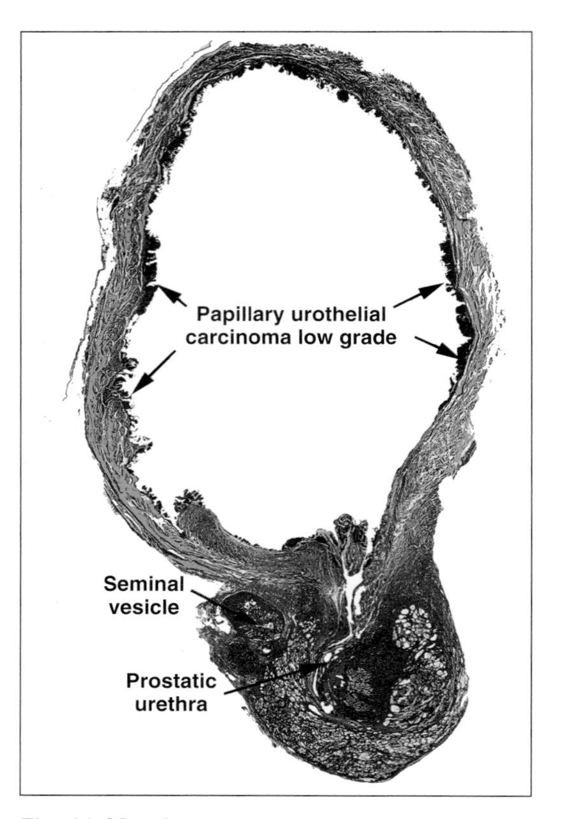

Fig. 11.23 Giant microtome section of the gross specimen from Fig. 11.22. Notice that the entire urothelial surface has multiple papillary urothelial tumors as well as invasive urothelial cancer in some foci (pT2 lesions).

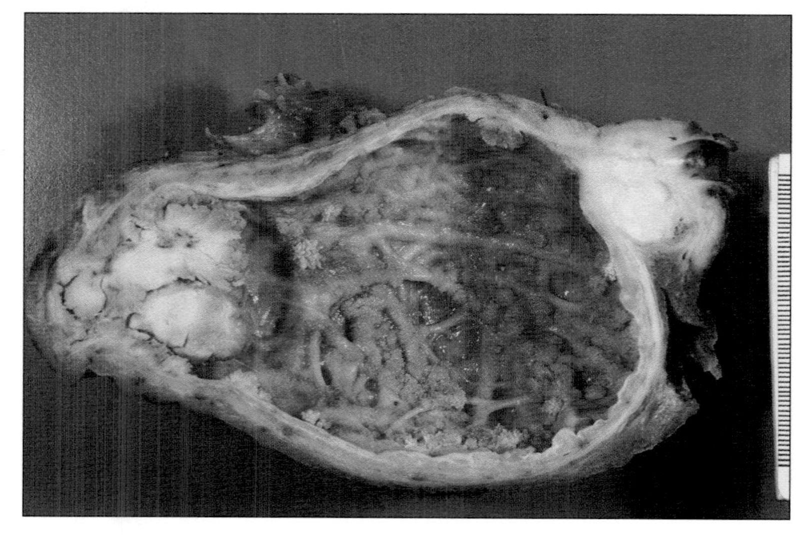

Fig. 11.24 Gross specimen of a radical cystoprostatectomy in which the entire urothelial surface has multiple papillary urothelial tumors as well as invasive urothelial cancer at the dome and other portions of the bladder wall.

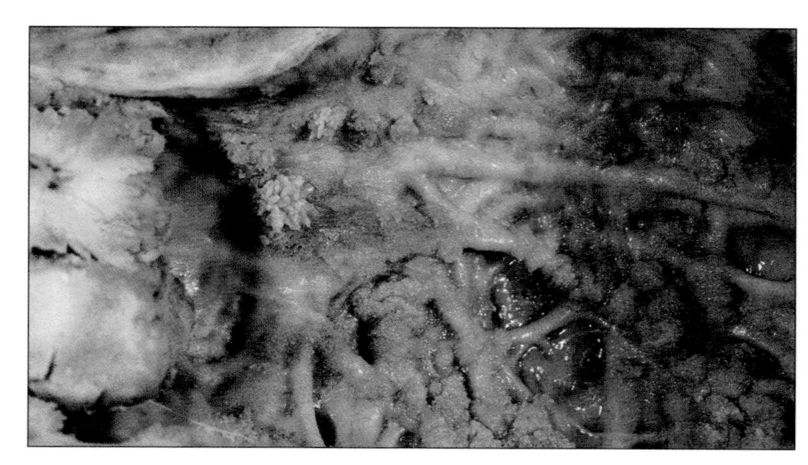

Fig. 11.25 A higher magnification of the specimen shown in Fig. 11.24.

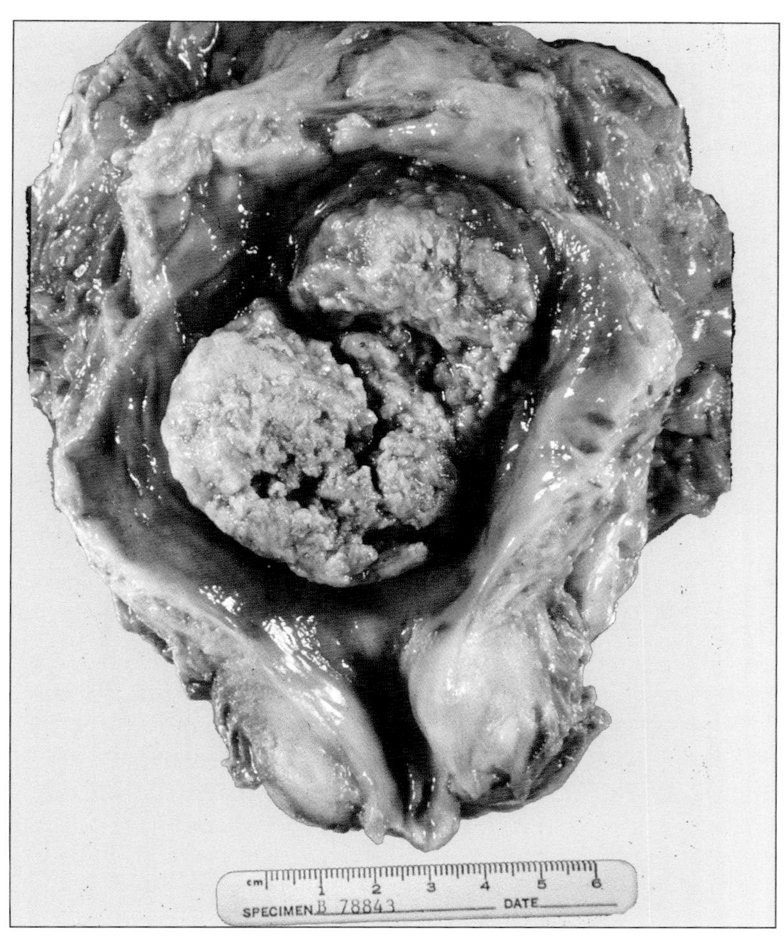

Fig. 11.26 Gross specimen of a radical cystoprostatectomy in which there is a large high-grade urothelial tumor filling the lumen of the urinary bladder. The entire urothelial surface has dysplasia and carcinoma in situ. The tumor in this patient was detected because of positive urinary cytology and high fever due to pyelonephritis.

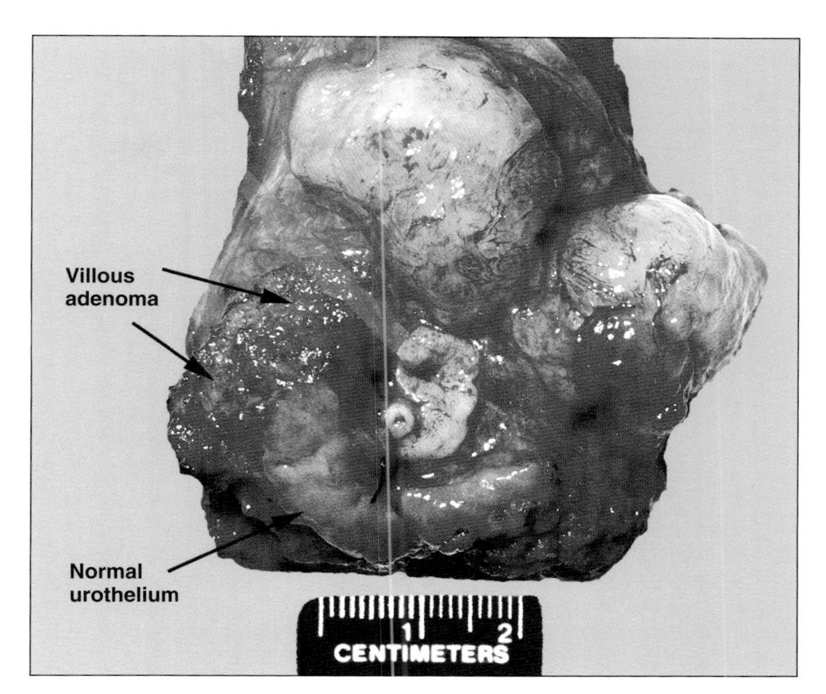

Fig. 11.27 Gross specimen of a partial cystectomy for a urachal carcinoma. The specimen has on its surface a villous adenoma as well as an invasive intramural mucinous adenocarcinoma.

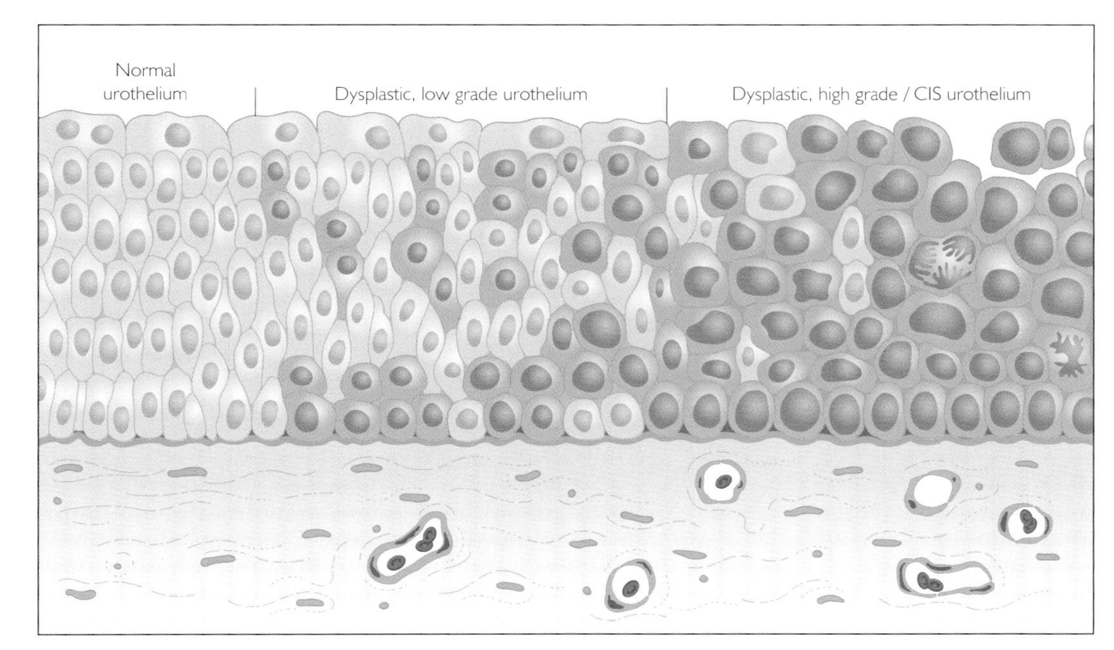

Fig. 11.28 Changes in the cellular arrangement of cytologically benign normal cells (pink cytoplasm and finely blue granular nuclei) and cytologically abnormal or neoplastic cells (the cytoplasm is dark red and the nuclei are coarsely granular blue). There is a progression of architectural and cytologic changes as we go from normal urothelium to low-grade dysplastic urothelium, and then finally into high-grade dysplasia. In the last of these, there are increasing percentages of dysplastic cells, with a final disappearance of the surface cells (which is carcinoma in situ; CIS). The last of these is seen also in Figs 11.15, 11.16, 11.18, and 11.19.

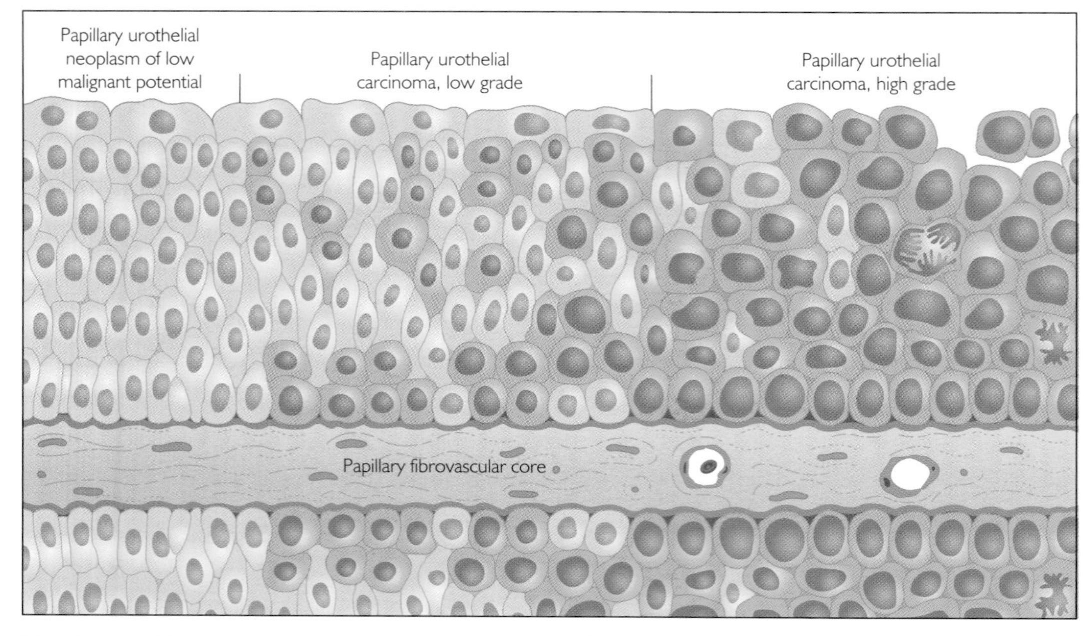

Fig. 11.29 The change in the cellular arrangement of cytologically benign normal cells (pink cytoplasm and finely blue granular nuclei) and cytologically abnormal or neoplastic cells (the cytoplasm is dark red and the nuclei are coarsely granular blue) surrounding both sides of a papillary fibrovascular stalk. There is a progression of changes in architecture and cytology of the cells when we examine urothelial neoplasms of low malignant potential, low-grade urothelial cancer, and then finally high-grade urothelial cancer. In the last of these, there are increasing percentages of pleomorphic and anaplastic cells, with a final disappearance of the surface or umbrella cells. This progression is the same as that shown in Fig. 11.28, except that there is a fibrovascular stalk here, which is surrounded on both sides by neoplastic urothelium.

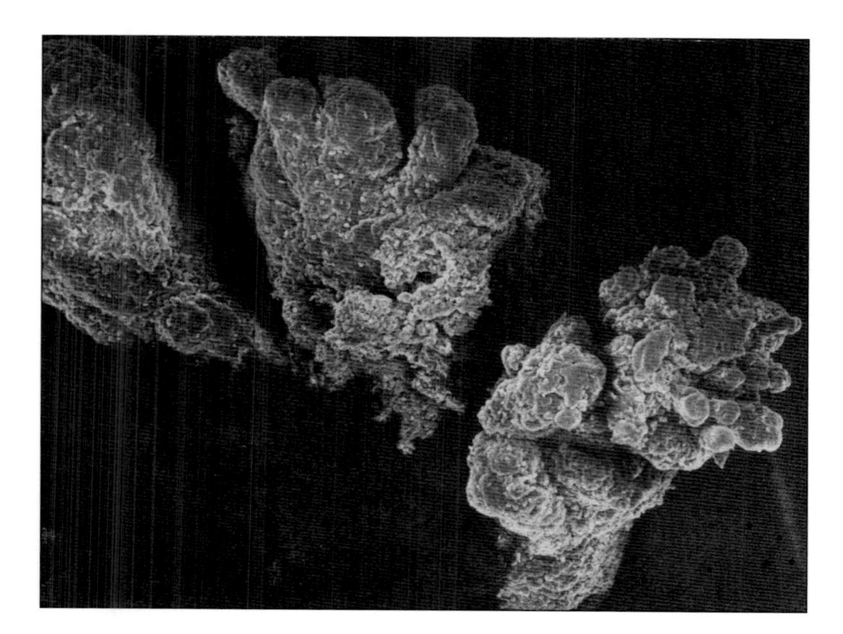

Fig. 11.30 Scanning electron microscopy of a papillary urothelial tumor of low malignant potential. This specimen was obtained from a patient with recurrent papillary tumors. The fibrovascular stalks are lined by urothelium that is cytologically benign. A graphic representation is seen in Fig. 11.29 and Figs 11.31–11.37.

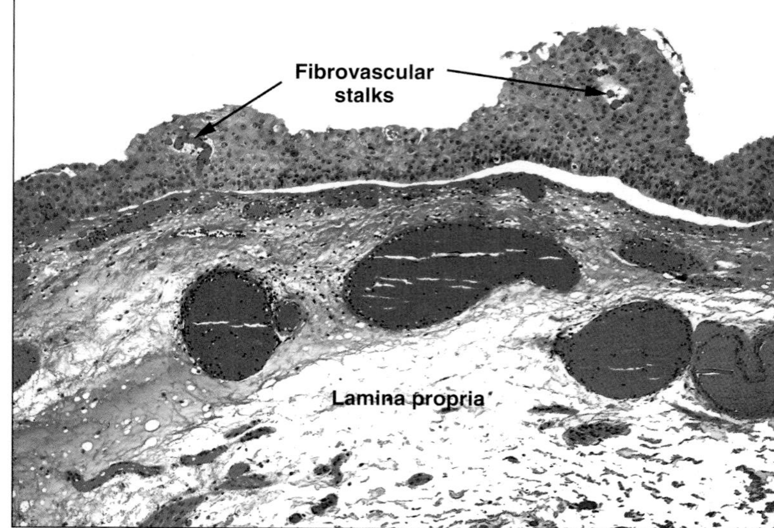

Fig. 11.31 A 'cold cup' biopsy of a erythematous area near the trigone. Intraepithelial fibrovascular stalks are visible only as an area of erythema.

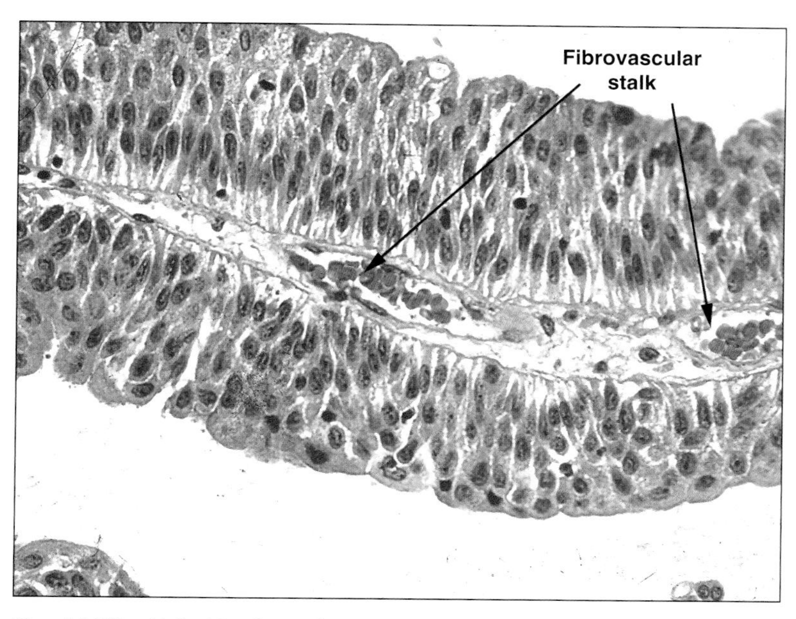

Fig. 11.32 Light histology photomicrograph of a papillary urothelial tumor of low malignant potential. This specimen was obtained from the same patient as in Fig. 11.22. The fibrovascular stalks are lined by urothelium that is cytologically non-malignant or normal.

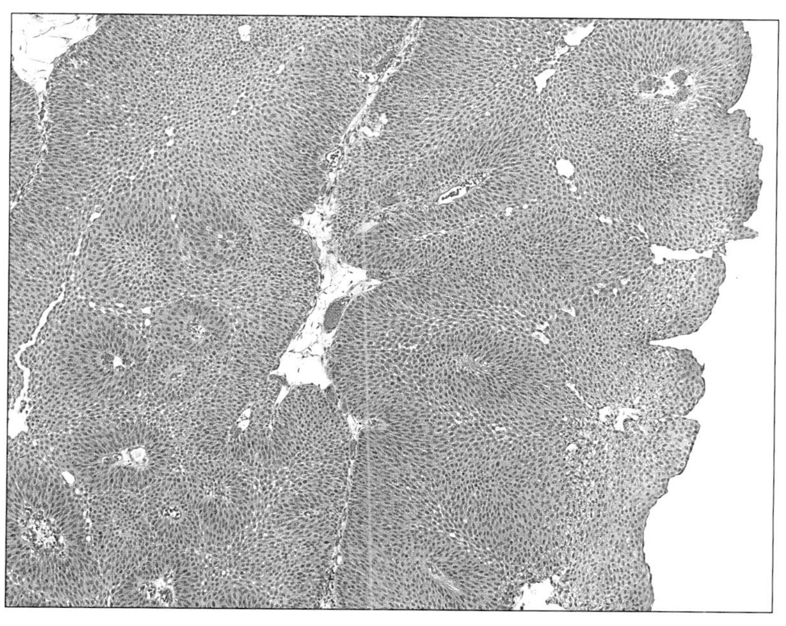

Fig. 11.34 Light histology photomicrograph, but at even higher magnification, of a confluent papillary urothelial tumor of low malignant potential. The fibrovascular stalks are lined by hyperplastic urothelium that is cytologically non-malignant.

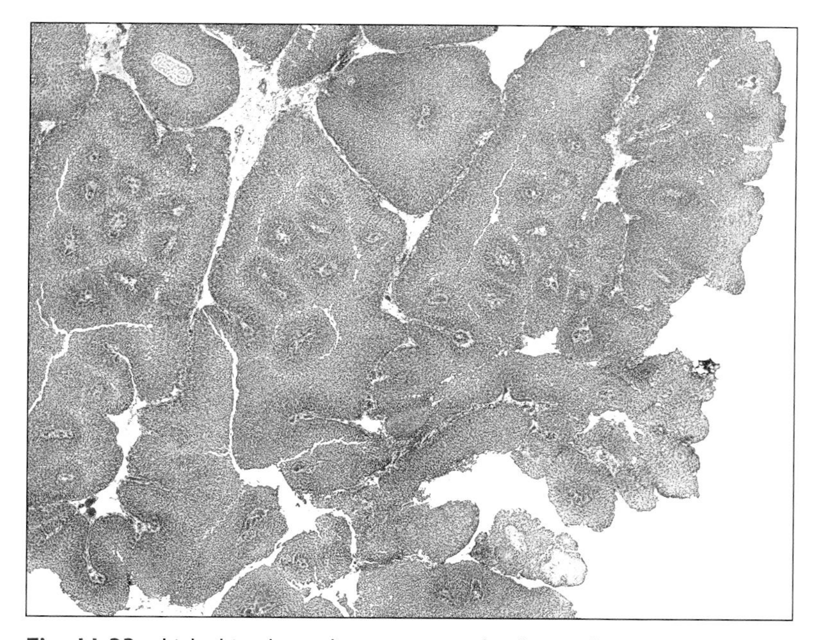

Fig. 11.33 Light histology photomicrograph of a confluent papillary urothelial tumor of low malignant potential (specimen obtained from the same patient as in Fig. 11.22). The fibrovascular stalks are lined by urothelium that is cytologically non-malignant or normal.

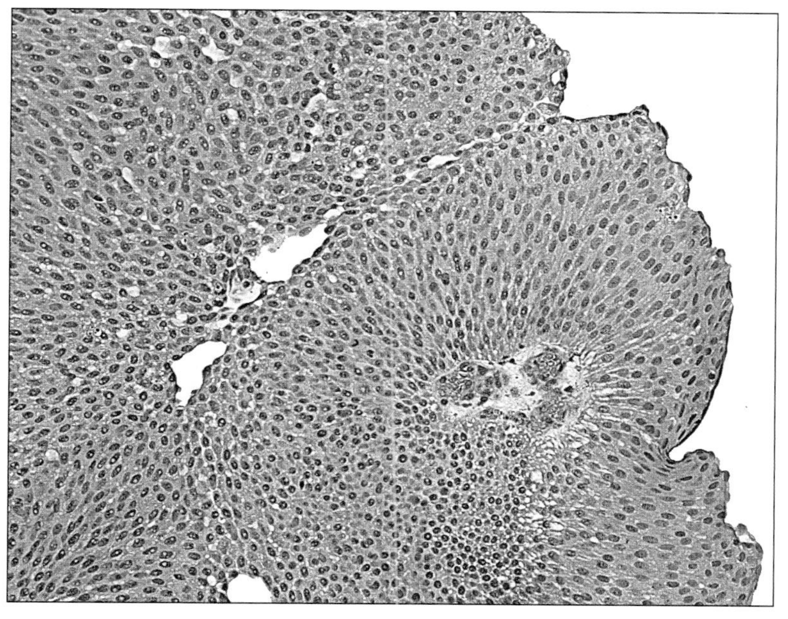

Fig. 11.35 Light histology photomicrograph, but at higher magnification, of a confluent papillary urothelial tumor of low malignant potential (specimen obtained from the same patient as in Fig. 11.22). The fibrovascular stalks are lined by cytologically non-malignant or normal urothelium.

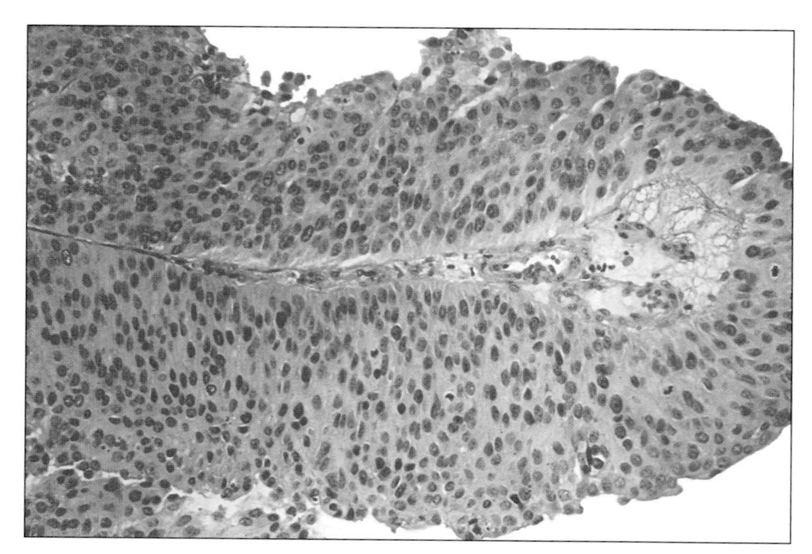

Fig. 11.36 Light histology photomicrograph of a papillary urothelial carcinoma (low grade). This specimen was obtained from the same patient as in Fig. 11.22. The fibrovascular stalks are lined by urothelium that is cytologically malignant (see Figs 11.28 and 11.29).

Table 11.3 Comparison of the modified Bergkvist, old and new World Health Organization (WHO), and WHO–International Society of Urological Pathology (ISUP) consensus classification systems[17]

Modified Bergkvist	*WHO 1972*	*WHO 1999*	*WHO–ISUP 1999 consensus*
Papilloma grade 0	Papilloma grade 0	Papilloma grade 0	Papilloma grade 0
Papilloma grade 1	Transitional cell cancer grade 1	Urothelial neoplasm of low malignant potential	
Cancer grade 2a	Transitional cell cancer grade 1	Urothelial cancer grade 1	Urothelial cancer, low grade
Cancer grade 2b	Transitional cell cancer grade 2	Urothelial cancer grade 2	Urothelial cancer, high grade
Cancer grade 3	Transitional cell cancer grade 3	Urothelial cancer grade 3	Urothelial cancer, high grade

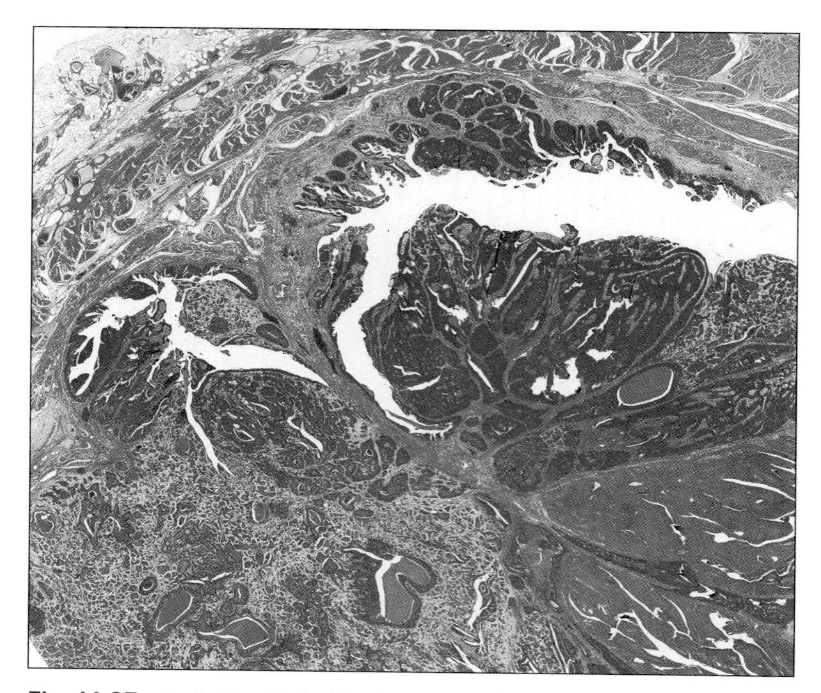

Fig. 11.37 A digitized light histology scan of a whole slide of high-grade papillary urothelial carcinoma found in the gross specimen from Fig. 11.26. There is a multicentric tumor of different cytologic grades and depth of invasion.

with multiple tumors, as well as in those with recurrence after the first 3–4-month follow-up period. The stage progressed in six patients (2.4%), all with low-grade papillary carcinoma at diagnosis. This study demonstrated that more than 90% of patients with stage Ta, WHO grade 1 have a benign form of bladder neoplasm, and few have truly malignant tumors. Future research should focus on reducing the number of recurrences and follow-up cystoscopies, and on finding methods to identify malignant tumors so that pertinent treatment can be instituted. Subgrouping of WHO grade 1 bladder tumors as papillary neoplasm of low malignant potential and low-grade papillary carcinoma seems to add valuable prognostic information.[16] A comparison of the various grading protocols is shown in Table 11.3.

A major goal is to reduce the large number of negative cystoscopies, which are costly and cause patient discomfort. Many have noted that patients with a negative cystoscopy at 3 months have a good prognosis,[18,19] and it has been suggested that such patients should undergo the next follow-up evaluation after 9 months.[20] Morris and coworkers noted that patients with a negative cystoscopy at 3 months rarely had recurrences and, if they did, these recurrences had a low malignant potential and were easily fulgurated. As a rule, intravesical therapy was not indicated in such patients.[19] The results of the study by Holmäng's group confirm these findings,[16] lending support for a change in endoscopic follow-up routines. It remains to be determined whether voided urine cytology or simple bladder tumor tests, such as the bladder tumor antigen (BTA) test (Bard Diagnostics, Redmond, Washington, USA), will be of value if follow-up routines are changed.[21]

In these and other studies, high-grade papillary tumors may be present that are often associated with a poorly differentiated and invasive component (see Figs 11.37–11.45). In addition to these invasive components, in the final specimen or in the bladder biopsies, there is often urothelium that is neither CIS nor normal. In these biopsies of the urothelium, a diagnosis of urothelial dysplasia must be considered.

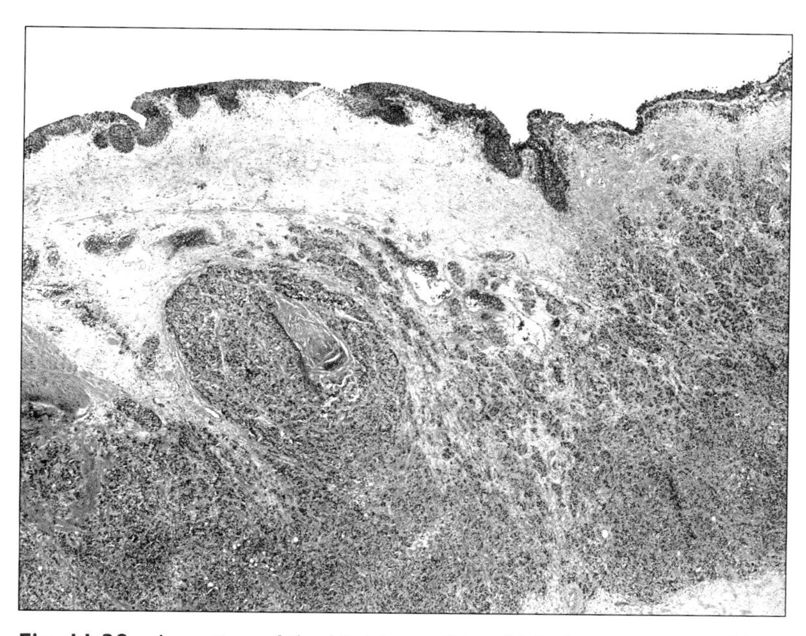

Fig. 11.38 A portion of the bladder wall in which there was no visible papillary tumor but a flat dysplastic urothelium overlying a poorly differentiated or high-grade urothelial cancer, which was invasive.

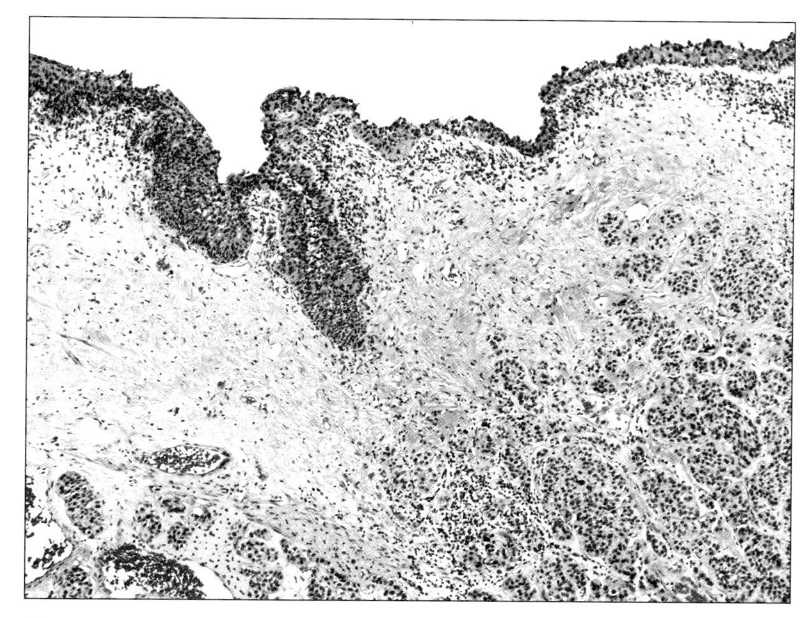

Fig. 11.39 A higher magnification of Fig. 11.38. Dysplastic intact urothelium over a lamina propria that contains a poorly differentiated invasive urothelial carcinoma.

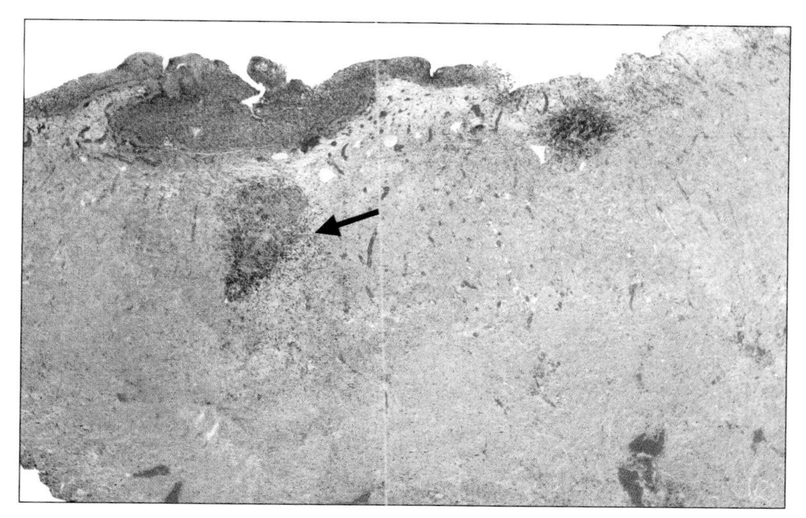

Fig. 11.40 Dysplastic and hyperplastic urothelium covering a granulomatous focus in the lamina propria (arrow). If this area is cauterized, it can be mistaken for carcinoma.

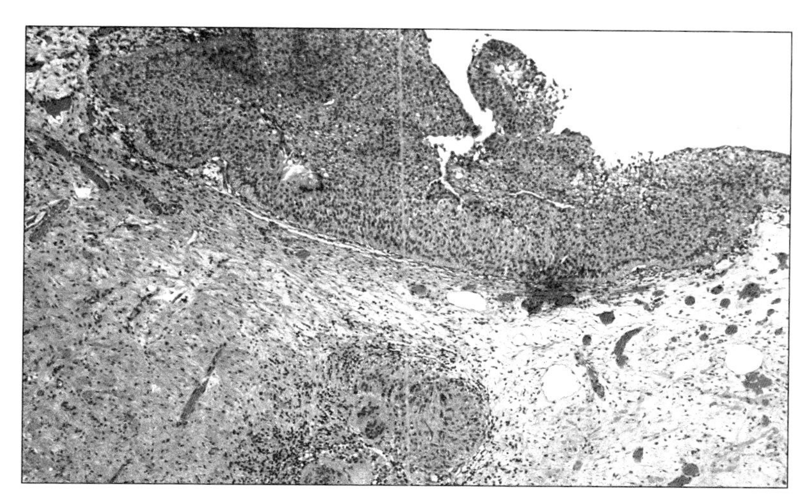

Fig. 11.41 A small low-grade papillary urothelial carcinoma and dysplastic urothelium overlying a granulomatous area in the lamina propria.

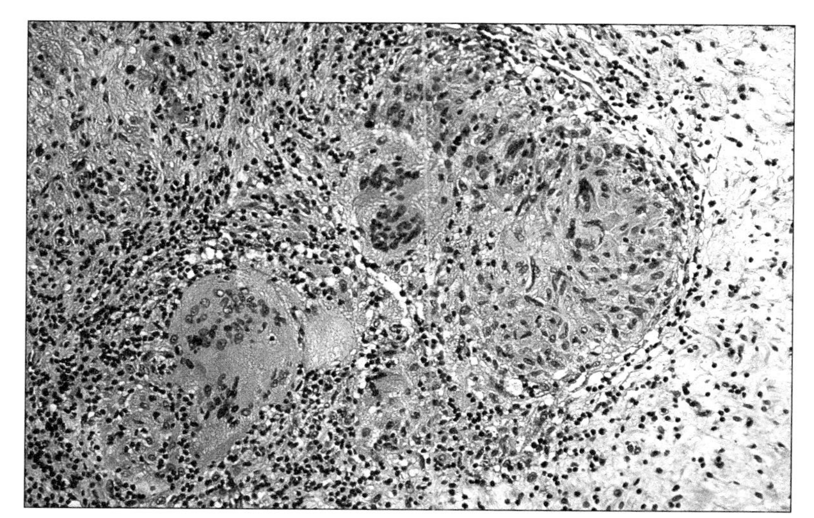

Fig. 11.42 A high-power photomicrograph of a granulomatous area in the lamina propria that can be due to previous biopsy, bacillus Calmette–Guérin therapy, and other chemotherapy.

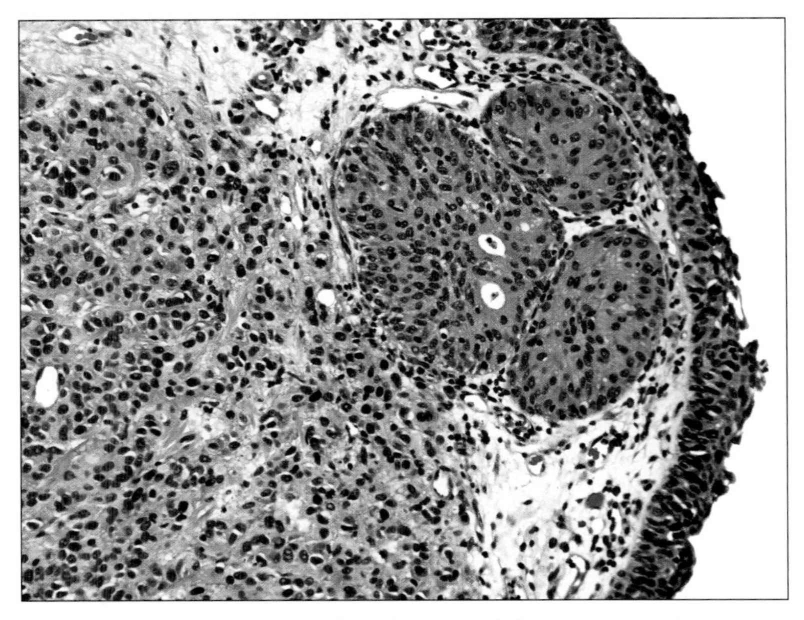

Fig. 11.43 Dysplastic urothelium (on the right) covers a neoplastic nest of von Brunn and also nests of high-grade invasive urothelial carcinoma (on the left).

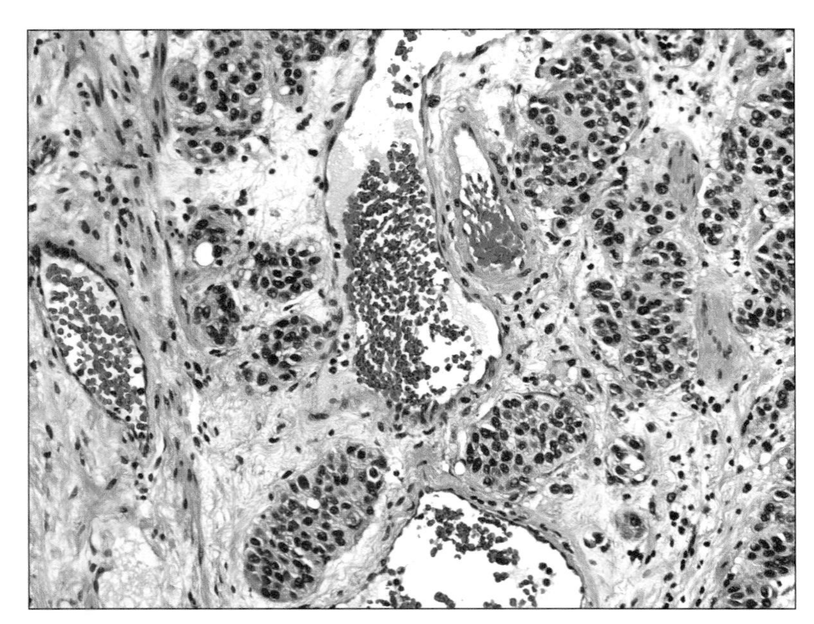

Fig. 11.44 Isolated nests of invasive high-grade urothelial carcinoma in the lamina propria.

UROTHELIAL DYSPLASIA

The clinical significance of urothelial dysplasia is beginning to be appreciated. There is good circumstantial evidence that, as a pathologic diagnosis, it may precede overt urothelial cancer. In a retrospective study of resected flat urothelium adjacent to exophytic urothelial cancer, Althausen and colleagues found that nine of 25 patients with urothelial dysplasia developed invasive cancers within a 5-year follow-up period.[22] Similarly, Murphy and coworkers studied prospectively selected urothelial biopsies from

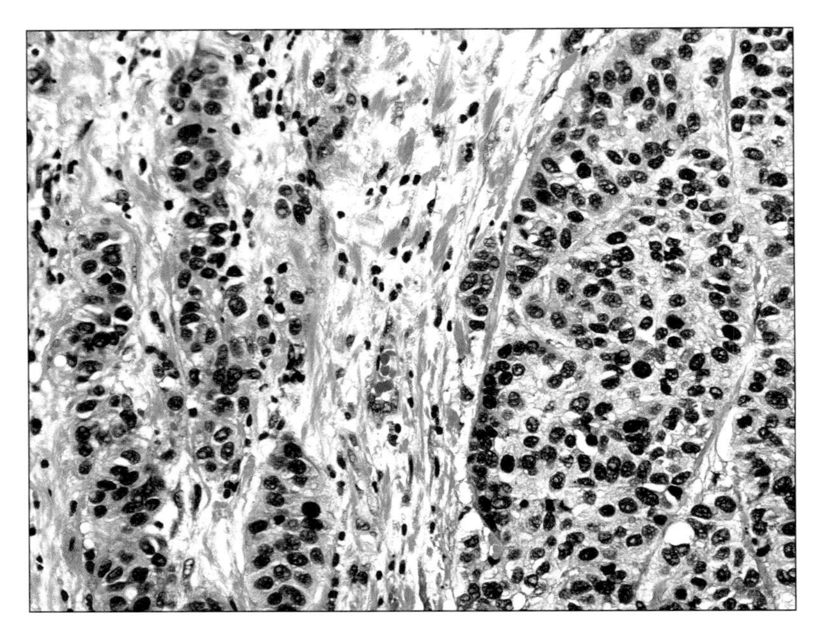

Fig. 11.45 Isolated nests of invasive high-grade urothelial carcinoma in the lamina propria (on the right) beginning to invade muscularis propria (on the left).

patients observed for urothelial cancer.[23] Eleven of 29 patients (38%) had documented recurrences after the appearance of these 'premalignant lesions', as compared with only five of 32 (16%) individuals with normal urothelium at the selected biopsy sites.

Urothelial dysplasia (or urothelial atypia) is a relatively recent pathologic term that will need further clinical definition with increasing pathologic recognition of this lesion. The disease is multifocal, and it is frequently encountered in those patients who are being observed for bladder cancer. The frequency of the disease in pathologic specimens varies considerably.[22,24-26] It is present with greater frequency in radical cystectomy specimens and can also be found in urothelial biopsies with no apparent clinical disease.[23,27] Many of the patients with urothelial dysplasia are middle-aged men without any history of urinary tract infection; however, they complain of frequency and dysuria. The urothelial atypia or dysplastic lesions cannot be localized endoscopically. These lesions, like CIS, commonly exfoliate cells into the urine. These cells cannot be readily differentiated from atypical cells commonly found with the urothelial atypia of regenerating urothelium associated with repair after trauma or infection.

Urothelial atypia or dysplasia describes a spectrum of histologic abnormalities between normal urothelium and CIS (see Fig. 11.28).[28] These lesions can be divided into two degrees of morphologic severity: low-grade dysplasia and high-grade dysplasia. Lesions of the lowest grade may not be readily distinguished from reactive, regenerating, and/or reparative urothelium. On occasion, the highest grade may be difficult to distinguish from unequivocal carcinoma.

CARCINOMA IN SITU

Five decades ago, Dr. M.M. Melicow at the Columbia-Presbyterian Medical Center coined the term carcinoma in situ. This term was applied to the neoplastic urothelium seen in histologic sections that was interposed (cystoscopically non-exophytic urothelium) between surrounding cystoscopically visible papillary tumors of the urinary bladder removed at cystectomy.[27,29,30]

More than 10 years later, employing urinary cytology, a group of patients was selected from an even larger group of patients who had urothelial cancer of the urinary bladder.[31] Patients in the former group showed evidence of positive cytology or cancer cells in the urine. When these patients were examined cystoscopically, they were found to be free of visible tumors, with the only evidence of malignancy being detected by urinary cytologic studies. They were then observed for varying periods of time, ranging from 3 months to 7 years, before there were any cystoscopically visible lesions or recurrences within the urinary bladder.

At Columbia-Presbyterian Medical Center, Memorial Hospital, and several other urologic oncology centers, this disease pattern began to be recognized.[27] It is now standard operational procedure to obtain selected biopsies of the bladder mucosa, especially from the lateral and posterior walls above the trigone, where the incidence of CIS is the highest. If multiple serial tissue levels are taken of the CIS, approximately 30% of the patients so examined will have an early invasive or early stage pT1 invading urothelial cancer. In some instances, the neoplastic urothelium may contain intraepithelial blood vessels that are not usually observed by the urologist on cystoscopic examination (see Fig. 11.31). The cytologic characteristics of the CIS cells can be pleomorphic when they are compared cytologically with normal cells that are present within the same microscopic field. In these early biopsy specimens, the CIS process is readily demonstrated to be present not only beneath the normal urothelium and above the basement membrane, but also in Brunn nests, cystitis cystica, and, in many instances, in the periurethral prostatic ducts. The nuclei of many of these CIS areas are usually two to three times the nuclear size of the normal urothelium. These urothelial lesions are usually found over a highly vascularized area of microcapillaries.

By mapping, Koss and colleagues studied this type of lesion in 20 surgically removed bladders.[32] They demonstrated CIS and related lesions, i.e. atypical hyperplasias, in those areas adjacent to or distant from visible tumors. They also found numerous areas of occult invasive carcinoma to be derived from such abnormal epithelium. These histologic findings suggest that the areas of the bladder most frequently involved by these precancerous lesions are the left and right lateral walls and the posterior wall. The trigone and dome regions are less frequently involved.

In a retrospective light histology study of CIS of the urinary bladder, Tannenbaum and Romas were able to observe 140 cases of CIS of the urinary bladder, with a follow-up period of 14–21 years.[33] The patient records in all their cases indicated no previous history of urothelial or bladder cancer. Eighty percent of the patients presented with symptoms of dysuria or microscopic hematuria. There was an initial histologic documentation of CIS for each of the patients before they were included in the study. In a period of 4–6 years, 40% of the patients progressed from a stage A to a stage B1 (pT1 to pT2a) lesion. Ten percent had stage B2 to stage C (pT2b to T3) disease. At the 10-year follow-up, 60% of these patients had stage A to B1 (pT1 to T2a) disease and 20% had B2 to C (pT2b to T3) disease; the remaining patients had died. When the same patients were examined 15–21 years after the initial documentation of their cystoscopically flat CIS, 40% had died from their disease, with the remaining majority being classified as having stage B2 to stage D (pT2 to T4) disease. This initial retrospective study strongly suggests that urothelial CIS is a biologically aggressive and non-retrogressive disease. It is only through cytologic studies and random biopsies of the cystoscopically normal urothelium under the most fastidious cystoscopic conditions and pathologic fixation that these early urothelial cancers can be documented.

Similar morphologic and clinical observations in lesions detected by positive urinary cytology in patients without any previous urothelial neoplasms have also been observed at the Mayo Clinic.[27] Researchers noted that the evolution of these tumors was considerably longer than they had previously documented.

The natural history of this lesion has yet to be resolved. On the basis of serial biopsies and mapping studies of cystectomy specimens,[34–36] it is readily recognized that there may be a progression of normal urothelium to flat CIS (cystoscopically flat erythematous areas) through the possible stages of hyperplasia and atypia (dysplasia of low grade and high grade), as illustrated in Fig. 11.28.[37] The various histologic features that exemplify CIS also cytologically characterize those features found in higher-grade papillary transitional cell tumors, i.e. grades 2 or 3. This clearly represents a loss of the superficial umbrella cells. With the sole utilization of light histology, there are no specific histologic features of the early phases of low-grade CIS (non-exophytic) that can be recognized. Perhaps it is the vascular pattern in the underlying lamina propria, a feature emphasized by Koss and colleagues,[36,38] that might provide valuable early histologic as well as cystoscopic identification of the potentially dangerous hyperplastic or atypical urothelium (dysplastic) that might progress into CIS.

After consideration of staging, grading, and the presence or absence of CIS and dysplasia, a consideration of multicentricity is of paramount importance before cystectomy is performed.

MULTICENTRICITY IN CARCINOMA OF THE URINARY BLADDER

When we discuss carcinoma of the urinary bladder, we have to include diverse pathologic entities with different biology and only two facts in common: that they are malignant epithelial tumors and that they originate in the vesical mucosa. Therefore when we refer to any of their characteristics, such as multicentricity, we have to consider the histologic types, because they all behave differently.

HISTOLOGIC TYPES OF BLADDER CANCER

The epithelium of the urinary bladder is designated as transitional (urothelial), because it is considered to be an intermediate (or transitional) variant between the stratified squamous epithelium and simple squamous epithelium. Its morphologic and functional peculiarities, however, justify the more precise term of urothelium.[39]

In 1954, Mostofi clearly established the potentialities of bladder urothelium transformation into squamous epithelium and glandular epithelium;[40] if we include the foci of squamous cells that are found in the trigone of 46% of normal female bladders and in 7% of normal male bladders,[41] as well as the existence of epithelial mucin-producing areas,[42] the histologic types of bladder carcinoma will be clearly understood.

Ninety percent of bladder carcinomas are transitional,[42] 6–7% are squamous cell carcinomas, 1–2% are vesical adenocarcinomas, and the remaining 1–2% are poorly differentiated carcinomas.[42,43]

GROWTH PATTERNS IN URINARY BLADDER CANCER

Three types of growth pattern may be recognized: the exophytic variant (mostly papillary but occasionally more polyploid), the flat or planophytic variant (without much excrescence toward the vesical lumen and with a wide implantation base), and the mixed type (a combination of the two patterns).[44]

Seventy percent of bladder tumors are papillary and non-infiltrating, 10% are flat infiltrating, and 20% are exophytic and infiltrating.[45] The flat or solid tumors are almost always infiltrating at the time of diagnosis, whereas papillary and exophytic tumors are usually of the superficial type.

CORRELATION BETWEEN HISTOLOGIC TYPES AND GROWTH PATTERNS

Urothelial (transitional) carcinoma

There is a close correlation between cellular malignant grade, degree of spread, and macroscopic growth pattern. Ninety-four percent of grade 1 transitional carcinomas are superficial, and only 6% are, or will be, infiltrating tumors, especially recurrent malignancies.[45] Grade 2 transitional carcinomas are infiltrating in 52% of cases; grade 3 carcinomas are infiltrating in 82% of cases,[44] and they usually exhibit a flat or planophytic growth pattern.

Squamous cell carcinoma

Seventy percent of all true squamous cell carcinomas show muscular invasion at the time of diagnosis.[46] They are often poorly differentiated solid tumors.[47]

Adenocarcinomas

Primary vesical adenocarcinomas are divided into two groups: those of urachal origin and those of urothelial origin. Urachal tumors have a vesical origin in 90% of cases and are most frequently located in the bladder dome and the anterior wall (87% of cases). Owing to their peculiar histologic type, urachal adenocarcinomas are always intraparietal and have a solid pattern.[48] Adenocarcinomas of urothelial origin can be classified as the signet ring type and the well-differentiated type. Primary signet ring cell adenocarcinomas (linitis plastica of the bladder) are more common on the posterior wall and are infiltrating. The papillary forms are exceptional.[49] Well-differentiated adenocarcinomas may range from papillary to solid tumors, although they are often solid and infiltrating.[47,50]

Poorly differentiated carcinomas

These are all solid and infiltrating tumors, regardless of having fusiform and/or giant cells.[47]

Carcinoma in situ

This variant deserves special mention, because it is a form of bladder carcinoma with marked anaplasia and a tendency to evolve into invasive undifferentiated carcinoma.[51] CIS shows a planophytic growth pattern (see Fig. 11.13).

MULTICENTRICITY OF URINARY TRACT TUMORS[52]

The concept of multicentricity in carcinoma of the urinary bladder cannot be restricted to urinary bladder mucosa, as a result of the entire urinary tract being lined by the same type of epithelium (with slight variations). The great majority of bladder carcinogens or their metabolites are transported to the bladder by the urine,[53] especially those that are responsible for transitional cell carcinoma.

As the word suggests, multicentricity connotes the presence of several foci of neoplastic growth. Although the concept is simple, identifying true multicentricity may be difficult, because this phenomenon is not always synchronous. For this reason, the differential diagnosis with recurrences caused by residual tumors should be considered (tumor persistence). In other respects, the criterion of multicentricity is usually established macroscopically (except in CIS). Thus apparent multiple neoplastic foci may have been microscopic neoplastic areas surrounding the initial tumor that were not detected by the endoscopist at the time of removal of the primary tumor.[54] There is a need for being as strict and as realistic as possible, as it is necessary to define a series of criteria of multicentricity to avoid diagnostic misinterpretations.

Synchronous urinary bladder multicentricity

If at the time of endoscopic diagnosis of a bladder carcinoma diverse areas of neoplastic growth are identified, then these should be considered as different and independent foci when macroscopic and microscopic findings of the intertumoral mucosa are normal (see Figs 11.22–11.25).

Asynchronous urinary bladder multicentricity

We should be sure that the following criteria are applied:

- certainty of the total resection or removal of the previous tumor;
- negativity of the standard biopsies of the macroscopically normal mucosa;
- the appearance of a new tumor must take place at least 1 month after the diagnosis of the previous tumor.[55]

The last criterion is questionable, because endoscopic follow-up examinations are not usually carried out before 3 months after resection.

Extraurinary bladder multicentricity

These criteria are not so well defined and depend only on the proximity or distance from the neoplastic involved bladder mucosa. If the neoplastic areas are far from the bladder (renal pelvis, calyces, lumbar and pelvic ureter, and distal urethra), they can be considered only as independent foci, unless there is a widespread CIS. If the neoplastic foci are closer to the bladder (terminal ureter and prostatic urethra), the characteristics of the neighboring vesical mucosa should be evaluated before the diagnosis of multicentricity.

UROTHELIAL CELL CARCINOMA MULTICENTRICITY

SYNCHRONOUS URINARY BLADDER MULTICENTRICITY

Algaba's group studied 72 consecutive cases of transitional cell carcinoma, with a mean follow-up period of 24.7 months. Twenty-five cases (34.7%) were multifocal at the beginning, with 80% of them being superficial tumors.[52] These findings are in accordance with those reported by Heney and colleagues.[56] Systematized multiple biopsies were carried out in 16 of these 25 cases, and in three of them (18.8%) concomitant sites of CIS were detected. Cellular dysplasia was noticed in one case (6.2%).

Sixty-eight percent of these multiple tumors recurred. Comparison of some characteristics of single tumors with multiple tumors revealed that the latter accounted for a higher incidence of associated CIS and rate of recurrence.

ASYNCHRONOUS URINARY BLADDER MULTICENTRICITY

Forty-four (61%) of 72 cases recurred. Recurrences usually occurred within approximately 15 months of complete excision of the initial tumor. Twenty-three (52%) of these 44 cases had a second recurrence within an average of 10.6 months of the first recurrence. Five cases (11%) had more than two recurrences. The chronologic relapses of Algaba's series are somewhat faster than in other studies, in which the average time was 31 and 13 months for the first and second recurrences, respectively.[55]

The following characteristics of the primary tumor have been correlated with further recurrence.

- The aforementioned initial multicentricity.
- The size of the tumor (1 cm with a 2% recurrence rate versus 5 cm with a 21% recurrence rate).[55]
- The grading, although the incidence was similar for grades 2 and 3 in Algaba's series.
- The staging, which in these reviewers' opinion is not easy to correlate, as infiltrating tumors are managed with radical surgery with no possibility of follow-up as far as recurrences are concerned.

- Chromosomes and chromosomal enzymes (telomerase activity) in the urine.[57–61]

UROTHELIAL EXTRAURINARY BLADDER MULTICENTRICITY

SYNCHRONOUS EXTRAURINARY BLADDER MULTICENTRICITY

In the Algaba series of 72 cases of transitional cell carcinoma, one case of pyelocalyceal carcinoma synchronous to the bladder cancer was detected (on the right side, grade 2, PI).[52] There was no case of ureteral tumor. In a larger series, Hvidi and Feldt-Rasmussen reported up to 4% of simultaneous bladder carcinomas in primary tumors of the renal pelvis and 2% in primary ureteral tumors.[62]

ASYNCHRONOUS EXTRAURINARY BLADDER MULTICENTRICITY

In a retrospective study of 188 cases of carcinoma of the upper urinary tract, 16.5% of cases had concomitant or previous bladder cancer.[63] The authors of this study and others usually did not record the overall number of bladder tumor cases treated over this period, and hence did not know the percentage of bladder cancer cases that developed a tumor in the upper urinary tract. Seven (8.6%) of 81 cases of bladder cancer presented with upper urinary tract tumors that developed after the vesical tumor had been diagnosed.[64]

This asynchronous extravesical multicentricity can be explained by the same causes already mentioned; however, many experimental[65] and clinical studies have shown a certain correlation between upper urinary tract tumors and ureteral reflux. In the series reported by Martinez-Piñeiro and coworkers,[64] 71.4% of tumors in the upper urinary tract occurred in patients with ureteral reflux, and in 80% of patients with ureteral reflux and upper urinary tract tumors who had undergone multiple surgical resections. These facts, together with the average latent period (2–3 years) elapsed between the diagnosis of the bladder cancer and the pyeloureteral tumor,[63] suggest the possible implantation of neoplastic cells that have flowed back from the vesical tumor. Nevertheless, the incidence of recurrence of prostatic urethral tumors in patients who have undergone a simultaneous resection of the prostate gland is similar to that of patients who have not undergone prostatic resection.[66] These events are in disagreement with the experimental pattern of cell implantation in humans, as well as with the hypothesis on the role of ureteral reflux and subsequent implantation of malignant cells in the upper urinary tract.

MULTICENTRICITY IN SQUAMOUS CELL CARCINOMA

Algaba and colleagues also reviewed 11 cases of true squamous cell carcinoma of the urinary bladder.[52] All cases were single and infiltrating at the time of diagnosis. Some extensive studies have found 6–10% of multifocal tumors.[67]

Squamous cell carcinomas have a solid cystoscopic appearance and a wide implantation base, and do not appear limited to a particular area of the urinary bladder. They may occur in any location, but were most frequently on the lateral walls (64%), bladder cupulae, and posterior wall. One case (9%) was intradiverticular. None of them presented with other tumors in the rest of the urinary tract. The tumors were infiltrating and were managed with radical surgery. Data on urinary bladder asynchronous multicentricity are not available.

MULTICENTRICITY IN ADENOCARCINOMAS

Seven (54%) of 13 cases of adenocarcinoma of the urinary bladder were secondary to invasion of an immediate vicinity tumor (rectosigmoid neoplasm in five cases, 71%, and prostatic cancer in two cases, 29%). There were five primary adenocarcinomas of the bladder (38%) and one case of undetermined origin (8%). None of the cases reported by Algaba's group arose from an exstrophic bladder.[52]

SUMMARY

The pathobiology of transitional or urothelial cancers in the genitourinary system is characterized by the many features enumerated in the above discussion. They include grade, multicentricity, and stage or depth of invasion into the bladder wall or muscularis propria. We have also noted that tumor size is of equal importance in the clinical progression of these urothelial cancers. We have included a discussion of a new and, it is hoped, clinically useful new grading system (Table 11.2) proposed by several different clinical pathology study groups. In the first part of the twenty-first century, this new system is already undergoing careful evaluation.[68] We are now in a new millennium of understanding, because of the application of molecular cell biology techniques arising from studies in cytogenetics and the DNA sequencing of human chromosomes.[57–61,69]

Before we consider a list of the variations of tumors, we will consider the embryology, anatomy, and again the histology of urothelium.

NORMAL EMBRYOLOGY, ANATOMY, AND HISTOLOGY[70-75]

EMBRYOLOGY

The urothelium develops from the urogenital sinus and wolffian ducts. The urothelial mucosa is derived from the lining of these structures. The anterior bladder wall is formed from mesenchyme induced by inferior regression of the cloacal membrane. Posterior and lateral walls develop from surrounding mesenchyme.

ANATOMY

- Retroperitoneal viscus in pelvis between symphysis pubis and rectum.
- The superior segment expands as a reservoir for urine collection. The inferior segment is fixed to the pelvic wall and urogenital diaphragm.
- In males, the bladder neck is closely associated with the prostate gland. Seminal vesicles adhere to its posteroinferior surface.
- Innervation is supplied by sympathetic and parasympathetic fibers originating from T11 to S4.
- Blood comes from hypogastric arteries and is drained by hypogastric veins. Lymphatics follow venous drainage.

HISTOLOGY

- The urothelium rests on a loose connective tissue lamina propria.
- The urothelial mucosa is a multilayered epithelium with a superficial layer that is ultrastructurally and morphologically different from the underlying intermediate and basal cells. Basal and intermediate cells cannot be distinguished, except by location.
- The exact number of cell layers constituting the normal bladder urothelium is unknown but probably does not exceed six.
- Superficial layer cells have abundant surface membranes, which are stored in folds when the bladder is contracted and unfold to expand the cell surface area when the bladder is distended.
- Superficial cells have apical plaques composed of unique proteins, uroplakins.
- The urothelium produces and secretes mucins.
- The urothelium rests on a basal lamina and overlies a layer of loose connective tissue, most accurately termed lamina propria, which is rich in thin-walled blood vessels closely applied to the epithelium.
- The lamina propria also contains scattered smooth muscle fibers, muscularis mucosae. It does not form a continuous anatomic structure.
- Muscle fibers of muscularis mucosae are distinguished from muscularis propria by size, arrangement, and configuration.
- Fibroadipose tissue covers smooth muscle wall, muscularis propria.
- Muscularis propria is interwoven to promote effective emptying of bladder urine.

GROSS PATHOLOGY OF PAPILLARY AND NONPAPILLARY UROTHELIAL CARCINOMA

- Exhibits a wide variety of growth patterns.
- Polypoid, may have a stalk, and is characteristic of sarcomatoid variant of urothelial carcinoma.
- Sessile.
- Ulcerated and infiltrative.

MICROSCOPIC PATHOLOGY OF PAPILLARY TUMORS

- Papillary urothelial carcinoma is exophytic, with papillae containing well-defined thin fibrovascular cores.
- The cores are covered by urothelium that varies from normal to anaplastic.
- There may be foci of squamous differentiation, which is more often seen in high-grade tumors.
- Numerous papillary fronds appear to float in the space above the mucosal surface.
- Mucinous cells may also be present, occasionally in large numbers.
- Oncocytic change is rarely encountered, with the cells having abundant, finely granular eosinophilic cytoplasm. These morphologic variations have no apparent clinical significance.
- Papillary tumors may have only small, short papillae, resulting in a micropapillary appearance.
- The cores are very fine, with scant stroma and only one or two thin vascular channels in the center.
- The papillae may be complex or branching, which is not seen in normal infolding of the bladder mucosa or in papillary hyperplasia.
- Cytology expresses the full range of grades.

CAUTION

- Bladder mucosa can produce normal folds that mimic papillae. In folds, the stroma appears normal but lacks fine vascular channels extending the length of the papillae of urothelial carcinoma.

- Polypoid cystitis has wider papillary structures with more stromal tissue and vascular structures than papillary carcinoma. In papillary cystitis, the surface epithelium may show reactive atypia. Severe cytologic atypia and disturbances of the papillary architecture are absent (see Figs 11.46–11.49).[76]
- Polypoid cystitis (papillary cystitis) is associated with indwelling catheters and can clinically mimic papillary neoplasia grossly. It consists of an exophytic lesion with edematous lamina propria covered by normal or hyperplastic urothelium. The stroma is wider and contains more inflammatory cells and capillaries than the cores of papillary carcinoma (Figs 11.50–11.60).[76]

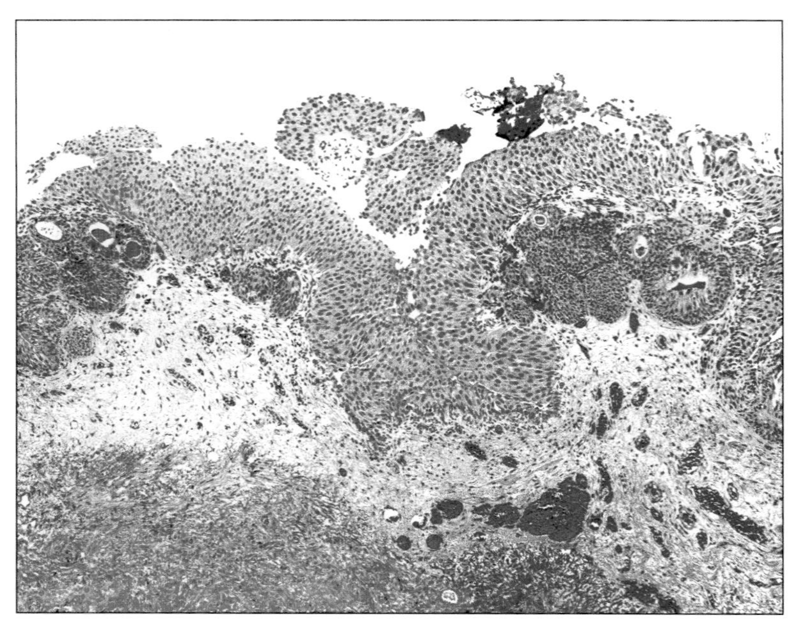

Fig. 11.46 Hyperplastic urothelial mucosa thrown up into folds. There are underlying glands of von Brunn both with and without lumens.

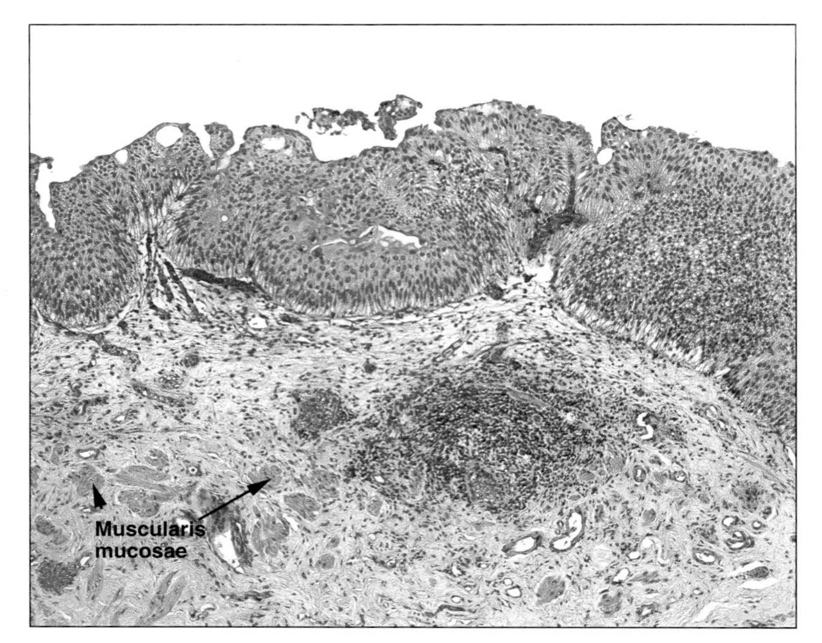

Fig. 11.48 Papillary hyperplastic urothelial mucosa with a von Brunn nest in the center and hyperplastic mucosa in the left of the photomicrograph.

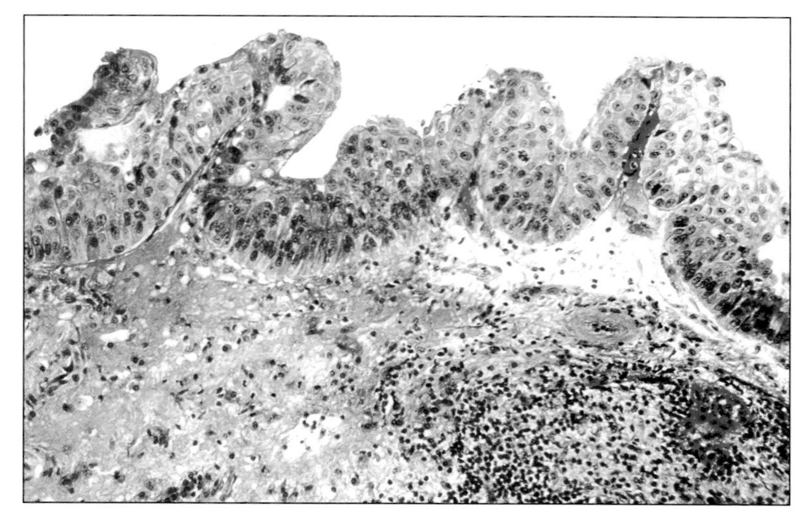

Fig. 11.47 Chronic cystitis with a pseudopapillary urothelial mucosa. Some broad and thickened papillary stroma are associated with the papillary urothelium hyperplasia.

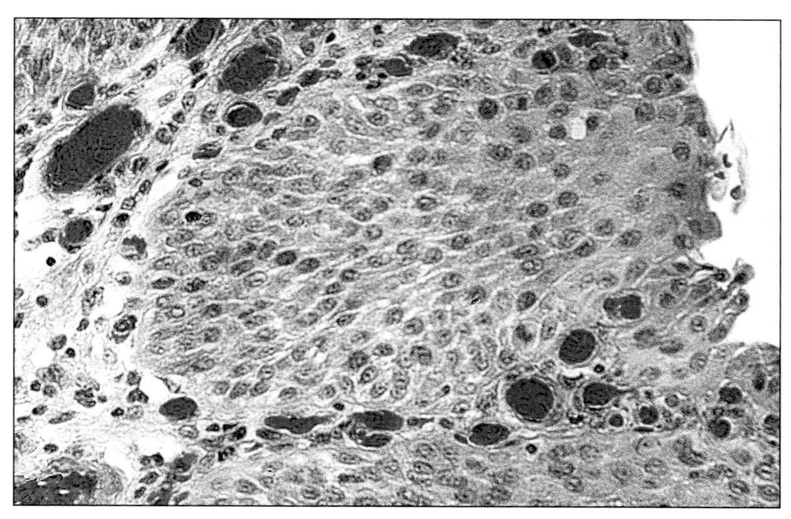

Fig. 11.49 Higher magnification of a portion of the Fig. 11.48 photomicrograph, in which there is intraurothelial microvasculature. We usually do not call these fields neoplasia.

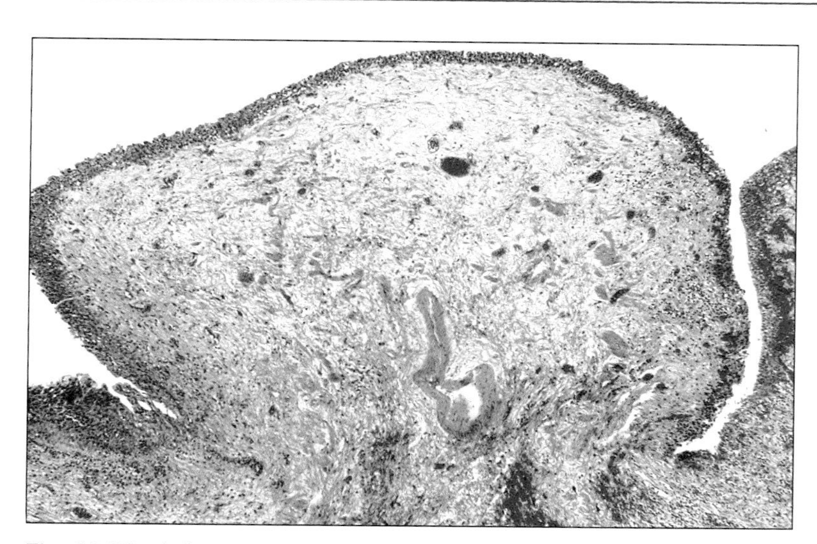

Fig. 11.50 Inflammatory polyp thought to be a tumor. Note the edematous lamina propria beneath the surface urothelium.

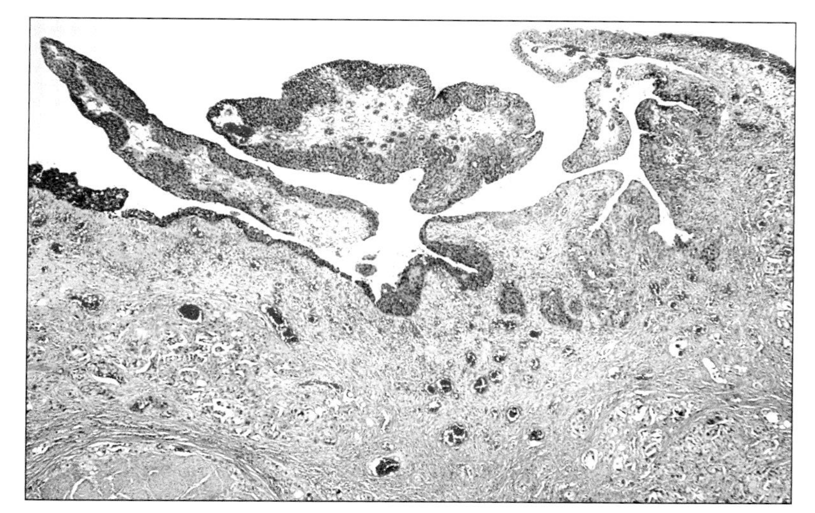

Fig. 11.51 Inflammatory polyp overlying the prostate in the prostatic urethra. This is not a rare phenomenon and appears cystoscopically as tumor.

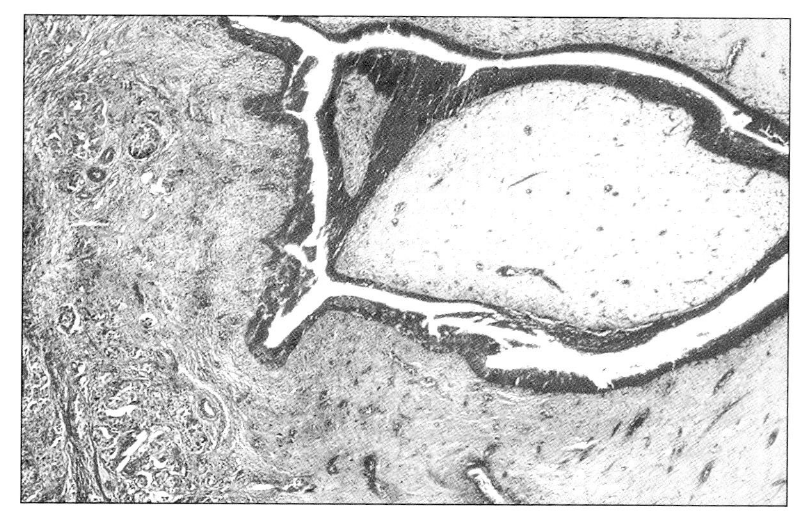

Fig. 11.52 Inflammatory polyp. Higher magnification of Fig. 11.51. The prostate glands are on the left.

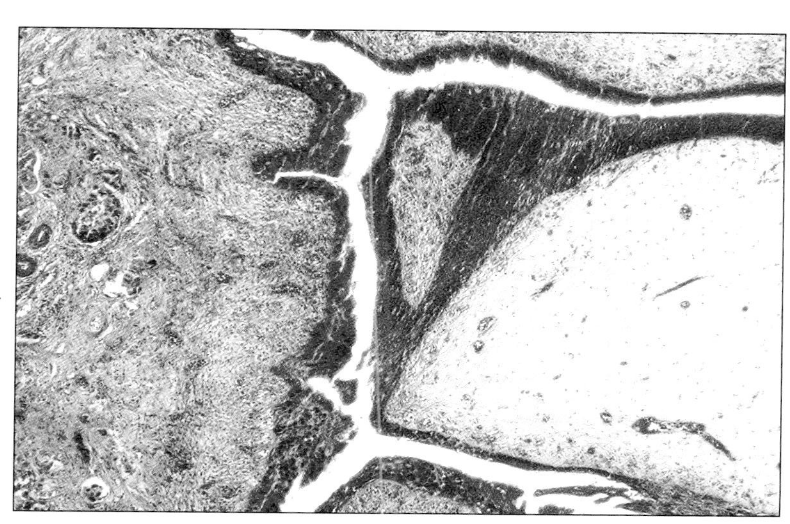

Fig. 11.53 Inflammatory polyp. Higher magnification of Fig. 11.52, with edematous stroma beneath the urothelium and the prostate glands on the left.

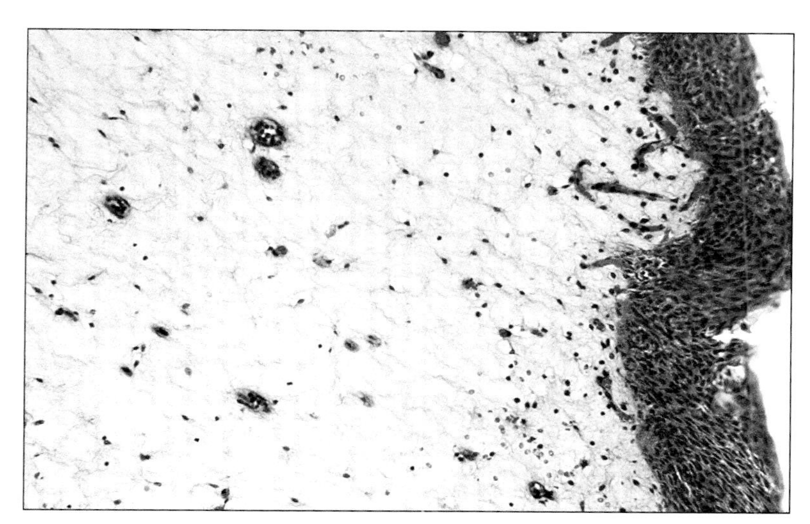

Fig. 11.54 Inflammatory polyp. Higher magnification of Fig. 11.53, with edematous stroma beneath the urothelium.

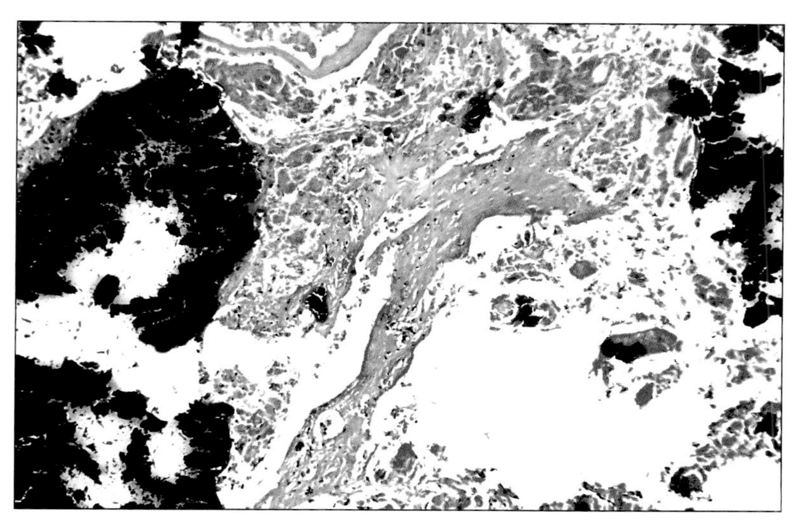

Fig. 11.55 Papillary tumor with necrosis and calcification. This occurs after radiation or chemotherapy and appears as polypoid lesions cystoscopically.

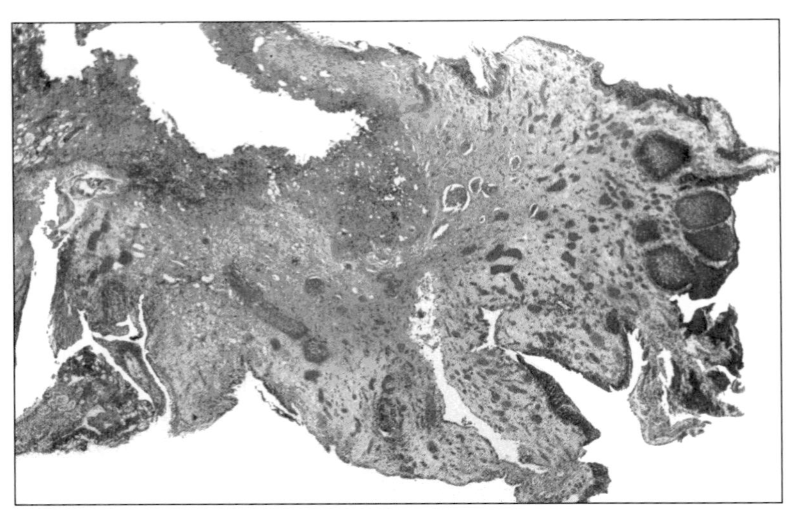

Fig. 11.56 Polypoid cystitis. Cystoscopically, this is a mass that is covered by urothelium that may be hyperplastic, with von Brunn nests on the right of this digital photo. The underlying stroma may be very vascularized or edematous.

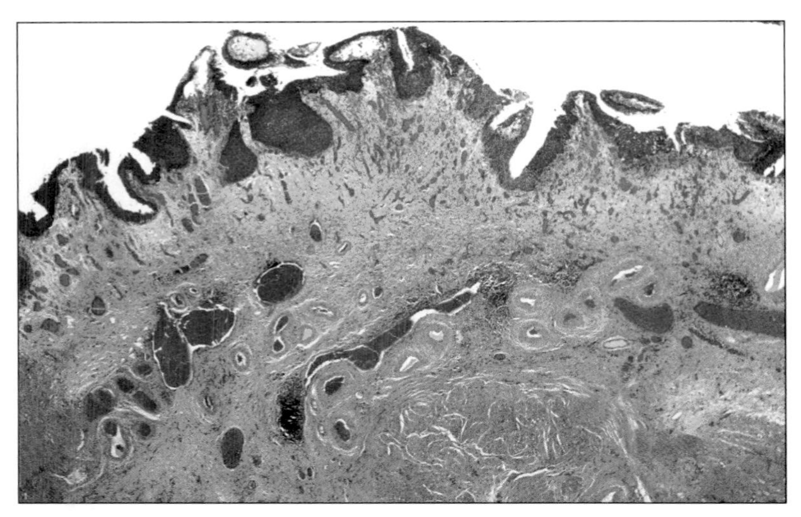

Fig. 11.57 Polypoid cystitis: a higher magnification of Fig. 11.56. Hyperplastic urothelium with solid urothelial nests of von Brunn. Numerous microcapillaries in the underlying stroma.

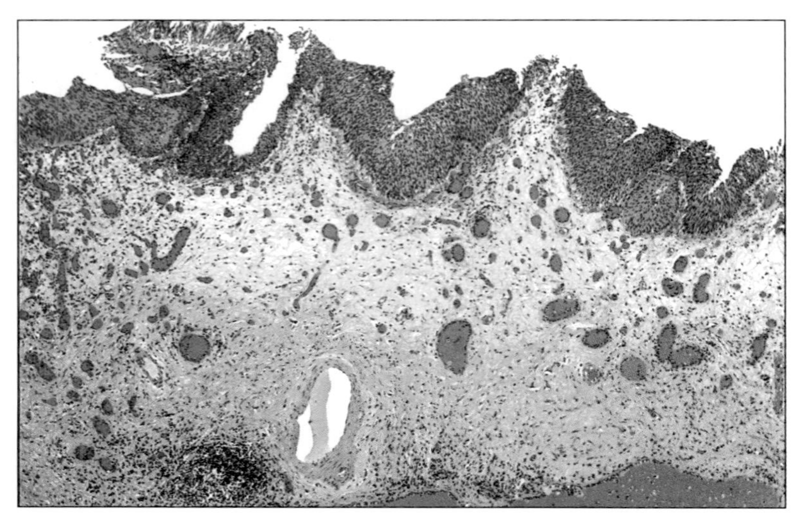

Fig. 11.58 Polypoid cystitis: a higher magnification of Fig. 11.56. Hyperplastic urothelium with pseudopapillary pattern.

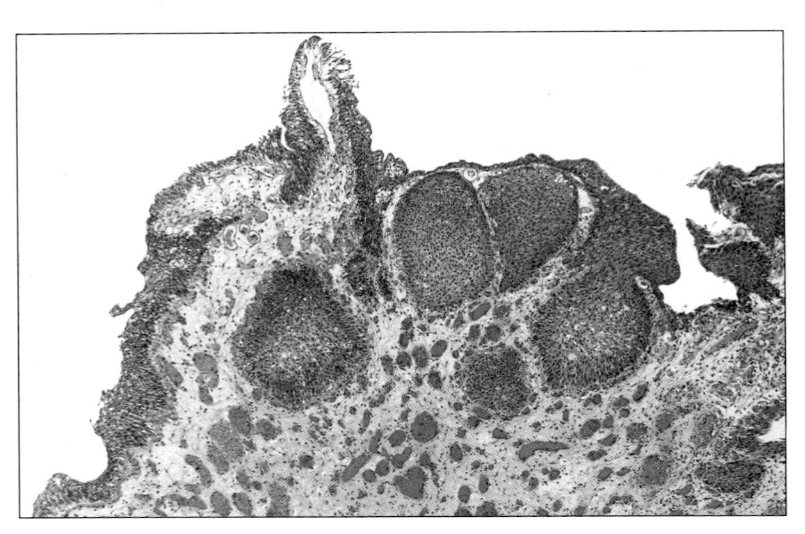

Fig. 11.59 Polypoid cystitis: a higher magnification of Fig. 11.56.

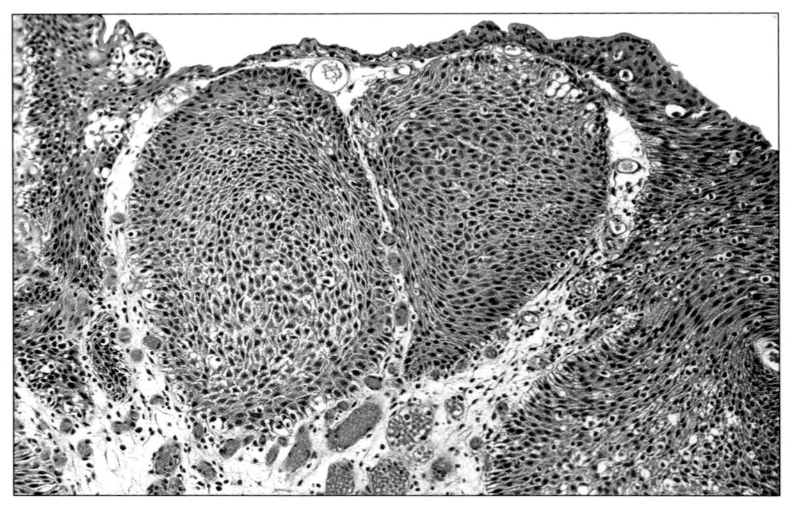

Fig. 11.60 Polypoid cystitis: a higher magnification of Fig. 11.56. Urothelial solid nests of von Brunn.

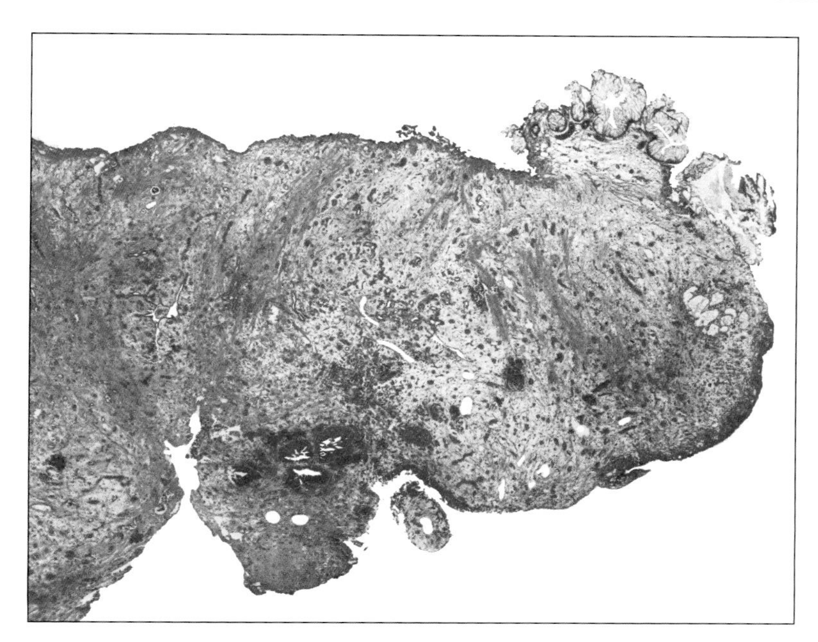

Fig. 11.61 Nephrogenic adenoma: metaplastic nephrogenic tubules found in stroma beneath the glandular metaplasia of the urothelium in the surface of the biopsy.

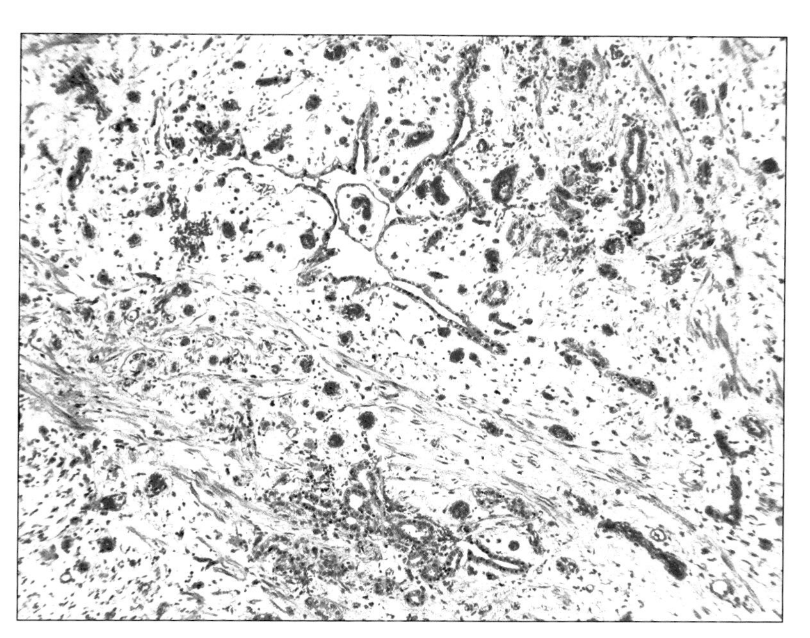

Fig. 11.63 Nephrogenic adenoma: a higher magnification of Fig. 11.61, with the nephrogenic tubules.

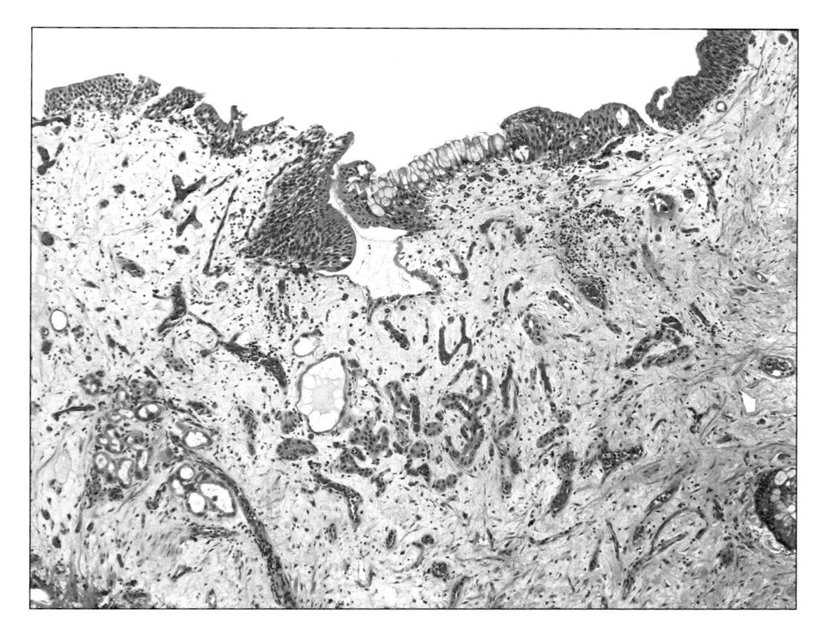

Fig. 11.62 Nephrogenic adenoma: a higher magnification of Fig. 11.61, with the metaplastic nephrogenic tubules found in stroma beneath the glandular metaplasia of the urothelium in the surface of the biopsy.

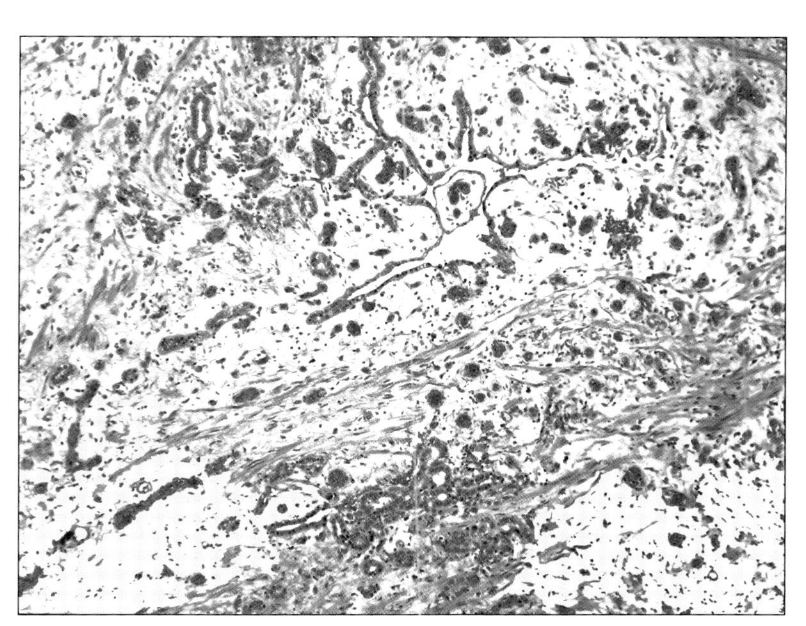

Fig. 11.64 Nephrogenic adenoma: a higher magnification of Fig. 11.61, showing nephrogenic tubules.

- Nephrogenic adenoma can have small papillary projections covered by cuboidal cells with tubular structures in the underlying lamina propria. Cystoscopically, this can simulate papillary urothelial carcinoma (see Figs 11.61–11.67).[77–84]

- Inverted papilloma can cystoscopically simulate papillary carcinoma but has a distinctive histologic picture that should not be confused with urothelial cancer (see Figs 11.68–11.82).[85–88]

Compare these figures (Figs. 11.68–11.82) to those showing the microscopic pathology of papillary tumors (Figs 11.83–11.112).

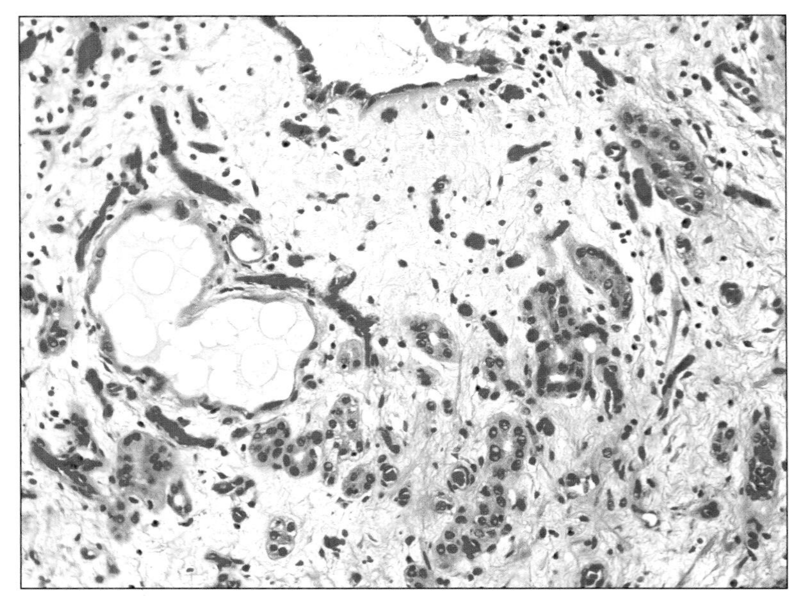

Fig. 11.65 Nephrogenic adenoma: a higher magnification of Fig. 11.61, with the nephrogenic tubules. There can be cystic dilatation of some of the tubules. The round tubules could be confused with prostatic carcinoma in either the bladder or the prostatic urethra.

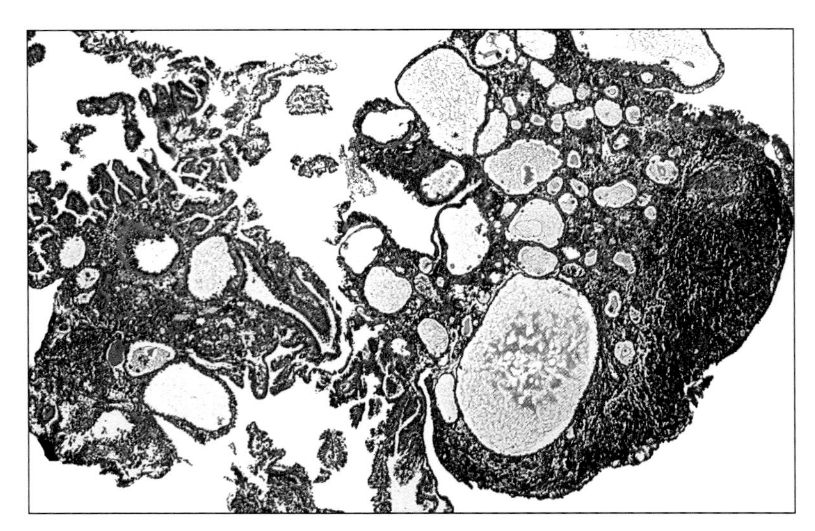

Fig. 11.67 Nephrogenic adenoma: low-power magnification of a papillary and cystic pattern.

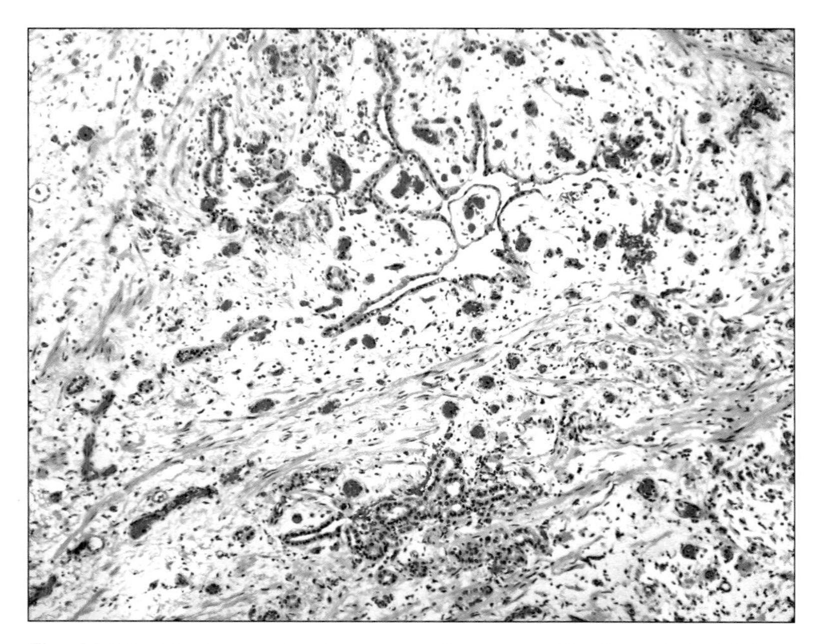

Fig. 11.66 Nephrogenic adenoma: a higher magnification of Fig. 11.61, with the nephrogenic tubules.

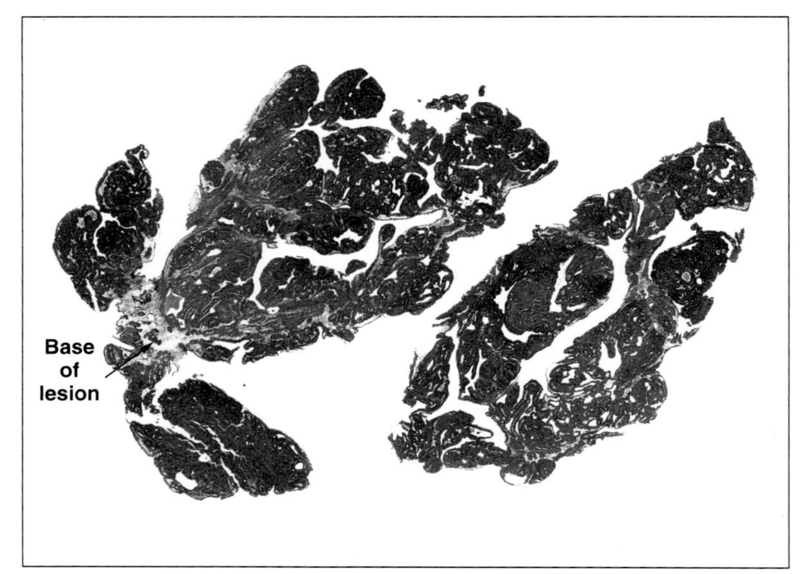

Fig. 11.68 Inverted papilloma: low-power magnification of the tumor and its base. Many have a 'golf tee' configuration at the base of the tumor.

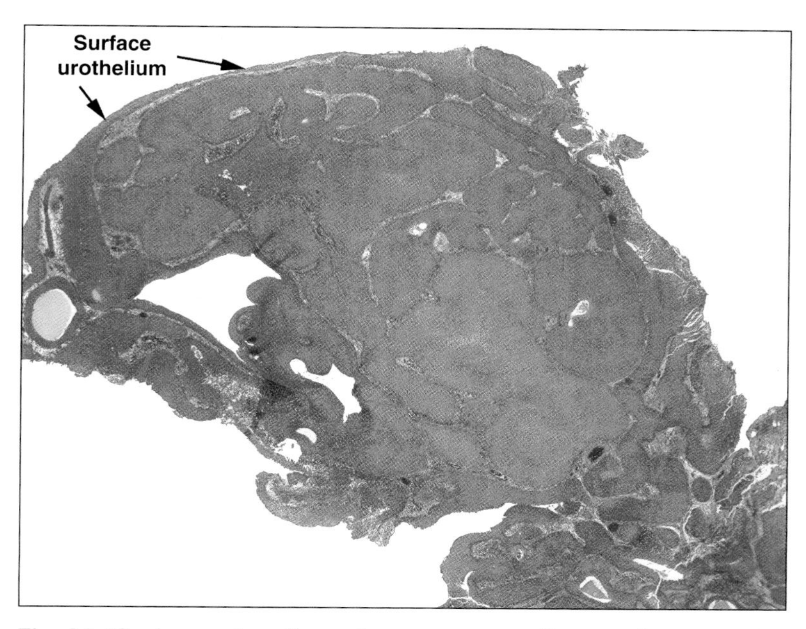

Fig. 11.69 Inverted papilloma: low-power magnification of tumor at the surface of the golf ball-sized tumor. Beneath the thin surface urothelium are numerous anastomosing sheets of urothelium composed of cells that are cytologically bland.

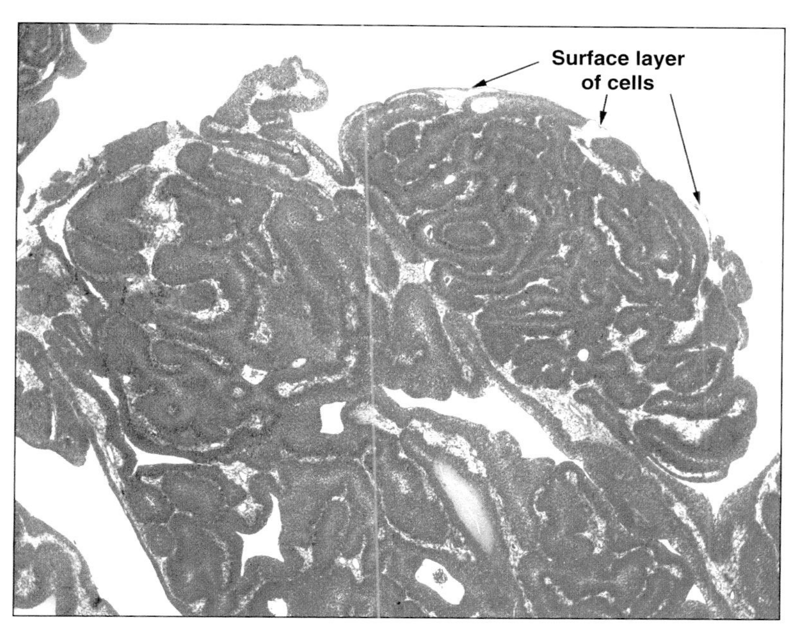

Fig. 11.71 Inverted papilloma: low-power magnification of tumor (Fig. 11.68) at its surface, where the urothelium forms a layer of two or three cells covering solid sheets or tubules of urothelium.

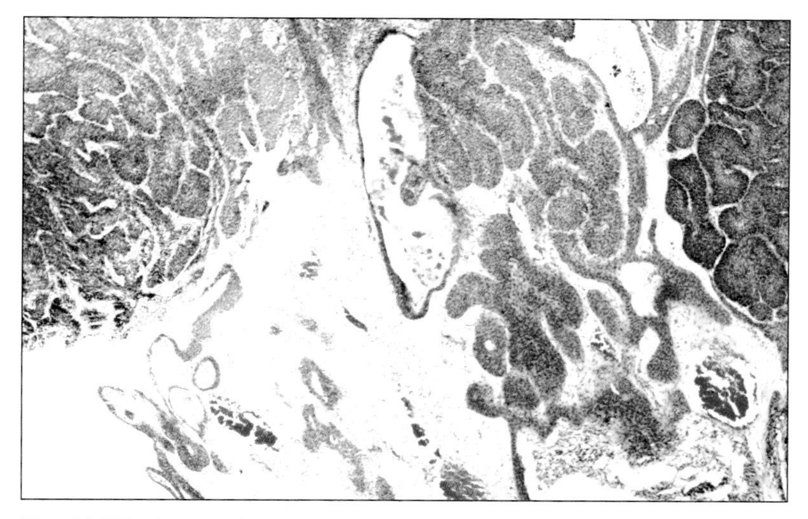

Fig. 11.70 Inverted papilloma: low-power magnification of tumor (Fig. 11.68) at its base, where some of the sheets form urothelial tubules.

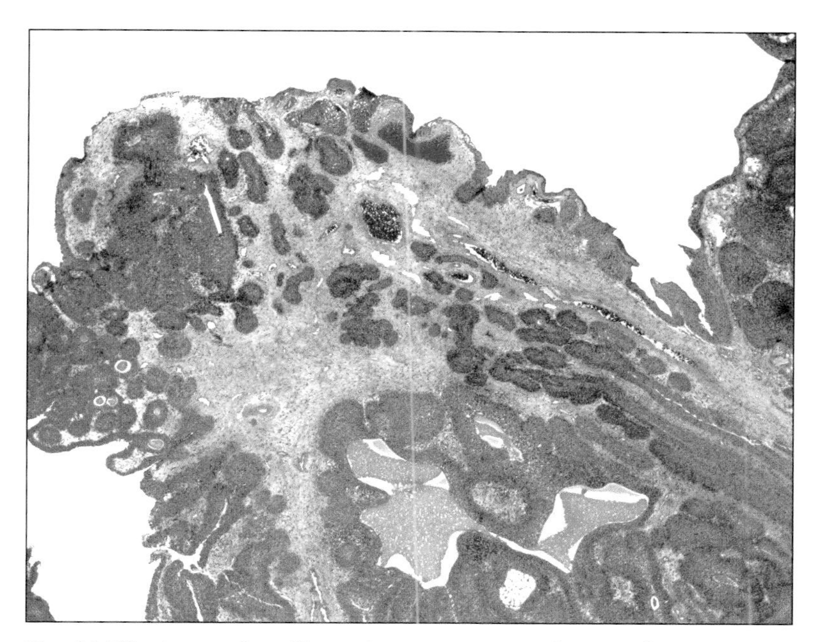

Fig. 11.72 Inverted papilloma: low-power magnification of a tumor in which there is both a cystic and a solid nest pattern to the urothelium beneath the surface urothelium.

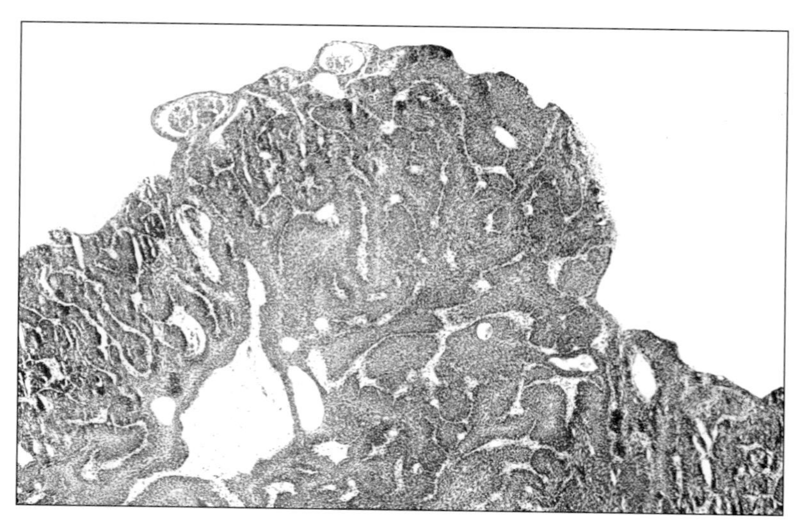

Fig. 11.73 Inverted papilloma: low-power magnification of a tumor in which there is both a cystic pattern and anastomosing sheets of urothelium beneath the surface urothelium.

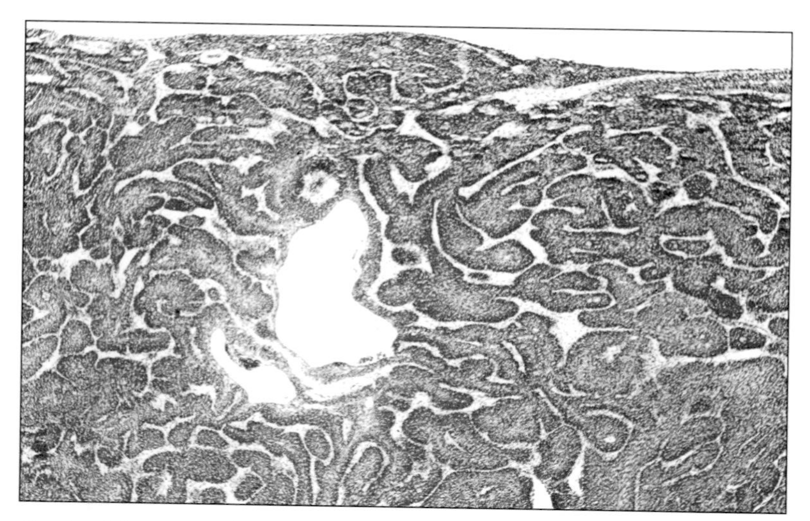

Fig. 11.74 Inverted papilloma: another low-power magnification of a tumor with a cystic pattern and anastomosing sheets of urothelium beneath the surface urothelium.

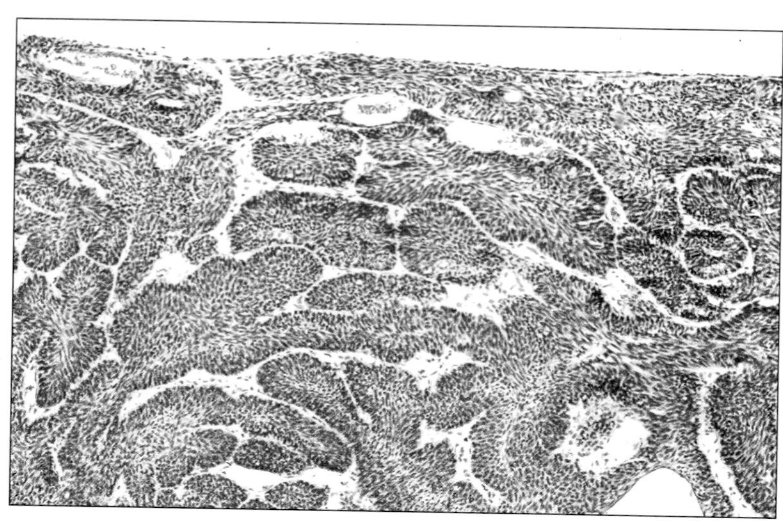

Fig. 11.75 Inverted papilloma: high-power magnification of tumor (Fig. 11.73) in which there is both a cystic pattern and anastomosing sheets of urothelium beneath the surface urothelium.

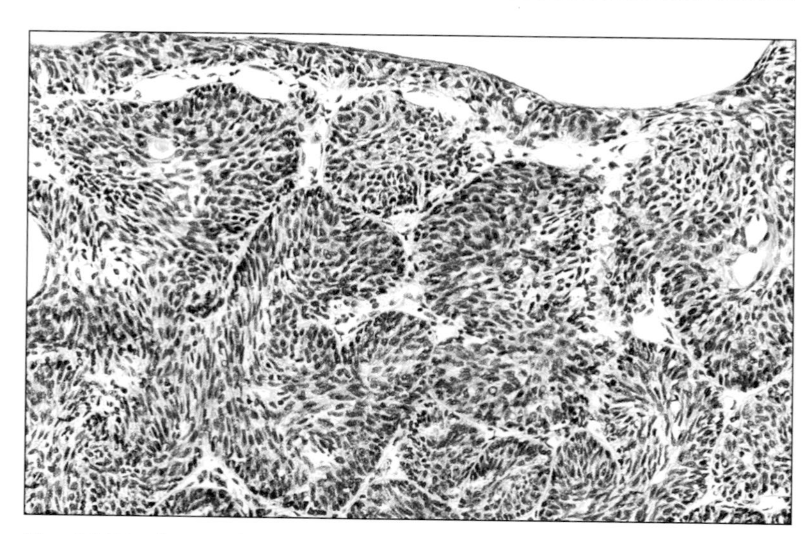

Fig. 11.76 Inverted papilloma: high-power magnification of tumor (Fig. 11.73) in which there are solid nests of urothelial cells with bland cytology. In some foci, these may be attached to the surface urothelium (upper right corner of the digital photomicrograph).

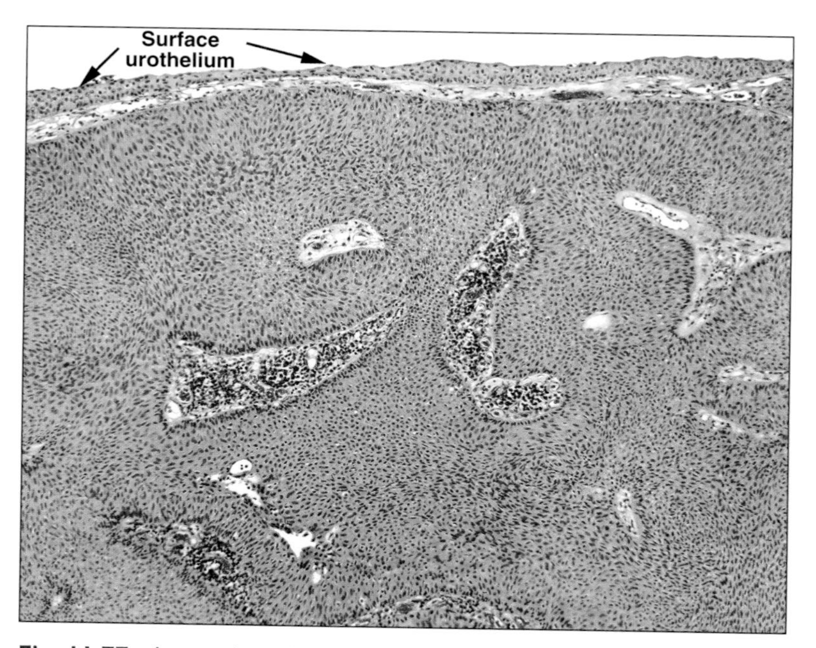

Fig. 11.77 Inverted papilloma. The solid nests of urothelial cells with bland cytology are in an anastomosing sheet of cells.

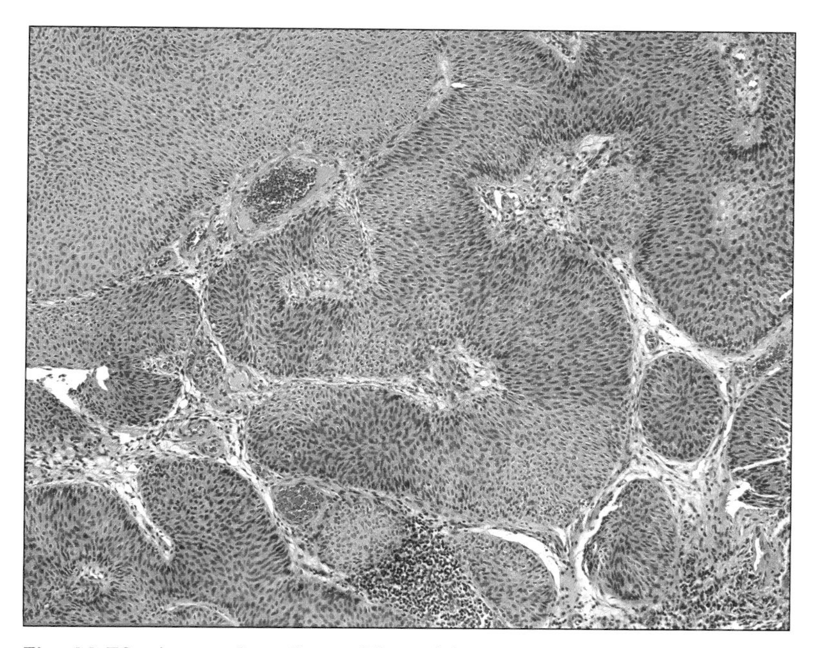

Fig. 11.78 Inverted papilloma. The solid nests of urothelial cells with bland cytology are in an anastomosing sheet of cells. This pattern was seen near the stalk base of the mass.

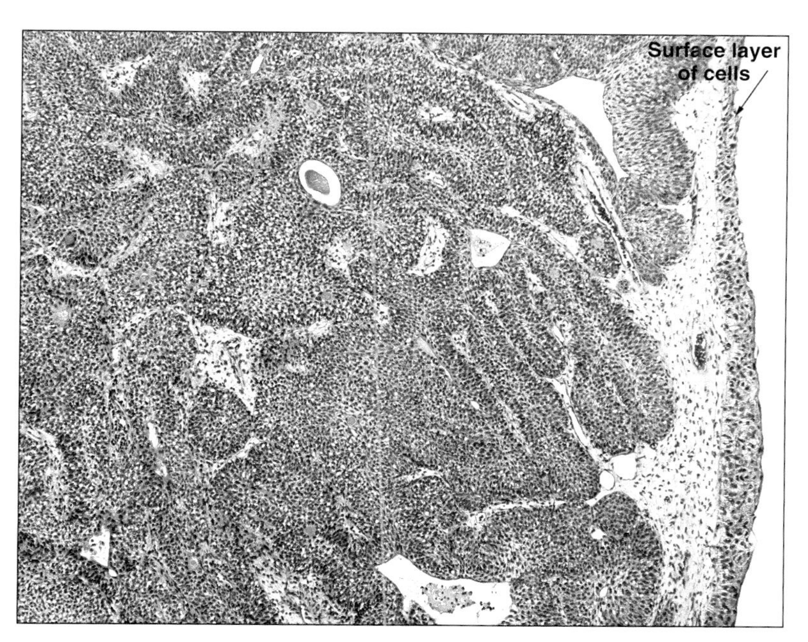

Fig. 11.80 Inverted papilloma. The solid anastomosing cords of urothelium near the urothelial surface of the polyp (arrow).

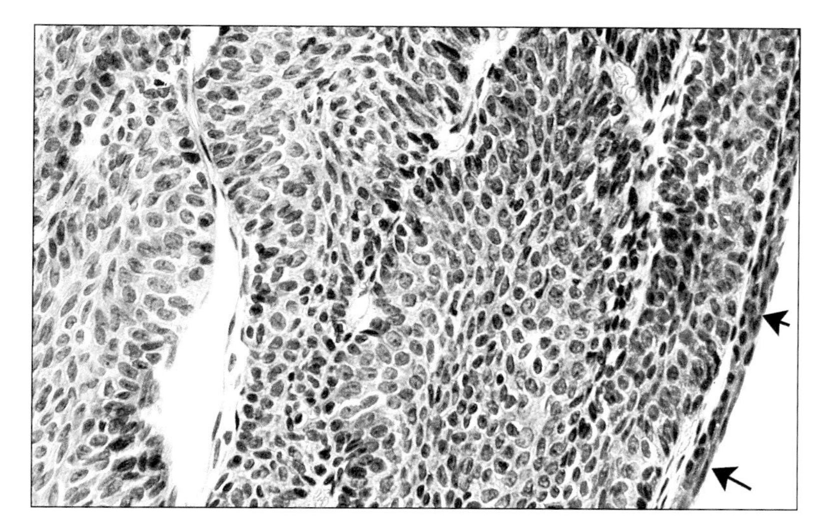

Fig. 11.79 Inverted papilloma. The solid nests of urothelial cells with bland cytology are pushing up against the urothelial surface of the polyp (arrows).

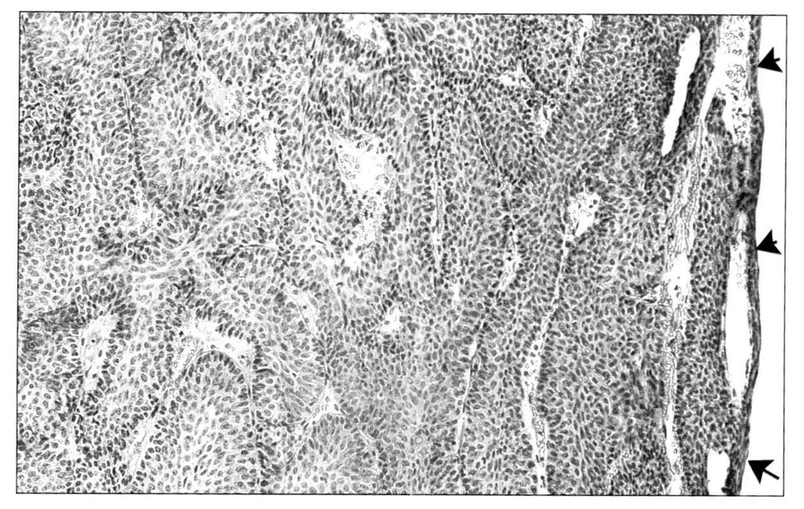

Fig. 11.81 Inverted papilloma: higher magnification. Solid anastomosing cords of bland urothelial cells near the urothelial surface of the polyp (arrows).

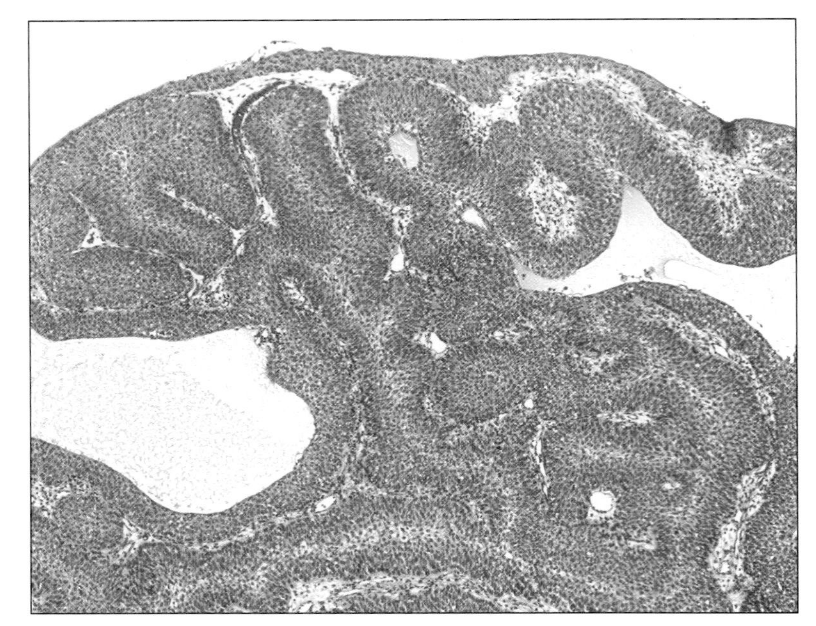

Fig. 11.82 Inverted papilloma: higher magnification. There are solid anastomosing cords of bland urothelial cells and cysts filled with clear fluid near the urothelial surface of the polyp.

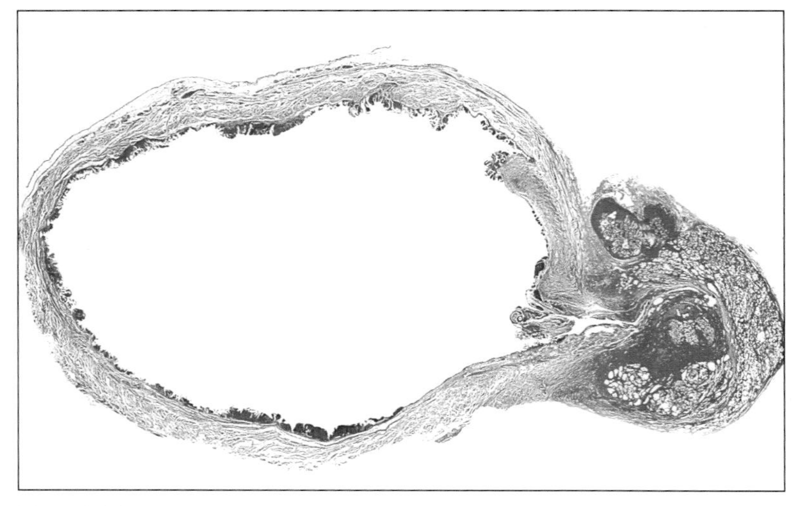

Fig. 11.83 Giant microtome section of a whole bladder taken out for multifocal bladder cancer. The prostate gland and the seminal vesicles are on the right. There are over 200 small papillary tumors in the bladder. One of them was a tumor of low malignant potential that was invading the muscularis propria. The following figures show the various grades that were found within this bladder.

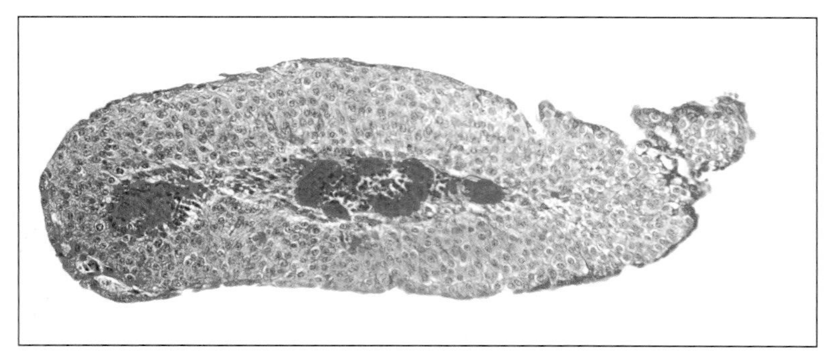

Fig. 11.84 Papillary urothelial neoplasm of low malignant potential. Cytologically bland-looking cells surround a fibrovascular stalk in this single frond tumor.

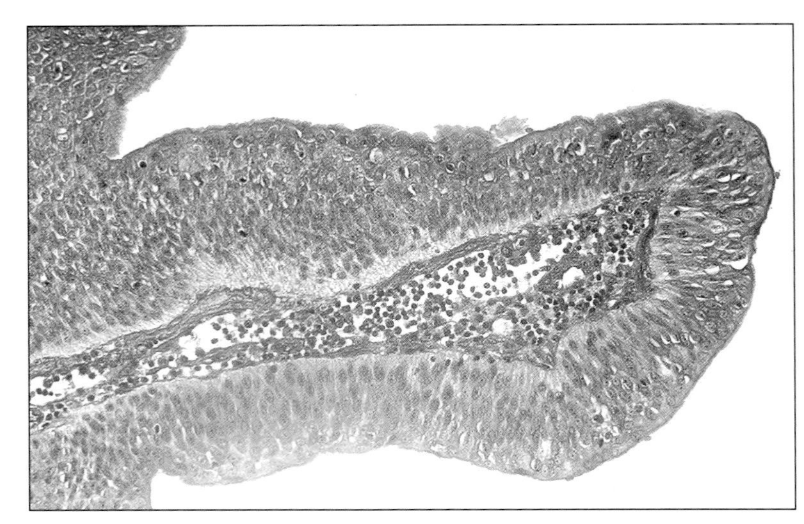

Fig. 11.85 Higher magnification of another papillary urothelial neoplasm of low malignant potential, again showing cytologically bland-looking cells surrounding a fibrovascular stalk in this single frond tumor.

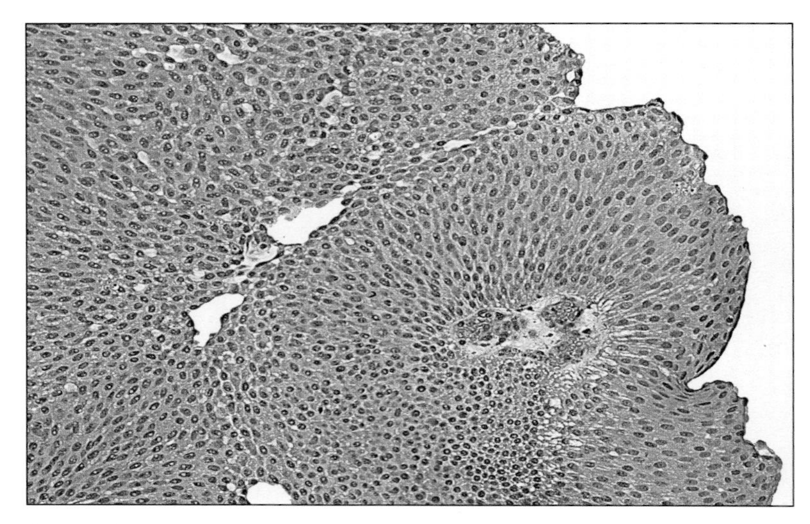

Fig. 11.86 Higher magnification of another papillary urothelial neoplasm of low malignant potential. There is no cytologic atypia, with numerous umbrella, intermediate, and basal cells. The fronds are fused together.

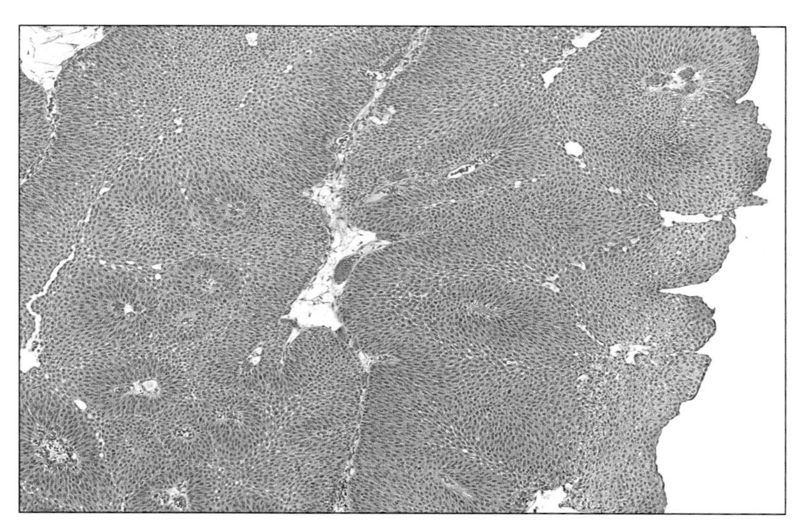

Fig. 11.87 A lower magnification of the Fig. 11.86 papillary urothelial neoplasm of low malignant potential to demonstrate that the fronds are fused together.

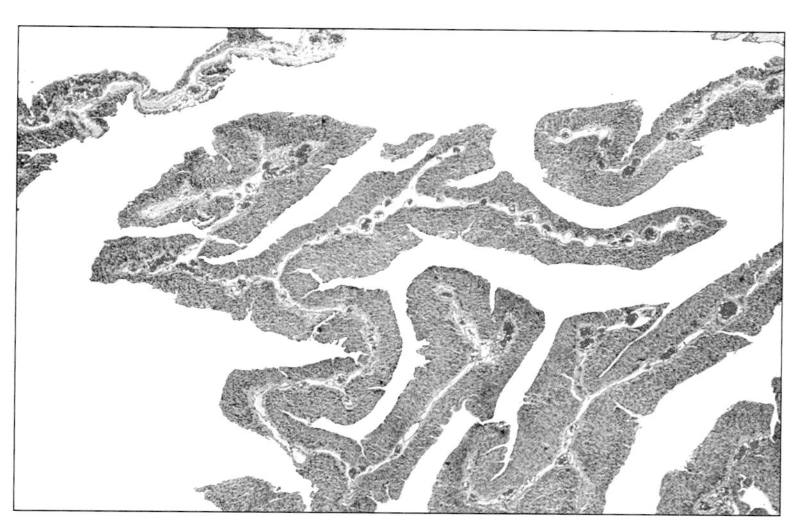

Fig. 11.88 A lower magnification of another papillary urothelial neoplasm of low malignant potential to demonstrate the multiplicity of the individual fronds.

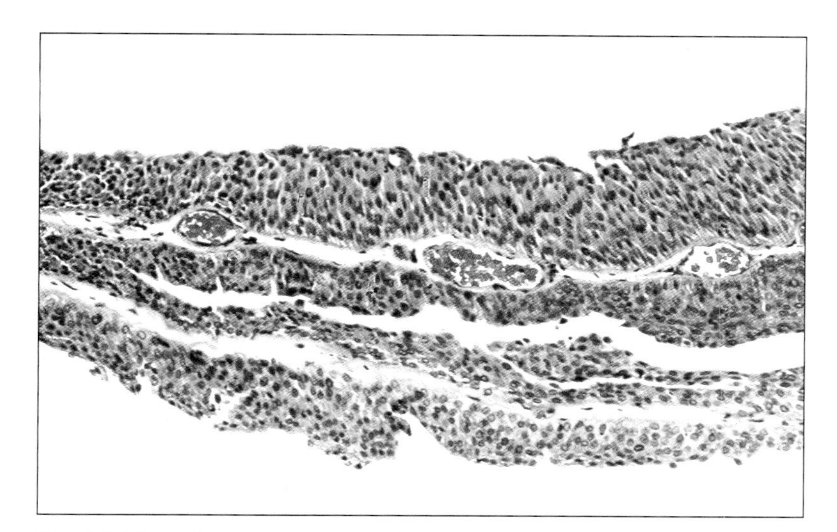

Fig. 11.89 A low magnification of papillary urothelial carcinoma, low grade, demonstrating the individual fronds.

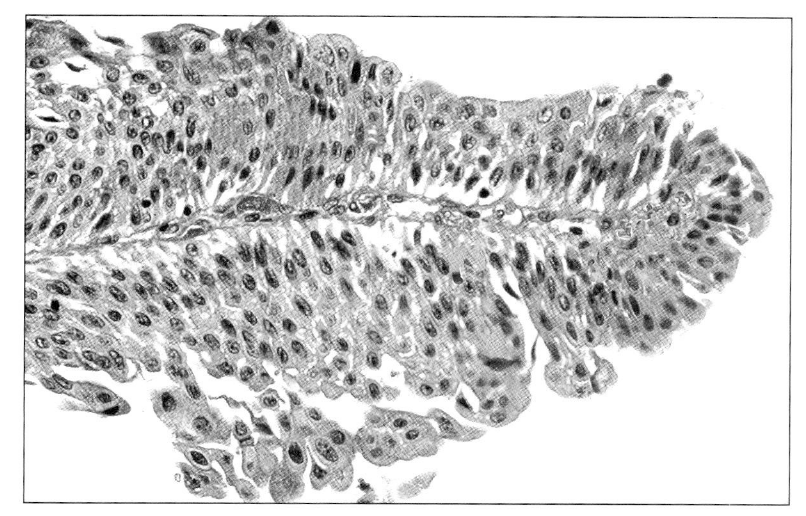

Fig. 11.90 A low magnification of papillary urothelial carcinoma, low grade, demonstrating an individual frond, which has several pleomorphic cells. There is no loss of polarity of differentiation.

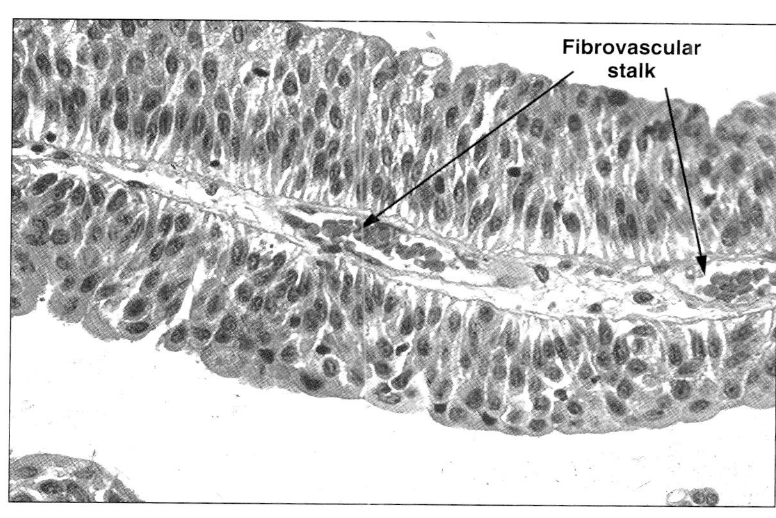

Fig. 11.91 A low magnification of papillary urothelial carcinoma, low grade, demonstrating an individual frond, which has several pleomorphic cells. There is no loss of polarity of differentiation.

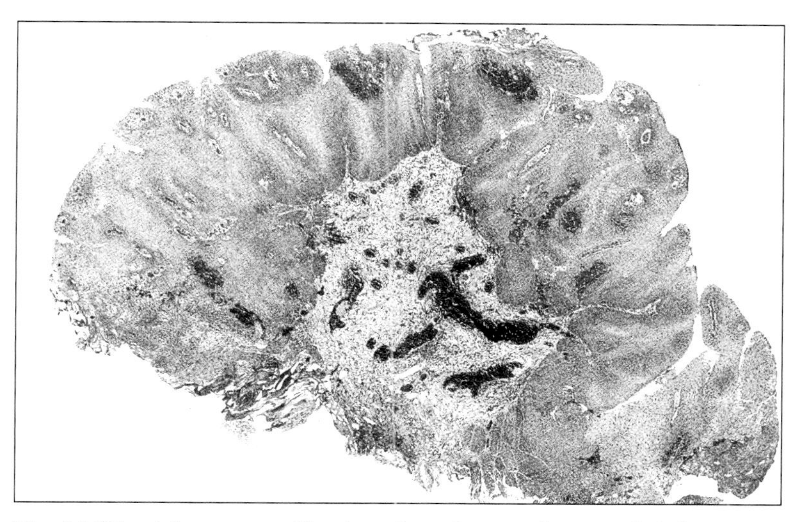

Fig. 11.92 A lower magnification of another papillary urothelial neoplasm of low malignant potential to demonstrate that it invades the lamina propria.

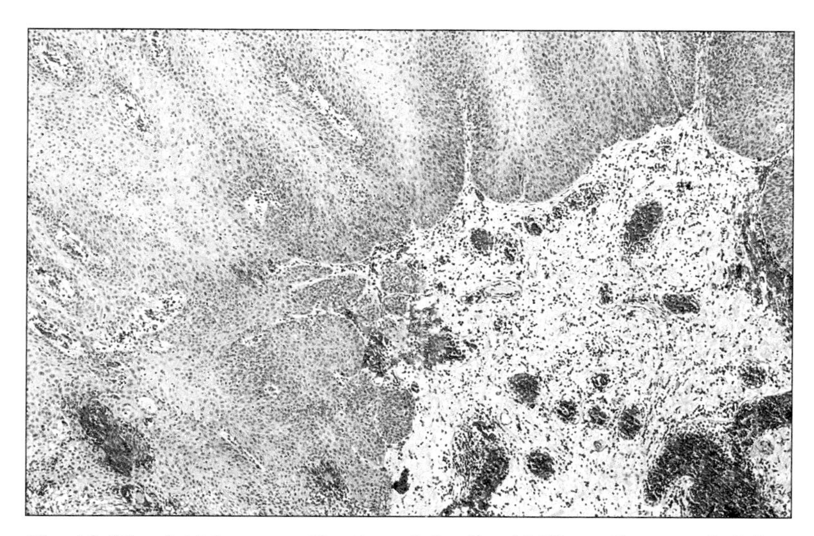

Fig. 11.93 A higher magnification of the Fig. 11.92 papillary urothelial neoplasm of low malignant potential to demonstrate that it invades the lamina propria.

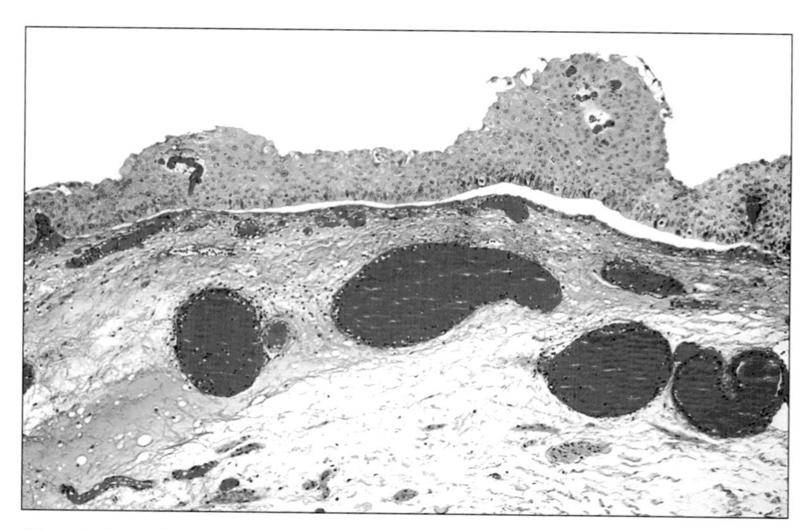

Fig. 11.94 A low magnification of papillary urothelial carcinoma, low grade, demonstrating intraepithelial capillary fronds. There is also a tendency of the neoplastic urothelium to detach from the basement membrane because of a loss of hemidesmosomes.

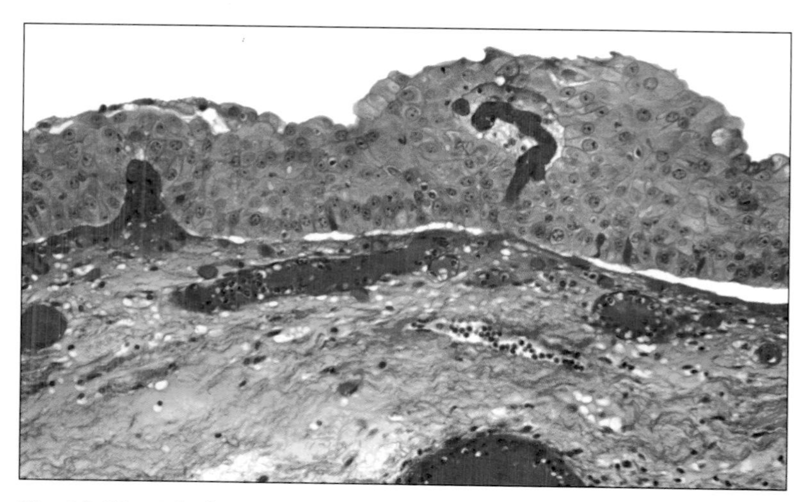

Fig. 11.95 A higher magnification of a portion of Fig. 11.94, where it appears more like a papillary urothelial neoplasia of low malignant potential. Here, too, the urothelium is lifting off from basement membrane.

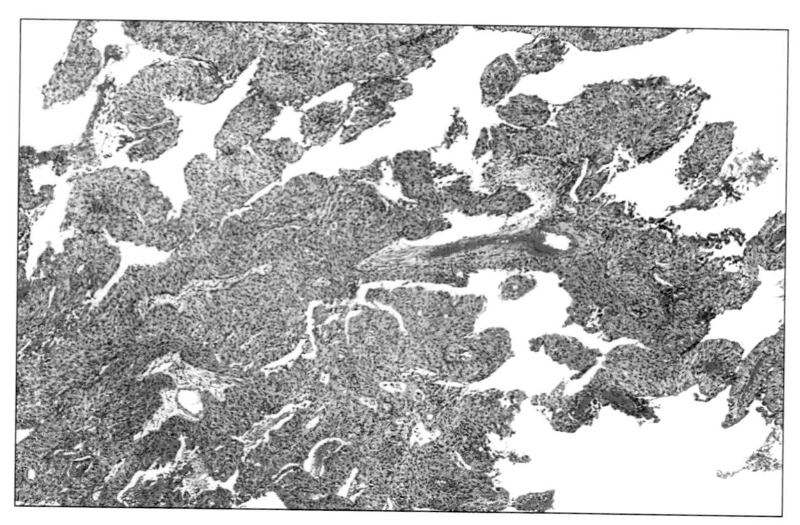

Fig. 11.96 A low magnification of papillary urothelial carcinoma, low grade, demonstrating numerous confluent and individual fronds. Each area has several pleomorphic cells, and there is no loss of polarity or differentiation. Some areas have glandular metaplasia.

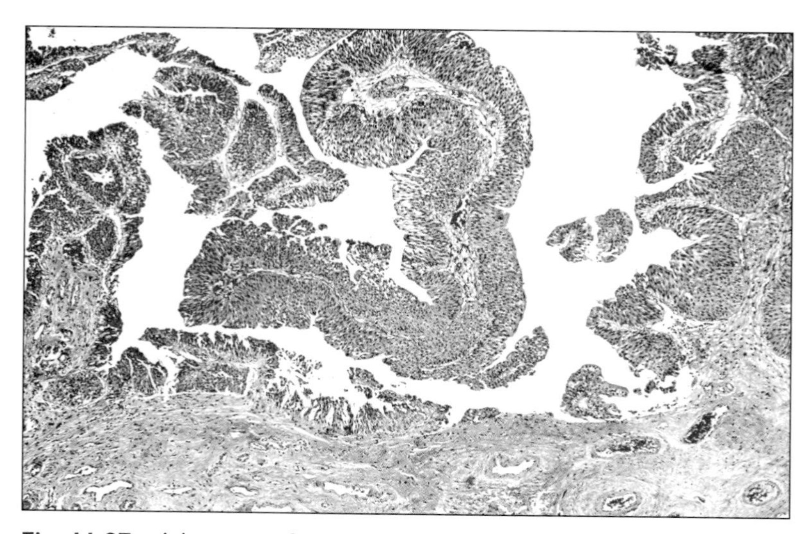

Fig. 11.97 A low magnification of papillary urothelial carcinoma, low grade, again demonstrating numerous confluent and individual fronds. There is a micropapillary pattern without fibrovascular stalks in the urothelium overlying the lamina propria in the lower third of the photomicrograph.

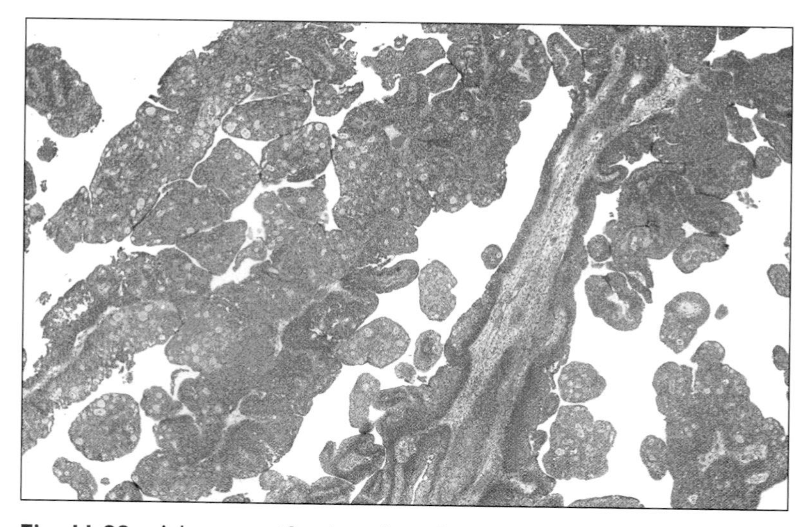

Fig. 11.98 A low magnification of papillary urothelial carcinoma, low grade. Numerous confluent and individual fronds in which there is microglandular metaplasia.

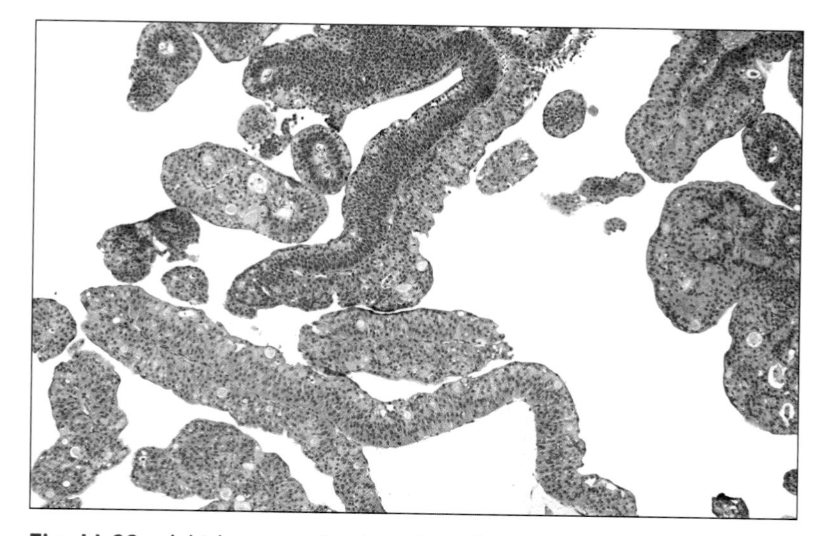

Fig. 11.99 A higher magnification of papillary urothelial carcinoma, low grade, demonstrating numerous confluent and individual fronds in which there is microglandular metaplasia (where there are pink secretions).

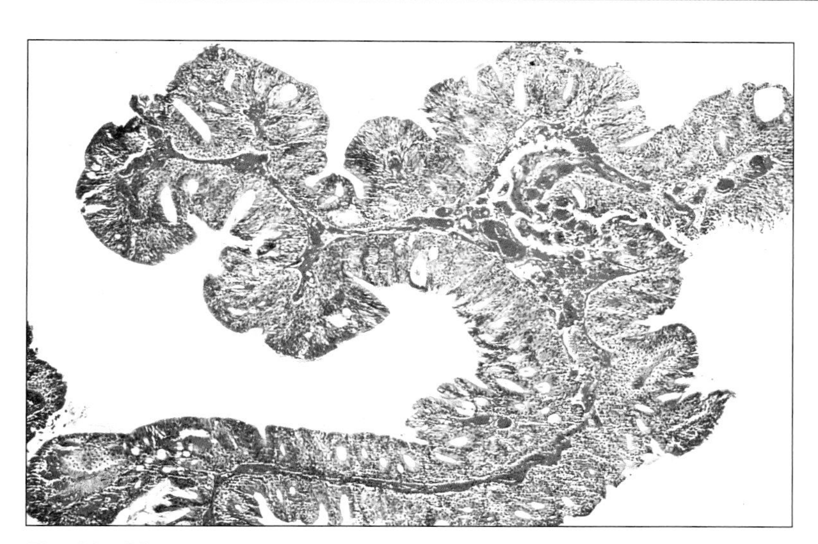

Fig. 11.100 A low magnification of papillary urothelial carcinoma, low grade, demonstrating microglandular metaplasia within the layers of urothelium.

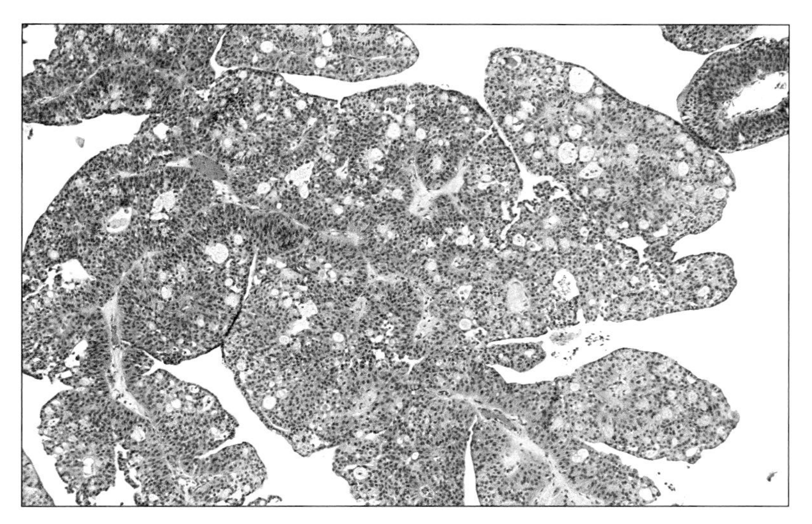

Fig. 11.101 A higher magnification of papillary urothelial carcinoma, low grade, in which there is microglandular metaplasia (where there are pink secretions).

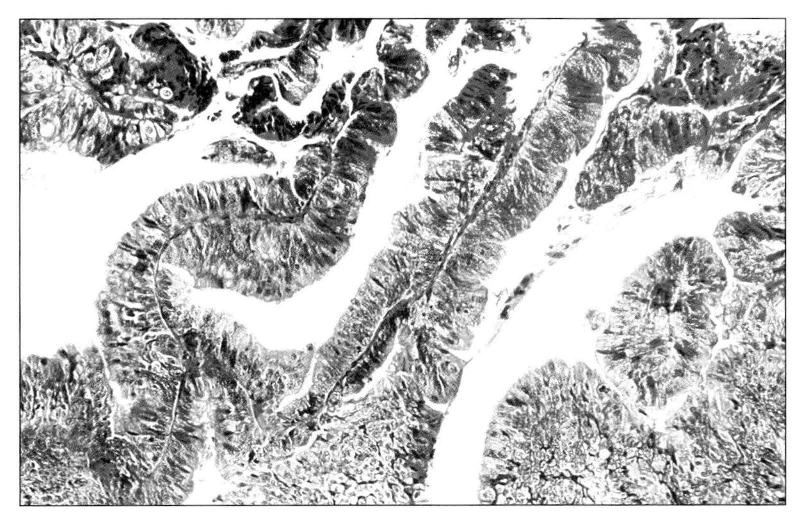

Fig. 11.102 A low magnification of papillary urothelial carcinoma, low grade, in which there is microglandular metaplasia.

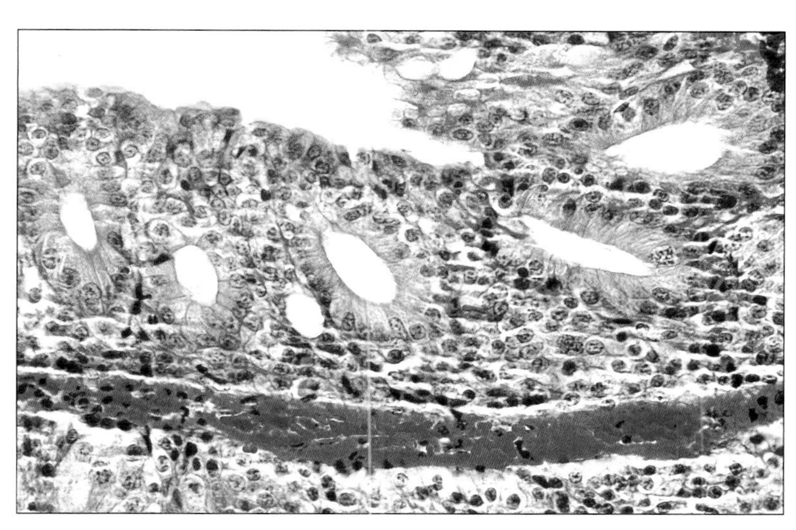

Fig. 11.103 A high magnification of papillary urothelial carcinoma, low grade, in which there are glands embedded in the urothelium.

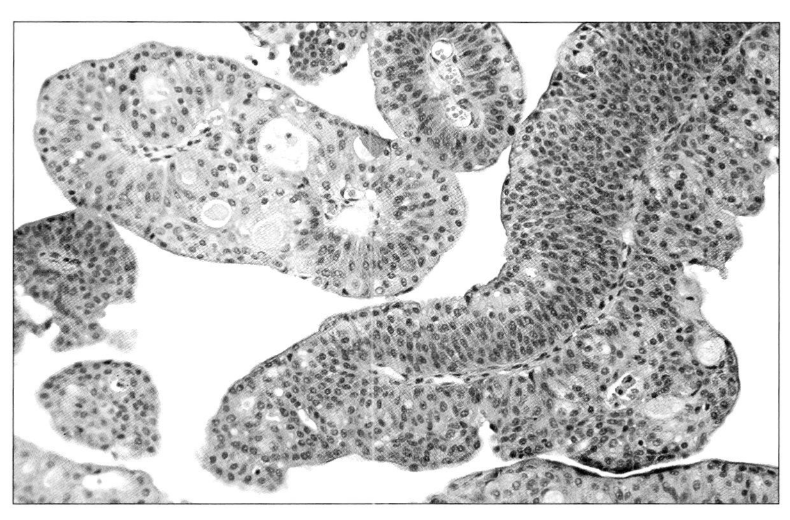

Fig. 11.104 A higher magnification of papillary urothelial carcinoma, low grade, in which there is microglandular metaplasia (where there are pink secretions).

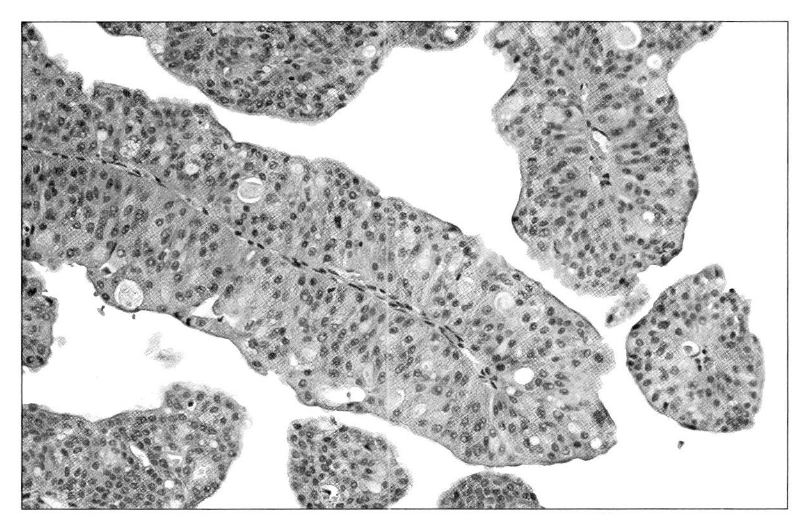

Fig. 11.105 An even higher magnification of papillary urothelial carcinoma, low grade, in which there is microglandular metaplasia (with pink luminal secretions).

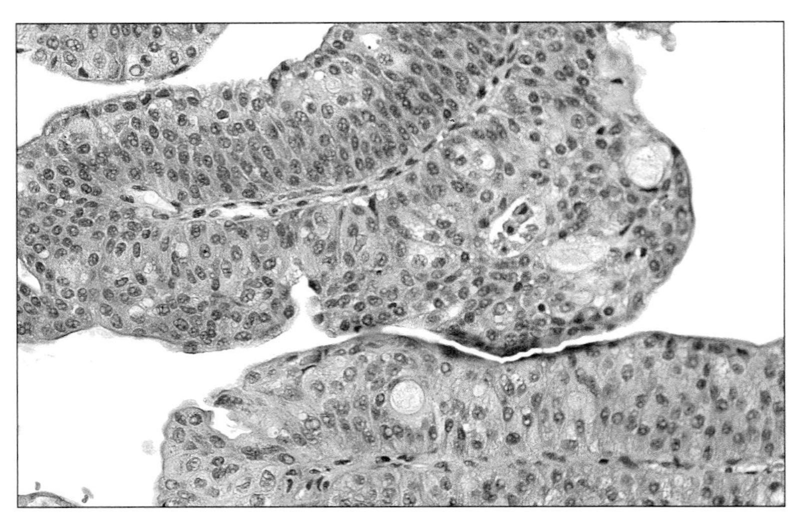

Fig. 11.106 An even higher magnification of papillary urothelial carcinoma, low grade, in which there is microglandular metaplasia that contains pink luminal secretions.

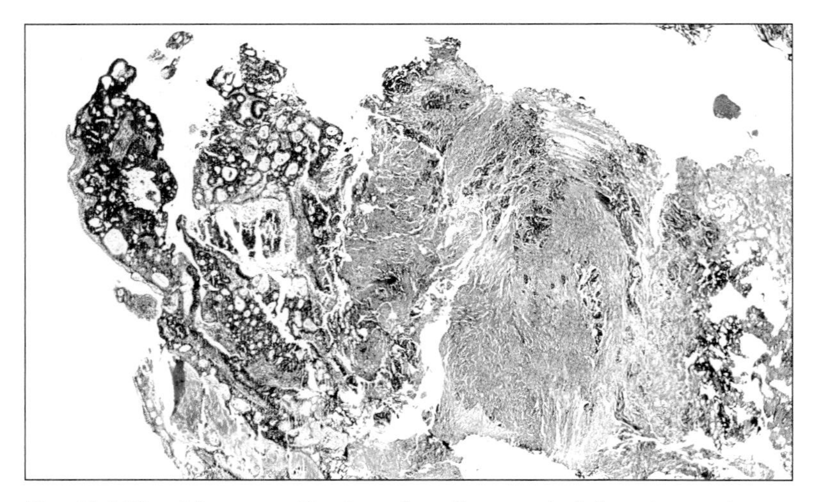

Fig. 11.107 A low magnification of papillary urothelial carcinoma, low grade, in which there are cystic glands within the urothelium.

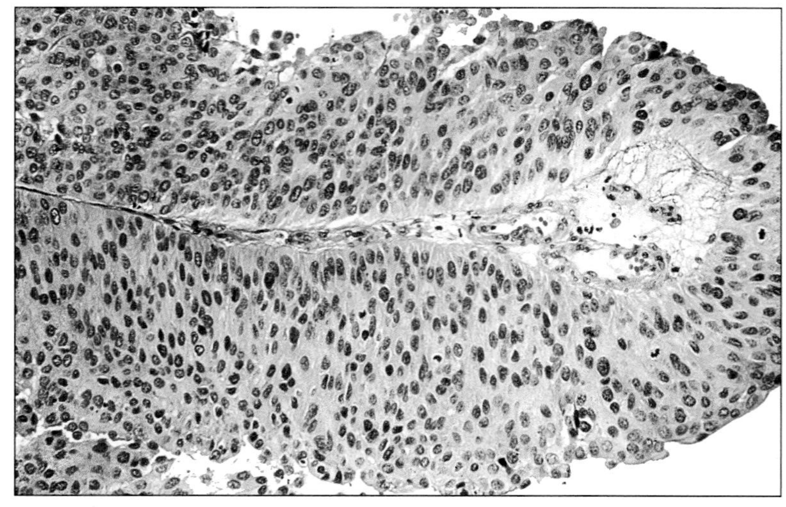

Fig. 11.108 A high magnification of papillary urothelial carcinoma, low grade, showing a frond. There are a few pleomorphic cells within the urothelial layers.

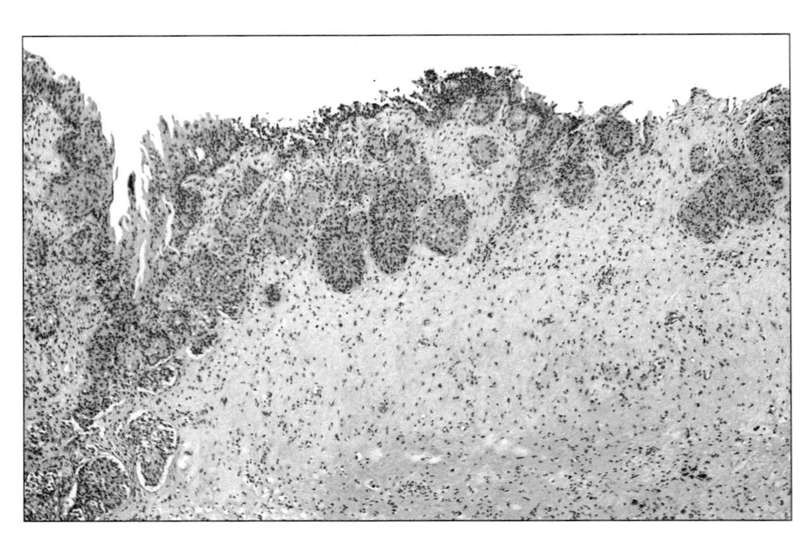

Fig. 11.109 Low magnification of papillary urothelial carcinoma, low grade, with a nesting pattern in the lamina propria. The urothelium over these neoplastic nests demonstrates an intraurothelial papillary carcinoma without fibrovascular cores.

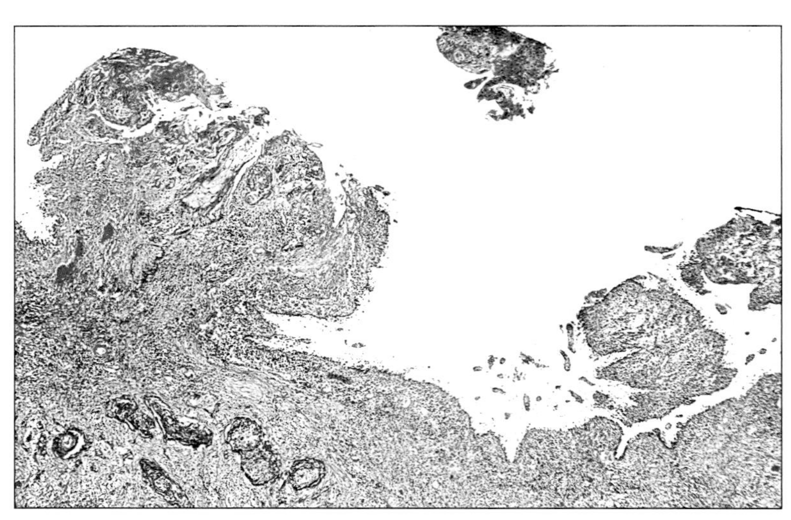

Fig. 11.110 Low magnification of papillary urothelial carcinoma, high grade, with numerous clusters of neoplastic nests with pseudoglandular spaces.

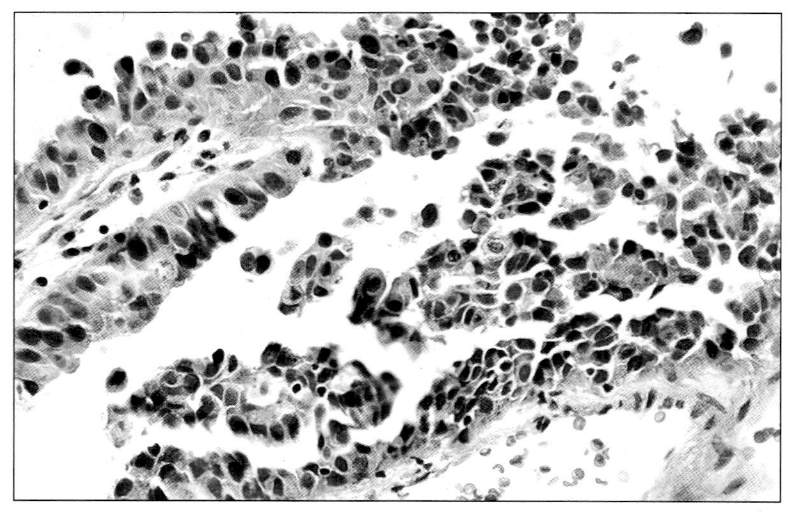

Fig. 11.111 Low magnification of papillary urothelial carcinoma, high grade, with numerous clusters of pleomorphic cells in a loose cohesive pattern.

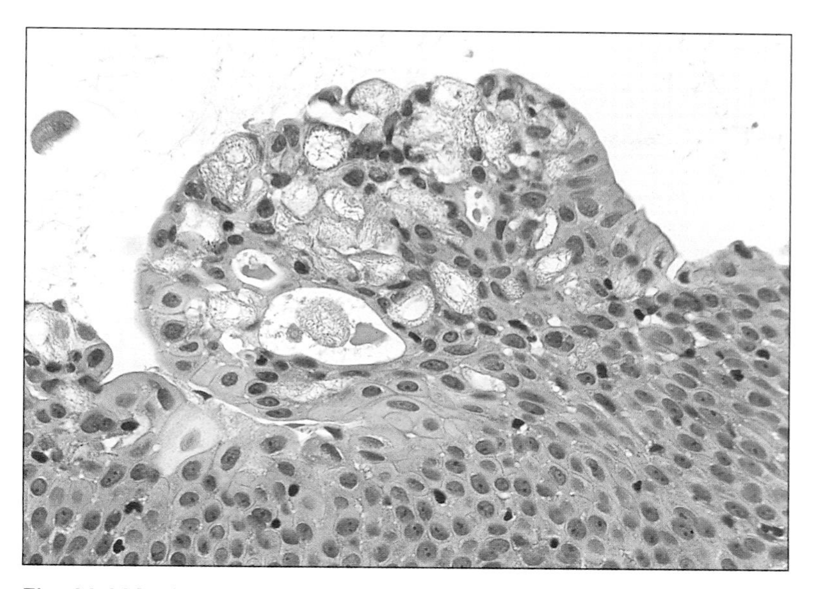

Fig. 11.112 Low magnification of papillary urothelial carcinoma, high grade, with pseudoglandular spaces surrounded by numerous pleomorphic cells.

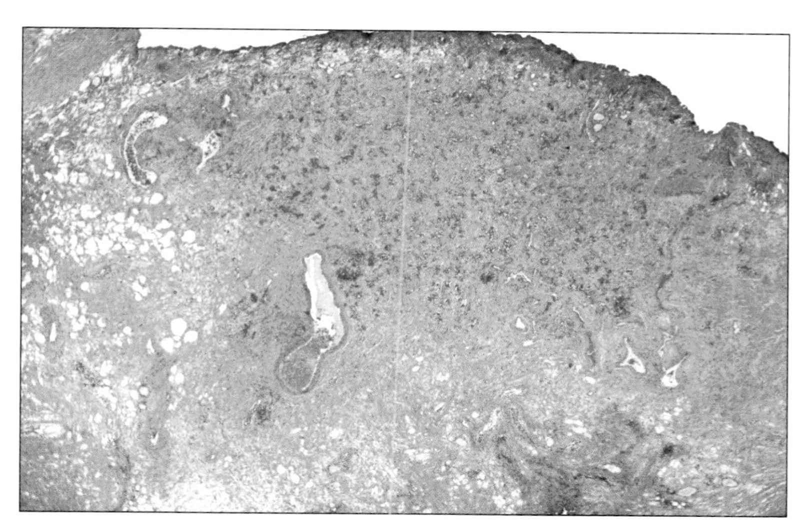

Fig. 11.113 Nesting pattern: low-power magnification of numerous neoplastic nests infiltrating the lamina propria beneath carcinoma in situ.

MICROSCOPIC PATHOLOGY OF NONPAPILLARY UROTHELIAL CARCINOMA

NESTED UROTHELIAL CARCINOMA PATTERN[89–96]

- This pattern (Figs 11.113–11.129) indicates an invasive urothelial carcinoma with a growth pattern of small nests of benign-appearing urothelial cells that resemble von Brunn nests.
- The nests invade the lamina propria.
- The nests may have small tubular lumens.
- Cytologically, nuclei may show little or no atypia, but the deeper portions of the lesion may have increasing cellular anaplasia.
- Some nuclei may be enlarged, with a coarse chromatin pattern.

CAUTION

This may be simulated by the following.

- Von Brunn nests: some nests will show central glandular differentiation.
- Cystitis cystica and glandularis.
- Inverted papilloma: this will have anastomosing cords of urothelium.

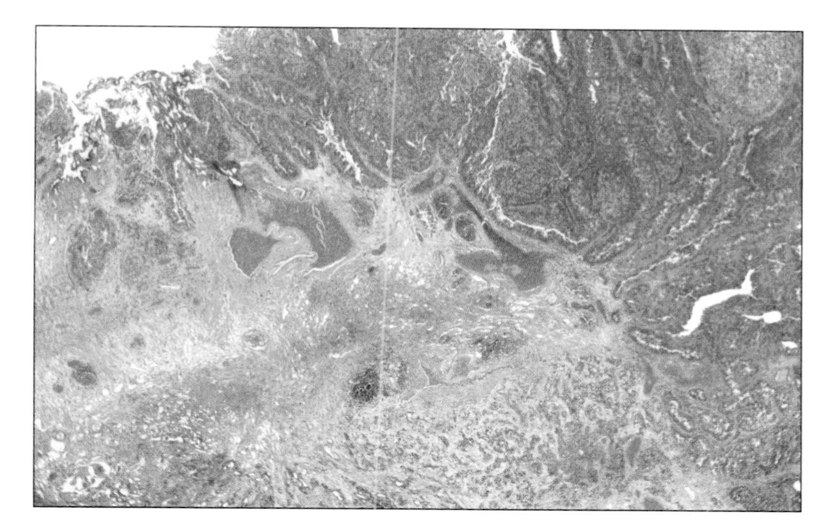

Fig. 11.114 Nesting pattern: low-power magnification of numerous neoplastic nests infiltrating the lamina propria beneath a papillary urothelial carcinoma, high grade.

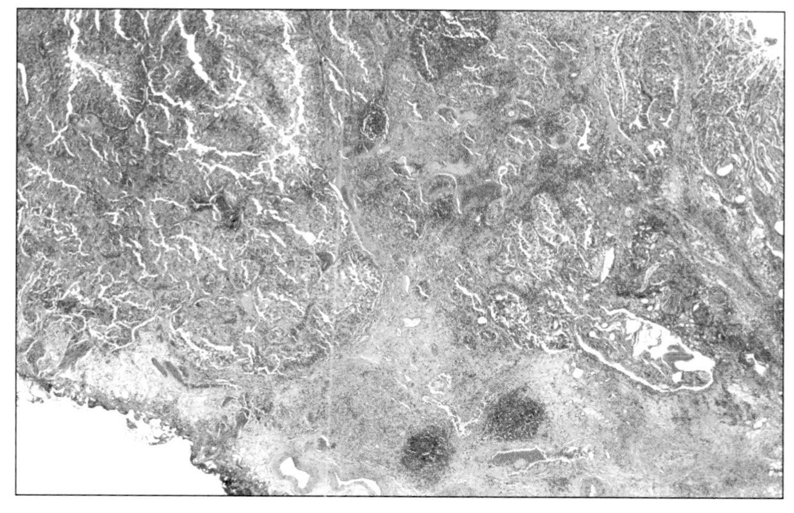

Fig. 11.115 Nesting pattern: a high-power magnification of Fig. 11.114.

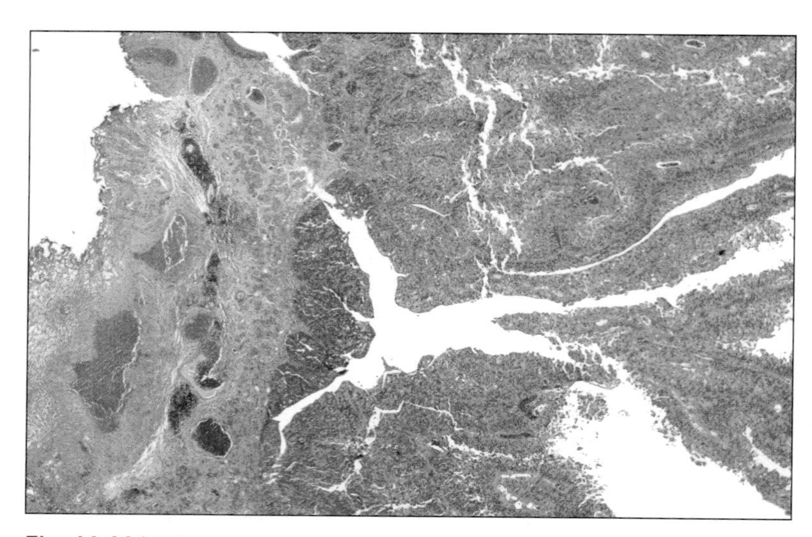

Fig. 11.116 Nesting patterns: low-power magnification of numerous neoplastic nests infiltrating the lamina propria (left) beneath a papillary urothelial carcinoma, high grade, with glandular metaplasia in the right half of the figure.

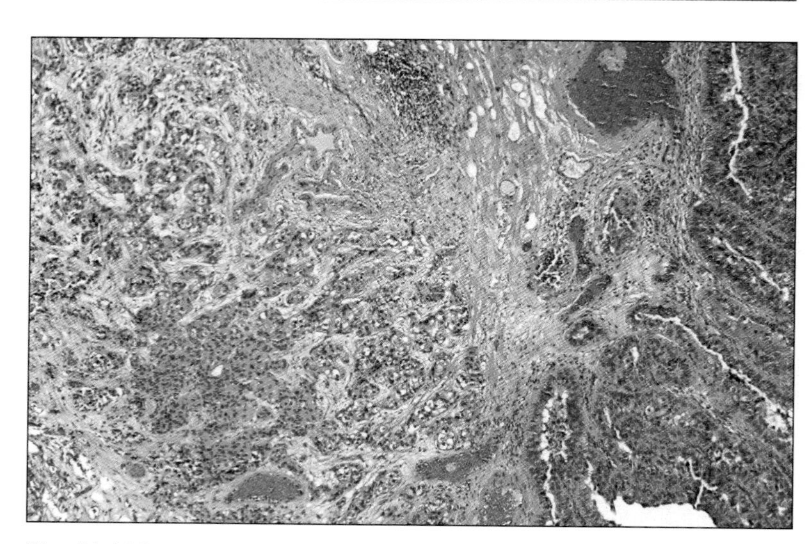

Fig. 11.119 Nesting patterns: a high-power magnification of Fig. 11.114. Small nests, cords, and glandular forms of pleomorphic cells cytologically.

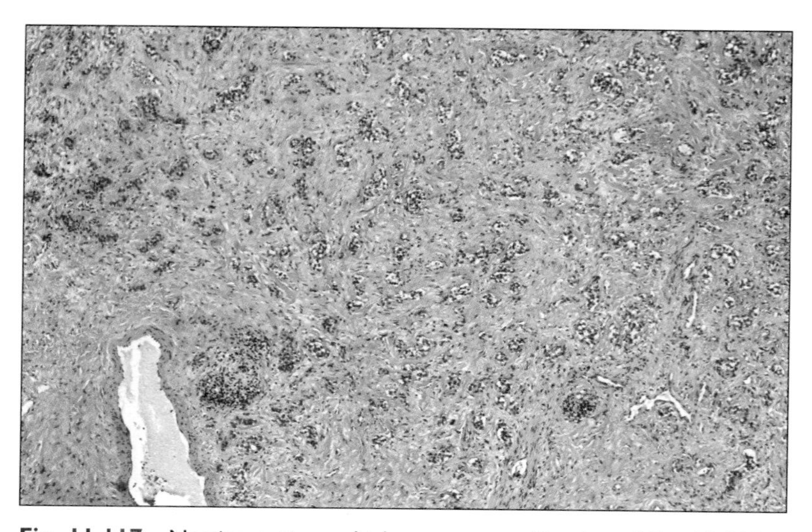

Fig. 11.117 Nesting patterns: high-power magnification of Fig. 11.113, with numerous neoplastic nests infiltrating the lamina propria beneath carcinoma in situ.

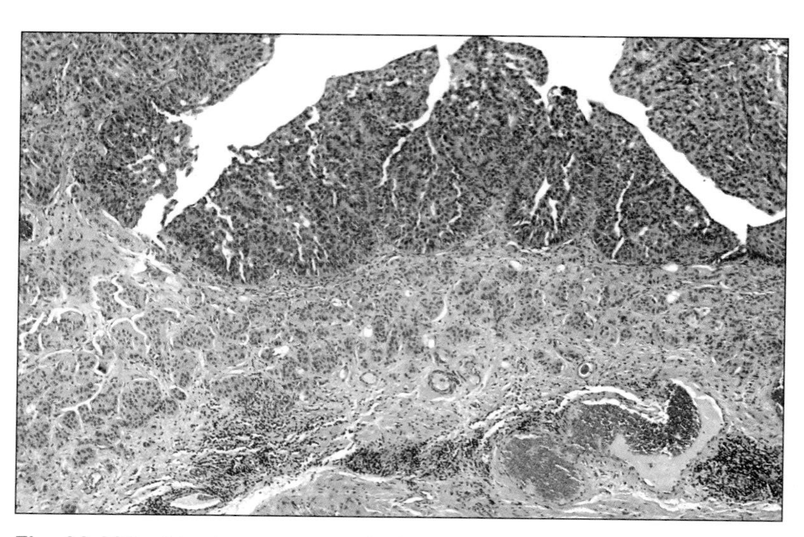

Fig. 11.120 Nesting patterns: a high-power magnification of Fig. 11.116. Small nests of bland-looking cells.

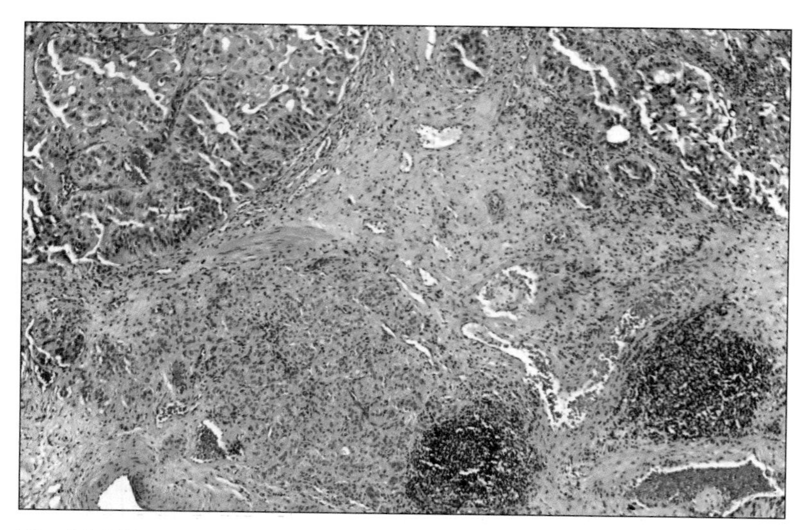

Fig. 11.118 Nesting patterns: a high-power magnification of Fig. 11.116. Small nests of bland cells cytologically.

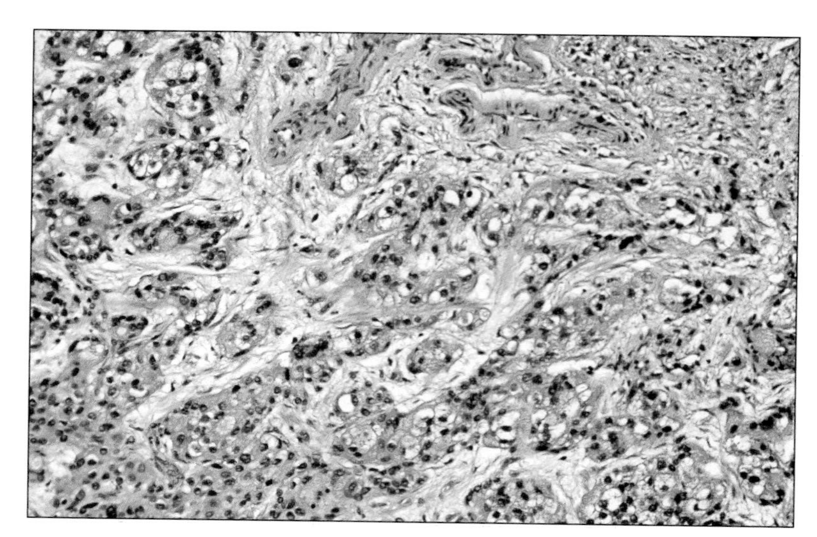

Fig. 11.121 Nesting patterns: a higher-power magnification of Fig. 11.119. Small nests, cords, and signet ring forms of pleomorphic cells cytologically.

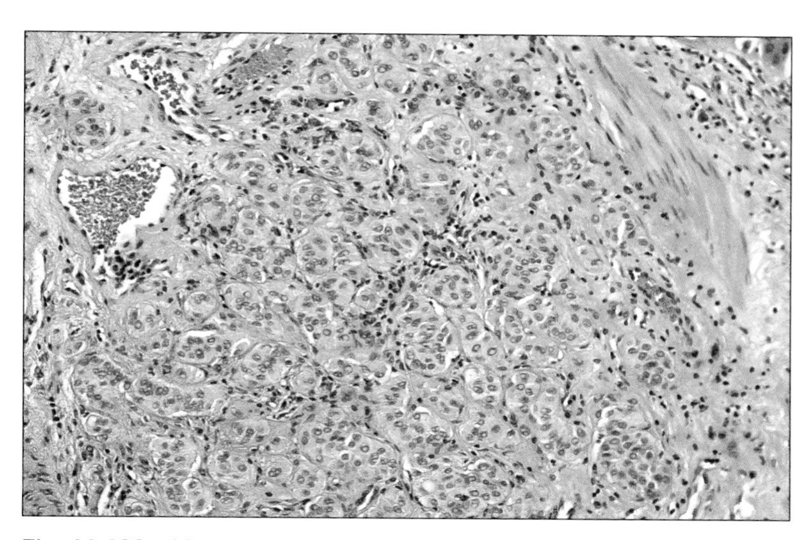

Fig. 11.122 Nesting patterns: a higher-power magnification of Fig. 11.116. Small nests of bland-looking cells.

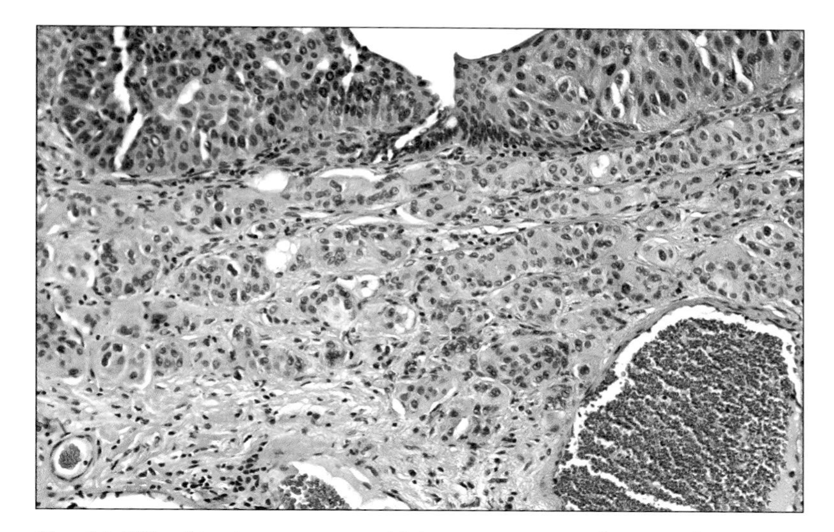

Fig. 11.123 Nesting patterns: a higher-power magnification of Fig. 11.116, again showing small nests of bland-looking cells.

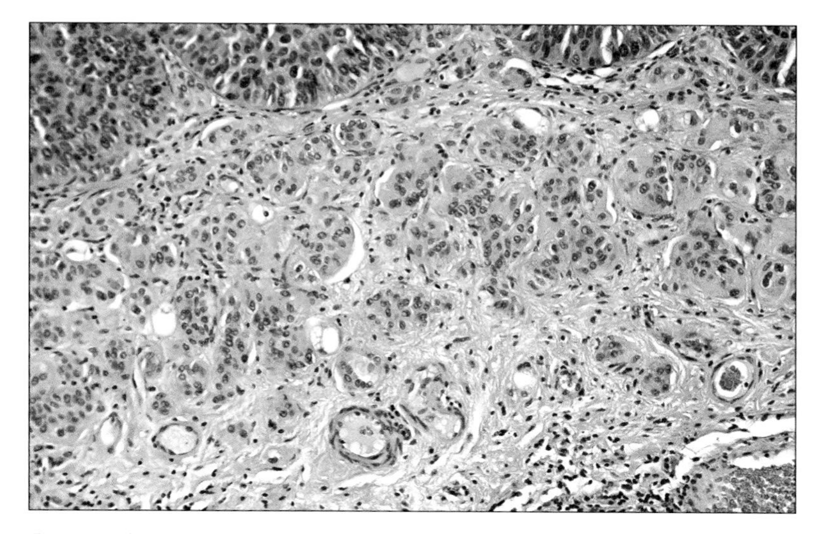

Fig. 11.124 Nesting patterns: an even higher-power magnification of Fig. 11.116. Small nests of bland-looking cells.

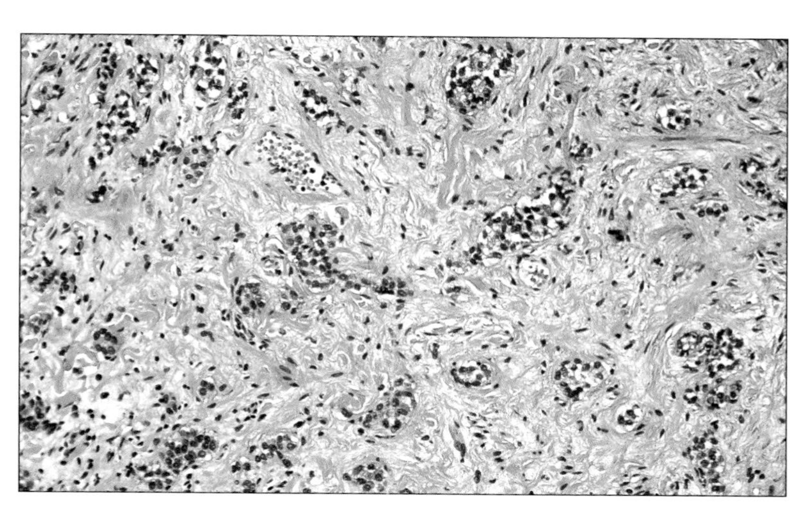

Fig. 11.125 Nesting patterns: higher-power magnification of numerous neoplastic nests infiltrating the lamina propria beneath carcinoma in situ. The cells in these nests are also bland in cytologic appearance.

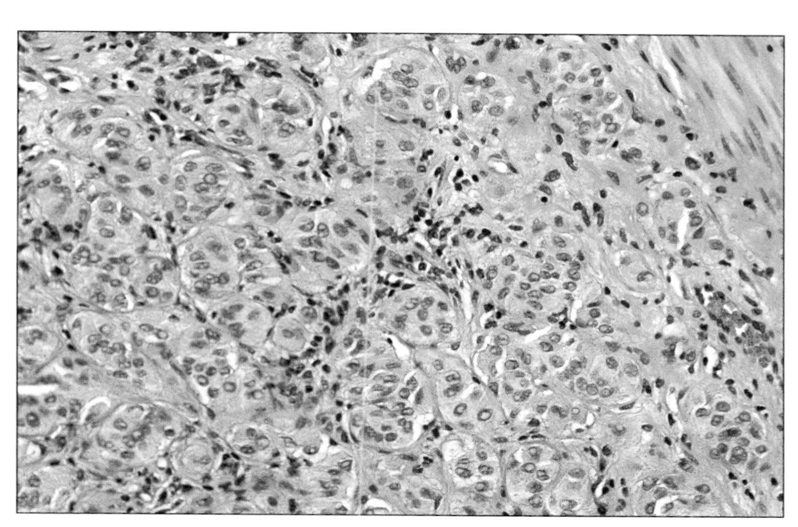

Fig. 11.126 Nesting patterns: a higher-power magnification of Fig. 11.116. Small nests of bland-looking cells. The morphology is very similar to that of a paraganglioma. The cells are synaptophysin-negative.

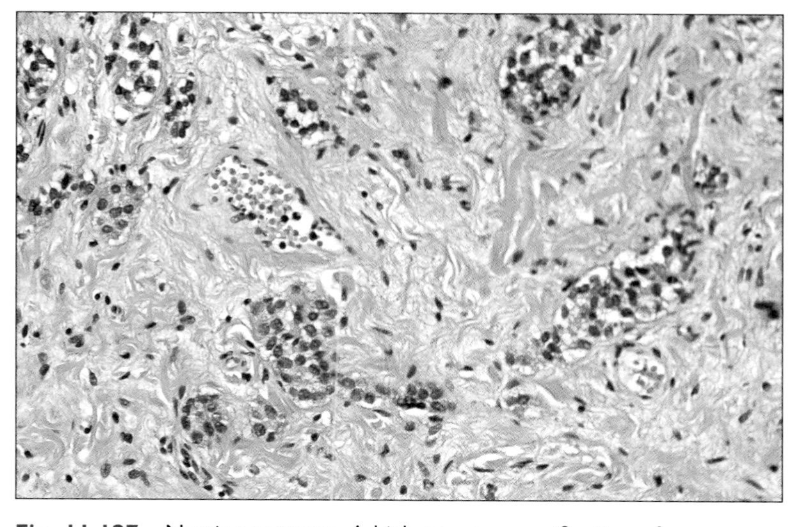

Fig. 11.127 Nesting patterns. A high-power magnification of Fig. 11.113, with numerous neoplastic nests infiltrating the lamina propria beneath carcinoma in situ. In a transurethral resection of the prostate of the bladder in which there is tumor, these cells can easily be overlooked.

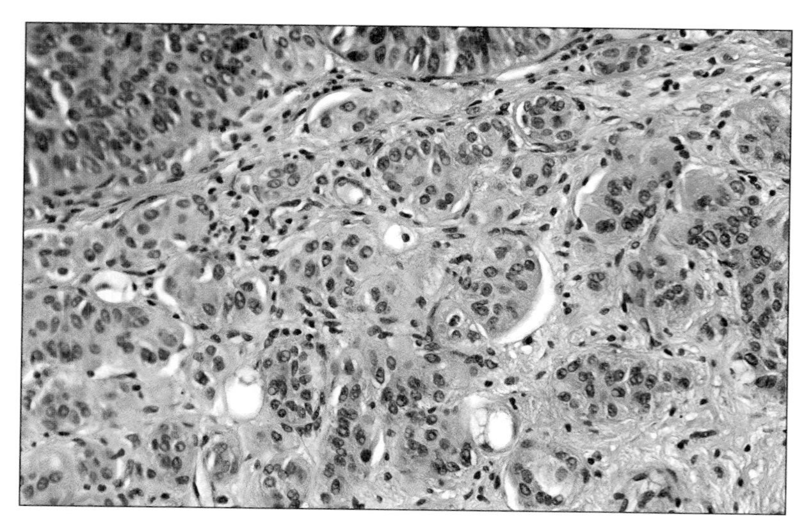

Fig. 11.128 Nesting patterns: a high-power magnification of Fig. 11.116. Numerous neoplastic nests infiltrating the lamina propria (left) beneath a papillary urothelial carcinoma, high grade. These balls of cells, which closely resemble a paraganglioma, are synaptophysin-negative.

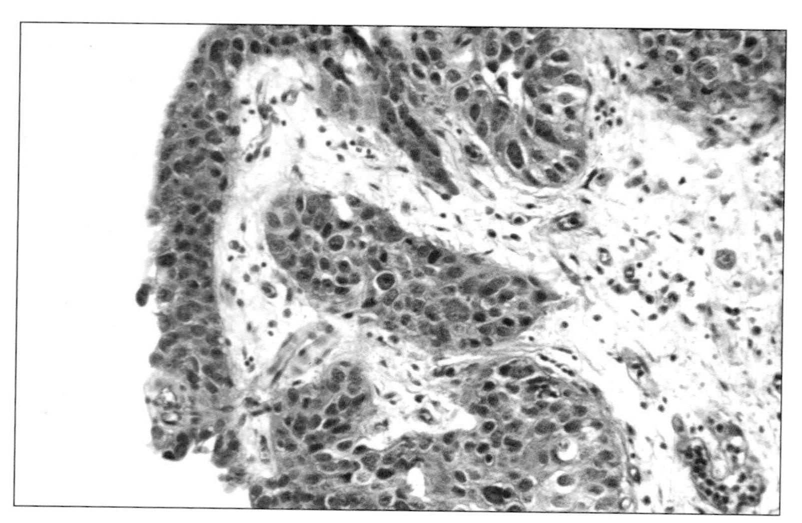

Fig. 11.130 Carcinoma in situ that extends into von Brunn nests. This is not a nesting pattern. The cells in surface epithelium and nests are pleomorphic, whereas in the nesting pattern they are more monomorphic.

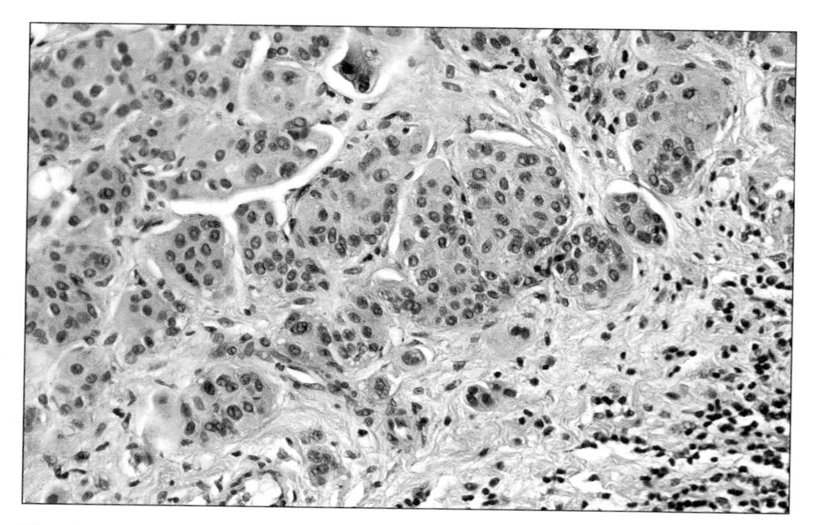

Fig. 11.129 Nesting patterns: a high-power magnification of Fig. 11.116. Numerous neoplastic nests infiltrating the lamina propria (left) beneath a papillary urothelial carcinoma, high grade. The spaces surrounding these balls of cells are artifact and stain negative for vascular endothelium.

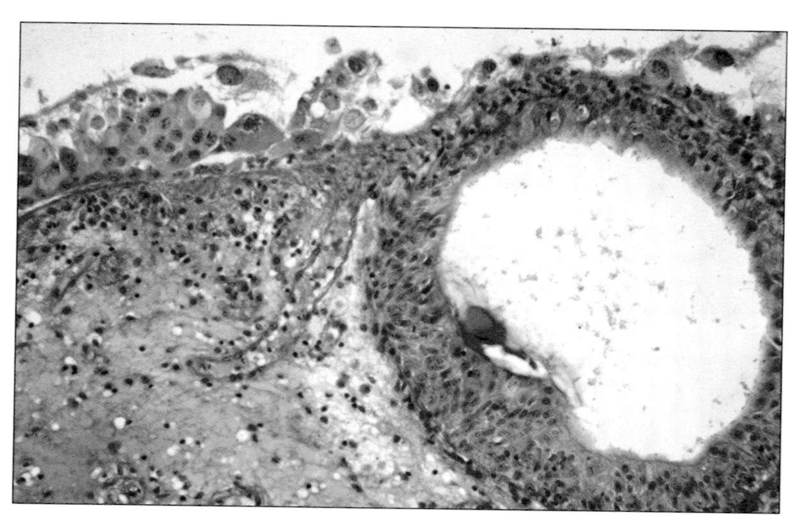

Fig. 11.131 Carcinoma in situ (CIS) that extends into von Brunn nests. The CIS is of the large cell type on the left side, and on the right it has partially desquamated off the basement membrane. The von Brunn nest is cystic but is lined by neoplastic cells.

- Nephrogenic adenoma: this has a papillary component and a prominent tubular growth pattern.
- Paraganglioma: this has a prominent vascular pattern, with cells that are immunohistochemically synaptophysin-positive. Urothelial carcinomas express cytokeratin and other epithelial markers.

CARCINOMA IN SITU[97–105]

This is a form of nonpapillary urothelial carcinoma that can present with or without an associated papillary or invasive carcinoma component in adjacent microscopic fields. Numerous patterns can be linked with it and are found on random biopsies from a urinary bladder associated with positive cytology (see Figs 11.130–11.151, Table 11.1).

TYPICAL NONPAPILLARY UROTHELIAL CARCINOMA PATTERN

- The majority of invasive urothelial carcinomas are high grade.
- They consist of cohesive nests or islands of cells with moderate to abundant amphophilic cytoplasm and large hyperchromatic nuclei.

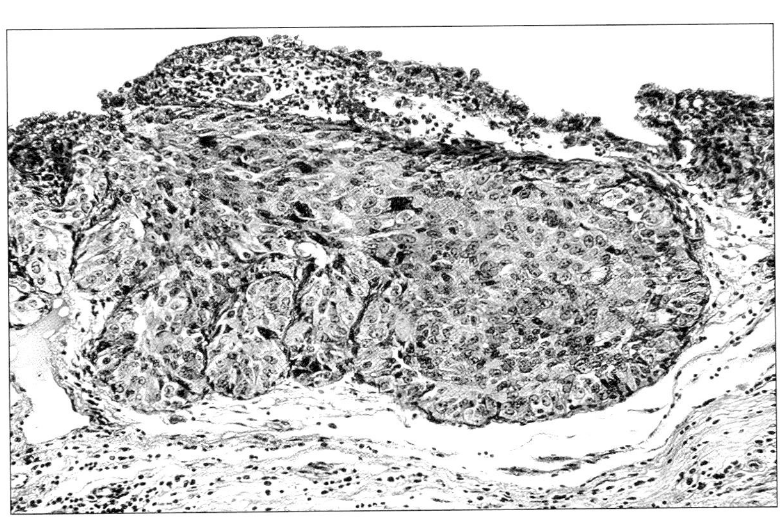

Fig. 11.132 Carcinoma in situ that extends into von Brunn nests. The surface epithelium has desquamated off. The surface is covered by ulcer debris, which covers the von Brunn nest. The von Brunn nest is composed of very pleomorphic neoplastic urothelial cells.

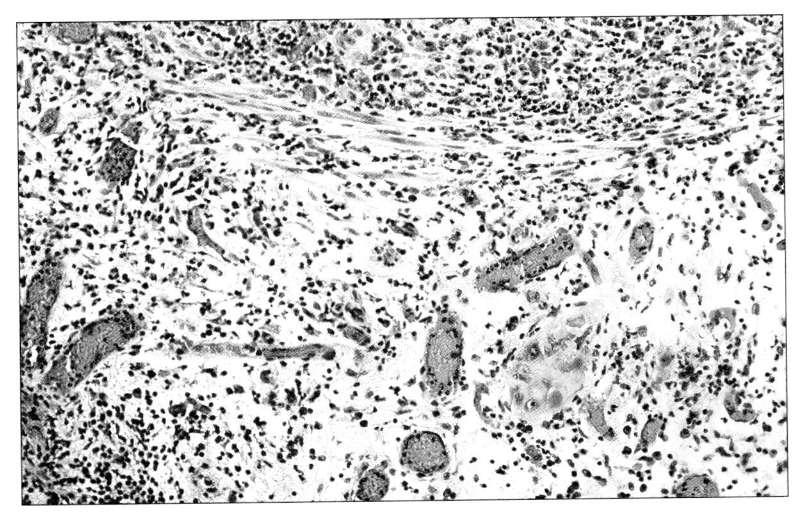

Fig. 11.133 Carcinoma in situ that extends into the inflamed and edematous lamina propria. There are two isolated clusters of large neoplastic urothelial cancer cells.

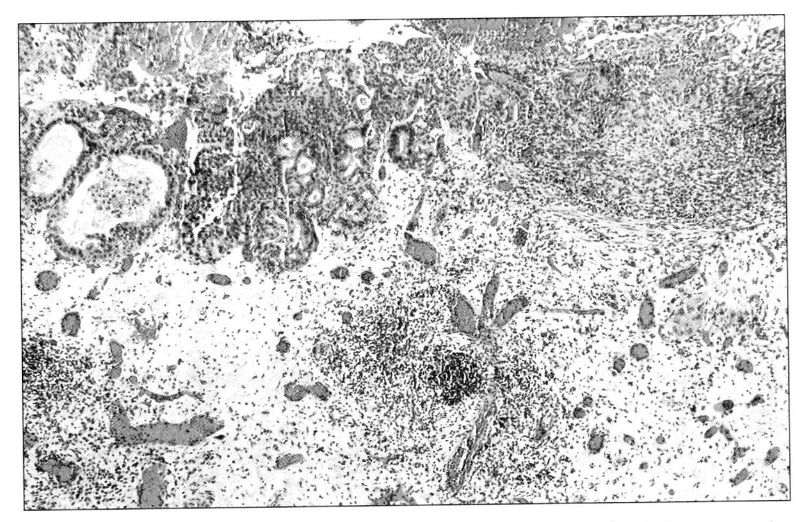

Fig. 11.134 Carcinoma in situ (CIS) that extends into the inflamed and edematous lamina propria. There are cystic carcinomatous von Brunn nests, as well as an area in which neoplastic glandular change is present. CIS has various morphologic forms: large cell, small cell, squamous, partially desquamated, and pagetoid.

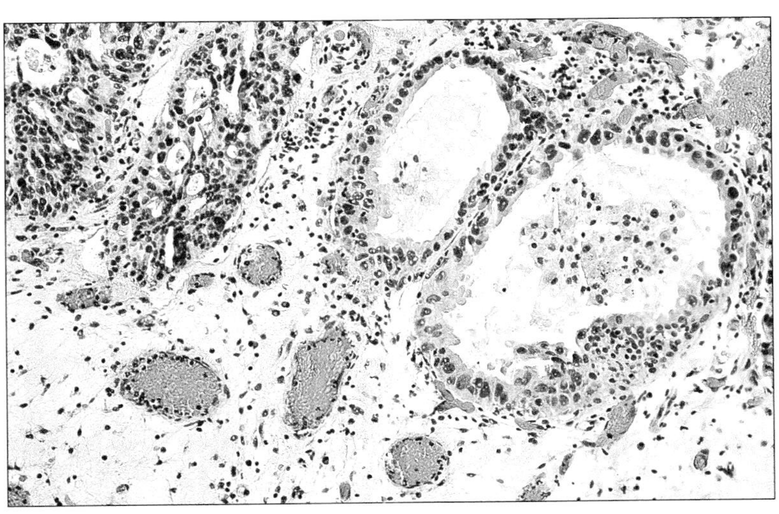

Fig. 11.135 Carcinoma in situ that extends into the inflamed and edematous lamina propria. A higher magnification of the left side of Fig. 11.134.

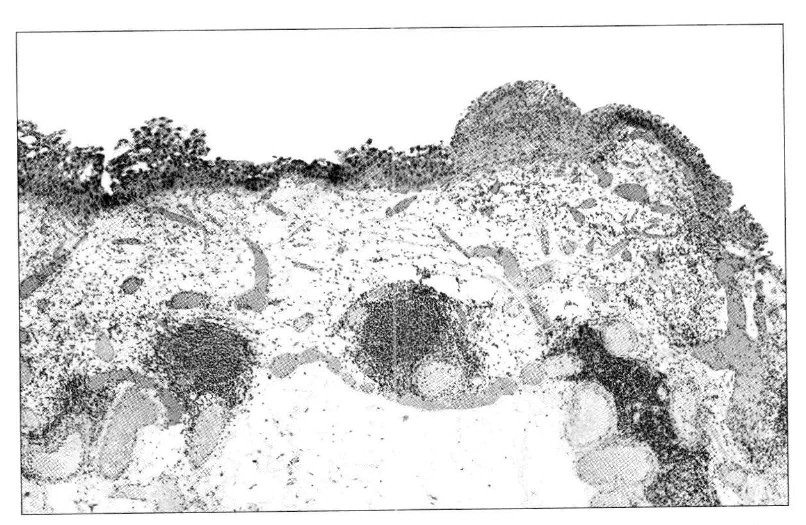

Fig. 11.136 Carcinoma in situ (CIS) that extends along the surface of the bladder above an inflamed and edematous lamina propria with cystitis follicularis. There is CIS in the left two-thirds of the photomicrograph, and then a mound of atypical urothelial hyperplasia next to normal urothelium on the right.

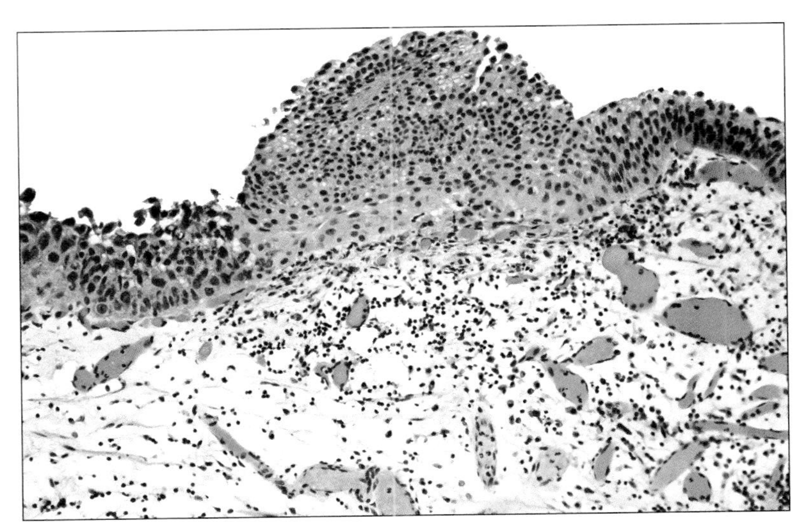

Fig. 11.137 Carcinoma in situ that extends along the surface of the bladder above an inflamed and edematous lamina propria with cystitis follicularis. A higher magnification of Fig. 11.136.

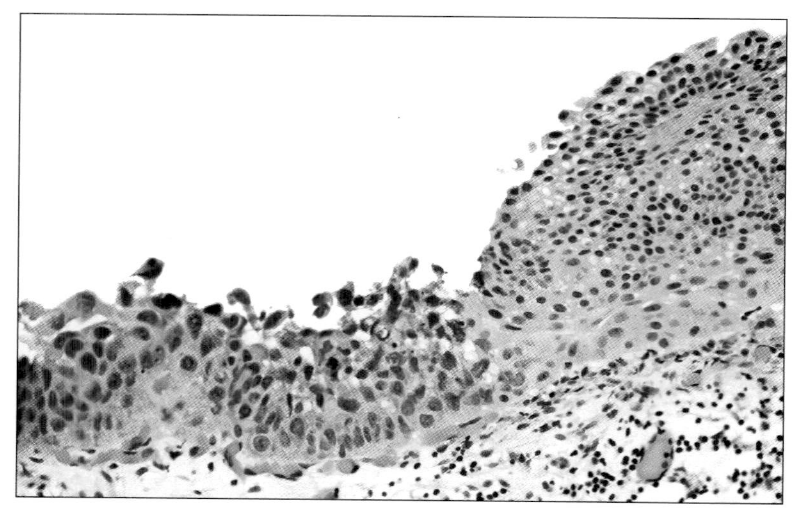

Fig. 11.138 Carcinoma in situ (CIS) that extends along the surface of the bladder above an inflamed and edematous lamina propria with cystitis follicularis. A higher magnification of Fig. 11.136, showing CIS next to a mound of atypical hyperplastic urothelium.

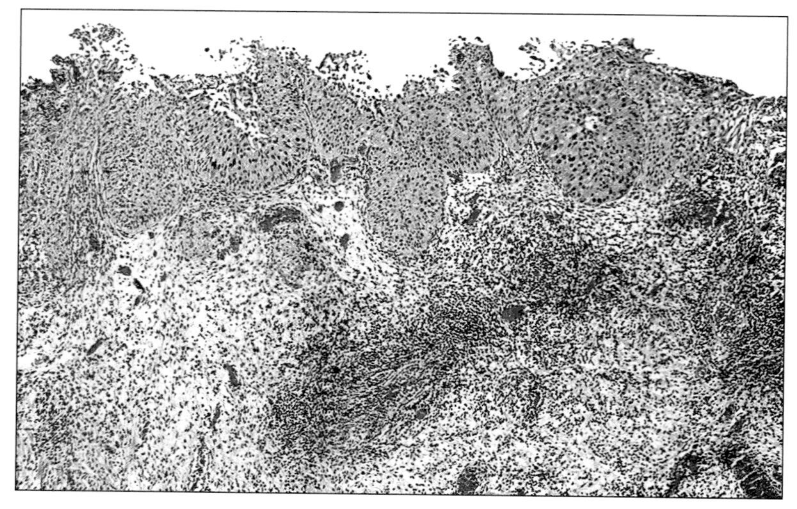

Fig. 11.139 Carcinoma in situ that extends along the surface of the bladder and into nests of von Brunn. Compare these nests to the nesting pattern seen in previous figures.

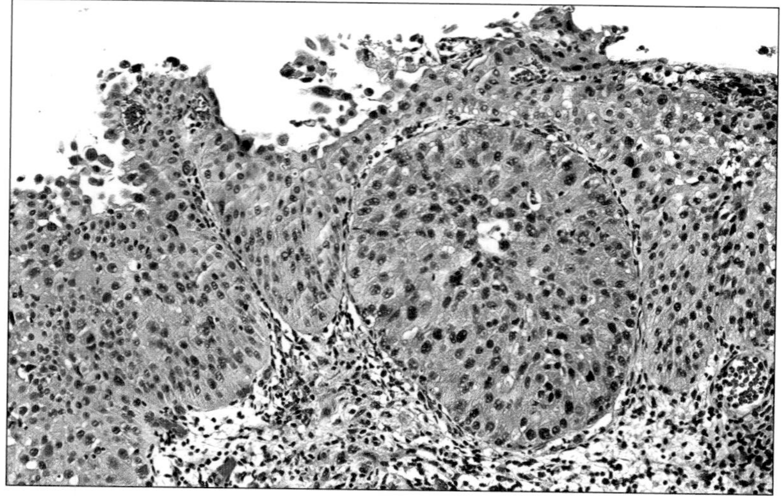

Fig. 11.140 A higher magnification of Fig. 11.139, in which the carcinoma in situ extends between the papillary, high-grade tumor compartment and the nests of von Brunn.

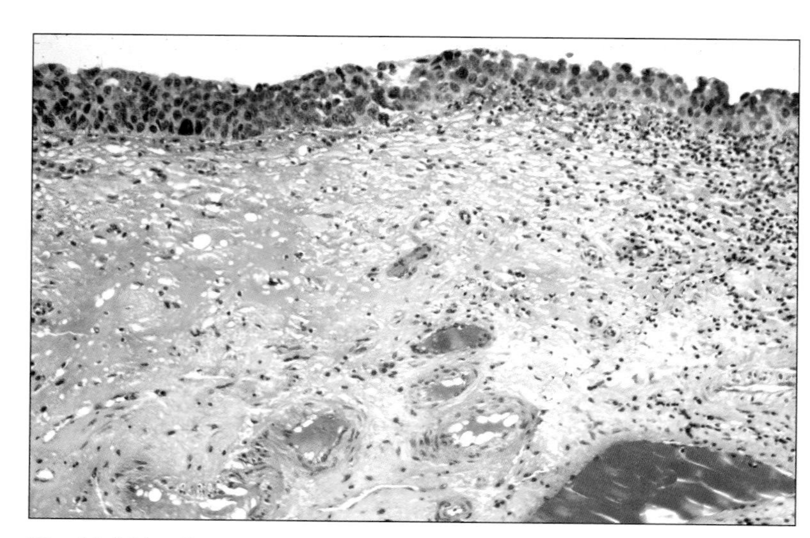

Fig. 11.141 Carcinoma in situ (CIS) extending along a flat surface between high-grade papillary tumors. Definitive CIS is on the left of the photomicrograph, and moderate to severe dysplasia is on the right.

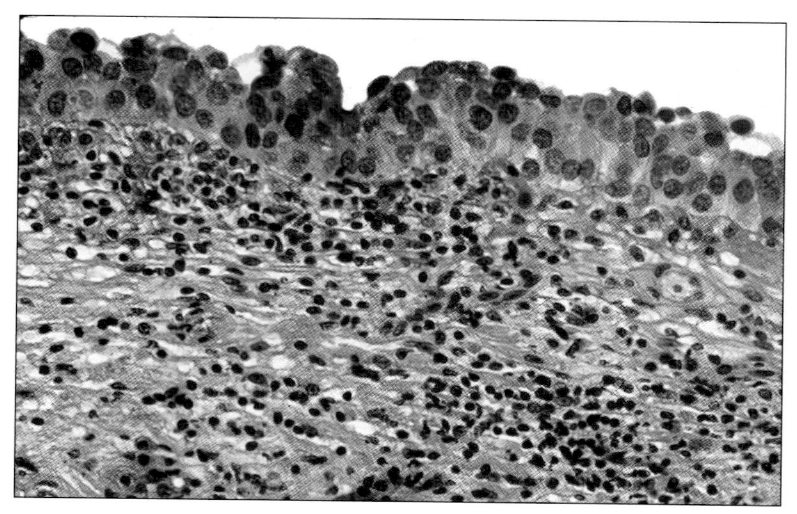

Fig. 11.142 Carcinoma in situ: the moderate to severe dysplasia from Fig. 11.141 at higher magnification (right side of photomicrograph).

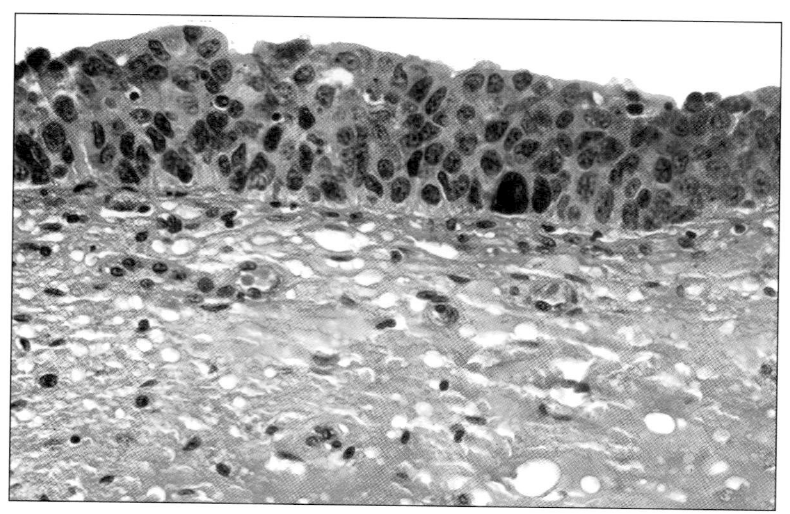

Fig. 11.143 Carcinoma in situ (CIS): the CIS from Fig. 11.141 at higher magnification (left side of photomicrograph).

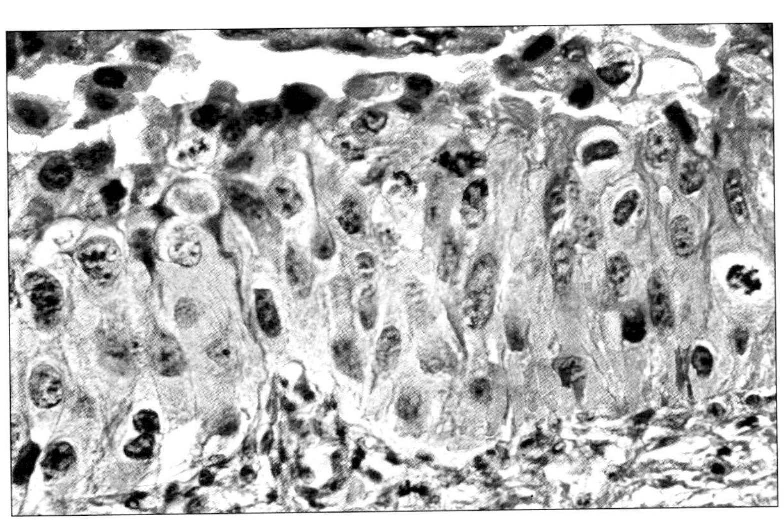

Fig. 11.144 Carcinoma in situ (CIS): another focus of CIS, at higher magnification, from another area of the bladder of the case shown in Fig. 11.141. When different areas of the bladder are biopsied, several different types of CIS can be found in the same patient.

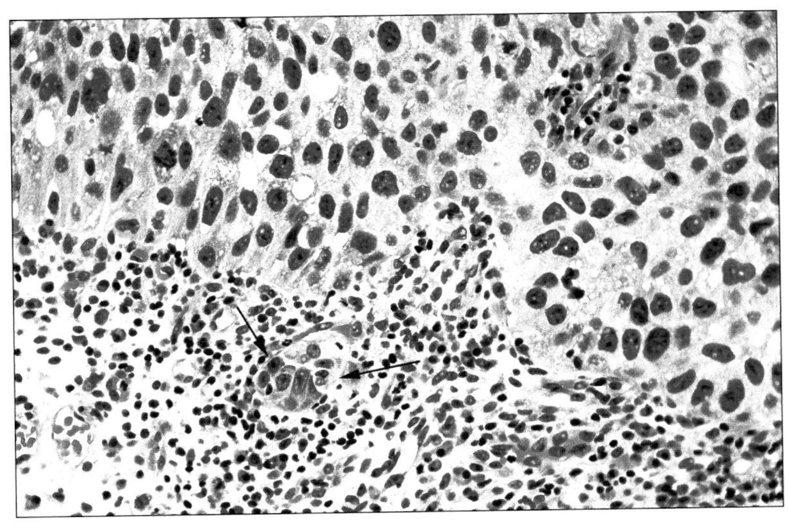

Fig. 11.145 Carcinoma in situ (CIS) with an invasive focus. Another focus of CIS, at higher magnification, from another area of the bladder of the case in Fig. 11.141. Further levels of the same block revealed an invasive focus (arrows).

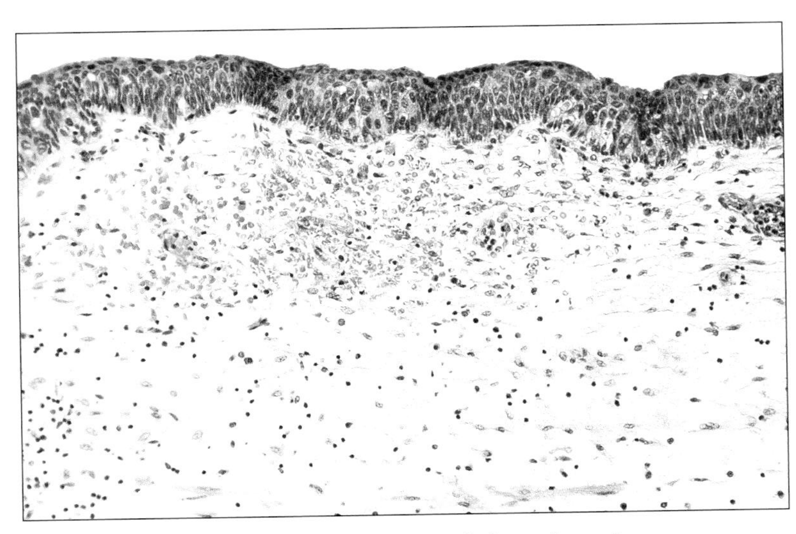

Fig. 11.146 Pagetoid changes in the urothelium: from the same case as in Fig. 11.141, 2 years before the bladder became extensively involved with carcinoma in situ.

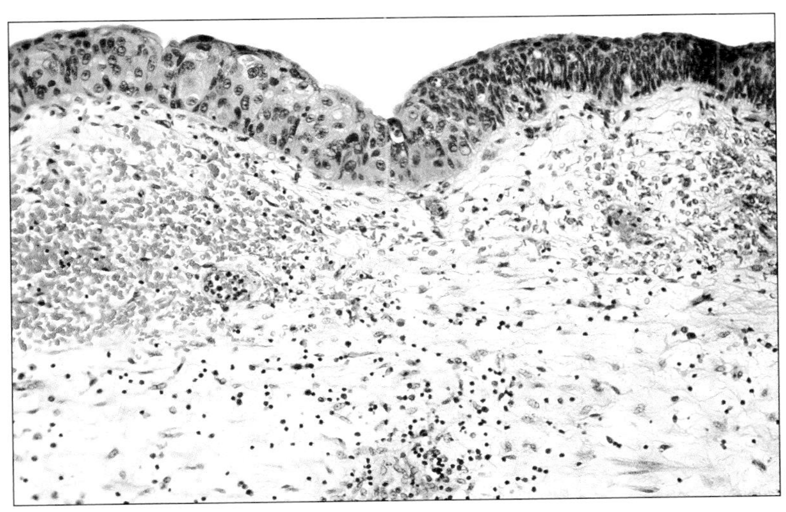

Fig. 11.147 Pagetoid changes in the urothelium: from the same case as in Fig. 11.146 but at higher magnification. The pagetoid area of carcinoma in situ is on the left of the photomicrograph, and the dysplastic urothelium is on the right.

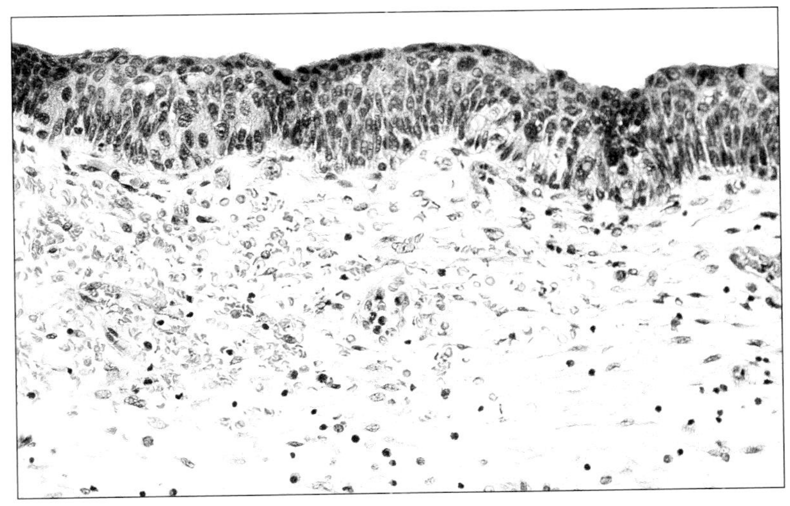

Fig. 11.148 Pagetoid changes in the urothelium: from the same case as in Fig. 11.146, in which the pagetoid cells are mixed with urothelial cells. There are atypical umbrella cells at the upper surface of the urothelium.

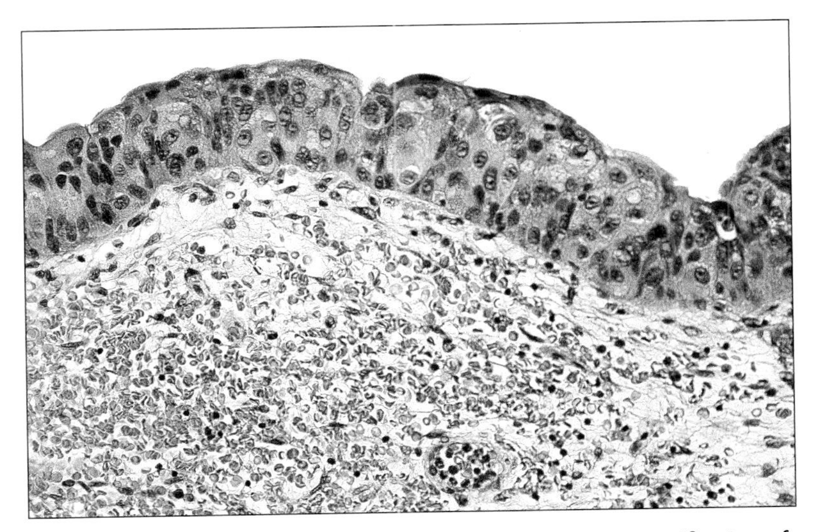

Fig. 11.149 Pagetoid changes in the urothelium: higher magnification of pagetoid cells in the urothelium, from the same case as in Fig. 11.146. The pagetoid cells are mixed with atypical umbrella cells at the upper surface of the urothelium.

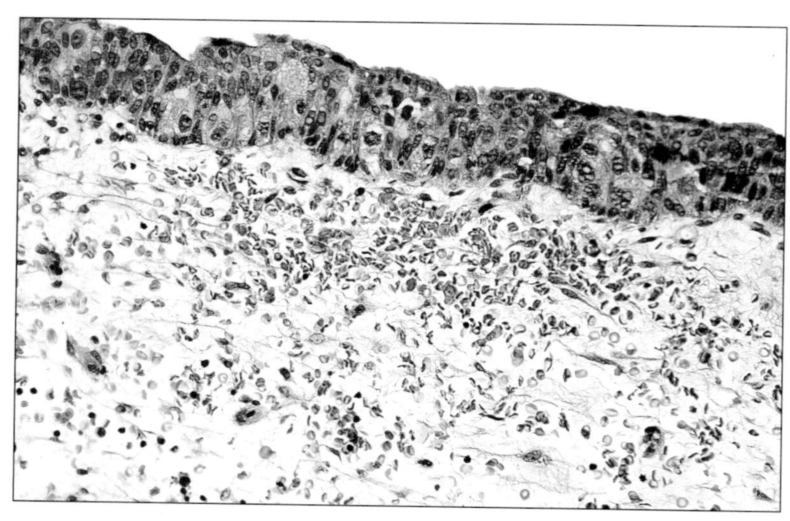

Fig. 11.150 Pagetoid changes in the urothelium: higher magnification of pagetoid cells in the urothelium, from the same case as in Fig. 11.146. Here, the atypical umbrella cells have been cast off, providing very atypical cells in the urinary cytology.

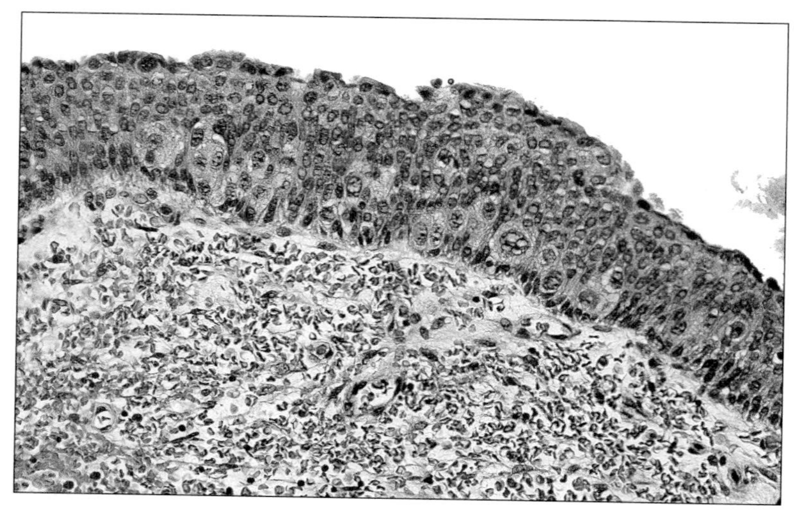

Fig. 11.151 Pagetoid changes in the urothelium: higher magnification of pagetoid cells in the urothelium from the same case as in Fig. 11.146. Here, the atypical umbrella cells and hyperplasia of the intermediate cells above the pagetoid cells is evident.

- A minority of invasive tumors have remnants of papillary architecture that persist, in larger nests with palisading nuclei at the edges of the nests and stratification toward the center.
- Commonly, carcinoma cells are arranged in small clusters or single cells.
- The tumor may invade as solid sheets with little intervening stroma.
- Nuclei are pleomorphic, with irregular contours and angular profiles.
- Nuclear grooves, characteristic of low-grade urothelial cancer, may be identified in some cells.
- Nucleoli are highly variable in number and appearance, with some cells containing single or multiple small nucleoli and others having large eosinophilic nucleoli.
- The foci of marked pleomorphism may be seen, with bizarre and multinuclear tumor cells in solid areas.
- Mitotic figures are common, with numerous abnormal forms.
- Invasive nests may induce a striking desmoplastic stromal reaction.
- The desmoplastic reaction may have a malignant spindle cell component.

CAUTION

- Artifactual clefts are often present around the nests of carcinoma cells, mimicking vascular invasion; avoid overdiagnosis of vascular invasion. Immunohistochemically, use factor VIII–related antigen to demonstrate the presence of endothelial cells around the nests of carcinoma.
- Squamous differentiation occurs in up to 20% of cases of invasive urothelial carcinoma. These consist of cells with more abundant eosinophilic or clear cytoplasm with glycogen.
- Urothelial carcinoma may have foci of squamous or glandular differentiation. High-grade urothelial carcinoma often shows foci of squamous, glandular, or small cell differentiation.
- Squamous differentiation is defined by the presence of intercellular bridges or keratinization; it occurs in up to 20% of urothelial carcinomas. The proportion of the squamous component may vary considerably.
- The diagnosis of squamous cell carcinoma is reserved only for pure lesions with no associated urothelial component or urothelial CIS.
- Tumors with a urothelial element are diagnosed as urothelial carcinoma with foci of squamous differentiation.
- Squamous differentiation is associated with a poor response to systemic chemotherapy and radiation.
- Glandular differentiation is less common than squamous differentiation.
- Mucin-containing cells are common in high-grade urothelial carcinoma.
- Glandular differentiation is indicated by the presence of true glandular spaces within the tumor.
- Pseudoglandular spaces caused by necrosis or artifact should not be considered evidence of glandular differentiation.
- The diagnosis of adenocarcinoma is reserved for pure tumors, and a tumor with mixed glandular and urothelial differentiation should be signed out as urothelial carcinoma with glandular differentiation.

- The clinical significance of glandular differentiation and mucin positivity in urothelial carcinoma remains uncertain.

MICROCYSTIC UROTHELIAL CARCINOMA PATTERN[106,107]

- This is characterized by the formation of microcysts.
- It includes lesions with intermediate- to high-grade urothelial carcinoma having areas of microcystic or macrocystic change, or tubular (glandular) differentiation.
- The cysts and tubules can be empty or contain necrotic debris or mucin.
- It is important to distinguish cystic change in urothelial carcinoma from benign and malignant mimics.

CAUTION

It may be confused with:

- benign proliferations such as cystitis cystica and glandularis;
- nephrogenic adenoma;
- adenocarcinoma of the bladder, which is restricted to tumors with true gland formation.

INVERTED UROTHELIAL CANCER PATTERN[108,109]

- An exophytic papillary and invasive component that is associated with the inverted element.
- Urothelial carcinoma can mimic inverted papilloma architecturally but possesses high-grade cytologic abnormalities.
- This variant of urothelial carcinoma has significant nuclear pleomorphism, mitotic figures, and architectural disruption. The overlying epithelium has similar abnormalities.

GIANT CELL UROTHELIAL CANCER PATTERN[110,111]

- Giant cells have been seen in a variety of instances.
- The giant cells stain positively for cytokeratin.
- This tumor type has a very poor prognosis.
- Giant cells are also seen in urothelial carcinoma and may be associated with human chorionic gonadotropin production.
- Osteoclast-like giant cells can be found in invasive high-grade urothelial carcinoma.
- There is no evidence that osteoclast-like giant cells indicate increased aggressiveness.
- Similar tumors have been seen as giant cell reparative granuloma and giant cell tumor. The giant cells probably reflect a stromal response to the tumor.
- Giant cells are also seen in patients who receive bacillus Calmette-Guérin therapy; a granulomatous response that includes Langerhans giant cells can be seen.
- Giant cells are also seen in patients who have undergone prior resection or biopsy; foreign body–type giant cells may be seen.
- The giant cells have abundant eosinophilic cytoplasm and numerous small, round, regular nuclei, and they stain positively for vimentin but not for epithelial markers.

LYMPHOEPITHELIOMA-LIKE VARIANT OF UROTHELIAL CARCINOMA[112–116]

- This is a carcinoma that histologically resembles lymphoepithelioma of the nasopharynx. It is more common in men than in women (3:1 ratio) and occurs in late adulthood, associated with hematuria.
- It has a sessile growth pattern that involves the dome, posterior wall, or trigone.
- Histologically, it may be pure or mixed with typical urothelial carcinoma, the latter being focal and inconspicuous in some instances.
- The tumor is composed of nests, sheets, or cords of undifferentiated cells with large nuclei and prominent nucleoli.
- The cytoplasmic borders are poorly defined and may appear as syncytial cells. The background consists of a prominent lymphoid stroma.
- Glandular and squamous differentiation can be seen.

CAUTION

Other diagnostic considerations are:

- poorly differentiated urothelial carcinoma;
- squamous cell carcinoma;
- lymphoma;
- severe chronic cystitis, unless there are immunohistochemically cytokeratin positive epithelial cells.

LYMPHOMA-LIKE VARIANT OF UROTHELIAL CANCER (Figs 11.152–11.161)

- Bladder carcinoma can diffusely permeate the bladder wall and mimic lymphoma.

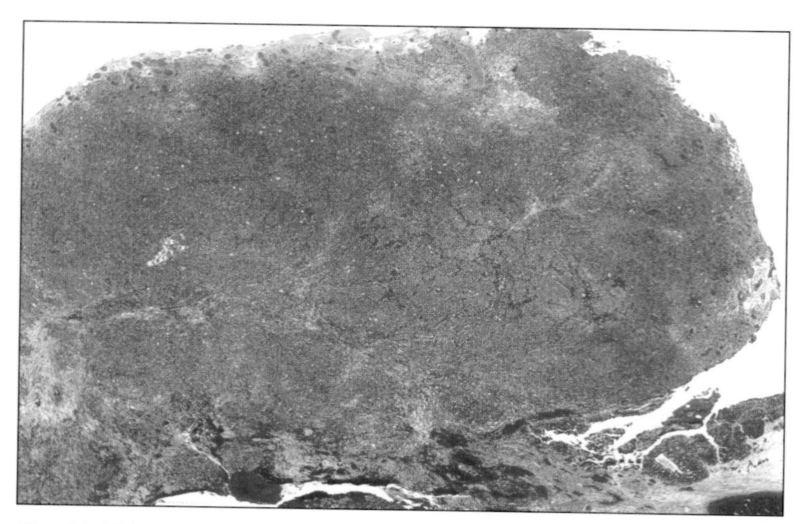

Fig. 11.152 A lymphoma-like variant of urothelial carcinoma in the bladder. A photograph of the whole slide of this mushroom-like mass in the bladder.

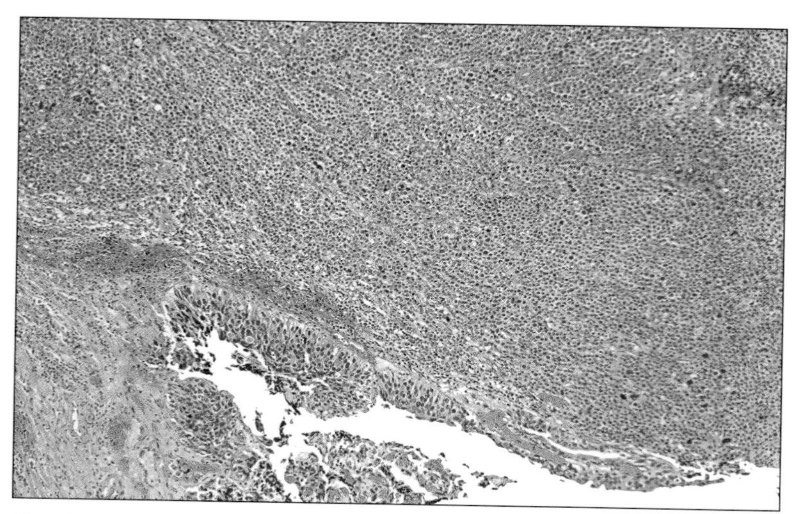

Fig. 11.153 A lymphoma-like variant of urothelial carcinoma in the bladder. The upper two-thirds of the photograph consist of a monotonous sea of cells that are loosely cohesive and suggestive of lymphoma. The lower third consists of high-grade urothelial carcinoma surrounding this mass.

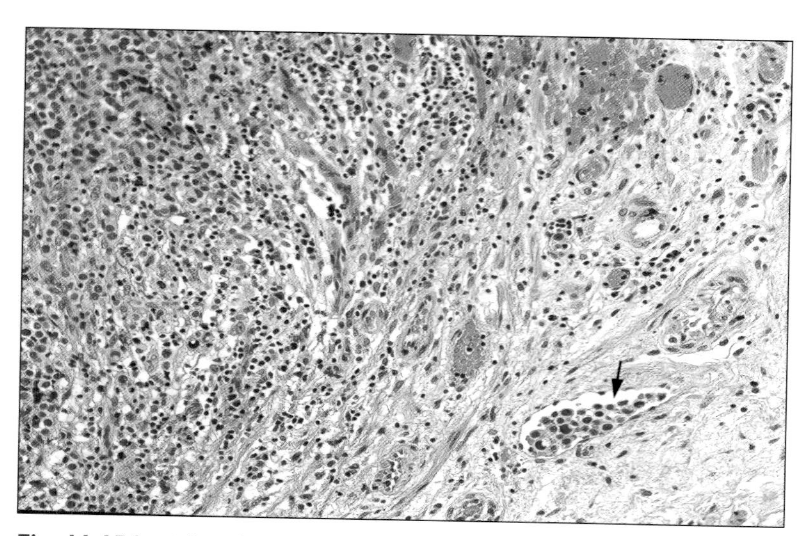

Fig. 11.154 A lymphoma-like variant of urothelial carcinoma in the bladder. At the periphery of this mass is an epithelial cluster of urothelial carcinoma in a vascular space (arrow).

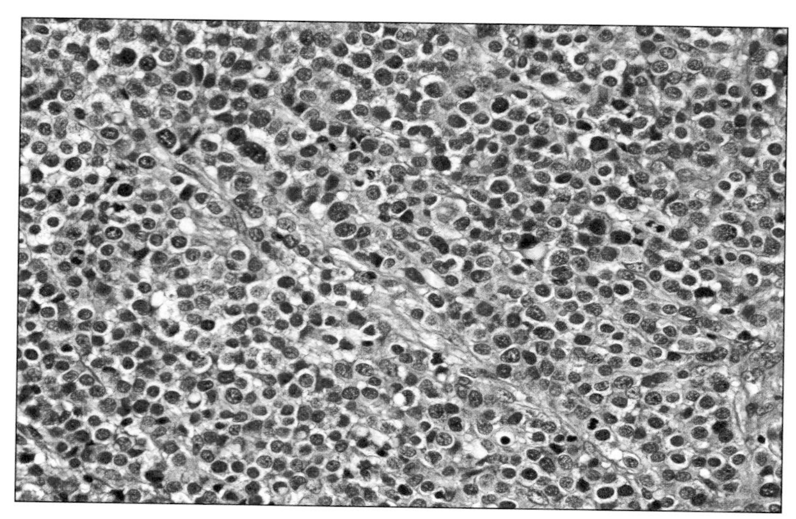

Fig. 11.155 A lymphoma-like variant of urothelial carcinoma in the bladder. A photomicrograph of the middle of this bladder mass. It consists of large non-cohesive cells.

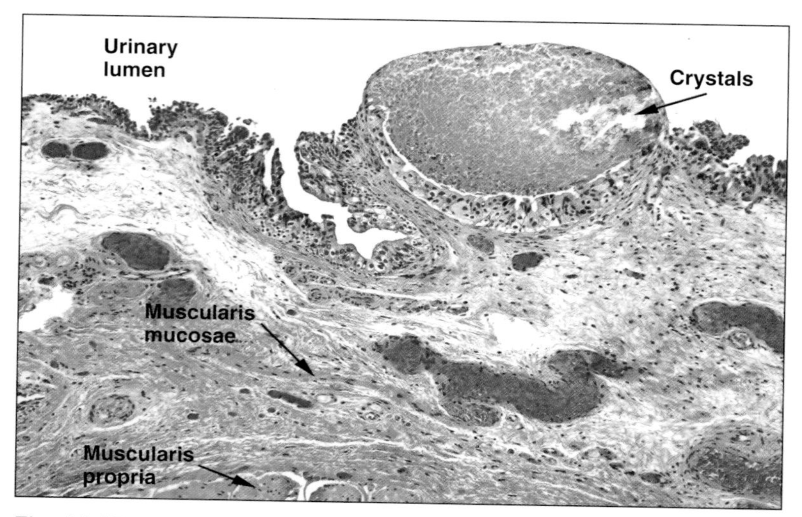

Fig. 11.156 A lymphoma-like variant of urothelial carcinoma in the bladder. A photomicrograph of the bladder mucosa at the periphery of this mass. The urothelium on the surface is in the form of a micropapillary urothelial high-grade carcinoma. There are also crystals in the lumen of a neoplastic von Brunn urothelial nest.

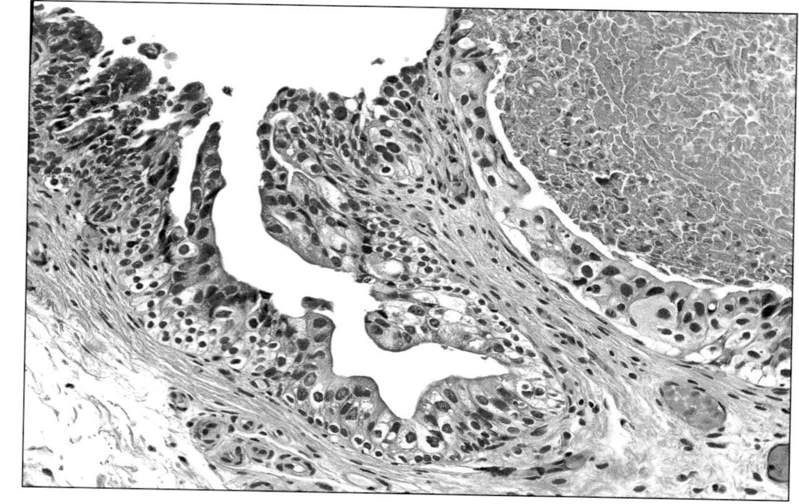

Fig. 11.157 A lymphoma-like variant of urothelial carcinoma in the bladder. A higher-power magnification of Fig. 11.156, in which there is a micropapillary urothelial high-grade carcinoma on the left and a lumen of a neoplastic von Brunn urothelial nest on the right.

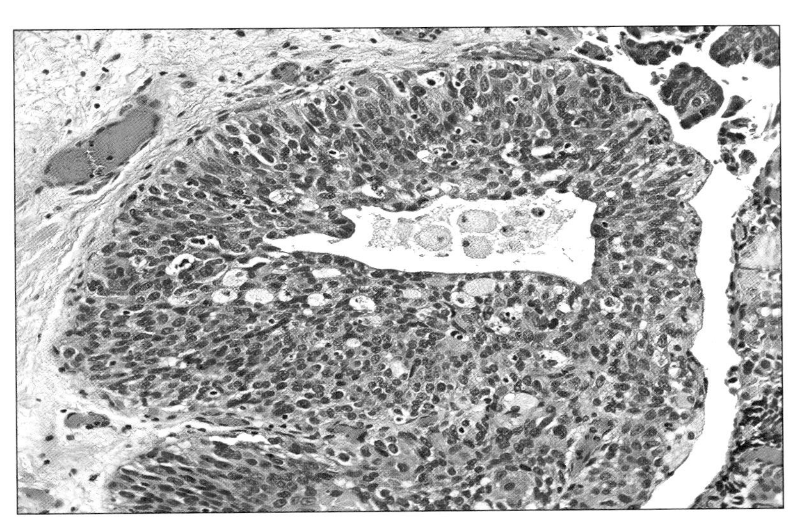

Fig. 11.158 A lymphoma-like variant of urothelial carcinoma in the bladder. A higher-power magnification of a portion of Fig. 11.152 in which there is a urothelial high-grade carcinoma of the von Brunn nest.

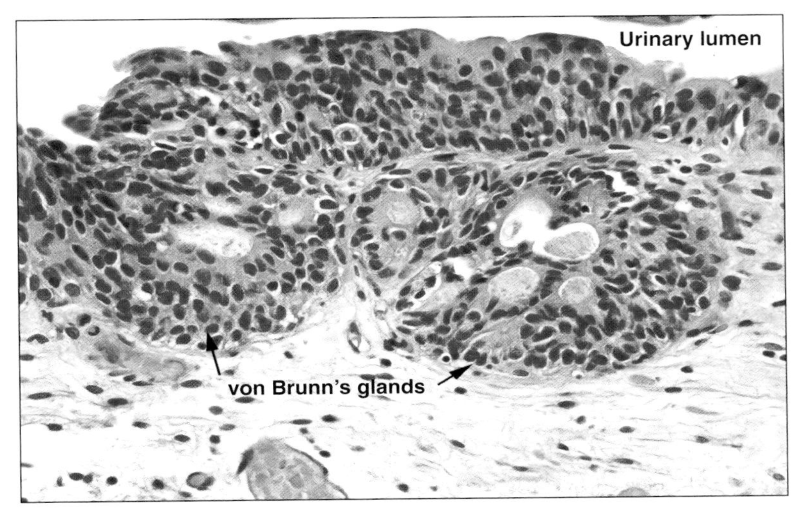

Fig. 11.159 A lymphoma-like variant of urothelial carcinoma in the bladder. A higher-power magnification of a portion of Fig. 11.152 in which there is a neoplastic urothelial carcinoma in situ covering two involved nests of von Brunn.

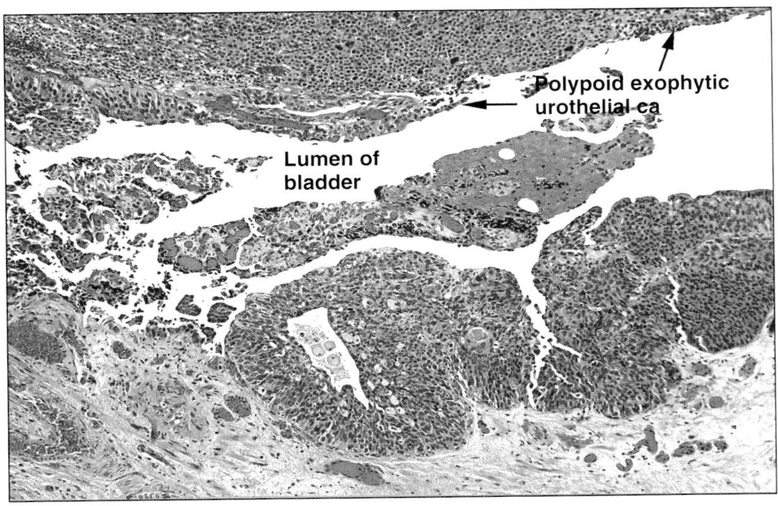

Fig. 11.160 A lymphoma-like variant of urothelial carcinoma in the bladder. A higher-power magnification of a portion of Fig. 11.152 in which there is the bottom part of the polypoid exophytic urothelial carcinoma and the surrounding neoplastically involved nests of von Brunn.

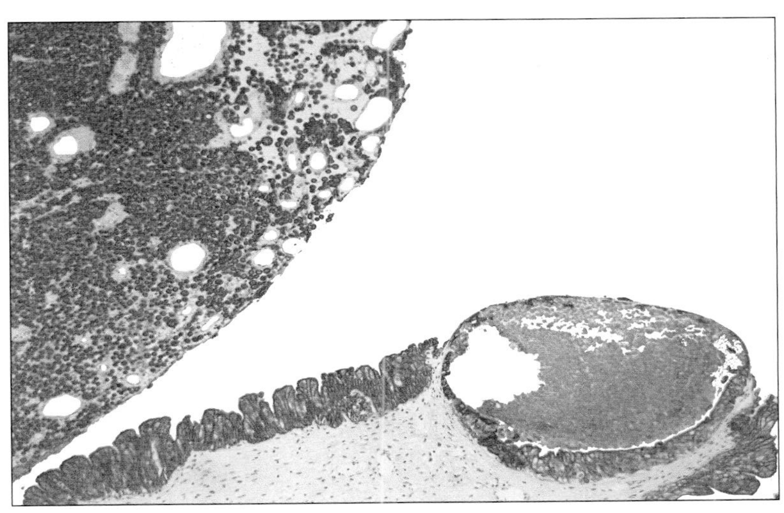

Fig. 11.161 A lymphoma-like variant of urothelial carcinoma in the bladder. A positive low molecular weight cytokeratin immunostain of the carcinoma shown in Fig. 11.152. Note that the cells of the polypoid mass are cytokeratin-positive. If it were lymphoma, it would not have stained.

- Tumor cells can have a plasmacytoid appearance.
- The diagnosis of carcinoma is confirmed by immunoreactivity for cytokeratin and carcinoembryonic antigen, and negative staining for lymphoid markers.

CAUTION

Consideration must be given to:

- plasmacytosis;
- lymphoma;
- multiple myeloma.

SARCOMATOID UROTHELIAL CARCINOMA AND CARCINOSARCOMA (Figs 11.162–11.175)[117–122]

- Some urinary bladder cancers contain both malignant epithelial and spindle cell patterns.
- In the literature, other names are carcinosarcoma, sarcomatoid carcinoma, pseudosarcomatous transitional cell carcinoma, malignant mesodermal mixed tumor, spindle cell and giant cell carcinoma, and malignant teratoma. We favor the term sarcomatoid carcinoma.
- Sarcomatoid carcinoma affects males more frequently than females (2:1). Patients are in the seventh and eighth decades. It can occur in patients below 50 years.
- Grossly, the tumor is usually exophytic, with a polypoid or pedunculated growth pattern. Many are large masses up to 12 cm in diameter.

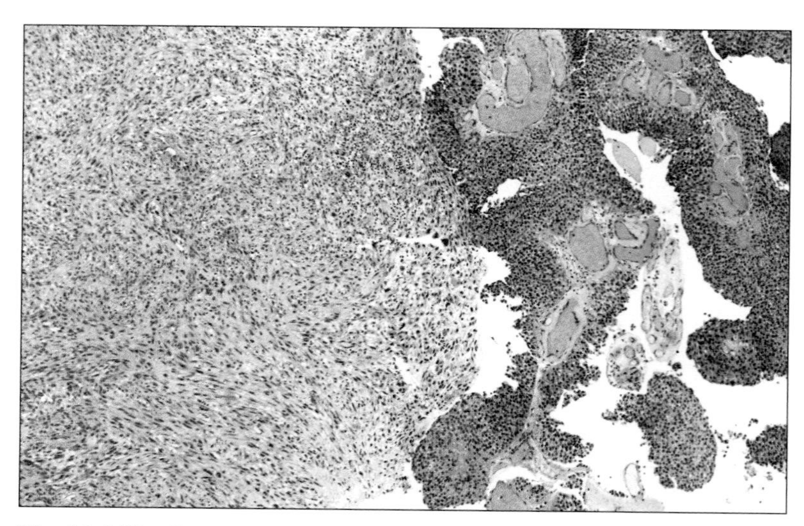

Fig. 11.162 Carcinosarcoma. A high-grade papillary urothelial cancer is on the right, whereas on the left there is a sarcoma. The latter has a spindle storiform pattern similar to that in malignant fibrous histiocytoma. The cells are cytokeratin-negative.

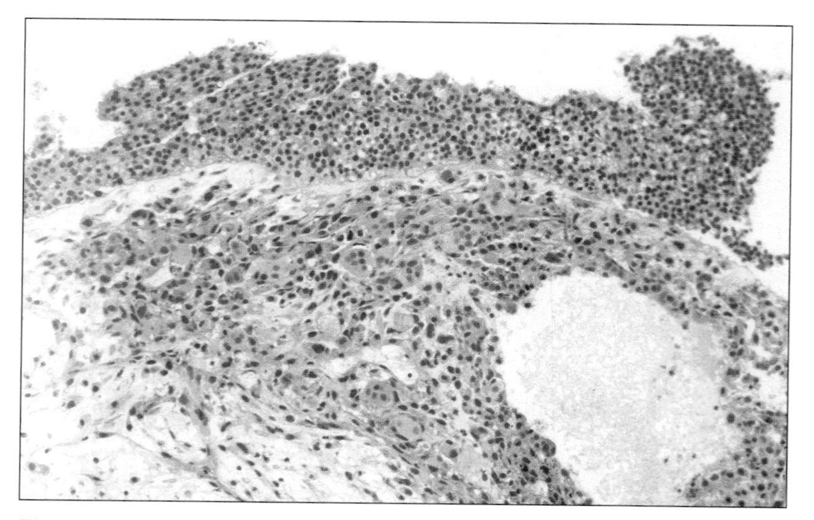

Fig. 11.163 Carcinosarcoma. A high-grade urothelial cancer in the lower two-thirds of the digital picture; above it is urothelial hyperplasia. The cytology in the urothelium is bland, whereas below the basement membrane there are numerous large tumor cells, some of which are multinucleated. These are cytokeratin-positive.

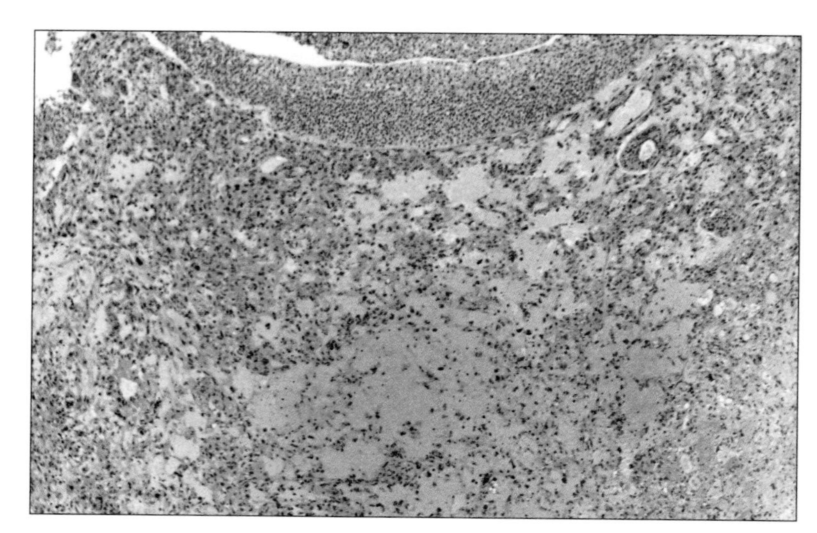

Fig. 11.164 Carcinosarcoma. A high-grade urothelial cancer in the lower two-thirds of the digital picture; above it is urothelial dysplasia or hyperplasia. The cytology in the urothelium is more pleomorphic than that shown in Fig. 11.163. Below the basement membrane are numerous large tumor cells, some of which are multinucleated, and one epithelial tumor nest in the right upper corner.

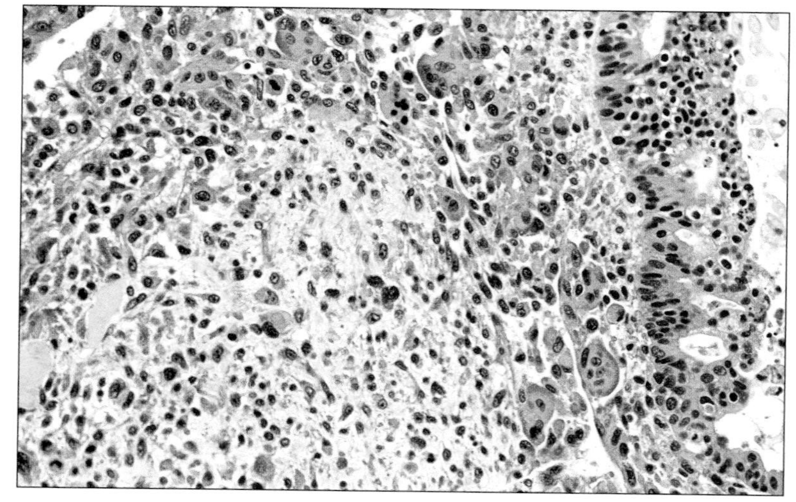

Fig. 11.165 Carcinosarcoma. A high-grade urothelial carcinoma in situ is shown on the right. Beneath it, to the left, is a pleomorphic sarcoma with multinucleated tumor cells that are cytokeratin-negative.

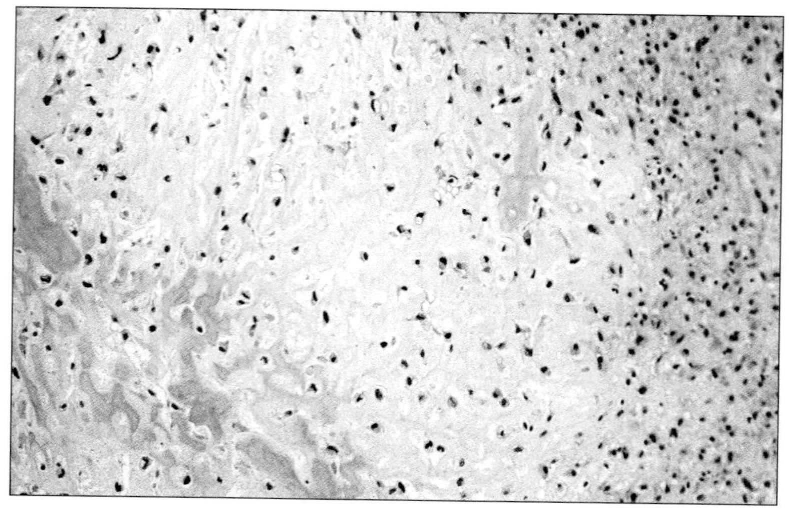

Fig. 11.166 Carcinosarcoma. An area of chondrosarcoma in the middle two-thirds, with osteoid on the left and an area of sarcoma on the right. No malignant urothelium is seen. All areas are cytokeratin-negative.

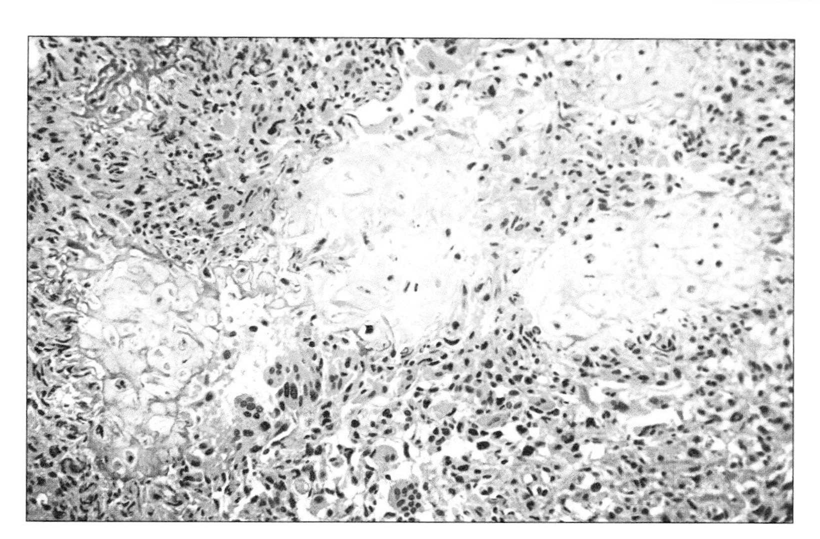

Fig. 11.167 Carcinosarcoma. Another area of chondrosarcoma in the middle third of the digital photo, surrounded by areas of sarcoma above and below. Multinucleated giant cells are scattered throughout the tumor. No malignant urothelium is seen. All areas are cytokeratin-negative.

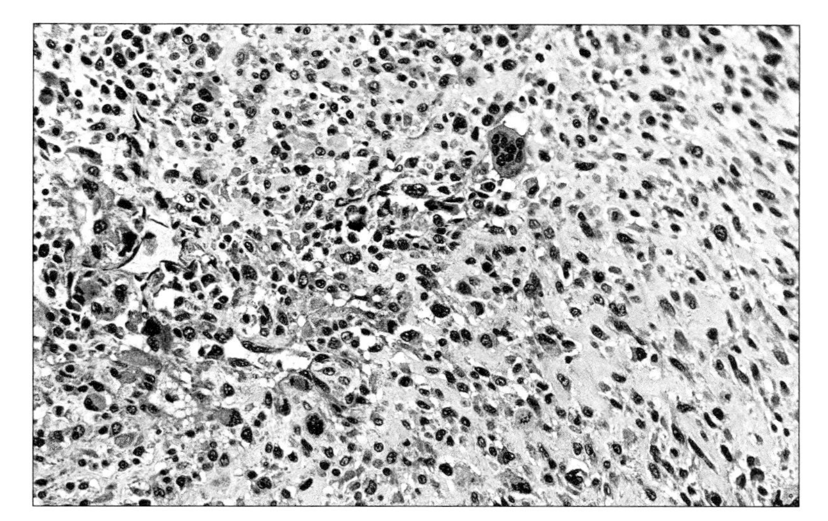

Fig. 11.168 Carcinosarcoma. Another area of sarcoma with a few multinucleated giant cells scattered throughout the tumor. No malignant urothelium is seen. All areas are cytokeratin-negative.

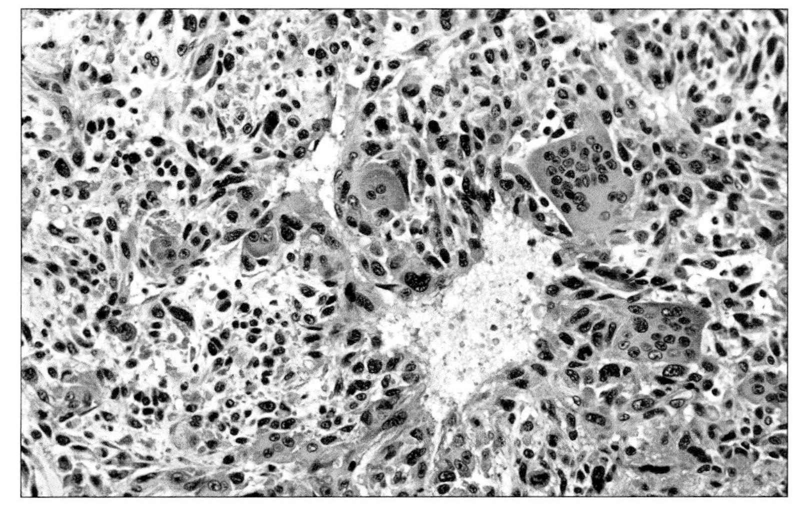

Fig. 11.169 Carcinosarcoma. Another area of sarcoma at higher magnification, with numerous multinucleated giant cells scattered throughout the tumor. No malignant urothelium is seen. All areas are cytokeratin-negative.

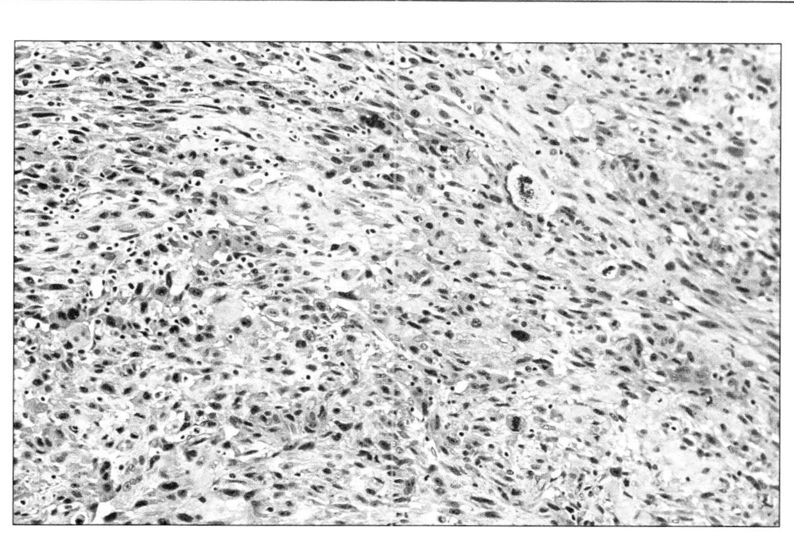

Fig. 11.170 Carcinosarcoma. Another area of sarcoma, with mitosis and an appearance of malignant fibrous histiocytoma. No malignant urothelium is seen. All areas are cytokeratin-negative.

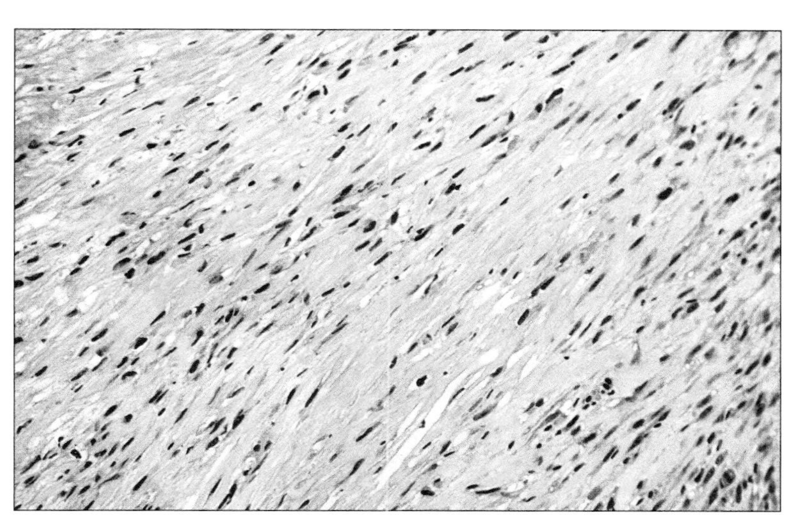

Fig. 11.171 Carcinosarcoma. Another area of sarcoma, with mitosis and an appearance of fibrosarcoma. No malignant urothelium is seen. All areas are cytokeratin-negative.

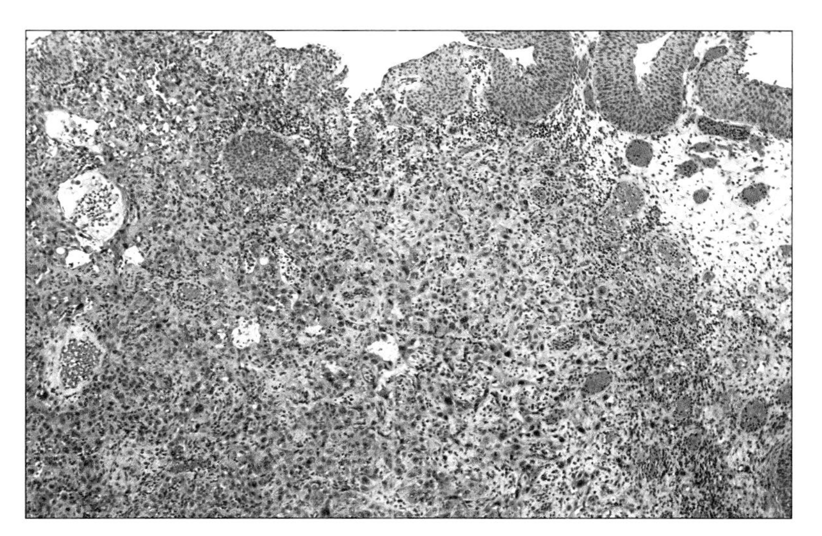

Fig. 11.172 High-grade urothelial carcinoma with an area of pseudosarcomatous change with mitosis, with malignant urothelium on the surface and in von Brunn nests. All areas are cytokeratin-positive.

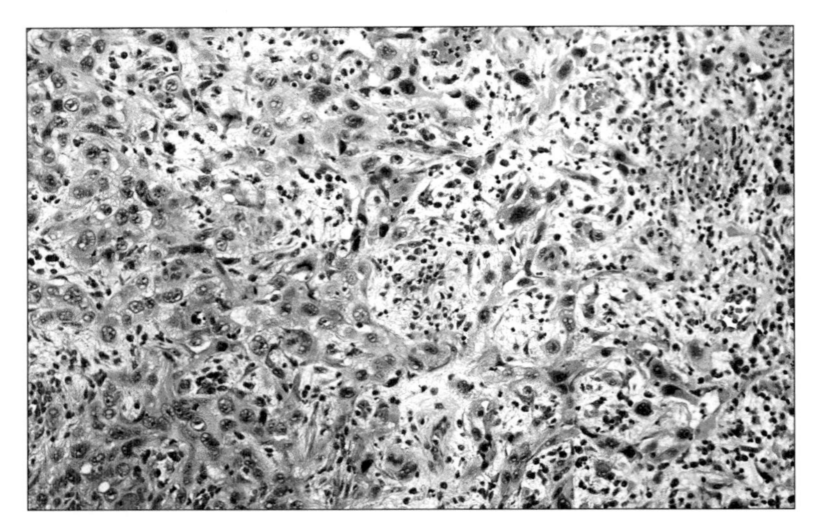

Fig. 11.173 High-grade urothelial carcinoma with an area of pseudosarcomatous change with mitosis. All areas are cytokeratin-positive.

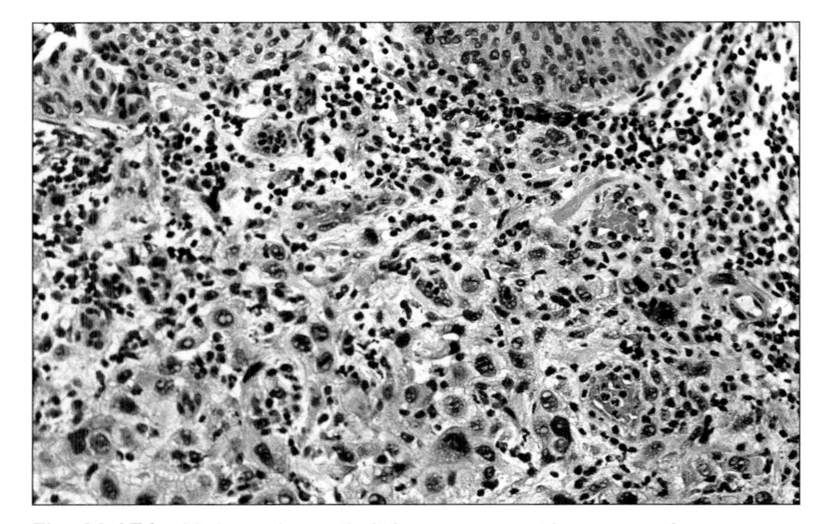

Fig. 11.174 High-grade urothelial carcinoma with an area of pseudosarcomatous change with mitosis, higher magnification. All areas are cytokeratin-positive.

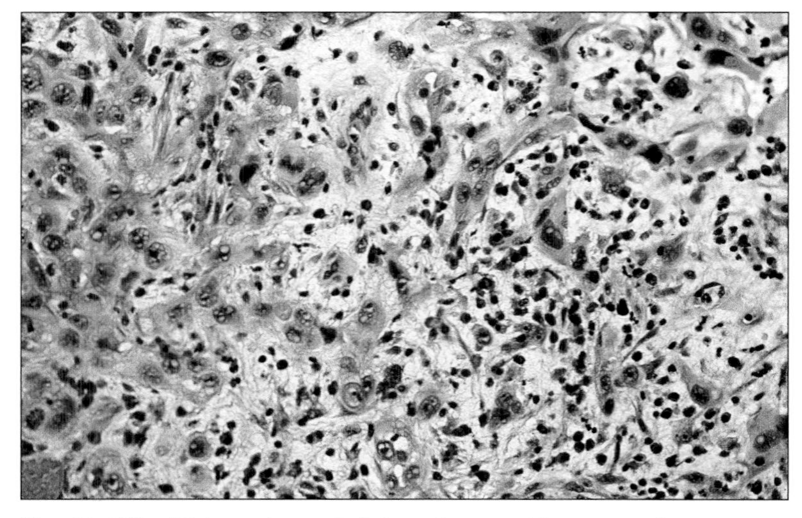

Fig. 11.175 High-grade urothelial carcinoma with an area of pseudosarcomatous change with mitosis. There are pleomorphic cells with a high Ki-67 count and multinucleated cells that are cytokeratin-positive.

- Histologically, the tumors contain a mixture of carcinoma and malignant spindle cells.
- The epithelial component is urothelial.
- A squamous component may also be seen.
- Adenocarcinoma is sometimes seen.
- Small cell carcinoma can also occur.
- Immunohistochemistry may be required to prove the epithelial nature of the spindle cells; the spindle cell element has been found to be focally cytokeratine positive. Epithelial membrane antigen may also be expressed.
- Heterologous differentiation may occur and consists of chondrosarcoma, osteosarcoma, or rhabdomyosarcoma.
- Sarcomatoid urothelial carcinoma stains immunohistochemically positive for cytokeratin, with strong cytoplasmic reactivity in the spindle cells.
- Vimentin in the spindle cell component is usually negative.

CAUTION

- In cases with carcinoma and a malignant spindle cell component, a major diagnostic consideration is urothelial carcinoma with a pseudosarcomatous stroma. There is a reactive stroma that demonstrates cellularity and atypia. The stroma may demonstrate myxoid areas with stellate or multinucleated cells. The stromal cells of pseudosarcoma immunohistochemically demonstrate fibroblastic and myofibroblastic differentiation. They lack cytokeratin.
- Osseous metaplasia may be present in urothelial carcinoma and should be differentiated from an osteosarcoma. This finding has also been described in metastatic urothelial carcinoma. The metaplastic bone is histologically benign, with a normal lamellar pattern; it is usually found adjacent to areas of hemorrhage.
- The giant cells of giant cell cystitis should not be confused with sarcomatoid carcinoma. These cells typically have several small, round, uniform nuclei and scant cytoplasm.
- Primary bladder sarcoma is rare, and a malignant spindle cell tumor in an adult should be considered sarcomatoid carcinoma until proven otherwise. Immunohistochemical studies with antibodies to low molecular weight cytokeratin may give evidence of epithelial differentiation.

SQUAMOUS CELL CARCINOMA PATTERN (Figs 11.176–11.183)[123–132]

- This varies in different parts of the world.
- In areas where schistosomiasis is endemic, squamous cell carcinoma accounts for up to 70% of bladder

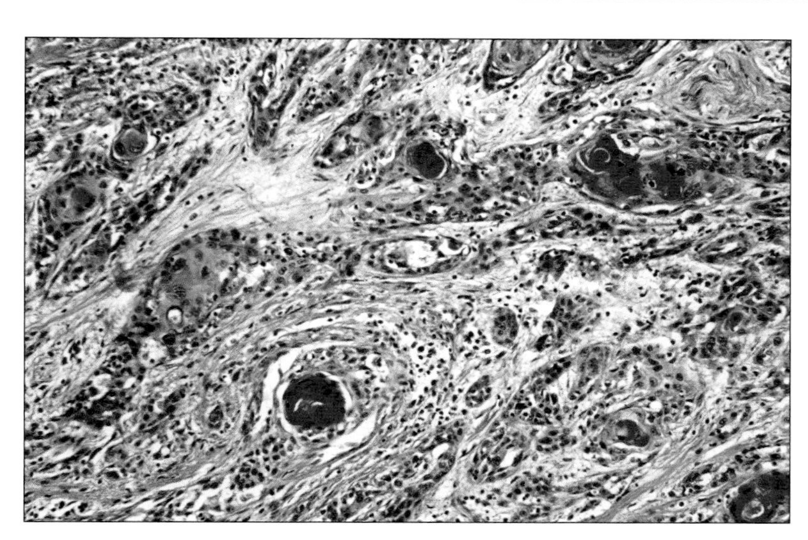

Fig. 11.176 High-grade urothelial carcinoma with areas of squamous cell change. It is difficult at times to differentiate, by this field alone, from a true squamous cell carcinoma of the bladder. There is keratohyaline and desmosomes between the cells.

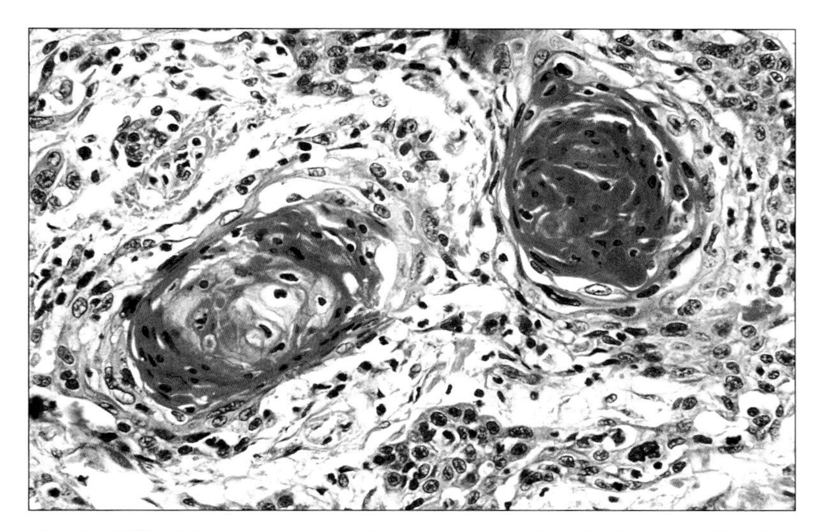

Fig. 11.177 High-grade urothelial carcinoma with a higher magnification of an area of squamous cell change. It is difficult at times to differentiate, by this field alone, from a true squamous cell carcinoma of the bladder. Here, there is keratohyaline and desmosomes between the cells.

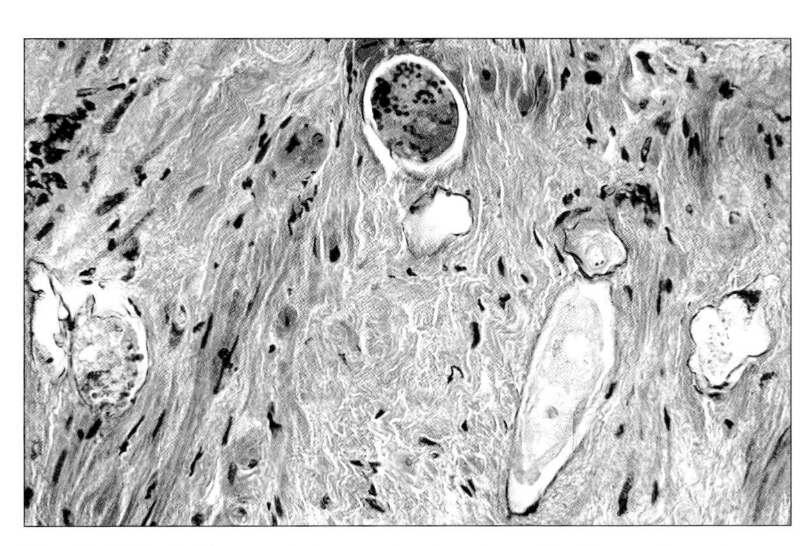

Fig. 11.178 Schistosomiasis: eggs in the urinary bladder wall, causing fibrosis. Over a long period of time, in some patients squamous cell carcinoma of the urinary bladder can result.

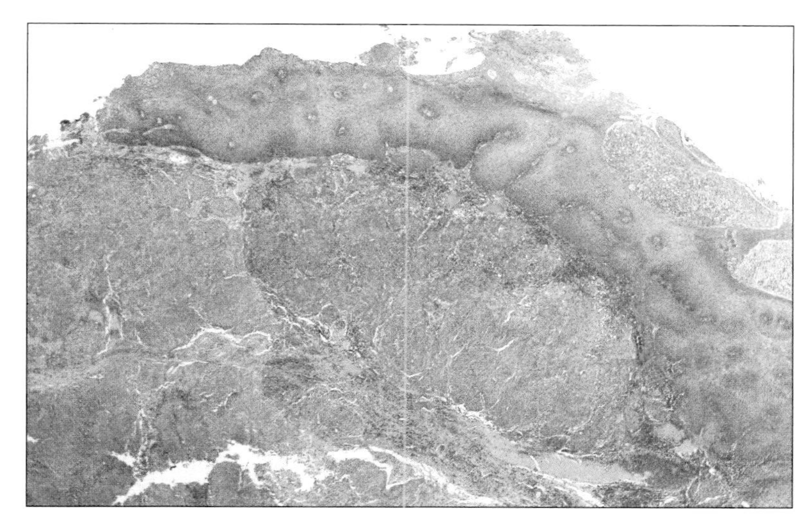

Fig. 11.179 Paraplegic bladder cancer. Beneath the basement membrane and the keratinizing urothelial mucosa is a high-grade urothelial carcinoma. Many of these bladders have multiple episodes of bacterial infection, with numerous inflammatory cells in the urine, long before the appearance of neoplastic cells.

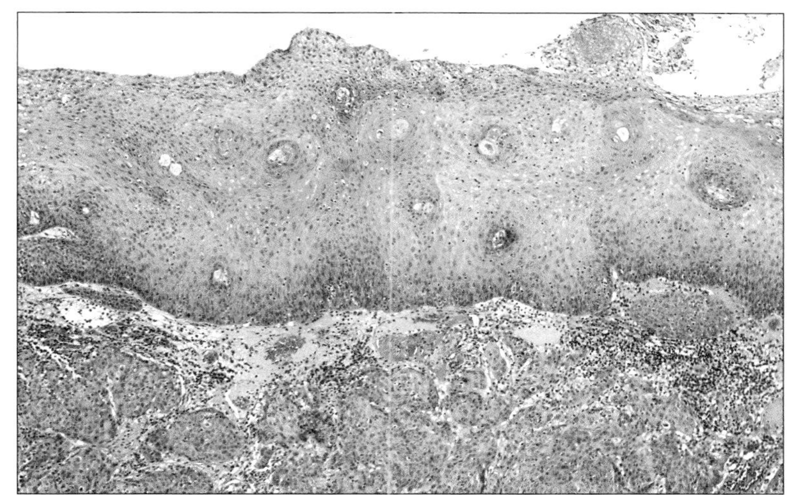

Fig. 11.180 Paraplegic bladder cancer. A high-grade urothelial carcinoma beneath the basement membrane and the keratinizing urothelial mucosa.

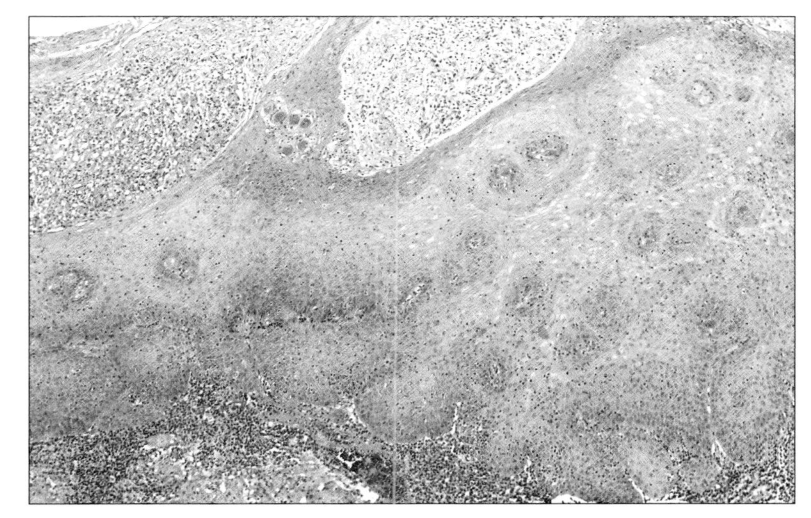

Fig. 11.181 Paraplegic bladder cancer. A higher magnification of the bladder mucosa of Fig. 11.179, in which there is marked squamous metaplasia of the normal urothelium. There are numerous intermediate cells and abnormal basal cells in this thickened mucosa.

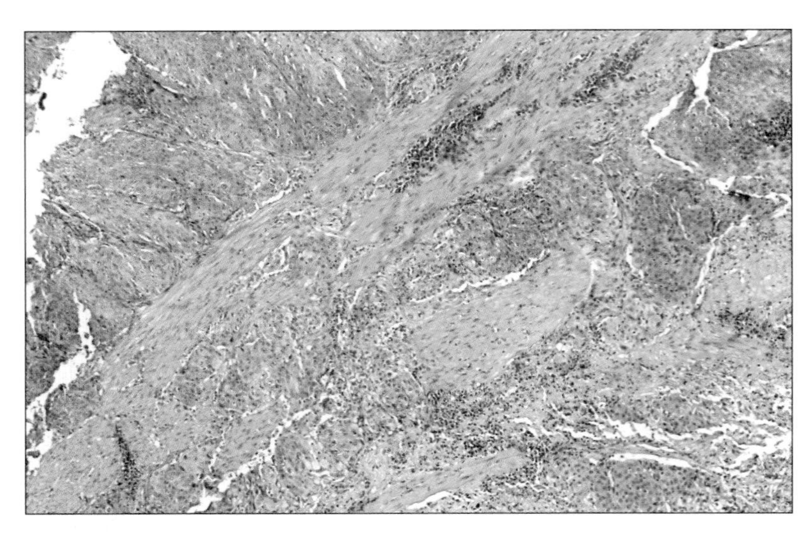

Fig. 11.182 Paraplegic bladder cancer. Beneath the basement membrane and the urothelial surface cancer are numerous islands of low-grade urothelial carcinoma. A higher magnification of bladder mucosa reveals low-grade urothelial cancer similar to that which is below the basement membrane.

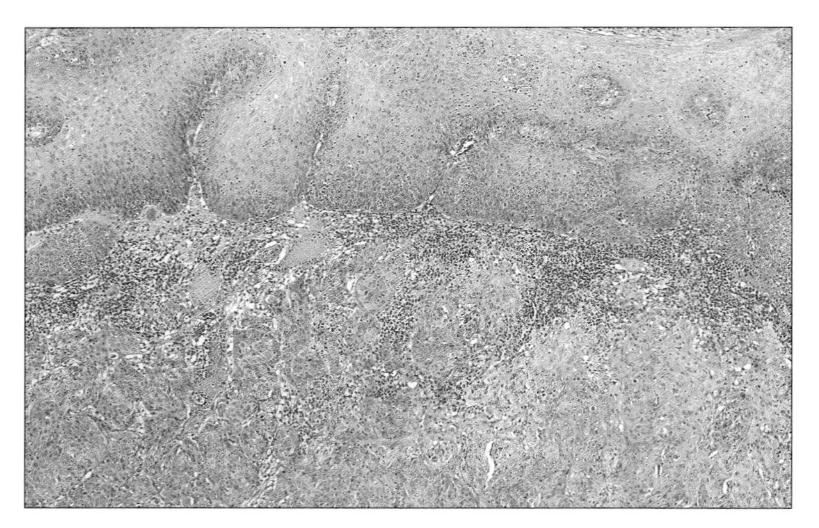

Fig. 11.183 Paraplegic bladder cancer. A higher magnification of Fig. 11.179, showing a high-grade urothelial carcinoma beneath the basement membrane and the keratinizing urothelial mucosa.

cancers. The *Schistosoma haematobium* life cycle begins with adult trematodes in the urogenital system, where eggs are produced, excreted into urine, and then hatched in fresh water. The larvae infect snails and produce cercaria, which are excreted back into the water. Cercaria are able to penetrate the skin of humans when it comes into contact with water. The schistosomes then migrate to the pelvic and mesenteric venous plexuses, where they mature, reproduce, and lay eggs, completing the life cycle.

- In western Europe and the USA, squamous cell carcinoma comprises only 3% of bladder malignancies.
- The male-to-female ratio is 1.7:1.
- The age range is from 30 to 90 years (mean 65.5 years).
- Most patients present with hematuria or irritative symptoms.
- The prognosis is poor for patients with squamous cell carcinoma.
- The biologic behavior of squamous cell carcinoma is different from that of urothelial carcinoma, and in most patients death is caused by local recurrence rather than metastasis.

ETIOLOGY AND PATHOGENESIS

- Many patients have a long history of bladder irritation caused by:
  infections;
  stones;
  indwelling catheters (e.g. in paraplegic patients with a 20-year history);
  intermittent self-catheterization;
  urinary retention.
- Keratinizing squamous metaplasia (leukoplakia) is an important risk factor that may be associated with the above variables (e.g. stones).
- With schistosomiasis, three major species are pathogenic in humans:
  S. mansoni;
  S. japonicum;
  S. haematobium.
  Only *S. haematobium* causes bladder cancer, and eggs can be identified in the bladder wall.
- The eggs are trapped within the muscularis and lamina propria of the bladder wall, where they are destroyed or become calcified.
- The eggs induce a severe inflammatory and fibrotic reaction.
- The calcified eggs cause a granular, yellow lesion known as a sandy patch.
- Bladder urothelial mucosa may demonstrate urothelial hyperplasia, metaplasia, dysplasia, polyposis, ulceration, or carcinoma.
- Squamous cell carcinoma is the most frequent type of cancer, but occasionally adenocarcinoma may also be seen.

GROSS PATHOLOGY

- The lesions are commonly found on the lateral wall and trigone of the bladder as bulky, polypoid, solid, necrotic masses; which may fill the lumen of the bladder.
- Some are flat with ulceration and infiltration.

- A constant finding is that of necrotic and keratin debris on the surface of the neoplasm.

MICROSCOPIC PATHOLOGY

- Squamous cell carcinoma should be restricted to those pure tumors without urothelial carcinoma being present.
- Well-differentiated carcinomas have islands of squamous cells with keratinization, prominent intercellular bridges, and minimal nuclear pleomorphism.
- Poorly differentiated squamous cell carcinomas have marked nuclear pleomorphism with some focal squamous differentiation.
- Squamous metaplasia of adjacent urothelial mucosa may be present in one-fifth to one-half of cases.
- Verrucous carcinoma or well-differentiated squamous cell carcinoma is more common in patients with schistosomiasis. This cancer appears as an exophytic, papillary, or warty mass and histologically has epithelial acanthosis, and minimal nuclear and architectural atypia. Verrucous carcinomas reported at other organ sites have been linked to human papilloma virus infection. Condyloma acuminata may occur in the bladder and has been shown to contain human papilloma virus. Those cases that have local aggressiveness may actually represent verrucous carcinoma.

CAUTION

- Secondary invasion from adjacent primary squamous cell carcinoma of the cervix or vagina must be considered and excluded clinically.
- The major differential diagnostic consideration for squamous cell carcinoma is urothelial carcinoma with squamous differentiation. If an identifiable urothelial carcinoma, even in situ, is found, the tumor should be classified as urothelial carcinoma with squamous differentiation.
- The presence of keratinizing squamous metaplasia favors the diagnosis of squamous cell carcinoma.

ADENOCARCINOMA PATTERN

- Primary adenocarcinomas comprise about 1% of malignant bladder tumors.
- Adenocarcinomas of the bladder are divided into those that develop as urachal tumors and those that arise in the bladder proper.

URACHAL ADENOCARCINOMA (Figs 11.184–11.187)[133–139]

ETIOLOGY AND PATHOGENESIS

- Intestinal metaplasia of the urachal epithelium accounts for the preponderance of adenocarcinomas of the urachus. Some may arise from villous adenoma.

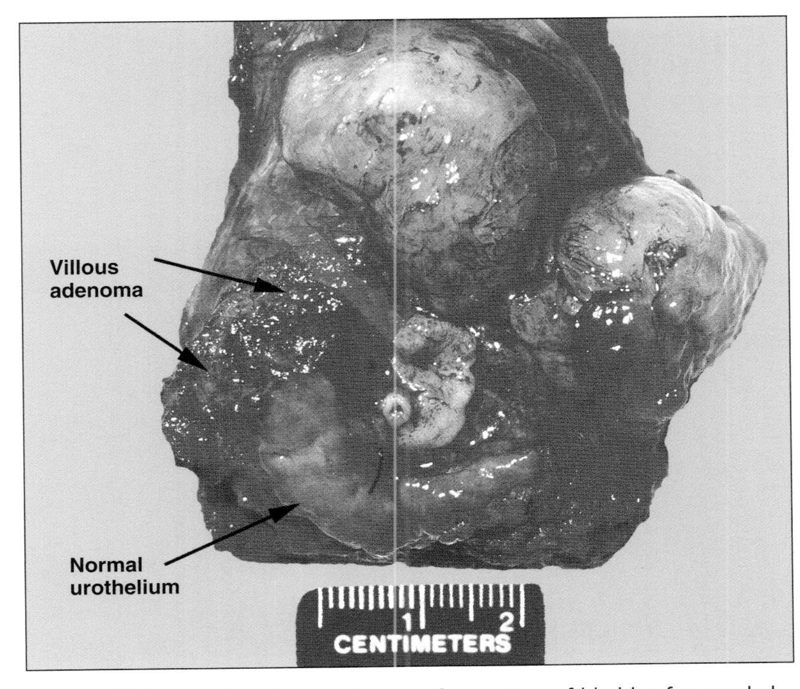

Fig. 11.184 Urachus. Gross picture of resection of bladder for urachal carcinoma and villous adenoma. The patient had mucus and multiple bacterial infection in the urine.

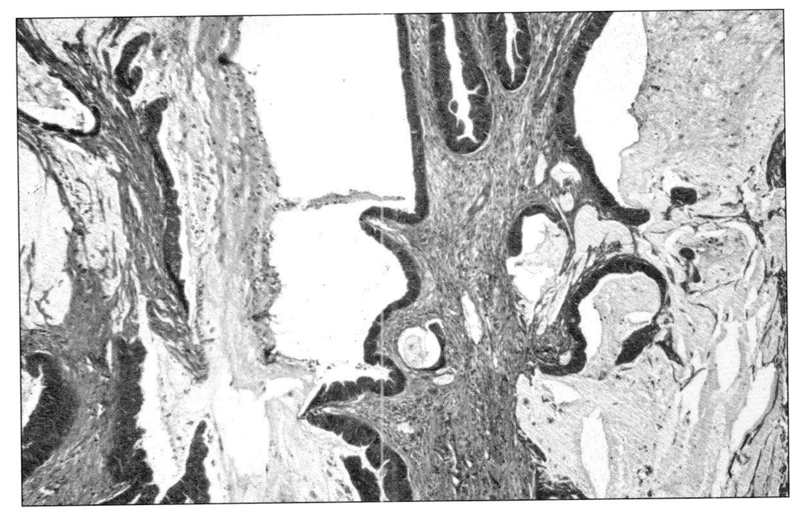

Fig. 11.185 Urachus. Urachal adenocarcinoma in which there is marked mucin production and epithelium that is histologically similar to that appearing in the lower gastrointestinal tract.

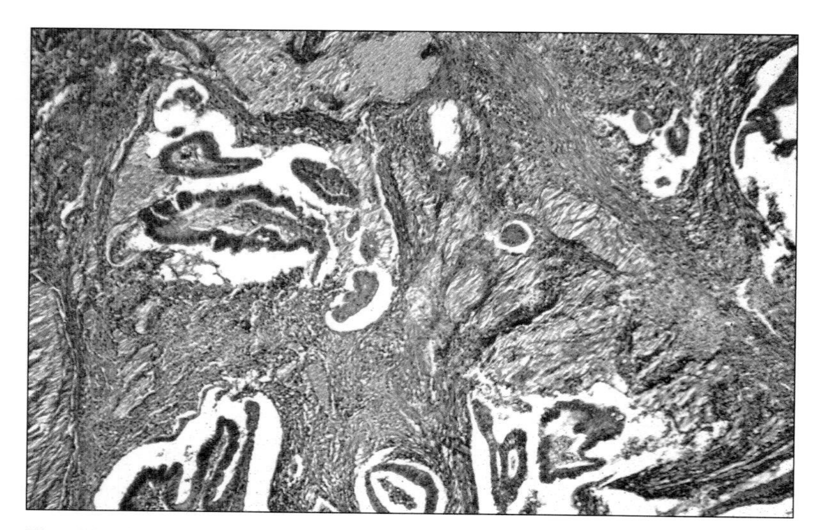

Fig. 11.186 Urachus. Urachal adenocarcinoma in which there is marked mucin production that is mucicarmine-positive.

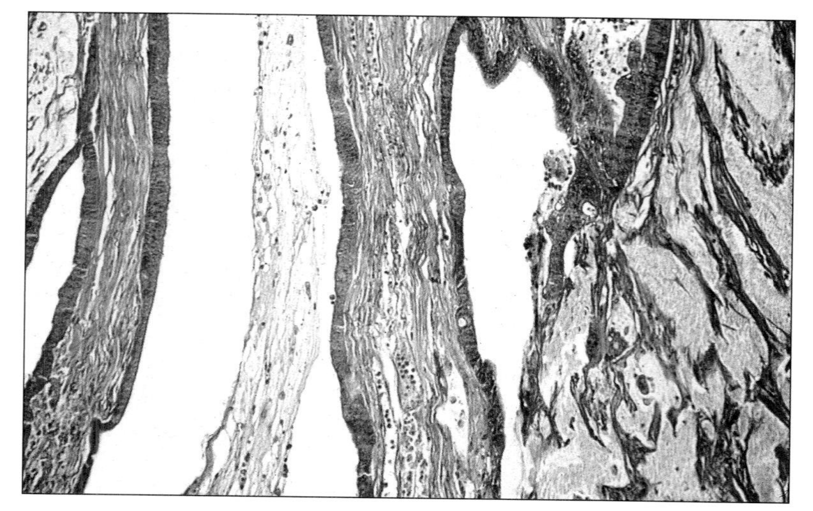

Fig. 11.187 Urachus. Urachal adenocarcinoma, at a higher magnification, in which there is marked mucin production that is mucicarmine-positive.

- The separation of urachal from non-urachal adenocarcinoma needs clinical and pathologic correlation.
- Urachal tumors arise in the bladder dome.
- Urachal adenocarcinoma primarily involves the deeper structures of the bladder wall.
- It may be present as a suprapelvic mass.
- The tumor grows in the bladder wall, extending into the space of Retzius. There is a sharp separation of the tumor from the normal surface epithelium.
- There is an absence of cystitis cystica and glandularis elsewhere in the bladder.
- The tumor is located anteriorly or in the dome.
- There should be a sharp demarcation between tumor and normal epithelium, and a primary urothelial tumor elsewhere must be excluded. In the adjacent urothelium, there is no cystitis glandularis or intestinal metaplasia.
- The majority of urachal tumors are mucinous (colloid), but there can be a similarity with non-urachal tumors.
- There are no differences in immunohistochemistry and mucin histochemistry between urachal and non-urachal adenocarcinomas.
- The majority of cases occur in the fifth and sixth decades, with a mean 10 years younger than the mean for adenocarcinoma elsewhere in the bladder.
- There is a predominance of men over women (2:1).
- The most frequent presenting symptoms are hematuria, pain, irritative symptoms, mucinuria, and umbilical discharge.

MACROPATHOLOGY

- Discrete masses are formed in the dome of the bladder and are in the wall of the bladder, rather than in the mucosa (which is more typical for non-urachal tumors). The cut surface of the tumor may be solid and has a glistening gelatinous appearance because of mucin production.

MICROSCOPIC PATHOLOGY

The most common pattern is mucinous (colloid) carcinoma, with nests and single cells appearing to float in pools of extracellular mucin. The cells may be of signet ring cell or columnar cell morphology. Another pattern is enteric adenocarcinoma, which resembles colorectal adenocarcinoma and may include Paneth cells and argyrophilic neuroendocrine cells.

CAUTION

Diagnostic consideration is given to non-urachal bladder adenocarcinoma, which requires clinicopathologic correlation. Urachal adenocarcinoma should be distinguished from urachal villous adenoma, histologically identical to those found in the gastrointestinal tract.

STAGING

Urachal adenocarcinoma is staged with the same system used for urothelial bladder cancer, but this is questionable, because urachal carcinomas, by virtue of their anatomic origin, are almost all muscle-invasive.

TREATMENT

The treatment advocated is en bloc cystectomy with pelvic lymphadenectomy and umbilectomy. Whether partial or radical cystectomy is performed, the inclusion of the entire urachal tract is important. Urachal adenocarcinoma appears to be resistant to radiation therapy.

NON-URACHAL ADENOCARCINOMA (Figs 11.188–11.201)[140–148]

- Non-urachal adenocarcinoma accounts for 75% of primary bladder adenocarcinomas.
- It occurs over a wide age range and is more common in males than in females (2.6:1).
- Hematuria is the most common symptom, followed by irritative symptoms and rarely mucinuria.

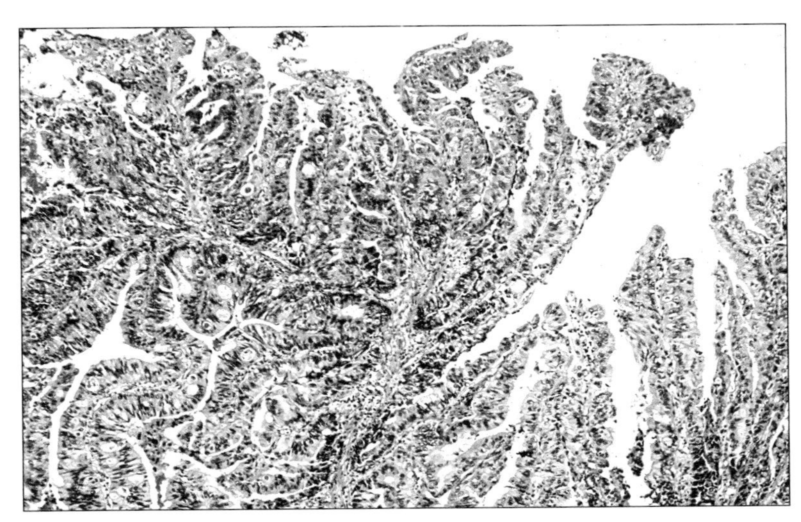

Fig. 11.190 Adenocarcinoma primary in the bladder, with an appearance similar to that of a papillary villous adenocarcinoma in the lower gastrointestinal tract.

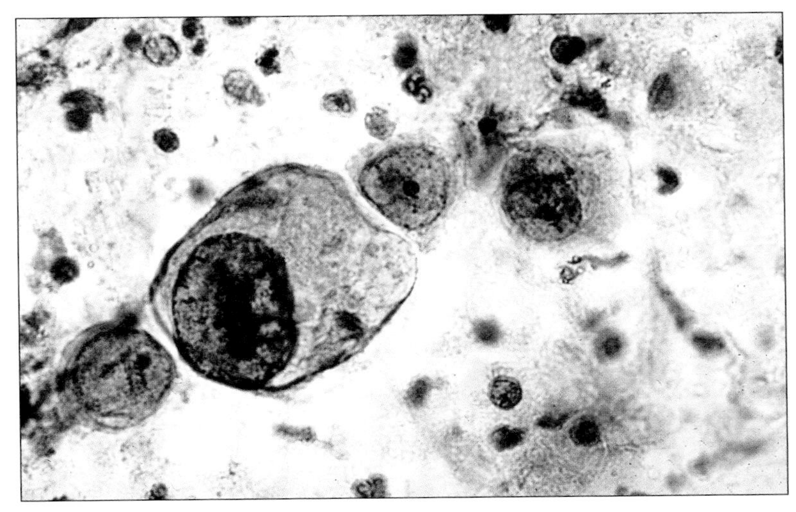

Fig. 11.188 Adenocarcinoma, urinary cytology. A large positive tumor cell in the center contains mucin in the cytoplasm and a large nucleolus.

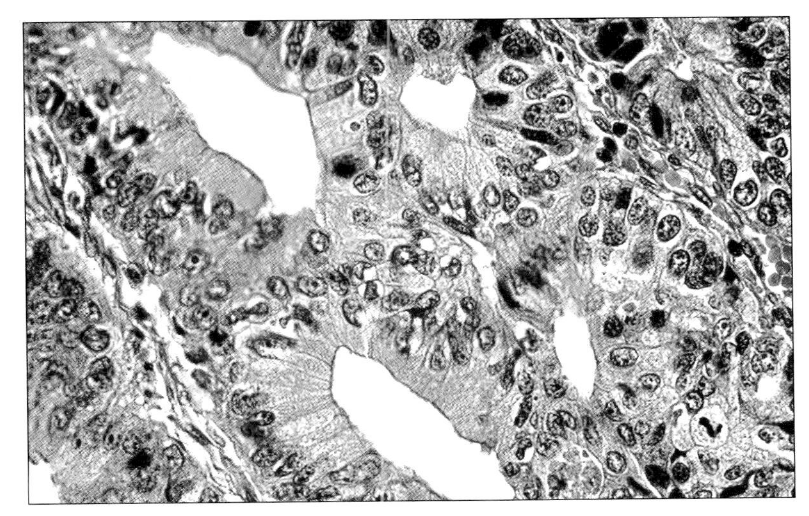

Fig. 11.191 Adenocarcinoma primary in the bladder: higher magnification of Fig. 11.190.

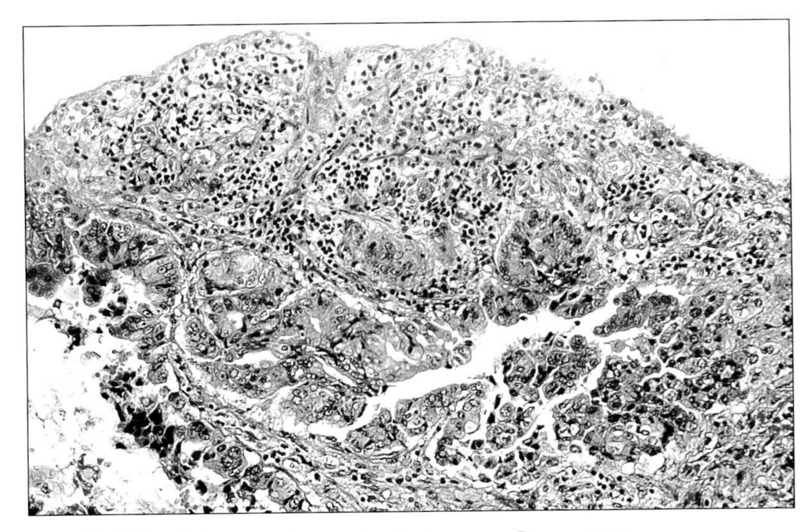

Fig. 11.189 Adenocarcinoma in situ in a von Brunn nest.

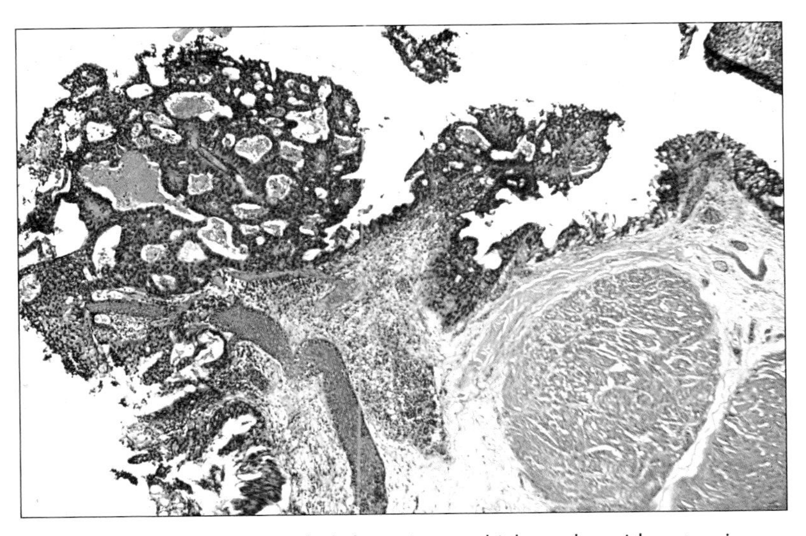

Fig. 11.192 Papillary urothelial carcinoma, high grade, with extensive gland formation.

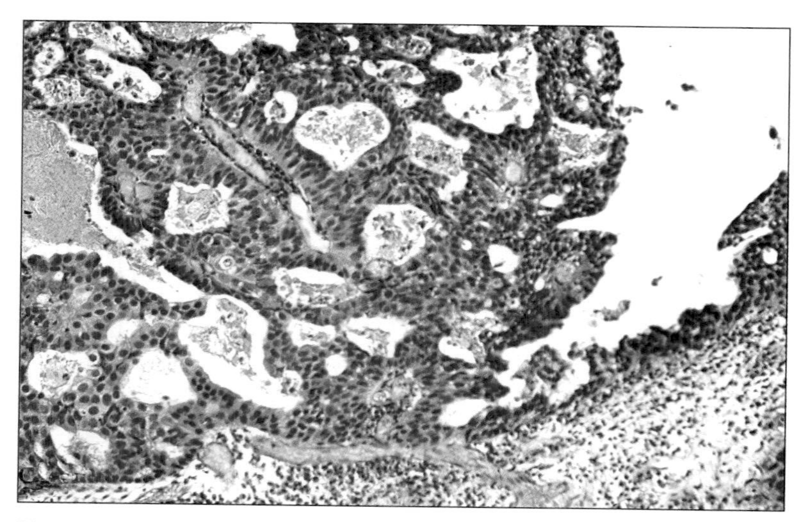

Fig. 11.193 Papillary urothelial carcinoma, high grade, with extensive gland formation: a higher magnification of Fig. 11.192.

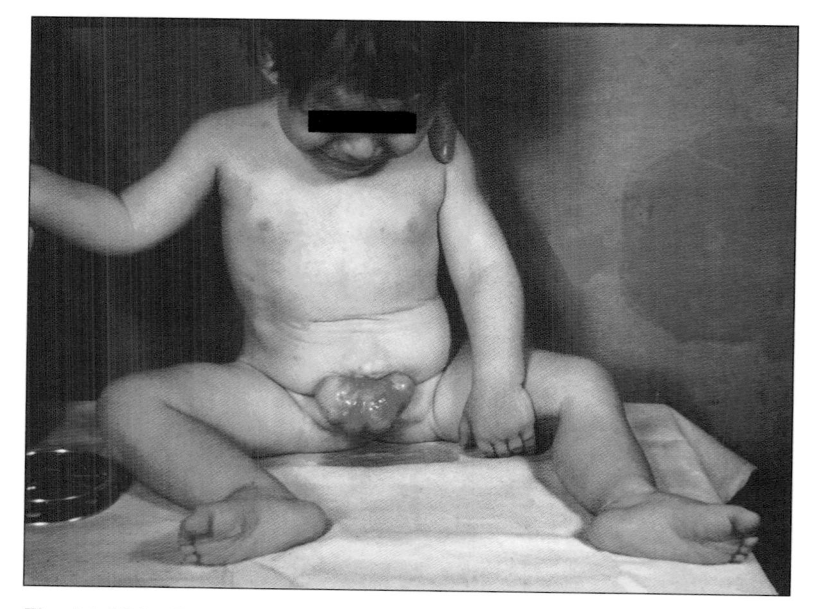

Fig. 11.194 Exstrophy in a 2-year-old boy.

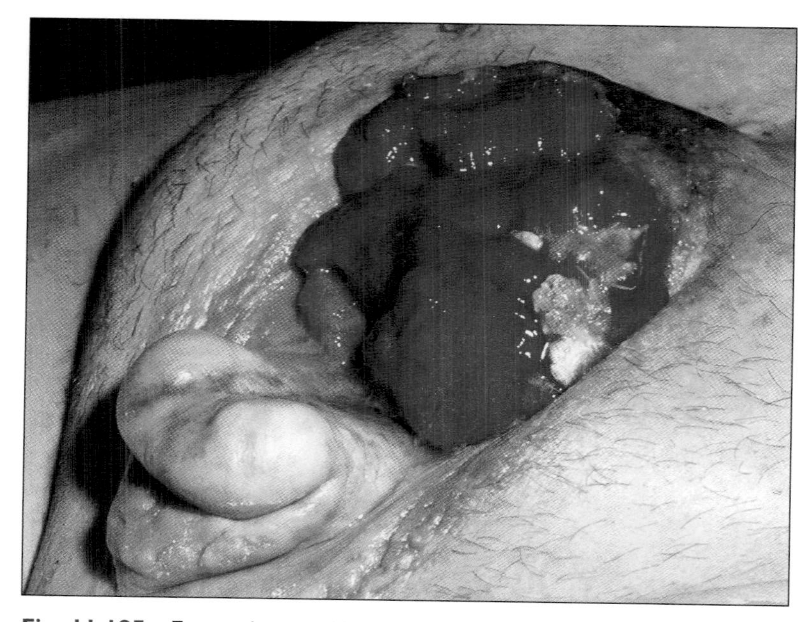

Fig. 11.195 Exstrophy in a 61-year-old man. An adenocarcinoma has developed in this exstrophy of the bladder.

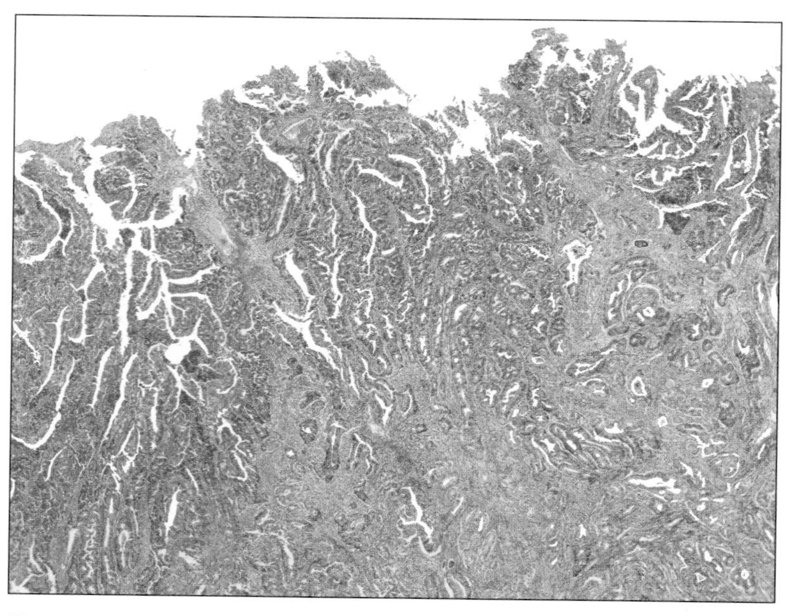

Fig. 11.196 Exstrophy in a 61-year-old man. A digital photomicrograph of the adenocarcinoma that has developed in this exstrophy of the bladder.

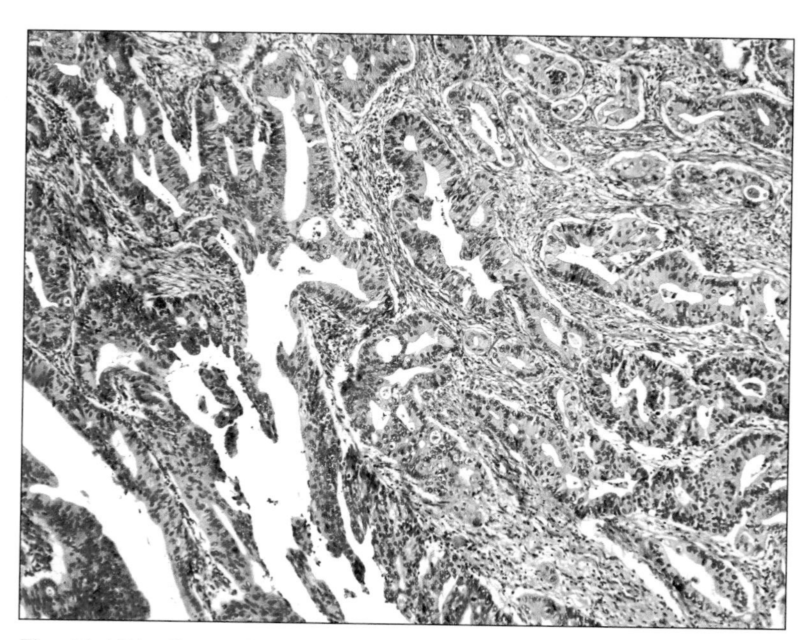

Fig. 11.197 Exstrophy in a 61-year-old man. A digital photomicrograph, at a higher magnification, of the adenocarcinoma seen in Fig. 11.195.

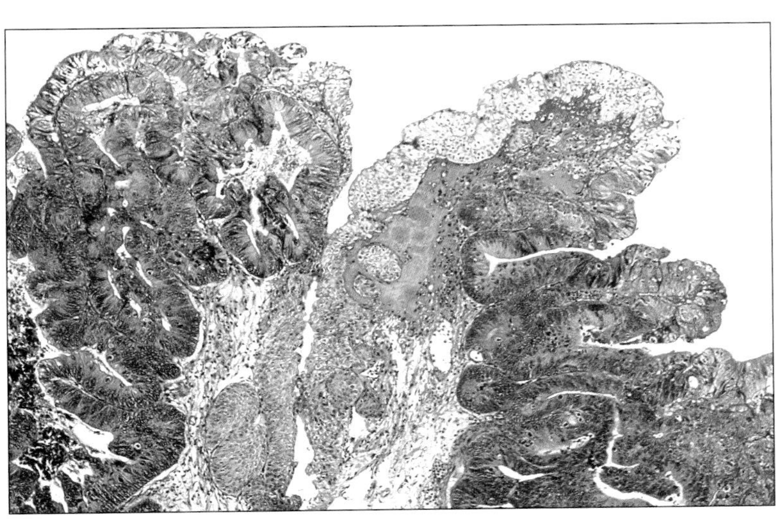

Fig. 11.198 Exstrophy in a 61-year-old man. A higher-magnification digital photomicrograph of the adenocarcinoma seen in Fig. 11.196. Histologically, the tumor appears identical to a colorectal adenocarcinoma. There is non-neoplastic urothelium in the middle third of the photomicrograph.

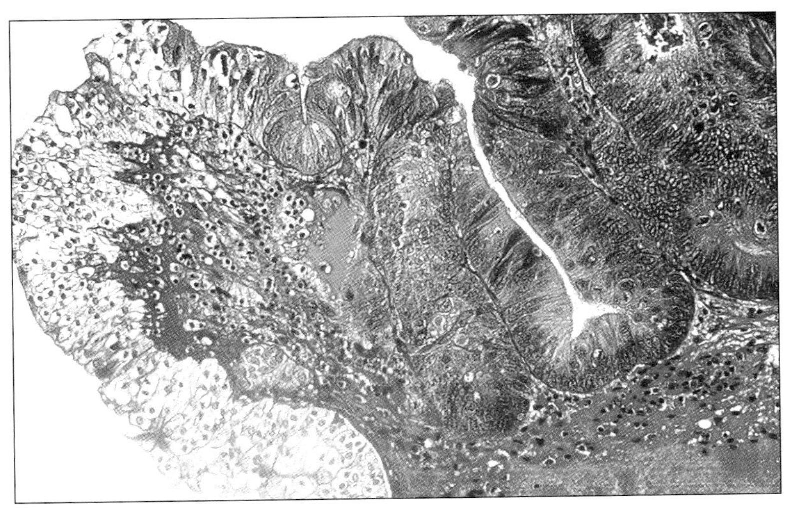

Fig. 11.199 Exstrophy in a 61-year-old man. A digital photomicrograph, at a higher magnification, of the adenocarcinoma seen in Fig. 11.196. A non-neoplastic urothelium is visible on the left of the photomicrograph.

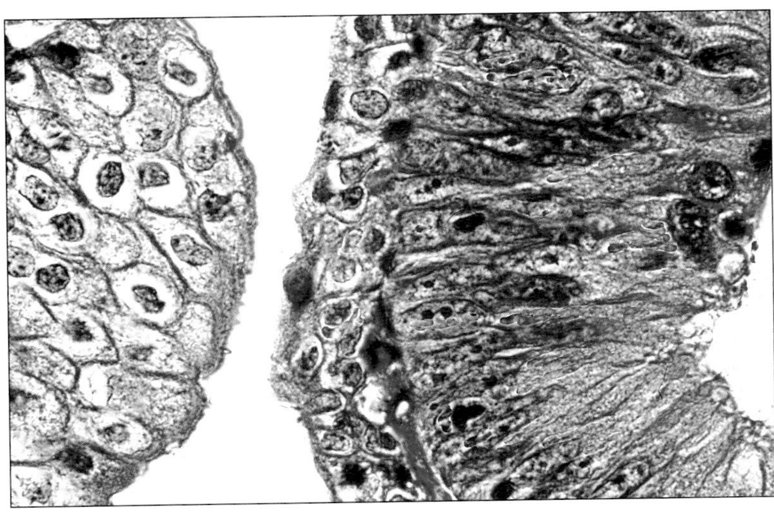

Fig. 11.200 Exstrophy in a 61-year-old man. A higher-magnification digital photomicrograph of the adenocarcinoma seen in Fig. 11.196. A non-neoplastic urothelium is visible on the left of the photomicrograph.

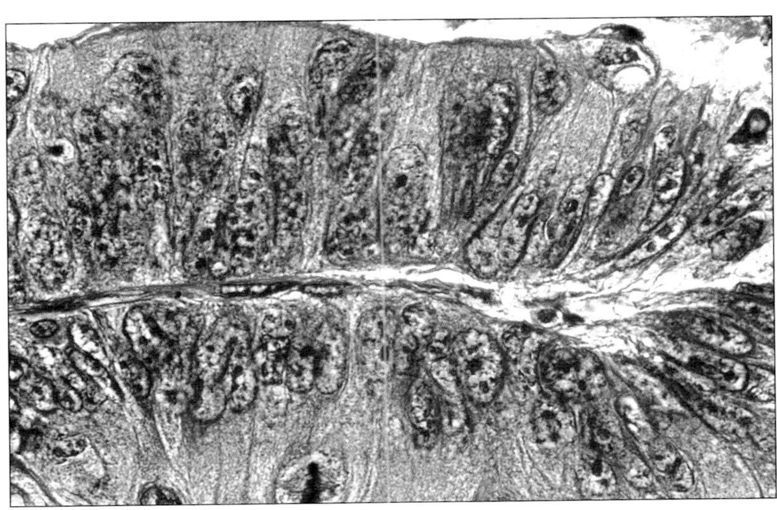

Fig. 11.201 Exstrophy in a 61-year-old man. A digital photomicrograph, at a higher magnification, of the adenocarcinoma seen in Fig. 11.196. Histologically, the tumor appears identical to a colorectal adenocarcinoma.

- Many cases arise from metaplasia of the urothelium, especially those with longstanding intestinalization of the urothelium associated with a nonfunctioning bladder, chronic irritation, and obstruction. Cystitis cystica and glandularis is present in the urothelium of one-sixth to two-thirds of cases.
- Metaplasia is also considered to be the mechanism in patients with exstrophy, where most cancers are adenocarcinoma. The risk of adenocarcinoma in patients with exstrophy is about 5%.
- Adenocarcinoma can occur with *S. haematobium* infection.

MACROPATHOLOGY

Tumors appear as an exophytic, papillary, solid, sessile, ulcerating, or infiltrating mass. The signet ring cell variant frequently shows diffuse thickening of the bladder wall, producing a linitis plastica-like appearance, and urothelial mucosal biopsies may be negative.

MICROSCOPIC PATHOLOGY

Any case including a urothelial carcinoma component is classified as urothelial carcinoma with glandular differentiation. Grignon et al recognized six histologic variants of adenocarcinoma of the urinary bladder:[146]

1. Adenocarcinoma of no specific type. The tumor did not resemble another recognized pattern.
2. Enteric. The cancer was composed of pseudostratified columnar cells forming glands, often with central necrosis, resembling colonic adenocarcinoma.

3. Mucinous (colloid). The tumor cells were single or in nests appearing to float in extracellular mucin.
4. Signet ring cell. The tumor consisted of signet ring cells diffusely infiltrating the bladder wall.
5. Clear cell. The tumor was composed of papillary and tubular structures with cytologic features similar to mesonephric adenocarcinoma of the female genital system.
6. Mixed: two or more of the described patterns were found.

The nonspecific and enteric types were the most common, with Paneth and argentaffin cells being present in the enteric-type tumors.

GRADING OF ADENOCARCINOMA

A uniform grading system has not been applied to adenocarcinoma of the bladder. The histologic patterns did not correlate with outcome.[146]

IMMUNOHISTOCHEMISTRY

Immunohistochemistry in urachal and non-urachal adenocarcinoma is identical, in that both groups express carcinoembryonic antigen and LeuM1. There can be focal reactivity to prostate-specific antigen and prostatic acid phosphatase in some non-urachal tumors.

CAUTION

The following are benign mimics of adenocarcinoma.

- Cystitis cystica and cystitis glandularis, which can produce pseudopapillary or polypoid lesions.
- Extracellular mucin is present.
- Longstanding intestinal metaplasia is at risk for the development of adenocarcinoma, and biopsies should be carefully evaluated for evidence of neoplastic transformation.
- Villous adenoma rarely occurs in the urinary bladder.
- Nephrogenic adenoma must be distinguished from adenocarcinoma, particularly the clear cell variant.
- Endometriosis can involve the bladder and should be distinguished from adenocarcinoma. The histology is similar to endometriosis elsewhere.

STAGING

In contrast to urachal adenocarcinoma, non-urachal adenocarcinoma is staged by using the standard American Joint Committee on Cancer tumor, node, metastasis (TNM) or Marshall modification of the Jewett staging system. There are few long-term survivors with transmural invasion.

TREATMENT

Radical cystectomy or cystoprostatectomy with pelvic lymph node dissection is the preferred therapy for adenocarcinoma of the bladder. The roles of radiation therapy and chemotherapy remain uncertain.

SIGNET RING CELL ADENOCARCINOMA

(Figs 11.202 and 11.203)[149–153]

- Grignon et al[146,153] reported 12 cases and reviewed 56 cases from the literature. They provided a detailed analysis of their 12 cases and 37 of the cases from the literature for which their criteria for diagnosis were met and sufficient clinical details were available.
- They required at least a focal component of diffuse linitis plastica-like signet ring cell adenocarcinoma, and there could not be an element of urothelial carcinoma.
- In 47% of cases, cystoscopy did not show a mucosal or mass lesion, with the mucosa most often described as edematous or bullous.
- Biopsies revealed diffuse permeation by single signet ring cells, some with single cytoplasmic vacuoles and others with bubbly cytoplasm.
- The significance of this subtype of adenocarcinoma is its extremely poor prognosis.

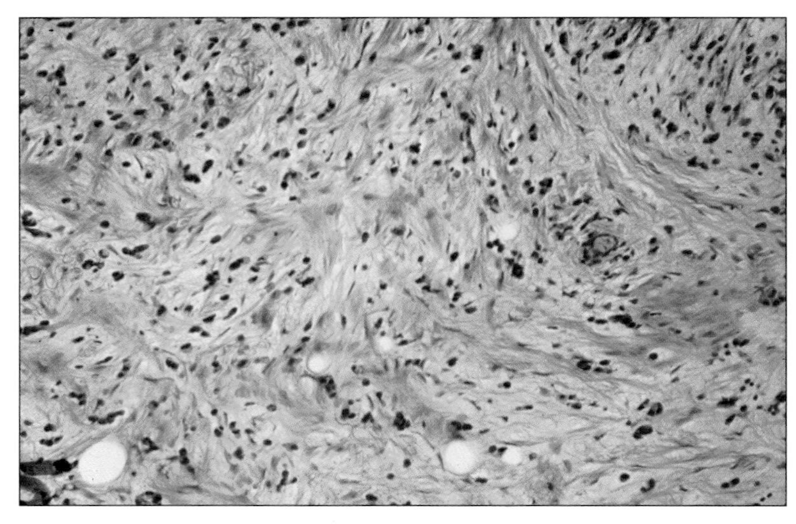

Fig. 11.202 Signet ring adenocarcinoma. Numerous small ring cells with mucin are scattered through the bladder wall. They can be readily missed on low-power scanning of the slide.

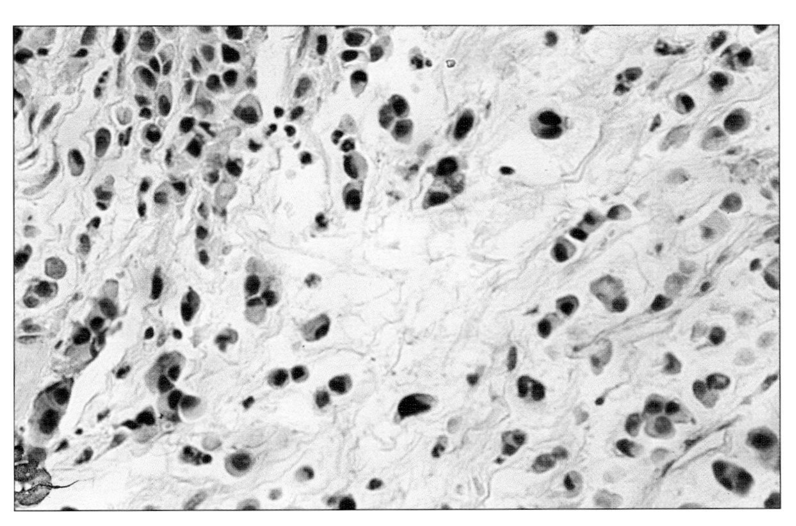

Fig. 11.203 Signet ring adenocarcinoma. Numerous small cells with mucin are scattered through the bladder wall. Higher-magnification examination of the slide reveals signet ring cells that contain mucicarmine material in their cytoplasm.

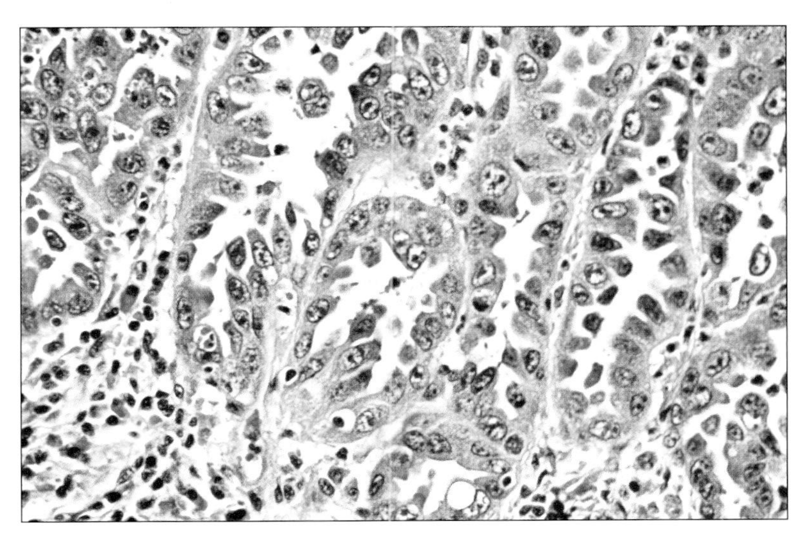

Fig. 11.205 Clear cell adenocarcinoma. Numerous glands are lined by cells that have a hobnail configuration. This digital photomicrograph, taken from Fig. 11.204, shows the bladder wall muscularis propria on the left of the image.

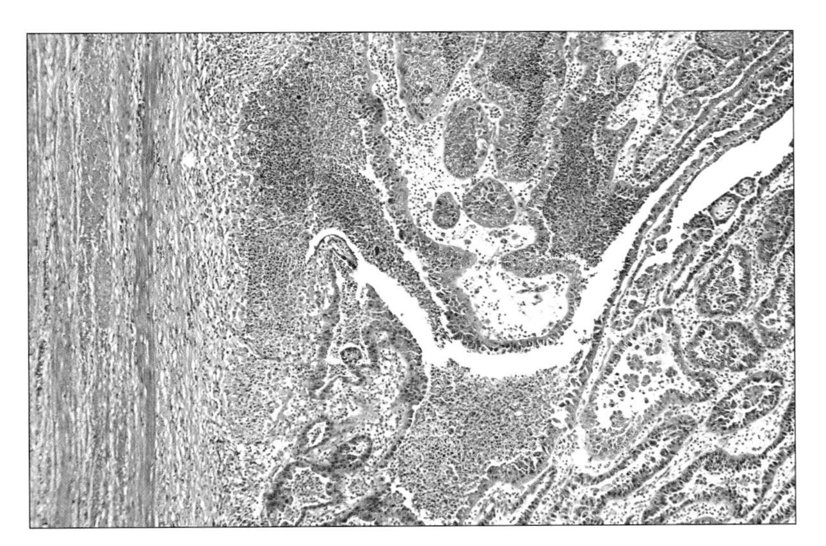

Fig. 11.204 Clear cell adenocarcinoma. There are numerous glands and papillary configurations where these structures are lined by cells that have a hobnail configuration. Bladder wall muscularis propria is on the left of the digital photomicrograph.

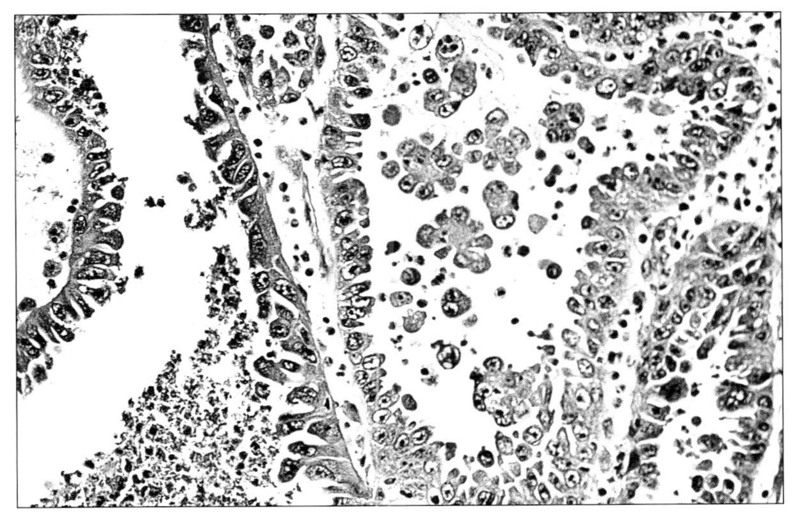

Fig. 11.206 Clear cell adenocarcinoma. Numerous glands and papillary structures are lined by cells that have a hobnail configuration. Digital photomicrograph taken from Fig. 11.204.

CLEAR CELL ADENOCARCINOMA (Figs 11.204–11.206)[154–157]

Primary clear cell adenocarcinoma of the urinary bladder is rare.

MACROPATHOLOGY

The tumors are solid or papillary, and located in the trigone or posterior wall.

HISTOPATHOLOGY

There is a tubular component, which may be cystically dilated. The lining cells are flattened, cuboidal, or columnar, with clear cytoplasm and, at least focally, the characteristic hobnail cells. The cells have significant nuclear pleomorphism, with frequent mitotic figures. Special stains demonstrate abundant cytoplasmic glycogen and, in most, focal cytoplasmic and luminal mucin.

CAUTION

These tumors must be differentiated from the following.

- Nephrogenic adenoma, which is typically small, has papillary and tubular components, but lacks solid

areas. There is usually a history of trauma or instrumentation. Cytologically, there is minimal cellular atypia.
- Metastatic clear cell carcinoma should be excluded in all female patients and requires clinical correlation. Renal cell carcinoma can metastasize to the bladder.

The pathogenesis of clear cell adenocarcinoma in the bladder remains unresolved.

SMALL CELL CARCINOMA
(Figs 11.207–11.212)[158–171]

CLINICAL FEATURES

- Histologically resembles the tumors that occur in the lung.
- The tumor represents 0.5% of bladder malignancies. It is more frequent in men than in women (ratio 4:1) and is found in patients between the ages of 20 and 85 years, with a mean of 66 years.
- Hematuria is the most frequent presentation (90% of cases).
- Paraneoplastic syndromes have been rarely reported, including ectopic adrenocorticotropic hormone production, hypercalcemia, and hypophosphatemia.

MACROPATHOLOGY

- There are no specific gross features separating small cell carcinoma from other carcinomas.
- The tumor ranges in size from 2-cm polypoid lesions to 10-cm solid masses.
- It can develop at any location, including the dome and within diverticula.
- The overlying mucosa may be ulcerated.

MICROSCOPIC PATHOLOGY

- This tumor cell type may be associated with other histologic variants, such as urothelial carcinoma and adenocarcinoma.

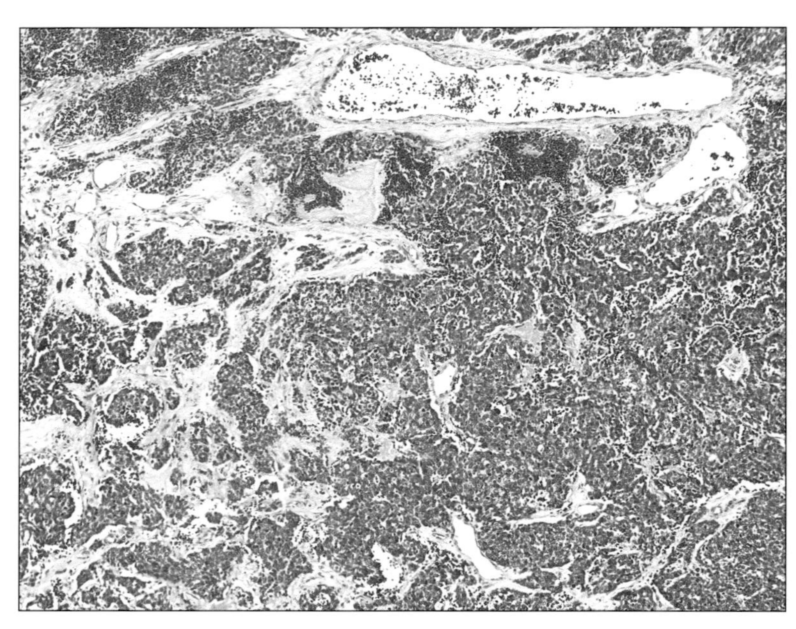

Fig. 11.208 Small cell carcinoma. The cells are synaptophysin-positive. A medium-power digital photomicrograph.

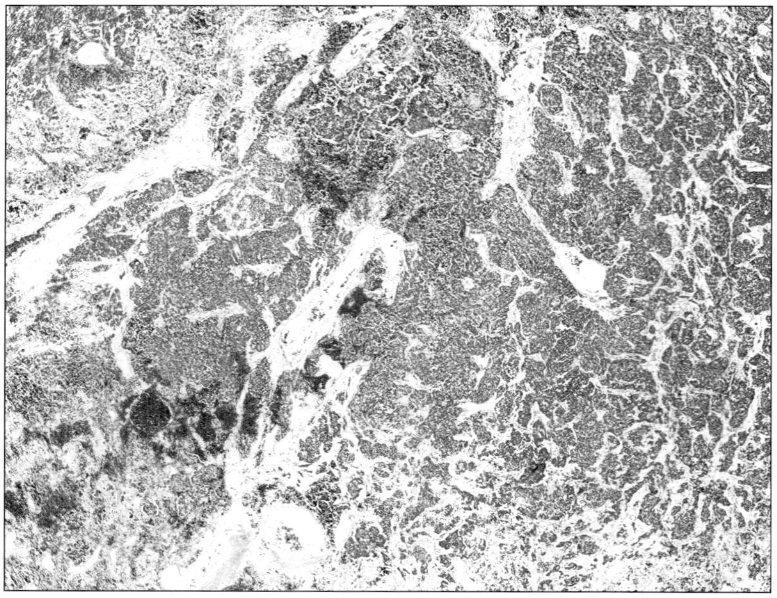

Fig. 11.207 Small cell carcinoma. Anastomosing cords of intermediate neuroendocrine cells in the bladder comprise this tumor. A low-power digital photomicrograph.

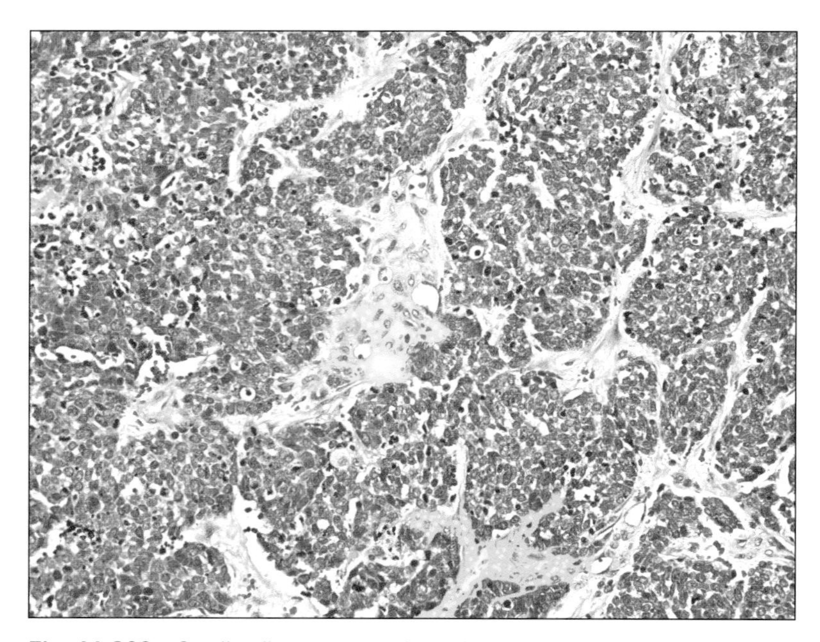

Fig. 11.209 Small cell carcinoma. A medium-power digital photomicrograph showing the numerous microcapillaries present in this tumor.

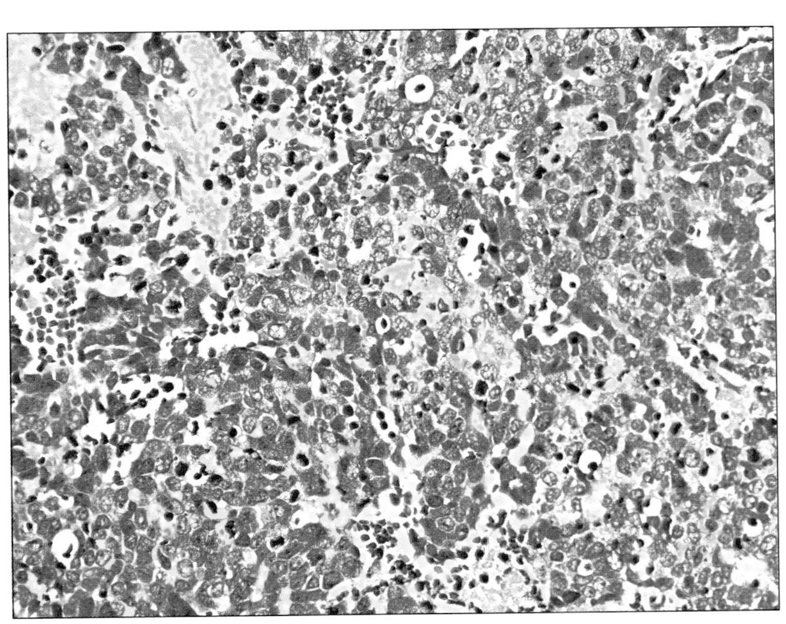

Fig. 11.210 Small cell carcinoma. A higher magnification of Fig. 11.209. Numerous microcapillaries are present in this tumor.

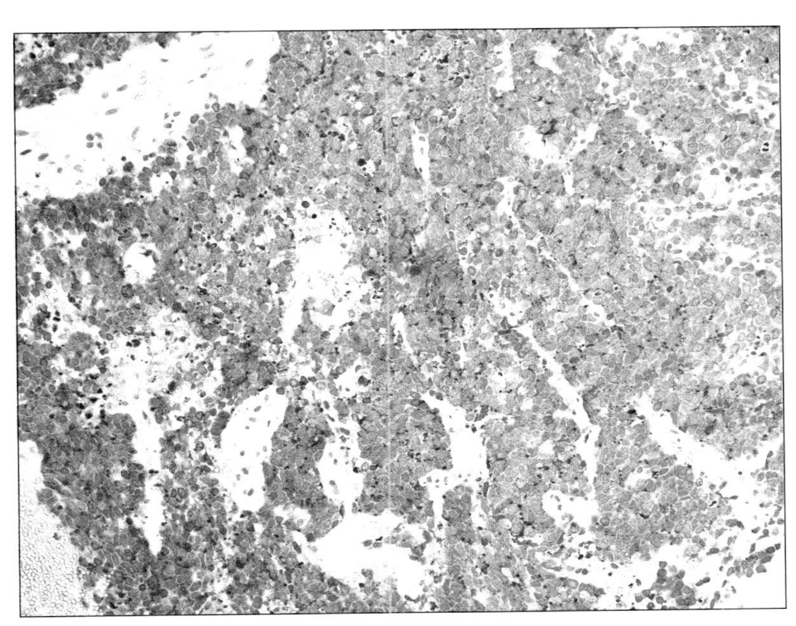

Fig. 11.212 Small cell carcinoma. A higher magnification of Fig. 11.209.

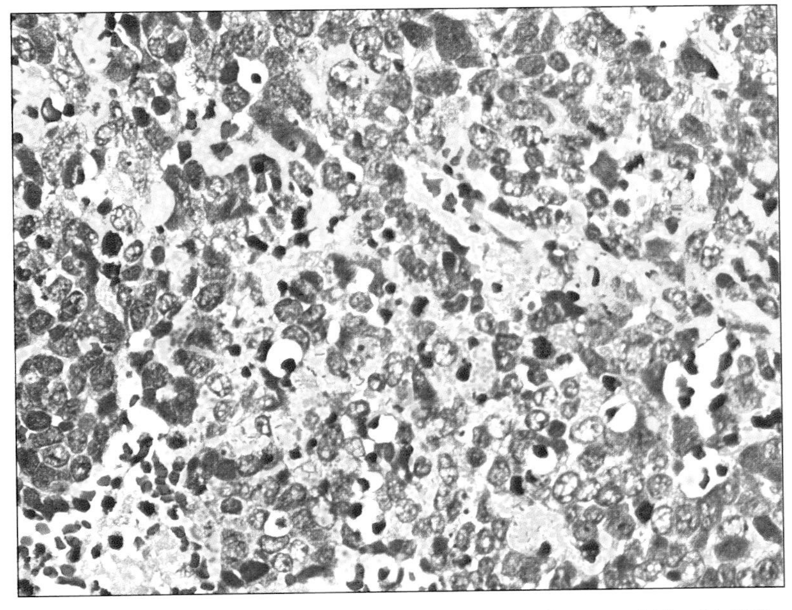

Fig. 11.211 Small cell carcinoma. A higher magnification of Fig. 11.209.

- The tumor demonstrates light microscopic criteria used for small cell carcinoma of the lung.
- Cytologically, the cell type is either a small cell or an intermediate cell pattern; both may be present in the same tumor.
- The small cell type consists of a relatively uniform population of cells with scant cytoplasm and hyperchromatic nuclei with dispersed chromatin. Nucleoli are absent or inconspicuous.
- The intermediate cell type has more cytoplasm, larger nuclei with less hyperchromasia, and a similar chromatin pattern and nucleolar features.
- Both cell types have extensive necrosis, prominent nuclear molding, and frequent mitotic figures, and they may have DNA encrustation of blood vessel walls (the Azzopardi phenomenon).
- A urothelial papillary or nonpapillary carcinoma component is common.
- A glandular and squamous component may also be noted. There may also be histologic features of carcinoid tumor.
- Mixed tumors are reported as small cell carcinoma with other histologic patterns, whereas urothelial carcinoma is reported as having squamous or glandular differentiation. This difference in terminology is related to therapy.
- Immunohistochemically, the cells stain for chromogranin, synaptophysin, and also cytokeratin, which demonstrates cytoplasmic reactivity (in some cells this has a dot-like pattern).

CAUTION

- Small cell carcinoma may arise in the prostate and invade the bladder neck.
- Major consideration has to be given to small cell carcinoma from another site and malignant lymphoma, in which immunohistochemical staining for cytokeratin and leukocyte common antigen in difficult cases should readily distinguish between the two.

TREATMENT

- The importance of recognizing this distinct form of bladder cancer is stressed because it may respond to multimodal therapy.

MALIGNANT MELANOMA

- Malignant melanoma is rarely primary in the bladder. Metastatic melanoma is much more common in the bladder than primary melanoma.
- It occurs more frequently in women than in men and appears in the sixth to seventh decades.

MACROPATHOLOGY

- It is a dark brown to black, polypoid or fungating, and solid or infiltrating lesion.
- Some cases have a flat or macular appearance.

MICROPATHOLOGY

- It consists of large cells in nests with varying amounts of pigment.
- Immunohistochemistry shows immunoreactivity for S-100 protein and HMB-45.
- Ultrastructural studies reveal typical melanosomes.

PARAGANGLIOMA (PHEOCHROMOCYTOMA)[172,173]

- Paraganglioma probably arises from paraganglionic tissue within the bladder wall.
- It occurs from childhood to old age.
- It is found equally in males and females.
- Patients show symptoms of catecholamine excess, including tachycardia, hypertension, headaches, fainting, and dizziness.
- Hematuria is common, with paroxysmal hypertension and painless hematuria at the time of micturition.
- The diagnosis is confirmed by the presence of catecholamines and their metabolites in urine and serum.
- The lesion in the urinary bladder is localized by ^{131}I metaiodobenzylguanidine (MIBG) scintigraphy.

MACROPATHOLOGY

- The paraganglioma is intramural in the trigone, anterior wall, or dome.
- The overlying mucosa may be intact or ulcerated.
- It is usually circumscribed, lobulated, and yellow-brown or pink.

MICROSCOPIC PATHOLOGY

- The tumor is identical to those occurring elsewhere.
- It is composed of cells arranged in discrete nests (*Zellballen*) separated by a prominent sinusoidal vascular network.
- Individual cells have abundant pale eosinophilic or clear cytoplasm with central nuclei.
- Nuclei usually have finely dispersed chromatin but may show considerable variation in size, with some nuclear atypia.
- Mitotic figures are infrequent, and necrosis is not prominent.
- In some cases, flattened sustentacular cells can be recognized around the cell nests.
- Pathologic predictors of behavior for these tumors are not well defined.

IMMUNOHISTOCHEMISTRY

- Lack of immunoreactivity for cytokeratin, epithelial membrane antigen, and carcinoembryonic antigen, and positive reaction with antibodies to neuroendocrine markers. These include neuron-specific enolase, chromogranin, serotonin, somatostatin, and synaptophysin.
- Sustentacular cells stain positively for S-100 protein.

CAUTION

- Urothelial carcinoma has a wide range of morphologic patterns, including a discrete nesting pattern. Here, the prominent sinusoidal vascular pattern of paraganglioma is a useful diagnostic clue.
- Immunohistochemistry can exclude urothelial carcinoma with positive cytokeratin and positive neuroendocrine markers.
- Adenocarcinoma.

GERM CELL NEOPLASMS[174–178]

- Choriocarcinoma can arise in the urinary bladder.
- There are no cases of pure choriocarcinoma of the bladder. This may indicate that a urothelial carcinoma component is present in these cases, supporting a metaplastic origin.
- Typical urothelial carcinoma develops the ability to produce human chorionic gonadotropin, and subsequently displays tumor giant cells and then syncytiotrophoblastic giant cells before complete evolution of choriocarcinoma.

- Most patients have symptoms typical of other bladder cancers, including hematuria, dysuria, and frequency.
- Gynecomastia has been reported in some men with increased levels of serum or urinary gonadotropins.
- The level of serum chorionic gonadotropin does not correlate with response to chemotherapy.
- Cases with morphologic evidence of trophoblastic differentiation are highly aggressive neoplasms with early metastases and death.

MACROPATHOLOGY

- Choriocarcinoma may have a large, exophytic, or fungating appearance.

MICROPATHOLOGY

- The histologic features of choriocarcinoma are a mixture of syncytiotrophoblastic and cytotrophoblastic elements.
- In more than two-thirds of reported cases, urothelial carcinoma is also present and should be classified as urothelial carcinoma with syncytiotrophoblastic differentiation rather than choriocarcinoma.
- Tumor giant cells and syncytiotrophoblastic giant cells may be seen without cytotrophoblasts, similar to those seen in testicular tumors.
- Some cases of urothelial carcinoma reveal immunoreactivity with chorionic gonadotropin in mononuclear cells without evidence of trophoblastic differentiation. This can also be seen in seminoma of the testis.

BENIGN MESENCHYMAL NEOPLASMS

- Benign mesenchymal neoplasms are uncommon in the bladder and were only 0.9% of primary bladder lesions studied at Columbia-Presbyterian Hospital.
- The majority are leiomyomas and hemangioma, neurofibroma constitute the rest.
- Other benign mesenchymal neoplasms that have been reported are granular cell tumor, lymphangioma, benign fibrous histiocytoma, and ganglioneuroma.

LEIOMYOMA[179–181]

- Leiomyoma is more common in women than in men, and the majority occur in adults.
- Obstructive symptoms are common, because of a ball-valve effect of the pedunculated tumor.

MACROPATHOLOGY

- The tumor is submucosal in two-thirds of cases, producing a polypoid or pedunculated mass.
- It can also arise within the wall or subserosally. The overlying epithelium is usually intact.
- Tumors usually vary in size from 1 to 4 cm in diameter, although some may be larger.

MICROPATHOLOGY

- The typical feature of leiomyoma is the presence of fascicles of spindle-shaped cells with fusiform, blunt-ended nuclei, and eosinophilic cytoplasm.
- There is minimal atypia and few mitotic figures.
- In tumors with atypical features, there are nuclear pleomorphism, frequent mitotic figures, and/or necrosis.
- If there is an infiltrative pattern, low-grade leiomyosarcoma must be considered.

TREATMENT

- Transurethral resection is indicated.
- In cases with cytologic features, mesenchymal tumors resection with frozen sections to ensure negative margins may be appropriate.

HEMANGIOMA[182,183]

- In Melicow's series, hemangioma accounted for 40% of benign soft tissue tumors and 0.6% of primary bladder tumors.
- It occurs at any age, with the majority presenting before the age of 30.
- Bladder hemangioma occurs in 3–6% of patients with Klippel–Trenaunay syndrome.
- Hemangioma appears as a purple, multilobulated, and sessile lesion cystoscopically.

MACROPATHOLOGY

- Hemangioma may be single or multiple, and be superficial or extend through the full thickness of the bladder wall.
- The majority are small, 1–2-cm lesions.

MICROPATHOLOGY

- It is composed of vascular spaces containing blood and thrombi.

- Hemangioma is classified as cavernous, capillary, venous, or racemose, with cavernous being most common.

CAUTION

- The major diagnostic consideration is angiosarcoma.
- Kaposi sarcoma in AIDS patients has been seen in the urinary bladder.
- Hemangiopericytoma can arise in the bladder.

TREATMENT

- Most urologists perform a partial cystectomy or local excision.
- Biopsy and transurethral resection of these lesions can cause massive hemorrhage.

NEUROFIBROMA[184]

- The majority of cases occur in patients with von Recklinghausen disease.
- In von Recklinghausen disease, the urinary bladder is the most frequent site of involvement in the genitourinary tract.
- Neurofibroma can appear at any age.
- The majority of patients complain of hematuria, dysuria, or irritative symptoms.
- There can be concomitant involvement of other genitourinary sites: the ureter, spermatic cord, penis, and scrotum.

MACROPATHOLOGY

- Can be single, multiple, or discrete variably sized nodules within the bladder wall or submucosa.
- Many are small but can measure up to several centimeters in diameter.
- Neurofibroma may also appear as diffuse thickening of the bladder wall without discrete margins.
- This pattern corresponds to the plexiform variant associated with von Recklinghausen disease. Here, it can extensively involve the muscularis propria, ureters, and adjacent soft tissues.

MICROPATHOLOGY

- Neurofibroma of the bladder is identical to neurofibroma found elsewhere. It is composed of fascicles of elongated, spindle-shaped cells with thin wavy nuclei in a collagenized and fibrillar background.
- Small nerve fibers are present within the mass; myxoid areas may also be present.
- Immunohistochemistry: results are similar to those for other neurofibromas; S-100 protein-positive.
- Malignant change in neurofibroma of the bladder is rare.

CAUTION

- Consider other benign spindle cell lesions, such as leiomyoma, and inflammatory pseudotumor.
- Immunohistochemistry: in leiomyoma, evidence of muscle differentiation.
- Immunohistochemistry: cells of inflammatory pseudotumor contain vimentin and actin, reflecting the fibroblastic and myofibroblastic nature.

TREATMENT

- Treatment of neurofibroma remains controversial.
- Most urologists advocate radical resection with urinary diversion because of the high rate of recurrence with partial resection.
- Neurofibroma often recurs and can cause death by urinary obstruction and renal failure.

GRANULAR CELL TUMOR (Figs 11.213–11.215)[185-187]

- Granular cell tumor is rare in the urinary bladder.
- It usually arises in adults, with equal sex distribution.
- All patients presented with hematuria.
- All cases have been benign, except for one reported by Ravich et al.[185]

MACROPATHOLOGY

- The tumor is circumscribed or encapsulated, appearing as single or multiple yellow-white nodules.

MICROPATHOLOGY

- The tumor is composed of spindle- to polygonal-shaped cells with abundant eosinophilic coarse granular cytoplasm.
- The granules are periodic acid–Schiff–positive and diastase-resistant.
- This tumor is considered to be neurogenic (Schwann cell) in origin.
- The tumor is S-100 protein-positive, similar to granular cell tumors elsewhere.

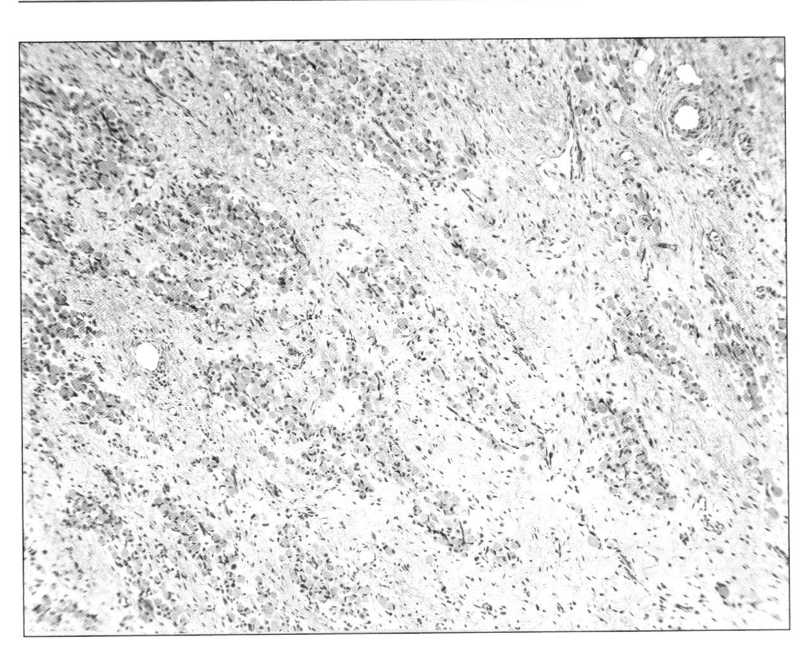

Fig. 11.213 Granular cell tumor in the bladder. A digital photomicrograph from slides of a malignant granular cell tumor described by Drs Stout and Ravich. The cells are S-100-positive.

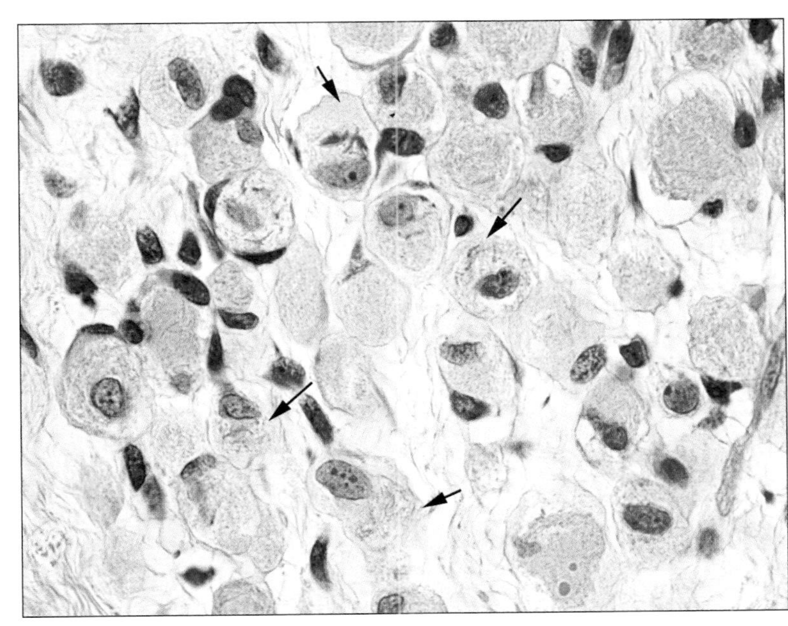

Fig. 11.215 Granular cell tumor in the bladder. A higher magnification of Fig. 11.213. Arrows point to crystalline inclusions.

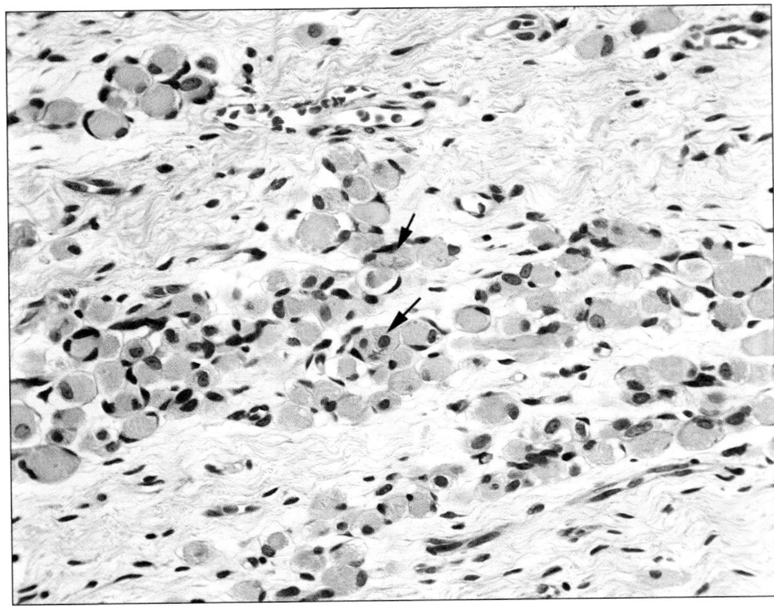

Fig. 11.214 Granular cell tumor in the bladder. A higher magnification of Fig. 11.213. Cells contain an ill-defined cytoplasmic crystalline inclusion. The cells are S-100-positive.

- A malignant case showed benign histologic features in the bladder lesion but subsequently recurred and metastasized (Ravich et al.[185]).

MALIGNANT SOFT TISSUE NEOPLASMS

- Sarcomas of the urinary bladder are rare.
- There is a distinctive age distribution according to histologic type. Rhabdomyosarcoma is more frequent in childhood.

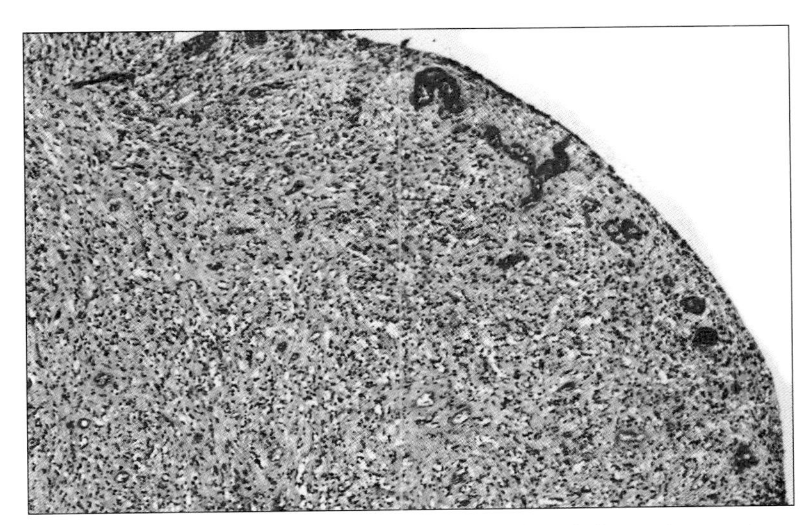

Fig. 11.216 Sarcoma botryoides: low-power digital photomicrograph. Small cells in the bladder submucosa similar to those found in rhabdomyosarcoma elsewhere.

- Leiomyosarcoma is more common in adults.
- Sarcomas accounted for 2.7% of all primary bladder neoplasms seen at Columbia-Presbyterian Hospital.

RHABDOMYOSARCOMA
(Figs 11.216–11.218)[188–191]

- Rhabdomyosarcoma can be seen in patients under the age of 15 years.
- In children, it occurs more frequently in boys, and most cases develop before the patient is 5 years old.
- It most often presents with hematuria and bladder neck obstruction.

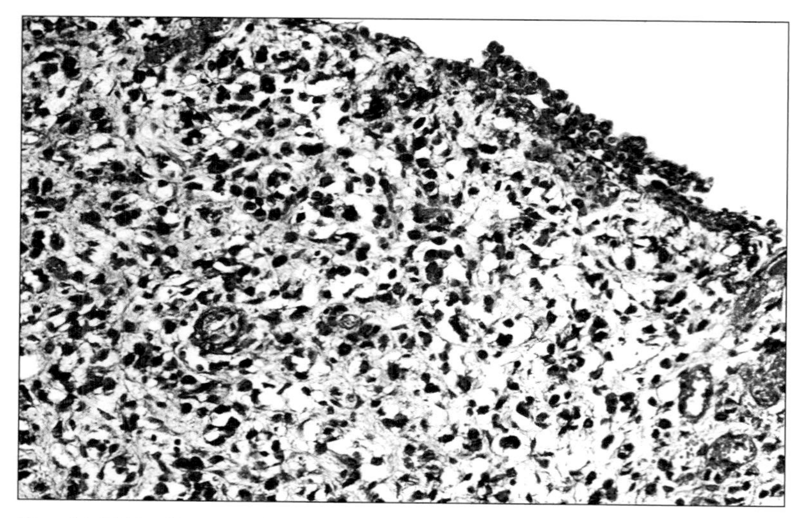

Fig. 11.217 Sarcoma botryoides: medium-power digital photomicrograph. Small cells in the bladder submucosa similar to those found in embryonal rhabdomyosarcoma elsewhere. Bladder mucosa is in the upper right corner.

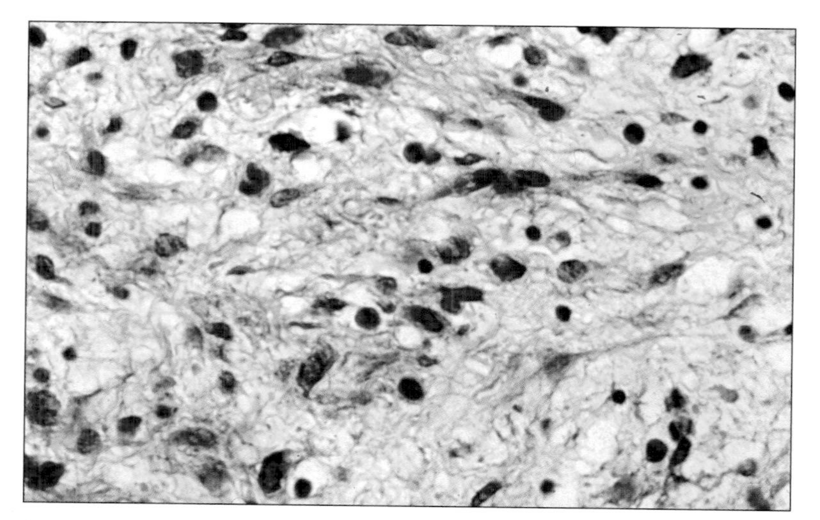

Fig. 11.218 Sarcoma botryoides, again showing small cells in the bladder submucosa similar to those found in embryonal rhabdomyosarcoma elsewhere.

MACROPATHOLOGY

- It is a polypoid mass, which may be single or multiple, and can fill the bladder lumen.
- Rhabdomyosarcoma forms polypoid masses that produce a sarcoma botryoides (grape-like clusters).
- The trigone is the most common location.

MICROPATHOLOGY

- The majority are embryonal rhabdomyosarcoma diffusely infiltrating as small round blue cells with scant cytoplasm.
- The sarcoma botryoides variant has cells that are scattered in a loose myxoid stroma, with a prominence of rhabdomyoblasts beneath the surface urothelium.
- Rhabdoid or strap cells containing cross striations may be found.
- Immunohistochemistry or electron microscopic studies are necessary for proving rhabdomyoblastic differentiation.

LEIOMYOSARCOMA[181,192–196]

- This is the most common sarcoma of the bladder in adults.
- Patients have a wide age range (7–81 years), with a mean age of 52 years.
- The most common presentation is hematuria and obstructive symptoms.

MACROPATHOLOGY

- The tumor is lobulated or polypoid, with possible ulceration.
- Most tumors vary in diameter, from 2 to 5 cm or more.

MICROPATHOLOGY

- Most tumors have the typical appearance of leiomyosarcoma, and are composed of interwoven fascicles of spindle-shaped cells with long blunt-ended nuclei and eosinophilic cytoplasm.
- Nuclear pleomorphism is variable, as is the mitotic rate.
- It may occur with urothelial CIS, and noninvasive and invasive urothelial papillary carcinoma.
- Some tumors are myxoid or have an epithelioid appearance.
- Electron microscopy reveals smooth muscle cells with thin filaments, and pinocytotic vesicles.

IMMUNOHISTOCHEMISTRY

- Cytokeratin-negative; vimentin- and muscle-specific actin-positive.

CAUTION

Sarcomatoid urothelial carcinoma

- This can mimic high-grade leiomyosarcoma.
- Extensive sampling usually demonstrates a recognizable epithelial component.
- Immunohistochemistry is invaluable when there are cases of sarcomatoid carcinoma without identifiable foci of carcinoma.

- Sarcomatoid carcinomas express cytokeratin (positive) focally in the spindle cells.
- Muscle markers such as actin and desmin are negative.

Leiomyoma

The separation of leiomyoma from leiomyosarcoma may be difficult. Leiomyosarcoma has:

- the presence of nuclear pleomorphism;
- high mitotic rate (five or more mitotic figures per 10 high-power fields);
- infiltrative growth.
- Necrosis suggests malignancy.

Inflammatory pseudotumor (pseudosarcomatous fibromyxoid tumor)

- It is most often an incidental finding and develops following surgery or trauma.
- It is a benign bladder pseudo-sarcoma that exhibits histologically a spindle cell proliferation pattern that is of great concern.

Macropathology
- A polypoid mass.

Micropathology
- It has a loose myxoid appearance, with slit-like blood vessels and a background of acute and chronic inflammatory cells.
- There are spindle-shaped or stellate cells with little nuclear pleomorphism.
- Occasional bizarre nuclei may be seen, but mitotic figures are infrequent and morphologically normal.
- The process may be infiltrative, and the muscularis propria may be difficult to separate from myxoid leiomyosarcoma of the bladder.

Immunohistochemistry
- Results have been variable, with vimentin and actin positive and desmin negative.

MALIGNANT FIBROUS HISTIOCYTOMA (Figs 11.219–11.226)[197,198]

- These are rare tumors that must be differentiated from sarcomatoid carcinoma.

MACROPATHOLOGY

- These tumors are large and necrotic.

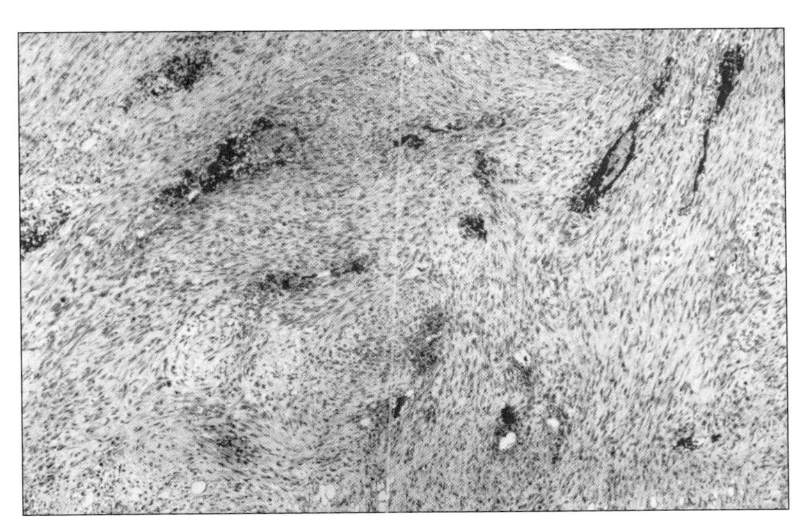

Fig. 11.219 Sarcoma. Spindle-shaped cells with a malignant fibrous histiocytoma pattern. Small spindle-shaped cells in the bladder submucosa, similar to those found in malignant fibrous histiocytoma elsewhere in the body. This pattern is cytokeratin-negative.

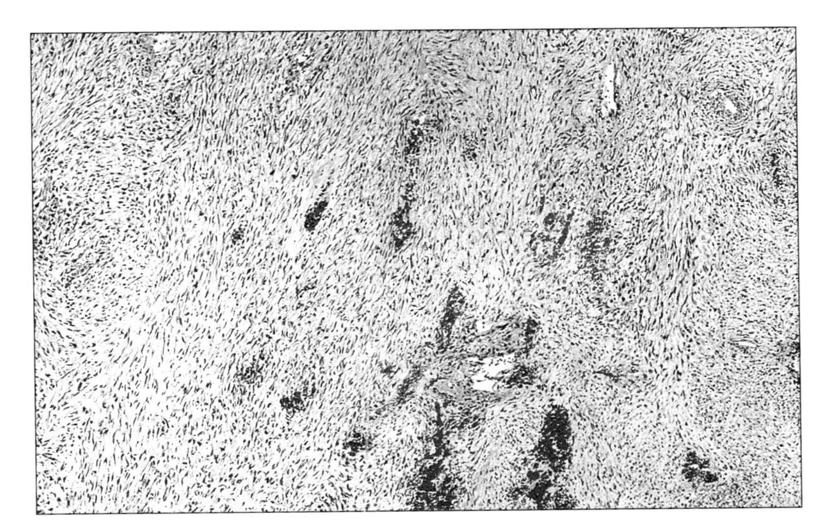

Fig. 11.220 Sarcoma.

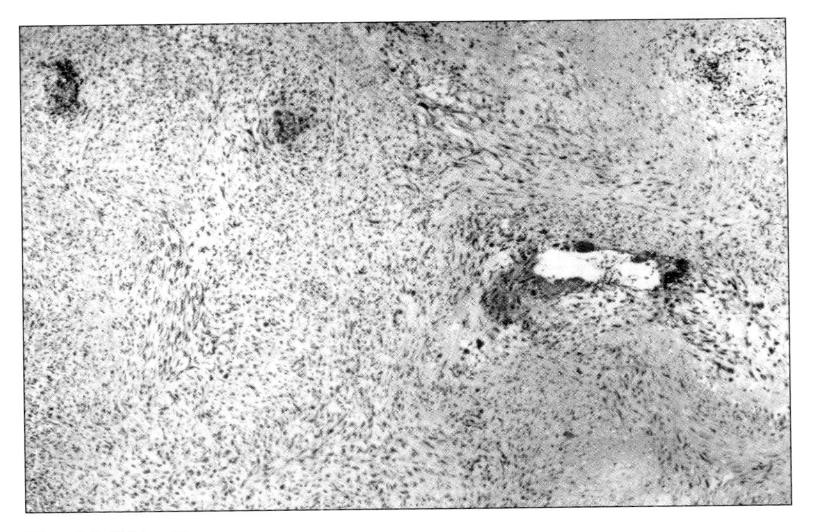

Fig. 11.221 Sarcoma.

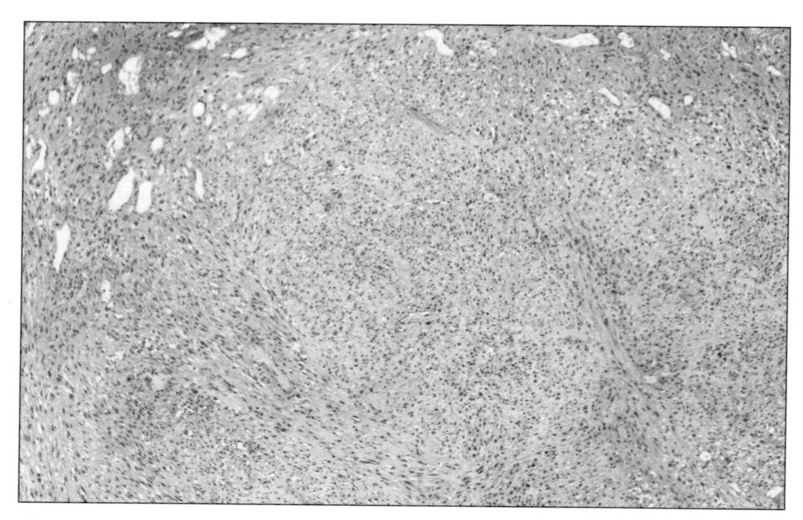

Fig. 11.222 Sarcoma. Low-power digital photomicrograph of spindle-shaped cells with a malignant fibrous histiocytoma pattern.

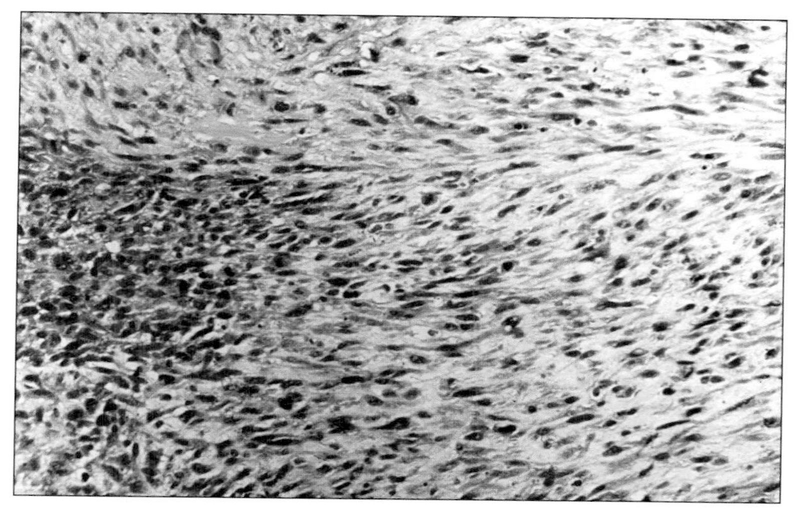

Fig. 11.223 Sarcoma. A higher-power image of spindle-shaped cells with a malignant fibrous histiocytoma pattern.

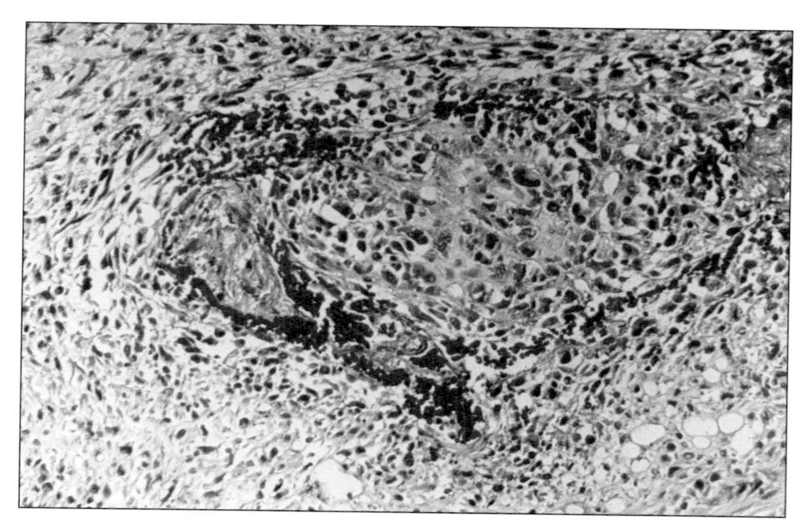

Fig. 11.224 Sarcoma. Another higher-power image of spindle-shaped cells with a malignant fibrous histiocytoma pattern; this pattern is cytokeratin-negative. However, there is an epithelioid-like area, which is also cytokeratin-negative, but CD34-positive.

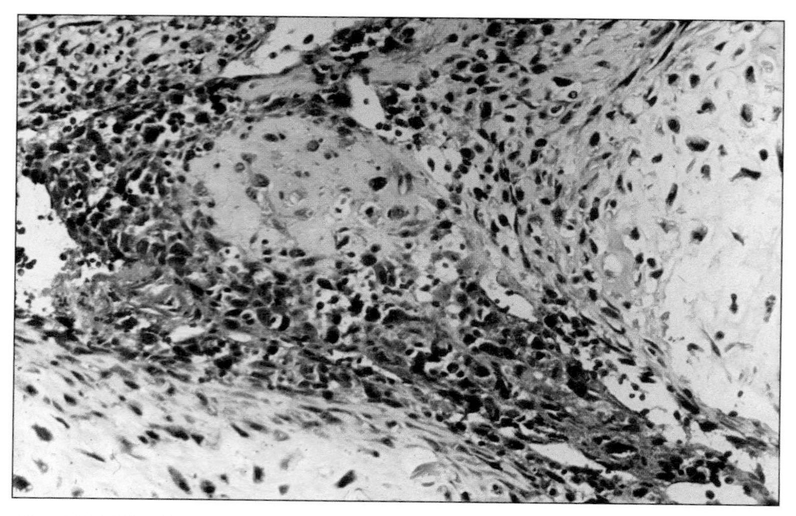

Fig. 11.225 Sarcoma. Malignant fibrous histiocytoma and chondrosarcoma with a higher-power magnification of spindle-shaped cells with a malignant fibrous histiocytoma pattern; this pattern is cytokeratin-negative. However, an epithelioid-like area, which is also cytokeratin-negative, surrounds cartilaginous areas that are malignant.

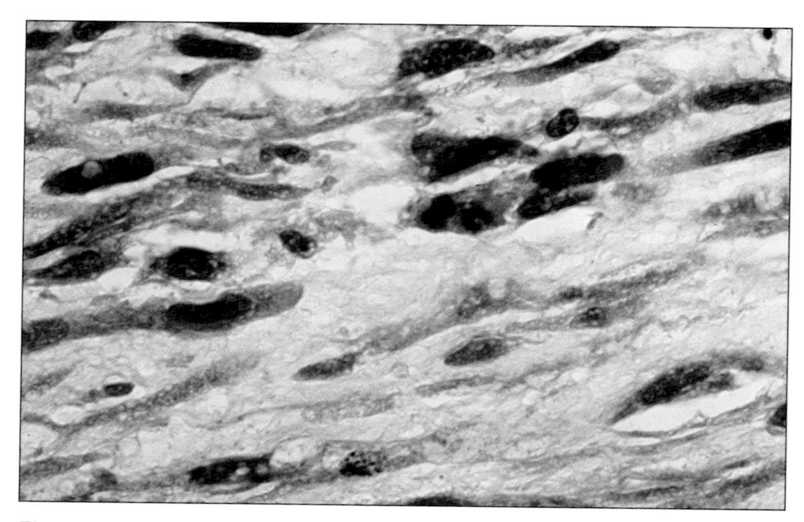

Fig. 11.226 Sarcoma. An oil immersion magnification of large spindle-shaped cells in the bladder that stain positive with skeletal muscle monoclonal antibodies.

MICROPATHOLOGY

- They have a variegated appearance.
- There is a storiform pattern, which may be mixed with areas that are myxoid, pleomorphic, or inflammatory.
- Immunohistochemistry is consistent with malignant fibrous histiocytoma arising in other organs.

CAUTION

- Must be differentiated from sarcomatoid carcinoma, which microscopically may reveal a malignant fibrous histiocytoma-like growth pattern.

- If there are no epithelial patterns found within the tumor, immunohistochemistry should be used to look for evidence of epithelial differentiation.

OSTEOSARCOMA[199]

- These are rare tumors that occur predominantly in men.
- Symptoms include hematuria and abdominal mass.

MACROPATHOLOGY

- The tumor is large, polypoid, and deeply infiltrative.

MICROPATHOLOGY

- The tumor is a high-grade sarcoma with osteoid production.

CAUTION

- Sarcomatoid urothelial carcinoma and urothelial carcinoma with osseous metaplasia must be considered. Osteoid formation can be seen in sarcomatoid carcinoma (carcinosarcoma), which is to be considered when there is an identifiable epithelial component within the tumor.
- Areas of osseous metaplasia have been described in urothelial carcinoma without a sarcomatous component, and the bone in these cases is mature, with a lamellar architecture and no cytologic atypia.
- Bone has been seen in malignant mesenchymoma of the bladder.
- The prognosis for patients with osteosarcoma is poor.

FIBROSARCOMA[200]

- Fibrosarcoma is very rare.
- To qualify for this diagnosis, a tumor should meet the criteria utilized for fibrosarcoma elsewhere in the body.

ANGIOSARCOMA[182,183]

- Angiosarcomas are very rare.
- The major differential diagnostic consideration is hemangioma, which is cavernous, and all types lack significant cytologic atypia.

HEMANGIOPERICYTOMA[201]

- These are rare tumors that occur in adults (male-to-female ratio 1:4).

MACROPATHOLOGY

- The tumor is solid, ovoid, and well circumscribed.

MICROPATHOLOGY

- Typical features of hemangiopericytoma are present.

CAUTION

- Hemangiopericytoma-like areas may be found in sarcomatoid carcinoma of the bladder.

RHABDOID TUMOR[202–204]

- This occurs in a young age group.

HISTOPATHOLOGY

- Rhabdoid morphology in cells of tumor.
- The tumor is a mixture of urothelial carcinoma, high-grade sarcoma, and rhabdoid tumor cells.
- Histochemistry: vimentin-positive with variable coexpression of cytokeratin.
- Electron microscopy: whorled cytoplasmic intermediate filaments.

LYMPHORETICULAR AND HEMATOPOIETIC NEOPLASMS

MALIGNANT LYMPHOMA[205,206]

- Malignant lymphoma in the bladder is usually secondary to systemic lymphoma. In patients with non-Hodgkin lymphoma, bladder involvement is present in about 13% of cases (autopsy cases).
- Primary malignant lymphoma in the bladder in the absence of systemic lymphoma accounts for only 0.2% of all cases of extranodal malignant lymphoma.
- Most patients present with gross hematuria, dysuria, or irritative symptoms.

Macropathology

- The tumor may be single or multiple, sessile or polypoid.
- Intact mucosa overlies the lymphoid mass.

Micropathology

- A diffuse and infiltrative proliferation of lymphoid cells permeating and surrounding normal structures rather than replacing them.
- The lymphoid cells are usually of the diffuse large cell or small lymphocytic lymphoma.
- Less commonly, there are follicular, plasmacytoid, mantle zone, and monocytoid lymphomas.
- A Hodgkin disease primary in the bladder is extremely rare.

Caution

- Chronic inflammatory process: lesions contain a polymorphous infiltrate without formation of a mass, and immunohistochemistry shows polyclonality.
- Small cell carcinoma: histologic features identical to small cell carcinoma elsewhere in the body. A cohesive growth pattern and prominent nuclear molding are present. Most cases have an identifiable urothelial or other epithelial component.
- Lymphoma-like carcinoma: cytokeratin-negative and leukocyte common antigen-positive. Most cases of small cell carcinoma are cytokeratin-positive and leukocyte common antigen-negative. There are also cases that resemble nasopharyngeal carcinoma and consist of syncytial groups of cytokeratin-positive carcinoma cells in a polymorphous inflammatory background.

PLASMACYTOMA[207]

- The bladder contains neoplastic plasma cells like those in disseminated multiple myeloma.
- It may also appear as a solitary plasmacytoma.

Gross pathology

- There may be polypoid or pedunculated tumors.
- The surface mucosa is typically intact.

Histopathology

- The tumor is composed of sheets of plasma cells with varying degrees of atypia.

Caution

- A differential diagnostic consideration is plasmacytoid urothelial carcinoma. The epithelial nature of the tumor is indicated by a cohesive growth pattern and/or the presence of CIS.
- Immunohistochemistry: staining for cytokeratin and light chains should distinguish the two.

LEUKEMIA

- Autopsy studies reveal bladder involvement in patients who died from chronic lymphocytic leukemia and chronic myelogenous leukemia.
- Infiltration of the bladder in patients with leukemia rarely presents clinically.

METASTASES[208–213]

- The majority (72%) were direct invasion from malignancies arising in adjacent organs.
- Secondary tumors accounted for 13.4% of bladder neoplasms.
- Distant metastases accounted for 3% of cases of bladder neoplasms; these would include:
  - malignant melanoma;
  - carcinomas of the stomach, breast, kidney, and lung (being the most common).

INFLAMMATION AND INFECTION (Figs 11.227–11.238)

- Cystitis occurs with a wide variety of bladder abnormalities that are associated with the normal aging processes and debilitating immunologic diseases.
- The pathologic lesions correlated poorly with the clinical disease.
- A single etiologic agent or clinical entity cannot be established from examination of the tissue samples alone.
- This inflammatory process is descriptive in the literature: gangrenous cystitis, membranous cystitis, and calcareous cystitis.
- In the inflammatory diseases of the bladder, the following factors must be considered.
  - The bladder has a limited capacity to react to injurious stimuli, and dissimilar etiologic events may result in the same histologic response.
  - The same stimuli may cause dissimilar reactions in different hosts.

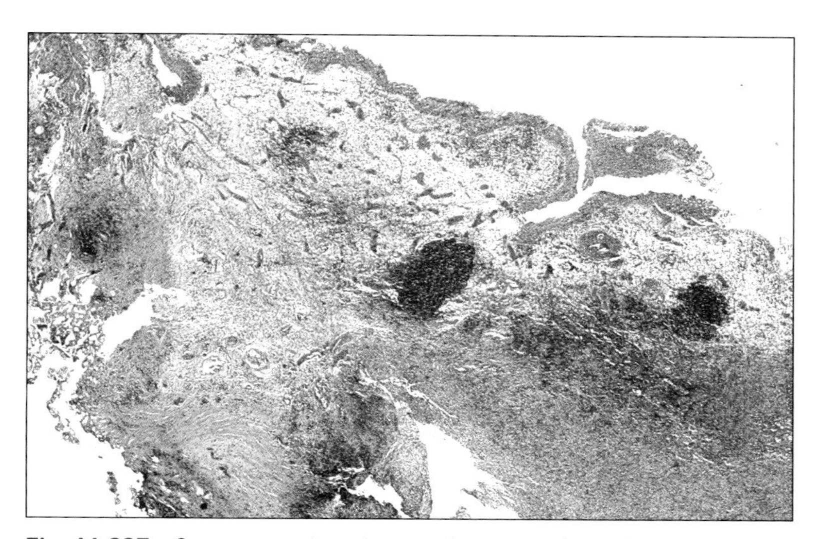

Fig. 11.227 Stone necrosis and stromal repair with marked cystitis follicularis. The urothelium is within normal limits. Sometimes, there are pseudopapillary configurations of the urothelial surface epithelium. There is fibrous stroma in the lower left third of the photograph.

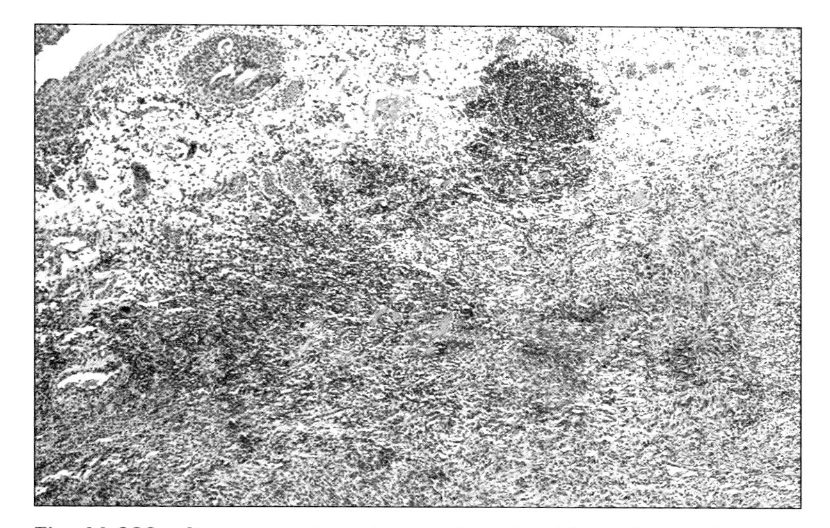

Fig. 11.228 Stone necrosis and stromal repair with marked cystitis follicularis. A higher magnification of Fig. 11.227.

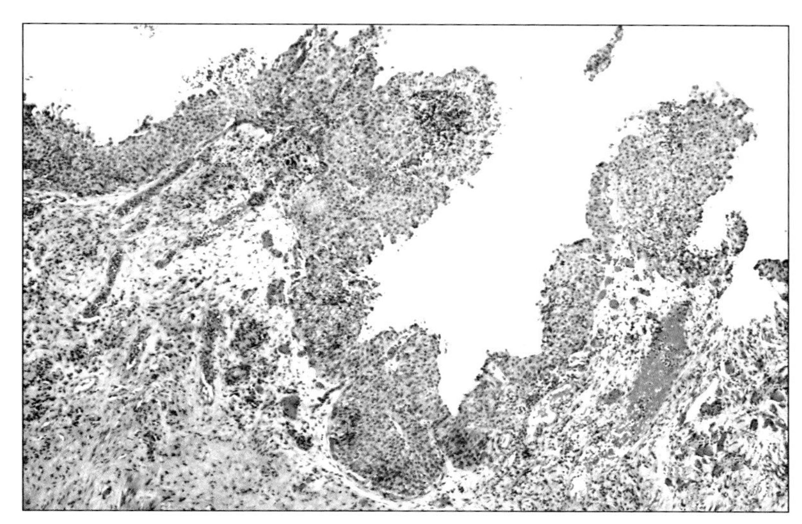

Fig. 11.229 Stone necrosis and stromal repair with marked cystitis follicularis. There is a pseudopapillary configuration of the urothelial surface epithelium.

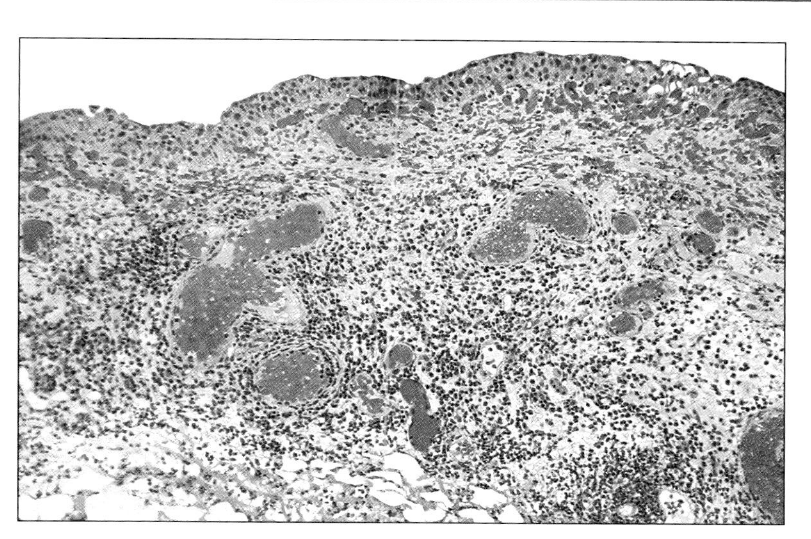

Fig. 11.230 A stone causing chronic eosinophilic cystitis with urothelial dysplasia.

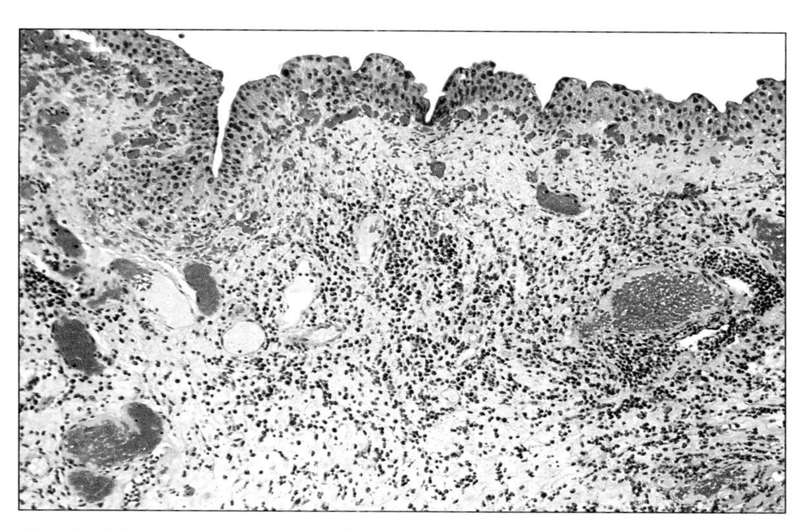

Fig. 11.231 A stone causing chronic eosinophilic cystitis with urothelial dysplasia. Higher magnification of Fig. 11.230.

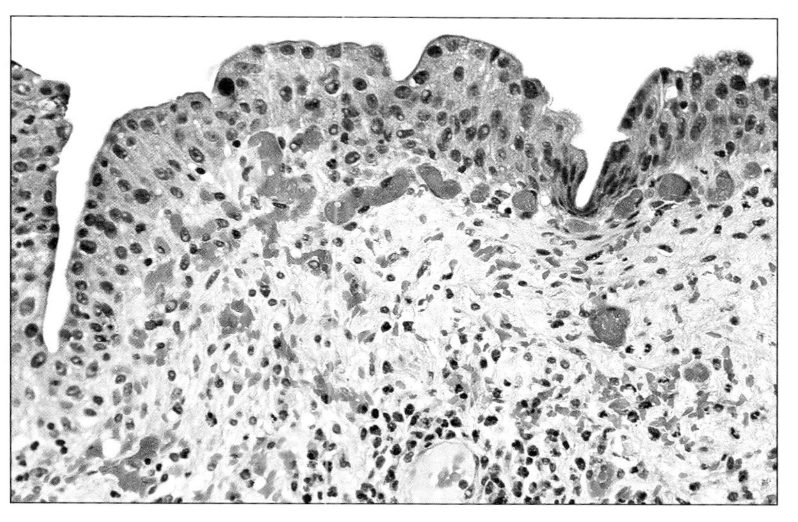

Fig. 11.232 A stone causing chronic eosinophilic cystitis with urothelial dysplasia. Another higher magnification of Fig. 11.230.

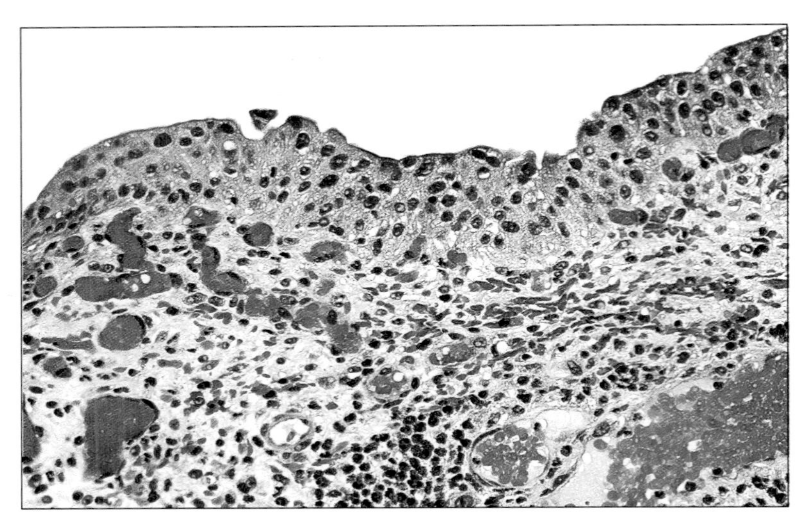

Fig. 11.233 Stone causing chronic eosinophilic cystitis with urothelial dysplasia. A higher magnification of Fig. 11.230.

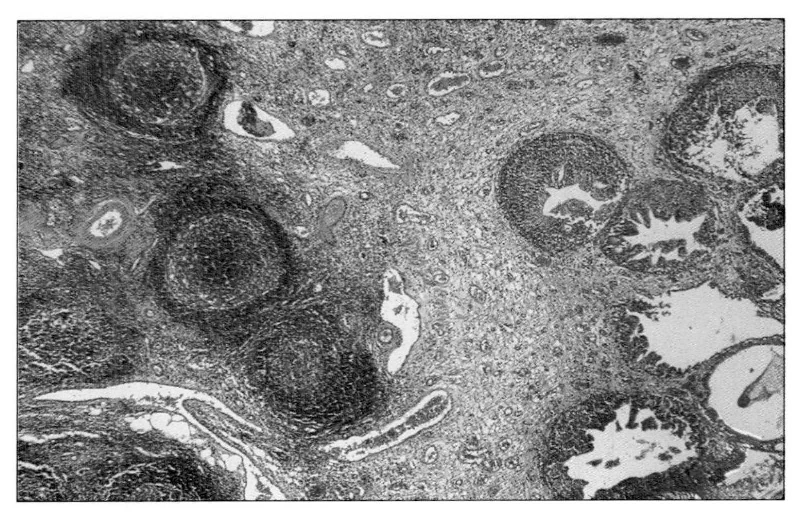

Fig. 11.234 Chronic cystitis with cystitis follicularis and cystitis glandularis.

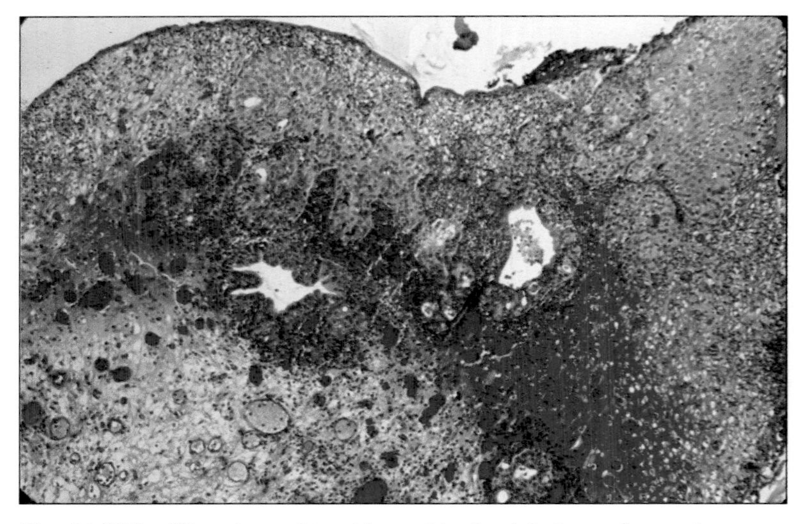

Fig. 11.235 Chronic cystitis with cystitis glandularis, nephrogenic metaplasia, and severely dysplastic urothelium associated with stones.

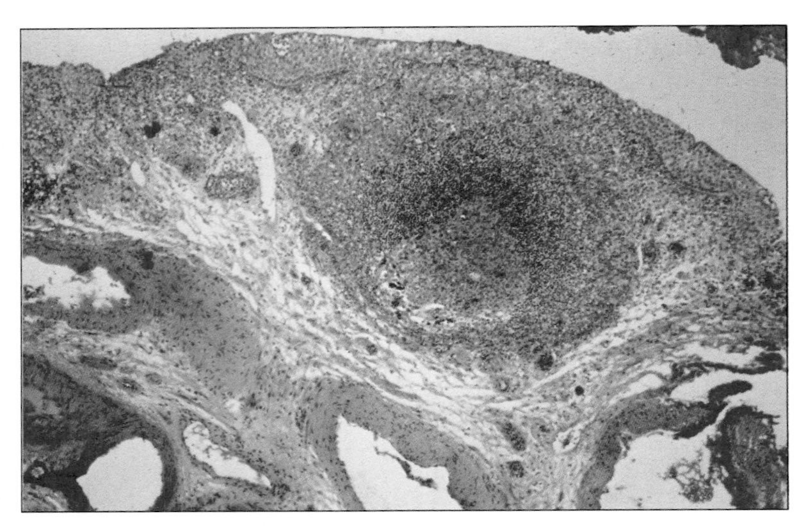

Fig. 11.236 Chronic cystitis with cystitis follicularis and severely dysplastic urothelium associated with stones.

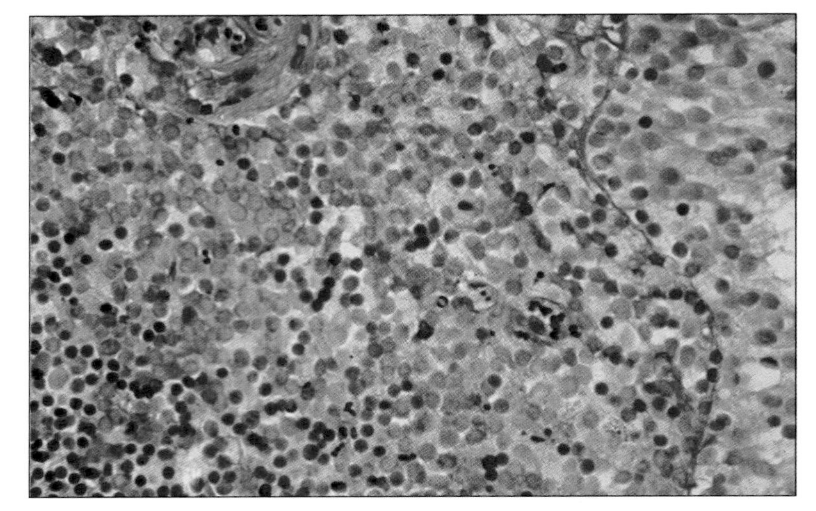

Fig. 11.237 Chronic cystitis with cystitis follicularis. A higher magnification of Fig. 11.236.

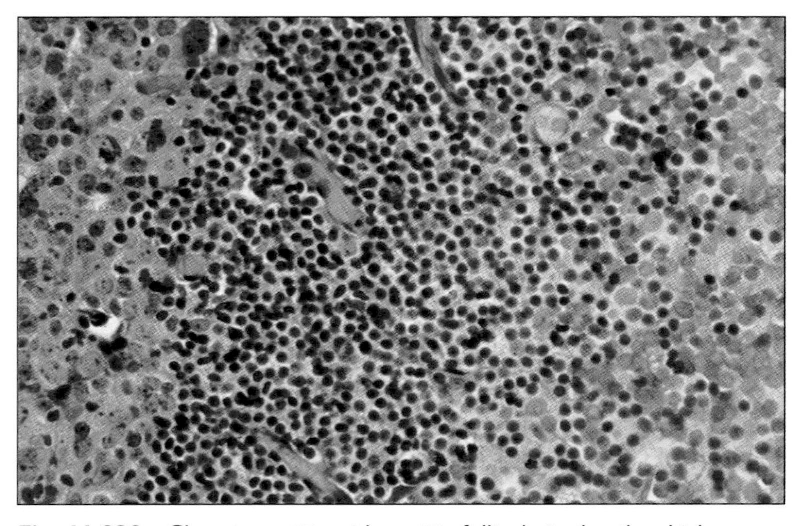

Fig. 11.238 Chronic cystitis with cystitis follicularis. Another higher magnification of Fig. 11.236.

Pathologic observations of inflammation and sequential biopsy depend on the onset, duration, and severity of the symptoms.

Inflammations resulting in the acute onset of severe symptoms will be biopsied earlier in the course of the symptoms than will those resulting in slow development of symptoms.

At any point in the time course of the inflammatory process, the leukocytic infiltration or fibrosis may predominate.

Bladder injury often results in denudation of the urothelium, and hematuria is a common but nonspecific event.

The subsequent reactive or regenerative epithelial changes tend to become part of the overall pathologic process and must be distinguished from dysplasia and neoplasia.

- Inflammations of the urinary bladder histologically can be seen to fit into distinctive histologic patterns.
- Distinctive histologic patterns are associated with various etiologic agents and nonspecific clinical features. This is manifested by Brunn nests and their derivatives, pseudosarcomatous fibromyxoid tumor or postoperative spindle cell nodule, and various manifestations of inflammation.
- Distinctive histologic patterns are associated with specific clinical entities such as malakoplakia, xanthogranulomatous cystitis, and interstitial cystitis.
- Histologic patterns are associated with specific etiologic agents such as infections and chemicals.
- Nonspecific histologic patterns can be associated with defined clinical entities such as immune disorders and lichen planus.

BRUNN NESTS

- Reactions to a variety of injurious agents result in urothelial lesions with distinctive histologic features.
- Many experts consider nests of Brunn to be variants of normal urothelium, which are rounded aggregates of transitional cells in the lamina propria.
- They may be attached to or separated from the overlying urothelium.
- They may contain a lumen, which is lined by superficial urothelial cells with the capacity to secrete mucin.
- Most common at the trigone, Brunn nests occur throughout the bladder.
- No sex predilection has been documented.
- Sometimes, the nesting pattern of urothelial cancer may be difficult to separate from Brunn nests, which often vary in both size and number.

CYSTITIS (Figs 11.239–11.257)

Cystitis glandularis (proliferative cystitis)[214–217]

- These are gland-like structures in the lamina propria of urinary bladders.
- The lesions of cystitis glandularis may represent proliferative reactions of Brunn nests.
- They are composed of layers of basal and intermediate transitional cells lined by superficial urothelial cells compressed into columnar shapes.
- Small amounts of mucin can be demonstrated in the glandular lumina along the luminal surfaces. Sometimes they appear as discrete intracellular vacuoles.
- Variable numbers of intestine-type goblet cells may occur.
- Cystitis glandularis is not primarily a lesion composed of colonic epithelium. Lesions of cystitis glandularis

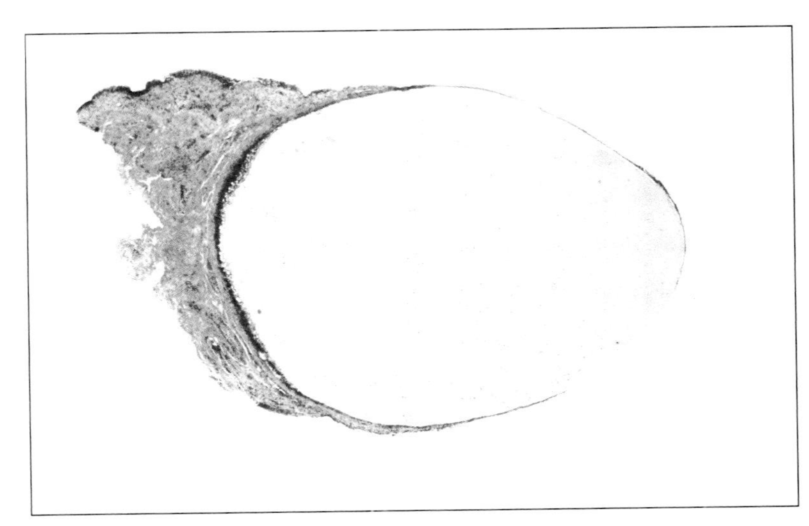

Fig. 11.239 Chronic cystitis with cystitis cystica.

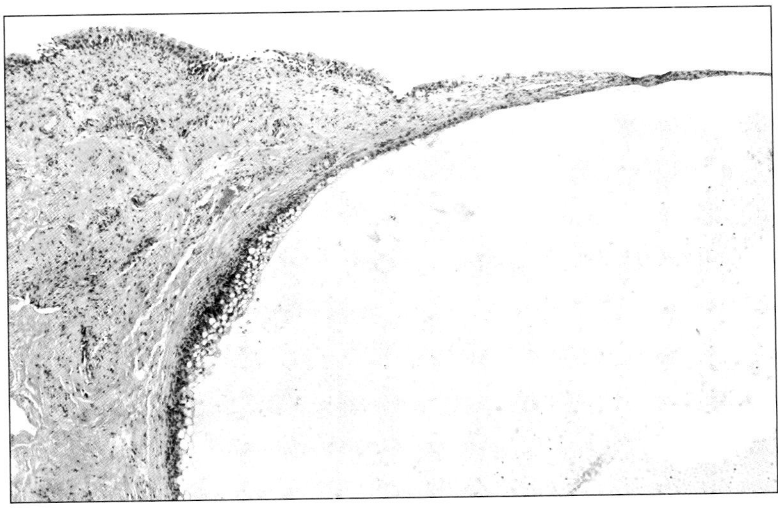

Fig. 11.240 Chronic cystitis with cystitis cystica. A high magnification of Fig. 11.239.

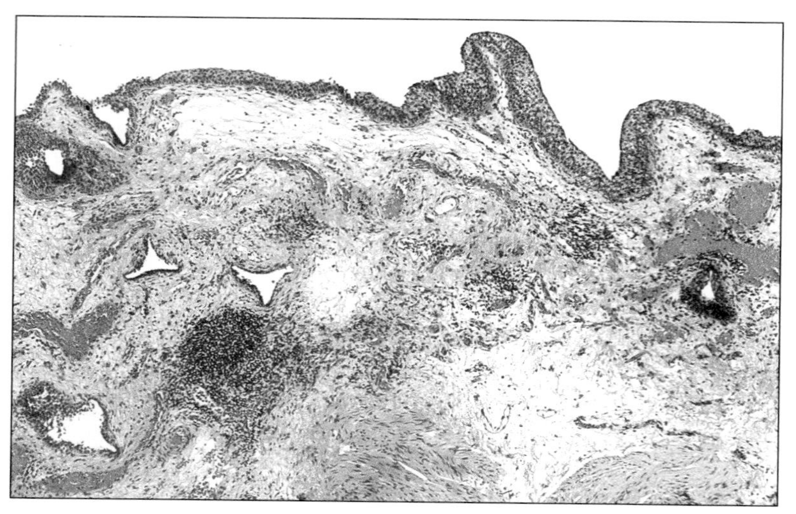

Fig. 11.241 Chronic cystitis with cystitis follicularis and pseudopapillary configuration: associated with prostatic obstructive uropathy.

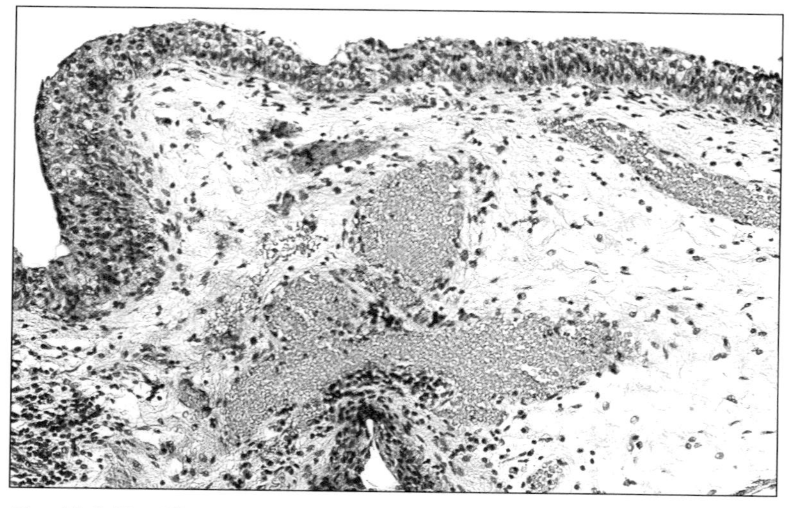

Fig. 11.242 Chronic cystitis associated with prostatic obstructive uropathy.

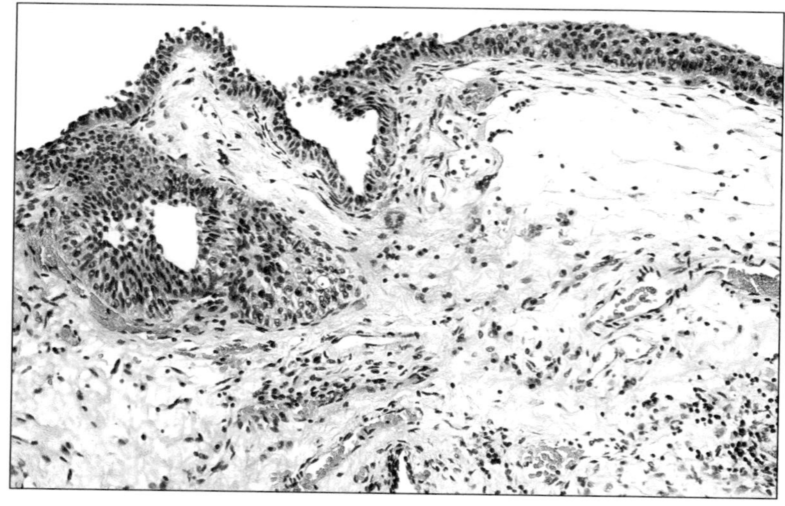

Fig. 11.243 Chronic cystitis associated with prostatic obstructive uropathy. There is atypical urothelium lining the bladder lumen. When these cells are exfoliated, there may be diagnostic difficulties in the urinary cytology.

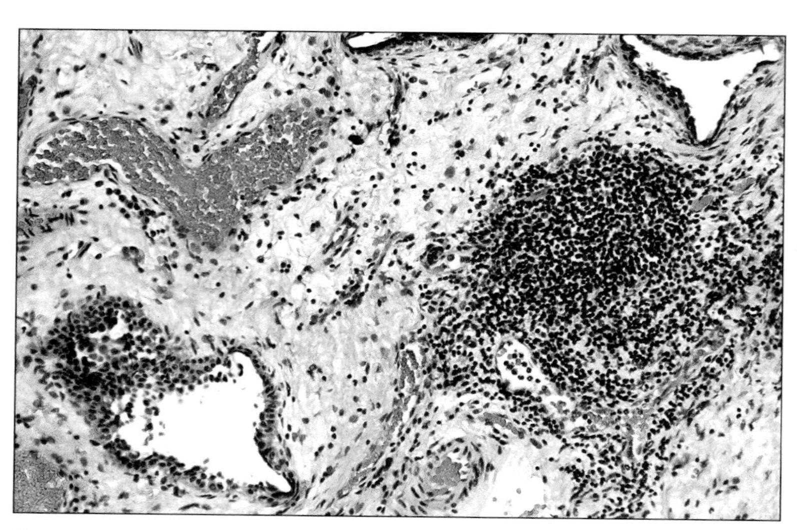

Fig. 11.244 Chronic cystitis associated with prostatic obstructive uropathy.

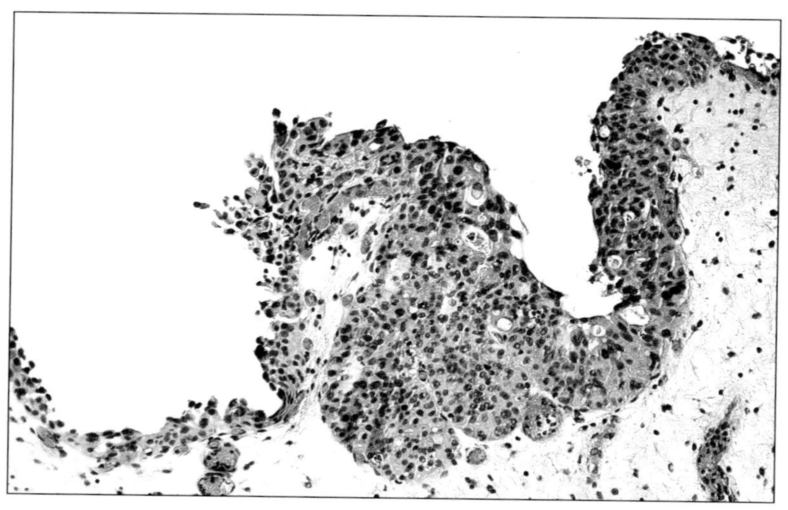

Fig. 11.245 Chronic cystitis associated with prostatic obstructive uropathy and stones. There is markedly dysplastic urothelium of carcinoma in situ. When the urothelial cells are exfoliated, this can give positive urinary cytology. The cystoscopy may not reveal any visible lesions, and hence random biopsies are taken.

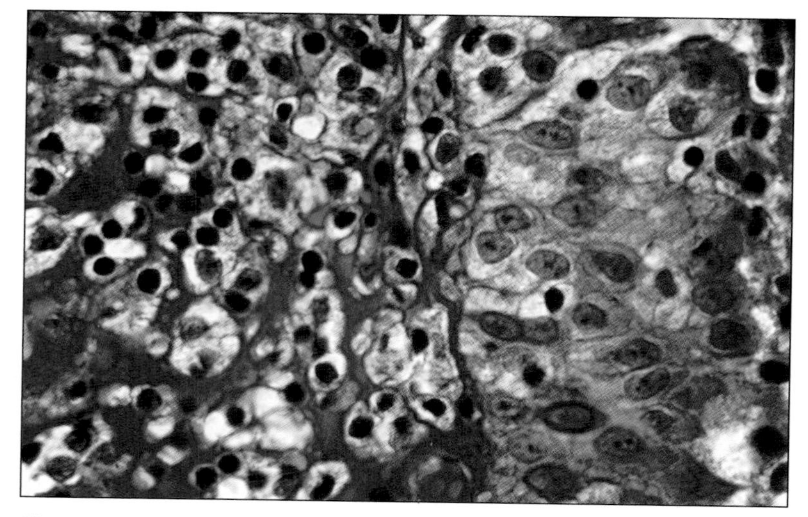

Fig. 11.246 Chronic cystitis associated with prostatic obstructive uropathy and stones. This was from a random area a few millimeters away from the area seen in Fig. 11.245. No neoplasia was present.

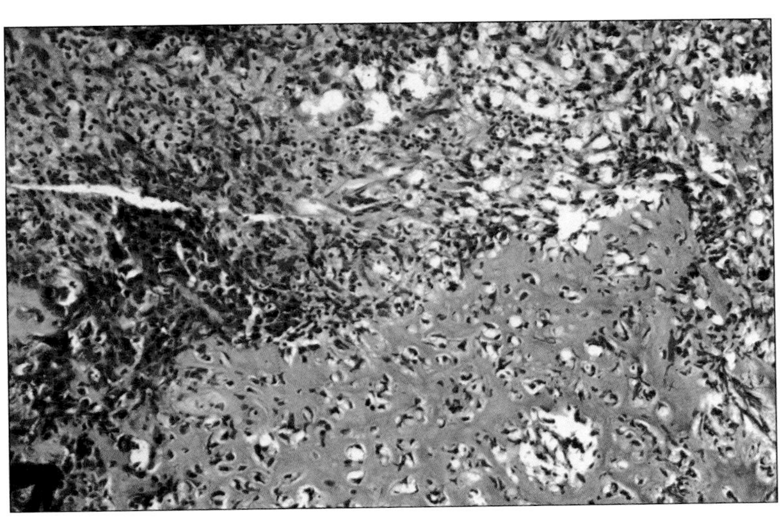

Fig. 11.247 Chronic cystitis associated with prostatic obstructive uropathy and stones. There is marked urothelial repair and cautery artifact resulting from the biopsy procedure. This was from a random area a few millimeters away from the area seen in Fig. 11.245. The histologic field is not readable.

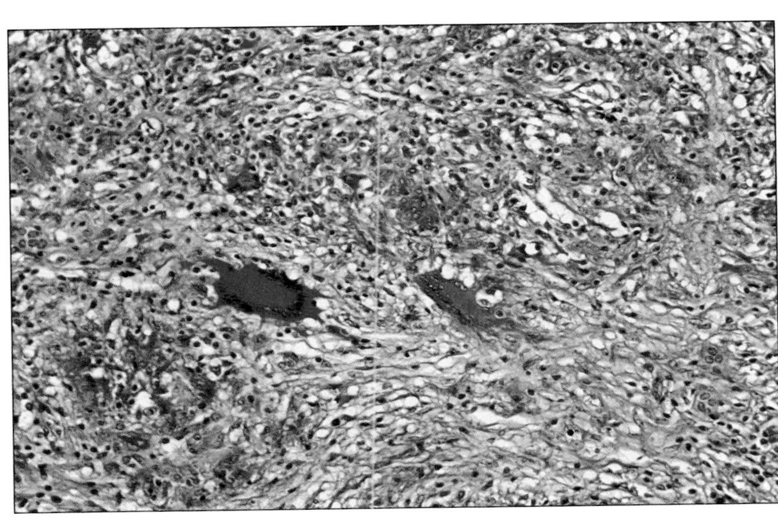

Fig. 11.248 Chronic granulomatous cystitis associated with a post transurethral resection done for visible bladder tumors.

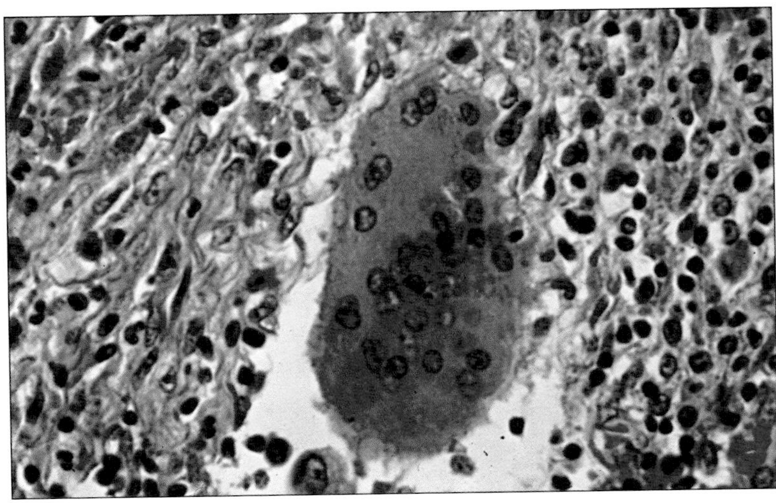

Fig. 11.249 Multinucleated giant cell commonly seen after TURP and BCG therapy.

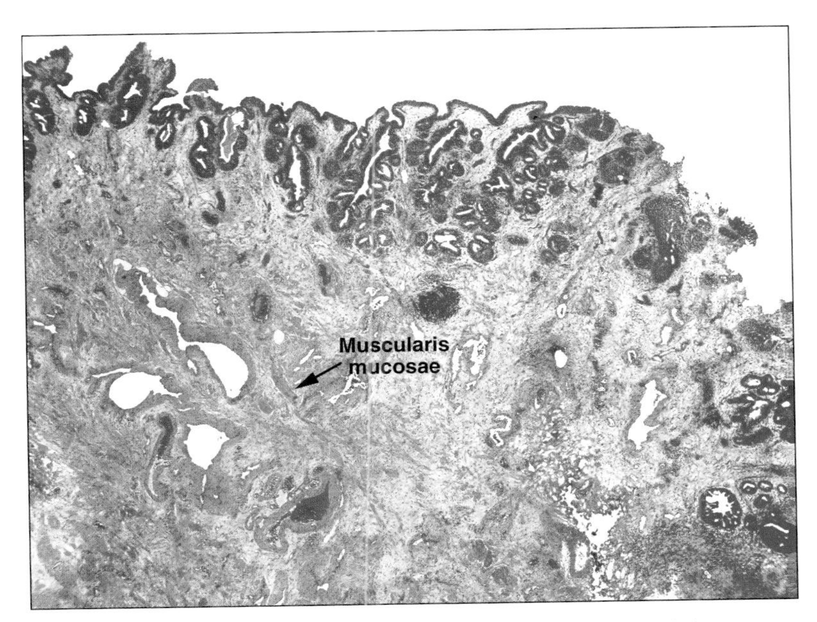

Fig. 11.250 Chronic cystitis-associated colonic metaplasia of the urothelium.

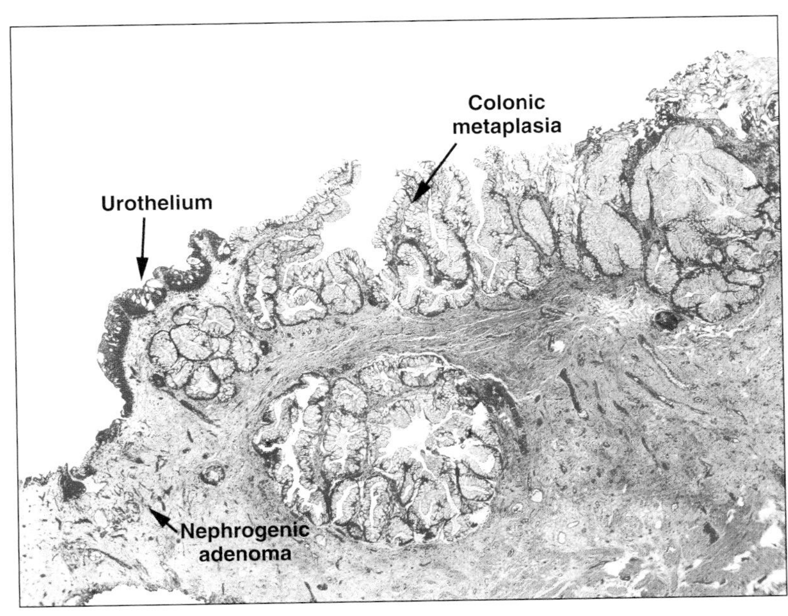

Fig. 11.251 Chronic cystitis-associated colonic metaplasia, and nephrogenic metaplasia of the urothelium.

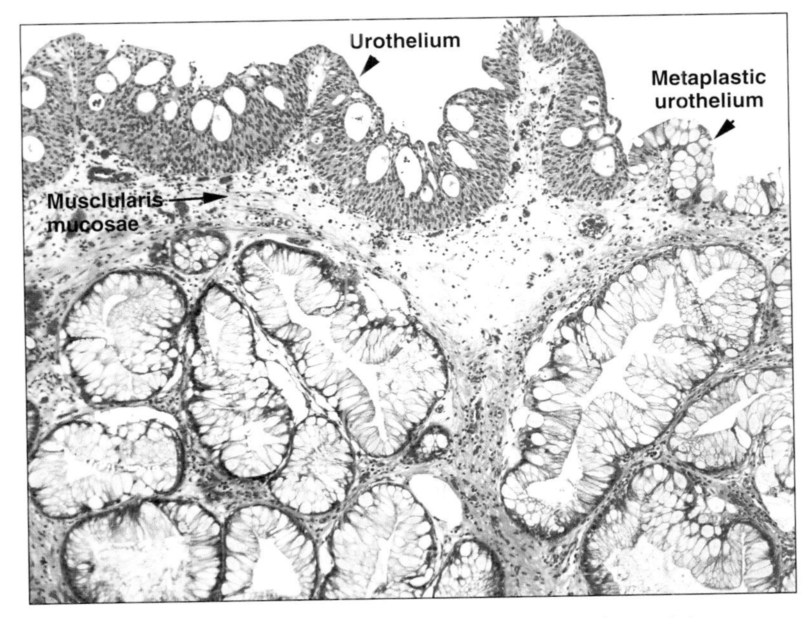

Fig. 11.252 Chronic cystitis-associated colonic metaplasia of the urothelium.

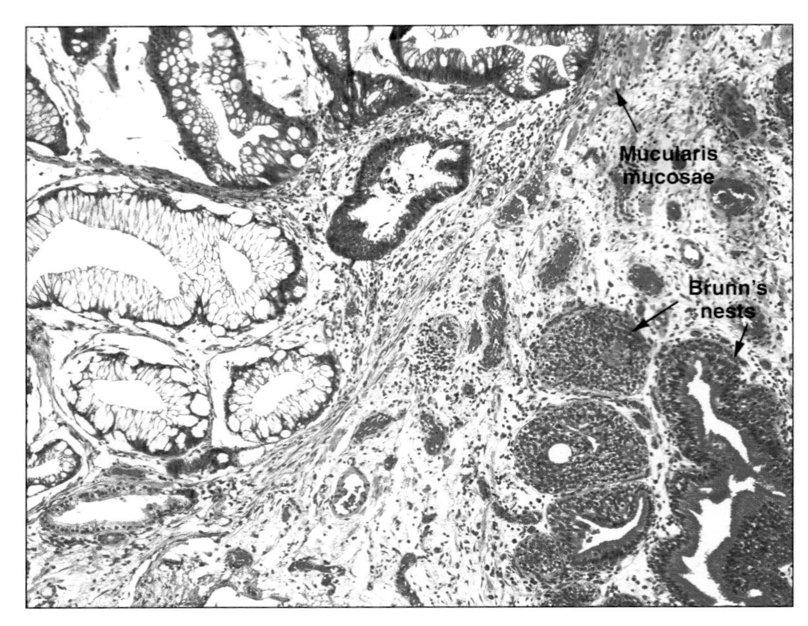

Fig. 11.253 Chronic cystitis-associated von Brunn nests and colonic metaplasia of the urothelium.

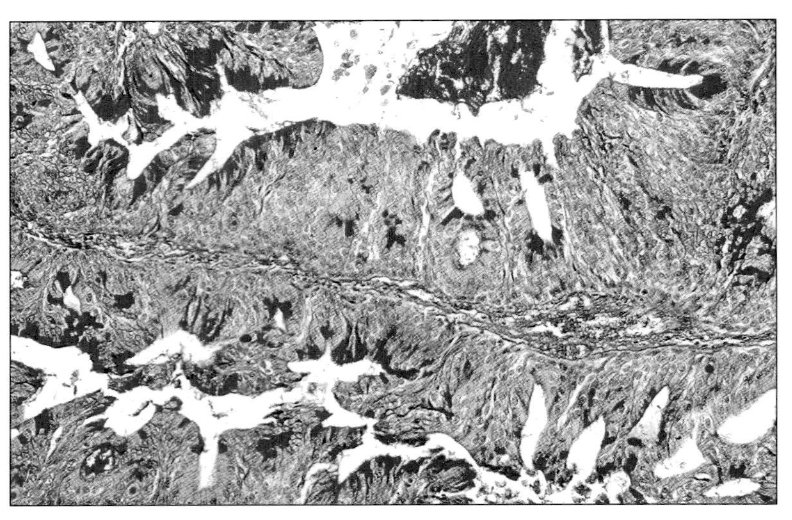

Fig. 11.256 Glandular metaplasia found in papillary urothelial carcinoma, low grade and stained with mucicarmine.

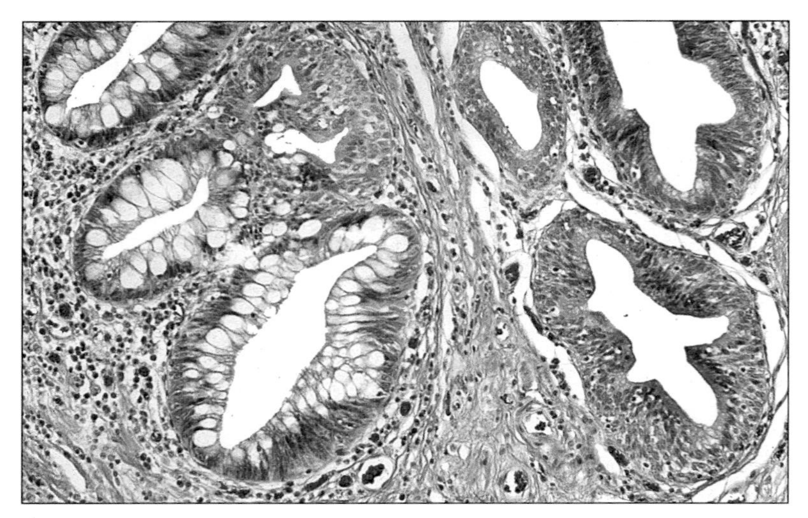

Fig. 11.254 Chronic cystitis-associated cystitis glandularis and colonic metaplasia of the urothelium.

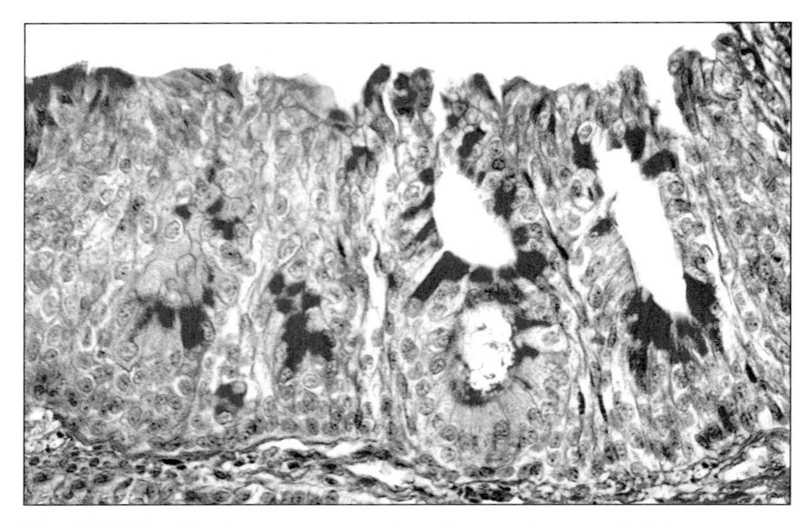

Fig. 11.257 Glandular metaplasia found in papillary urothelial carcinoma, low grade, stained with mucicarmine. A higher magnification.

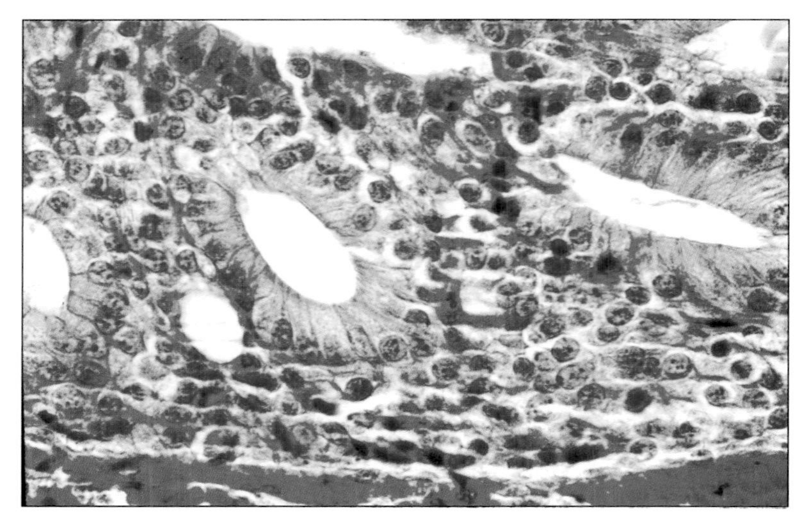

Fig. 11.255 Glandular metaplasia found in papillary urothelial carcinoma of low grade.

increase in frequency with age and occur predominantly at the trigone.

- Experimentally, they can be produced by chronic irritation of the urothelium and may represent a regenerative or reparative phenomenon.
- When the bladder contains a lot of these lesions, it may be difficult cystoscopically to differentiate these lesions from low-grade urothelial neoplasms such as inverted papilloma. However, benign urothelial proliferations are never found in the muscular wall of the bladder in the absence of congenital anomalies or previous surgery.
- Cystitis glandularis is a sign of a stimulated urothelium, and regenerative activity may be accompanied by any type of metaplasia.
- The controversy over the premalignant potential of cystitis glandularis probably relates to the amount of

intestinal metaplasia within the lesions. When transitional cell epithelium is replaced by colonic-type glands, the degree of disturbance in normal growth is apparently great, and the risk of subsequent cancer probably increases over time.
- Cystitis glandularis harbors few if any goblet cells and no colonic glands.
- The benign nature of the very common lesion cystitis glandularis overshadows the slightly increased risks associated with the rare metaplastic disease, intestinal metaplasia.
- Any bladder injury eliciting a prolonged regenerative response may result in the growth of proliferations of Brunn nests, metaplasias, or cancers.

Cystitis cystica[218–221]

- This differs from cystitis glandularis only in the prominence of dilated glandular lumina.
- Cystitis cystica represents part of the spectrum of changes associated with proliferations of Brunn nests and may be a normal variant in some individuals. The cysts are a result of obstruction to luminal outflow in Brunn nests and/or cystitis glandularis.
- The lining cells may be compressed to form a single layer of columnar, cuboidal, or flat cells.
- Calcification is a rare complication but can occur among patients infected with *S. haematobium* parasites.

Follicular cystitis[222]

- This involves lymphoid follicles complete with germinal centers in the lamina propria. The follicles are most numerous in the trigone.
- They elevate and attenuate the overlying urothelium and appear cystoscopically as submucosal nodules.
- Extensive follicle formation has been associated with *Salmonella* infection.
- The overlying urothelium often contains cells with many of the features of dysplasia.
- Dysplastic changes can be seen in any situation in which the urothelium is elevated into the bladder lumen.
- These dysplastic reactions are rarely so severe as to suggest an in situ neoplasm.

Bullous cystitis[76]

- Lamina propria edema is very common after physical trauma that is produced by indwelling catheters and radiation therapy. It can also be associated with neoplasms.
- If the edema is localized, the overlying urothelium may be elevated into the lumen, creating polypoid cystitis.
- Protrusion of urothelium into the bladder lumen may result in the appearance of slightly dysplastic, hyperplastic, or metaplastic cells.
- The lamina propria may contain multinucleated cells in response to various stimuli: surgery, topical chemotherapy, and radiation therapy.
- The giant cells are distinctive where they have star-shaped rather than rounded cell borders. The nuclei tend to cluster in one area rather than being arranged around the periphery. When numerous giant cells occur, the condition has been called giant cell cystitis. These cells are probably reactive fibroblasts, but both endothelial and histiocytic origins have been postulated.

Encrusted cystitis (calcareous, calculous cystitis)[223]

- If the bladder is infected with urea-splitting organisms, the urothelium may ulcerate, and salts of calcium phosphate and/or calcium magnesium phosphate may be embedded in the ulcer.

Emphysematous cystitis (pneumatosis cystica)[223,224]

- Gas-filled cysts are in the bladder.
- This lesion is identical to pneumatosis cystoides intestinalis of the bowel and results from trauma, fistulas, and/or bacterial infections.
- It occurs in patients with diabetes mellitus, neurogenic bladder, or chronic urinary infections. *Escherichia coli* and *Enterobacter aerogenes* are the most common infectious agents, but there are rare cases associated with *Clostridium perfringens* infections.
- The cysts may be lined with multinucleated giant cells.

Hemorrhagic cystitis[225,226]

- Focal or diffuse hemorrhages of the lamina propria resulting from indwelling catheters, exposure to organic chemicals, drugs, and viruses.
- There is usually urothelial denudation with lamina propria hemorrhage and inflammation.
- Rarely, bizarre urothelial cells may appear.

Eosinophilic cystitis[227]

- Bladder infiltration by eosinophils has been reported in individuals with asthma, allergies, eosinophilic gastroenteritis, periarteritis nodosa, systemic lupus erythematosus, prostatic hyperplasia, bladder trauma, neurogenic bladder, and carcinoma.

- The infiltrate is usually diffuse but may be nodular, masquerading as a neoplasm.
- Leukocytic infiltrates rich in eosinophils are common after transurethral resection.
- The process can be self-limiting but is usually chronic.
- Cystoscopy may reveal erythema, edema, bladder wall thickening, discrete masses, or mucosal ulcers, depending on the severity and age of the process.

Histologic pathology

- A polymorphous infiltrate rich in eosinophils but also including lymphocytes, plasma cells, histiocytes, giant cells, and mast cells has been described in the lamina propria, between muscle fascicles, and even in the distal ureters.
- Bladders may be fibrotic and contracted.
- Pathologists may find *eosinophilic cystitis* a useful term for bladder tissues having a transmural chronic leukocytic infiltrate, fibrosis, and focal necrosis of the muscularis propria.

PSEUDOSARCOMATOUS FIBROMYXOID TUMOR–INFLAMMATORY PSEUDOTUMOR (PFMT–IP) AND POSTOPERATIVE SPINDLE CELL NODULE (PSCN) (Figs 11.258–11.264)[228–238]

- These are myofibroblastic proliferations that occasionally arise in the genitourinary tracts of both sexes.
- These lesions differ slightly in their reported sex frequency, histology, and immunohistochemistry but are essentially the same in their histogenesis, cell type, and biologic behavior.

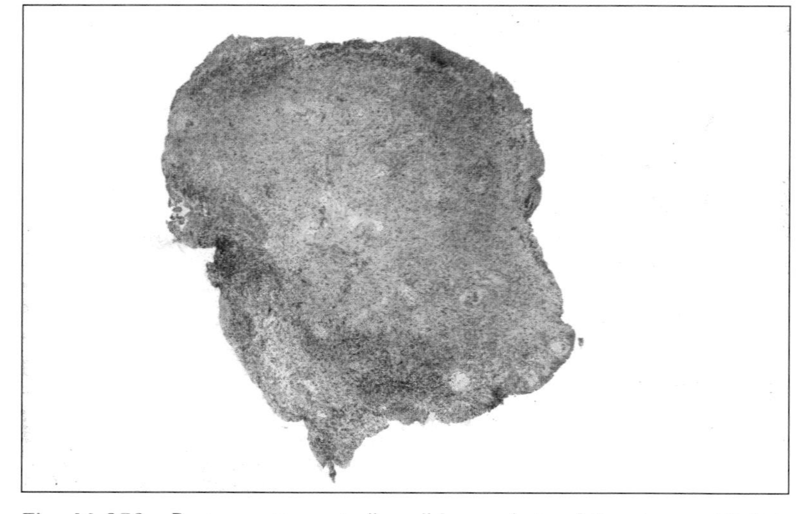

Fig. 11.258 Postoperative spindle cell hyperplasia of the stroma. Digital scan of the whole glass slide. Numerous spindle cells that are cytokeratin-negative are present. There is a history of previous surgery on the bladder.

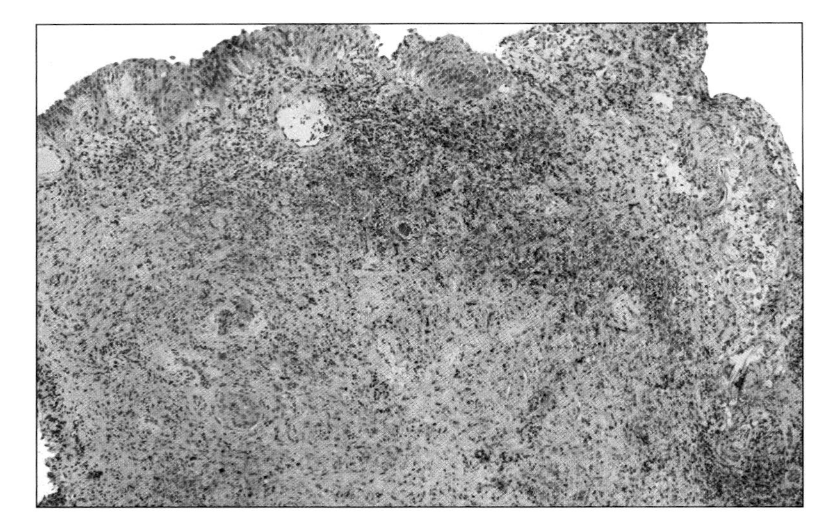

Fig. 11.259 Postoperative spindle cell tumor or hyperplasia of the stroma.

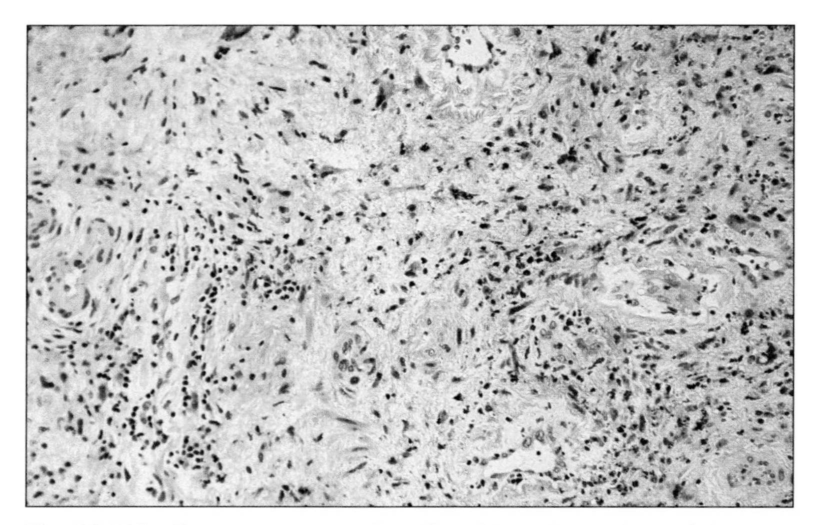

Fig. 11.260 Postoperative spindle cell nodule or hyperplasia of the stroma. There are areas of hemosiderin pigment.

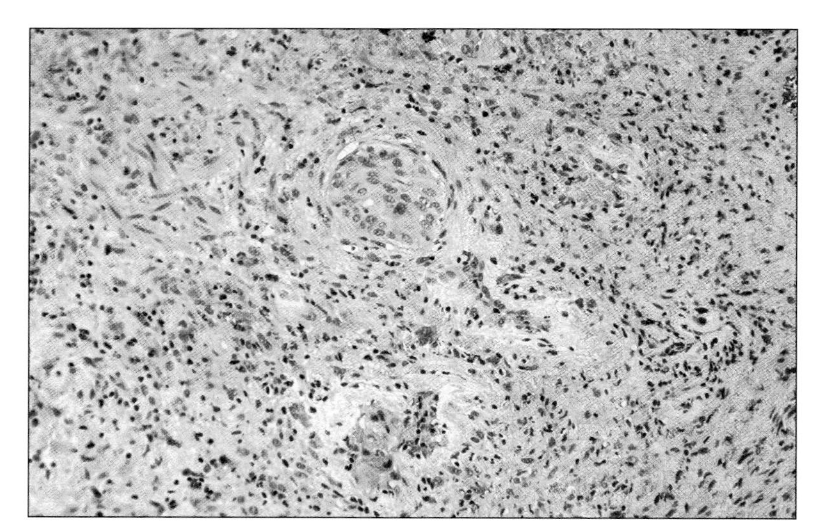

Fig. 11.261 Postoperative spindle cell nodule or hyperplasia of the stroma. As well as areas of hemosiderin pigment, an entrapped island of urothelium that is not neoplastic is present.

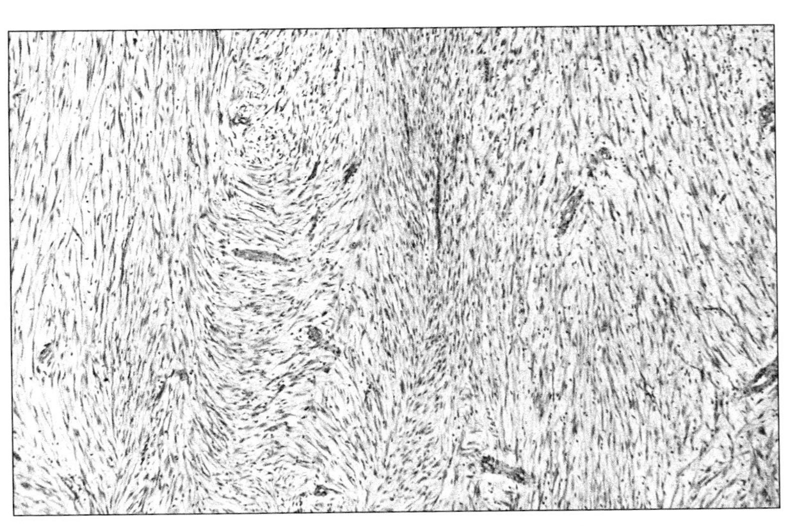

Fig. 11.262 Inflammatory myofibroblastic spindle cell tumor. Cytokeratin stains are negative. There are no areas of hemosiderin pigment and no areas of entrapped island urothelium. There is no history of previous trauma or surgery.

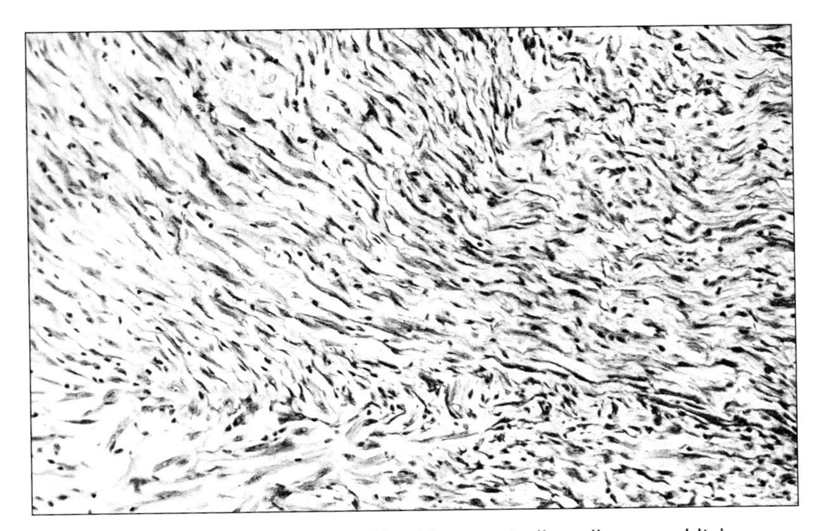

Fig. 11.263 Inflammatory myofibroblastic spindle cell tumor. Higher magnification. Cytokeratin stains are negative.

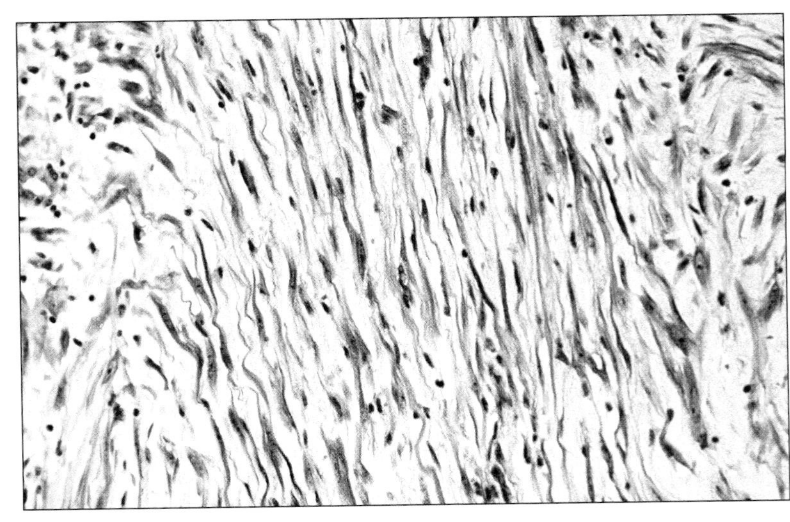

Fig. 11.264 Inflammatory myofibroblastic spindle cell tumor, again at higher magnification. The pattern is like a tissue culture growth of fibroblasts.

- PSCN occurs only after tissue injury, whereas PFMT–IP appears de novo.
- PSCN is rare but most often appears in the prostatic fossa within a few months of a transurethral resection for prostatism.
- Surgery for prostatism most likely accounts for the predominance of this lesion in men.
- Most tumors are less than 1 cm in their greatest dimension and are poorly circumscribed.

Histopathology

- Most PSCNs resemble nodular or proliferative fasciitis.
- Characteristic changes include a fascicular growth pattern, uniform but marked cellularity, a scattered leukocytic infiltrate, and numerous mitoses.
- Histologic variations may occur, and PSCNs may infiltrate adjacent stroma and muscle, but the differential diagnosis from sarcoma is not a problem, especially when there is previous surgery or trauma.
- Many cases of PFMT–IP in the female genital tract in young girls have been reported, and in the bladder the lesions have ordinarily arisen at the dome.
- Histopathology tends to resemble a tissue culture, with myofibroblasts associated with abundant thin-walled blood vessels.
- Variations in histology are common but with a wider range of nuclear pleomorphism than occurs in PSCN.

Gross pathology

- PFMT–IPs are large, and infiltration of the adjacent muscularis propria is common.
- Necrosis is also common, although it does not involve the bladder wall muscles.
- It can be separated from a sarcoma by lack of significant nuclear pleomorphism, lack of bizarre mitoses, and absence of necrosis at the interface between the lesion and the adjacent detrusor muscles.
- Most PFMT–IPs can be distinguished from well-differentiated myosarcomas.

MALAKOPLAKIA (Figs 11.265-11.268)[239-247]

- Malakoplakia has been found in individuals aged 6 weeks to 96 years but is much more common in adults than in children.
- The male-to-female ratio is 1:4.
- Most patients complain of bladder irritability and hematuria, but symptoms are nonspecific.
- At cystoscopy, lesions are most common at the bladder base, where they appear as soft, light brown or yellow

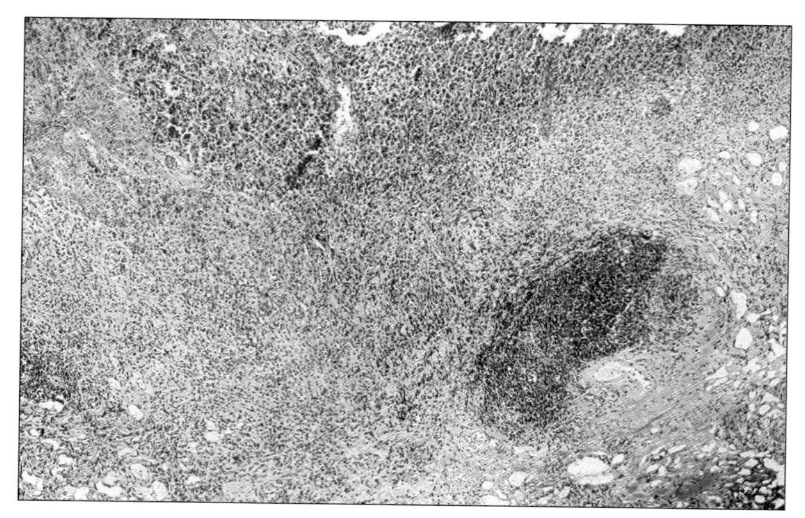

Fig. 11.265 Chronic granulomatous cystitis (malakoplakia) associated with numerous histiocytes. Low magnification.

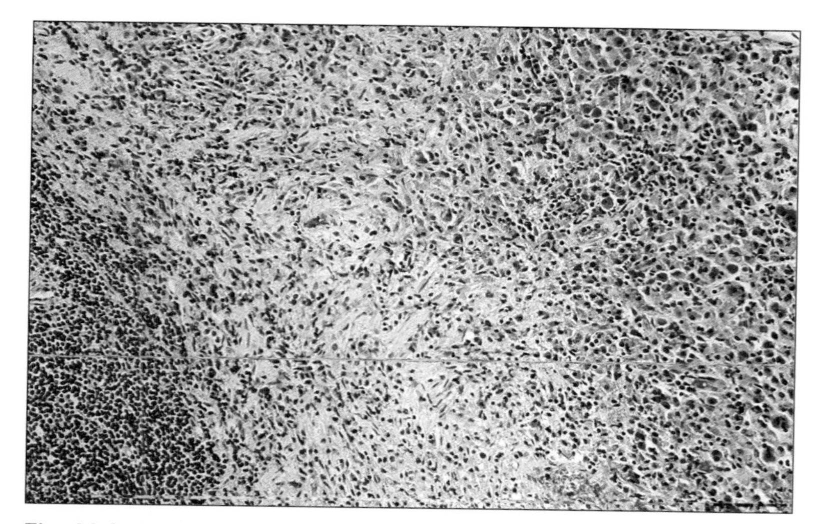

Fig. 11.266 Chronic granulomatous cystitis (malakoplakia) associated with numerous eosinophilic histiocytes that are not multinucleated. See figures 11.267 and 11.268 for higher magnifications of this figure.

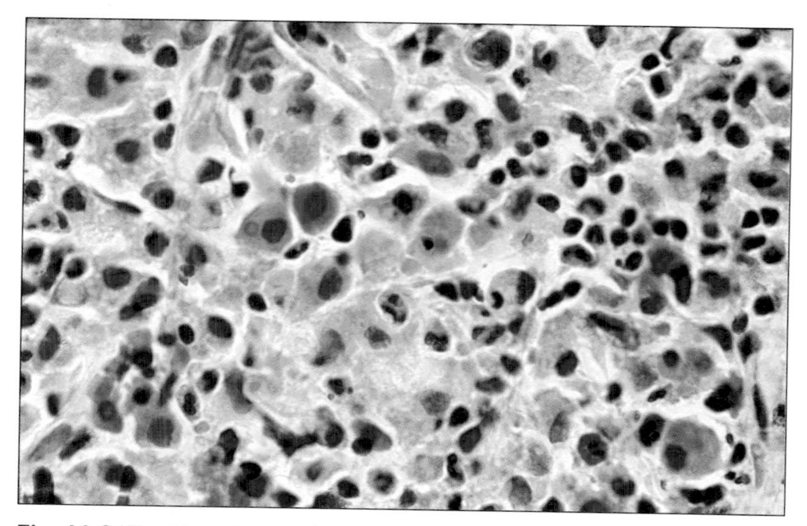

Fig. 11.267 Chronic granulomatous cystitis (malakoplakia) associated with numerous eosinophilic histiocytes that are not multinucleated. Under higher magnification, they can be seen to contain cytoplasmic inclusions, which are Michaelis–Gutmann bodies.

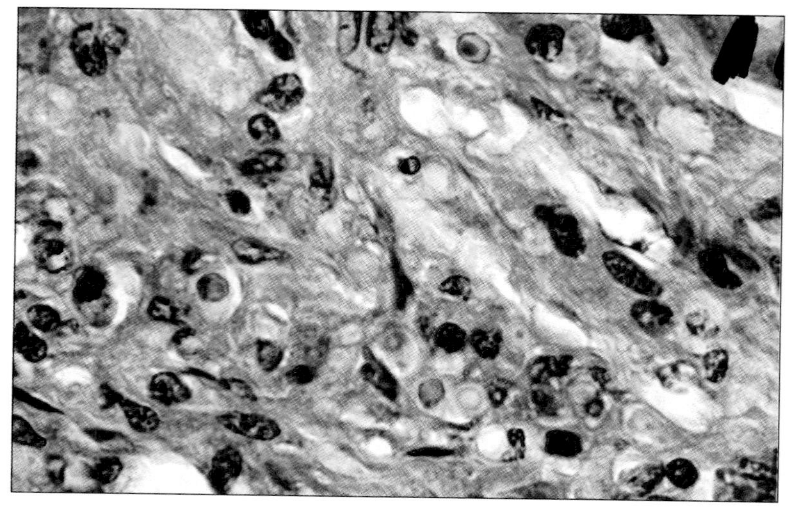

Fig. 11.268 Chronic granulomatous cystitis (malakoplakia) associated with numerous eosinophilic histiocytes that are not multinucleated. Blue Michaelis–Gutmann bodies under higher magnification.

plaques or nodules with erythematous borders and occasionally umbilicated centers.
- Malakoplakia has been identified throughout the genitourinary system. The bladder has been involved in 69% of cases, ureters in 19%, renal pelvis and ureteropelvic junctions in 22%, and urethras in 5%.
- Malakoplakia is a host reaction to chronic infection manifested by accumulation of histiocytes and other inflammatory elements appearing grossly as soft yellow plaques or nodules.
- Subsequent researchers have suggested a variety of etiologic factors and pathogenetic mechanisms, including infections with abnormal strains of bacteria.
- There is an inability of histiocytes to kill bacteria.
- There is an inability of tissue monocytes to expel lysosomes containing partially digested bacteria.
- The only consistent etiologic factor has been the relationship of malakoplakia to bacterial infection, predominantly with *E. coli*.

Histopathology

- The overlying urothelium is intact.
- As they age, lesions may become firm, fungating, ulcerated, and associated with ureteral strictures.
- Malakoplakia occurs in the lamina propria, where it consists of sheets of histiocytes (von Hansemann cells) intermixed with variable numbers of lymphocytes, plasma cells, neutrophils, and eosinophils.
- Well-delineated granulomas and giant cells are unusual, despite the usual classification of malakoplakia as a granulomatous disease.
- The inflammatory process progresses very slowly, and fibrosis is not a prominent feature in most cases.

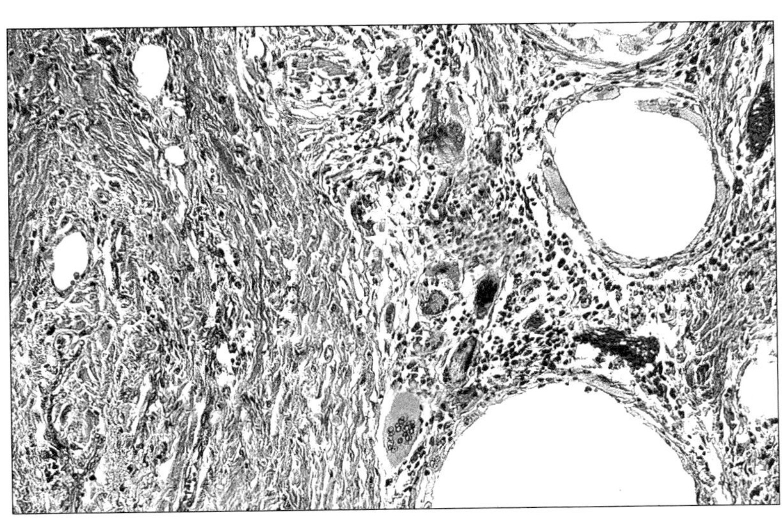

Fig. 11.269 Chronic granulomatous cystitis associated with foreign bodies and foreign body giant cell reaction. This is usually the result of previous surgery.

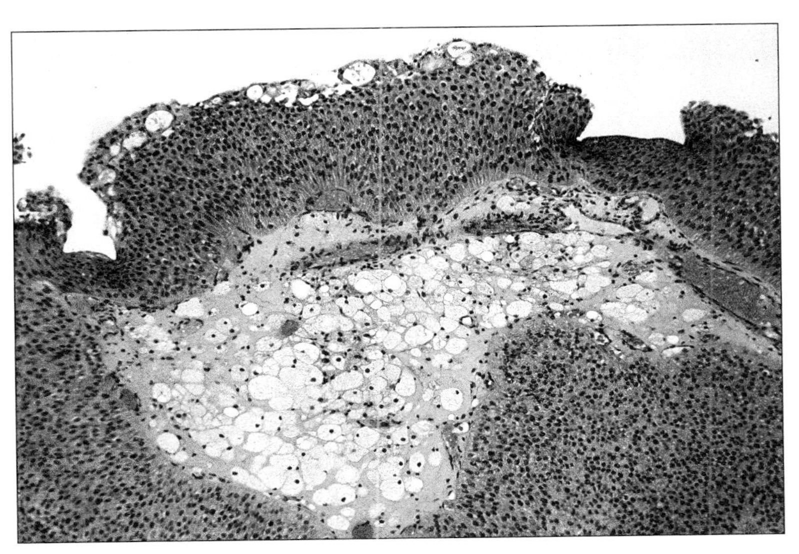

Fig. 11.270 Chronic granulomatous cystitis-associated xanthoma cells. This created a mass in the bladder wall. There was an associated urothelial hyperplasia.

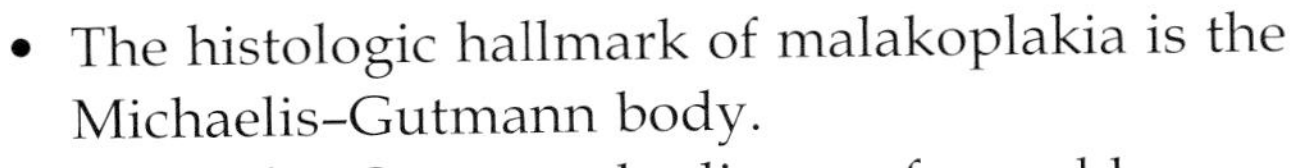

- The histologic hallmark of malakoplakia is the Michaelis–Gutmann body.
- Michaelis–Gutmann bodies are formed by mineralization of the phagolysosomes of histiocytes. Deposition of iron and calcium phosphate (apatite) probably occurs on a nidus of partially digested bacteria.
- Michaelis–Gutmann bodies may be intracellular or extracellular, range in size from 2 to 10 μm, and often have a target-like appearance, with a central density surrounded by a lucent space enclosed by a ring.
- These structures are usually slightly basophilic with hematoxylin and eosin, and stain positively with periodic acid–Schiff, von Kossa, Prussian blue, alizarin red, and Gomori reagents.

XANTHOGRANULOMATOUS INFLAMMATION (Figs 11.269–11.276)

- The few documented cases have been in men 16–51 years old.
- Most cases of xanthogranulomatous inflammation have been associated with urachal adenomas.
- Pathologically, the lesions resemble those of malakoplakia, but they lack the characteristic Michaelis–Gutmann bodies.
- They have more Touton-type giant cells and exhibit cholesterol clefts.

PLASMA CELL GRANULOMA

- This presents as a large, moderately well-circumscribed mass involving the entire bladder wall and adjacent soft tissue but sparing the urothelium.

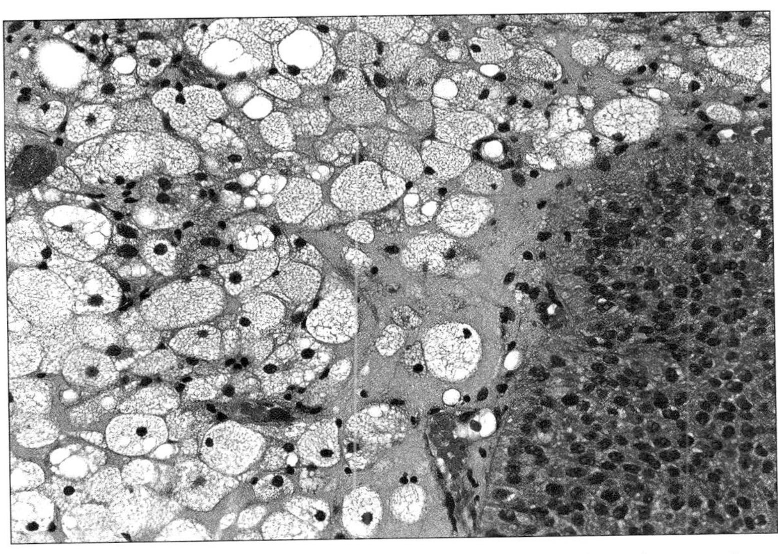

Fig. 11.271 Chronic granulomatous cystitis-associated xanthoma cells. A higher magnification of Fig. 11.270.

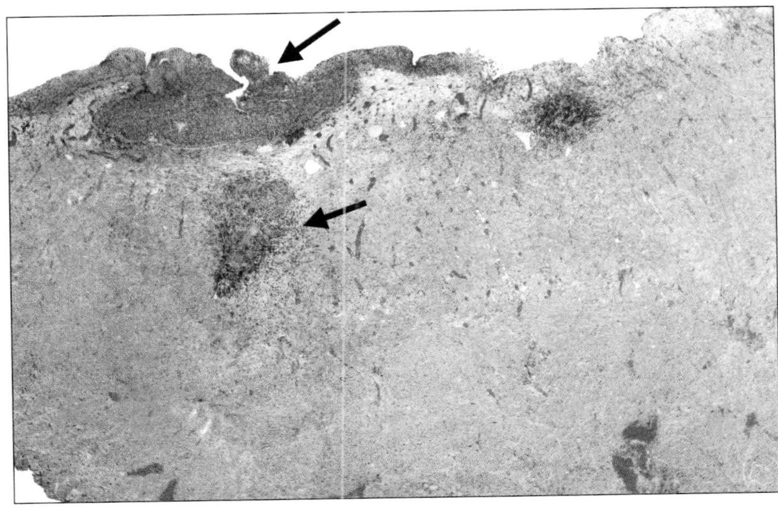

Fig. 11.272 Granulomatous cystitis-associated papilloma. There is a foreign body giant cell reaction beneath the papillary tumor.

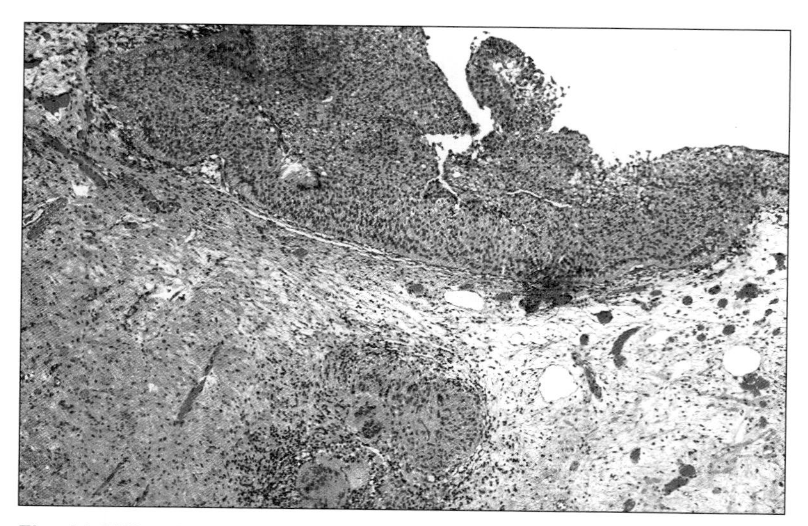

Fig. 11.273 Granulomatous cystitis-associated papilloma. A higher magnification of Fig. 11.272.

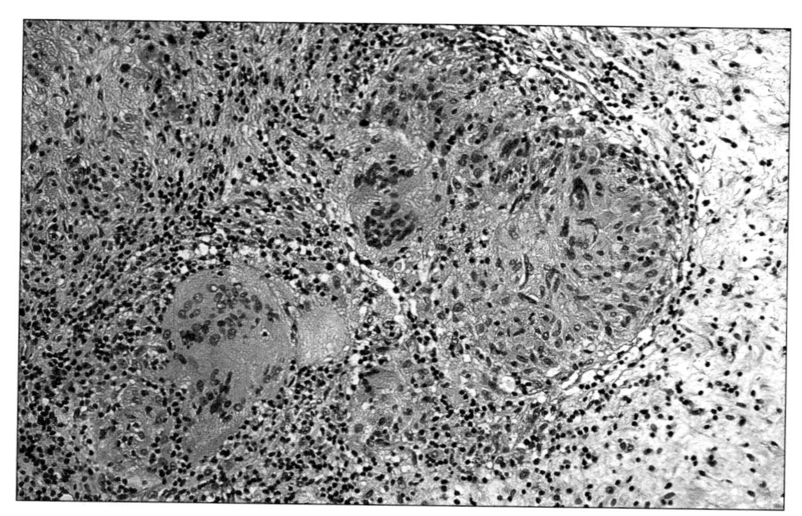

Fig. 11.274 Granulomatous cystitis-associated papilloma. A higher magnification of Fig. 11.272.

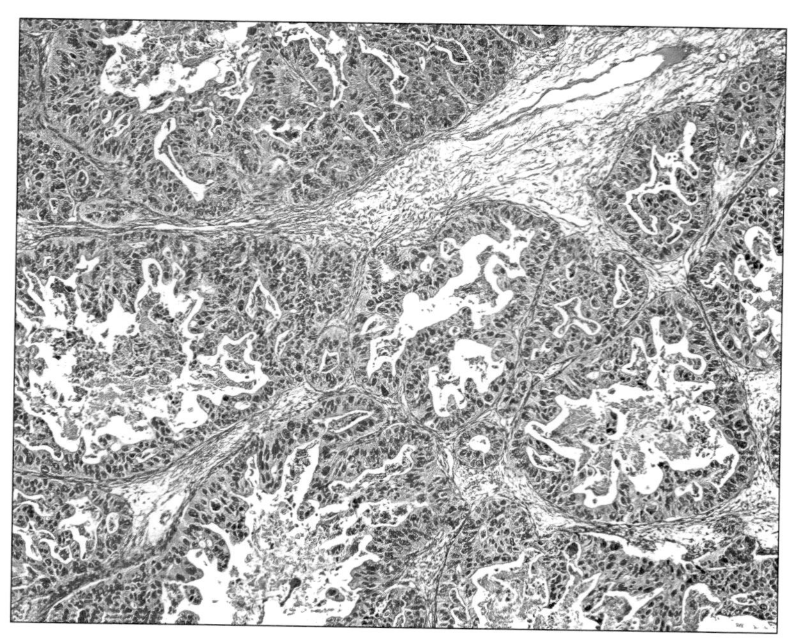

Fig. 11.275 Granulomatous cystitis-associated Crohn disease. This is very similar to Fig. 11.274. In this case, it was also associated with an adenocarcinoma of the small bowel, of which this is an example.

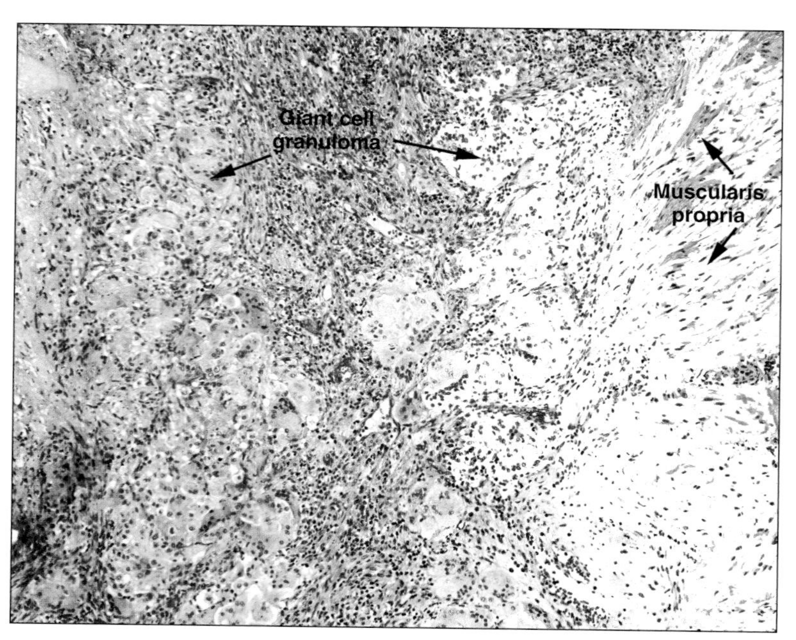

Fig. 11.276 Granulomatous cystitis-associated Crohn's disease. This is very similar to the granulomatous area in Fig. 11.274. In this case, the granulomatous reaction produced a mass clinically, which was believed to be an extension of the adenocarcinoma from the intestine.

Histopathology

- The lesion was composed of an almost pure population of polyclonal plasma cells intermixed with fibrous tissue.

INTERSTITIAL CYSTITIS[248–258]

- Interstitial cystitis (Hunner ulcer, elusive ulcer, paracystitis, cystitis lymphopathia) is an uncommon disease.
- The entity has been poorly defined clinically.
- Clinically, this is a primary bladder disorder characterized by:
  a history of intermittent or continuous suprapubic or retropubic pain of over 6 months' duration;
  urinary frequency, urgency, dysuria, or hematuria in the absence of urinary tract infection;
  mucosal erythema with blanching and fissuring during luminal distension or linear ulceration, and scarring.
- Etiology: infection, trauma, and structural defects in bladder mucosa have all been implicated.
- The female-to-male ratio varies up to 11:1. It is most common among middle-aged white women.
- Laboratory tests have been important primarily in excluding urinary tract infections and urothelial CIS. The fluorescent antinuclear antibody test is positive in low titer in approximately 50% of patients, but the significance of this finding is obscure.
- Two different histopathologic forms of interstitial cystitis can be seen. Both forms spare the trigone but are found in bladder tissues in all other parts.

Ulcer

- Ulcer form (Hunner ulcer) is characterized by:
  wedge-shaped mucosal ulcers associated with granulation tissue, hemorrhage, and detached fragments of urothelium;
  intense mononuclear infiltrate lymphocytes, and plasma and mast cells in the lamina propria;
  scattered, interstitial infiltrate in the muscular wall surrounding blood vessels and nerves.

Non-ulcer

- Fissures, cracks, and ruptures of the urothelium without significant inflammation.
- Hemorrhage in the adjacent lamina propria; this may not always be found.
- An increased number of mast cells is not constantly identified.
- In bladder biopsies evaluated for interstitial cystitis, urothelial CIS should be excluded. This can be done by tissue and urinary cytology assessment.

Interstitial cystitis is a clinical syndrome, and its diagnosis requires assessment of multiple factors, of which the histopathologic changes in the bladder are only a part.

INFECTIONS OF BLADDER

BACTERIA

- The most common specific etiologic agents associated with cystitis are bacteria.
- Bacterial colonization of urine is asymptomatic, especially in schoolchildren. Its prevalence has been documented as 1.2% in girls and 0.03% in boys.
- The frequency of bacteriuria increases with age, reaching levels of 3–7% in adult women compared with 0.5% in men. After middle age, urinary tract infection rates increase in men because of bladder outlet obstruction secondary to nodular prostatic hyperplasia.
- The histopathologic features are inflammation, hyperemia, edema, infiltration of leukocytes, fibrin deposition, capillary proliferation, and fibrosis. This occurs after any bacterial infection.
- These features may be arrested at any stage of its development.
- Recognizing various stages or degrees of severity of the inflammatory process and describing them as if they were specific pathologic entities or manifestations of specific bacterial infections, such as suppurative cystitis, ulcerative cystitis, and gangrenous cystitis, has added little to our understanding of bacterial infections of the bladder.
- Organisms can be much better identified by culture of the urine than by examination of the tissue. Early stages of infection, i.e. bacterial colonization and adherence, are often asymptomatic and usually unassociated with abnormalities at the light microscopic level. Even when severe reactions appear histologically, knowledge of the pathology is rarely an important factor in determining the treatment.
- The normal urinary bladder is resistant to infection. The mucopolysaccharide coating of the urothelium may mechanically entrap organisms, impeding adherence to the mucosa and facilitating removal during voiding.
- Bacterial cystitis is associated with intestinal flora (*E. coli*) carried directly from the gastrointestinal tract. The concentration of bacteria necessary to cause disease is unclear. Most experts agree that fewer than 100 000 colonies per milliliter can be pathogenic.
- Bladder infections are more common in the presence of certain predisposing factors. The shorter female urethra has long been cited as the primary reason for greater urinary tract infection rates in this group. Any injury, malformation, or obstructive process may prevent complete emptying and increases the likelihood of urinary tract infection. Among the most common of these conditions are neurogenic bladder and nodular prostatic hyperplasia. Foreign bodies such as stones and catheters can be a nidus on which bacteria can grow, as well as an agent of mechanical destruction of the bladder mucosa, providing direct access of urinary material to the bladder wall.

Actinomycosis

- This is a rare bladder infection caused by *Actinomyces israelii*.
- Bladder involvement usually occurs via direct extension from primary infections of the pelvic organs.
- The usual presentation is that of a moderately circumscribed mass centered in the lamina propria attenuating the overlying mucosa.
- The gross pathology is of a tumor that is firm and pale gray, and resembles carcinoma.
- On gross sectioning of the specimen, the characteristic yellow 'sulfur' granules are visible.
- Histopathology: the actinomycetes often exist as tangled masses lying in abscesses surrounded by organizing and chronic inflammation. Gram stains reveal central Gram-positive 'mycelia' with Gram-negative terminal clubs.
- The clinical course may be complicated by formation of fistulas.

Nocardia asteroides

- The urine may be colonized by *Nocardia asteroides*.
- The patients have usually been immunosuppressed or had conditions such as diabetes mellitus that predispose them to chronic infections.

Chlamydia (*C. trachomatis*) and *Mycoplasma* (*M. hominis*, *M. urealyticum*)

- These organisms can be cultured from bladder urine.
- They are more important pathogens in the urethra, kidney, and genital system. There is an increased tendency toward urinary stones in patients with mycoplasmal infections.
- Chlamydiae have been identified by both culture and immunohistochemistry in inflamed bladders.
- The histopathologic changes are nonspecific.

Tuberculosis[258]

- This involves the urinary tract through the kidney, with bladder involvement being the result of passage of tubercle bacilli in the urine.
- Tuberculosis is not associated with bladder cancer therapy.
- Tubercular lesions can also be associated with topical therapy using bacillus Calmette–Guérin.
- Non-iatrogenic bladder tuberculosis is more common in women than in men (2:1).
- Onset is insidious, with most patients complaining of frequency without pain or hematuria.
- Detection is best accomplished by culture of five early-morning urine samples. Bladder biopsies for the diagnosis of tuberculosis are not currently recommended in the urologic literature.
- Mucosal ulcers occur early and are usually the primary cystoscopic finding.
- Tuberculosis of the urinary bladder initially centers in the lamina propria around the ureteral orifices, where it appears as an erythematous area cystoscopically.
- The disease progresses through all the stages of inflammation, with eventual fibrosis and bladder contracture.
- Granulomas are not cystoscopically visible and can present rarely as a space-occupying mass.

Histopathology

- The earliest lesions consist of only denudation and edema of the lamina propria.
- The more characteristic early lesions consist of superficial necrosis with underlying acute and chronic inflammation, as well as capillary proliferation rather than typical tubercles with central caseous necrosis surrounded by epithelioid histiocytes, lymphocytes and with Langhans giant cells.
- Progressive lesions involve larger areas of mucosa as well as the bladder wall and contain more fibrous tissue, but the superficial ulcers tend to persist.
- Accurate histologic diagnosis depends on the identification of tubercle bacilli in tissues.
- If untreated, fistulas may form or the bladder may become contracted and even rupture.
- Even though there is an initial paraureteral location of the lesions, ureteral obstruction is a late phenomenon.

Syphilis

- It rarely involves the urinary bladder and then only in the secondary and tertiary forms.
- The clinical signs are nonspecific and reflect neither the onset nor the severity of the disease.
- The organism *Treponema pallidum* has not been identified in the bladder.
- Syphilitic bladder lesions can occur either as papillomatous reactions of the urothelium and lamina propria, or as gummas with a predilection for the trigone and ureteral orifices.
- Gummas range in size from a few millimeters to more than 5 cm; the larger ones occupy the entire thickness of the bladder wall. Although not well described histologically, the gummas have a necrotic core, an ulcerated surface, and are similar to granulomatous inflammation characteristic of gummas elsewhere.

FUNGI[259]

- *Candida* species (monilia, thrush) account for almost all human fungal infections of the urinary bladder.
- Several types of *Candida* organisms have been cultured from the genitourinary tract, but *Candida albicans* is by far the most common.
- Organisms gain access from the intestines, where they make up part of the normal flora, and spread to the genitourinary tract via the lymphatics and bloodstream.
- Patients may be at increased risk of candidal infection in the following situations:
  antibiotic therapy, especially when given with aminoglycosides and cephalosporins;
  indwelling catheters;
  diabetes mellitus;
  cirrhosis;
  steroid or immunosuppressive therapy.
- *Candida* organisms are commonly found in urinary specimens and have been cultured from the bladders of

a small percentage of healthy asymptomatic individuals of both sexes.
- *Candida* species may inhabit the urinary system for years without causing symptoms.
- Clinical infections are common when more than 10 000 colonies per milliliter of urine are present.
- Candidal cystitis cystoscopically appears as slightly elevated white or brown patches, which are intimately attached to the mucosa. They leave a hemorrhagic area when disturbed.
- Histologically, the urothelium is replaced by an inflammatory exudate containing characteristic yeast and pseudohyphal forms.
- Squamous metaplasia is common in urothelium adjacent to the lesions.
- Fungus balls (bezoars), ranging in size from less than 1 mm to 10 cm, are especially likely in candidal cystitis.

VIRUSES

- A variety of viruses of RNA and DNA (herpes group, papova) types have been identified in urinary cytology specimens.
- Patients with immunosuppressed renal or bone marrow allografts suffer from herpes genitalia. Despite the frequency of viruria in these patients, viral infections of the bladder itself have rarely been documented and histologic descriptions are sparse.
- Certain types of adenoviruses have been associated with a high frequency of hemorrhagic inflammation, especially among patients receiving cyclophosphamide.
- Papovaviruses are generally credited with the induction of squamous papillomas and condylomas of the urothelium.
- The relationship of viruses to bladder diseases centers on the ability of certain organisms to influence the development of urothelial carcinoma.

PARASITES

- Parasitic infestations of the urinary bladder are rare, with the exception of schistosomal and trichomonal infections.
- Factors predisposing to human parasitic disease, such as poor nutrition, sanitation, and personal hygiene, are prevalent in underdeveloped countries.
- Various organisms have been described and include:
  Schistosoma haematobium and *S. mansoni*;
  Trichomonas vaginalis;
  Echinococcus granulosus;
  Entamoeba histolytica;
  Wuchereria bancrofti;
  Strongyloides stercoralis;
  Toxocara canis.

SCHISTOSOMAL INFECTIONS (BILHARZIASIS)[260,261]

- *Schistosoma haematobium* has been a major health hazard in eastern Africa, the Middle East, and Southwest Asia for centuries.
- The urogenital tract is the preferred human habitat for *S. haematobium*, and bladder infections with this organism are common in endemic areas.
- The life cycle of the parasite worm has been well established. Briefly, adult trematode worms living in the urogenital tract of mammals lay eggs in multiple cycles.
  - The eggs are deposited into fresh water, where they swell and burst, releasing ciliated larvae (miracidia) that penetrate a type of snail living in the area. Asexual reproduction occurs in the snail, with the excretion of forked-tailed cercariae.
  - The cercariae penetrate the skin of humans standing in the water (usually tending crops irrigated by flooding techniques) and migrate to the urogenital tract.
  - Here they mature into adult worms and begin the cycle again.
- The first manifestations of *S. haematobium* infection usually occur as gross hematuria in pubescent children, accounting for the well-known description of Egypt by Napoleon's troops as 'the land of menstruating men'.
- The pathologic changes of *S. haematobium* infections are related to deposition of the eggs in the urinary bladder.
- Initially, there is edema and hyperemia in the lamina propria with elevation and attenuation of the overlying mucosa, appearing as reddened plaques or papules grossly.
- Various parts of the bladder may be involved, but there is a predilection for the trigone and ureteral orifices.
- As the eggs die, they become calcified and elicit a granulomatous tissue response characterized by typical foreign body cells. Early granulomas are rich in eosinophils, and the lesions are confined to the lamina propria until late in the disease.
- Superficial sandy patches (the calcified eggs) are the characteristic changes that occur in patients aged 10–30 years.
- The diagnosis is dependent on identification of *Schistosoma* eggs with terminal spines. With the continual deposition of parasitic eggs, the

granulomatous inflammation becomes widespread. As the lesions grow, they result in ulceration of the overlying mucosa and exposure of the bladder wall to bacterial infection.
- These inflammatory reactions heal with fibrosis and retraction, with subsequent diminution in bladder capacity and difficulties in voiding.
- There may be obstruction of the ureteral orifices with hydronephrosis, obstruction of the bladder neck and urethra, abscesses, and epithelial metaplasia and hyperplasia.
- There are significant epithelial abnormalities, often developing into carcinoma.

TRICHOMONAS (VAGINAL)

- *Trichomonas* is a common parasite usually found in the female genital tract, and male infection occurs by sexual transmission. The male urethra is involved, but bladder infections are rare.
- The organism, which is pear-shaped with anterior and posterior flagella, is easily identified in wet preparations or urinary cytology.
- There is an inability of the organisms to penetrate the undamaged mucosa. Histopathology reveals, on biopsy of the bladder, edema and hyperemia without leukocytic infiltration of the lamina propria. There is focal hyperplasia of the urothelium.

HYDATID CYSTS

- Hydatid cysts represent the larval forms of *Echinococcus granulosus*.
- The definitive host is the dog, with sheep as intermediary hosts. Most cases are reported from sheep-raising areas.
- In humans, the common site of infection is the kidney, but the bladder is involved when the scolices are excreted.
- Cysts grow slowly and may be asymptomatic for long periods. They are composed of the wall of the parasite and are surrounded by an inflammatory fibrous reaction.
- The diagnosis is readily made by radiography or computed tomography rather than biopsy.

AMEBIC CYSTITIS

- Amebic cystitis results from drinking water contaminated by *Entamoeba histolytica*. Bladder involvement is part of a disseminated disease pattern.
- The preferred human site of infection is the kidney, but the bladder is involved through the bloodstream.
- The organisms are most easily identified by examination of excreta rather than by biopsy of tissue.
- Similar to those lesions found in the rectum, the amebae cause shaggy ulcers with undermining of normal bladder mucosa.

WUCHERERIA

- *Wuchereria bancrofti* microfilariae can be identified in urine samples.
- The organisms gain access to the bladder by way of the lymphatics. In the bladder, they cause a nonspecific inflammatory reaction.
- Chyluria is an often-associated condition.

CHEMICAL CYSTITIS

Chemical cystitis has been associated with various chemicals, including formalin, turpentine, ether, and acetic acid.

- Formalin has been instilled directly into the bladder in doses of 1–10% for the treatment of unrelenting hemorrhage secondary to cyclophosphamide, radiation, or infiltrating carcinomas. If introduced into the bloodstream, formalin is metabolized to formic acid and formate, which exert toxic effects on multiple organs.
- Turpentine, when ingested either intentionally or accidentally, has its metabolic products excreted into the urine via the kidney. The combination of terpinol and glucuronic acid produces a distinct odor of violets in the urine. The effects on urothelium are generally reversible.
- Ether has been used to dissolve the balloons of Foley catheters when other means of deflation have failed. Prolonged contact of ether with the urothelium has resulted in permanent bladder dysfunction.
- Acetic acid has been instilled to control bladder infection, especially in patients on bladder catheterization programs. As with other chemicals, concentrations greater than recommended can produce adverse consequences.
- The pathologic effects of these chemicals and drugs are similar. All cause hemorrhagic necrosis of the urothelium, with marked edema and moderate leukocytic infiltration of lamina propria and underlying muscularis propria. These effects may be reversible or result in scarring, with reduced bladder

capacity and persistent frequency, dysuria, and suprapubic pain.

IMMUNE DISORDERS

- Bladder involvement has been reported in various systemic diseases:
  - Lupus erythematosus;
  - Progressive systemic sclerosis;
  - Rheumatoid arthritis;
  - Stevens–Johnson syndrome;
  - Chronic granulomatous disease of childhood;
  - Pemphigus vulgaris.
- The signs and symptoms of these diseases in the bladder usually occur with advanced disease.
- Primary manifestation of these disorders is not seen, and many patients with immune disorders have received drugs (e.g. cyclophosphamide) that obscure the relationship of the bladder pathology to the primary disease.

SYSTEMIC LUPUS ERYTHEMATOSUS

- Cystitis can occur in women over 50 years old who have advanced systemic disease.
- Clinical symptoms are similar to those of interstitial cystitis.
- The histopathology demonstrates a thickening of the bladder wall, with decreased luminal capacity and a chronic inflammatory infiltrate. Vascular lesions have not been identified with any consistency.

PROGRESSIVE SYSTEMIC SCLEROSIS (SCLERODERMA)

- Bladder involvement is a rare manifestation of advanced disease and may be found in patients with or without urinary symptoms.
- The bladder is thickened, and there is both lamina propria and interstitial fibrosis beyond what would be expected for patients of this age.

STEVENS–JOHNSON SYNDROME

- Urogenital mucosal involvement (primarily penis and urethra) is common in this rare disease characterized by systemic toxicity, erythema multiforme, and vesicular lesions of the mucous membranes.
- Bladder involvement is similar to that in the gastrointestinal tract.

CHRONIC GRANULOMATOUS DISEASE OF CHILDHOOD

- A genetic defect in the leukocytes, which cannot destroy phagocytized bacteria.
- This manifests itself in the urinary tract; young male patients have draining abscesses in the bladder. These are surrounded by granulomatous inflammation.

PEMPHIGUS VULGARIS

- This consists of a vesicular eruption of skin and mucous membranes characterized by dissolution of the intercellular cement substance, associated with circulating autoantibodies.
- Bladder lesions, which are rare, are never a primary manifestation of this disease. They are characterized by a nonspecific inflammation.

LICHEN PLANUS

- A chronic dermatosis with lymphocytic band-like dermal infiltrate beneath basal cell degeneration of the epidermis. It has been reported in the bladder of a patient with lichen planus of the skin.
- Seen in the glans penis and terminal urethra.
- A specific diagnosis of bladder involvement is probably not possible in the absence of the characteristic skin lesions.

METAPLASIA OF UROTHELIUM

Trauma, chemotherapy, surgery, and the above-mentioned infections may initiate morphologic changes in the urothelium that must be differentiated from morphologic patterns that are characteristic histologically of aggression. These include:

- squamous;
- intestinal;
- nephrogenic.

These are three common types of urinary bladder metaplasia.

Metaplasia of mature bone and cartilage, which are called osseous and cartilaginous metaplasia, respectively, can occur in urinary bladders.

- Metaplastic changes are a manifestation of a urothelial response to injurious stimuli. There is an increased risk for neoplasia.

- They are often seen in recurrent urinary tract infections.
- Metaplastic epithelium is associated with different proliferative reactions:
  cystitis glandularis et cystica;
  intestinal;
  nephrogenic.
- Metaplasia marks an epithelium as unstable or unregulated.
- Squamous carcinoma and adenocarcinoma can occur in association with metaplasias of a similar cell type in the urinary bladder.
- When a carcinogenic stimulus is applied to urothelium that responds abnormally, both metaplastic and neoplastic lesions occur simultaneously rather than sequentially. The fact that squamous carcinomas and adenocarcinomas occur much less frequently subsequent to metaplasia indicates that the metaplasias are not precursor lesions.

SQUAMOUS METAPLASIA[262–266]

- Squamous metaplasia (leukoplakia, vaginal metaplasia, trigonal cystitis, or pseudomembranous trigonitis) describes the histologic appearance. Keratinizing or nonkeratinizing squamous epithelium replaces portions of normal urothelium.
- Its clinical significance remains unclear.
- Keratinizing (cornifying) lesions apparently have a different biologic potential from that of nonkeratinizing (vaginal-type) epithelia. Nonkeratinizing vaginal-type epithelium is the usual finding. Squamous metaplasia is six times more frequent in women than in men.
- The incidence of squamous metaplasia in normal adult bladders varies from 36% to 72%. This type of metaplasia has not been observed in normal prepubertal females, nor is it often associated with inflammation.
- Squamous metaplasia associated with chronic irritation (caused by stones or indwelling catheters) is usually of the keratinizing type.
- Most lesions are uncovered incidentally during cystoscopy for other problems, and cystoscopically the areas of squamous metaplasia appear as irregular, opaque, pale gray, often roughened lesions.
- Although the entire urothelium is susceptible, squamous changes are most common in the trigone and tend to spare the ureteral orifices.
- Histopathology: lesions consist more often of stratified nonkeratinizing squamous epithelium rich in glycogen. Less frequently, there is keratosis, with or without a granular layer, and little or no cellular glycogen. Cells at the basal layers may have enlarged, irregular nuclei, but significant cellular atypia in the absence of invasive carcinoma is unusual.
- Metaplastic squamous cells exfoliated into urine cannot be consistently distinguished from vaginal epithelial cells in voided urine.
- The relationship of keratinizing squamous metaplasia to urothelial carcinoma is of more concern than that of nonkeratinizing cases.
- Urothelial carcinoma has developed in bladders harboring squamous metaplasia of the keratinizing type. It is keratinizing squamous metaplasia that is most often associated with sources of chronic irritation.
- The nonkeratinizing vaginal type of squamous metaplasia is apparently a benign lesion carrying little risk of future neoplasia.
- Squamous cell bladder cancers coexist with areas of squamous metaplasia, but the subsequent occurrence of cancer in a bladder with squamous metaplasia is unusual.
- Cancer risk is greatest when squamous metaplasia results from chronic irritation, such as from an indwelling catheter in patients with spinal cord injury.
- Almost all neoplasms arising after keratinizing squamous metaplasia are squamous carcinomas.
- Carcinomas associated with squamous metaplasia have had essentially the same prognosis as other high-grade bladder cancers.

INTESTINAL METAPLASIA[267–273]

- Intestinal metaplasia has the appearance of colonic-type glands and/or mucin-containing goblet cells in the bladder.
- It has also been called cystitis glandularis, glandular metaplasia, goblet cell metaplasia, cystitis glandularis of gastrointestinal type, mucous metaplasia, and aberrant gastrointestinal tissue.
- Goblet cells and/or small colonic glands are commonly mixed with proliferations of Brunn nests. This type of lesion has been called cystitis glandularis to emphasize the intestinal metaplasia.[267]
- Similar lesions occur in exstrophy or adjacent to bladder adenocarcinomas. In this instance, they are called intestinal or glandular metaplasia.
- The term *intestinal metaplasia* should be restricted to cases in which portions of the surface urothelium have been completely replaced by colonic glands. There may even be Paneth cells.
- Intestinal metaplasia is usually a focal phenomenon arising as a reactive process to urothelial injury.

- When the lesion is large enough, it appears cystoscopically as a glistening, erythematous, and mucin-secreting area in the bladder mucosa. However, most intestinal metaplasias are too small for endoscopic detection.
- Clinically detectable mucus in the urine is uncommon, because mucus is produced by the goblet cells, and these lesions are small. Cytologically benign columnar cells can occasionally be detected in urinary samples.
- Intestinal metaplasia is commonly seen in association with urothelial carcinomas of the adenocarcinomatous type, but urothelial adenocarcinomas occurring subsequent to intestinal metaplasia are rare. These rare tumors appear in patients over 70 years old who have long histories of bladder outlet obstruction and chronic urothelial irritation. This occurs in paraplegic patients and also in patients with longstanding exstrophy with or without closure.

NEPHROGENIC METAPLASIA[77–84]

- This is the result of a reactive process that may occur anywhere in urothelium-lined organs but is most common in the urinary bladder.
- It is also called nephrogenic adenoma, nephrogenic metaplasia, hamartoma, adenomatoid tumor, and adenomatoid metaplasia.
- Most investigators consider it to be of metaplastic origin, while others consider it to be a choristoma, hamartoma, or congenital anomaly.
- There is a constant relationship of nephrogenic metaplasia to urothelial injury in the forms of previous surgery, chronic irritation, chronic infection, or structural defects.
- Small areas of metaplasia are confused with urothelial regeneration or repair, and only the florid, tumorous conditions have been documented.
- Nephrogenic metaplasia is not a rare entity, and is twice as common in men as in women. It is found in patients aged between 3 weeks and 83 years.

DIFFERENTIAL DIAGNOSIS

Gross pathology

- Can appear as papillary or polypoid tumors similar to transitional cell carcinomas.
- They most often appear as single lesions at the bladder base.
- Multiple lesions can involve the lateral walls, dome, and ureteral orifices.

Histopathology

- Composed of papillary fronds, tubules, or both.
- Papillary components are exophytic, but the tubules lie predominantly in the lamina propria.
- Involvement of the muscular wall of the bladder is very rare.
- Nephrogenic metaplasia cells form a single layer lining the papulations and tubules. They are cuboidal cells with bland nuclei.
- Atypical nuclei usually appear in the tubular component and are focal.
- Nephrogenic metaplasia is distinguished from papillary carcinoma by its single layer of bland cells.
- Similar features can distinguish the tubular component from prostatic carcinoma. The cells of nephrogenic metaplasia react with antibodies to high molecular weight cytokeratins such as 34βE12 and do not react with antibodies to prostate-specific antigen or prostatic acid phosphatase.
- The nested variant of transitional cell carcinoma shares some features with nephrogenic metaplasia.
- Portions of the clear cell variant of adenocarcinoma may appear histologically indistinguishable from nephrogenic metaplasia.
- Recurrences after treatment for nephrogenic metaplasia have been documented.
- This type of metaplasia does not have carcinogenic potential.

ENDOMETRIOSIS (Figs 11.277–11.283)[274–281]

- The urothelial surface has the ability to undergo metaplasia to form the glandular lesions mentioned earlier. This is not the cause of endometriosis of the urinary bladder.

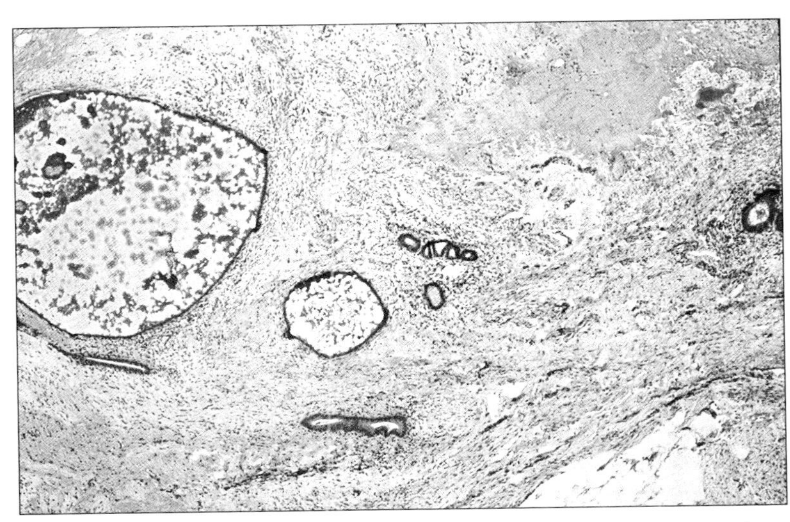

Fig. 11.277 Endometriosis. This produced a mass in the bladder and the ureter, which clinically was believed to be a urothelial tumor. On resection, it turned out to be endometriosis with fibrosis.

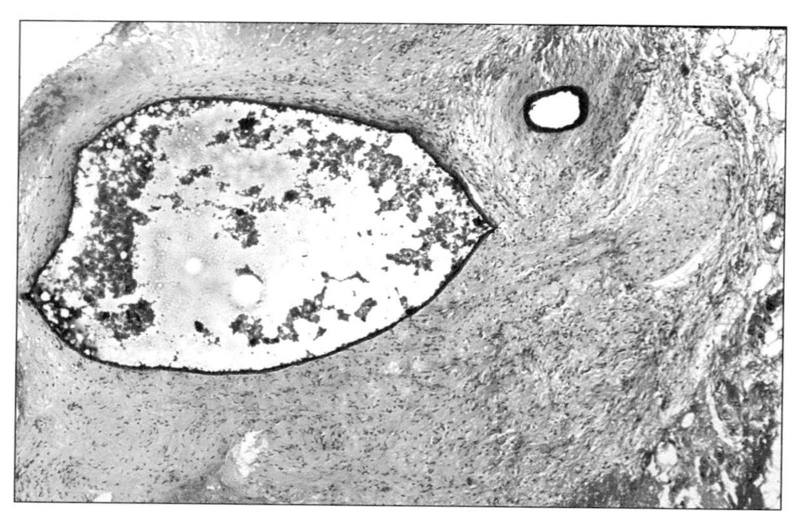

Fig. 11.278 Endometriosis. There are sometimes cysts filled with blood and sometimes with cloudy white fluid.

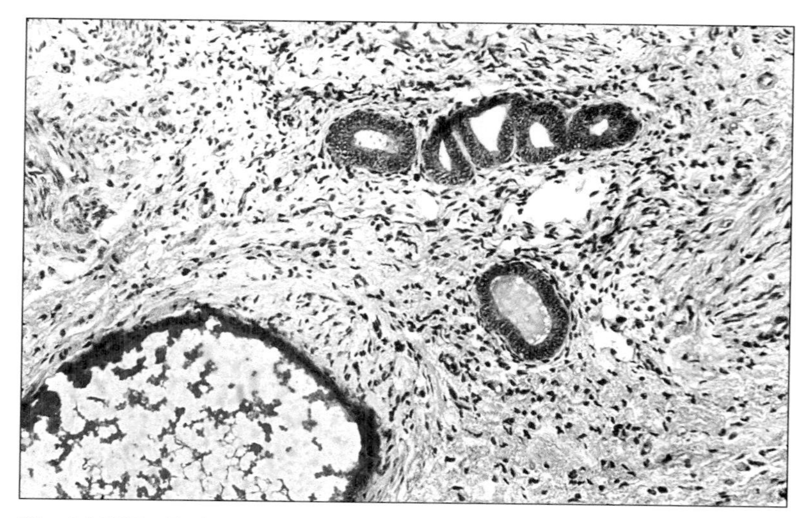

Fig. 11.279 Endometriosis. There is a cyst and endometrial glands surrounded in this instance by fibrosis and not endometrial stroma.

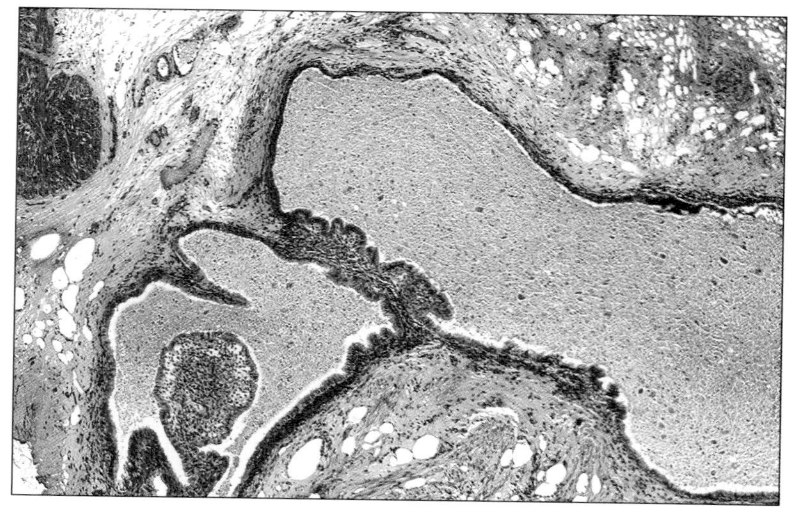

Fig. 11.280 Endometriosis. There are cysts filled with proteinaceous fluid. Endometrial glands are associated with endometrial stroma.

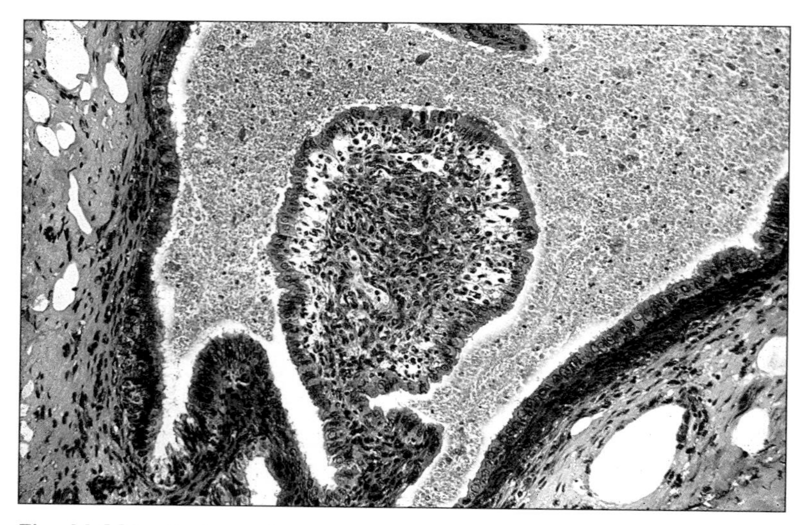

Fig. 11.281 Endometriosis. An endometrial papillary structure associated with endometrial glands and stroma.

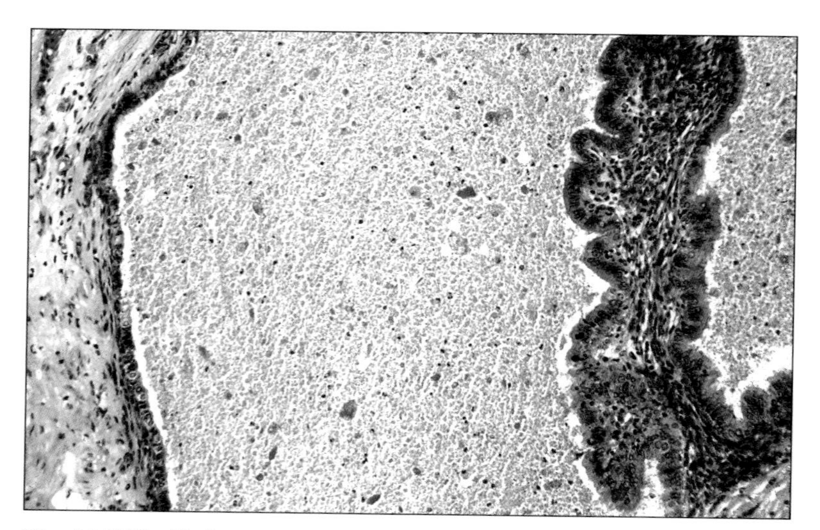

Fig. 11.282 Endometriosis. Endometrial epithelium associated with endometrial glands and stroma.

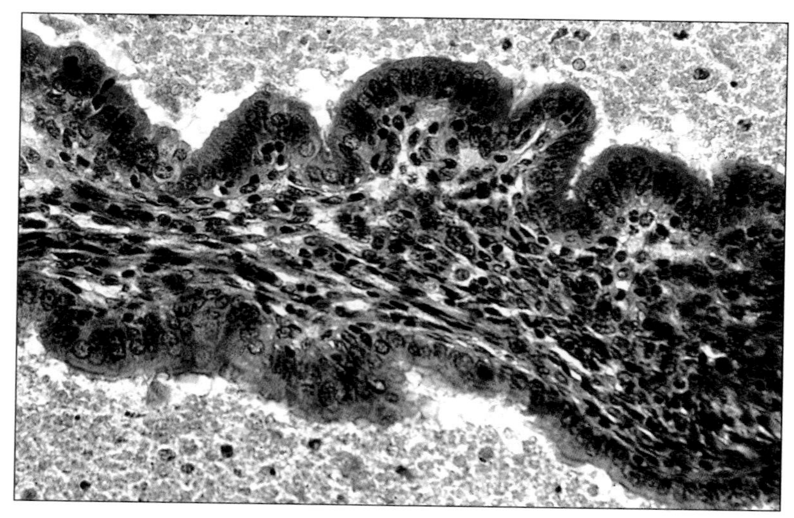

Fig. 11.283 Endometriosis. A higher magnification of Fig. 11.282. A cyst filled with proteinaceous fluid and endometrial epithelium associated with endometrial glands and stroma.

- It involves more commonly the urinary bladder but may involve other parts of the genitourinary system, such as the ureter.
- It affects women between the second and fifth decades but may be seen in postmenopausal women receiving exogenous estrogen therapy.
- Rare cases have been reported in men with prostate cancer receiving exogenous estrogen therapy.
- Clinically, the patient presents with suprapubic pain, frequency, and urgency, and occasionally with hematuria.
- By palpation or cystoscopic examination, there may be a mass.
- Histologically, the lesion is often seen in the superficial or deep layers of the bladder wall or in the adjacent perivesical soft tissue.
- The lesion resembles endometriosis elsewhere.
- The endometrium-like glands are often present with endometrial stromal cells.
- There may be old or recent hemorrhage.
- There may be only stroma or glands. When there are only glands, a differential diagnosis of an infiltrating carcinoma must be considered.

REFERENCES

1. Pow-Sang JM. Prostate cancer: of turtles, birds, and rabbits [editorial]. Cancer Control 1998; 5:483–484.
2. Wynder EL, Goldsmith R. The epidemiology of bladder cancer: a second look. Cancer 1977; 40:1246–1268.
3. Koss LG. Tumors of the urinary bladder. In: Atlas of tumor pathology, second series, part II, fascicle 8. Washington: Armed Forces Institute of Pathology; 1985.
4. Mostofi FK. Pathology of malignant tumors of urinary bladder. In: Cooper EH, Williams RE, eds. The biology and clinical management of bladder cancer. Oxford: Blackwell Scientific; 1975.
5. Murphy WM, et al. Tumors of the kidney, bladder, and related urinary structures. In: Atlas of tumor pathology, third series, fascicle 11. Washington: Armed Forces Institute of Pathology; 1993:193–297.
6. Fawcett DW. The urinary system. In: A textbook of histology. 12th edn. Philadelphia: Saunders; 1994:758–764.
7. Koss LG. Diagnostic cytology and its histopathologic basis. Philadelphia: JB Lippincott; 1972.
8. Fleming ID, ed. AJCC cancer staging manual. 5th edn. Philadelphia: Lippincott-Raven; 1998:223–226
9. Younes M, Sussman J, True LD. The usefulness of the level of the muscularis mucosae in the staging of invasive transitional cell carcinoma of the urinary bladder. Cancer 1990; 66:543–548.
10. Hasui Y, Osada Y, Kitada S, et al. Significance of invasion to the muscularis mucosae on the progression of superficial bladder cancer. Urology 1994; 43:782–786.
11. Angulo JC, Lopez JI, Grignon DJ, et al. Muscularis mucosa differentiates two populations with different prognosis in stage T1 bladder cancer. Urology 1995; 45:47–53.
12. Melicow MM. Tumors of the bladder: a multifaceted problem. J Urol 1974; 112:467–478.
13. Tannenbaum M. Pathology of urothelial cancers. In: Javadpour N, ed. Bladder cancer. Baltimore: Williams & Wilkins; 1984:50–57.
14. Ooms ECM, Anderson WAD, Alons CL, et al. Analysis of the performance of pathologists in the grading of bladder tumors. Hum Pathol 1983; 14:140–143.
15. Ooms ECM, Kurver PHJ, Veldhuizen RW, et al. Morphometric grading of bladder tumors in comparison with histologic grading by pathologists. Hum Pathol 1983; 14:144–149.
16. Holmäng S, Hedelin H, Anderström C, et al. Recurrence and progression in low grade papillary urothelial tumors. J Urol 1999; 162:702–707
17. Epstein JI, Amin MB, Reuter VR, et al. The World Health Organization/International Society of Urological Pathology consensus classification of urothelial (transitional cell) neoplasms of the urinary bladder. Am J Surg Pathol 1998; 22:1435–1448.
18. Fitzpatrick JM, West AB, Butler MR, et al. Superficial bladder tumors (stage pTa, grade 1 and 2). The importance of recurrence pattern following initial resection. J Urol 1986; 135:920–923.
19. Morris SB, Shearer RJ, Gordon EM, et al. Superficial bladder cancer: timing of check cystoscopies in the first year. Br J Urol 1993; 72:446–449.
20. Hall RR, Parmar MK, Richards AB, et al. Proposal for changes in cystoscopy follow up of patients with bladder cancer and adjuvant intravesical chemotherapy. Br Med J 1994; 308:257–258.
21. Murphy WM, Rivera-Ramirez I, Medina CA, et al. The bladder tumor antigen (BTA) test compared to voided urine cytology in the detection of bladder neoplasms. J Urol 1997; 158:2102-2106.
22. Althausen AF, Prout GR Jr, Daly JJ. Non-invasive papillary carcinoma in situ. J Urol 1976; 116:575–580.
23. Murphy WM, Nagy GK, Rao MK, et al. 'Normal' urothelium in patients with bladder cancer. Cancer 1979; 44:1050–1056.
24. Schade ROK, Swinney J. Pre-cancerous changes in bladder epithelium. Lancet 1968; 2:943–945.
25. Eisenberg RB, Roth RR, Schweinberg MH. Bladder tumors and associated proliferative mucosal lesions. J Urol 1960; 84:544–553.
26. Soloway MS, Murphy WM, Rao MK, et al. Serial multiple site biopsies in patients with bladder cancer. J Urol 1978; 120:57–59.
27. Farrow GM, Utz DC, Rife CC. Morphological and clinical observations of patients with early bladder cancer treated with total cystectomy. Cancer Res 1976; 36:2495–2502.
28. Murphy WM, Soloway MS. Developing carcinoma (dysplasia) of the urinary bladder. In: Sommers SC, Rosen PP, eds. Pathology annual, vol 17. New York: Appleton-Century-Crofts; 1982.
29. Melicow MM. Histological study of vesical urothelium intervening between gross neoplasms in total cystectomy. J Urol 1952; 68:261–273.
30. Melicow MM, Hollowell JW. Intraurothelial cancer, carcinoma in situ, Bowen's disease of the urinary system: discussion of thirty cases. J Urol 1952; 68:763–784.
31. Melamed MD, Vousta NG, Grabstaid H. Natural history and clinical behavior of in situ carcinoma of the human urinary bladder. Cancer 1964; 17:1533–1541.
32. Koss LG, Nakanishi I, Freed SZ. Non-papillary carcinoma in situ and atypical hyperplasia in cancerous bladders. Further studies of surgically removed bladders by mapping. Urology 1977; 9:442–450.
33. Tannenbaum M, Romas NA. The pathobiology of early urothelial cancers. In: Skinner DG, deKernion JB, eds. Genitourinary cancer. Philadelphia: Saunders; 1978.
34. Cooper PH, Waisman J, Johnston WH, et al. Severe atypia of transitional epithelium and carcinoma of the urinary bladder. Cancer 1973; 31:1055–1061.
35. Koss LG. Cytology in the diagnosis of bladder cancer. In: Cooper EH, Williams RE. The biology and clinical management of bladder cancer. Oxford: Blackwell; 1975.
36. Koss LG. Mapping of the urinary bladder: its impact on the concept of bladder cancer. Hum Pathol 1979; 10:533–548.
37. Melicow MM. The urothelium: a battleground for oncogenesis. J Urol 1978; 120:43–47.
38. Pugh RCB. Histological staging and grading of bladder tumours. In: Oliver RTD, Bloom HJG, Hendry WF. Bladder cancer: principles of combination therapy. London: Butterworths; 1981.
39. Wiener DP, Koss LG, Sablay B, et al. The prevalence and significance of Brunn's nests, cystitis cystica and squamous metaplasia in normal bladders. J Urol 1979; 122:317–321.
40. Mostofi FK. Potentialities of bladder epithelium. J Urol 1954; 71: 705–714.
41. Koss LG. Diagnostic cytology and its histopathologic bases, vol 2. 4th edn. Philadelphia: Lippincott; 1992:934–1017.
42. Corwin SH, Tassy F, Malament M, et al. Signet ring cell variant of mucinous adenocarcinoma of the bladder. J Urol 1971; 106:697–700.
43. Mostofi FK, Dorris CJ. Pathology of urologic cancer. In: Javadpour N, ed. Principles and management of urologic cancer. Baltimore: Williams & Wilkins; 1979:55.

44. Friedell GH. Current concepts of the aetiology, pathogenesis and pathology of bladder cancer. Urol Res 1978; 6:179–182.
45. Greene LF, Hanash KA, Farrow GM. Benign papilloma or papillary carcinoma of the bladder? J Urol 1973; 110:205–207.
46. Johnson DE, Schoenwald MB, Ayala AG, et al. Squamous carcinoma of the bladder. J Urol 1976; 115:542–547.
47. Koss LG. Tumors of the urinary bladder. In: Atlas of tumor pathology, fascicle 11. Washington: Armed Forces Institute of Pathology; 1975:46–54.
48. Beck AD, Gaudin HJ, Bonham DG. Carcinoma of the urachus. Br J Urol 1970; 42:555–562.
49. Gonzalez E, Fowler MR, Venable DD. Primary signet ring cell adenocarcinoma of the bladder (linitis plastica of the bladder): report of a case and review of the literature. J Urol 1982; 128:1027–1030.
50. Jones WA, Gibbons RP, Correa RJ Jr, et al. Primary adenocarcinoma of bladder. Urology 1980; 15:119–122.
51. Koss LG, Tiamson EM, Robbins MA. Mapping cancerous and precancerous bladder changes. A study of the urotheliurn in ten surgically removed bladders. JAMA 1974; 227:281–286.
52. Algaba F, Zungri E, Vicente J, et al. Multicentricity in carcinoma of the urinary bladder. In: Javadpour N, ed. Bladder cancer. International perspectives in urology, vol 12. Baltimore: Williams & Wilkins; 1984:86–99.
53. Paulson DF. Carcinogenesis in urogenital sites. Invest Urol 1978; 16:77–86.
54. Friedell GH, Parija GC, Nagy GK, et al. The pathology of human bladder cancer. Cancer 1980; 45:1823–1831.
55. Cutler SJ, Heney NM, Friedell GH. Longitudinal study of patients with bladder cancer: factors associated with disease recurrence and progression. In: Bonney WW, Prout GR Jr, eds. Bladder cancer, AUA monographs, vol 1. Baltimore: Williams & Wilkins; 1982:37–46.
56. Heney NM, Nocks BN, Daly JJ, et al. Ta and T1 bladder cancer: location, recurrence and progression. Br J Urol 1982; 54:152–157.
57. Javadpour N. Chromosomes in urologic cancers. In: Recent advances in urologic cancer (Libertino's series of international perspectives in urology), vol 2. Baltimore: Williams & Wilkins; 1982:31.
58. Martorana G, Giberti C, Ferrari M, et al. Cytogenetic analysis of transitional cell carcinoma of the bladder. Clinical implications. Eur J Urol 1983; 9:28–31.
59. Landman J, Chang Y, Kavaler E, et al. Sensitivity and specificity of NMP-22, telomerase, and BTA in the detection of human bladder cancer. Urology 1998; 52:398–402.
60. Muller M, Keine H, Heicappell R, et al. Comparison of human telomerase RNA and telomerase activity in urine for diagnosis of bladder cancer. Clin Cancer Res 1998; 4:1949–1954.
61. Hoshi S, Takahashi M, Satoh M, et al. Telomerase activity: simplification of assay and detection in bladder tumor and urinary exfoliated cells. Urol Oncol 2000; 5:25–30.
62. Hvidi V, Feldt-Rasmussen K. Primary tumours in the renal pelvis and ureter with particular attention to the diagnostic problems. Acta Chir Scand (Suppl) 1973; 433:91–101.
63. Sole-Balcells F, Zungri E. Les tumeurs de la voie excréto-urinaire haute. Journées urologiques du Necker. Paris: Masson; 1981:93–105.
64. Martinez-Piñeiro JA, Pertusa C, Torrenteras J, et al. Tumeurs urothéliales du haut appareil urinaire apparaissant après le traitement d'un carcinome de vessie. Journées urologiques du Necker. Paris: Masson; 1981:22–29.
65. Edwards L, Rosin D, Leaper D, et al. The induction of cystitis and the implantation of tumours in rat and rabbit bladders. Br J Urol 1978; 50:502–504.
66. Laor E, Grabstald H, Whitmore WF. The influence of simultaneous resection of bladder tumors and prostate on the recurrence of prostatic urethral tumors. J Urol 1981; 126:171–172.
67. Rundle JSM, Hart AJL, McGeorge A, et al. Squamous cell carcinoma of bladder. A review of 114 patients. Br J Urol 1982; 54:522–526.
68. Harnden P, Southgate J. Revised classification of urothelial neoplasms [letter]. Am J Surg Pathol 2000; 24;160–161.
69. Grossman HB, Dinney CPN. Markers of bladder cancer: state of the art. Urol Oncol 2000; 5:3–10.
70. Moore KL. The developing human. 3rd edn. Philadelphia: Saunders; 1982:267.
71. Moore KL. Clinically oriented anatomy. 2nd edn. Baltimore: Williams & Wilkins; 1985:265.
72. Fawcett DW. Bloom and Fawcett: a textbook of histology. 11th edn. Philadelphia: Saunders; 1986:787–790.
73. Reuter VE. Urinary bladder and ureter. In: Sternberg SS, ed. Histology for pathologists. 2nd edn. New York: Raven Press; 1997:835–847.
74. Ro JY, Ayala AG, El-Naggar A. Muscularis mucosa of urinary bladder: importance for staging and treatment. Am J Surg Pathol 1987; 11:668–673.
75. Philip AT, Amin MB, Tamboli P, et al. Intravesical adipose tissue. Quantitative study of its presence and location with implications for therapy and prognosis. Am J Surg Pathol 2000; 24:1286–1290.
76. Young RH. Papillary and polypoid cystitis: a report of 8 cases. Am J Surg Pathol 1988; 12:542–546.
77. Baghavan BS, Tiamson EM, Wenk RE, et al. Nephrogenic adenoma of the urinary bladder and urethra. Hum Pathol 1981; 12:907–916.
79. Molland EA, Trott PA, Paris MI, et al. Nephrogenic adenoma: a form of adenomatous metaplasia of the bladder. A clinical and electron microscopical study. Br J Urol 1976; 48:453–462.
80. Navarre RJ, Loening SA, Narayana A. Nephrogenic adenoma: a report of nine cases and review of the literature. J Urol 1982; 127:775–779.
81. Ford TF, Watson GM, Cameron KM. Adenomatous metaplasia (nephrogenic adenoma) of urothelium: an analysis of 70 cases. Br J Urol 1985; 57:427–433.
82. Newman J, Antonakopoulos GN. Widespread mucus metaplasia of the urinary bladder with nephrogenic adenoma. Arch Pathol Lab Med 1985; 109:560–563.
83. Allen CH, Epstein JI. Nephrogenic adenoma of the prostatic urethra: a mimicker of prostate adenocarcinoma. Am J Surg Pathol 2001; 25:802–808.
84. Stilment MM, Sivoky MB. Nephrogenic adenoma associated with intravesical bacillus Calmette-Guérin treatment: a report of two cases. J Urol 1986; 135:359–361.
85. Yagi H, Igawa M, Shiina H, et al. Inverted papilloma of the urinary bladder in a girl. Urol Int 1999; 63:258–260.
86. DeMeester LJ, Farrow GM, Utz DC. Inverted papilloma of the urinary bladder. Cancer 1975; 36: 505–513.
87. Kunze E, Schauer A, Schmitt M. Histology and histogenesis of two different types of inverted urothelial papillomas. Cancer 1983; 51:348–358.
88. Amin MB, Gomez JA, Young RH. Urothelial transitional cell carcinoma with endophytic growth patterns: a discussion of patterns of invasion and problems associated with assessment of invasion in 18 cases. Am J Surg Pathol 1997; 21:1057–1068.
89. Murphy WM, Deana DG. The nested variant of transitional cell carcinoma: a clinicopathologic and immunohistochemical study of 44 cases. Mod Pathol 1992; 5:240–243.
90. Drew PA, Furman J, Civantos F, et al. The nested variant of transitional cell carcinoma: an aggressive neoplasm with innocuous histology. Mod Pathol 1996; 9:989–994.
91. Talbert WM, Young RH. Carcinomas of the urinary bladder with deceptively benign appearing foci – a report of three cases. Am J Surg Pathol 1989; 13:374.
92. Cardillo M, Reuter VE, Lin O. Cytologic features of the nested variant of urothelial carcinoma: a study of seven cases. Cancer 2003; 99:23–27.
93. Young RH, Oliva E. Transitional carcinomas of the urinary bladder that may be underdiagnosed: a report of four cases exemplifying the homology between neoplastic and non-neoplastic transitional cell lesions. Am J Surg Pathol 1996; 20:1148–1154.
94. Holmäng S, Johansson SL. The nested variant of transitional cell carcinoma – a rare neoplasm with poor prognosis. Scand J Urol Nephrol 2001; 35:102–105.
95. Ro JY, Lapham R, Amin MB. Deceptively bland transitional cell carcinoma of the urinary bladder: further characterization of subtle and diagnostically treacherous patterns of invasion in urothelial neoplasia. Adv Anat Pathol 1997; 4:244–251.
96. Amin MB, Young RH. Intraepithelial lesions of the urinary bladder with a discussion of the histogenesis of urothelial neoplasia. Semin Diagn Pathol 1997; 14:84–97.
97. Tannenbaum M. Inflammatory proliferative lesion of the urinary bladder: squamous metaplasia. Urology 1976; 7:428–429.
98. Althausen AF, Prout GRJ, Daly J. Noninvasive papillary carcinoma of the bladder associated with carcinoma-in-situ. J Urol 1976; 116:575–580.
99. Lamm DL. Carcinoma in situ. Urol Clin North Am 1992; 19:499–508.
100. Smith G, Elton RA, Beynon LL. Prognostic significance of biopsy results of normal-looking mucosa in cases of superficial bladder cancer. Br J Urol 1983; 55:665–669.
101. Milford RA, Lecksell K, Epstein JI. An objective morphologic parameter to aid in the diagnosis of flat urothelial carcinoma in situ. Hum Pathol 2001; 32:997–1002.
102. Cheng L, Cheville JC, Neumann RM, et al. Flat intraurothelial lesions of the urinary bladder. Cancer 2000; 88:625–631.
103. Levi AW, Potter SR, Schoenberg MP, et al. Clinical significance of denuded urothelium in bladder biopsy. J Urol 2001; 166:457–460.
104. Kenney JK, Gomez JA, Desai S, et al. Morphologic expressions of urothelial carcinoma in situ: a detailed evaluation of its histologic patterns

with emphasis on carcinoma in situ with microinvasion. Am J Surg Pathol 2001; 25:356–362.
105. Amin MB, McKenney JK. An approach to the diagnosis of flat intraepithelial lesions of the urinary bladder using the World Health Organization/International Society of Urological Pathology (WHO/ISUP) consensus classification system. Adv Anat Pathol 2002; 9:222–232.
106. Young RH, Zukerberg LR. Microcystic transitional cell carcinomas of the urinary bladder: a report of four cases. Am J Clin Pathol 1991; 96:635–639.
107. Paz A, Rath-Wolfson L, Lask D, et al. The clinical and histological features of transitional cell carcinoma of the bladder with microcysts: analysis of 12 cases. Br J Urol 1997; 79:722–725.
108. Terai A, Tamaki M, Hayashida H, et al. Bulky transitional cell carcinoma of bladder with inverted proliferation. Int J Urol 1996; 3:316–319.
109. Amin MB, Gomez JA, Young RH. Urothelial transitional cell carcinoma with endophytic growth patterns: a discussion of patterns of invasion and problems associated with assessment of invasion in 18 cases. Am J Surg Pathol 1997; 21:1057–1068.
110. Amin MB, Murphy WM, Reuter VE, et al. Controversies in the pathology of transitional cell carcinoma of the urinary bladder. Part I, chapter 1. In: Rosen PP, Fechner RE, eds. Reviews of pathology, vol 1. Chicago: ASCP Press; 1996:1–39.
111. Eble JN, Young RH. Carcinoma of the urinary bladder: a review of its diverse morphology. Semin Diagn Pathol 1997; 14:98–108.
112. Young RH, Eble JN. Lymphoepithelioma-like carcinoma of urinary bladder. J Urol Pathol 1993; 1:63–67.
113. Amin MB, Ro JY, Lee KM, et al. Lymphoepithelioma-like carcinoma of urinary bladder. Am J Surg Pathol 1994; 18:466–473.
114. Holmäng S, Borghede G, Johansson SL. Bladder carcinoma with lymphoepithelioma-like differentiation: a report of 9 cases. J Urol 1998; 159:779–782.
115. Lopez-Beltran A, Luque RJ, Vicioso L, et al. Lymphoepithelioma-like carcinoma of the urinary bladder: a clinicopathologic study of 13 cases. Virchows Arch 2001; 438:552–557.
116. Ward JN, Dong WF, Pitts WR Jr. Lymphoepithelioma-like carcinoma of the bladder. J Urol 2002; 167:2523–2524.
117. Ro JY, Ayala AG, Wishnow K, et al. Sarcomatoid bladder carcinoma: clinicopathological and immunohistochemical study of 44 cases. Surg Pathol 1988; 1:359.
118. Young RH, Wick MR, Mills SE. Sarcomatoid carcinoma of the urinary bladder: a clinicopathological analysis of 12 cases and review of literature. Am J Clin Pathol 1988; 90:653–661.
119. Torenbeek R, Blomjous CE, de Bruin PC, et al. Sarcomatoid carcinoma of the urinary bladder. Clinicopathologic analysis of 18 cases with immunohistochemical and electron microscopic findings. Am J Surg Pathol 1994; 18:241–249.
120. Jones EC, Young RH. Myxoid and sclerosing sarcomatoid transitional cell carcinoma of the urinary bladder: a clinicopathologic and immunohistochemical study of 25 cases. Mod Pathol 1997; 10:908–916.
121. Lopez-Beltran A, Pacelli A, Rothenberg HJ, et al. Carcinosarcoma and sarcomatoid carcinoma of the bladder: clinicopathological study of 41 cases. J Urol 1998; 159:1497–1503.
122. Ikegami H, Iwasaki H, Ohjimi Y, et al. Sarcomatoid carcinoma of the urinary bladder: a clinicopathologic and immunohistochemical analysis of 14 patients. Hum Pathol 2000; 31:332–340.
123. Newman DM, Brown JR, Jay AC, et al. Squamous cell carcinoma of the bladder. J Urol 1968; 112:66–67.
124. Bissada NK, Cole AT, Fried FA. Extensive condyloma acuminata of the entire male urethra and the bladder. J Urol 1974; 112:201–203.
125. El Sebai I, Sherif M, El Bolkaimy MN, et al. Verrucous squamous carcinoma of the bladder. Urology 1974; 4:407–410.
126. Zahran MM, Kamel M, Mooro H, et al. Bilharziasis of urinary bladder and ureter: comparative histopathologic study. Urology 1976; 8:73–79.
127. DeBenedictis TJ, Marmar JL, Praiss DE. Intraurethral condyloma acuminata: management and review of the literature. J Urol 1977; 118:767–769.
128. Wyatt JK, Craig I. Verrucous carcinoma of urinary bladder. Urology 1980; 16:97–99.
129. Faysal MH. Squamous cell carcinoma of the bladder. J Urol 1981; 126:598–599.
130. Keating MA, Young RH, Carr CP, et al. Condyloma acuminatum of the bladder and ureter: case report and review of the literature. J Urol 1985; 133:465–467.
131. Walther M, O'Brien D, Birch HW. Condyloma acuminata and verrucous carcinoma of the bladder: case report and literature review. J Urol 1986; 135:362–365.
132. Khan MS, Thornhill JA, Gafney E, et al. Keratinizing squamous metaplasia of the bladder: natural history and rationalization of management based on review of 54 years' experience. Eur Urol 2002; 42:469–474.
133. Jakse G, Schneider HM, Jacobi GH. Urachal signet-ring cell carcinoma, a rare variant of vesical adenocarcinoma: incidence and pathological criteria. J Urol 1978; 120:764–766.
134. Schubert GE, Paukovic MB, Bethke-Bedurftig BA. Tubular urachal remnants in adult bladders. J Urol 1982; 127:40–42.
135. Ghazizadeh M, Yamamoto S, Kurokawa K. Clinical features of urachal carcinoma in Japan: review of 157 patients. Urol Res 1983; 11:235–238.
136. Hayman J. Carcinoma of the urachus. Pathology 1984; 16:167–171.
137. Johnson DE, Hodge GB, Abdul-Karim FW, et al. Urachal carcinoma. Urology 1985; 26:218–221.
138. Alonso-Gorrea M, Mompo-Sanchis JA, Jorda-Cuevas M, et al. Signet ring cell adenocarcinoma of the urachus. Eur Urol 1985; 11:282–284.
139. Eble JN, Hull MT, Rowland RG, et al. Villous adenoma of the urachus with mucosuria: a light and electron microscopic study. J Urol 1986; 135:1240–1244.
140. Wheeler JD, Hill WT. Adenocarcinoma involving the urinary bladder. Cancer 1954; 7:119–135.
141. Mostofi FK, Thomson RV, Dean AL. Mucous adenocarcinoma of the urinary bladder. Cancer 1955; 8:741–758.
142. Jones WA, Gibbons RP, Correa RJ, et al. Primary adenocarcinoma of the bladder. Urology 1980; 15:119–122.
143. Nocks BN, Heney NM, Daly JJ. Primary adenocarcinoma of urinary bladder. Urology 1983; 21:26–29.
144. Anderstrom C, Johansson SL, von Schultz L. Primary adenocarcinoma of the urinary bladder: a clinicopathologic and prognostic study. Cancer 1983; 52:1273–1282.
145. Malek RS, Rosen JS, O'Dea MJ. Adenocarcinoma of the bladder. Urology 1983; 20:357–359.
146. Grignon DJ, Ro JY, Ayala AG, et al. Primary adenocarcinoma of the urinary bladder: a clinicopathologic analysis of 72 cases. Cancer 1991; 67:2165–2172.
147. Shaaban AA, Elbaz MA, Tribukait. Primary nonurachal adenocarcinoma in the bilharzial urinary bladder: deoxyribonucleic acid flow cytometric and morphologic characterization in 93 cases. Urology 1998; 51:469–476.
148. El-Mekresh MM, El-Baz MA, Abol-Enein H, et al. Primary adenocarcinoma of the urinary bladder: a report of 185 cases. Br J Urol 1998; 82:206–212.
149. Braun EV, Ali M, Fayemi O, et al. Primary signet-ring cell carcinoma of the urinary bladder: review of the literature and report of a case. Cancer 1981; 47:1430–1435.
150. Poore TE, Egbert B, Jahnke R, et al. Signet ring cell adenocarcinoma of the bladder: linitis plastica variant. Arch Pathol Lab Med 1981; 105: 203–204.
151. Choi H, Lamb S, Pintar K, et al. Primary signet-ring cell carcinoma of the urinary bladder. Cancer 1984; 53:1985–1990.
152. Bernstein SA, Reuter VE, Carroll PR, et al. Primary signet ring cell carcinoma of the urinary bladder. Urology 1988; 31:432–436.
153. Grignon DJ, Ro JY, Ayala AG, et al. Primary signet ring cell carcinoma of the urinary bladder. Am J Clin Pathol 1991; 95:13–20.
154. Skor AB, Warren MM. Mesonephric adenocarcinoma of the bladder. Urology 1977; 10:64–65.
155. Schultz RE, Block MJ, Tomaszewski JE, et al. Mesonephric adenocarcinoma of the bladder. J Urol 1984; 132:263–265.
156. Young RH, Scully RE. Clear cell adenocarcinoma of the bladder and urethra: a report of three cases and review of the literature. Am J Surg Pathol 1985; 9:816–826.
157. Oliva E, Amin MB, Jimenez R, et al. Clear cell carcinoma of the urinary bladder. A report and comparison of four tumors of Müllerian origin and nine of probable urothelial origin with discussion of histogenesis and diagnostic problems. Am J Surg Pathol 2002; 26:190–197.
158. Mills SE, Wolfe JT 3rd, Weiss MA, et al. Small cell undifferentiated carcinoma of the urinary bladder. A light-microscopic, immunocytochemical, and ultrastructural study of 12 cases. Am J Surg Pathol 1987; 11:606–617.
159. Blomjous CE, Vos W, De Voogt HJ, et al. Small cell carcinoma of the urinary bladder. A clinicopathologic, morphometric, immunohistochemical, and ultrastructural study of 18 cases. Cancer 1989; 64:1347–1357.
160. Grignon DJ, Ro JY, Ayala AG, et al. Small cell carcinoma of the urinary bladder. A clinicopathologic analysis of 22 cases. Cancer 1992; 69:527–536.
161. Weiss MA. Small cell carcinomas of the urinary tract. Arch Pathol Lab Med 1993; 117:237–238.

162. Lopez JL, Angulo JC, Flores N, et al. Small cell carcinoma of the urinary bladder. A clinicopathological study of six cases. Br J Urol 1994; 73: 43–49.
163. Holmäng S, Borghede G, Johansson SL. Primary small cell carcinoma of the bladder: a report of 25 cases. J Urol 1995; 153:1820–1822.
164. Angulo JC, Lopez JI, Sanchez-Chapado M, et al. Small cell carcinoma of the urinary bladder. J Urol Pathol 1996; 5:1–19.
165. Hailemariam S, Gaspert A, Komminoth P, et al. Primary, pure, large-cell neuroendocrine carcinoma of the urinary bladder. Mod Pathol 1998; 11:1016–1020.
166. Lohrisch C, Murray N, Pickles T, et al. Small cell carcinoma of the bladder: long term outcome with integrated chemoradiation. Cancer 1999; 86:2346–2352.
167. Bastus R, Caballero JM, Gonzalez G, et al. Small cell carcinoma of the urinary bladder treated with chemotherapy and radiotherapy: results in five cases. Eur Urol 1999; 35:323–326.
168. Agoff SN, Lamps LW, Philip AT, et al. Thyroid transcription factor-1 is expressed in extrapulmonary small cell carcinomas but not in other extrapulmonary neuroendocrine tumors. Mod Pathol 2000; 13:238–242.
169. Eusebi V, Damiani S, Pasquinelli G, et al. Small cell neuroendocrine carcinoma with skeletal muscle differentiation: report of three cases. Am J Surg Pathol 2000; 24:223–230.
170. Trias I, Algaba F, Condom E, et al. Small cell carcinoma of the urinary bladder. Presentation of 23 cases and review of 134 published cases. Eur Urol 2001; 39:85–90.
171. Fujita K, Nishimura K, Nonomura N, et al. Early stage small cell carcinoma of the urinary bladder. Int J Urol 2001; 8:643–644.
172. Cheng L, Leibovieh BC, Cheville JC, et al. Paraganglioma of the urinary bladder: can biologic potential be predicted? Cancer 2000; 88:844–852.
173. Nakatani T, Hayama T, Uchida J, et al. Diagnostic localization of extra-adrenal pheochromocytoma: comparison of ^{123}I-MIBG imaging and ^{131}I-MIBG imaging. Oncol Rep 2002; 9:1225–1227.
174. Ozkardes H, Ergen A, Ozen HA, et al. Immunohistochemical detection of beta-human chorionic gonadotropin in urothelial carcinoma. Int Urol Nephrol 1991; 23:5–11.
175. Yokoyama S, Hayashida Y, Nagaharna J, et al. Primary and metaplastic choriocarcinoma of the bladder. A report of two cases. Acta Cytol 1992; 36:176–182.
176. Tinkler SD, Roberts JT, Robinson MC, et al. Primary choriocarcinoma of the urinary bladder: a case report. Clin Oncol (R Coll Radiol) 1996; 8:59–61.
177. Dirnhofer S, Koessler P, Ensinger C, et al. Production of trophoblastic hormones by transitional cell carcinoma of the bladder: association to tumor stage and grade. Hum Pathol 1998; 29:377–382.
178. Sievert K, Weber EA, Heiwig R, et al. Pure primary choriocarcinoma of the urinary bladder with long-term survival. Urology 2000; 56:856.
179. Lake MH, Kossow AS, Bokinsky G. Leiomyoma of the bladder and urethra. J Urol 1981; 125:742–743.
180. Yusim IE, Neulander EZ, Eidelberg I, et al. Leiomyoma of the genitourinary tract. Scand J Urol Nephrol 2001; 35:295–299.
181. Martin SA, Sears D, Sebo TJ, et al. Smooth muscle neoplasms of the urinary bladder. A clinicopathologic comparison of leiomyoma and leiomyosarcoma. Am J Surg Pathol 2002; 26:292–300.
182. Fuleihan FM, Cordonnier JJ. Hemangioma of the bladder: report of a case and review of the literature. J Urol 1969; 102:581–585.
183. Proca E. Haemangioma of the bladder. Br J Urol 1977; 49:60.
184. Winfield HN, Catalona WJ. An isolated plexiform neurofibroma of the bladder. J Urol 1985; 134:542–543.
185. Ravich A, Stout AP, Ravich RA. Malignant granular cell myoblastoma involving the urinary bladder. Ann Surg 1945; 121:361–372.
186. Fletcher MS, Aker M, Hill JT, et al. Granular cell myoblastoma of the bladder. Br J Urol 1985; 57:109–110.
187. Mouradian JA, Coleman JW, McGovern JH, et al. Granular cell tumor (myoblastoma) of the bladder. J Urol 1974; 112:343–345.
188. Maurer HM. The intergroup rhabdomyosarcoma study (NIH). Objectives and clinical staging classification. J Pediatr Surg 1975; 10:977–978.
189. Scholtmeijer RJ, Tromp CG, Hazebroeck FWJ. Embryonal rhabdomyosarcoma of the urogenital tract in childhood. Eur Urol 1983; 9:69–74.
190. Hendricksson C, Zetterlund CG, Boisen P, et al. Large rhabdomyosarcoma of the urinary bladder in an adult. Scand J Urol Nephrol 1985; 19:237–239.
191. Leuschner I, Harms D, Mattke A, et al. Rhabdomyosarcoma of the urinary bladder and vagina. A clinicopathologic study with emphasis on recurrent disease: a report from the Kiel pediatric tumor registry and the German CWS study. Am J Surg Pathol 2001; 25:856–864.
192. Mackenzie AR, Whitmore WF, Melamed MR. Myosarcomas of the bladder and prostate. Cancer 1968; 22:833–844.
193. Weitzner S. Leiomyosarcoma of urinary bladder in children. Urology 1978; 12:450–452.
194. Swartz DA, Johnson DE, Ayala AG, et al. Bladder leiomyosarcoma: a review of 10 cases with five year followup. J Urol 1985; 133:200–202.
195. Russo P, Brady MS, Conlon K, et al. Adult urological sarcoma. J Urol 1992; 147:1032–1037.
196. Watanabe K, Baba A, Hoshi N, et al. Pseudosarcomatous myofibroblastic tumor and myosarcoma of the urogenital tract. Immunohistochemical characteristics and differential diagnosis. Arch Pathol Lab Med 2001; 125:1070–1073.
197. Henriksen OB, Mogensen P, Engelholm AJ. Inflammatory fibrous histiocytoma of the bladder. Acta Pathol Microbiol Immunol Scand [A] 1982; 90:333–337.
198. Turner AG. Malignant fibrous histiocytoma involving the bladder. Br J Urol 1985; 57:237–238.
199. Berenson RJ, Flynn S, Freiha FS, et al. Primary osteogenic sarcoma of the bladder. Cancer 1986; 57:350–355.
200. Foote JW, Seemayer TA, Duigan JP. Desmoid tumor involving the bladder: case report. J Urol 1975; 114:147–149.
201. Baumgartner G, Gaeta J, Wajsman Z, et al. Hemangiopericytoma of the urinary bladder: a case report and review of the literature. J Surg Oncol 1976; 8:281–286.
202. Harris M, Eyden BP, Joglekar VM. Rhabdoid tumour of the bladder: a histological, ultrastructural and immunohistochemical study. Histopathology 1987; 11:1083–1092.
203. Egawa S, Uchida T, Koshiba K, et al. Malignant fibrous histiocytoma of the bladder with focal rhabdoid tumor differentiation. J Urol 1994; 151:154–156.
204. Inagaki T, Nagata M, Kaneko M, et al. Carcinosarcoma with rhabdoid features of the urinary bladder in a 2-year-old girl: possible histogenesis of stem cell origin. Pathol Int 2000; 50:973–978.
205. Kempton CL, Kurtin PJ, Inwards DJ, et al. Malignant lymphoma of the bladder: evidence from 36 cases that low-grade lymphoma of the MALT type is the most common primary bladder lymphoma. Am J Surg Pathol 1997; 21:1324–1333.
206. Wazait HD, Chahal R, Sundurum SK, et al. MALT type primary lymphoma of the urinary bladder: clinicopathological study of 2 cases and review of the literature. Urol Int 2001; 66:220–224.
207. Ho DS, Patterson AL, Orozco RE, et al. Extramedullary plasmacytoma of the bladder: case report and review of the literature. J Urol 1993; 150:473–474.
208. Chalbaud RA, Johnson DE. Adenocarcinoma of tongue metastatic to bladder. Urology 1974; 4:454–455.
209. Van Driel MF, Ypma AFGVM, Van Gelder B. Gastric carcinoma metastatic to the bladder. Br J Urol 1987; 59:193–194.
210. Silverstein LI, Plaine L, Davis JE, et al. Breast carcinoma metastatic to bladder. Urology 1987; 29:544–547.
211. Silver SA, Epstein JI. Adenocarcinoma of the colon simulating primary urinary bladder neoplasia. A report of nine cases. Am J Surg Pathol 1993; 17:171–178.
212. Wang HI, Lu DW, Yerian LM, et al. Immunohistochemical distinction between primary adenocarcinoma of the bladder and secondary colorectal adenocarcinoma. Am J Surg Pathol 2001; 25:1380–1387.
213. Tamboli P, Mohsin SK, Hailemariam S, et al. Colonic adenocarcinoma metastatic to the urinary tract versus primary tumors of the urinary tract with glandular differentiation: a report of 7 cases and investigation using a limited immunohistochemical panel. Arch Pathol Lab Med 2002; 126:1057–1063.
214. Davies G, Castro JE. Cystitis glandularis. Urology 1977; 10:128–129.
215. Young RH, Bostwick DG. Florid cystitis glandularis of intestinal type with mucin extravasation: a mimic of adenocarcinoma. Am J Surg Pathol 1996; 20:1462–1468.
216. Corica FA, Husmann DA, Churchill BM, et al. Intestinal metaplasia is not a strong risk factor for bladder cancer: study of 53 cases with long-term follow up. Urology 1997; 50:427–431.
217. Jacobs LB, Brooks JD, Epstein JI. Differentiation of colonic metaplasia from adenocarcinoma of urinary bladder. Hum Pathol 1997; 28: 1152–1157.
218. Morse HD. The etiology and pathology of pyelitis cystica, ureteritis cystica and cystitis cystica. Am J Pathol 1928; 4:33–50.
219. Edwards PD, Hurm RA, Jaeschke WH. Conversion of cystitis glandularis to adenocarcinoma. J Urol 1972; 108:568–580.
220. Davies G, Castro JE. Cystitis glandularis. Urology 1977; 10:128–129.

221. Wiener DP, Koss LG, Sablay B, et al. The prevalence and significance of Brunn's nests, cystitis cystica and squamous metaplasia in normal bladders. J Urol 1979; 122:317–321.
222. Hansson S, Hanson E, Hjälmås K, et al. Follicular cystitis in girls with untreated asymptomatic or covert bacteriuria. J Urol 1990; 143:3311–332.
223. Patel NP, Lavengood RW, Fernandes M, et al. Gas-forming infections in genitourinary tract. Urology 1992; 39:341–345.
224. Quint I-IJ, Drach GW, Rappaport WD, et al. Emphysematous cystitis: a review of the spectrum of disease. J Urol 1992; 147:134–137.
225. Lawrence HJ, Simone J, Aur RJA. Cyclophosphamide-induced hemorrhagic cystitis in children with leukemia. Cancer 1975; 36: 1572–1576.
226. Pode D, Perlberg S, Steiner D. Busulfan-induced hemorrhagic cystitis. J Urol 1983; 130:347–348.
227. Verhagen PCMS, Nikkels PGJ, de Jong TPVM. Eosinophilic cystitis. Arch Dis Child 2001; 84:344–346.
228. Roth JA. Reactive pseudosarcomatous response in urinary bladder. Urology 1980; 16:635–637.
229. Proppe KH, Scully RE, Rosai J. Postoperative spindle-cell nodules of the genitourinary tract resembling sarcomas: a report of eight cases. Am J Surg Pathol 1985; 8:101–108.
230. Nochomovitz LE, Orenstein JM. Inflammatory pseudotumor of the urinary bladder—possible relationship to nodular fasciitis. Am J Surg Pathol 1985; 9:366–373.
231. Wick MR, Brown BA, Young RH, et al. Spindle-cell proliferations of the urinary tract: an immunohistochemical study. Am J Surg Pathol 1988; 12:379–389.
232. Ro JY, Ayala AG, Ordonez NG, et al. Pseudosarcomatous fibromyxoid tumor of the urinary bladder. Am J Clin Pathol 1986; 86:583–590.
233. Mahadevia PS, Alexander JE, Rojas-Corona R, et al. Pseudosarcomatous stromal reaction in primary and metastatic urothelial carcinoma: a source of diagnostic difficulty. Am J Surg Pathol 1989; 13:782–790.
234. Young RH. Spindle cell lesions of the urinary tract. Histol Histopathol 1990; 5:505–512.
235. Albores-Saavedra J, Manivel JC, Essenfeld H, et al. Pseudosarcomatous myofibroblastic proliferations in the urinary bladder of children. Cancer 1990; 66:1234–1241.
236. Jones EC, Clement PB, Young RH. Inflammatory pseudotumor of the urinary bladder. A clinicopathological, immunohistochemical, ultrastructural, and flow cytometric study of 13 cases. Am J Surg Pathol 1993; 17:264–274.
237. Reuter VE. Sarcomatoid lesions of the urogenital tract. Semin Diagn Pathol 1993; 10:188–201.
238. Iczkowski KA, Shanks JH, Gadaleanu V, et al. Inflammatory pseudotumor and sarcoma of the urinary bladder: differential diagnosis and outcome in thirty-eight spindle cell neoplasms. Mod Pathol 2001; 14:1043–1051.
239. Melicow MM. Malakoplakia. Report of case, review of literature. J Urol 1957; 78:33–40.
240. Smith BH. Malakoplakia of the urinary tract. A study of 24 cases. Am J Clin Pathol 1965; 43:409–417.
241. Lou TY, Teplitz C. Malakoplakia: pathogenesis and ultrastructural morphogenesis. A problem of altered macrophage (phagolysomal) response. Hum Pathol 1974; 5:191–207.
242. Lewin KJ, Fair WR, Steigbigel RT, et al. Clinical and laboratory studies into the pathogenesis of malakoplakia. J Clin Pathol 1976; 29:354–363.
243. Abdou NI, NaPornbejara C, Sagawa A, et al. Malakoplakia: evidence for monocyte lysosomal abnormality correctable by cholinergic agonist in vitro and in vivo. N Engl J Med 1977; 297:1413–1419.
244. Stanton MJ, Maxted W. Malakoplakia: a study of the literature and current concepts of pathogenesis, diagnosis and treatment. J Urol 1981; 125:139–146.
245. Steven S, McClure J. The histochemical features of the Michaelis–Gutmann body and a consideration of the pathophysiological mechanisms of its formation. J Pathol 1982; 137:119–127.
246. McClure J. Malakoplakia. J Pathol 1983; 140:275–330.
247. Qualman SJ, Gupta PK, Mendelsohn G. Intracellular *Escherichia coli* in urinary malakoplakia: a reservoir of infection and its therapeutic implications. Am J Clin Pathol 1984; 81:35–42.
248. Larsen S, Thompson SA, Hald T, et al. Mast cells in interstitial cystitis. Br J Urol 1982; 54:283–286.
249. Gillenwater JY, Wein AJ. Summary of the National Institute of Arthritis, Diabetes, Digestive, and Kidney Diseases Workshop on Interstitial Cystitis. National Institute of Health, Bethesda, Maryland, August 28–29, 1987. J Urol 1988; 140:203–206.
250. Johansson SL, Fall M. Clinical features and spectrum of light microscopic changes in interstitial cystitis. J Urol 1990; 143:1118–1124.
251. Johannsson SL. Interstitial cystitis. Mod Pathol 1993; 6:738–742.
252. Elbadawi A. Interstitial cystitis: a critique of current concepts with a new proposal for pathologic diagnosis and pathogenesis. Urology 1997; 49:14–40.
253. Sant GR. Interstitial cystitis. Curr Opin Obstet Gynecol 1997; 9:332–336.
254. Ochs RL. Autoantibodies and interstitial cystitis. Clin Lab Med 1997; 17:571–579.
255. Sant GR, Hanno PM. Interstitial cystitis: current issues and controversies in diagnosis. Urology 2001; 57(Suppl 6A):82–88.
256. Tomaszewski JE, Landis JR, Russack V, et al. Biopsy features are associated with primary symptoms in interstitial cystitis: results from the interstitial cystitis database study. Urology 2001; 57(Suppl 6A):67–81.
257. Theoharides TC, Duraisamy K, Sant GR. Mast cell involvement in interstitial cystitis: a review of human and experimental evidence. Urology 2001; 57(Suppl 6A):47–55.
258. Christensen WI. Genitourinary tuberculosis: review of 102 cases. Medicine 1974; 53:377–390.
259. Wise GJ, Silver DA. Fungal infections of the genitourinary system. J Urol 1993; 149:1377–1388.
260. Zahran MM, Kamel M, Mooro H, et al. Bilharziasis of urinary bladder and ureter: comparative histopathologic study. Urology 1976; 8:73–79.
261. Ghoneim MA. Bilharziasis of the genitourinary tract. BJU Int 2002; 89(Suppl 11):22–30.
262. Kertsschmer HL. Diverticula of the urinary bladder. A clinical study of 236 cases. Surg Gynecol Obstet 1940; 71:491–503.
263. Tannenbaum M. Inflammatory proliferative lesion of the urinary bladder: squamous metaplasia. Urology 1976; 7:428–429.
264. Zahran MM, Kamel M, Mooro H, et al. Bilharziasis of urinary bladder and ureter: comparative histopathologic study. Urology 1976; 8:73–79.
265. Godwin JT, Hanash K. Pathology of bilharzial bladder cancer. In: Bladder cancer, part A: pathology, diagnosis and surgery. New York: Alan R. Liss; 1984:95–143.
266. Khan MS, Thornhill JA, Gafney E, et al. Keratinizing squamous metaplasia of the bladder: natural history and rationalization of management based on review of 54 years' experience. Eur Urol 2002; 42:469–474.
267. Mostofi FK. Potentialities of bladder epithelium. J Urol 1954; 71:705–714.
268. Engel RM, Wilkson HA. Bladder extrophy. J Urol 1970; 104:699–704.
269. Davies G, Castro JE. Cystitis glandularis. Urology 1977; 10:128–129.
270. Nielsen K, Nielson KK. Adenocarcinoma in extrophy of the bladder—the last case in Scandinavia? A case report and review of literature. J Urol 1983; 130:1180–1182.
271. Young RH, Bostwick DG. Florid cystitis glandularis of intestinal type with mucin extravasation: a mimic of adenocarcinoma. Am J Surg Pathol 1996; 20:1462–1468.
272. Jacobs LB, Brooks JD, Epstein JI. Differentiation of colonic metaplasia from adenocarcinoma of urinary bladder. Hum Pathol 1997; 28:1152–1157.
273. Corica FA, Husmann DA, Churchill BM, et al. Intestinal metaplasia is not a strong risk factor for bladder cancer: study of 53 cases with long-term follow up. Urology 1997; 50:427–431.
274. Nixon WCW. Endometriosis of the bladder. Lancet 1940; 1:405–406.
275. Lichtenfeld FR, McCauley RT, Staples PP. Endometriosis involving the urinary tract. A collective review. Obstet Gynecol 1961; 17:762–768.
276. Fein RL, Morton BF. Vesical endometriosis: a case report and review of the literature. J Urol 1966; 95:45–50.
277. Stewart WW, Ireland GW. Vesical endometriosis in a postmenopausal woman: a case report. J Urol 1977; 118:480–481.
278. Pinkert TC, Catlow CE, Straus R. Endometriosis of the urinary bladder in a man with prostatic carcinoma. Cancer 1979; 43:1562–1567.
279. Randolph Schrodt G, Alcorn MO, Ibanez J. Endometriosis of the male urinary system: a case report. J Urol 1980; 124:722–723.
280. Lenaine WO, Admundsen CL, McGuire EJ. Bladder endometriosis: conservative management. J Urol 2000; 163:1814–1817.
281. Comiter CV. Endometriosis of the urinary tract. Urol Clin North Am 2002; 29:625–635.

URETHRA

Maria M. Shevchuk and Myron Tannenbaum

ANATOMY

Male urethra

The male urethra is approximately 16 cm long and is divided into three segments.

- The *prostatic* urethra extends from the bladder neck to the apex of the prostate. Ejaculatory ducts open laterally into the verumontanum, and prostatic ducts open along the lateral and posterior aspects of the prostatic urethra.
- The *membranous* urethra extends a short distance from the prostatic apex, through the urogenital diaphragm with the sphincter muscle, to the bulb of the penis. Cowper's glands (bulbourethral glands) are located laterally to this urethral segment.
- The *penile* urethra extends from the penile bulb to the urethral meatus, within the corpus spongiosum of the penis. There are periurethral glands (glands of Littré) along the course of this segment.

Urothelium lines the prostatic urethra, and is sometimes present in the membranous and penile urethra. More commonly, these two lower segments are lined by a pseudostratified columnar epithelium. Occasionally, the lining epithelium is focally glandular. The distal fossa navicularis in the glans and the orifice are lined by a nonkeratinizing squamous epithelium.

Female urethra

The female urethra is approximately 4 cm long and its periurethral glands are known as Skene's glands. Urothelium lines the proximal one-third and nonkeratinizing squamous epithelium lines the distal two-thirds.

CONGENITAL ANOMALIES

- *Duplication of the urethra* can consist of a complete, dorsally located, second urethra or a partial structure that ends blindly.
- *Congenital urethral polyps* are seen in males during childhood, are usually located in the prostatic urethra near the verumontanum, and can cause obstruction.
- *Urethral valves* are redundant folds of urethral mucosa that are usually asymptomatic.

NON-NEOPLASTIC LESIONS

Diverticula

- Diverticula of the urethra usually affect women and often are asymptomatic. They can frequently be palpated in the vaginal wall.
- Most are lined by urothelium, but squamous and glandular metaplasia can be seen. (Figs 12.1 & 12.2)
- Nephrogenic adenoma has been reported in diverticula.
- There is an increased risk (up to 15%) of carcinoma developing in diverticula.[1] Urothelial, squamous, and clear cell carcinoma, as well as intestinal-type adenocarcinoma, have been reported.

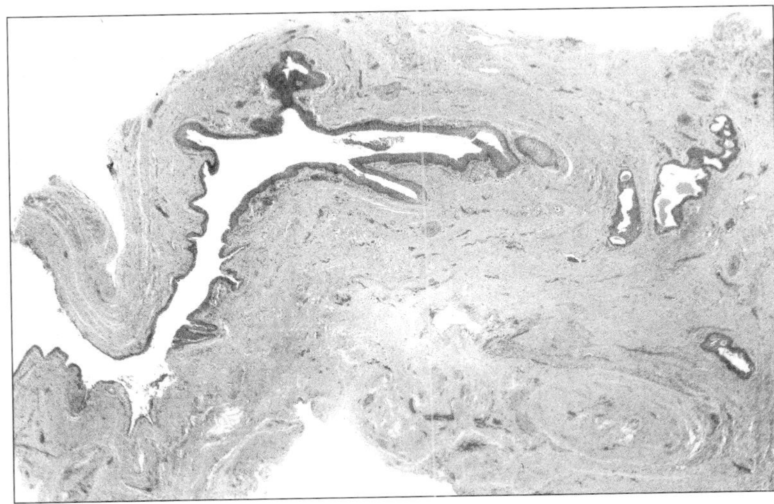

Fig. 12.1 Urethral diverticulum: an extension from the urethra. It may have a very narrow opening and is lined by epithelium that is either urothelial or squamoid.

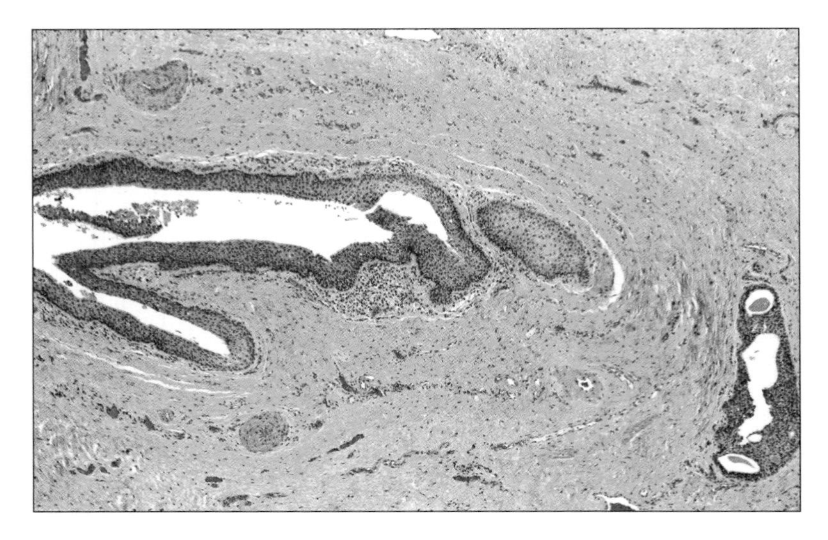

Fig. 12.2 Urethral diverticulum. A higher magnification of Fig. 12.1, reveals urothelium lining the diverticulum without dysplasia or neoplasia.

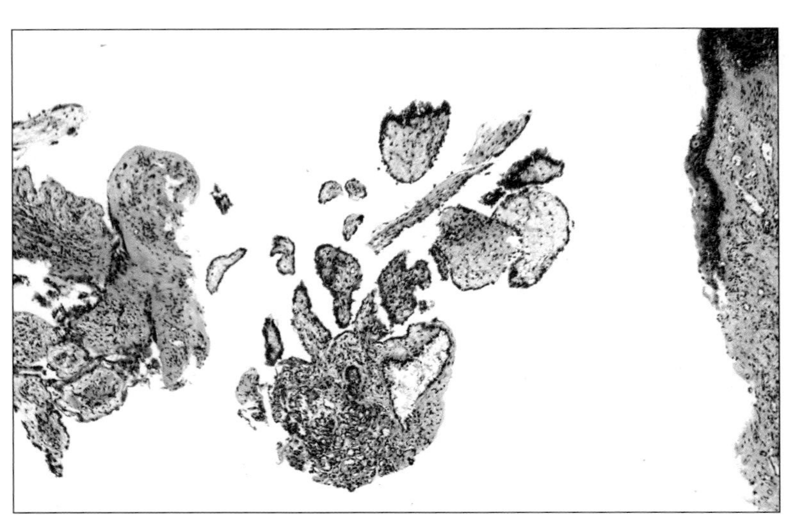

Fig. 12.4 Urethral polypoid urethritis. Higher magnification of Fig. 12.3. There may be some urethral glands in the stroma. The urethral wall is on the right.

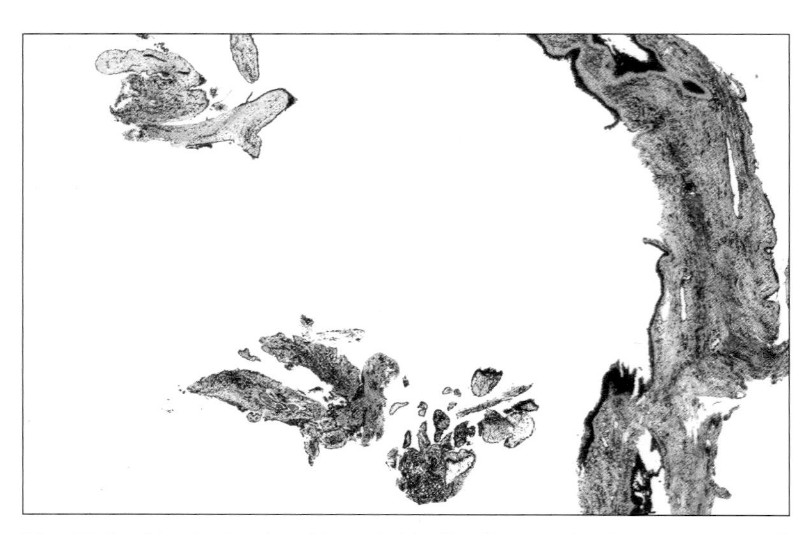

Fig. 12.3 Urethral polypoid urethritis. Papillary projections consisting of thickened stromal stalks lined by one or more layers of urothelial cells can be seen. The urethral wall is on the right.

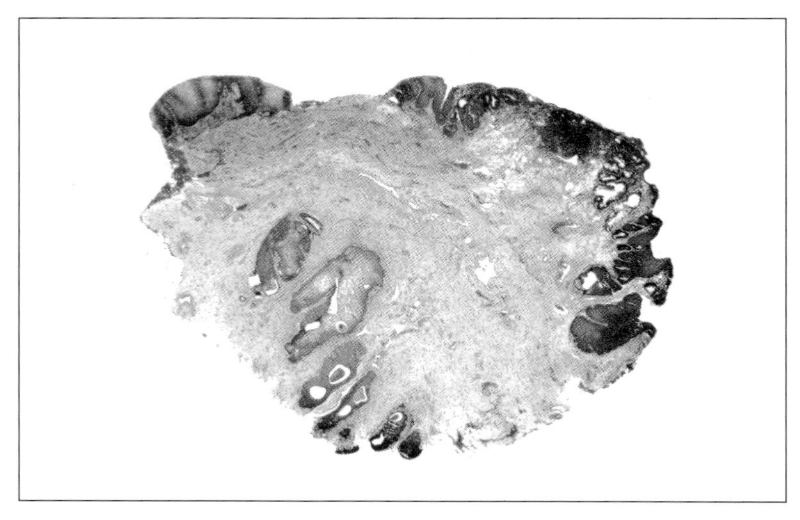

Fig. 12.5 Urethral caruncle. Low-power example of an exophytic growth in the female urethra. The fibrovascular stroma is lined in part by urothelium, squamous and glandular epithelium. No neoplasia is present.

Polypoid urethritis

- Polypoid urethritis is a reactive change, often near the verumontanum, that presents as multiple polyps or papillae.
- Histologically, there is a polypoid edematous stroma with prominent blood vessels, usually lined by urothelium. The surface may be ulcerated, show metaplastic changes, or contain ureteritis cystica. (Figs 12.3 & 12.4)

Caruncle

- Caruncle is a polypoid reactive mass of the distal urethra in women.
- The epithelium may be hyperplastic, resembling a urothelial or squamous papilloma. Glandular epithelium has also been reported.
- The stroma may be polypoid, edematous, or fibrotic, and is usually inflamed.
- The blood vessels can proliferate and the caruncle may resemble a hemangioma. (Figs 12.5–12.7)

Stricture

- Stricture is most common in the membranous portion of the male urethra, and is usually the consequence of repeated infections.

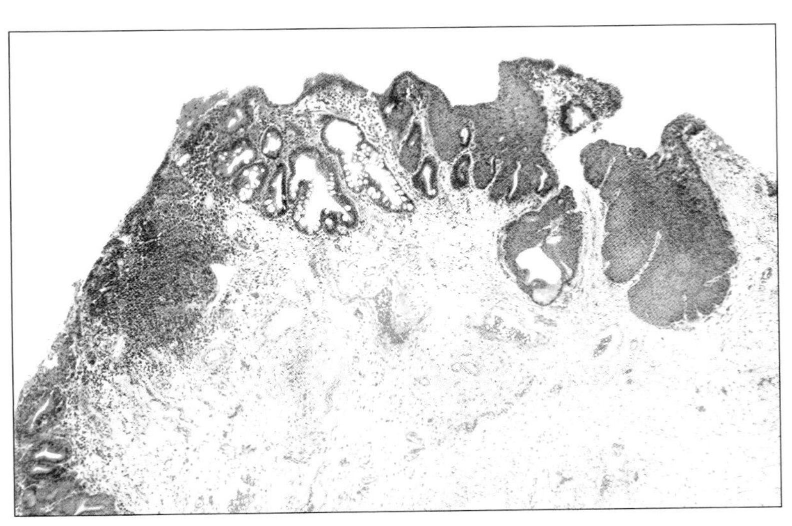

Fig. 12.6 Urethral caruncle. Higher magnification of Fig. 12.5, with prominent glandular and squamous epithelium.

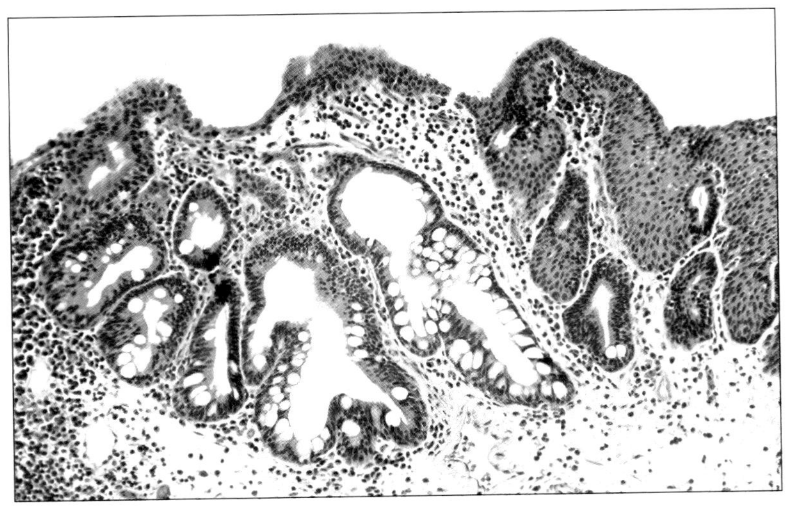

Fig. 12.7 Urethral caruncle. Higher magnification of Fig. 12.5, with prominent glandular and squamous epithelium.

- The most common histology is hyalinized fibrosis of urethral wall. (Fig 12.8–12.11)
- Stricture is a risk factor for carcinoma of the urethra.

Prostatic urethral polyps

- These consist of ectopic benign prostatic epithelium growing as papillary fronds or acini.

BENIGN TUMORS

Nephrogenic adenoma

- Nephrogenic carcinoma is not very common in the urethra.
- The presenting symptom is hematuria.

Villous adenoma

- Villous carcinoma resembles the colonic counterpart, and occurs primarily near the verumontanum of the male urethra and occasionally in the female urethra.[2]

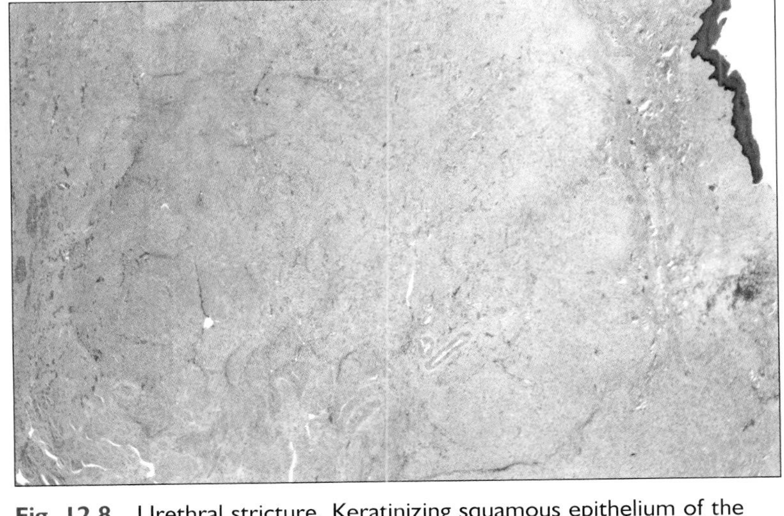

Fig. 12.8 Urethral stricture. Keratinizing squamous epithelium of the urethra is covering a scarred stroma.

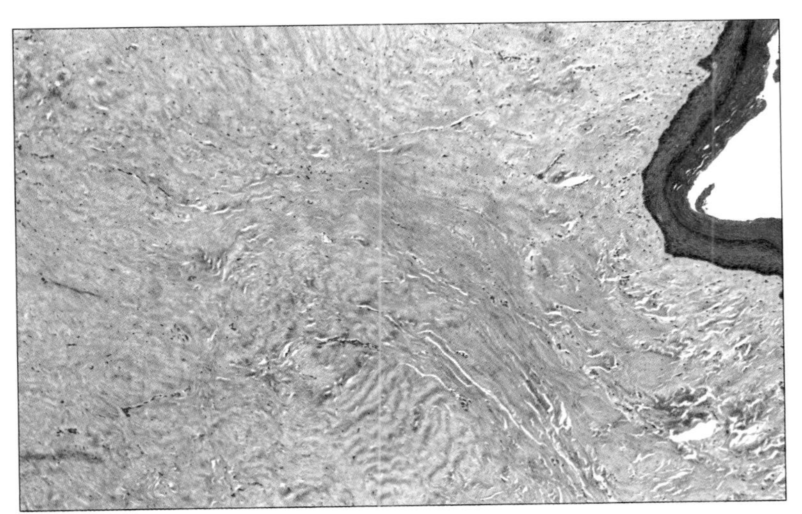

Fig. 12.9 Urethral stricture. A higher magnification of Fig. 12.8, showing, on the right, keratinizing squamous epithelium of the urethra covering a scarred stroma.

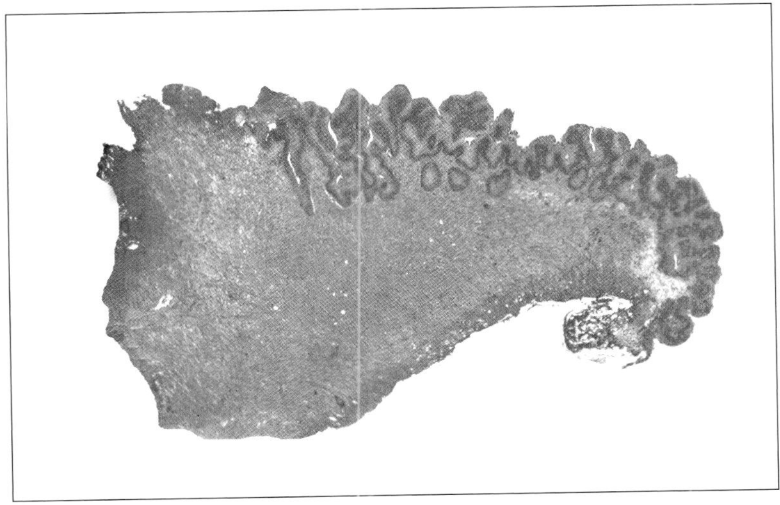

Fig. 12.10 Urethral stricture. Pseudopapillary nonkeratinizing squamous epithelium of the urethra covering a scarred stroma in a female urethra.

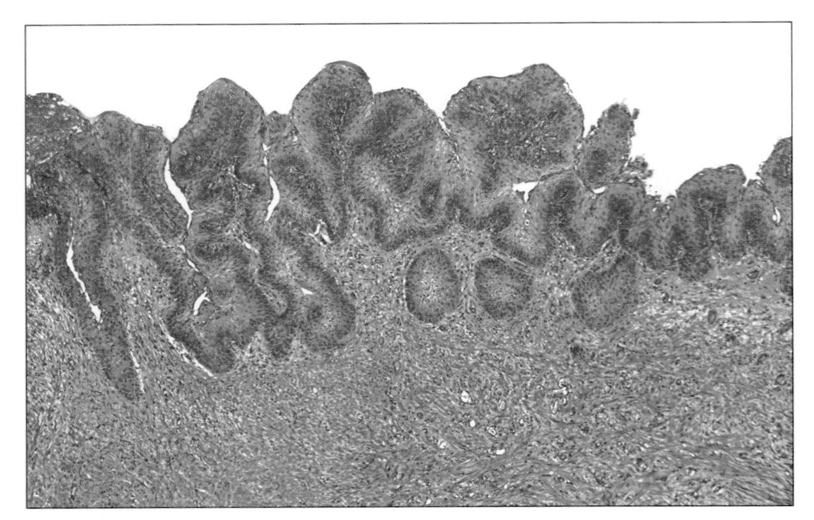

Fig. 12.11 Urethral stricture. Higher magnification of Fig. 12.10.

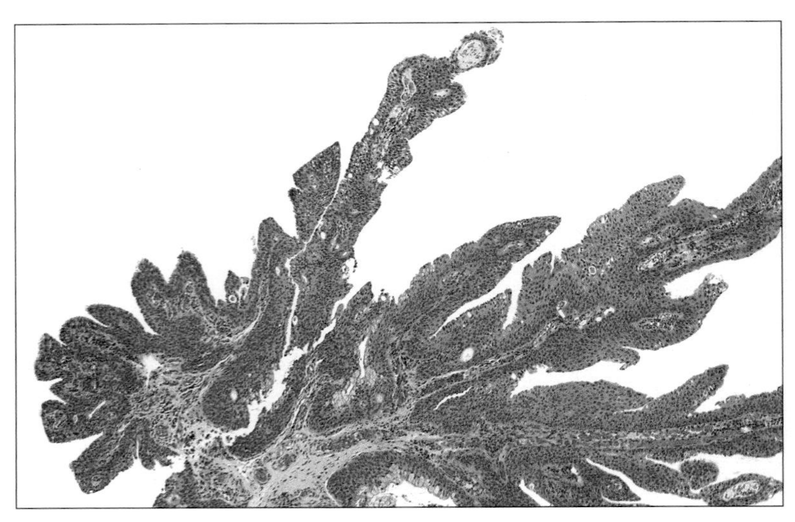

Fig. 12.13 Papilloma of urethra. Higher magnification of a portion of Fig. 12.12, where there is a papillary urothelial neoplasm in the center of the female urethra. There are no areas of cytologic atypia.

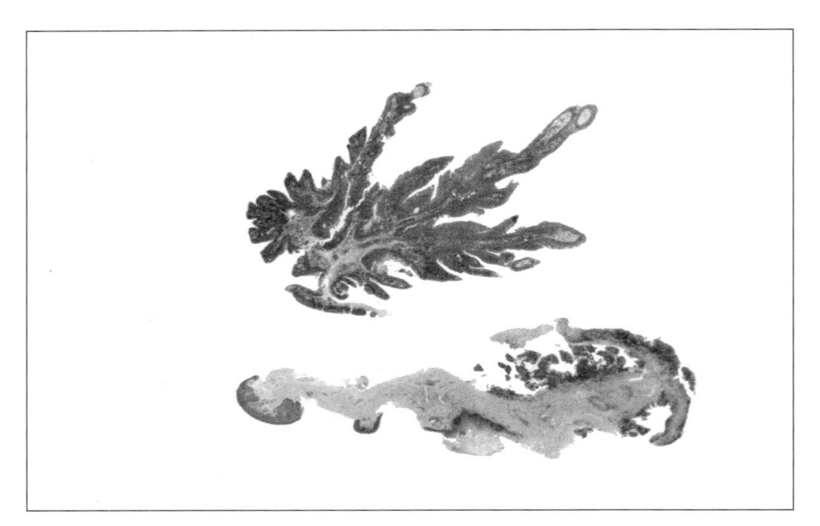

Fig. 12.12 Papilloma of urethra. Low magnification of a papillary urothelial neoplasm covering large areas of fibrovascular stroma. There are no areas of cytologic atypia.

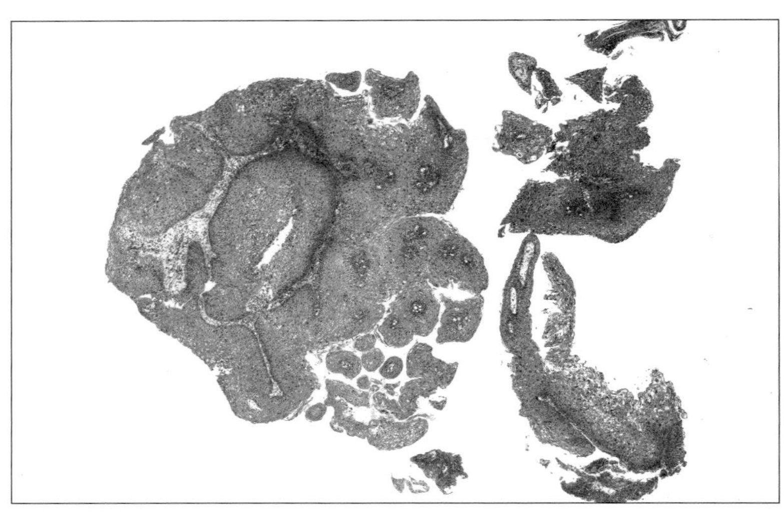

Fig. 12.14 Condyloma acuminatum. In the urethra, there was an elevated firm lesion on cystoscopy. It was biopsied and low-power magnification revealed a papillary nonkeratinizing squamous cell lesion.

Papilloma

- Papilloma of the urethra consists of fibrovascular cores, lined by benign or reactive-appearing, hyperplastic urothelium. Mitoses can be present, but are usually basal. The histology corresponds to papilloma or low-malignant-potential papillary urothelial tumor (grade 1) of the bladder. (Figs 12.12 & 12.13)
- Although papilloma of the urethra may recur, it usually follows a benign course. Occasionally, it can be continuous with a condyloma of the distal urethra. Many studies, however, have failed to identify human papillomavirus in urethral papillomas.

Condyloma acuminatum

- Condyloma acuminatum consists of a papillary hyperplasia of squamous epithelium, with frequent hyperkeratosis, mildly atypical hyperchromatic nuclei, and at least focal perinuclear clearing.
- Condylomas occur most commonly in the distal urethra of males and females, although they can be multifocal and can be found anywhere in the urethra, including the prostatic urethra.
- Human papillomavirus has been identified in these lesions (types 6 and 11, and to a lesser degree types 16 and 18, and others). (Figs 12.14–12.17)

Inverted papilloma

- Inverted papilloma is rare in the urethra.
- It presents with hematuria.
- The histology is identical to that of inverted papilloma elsewhere in the urothelial tract.

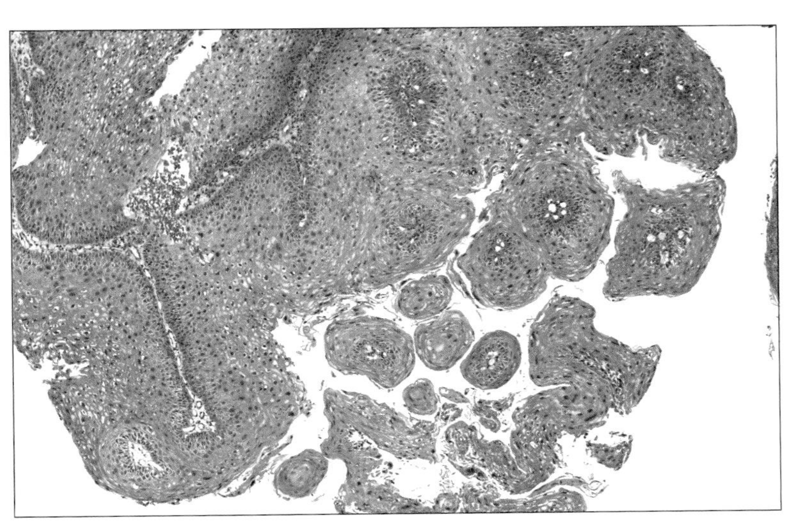

Fig. 12.15 Condyloma acuminatum. Higher magnification of Fig. 12.14 reveals papillary fronds with delicate fibrovascular cores covered by acanthotic epithelium.

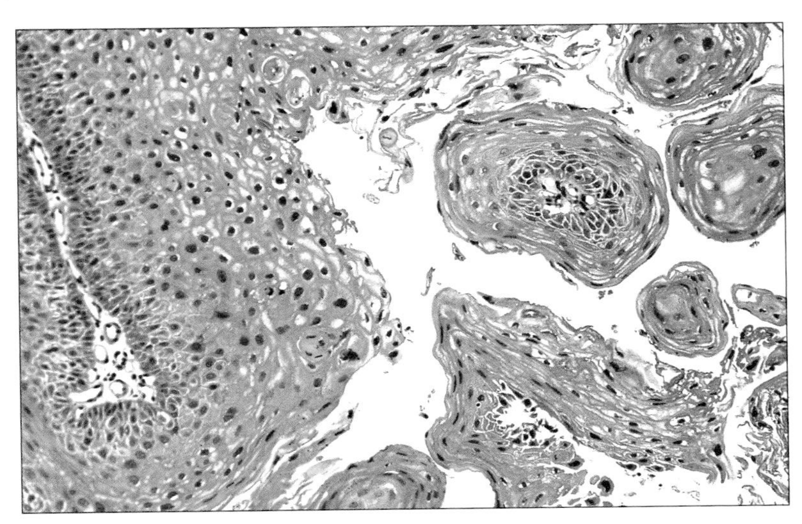

Fig. 12.16 Condyloma acuminatum. Higher magnification of Fig. 12.15. There are papillary fronds with delicate fibrovascular cores covered by acanthotic epithelium. There are superficial koilocytes with irregular nuclear contours and characteristic perinuclear clear spaces.

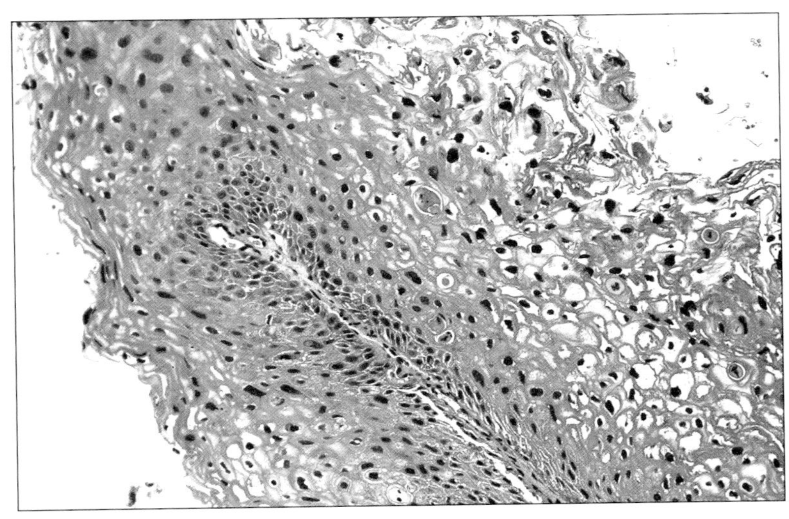

Fig. 12.17 Condyloma acuminatum. Higher magnification of Fig. 12.15. There are papillary fronds with a delicate fibrovascular core covered by acanthotic epithelium. There are superficial koilocytes with irregular nuclear contours and characteristic perinuclear clear spaces.

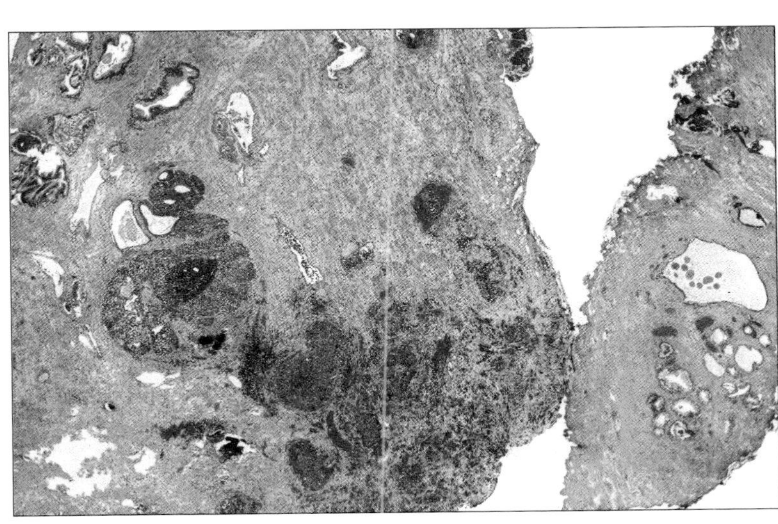

Fig. 12.18 Urothelial carcinoma from the prostatic urethra spreading up the periurethral prostatic ducts. The tumor is contained within the ducts on the left but is seen to spread out into the stroma in the middle of the image.

MALIGNANT TUMORS

UROTHELIAL CARCINOMA, ASSOCIATED WITH CARCINOMA OF BLADDER AND PROSTATE

Urothelial carcinoma of the bladder can spread by contiguity into the urethra. This occurs in up to 20% of patients with bladder cancer, and is in fact the most frequent urethral malignancy. It occurs most often in men,[3] and in patients with multifocal disease.

Histology

Urothelial carcinoma of the bladder can involve the urethra in the following ways.

- Urothelial carcinoma in situ may line the urethra.
- It can extend into periurethral prostatic ducts and give rise to prostatic gland involvement. This is still not an invasive tumor, but has graver consequences because secondary invasion of the prostate from these involved ducts cannot be easily identified. (Figs 12.18–12.20)
- Lastly, urothelial carcinoma may present as a papillary carcinoma of the urethra, with or without direct prostatic invasion.

Urothelial carcinoma of the urethra can also be continuous with *periurethral ductal (prostatic duct) carcinoma* of the prostate. This is a prostatic primary arising in the major periprostatic ducts, with urothelial or a glandular histology. It often shows involvement of overlying urethra. A higher

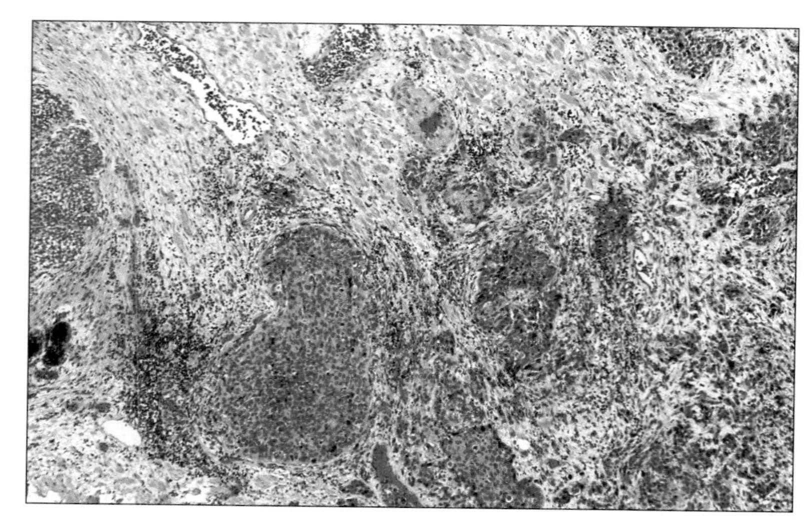

Fig. 12.19 Periurethral urothelial carcinoma. The tumor is contained within the ducts on the left but is seen to spread out into the stroma on the right side of the image.

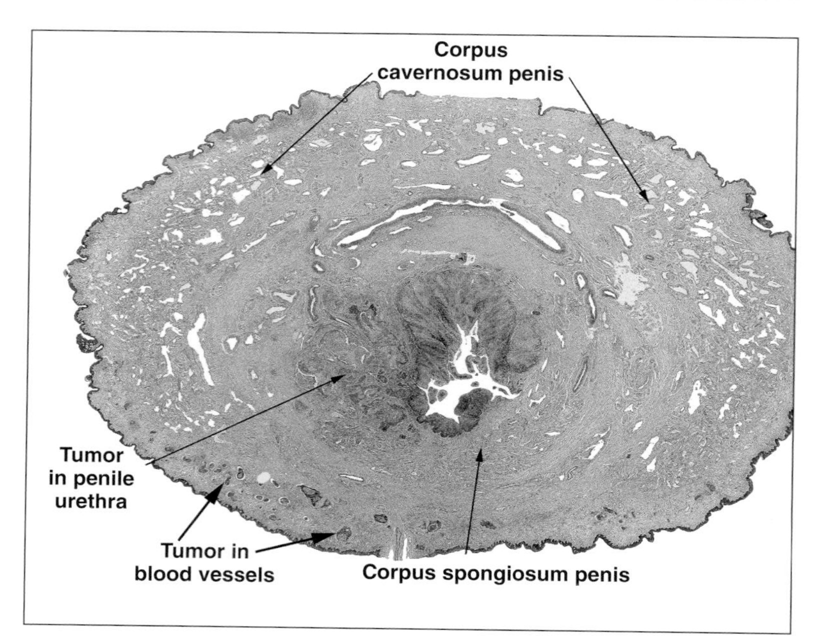

Fig. 12.21 Urothelial carcinoma of penile urethra. It has spread outside into the corpus spongiosum of the penis and peripheral subepidermal blood vessels. Whole-mount cross-section.

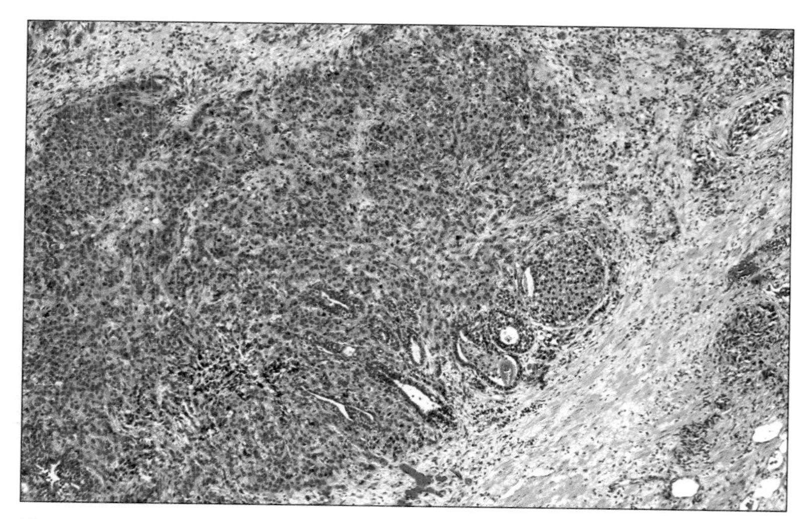

Fig. 12.20 Periurethral urothelial carcinoma. The tumor has spread out into the stroma. It is seen as small clusters of undifferentiated tumor cells spreading out in the stroma in a random pattern.

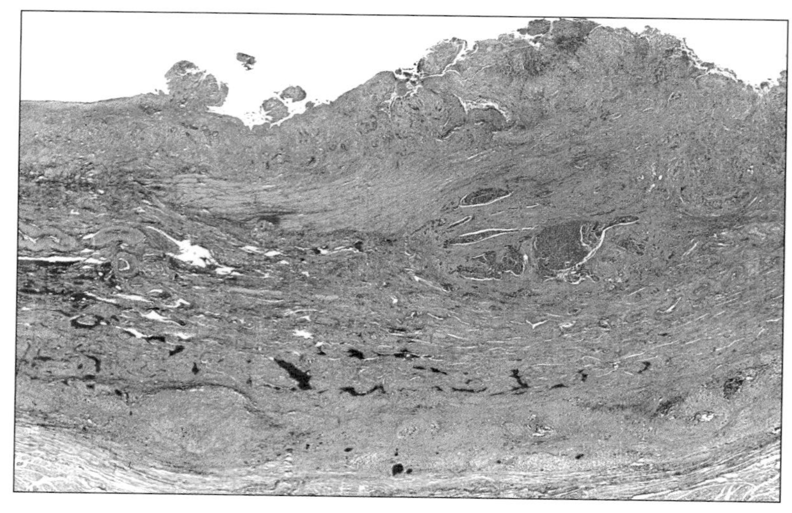

Fig. 12.22 Urothelial carcinoma of penile urethra. It has spread into the blood vessels of the corpus spongiosum. Low magnification.

incidence of associated urothelial bladder tumors has also been reported in these cases.

PRIMARY CARCINOMA OF THE URETHRA

Male urethra

- Primary *urothelial carcinomas* of the urethra are uncommon. They usually arise in the proximal segment. (Figs 12.21–12.29)
- *Squamous cell carcinoma* is usually found in the penile urethra. (Figs 12.30–12.32)
- Most tumors of the penile urethra are *nonkeratinizing squamous cell carcinomas*, often well differentiated.
- *Verrucous carcinoma* is most common in the distal penile urethra, and is histologically identical to this tumor in the penis. Human papillomavirus has been implicated in these lesions.
- *Adenocarcinomas* are uncommon in the male urethra. They are associated with strictures, diverticula, and infections (see discussion below). A few cases of Cowper's gland adenocarcinoma have been reported, and they are usually mucinous.[4]
- Prognosis of primary urethral carcinoma is dependent on stage. Distal urethral tumors have a better

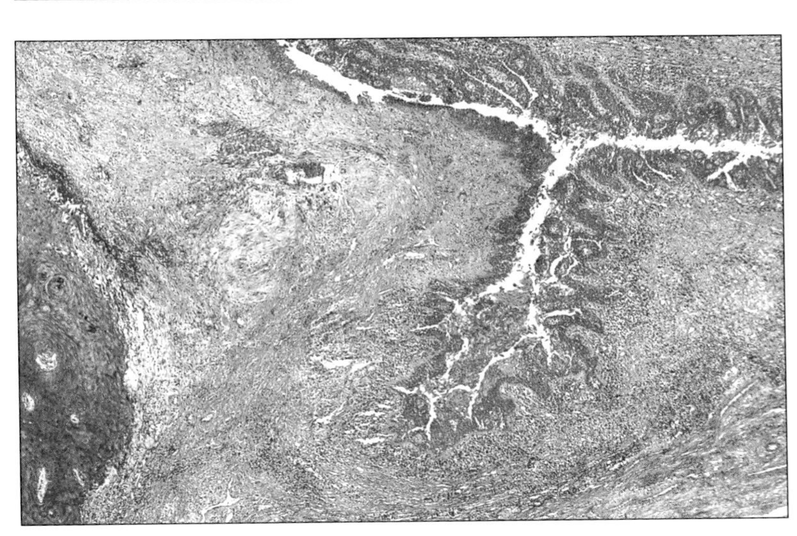

Fig. 12.23 Urothelial carcinoma of penile urethra. Cancer extends into the ducts of the submucosal glands. There is a marked inflammatory cell reaction beneath the neoplasm.

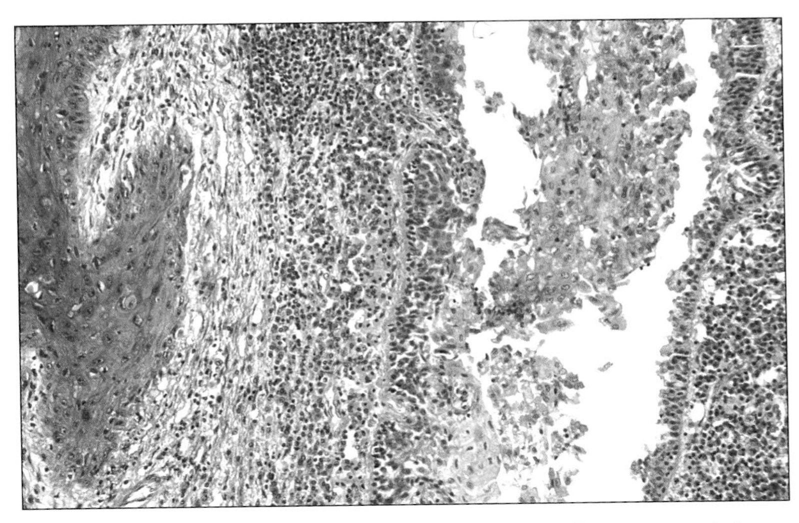

Fig. 12.24 Urothelial carcinoma of penile urethra. Cancer extends into the ducts of the submucosal glands. There is a marked inflammatory cell reaction beneath the neoplasm. There may be a squamous cell component (right) mixed with the urothelial cancer.

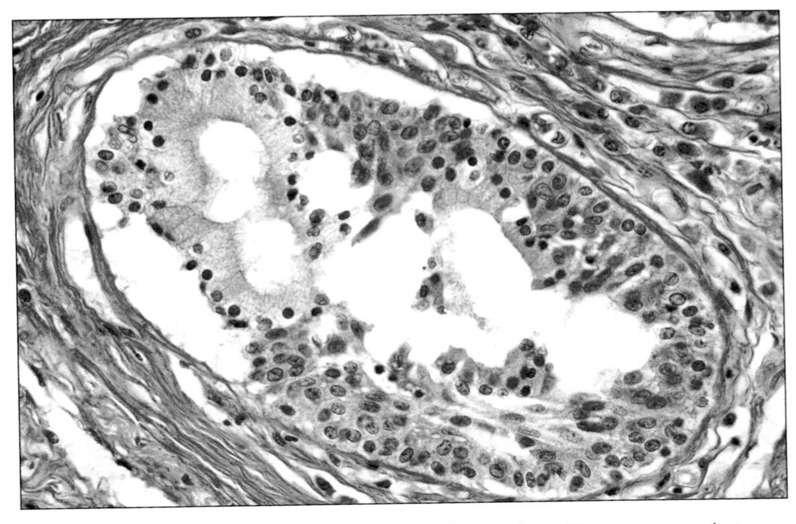

Fig. 12.25 Urothelial carcinoma of penile urethra. Cancer extends into the ducts and glands of the submucosa.

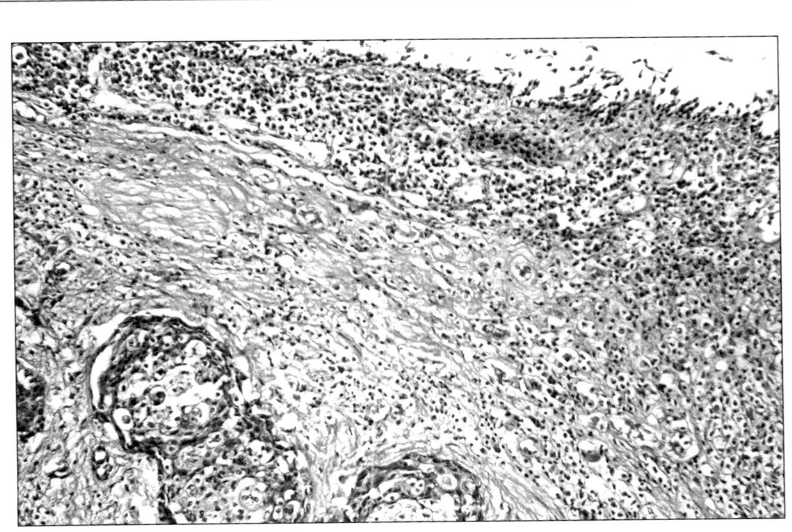

Fig. 12.26 Urothelial carcinoma of penile urethra. Cancer often detaches but extends into the ducts, where there is squamous cell change.

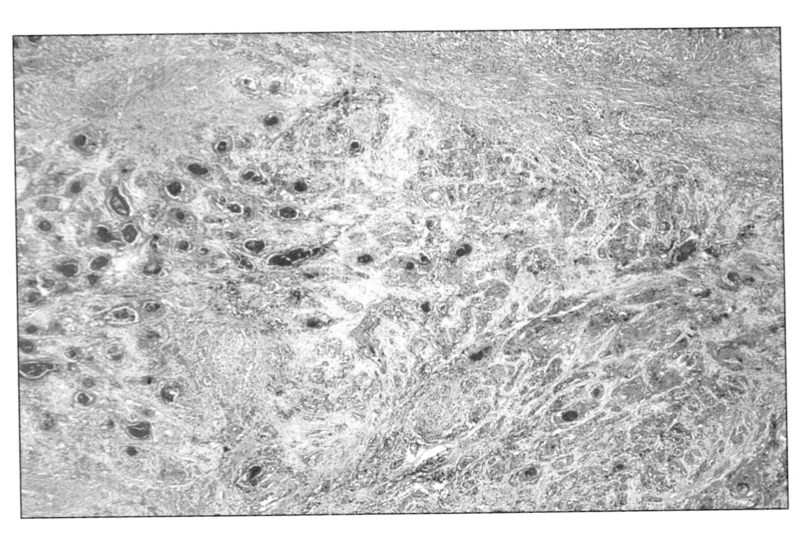

Fig. 12.27 Urothelial carcinoma of penile urethra. Low-power photomicrograph of the urothelial cancer spread into the corpora. There is extensive squamous cell change but the surface was a well-differentiated urothelial cancer.

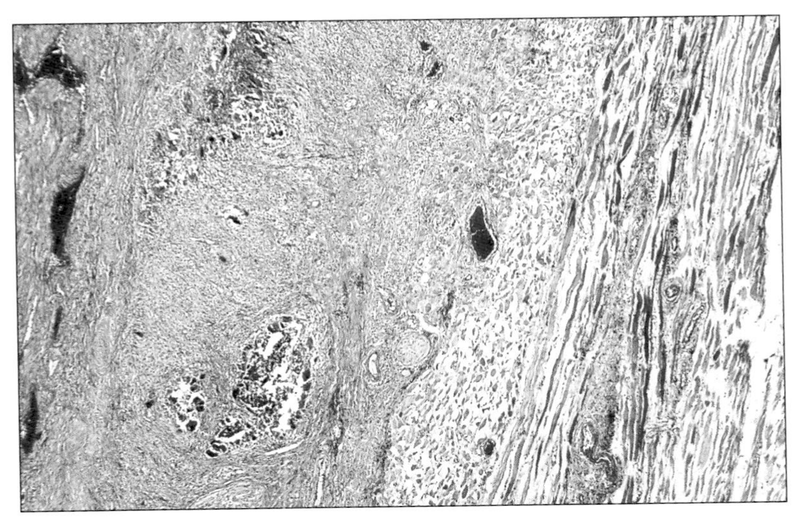

Fig. 12.28 Urothelial carcinoma of penile urethra. High-power magnification of the poorly differentiated urothelial cancer spreading into the corpora.

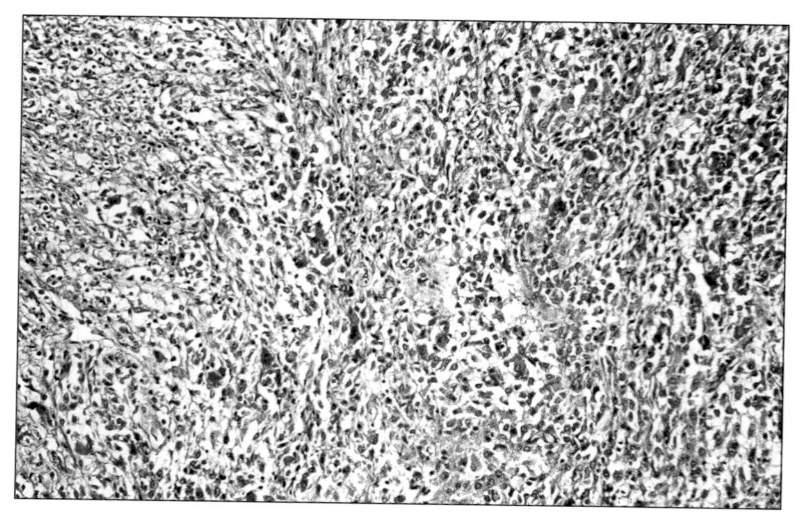

Fig. 12.29 Urothelial carcinoma of penile urethra. High-power magnification of the poorly differentiated urothelial cancer spreading into the corpora. Spindle and strap-like cancer cells are seen.

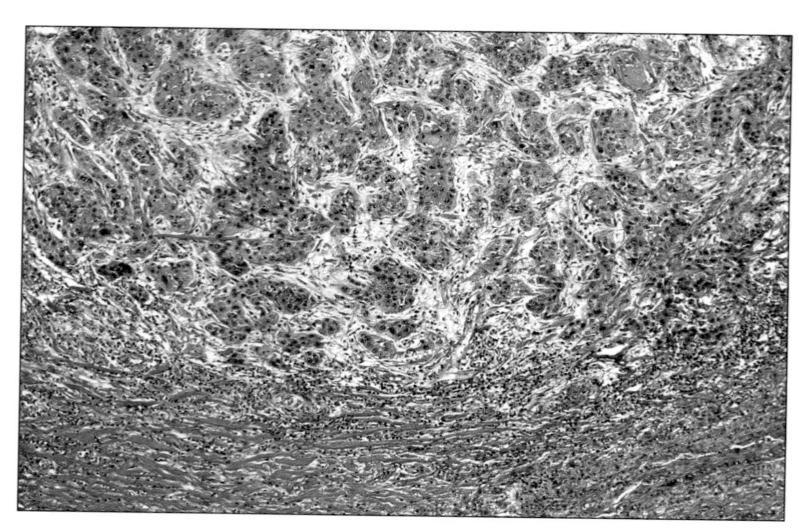

Fig. 12.31 Photomicrograph of an invading squamous cell carcinoma of the bulbourethral glands.

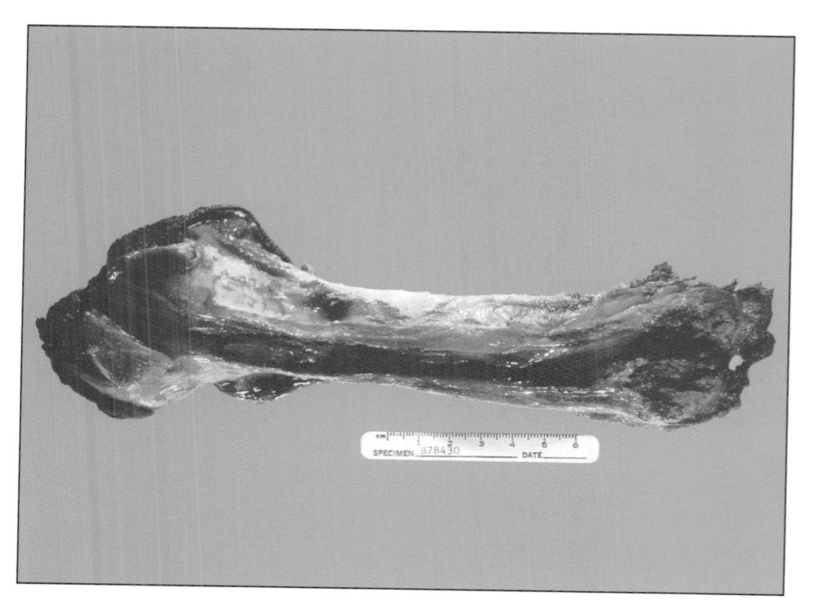

Fig. 12.30 Squamous cell carcinoma of the bulbourethral glands. This is a longitudinal section of the penis, with the glans penis on the left and the tumor in the bulbourethral glands on the right.

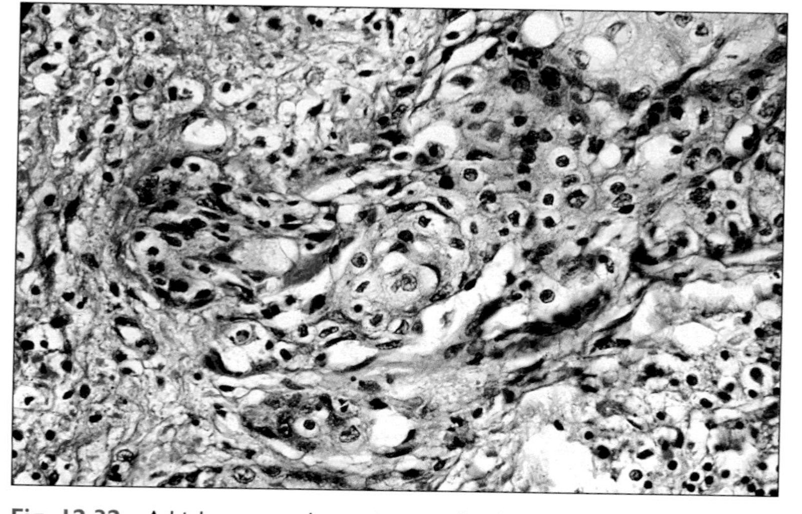

Fig. 12.32 A high-power photomicrograph of an invading squamous cell carcinoma of the bulbourethral glands.

prognosis, because they tend to be detected sooner. Urethral carcinomas metastasize to inguinal lymph nodes, and proximal tumors also metastasize to pelvic lymph nodes.

Female urethra

- Primary carcinoma of the urethra is more common in women than men. Many of these tumors appear clinically as caruncles.
- Approximately three-quarters of the tumors are squamous carcinomas, including *verrucous carcinoma*, and *nonkeratinizing* and *keratinizing squamous cell carcinoma*.
- *Urothelial carcinoma* comprises about 15% of the tumors and is usually proximal.
- *Adenocarcinoma* of the urethra occurs in both sexes, and is associated with diverticula and strictures. Adjacent mucosa may show urethritis cystica or glandular metaplasia. Often, they resemble colonic carcinoma.[2] (Figs 12.33–12.37)
- *Clear cell carcinoma* of the urethra almost always occurs in females, and often arises in diverticula. These tumors are frequently identified within the

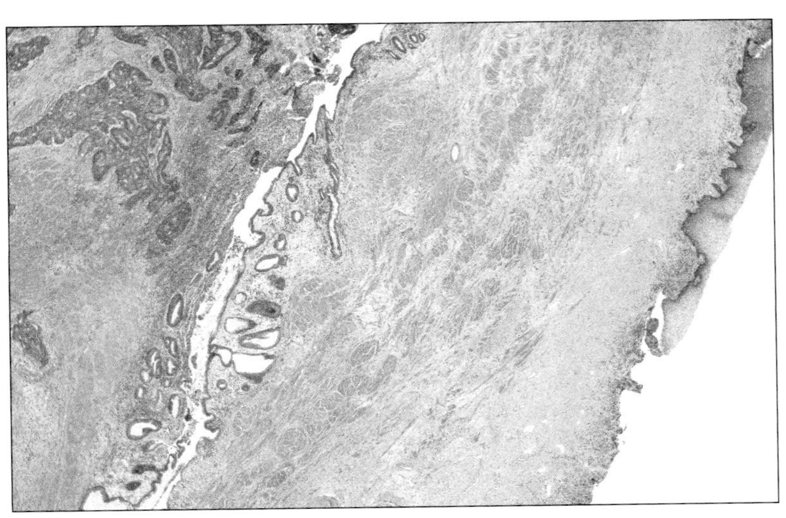

Fig. 12.33 Adenocarcinoma of the female urethra. The adenocarcinoma is on the left of the urethra.

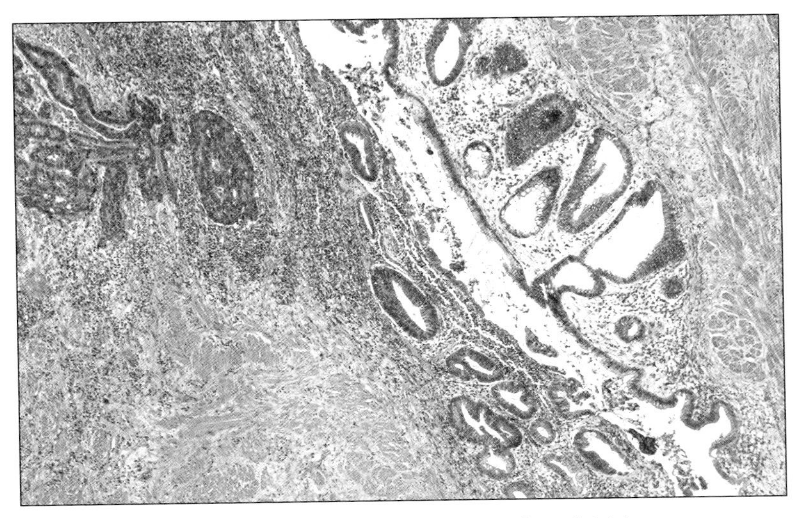

Fig. 12.34 Adenocarcinoma of the female urethra. A higher-magnification photomicrograph of Fig. 12.33. The adenocarcinoma is on the left of the urethra.

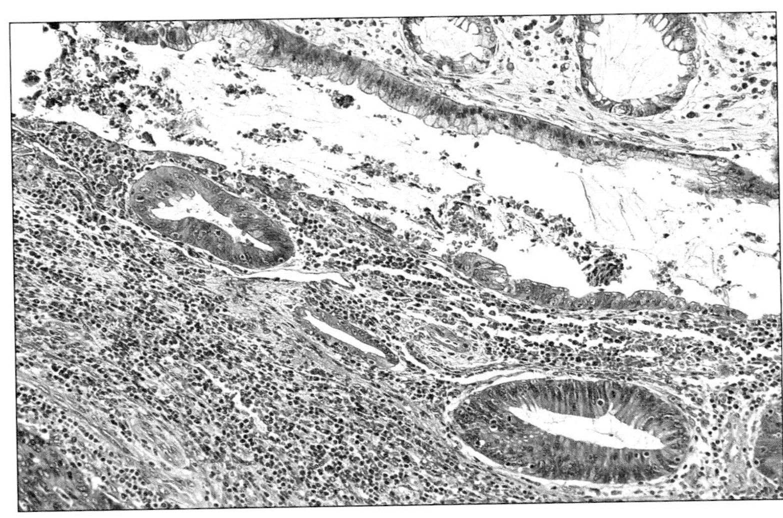

Fig. 12.35 Adenocarcinoma of the female urethra. A higher-magnification photomicrograph of Fig. 12.33. The adenocarcinoma is in the lower half of the photomicrograph. Non-neoplastic mucin-secreting glands are in the upper half.

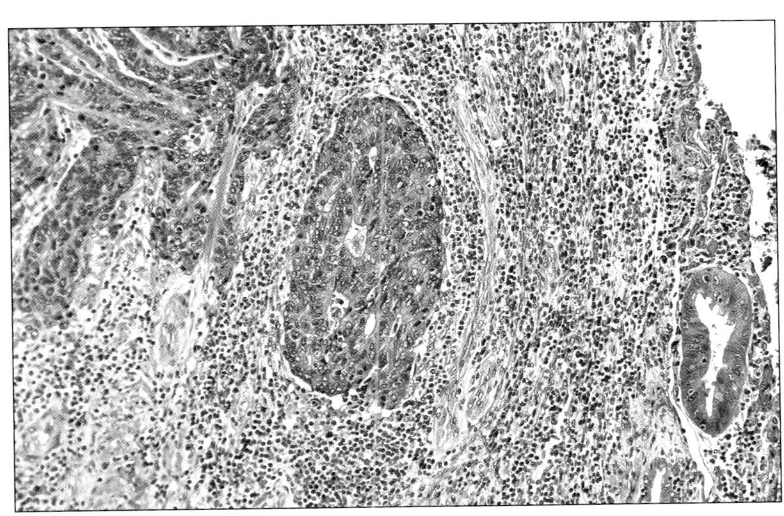

Fig. 12.36 Adenocarcinoma of the female urethra. A high-magnification photomicrograph of Fig. 12.33.

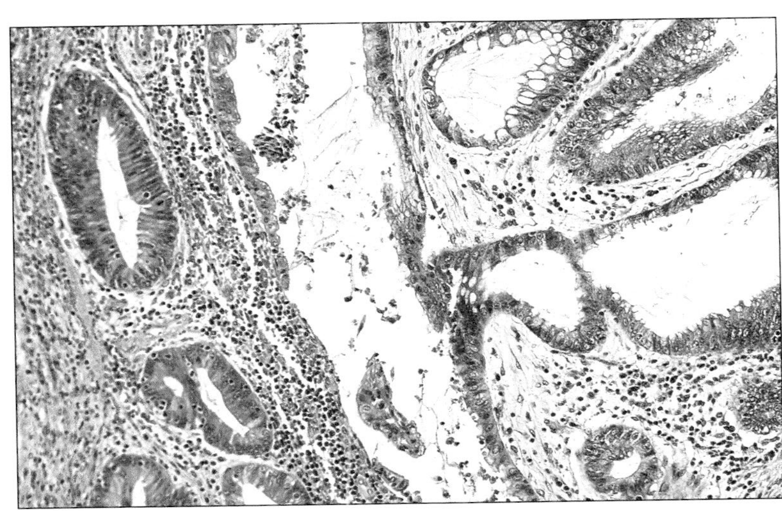

Fig. 12.37 Adenocarcinoma of the female urethra. A higher-magnification photomicrograph of Fig. 12.33. The adenocarcinoma is on the left of the urethra, and the non-neoplastic glands are on the right.

urethrovaginal wall, and the primary site of origin may be difficult to ascertain. Clear cell carcinoma of the vagina occurs in women exposed to diethylstilbestrol (DES) in utero, and rarely in elderly patients. Clinical history and tumor location are helpful. The muscularis of the vagina can serve as a helpful landmark. If most of the tumor is found on the urethral side of this muscle, whether in continuity with urethral lining or in a diverticular pocket, the tumor is a urethral primary.

- The histology of clear cell carcinoma of the urethra is identical to its counterpart in the female genital tract, consisting of clear or hobnail cells arranged in sheets, glands, and micropapillae.[5] These tumors are positive for glycogen, but mucicarmine reactivity is seen only on luminal membranes, not in the cytoplasm. (Figs 12.38–12.41)

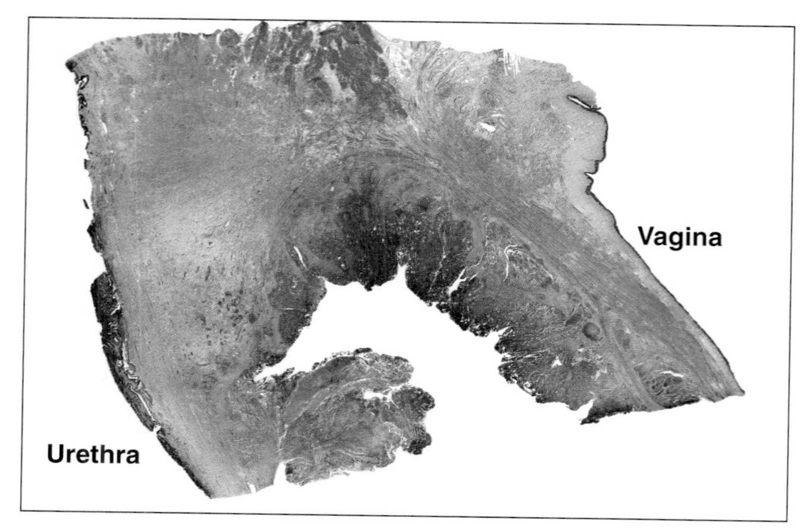

Fig. 12.38 Clear cell adenocarcinoma of the female urethra.

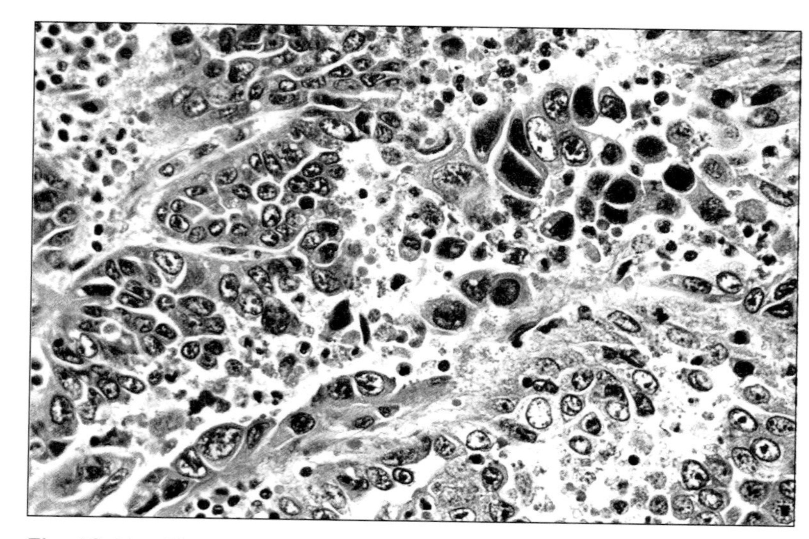

Fig. 12.41 Clear cell adenocarcinoma of the female urethra. Cells have a hobnail appearance and the nuclei are very pleomorphic.

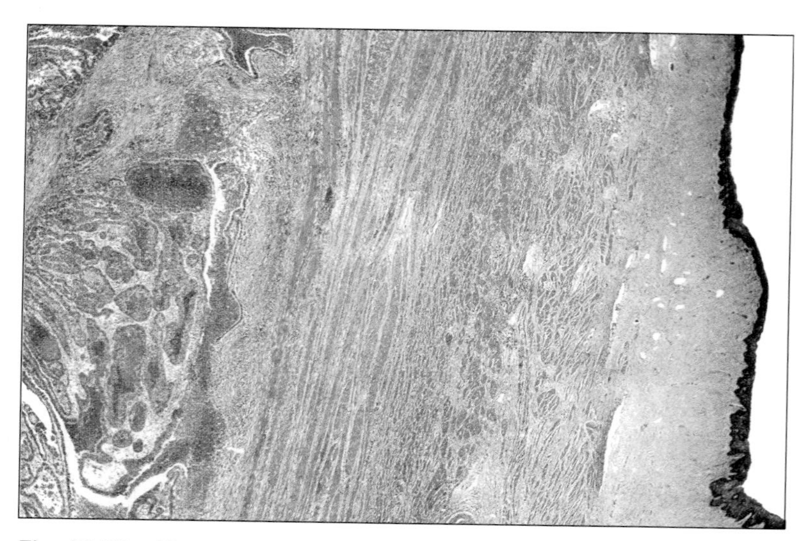

Fig. 12.39 Clear cell adenocarcinoma of the female urethra. Tumor is on the left and vaginal epithelium is on the right of the photomicrograph.

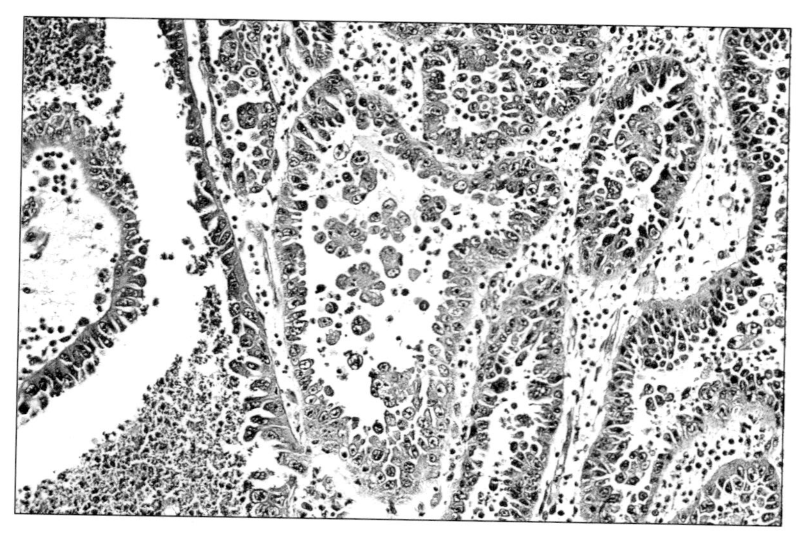

Fig. 12.40 Clear cell adenocarcinoma of the female urethra. The tumor has a papillary pattern and is composed of cells that have an apical hobnail appearance. The nuclei are pleomorphic.

Other rare carcinomas

Single cases of other rare carcinomas have been described:

- carcinoid;[6]
- adenoid cystic carcinoma;[7]
- adenosquamous carcinoma;[8]
- cloacogenic carcinoma.[9]

SKENE'S GLANDS CARCINOMA

Clinical Skene's gland adenocarcinoma is an uncommon tumor, usually presenting as a perineal abscess or mass. Prognosis is dependent on stage.

Histology These tumors may produce mucin. The malignant cells grow in glands, papillary formations, and sheets. The distinction from primary adenocarcinoma may be very difficult. The diagnosis of primary Skene's glands carcinoma is appropriate if residual benign Skene's glands are identified, particularly if they show in-situ changes. Reactivity for prostate-specific antigen (PSA) and prostatic acid phosphatase are helpful, since most Skene's glands carcinomas are positive, especially for PSA. (Figs 12.42–12.46)

MALIGNANT MELANOMA

Clinical Primary malignant melanoma of the urethra is rare, affects both sexes, and has been reported in dark-skinned individuals. These lesions are frequently amelanotic and may present with hematuria and obstruction. Significant radial spread is common.

Histology Malignant melanoma of the urethra has the same histology as that of other mucous membranes. Epithelial

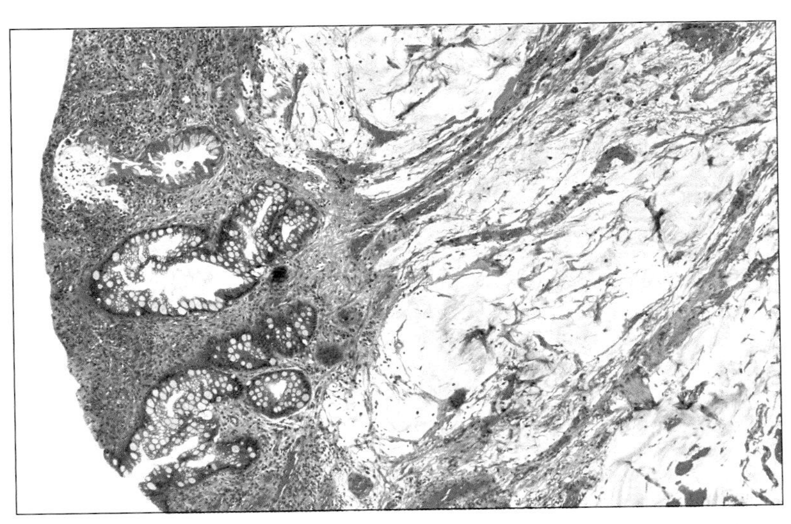

Fig. 12.42 Glands of Skene. The glands are composed of cells that have a goblet cell structure. There is extracellular mucin on the right of the photomicrograph. This results from urethral obstruction and inflammation.

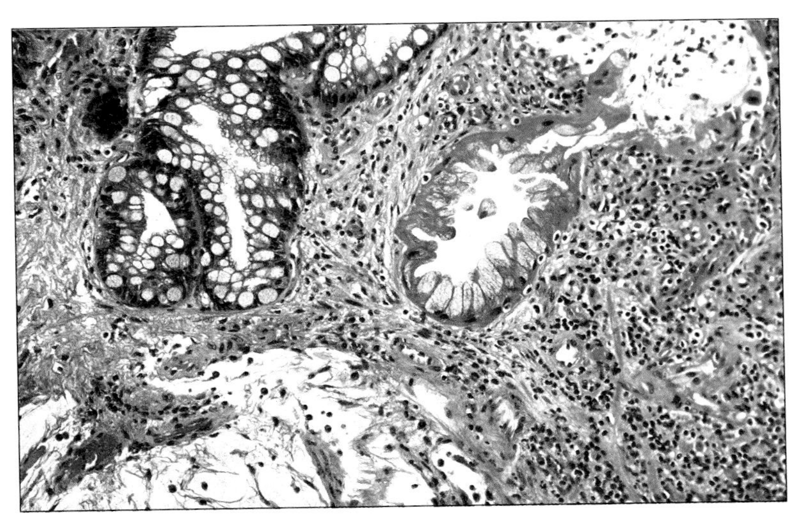

Fig. 12.43 Glands of Skene. Higher magnification of Fig. 12.42. The glands are composed of cells that have a goblet cell structure. There is extracellular mucin at the bottom of the photomicrograph.

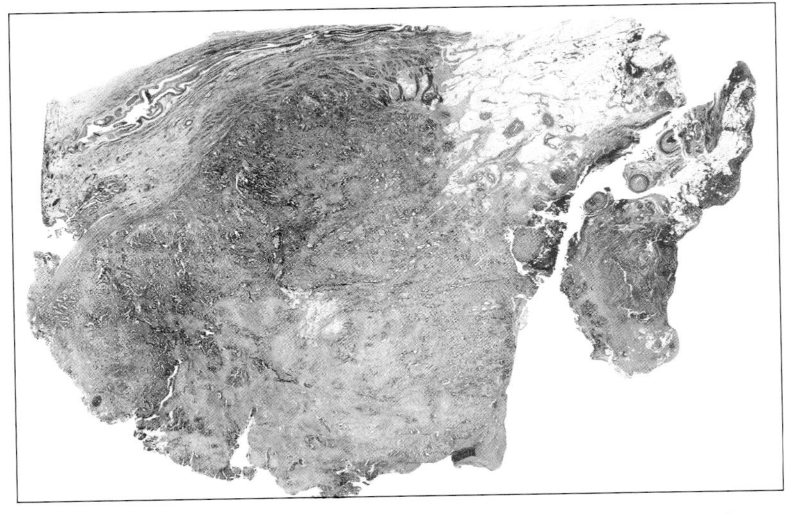

Fig. 12.44 Adenocarcinoma of Skene's glands. Photomicrograph of whole slide, where the urethra is at the top and beneath it are the infiltrating glands of the carcinoma. There is extracellular mucin in the stroma in the upper right corner of the tissue.

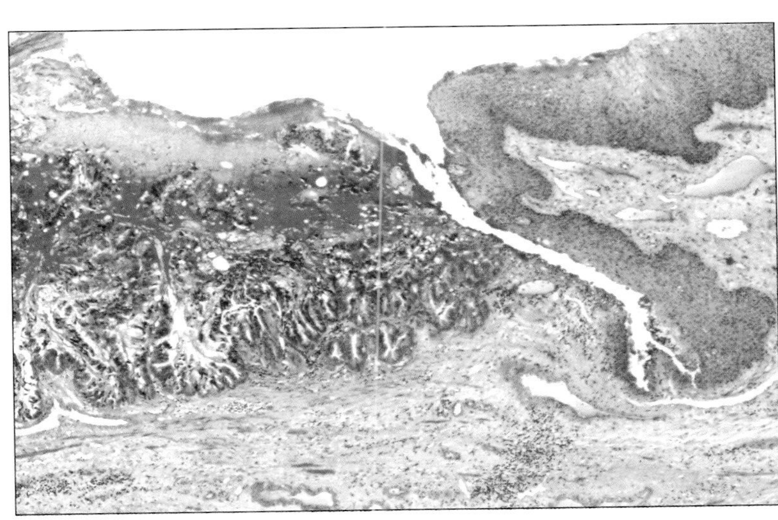

Fig. 12.45 Adenocarcinoma of Skene's glands. There is, in the left half of the photomicrograph, an adenocarcinoma at the surface of the urethra. The normal urethral lining is on the right side.

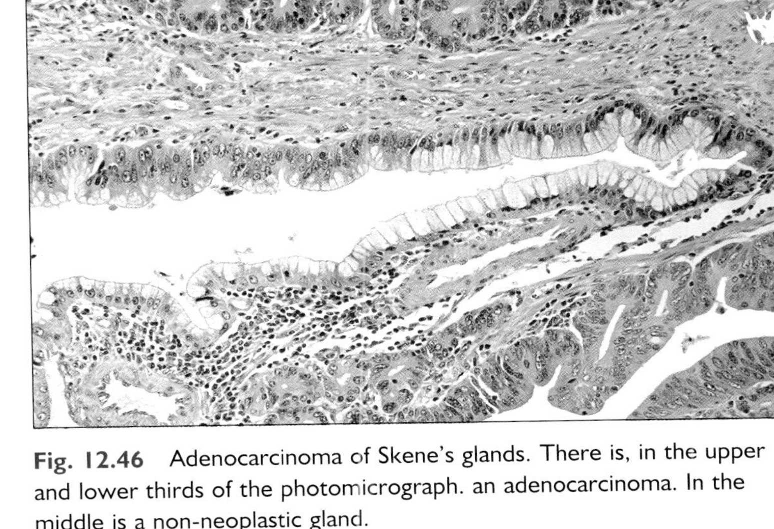

Fig. 12.46 Adenocarcinoma of Skene's glands. There is, in the upper and lower thirds of the photomicrograph. an adenocarcinoma. In the middle is a non-neoplastic gland.

lesions are seen, but spindle cell melanoma is more common. Particularly when they are amelanotic, spindle cell melanomas need to be distinguished from sarcomas. (Figs 12.47–12.53)

STROMAL TUMORS

Leiomyoma is the most common uretheral mesenchymal tumor, and can range in size from 1 to 40 cm.[10] Other tumors include *hemangioma, neurofibroma, paraganglioma,* and *aggressive angiomyxoma.*[11]

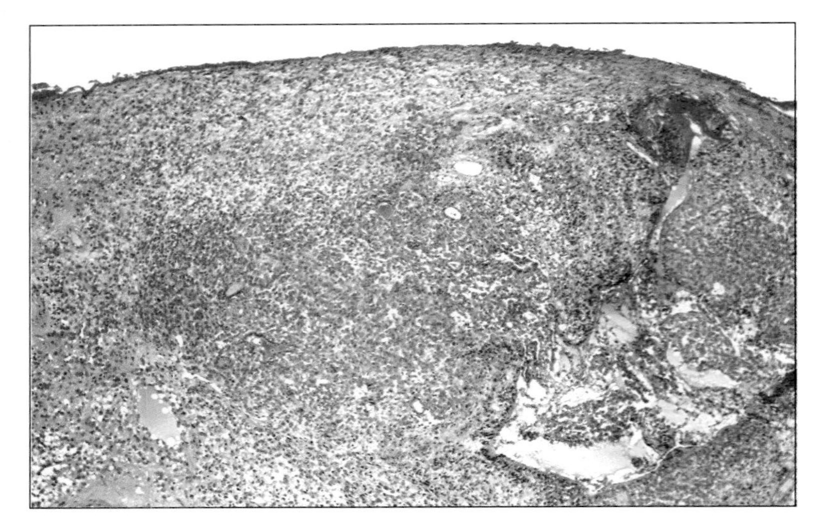

Fig. 12.47 Malignant melanoma of the urethra. Beneath the urethral surface (upper part of photomicrograph), there is a malignant melanoma.

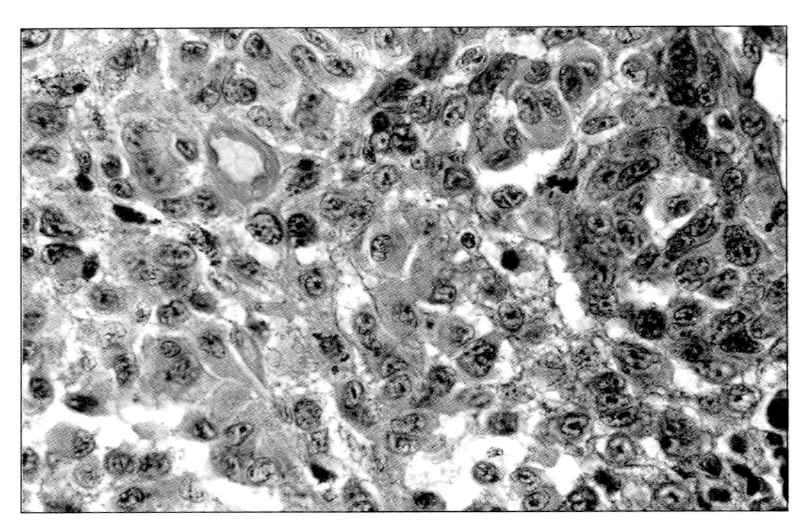

Fig. 12.49 Malignant melanoma of the urethra. Higher magnification of Fig. 12.47. Many malignant melanoma nuclei with prominent nucleoli can be seen. There are many abnormal mitoses and a rare cell with S-100-positive pigment in the cytoplasm.

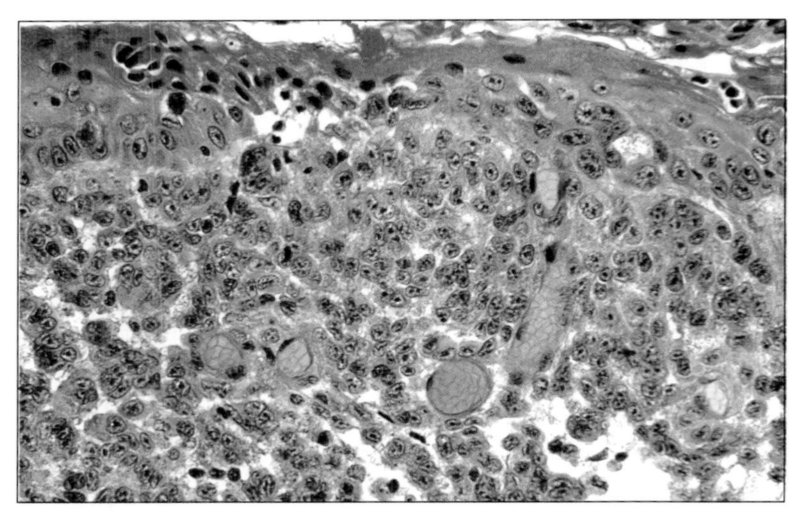

Fig. 12.48 Malignant melanoma of the urethra. Higher magnification of Fig. 12.47. Beneath the urethral surface (upper part of photomicrograph), there is a malignant melanoma.

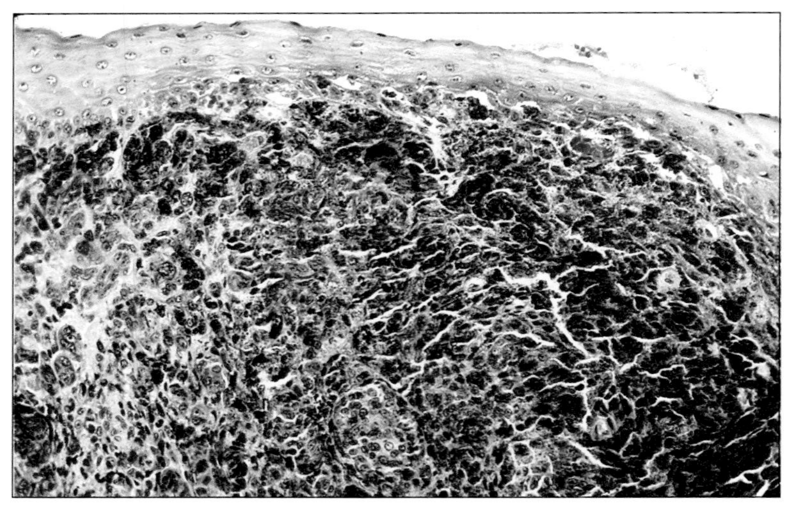

Fig. 12.50 Malignant melanoma of the urethra. Many malignant melanoma nuclei with prominent nucleoli can be seen. There are many cells with S-100-positive pigment in the cytoplasm. Here, the pigmentation is obvious on a slide stained with hematoxylin–eosin.

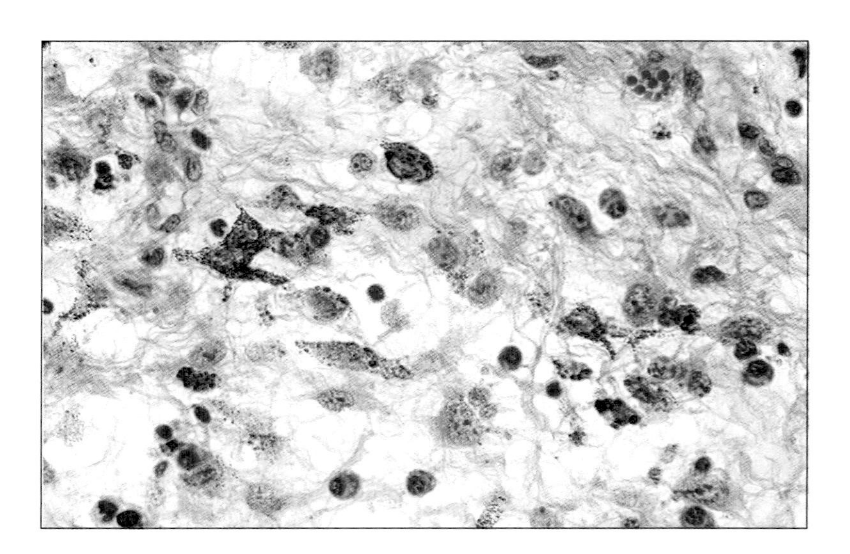

Fig. 12.51 Malignant melanoma of the urethra shows nuclei with prominent nucleoli and with S-100-positive pigment in the cytoplasm. Pigmentation is obvious.

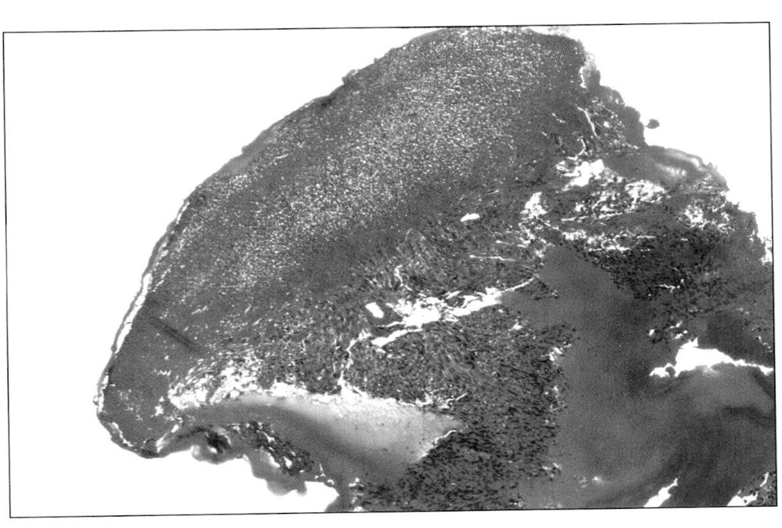

Fig. 12.52 Spindle cell malignant melanoma of the urethra. A biopsy of a necrotic portion of the distal urethra. A spindle cell malignant melanoma is present beneath the necrotic ulcerating urethral surface. Low-power digital photomicrograph.

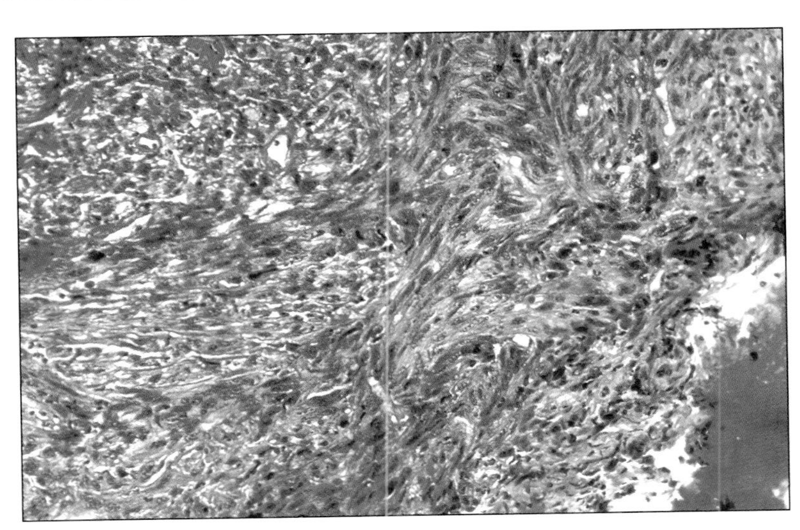

Fig. 12.53 Spindle cell malignant melanoma of the urethra. Higher magnification of Fig. 12.52. A spindle cell malignant melanoma is present beneath the necrotic ulcerating urethral surface. Immunohistochemistry is of help in distinguishing it from leiomyosarcoma and fibrous histiocytoma.

REFERENCES

1. Marshall S, Hirsch K. Carcinoma within urethral diverticula. Urology 1977;10:161–163.
2. Powell I, Cartwright H, Jano F. Villous adenoma and adenocarcinoma of female urethra. Urology 1981;18:612–614.
3. Gowing NFC. Urethral carcinoma associated with cancer of the bladder. Br J Urol 1960;32:428–430.
4. Keen MR, Golden RL, Richardson JF, Melicow MM. Carcinoma of Cowper's gland treated with chemotherapy. J Urol 1970;104:854–859.
5. Oliva E, Young RH. Clear cell adenocarcinoma of the urethra: a clinopathologic analysis of 19 cases. Mod Pathol 1996;9:513–520.
6. Sylora HO, Diamond HM, Kaufman M, et al. Primary carcinoid of the urethra. J Urol 1975;114:150–153.
7. Aronson P, Ronan SG, Briele HA, et al. Adenoid cystic carcinoma of female periurethral area. Light and electron microscopic study. Urology 1982;20:312–315.
8. Saito R. An adenosquamous carcinoma of the male urethra with hypercalcemia. Hum Pathol 1981;12:383–385.
9. Diaz-Cano SJ, Rios JJ, Rivera-Hueto F, et al. Mixed cloacogenic carcinoma of male urethra. Histopathology 1992;20:82–84.
10. Cheng C, Mac-Moune Lai F, Chan PS. Leiomyoma of the female urethra: a case report and review. J Urol 1991;148:1526–1527.
11. Steeper TA, Rosai J. Aggressive angiomyxoma of the female pelvis and perineum: report of nine cases of a distinctive type of gynecologic soft tissue neoplasm. Am J Surg Pathol 1983;7:463–475.

13

PATHOLOGY OF THE ADRENAL GLAND

Bruce M. Wenig

NON-NEOPLASTIC LESIONS OF THE ADRENAL GLAND (Table 13.1)

ADRENAL HETEROTOPIA AND ACCESSORY ADRENAL TISSUE[1-8]

Definition

True adrenal heterotopia refers to the presence of the entire adrenal gland in an abnormal location; in contrast, accessory adrenal tissue usually consists of small rests of cortical cells.

Clinical

- Patients with adrenal heterotopia or adrenal rests rarely have any symptoms related to the abnormality; most examples of adrenal heterotopia are incidental, found following surgery for unrelated problems.
- Heterotopia and accessory adrenal tissue are found anywhere along the path of descent of the gonads, but typically localize in the upper abdomen in relationship to the kidney; the latter finding is explained by the embryologic development of the adrenal gland in close spatial relationship with the kidneys (Table 13.2).
- Heterotopic adrenal usually occurs in the upper abdomen and typically localizes to the upper pole of the kidney beneath the renal capsule; rare examples are located in the capsule of the liver.
- Accessory adrenal tissue or adrenal rests are most often seen along the migration path of the gonads, the most common site being the area of the celiac axis; adrenal rests also are frequently found around the kidney, in the broad ligament, in and around the spermatic cord, and in hernia sacs; accessory adrenal tissue may also be found in rather unusual locations, including the ovary, placenta, gallbladder wall, lungs, and in the cranial cavity.
- Accessory adrenal tissue is a very common finding, present in almost one-third of individuals at autopsy.

Pathology

Gross

- Heterotopia is usually bilateral; the adrenal may be flattened and atrophic in appearance, though functionally it seems to be adequate to maintain normal cortisol levels.
- Accessory tissue appears as small, rounded, yellow, encapsulated nodules, a few millimeters in diameter.

Histology

- Adrenal rests are composed of lipid-rich cortical cells, usually without a medullary component; some degree of zonal differentiation is present.
- In complete adrenal heterotopia, a medullary component is not present.

Treatment and prognosis

- Adrenal heterotopia is not associated with any endocrine abnormality.
- Adrenal cortical rests require no treatment except in the rare instance of a cortical neoplasm arising in them. The rests may also be affected by any hyperplastic phenomenon resulting from adrenocorticotropic hormone (ACTH) stimulation.

CONGENITAL ADRENAL HYPOPLASIA[5,10-13]

Definition

Congenital adrenal hypoplasia is a sporadic or familial disorder characterized by a reduced volume of adrenal cortical tissue.

Clinical

- Congenital adrenal hypoplasia may occur sporadically or may be an autosomal recessive or X-linked inherited disorder. Other cases are associated with glycerol kinase enzyme deficiency.
- The most common form, the cytomegalic type, is X-linked; a rarer form is the 'miniature type'.

Table 13.1 Classification of non-neoplastic lesions of the adrenal gland	
1.	Heterotopic adrenal and accessory adrenal tissue
2.	Congenital hypoplasia
3.	Adrenal cytomegaly
4.	Congenital adrenal hyperplasia
5.	Addison's disease
6.	Infections affecting the adrenal gland
7.	Amyloidosis
8.	Waterhouse–Friderichsen syndrome
9.	Adrenal cysts
10.	Adrenal cortical nodules (nonhyperfunctioning)
11.	Adrenal cortical hyperplasia with hypercortisolism
12.	Adrenal cortical hyperplasia with hyperaldosteronism

Table 13.2 Location of accessory and heterotopic adrenal tissue	
Area of celiac axis	32%
Broad ligament	23%
Spermatic cord	4–9%
Adnexa of testes	8%
Kidney (subcapsular upper pole)	6%
Other sites	Rare
Adapted from Lack.[9]	

- Infants with congenital hypoplasia present with typical signs of adrenal cortical insufficiency, including vomiting, dehydration, weight loss, hyponatremia, and hyperkalemia.
- The onset of symptoms after birth is dependent on the amount of cortical tissue that is present.
- Males with X-linked cytomegalic-type hypoplasia also manifest a hypothalamic form of hypogonadism due to gonadotropin-releasing hormone deficiency.
- The cause of adrenal cortical insufficiency is unknown, but may be related to injury to the adrenal primordia in fetal life or lack of some key induction factor for the normal development of the cortex.
- Other causes of congenital adrenal insufficiency include anencephaly that results in agenesis or marked hypoplasia of the adrenals, familial glucocorticoid deficiency in which a selective deficiency of glucocorticoids due to an unknown cellular defect is found in the presence of high ACTH levels, glycerol kinase deficiency resulting in decreased glucocorticoid and mineralocorticoid levels, and adrenoleukodystrophy.
- Adrenoleukodystrophy is a demyelinating neurologic disorder associated with adrenal cortical atrophy and hypoadrenalism. It is caused by a defect in oxidation of fatty acids, resulting in accumulation of cholesterol esters in tissues. The neonatal form is usually an autosomal recessive disorder presenting with hypotonia, seizures, and rapid deterioration of sight and hearing at birth; mental and growth retardation are severe, and the children rarely live beyond 5 years. An X-linked childhood form becomes evident around 10 years of age, and an adult form may be seen in young men; these patients may present with adrenal insufficiency before neurologic disease is evident.

Pathology

Gross

- The 'miniature-type' congenital adrenal hypoplasia is characterized by very small, but normally formed, adrenal glands; the size is variable, and affects the clinical severity of disease.
- The cytomegalic type is characterized by small and dysmorphic glands.

Histology

- The histologic appearance of the 'miniature-type' hypoplasia is similar to that of a normal gland for the patient's age, with normal zonation and cytologic features.
- The cytomegalic type is very abnormal, with a distorted architectural pattern and strikingly atypical cytology. The cortical cells are large and vacuolated, with anisonucleosis, variable hyperchromasia, and frequent intranuclear cytoplasmic inclusions.
- The histology of adrenoleukodystrophy is characterized by large ballooned cortical cells containing lamellar inclusions; the lipid inclusions have a unique bilamellar and lamellar appearance ultrastructurally.

Treatment and prognosis

- In the past, congenital adrenal hypoplasia was uniformly fatal; however, with the availability of replacement glucocorticoid and mineralosteroid therapy, the prognosis is very good.
- Important to successful therapy is the early recognition of hypoadrenalism.

ADRENAL CYTOMEGALY AND BECKWITH–WIEDEMANN SYNDROME[5,14–18]

Definition

Adrenal cytomegaly represents the cellular enlargement, both cytoplasmic and nuclear, with nuclear pleomorphism and hyperchromasia, involving the adrenal cortical cells. It can be seen in the Beckwith–Wiedemann syndrome (BWS), which is characterized by exophthalmos, macroglossia, and gigantism.

Clinical

- Usually, adrenal cytomegaly is an incidental finding in a small percentage of neonates.
- Adrenal cytomegaly is seen in BWS. BWS has an estimated frequency of 1 in 13 000 live births. The majority of cases occur sporadically (85% in reported cases); a small percentage are inherited (in one report, in an autosomal dominant pattern with incomplete penetration). In addition to exophthalmos, macroglossia, and gigantism, BWS also may include a variety of abnormalities such as craniofacial abnormalities (midfacial hypoplasia, ear creases and pits, nevus flammeus, abdominal wall defects, and visceromegaly). Approximately 7.5% of children with BWS develop malignant tumors. The most common include nephroblastoma (Wilms' tumor) and adrenal cortical carcinoma; other malignant tumors that may occur in BWS include neuroblastoma, pancreatoblastoma, and pheochromocytoma. Loss of heterozygosity (LOH) for a locus on chromosome 11 in adrenal cortical neoplasms has been reported in BWS, and the gene involved in the predisposition to adrenal cortical neoplasms has been mapped to the 11p15.5 region.

Pathology

Gross

- The adrenals are enlarged in BWS, with expansion of the cortex, and, in some cases, the medulla as well.
- In incidental cytomegaly, the adrenal glands have a normal gross appearance.

Histology

- The cytomegalic cells are located in the fetal cortex; they are variable in number in incidentally discovered cases in infants, but are more numerous and diffusely distributed in BWS.
- The cells have increased cytoplasmic volume, as well as enlarged nuclei, nuclear pleomorphism, and hyperchromasia; intranuclear cytoplasmic inclusions are often seen. Mitoses are exceptional.

(Fig. 13.1)

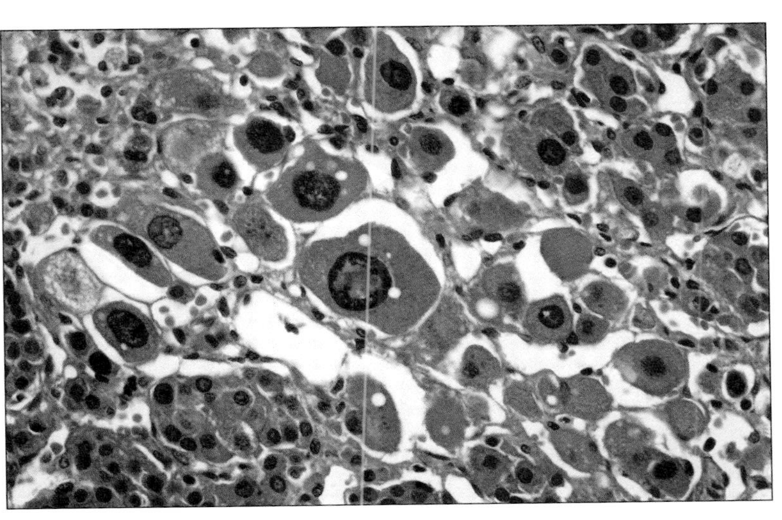

Fig. 13.1 Adrenal cytomegaly in a patient with Beckwith–Wiedemann syndrome. The cells have increased cytoplasmic volume, with enlarged nuclei, nuclear pleomorphism, and hyperchromasia; intranuclear cytoplasmic inclusions can be seen.

Treatment and prognosis

- Adrenal cytomegaly is of little clinical significance; however, there has been some association with Addison's disease.
- The association with BWS has more serious implications, including hypoglycemia in the neonatal period and the later increased risk of malignant neoplasms, particularly nephroblastoma (Wilms' tumor) and adrenal cortical carcinoma. The infant death rate in BWS is approximately 20% and failure to recognize the presence of hypoglycemia may result in permanent brain damage or death.

CONGENITAL ADRENAL HYPERPLASIA (ADRENOGENITAL SYNDROME)[5,19–25]

Definition

This is an autosomal recessive disorder resulting from defects in one of several enzymes necessary for the synthesis of cortisol and other steroid hormones from cortisol, with the resultant increase in other steroid products, usually androgenic, leading to virilization, in addition to deficiencies of various corticosteroids and mineralocorticoids.

Clinical

- The enzyme defects in congenital adrenal hyperplasia (CAH) include:
  21-hydroxylase;
  11-β-hydroxylase;
  17-hydroxylase;
  3-β-hydroxysteroid dehydrogenase;
  cholesterol desmolase.
- All of these defects are associated with deficiency of cortisol; additional manifestations vary.
- Virilization affects both males and females.

21-Hydroxylase deficiency

- This is responsible for 95% of cases of CAH.
- The classic form is seen in between 1:5000 and 1:15 000 live births in the Caucasian population, with a much higher incidence in Alaskan Eskimos.
- It is characterized by deficient cortisol production, resulting in hypersecretion of ACTH, which in turn stimulates the adrenal cortex. The end result is the excessive production of cortisol precursors, particularly 17-hydroxyprogesterone. The virilization results from the accumulation of 17-hydroxypregnenolone, which is metabolized to androgenic steroids (dehydroepiandrosterone and androstenedione).
- Aldosterone production may also be reduced, in some cases producing a more acutely threatening clinical syndrome of hypotension and salt-wasting. Aldosterone deficiency occurs in two-thirds of patients.
- Males appear normal at birth, while females have ambiguous genitalia characterized by clitoromegaly with fusion of labioscrotal folds (Fig. 13.2). Acne, development of genital hair, and bronzing of the skin are common. If treatment is delayed, the epiphyseal plates close prematurely.
- A non-classic form of 21-hydroxylase deficiency presents later in childhood or at puberty with virilization. Rare patients with the enzyme defect may be asymptomatic.

11-β-Hydroxylase deficiency

- This is the cause of approximately 5% of cases of CAH.
- It results in the deficient metabolism of 11-deoxycortisol to cortisol, with secondary overproduction of androgens, as in the 21-hydroxylase defect. Accumulation of deoxycorticosterone in the pathway for mineralocorticoid production may lead to hypertension and hypokalemia in addition to the signs of hypocortisolism and virilization.

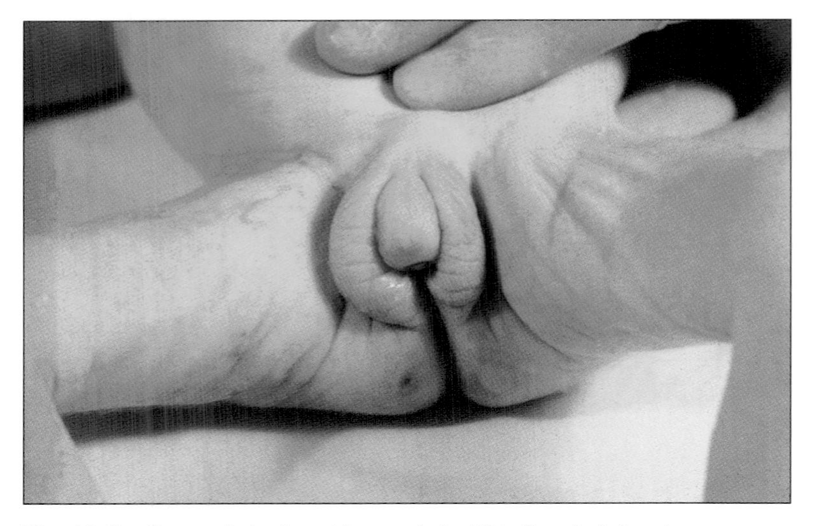

Fig. 13.2 Congenital adrenal hyperplasia. This female infant has ambiguous genitalia characterized by clitoromegaly with fusion of labioscrotal folds.

3-β-Hydroxysteroid dehydrogenase deficiency

- This affects synthesis of glucocorticoids, mineralocorticoids, and sex steroids (both testosterone and estrogens).
- The androgen accumulated is weak, and results in milder virilization of females and incomplete masculinization of male genitalia (hypospadias).
- Salt-wasting is present in severe forms.

17-Hydroxylase deficiency

- Deficiency of this enzyme interrupts the synthesis of glucocorticoids and sex steroids.
- This results in incomplete masculinization with hypospadias in males and amenorrhea in females, and in manifestations of hypocortisolism.

Cholesterol desmolase deficiency

- This is usually fatal in childhood, due to severe hypoadrenalism.
- Males have incomplete masculinization, while females lack virilization.

Pathology

Gross

- The adrenal glands in untreated CAH are several times the normal size, with weight dependent on age.
- The glands are brown, with a cerebriform surface, except in cholesterol desmolase deficiency, which is characterized by yellow areas and diffuse nodularity.

Histology

- The hyperplastic cerebriform appearance is noted microscopically, as well as grossly. The proliferating cells are eosinophilic, compact, and lipid-poor, with a few lipid-rich cells in some cases. Cholesterol clefts, with foreign body reaction and calcifications, are seen in cholesterol desmolase-deficient cases.
- Rarely, males with CAH have developed a peculiar form of testicular tumor in adolescence or young adulthood. These tumors are:
  frequently bilateral;
  responsive to ACTH stimulation, and produce cortisol;
  possibly up to several centimeters in diameter, and decrease in size with suppression of ACTH by dexamethasone.
- These lesions bear a striking histologic resemblance to Leydig cell tumors, but the lack of crystalloids of Reinke and the ACTH dependence are more suggestive of an adrenal cortical origin, possibly from adrenal cortical rests.

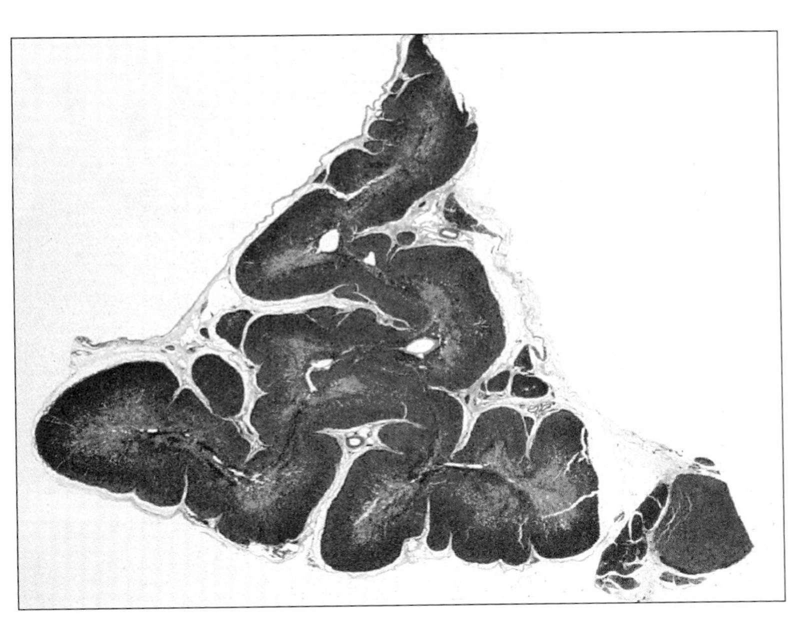

Fig. 13.3 Congenital adrenal hyperplasia showing characteristic cerebriform appearance.

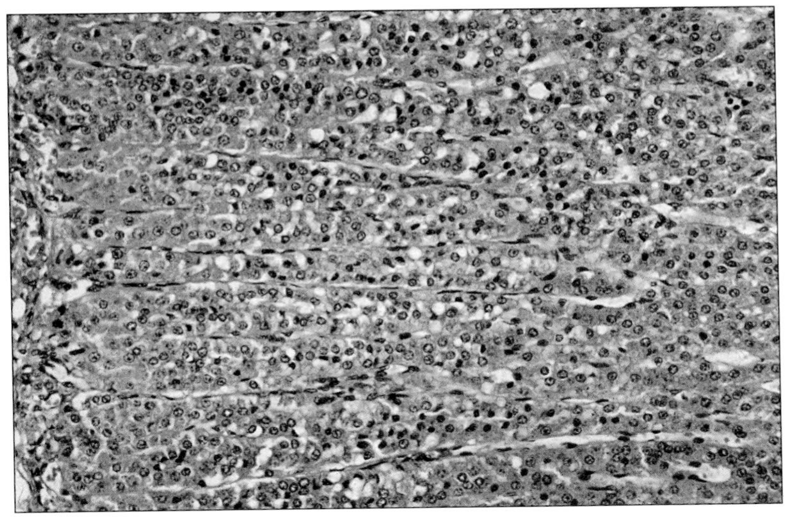

Fig. 13.4 Congenital adrenal hyperplasia with compact eosinophilic (lipid-poor) cells.

- It is not clear whether these tumors represent true neoplasms or hyperplastic nodules; they have a benign course.

(Figs 13.3 & 13.4)

Treatment and prognosis

- Replacement therapy is directed toward the deficient steroid group(s):
  cortisol is deficient in all of the enzyme defects;
  mineralocorticoids and sex steroids are administered according to need.
- Surgical correction of ambiguous external genitalia or hypospadias is necessary in many instances.
- Prognosis is dependent on the severity of the steroid deficiency and on time of diagnosis. The diagnosis is usually more obvious in females, due to the ambiguous genitalia; males are more likely to suffer longer effects of hypoadrenalism prior to recognition of CAH.
- Rare instances of benign and malignant adrenal cortical neoplasms arising in patients with CAH have been reported.

Table 13.3 Causes of Addison's disease
Idiopathic, or autoimmune
Infectious
Tuberculosis
Histoplasmosis
Coccidioidomycosis
North American blastomycosis
South American blastomycosis
Cryptococcosis
Cytomegalovirus
Herpes simplex virus
Varicella zoster
Visceral leishmaniasis
Infiltrative processes
Amyloidosis
Metastatic carcinoma
Lung
Breast
Stomach
Colon
Malignant lymphoma

ADDISON'S DISEASE (CHRONIC ADRENAL INSUFFICIENCY)[5,26–31]

Definition

This is a chronic deficiency of glucocorticoids and mineralocorticoids due to a variety of causes, including autoimmune adrenalitis, infectious diseases, metastatic malignant neoplasms, and accumulation of substances such as amyloid.

Clinical

- Addison's disease affects individuals of any age.
- The most common type of Addison's disease today is the idiopathic, or autoimmune, type; however, tuberculosis was the most common etiology until the past few decades (Table 13.3).
- Patients present with weakness, weight loss, and bronzing of the skin; left untreated, dehydration, hypotension, and shock may develop, especially when

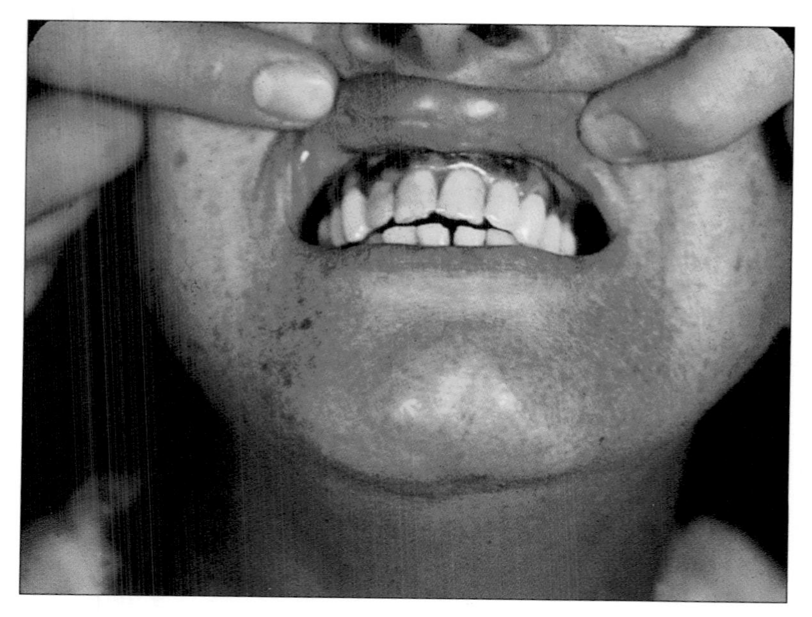

Fig. 13.5 Addison's disease patient with mucosal hyperpigmentation that is due to melanocyte-stimulating activity of ACTH.

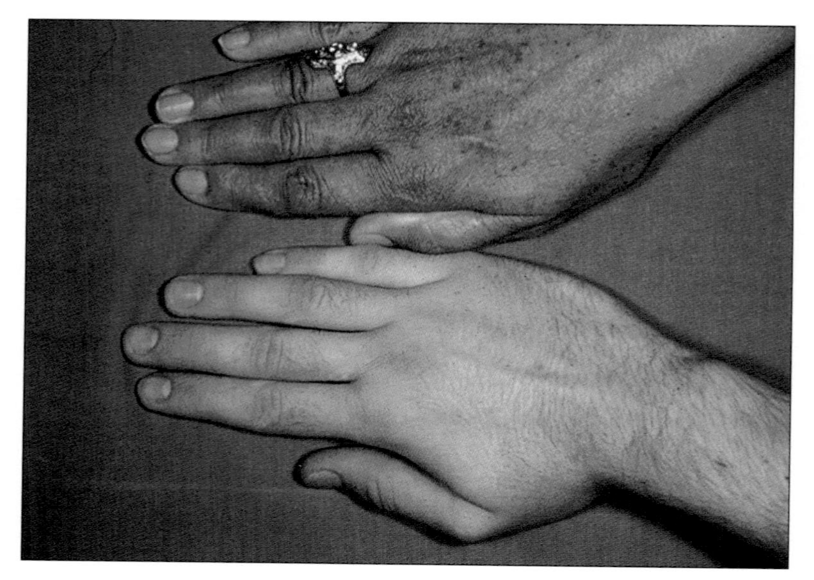

Fig. 13.6 The hand at the top belongs to an Addison's disease patient with cutaneous 'bronzing' in comparison to the lower hand of a patient without Addison's disease.

the patient encounters other physiologic stresses, such as an infection.

- Bronzing of the skin in Addison's disease is due to high levels of ACTH resulting from the lack of feedback inhibition on the pituitary by the incompetent adrenal glands.
- The mechanism of autoimmune Addison's disease is not clear but is related to an autoimmune form of adrenalitis.
- Other endocrine associations are seen in two subsets of idiopathic Addison's disease, known as polyglandular autoimmune (PGA) syndromes:
  PGA I is defined as the presence of at least two of the following: Addison's disease, hypoparathyroidism, or chronic mucocutaneous candidiasis. A related disorder has additional associations of dental and nail dystrophy, and a high incidence of juvenile diabetes, primary hypogonadism, and chronic active hepatitis.
  PGA II is an association of Addison's disease, autoimmune disease of the thyroid, and insulin-dependent diabetes.
- Adrenal insufficiency may also be pituitary in origin, as in Sheehan's syndrome or lymphocytic hypophysitis; such patients do not have the hyperpigmentation seen in Addison's disease.

(Figs 13.5 & 13.6)

Pathology

Gross

- The adrenal glands do not manifest hypofunction clinically until most of the cortical tissue is destroyed (as much as 90%). The glands, therefore, in clinically apparent Addison's disease are extremely small, and may be difficult to identify.
- The gland is often only a wisp of fibrovascular tissue, brown to gray in color, without the usual orange rim of cortex.

Histology

- The cortex is thin and discontinuous, appearing as sparsely distributed patches of eosinophilic, lipid-poor cells.
- A lymphoplasmacytic infiltrate is scattered through the remnant of the cortex. Lymphoid follicles may be present, similar to the pattern seen in lymphocytic thyroiditis. Unlike the infiltrate commonly seen as 'nonspecific' adrenalitis, often an incidental autopsy or surgical observation, the inflammatory cells are centered on the residual islands of cortex. In nonspecific adrenalitis they are distributed around blood vessels and as aggregates in the cortex, unassociated with evidence of tissue damage.
- Cytomegaly is present in some cases.

(Fig. 13.7)

Differential diagnosis

- Nonspecific adrenalitis.

Treatment and prognosis

Therapy is directed at replacement of cortical steroid products, and has dramatically altered the prognosis of Addison's disease.

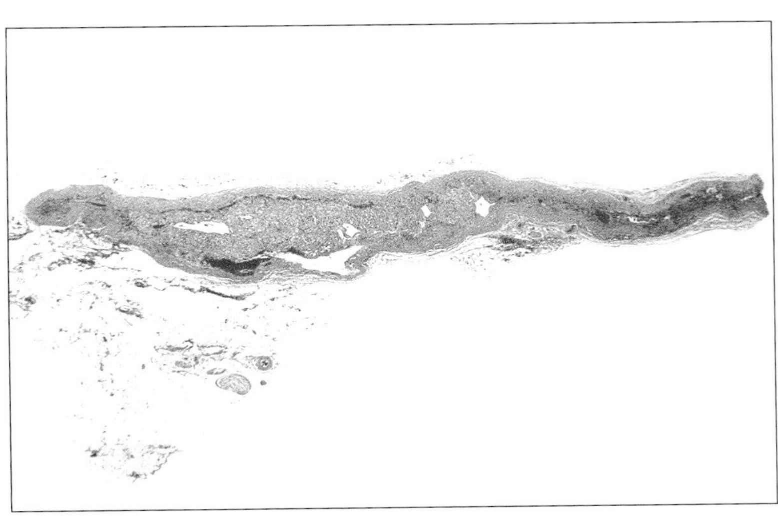

Fig. 13.7 Atrophic adrenal gland in a patient with Addison's disease. Note the thinness of the cortical ribbon.

INFECTIOUS DISEASES AFFECTING THE ADRENAL GLAND[5,26,29,32–36]

Definition

Infections involving the adrenal gland are usually secondary to a systemic infection. Although many infections are capable of producing Addison's disease, destruction of most of the cortex is usually required before manifestations of hypoadrenalism are seen.

Tuberculosis

- Tuberculosis was the most common cause of Addison's disease during the first part of the twentieth century, causing about 70% of cases, while a minority of cases were considered idiopathic. With the advent of effective antituberculous drugs, the statistics have reversed.
- In contrast to the findings in idiopathic Addison's disease, computed tomography (CT) and magnetic resonance imaging (MRI) show bilateral adrenal enlargement, often with calcification.
- The histologic pattern in adrenal tuberculosis is quite different from that of other organs, as seen by the presence of caseating necrosis with a diminished granulomatous reaction, as compared with well-developed granulomata in other sites.
- The causative microorganisms may be identified by acid-fast bacilli (AFB) staining.

Histoplasmosis

- Adrenal involvement is present in most cases of disseminated histoplasmosis, though less than 10% develop Addison's disease.

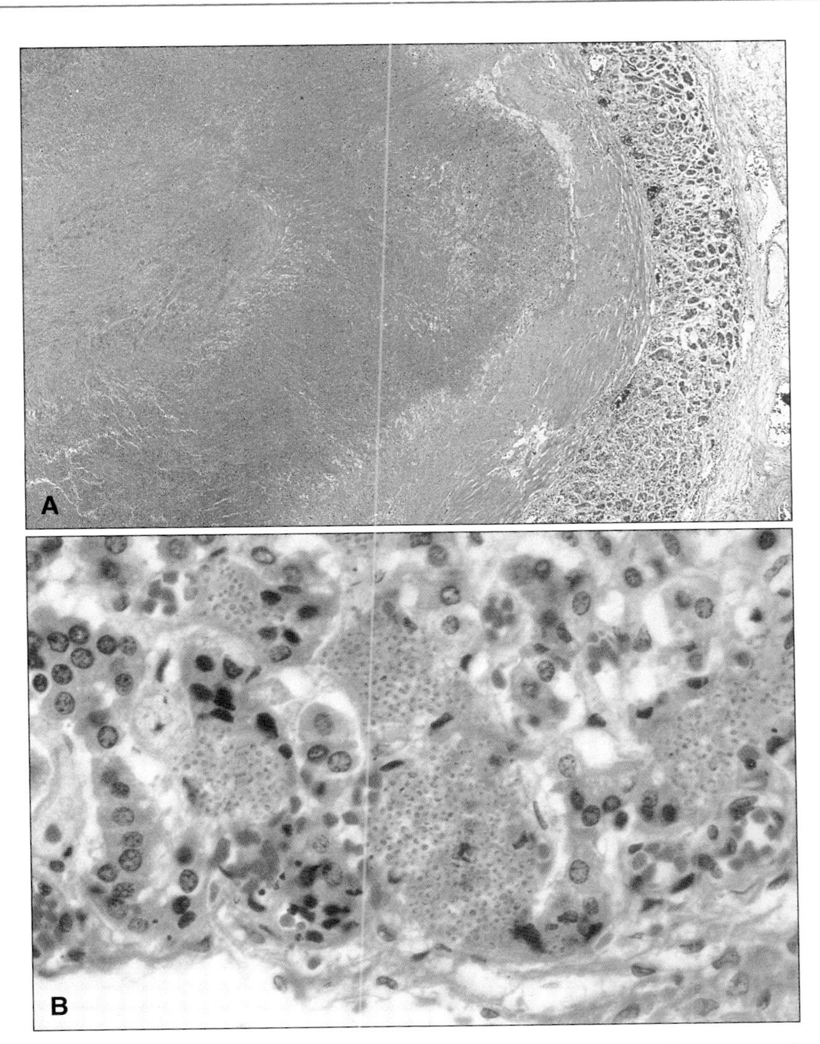

Fig. 13.8 The adrenal gland from a patient who died from disseminated histoplasmosis. (A) The adrenal glands were enlarged with effacement of the normal parenchyma and replacement by caseating necrosis, but absence of well-formed granulomas; residual adrenal parenchyma is seen to the left side of the illustration. (B) *Histoplasma capsulatum* is seen in macrophages in the adrenal gland; the microorganisms are tiny and ovoid, and distinction from amastigotes of leishmania is readily accomplished with Gomori's methenamine silver stain (GMS).

- As in tuberculosis, necrosis is usually prominent, while well-formed granulomata are not seen; in some cases the necrosis is not extensive.
- Aggregates of histiocytes containing the causative microorganisms can be found by hematoxylin–eosin (H&E) staining.

(Fig. 13.8)

Viral infections

- Neonatal herpes simplex viral infection causes necrosis in the adrenal and in the liver that may be patchy or confluent, but invokes little or no inflammatory reaction. Eosinophilic Cowdry A inclusions are easily found.
- Neonatal cytomegalovirus (CMV) infection is associated with multiple organ involvement. The

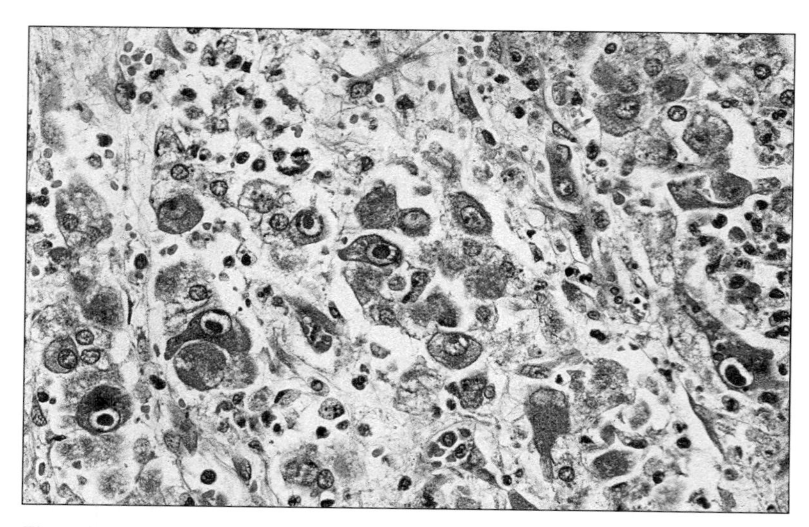

Fig. 13.9 AIDS-associated cytomegalovirus infection of the adrenal gland, characterized by the presence of intranuclear and cytoplasmic inclusions, including large eosinophilic nuclear inclusions with a peripheral halo and small basophilic cytoplasmic inclusions.

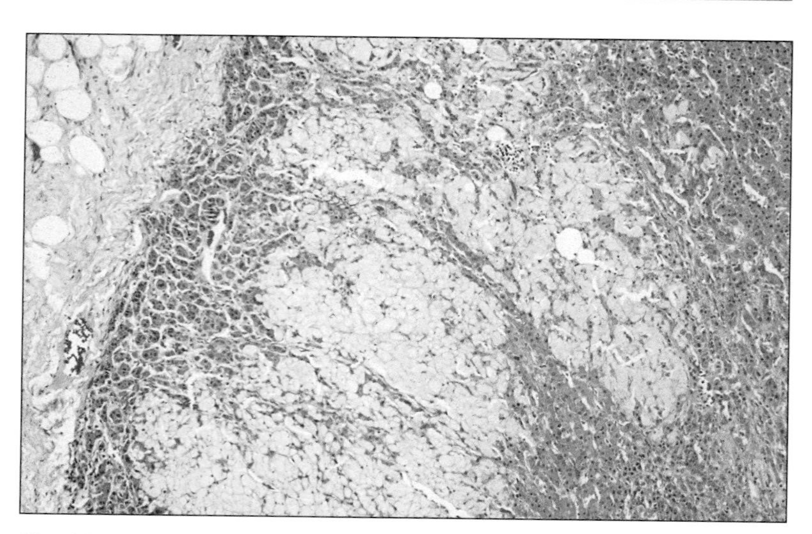

Fig. 13.10 Adrenal amyloidosis. Amorphous eosinophilic amyloid deposits are present in the cortex of a patient with the secondary form of amyloidosis, which is more common than primary amyloidosis as a cause of Addison's disease. The adjacent cortical cells are compact and eosinophilic.

adrenal lesions are similar to those in herpes simplex infection, with the exception of the characteristic intranuclear and cytoplasmic inclusions seen in CMV disease: large eosinophilic nuclear inclusions with a peripheral halo, and small basophilic cytoplasmic inclusions.
- AIDS-associated CMV infection has a predilection for adrenal involvement – it is the most commonly involved organ. In some patients, confluent necrosis is severe enough to cause Addison's disease.

(Fig. 13.9)

AMYLOIDOSIS[5,37]

Definition

Amyloidosis is abnormal accumulation of filamentous protein deposits in the interstitial tissue of the adrenal. Amyloidosis affecting the adrenal is most often of the secondary type, related to chronic inflammatory disease, particularly granulomatous infections.

Clinical

- Amyloidosis is quite rare as a cause of Addison's disease. It is usually associated with chronic inflammatory diseases (secondary amyloidosis). Primary amyloidosis, associated with plasma cell dyscrasias and caused by abnormal immunoglobulins, usually affects the blood vessels but does not accumulate in the parenchyma, and, therefore, is not a significant cause of adrenal insufficiency.
- Accumulation of amyloid in the adrenal is silent until adequate replacement of the cortex has occurred to cause adrenal insufficiency.

Pathology

Gross

- The accumulation of amyloid may greatly enlarge the gland; in such cases, the cut surface is yellow–white, smooth, and waxy.
- The loss of adrenal function is dependent on the distribution of the amyloid; if the deposits are concentrated in the inner cortex, adrenal insufficiency may occur before the glands are noticeably enlarged.

Histology

- Amorphous smudgy-appearing pink deposits are seen in H&E-stained sections, largely in the zona fasciculata and zona reticularis, crowding out the cortical tissue.
- The deposits are positive for Congo red, with apple-green birefringence, as well as for crystal violet and amyloid-specific immunohistochemistry.
- Electron microscopy shows deposits consisting of fine non-branching filaments.

(Fig. 13.10)

Treatment and prognosis

If amyloid deposition is extensive enough to cause Addison's disease, glucocorticoid and mineralocorticoid replacement is required.

WATERHOUSE–FRIDERICHSEN SYNDROME[38–40]

Definition

This is a form of septicemic shock associated with sudden vascular collapse, disseminated intravascular coagulation, and adrenal hemorrhage.

Clinical

- A variety of organisms have been associated with the syndrome, although it has historically been linked to meningococcemia; other causes include *Streptococcus pneumoniae, Hemophilus influenzae,* and neonatal echovirus infections.
- Rapid onset characterizes Waterhouse–Friderichsen syndrome, which is almost uniformly fatal.
- The disseminated intravascular coagulation is usually accompanied by a petechial rash.
- It is unlikely that the cause of shock in this syndrome is acute adrenal insufficiency; the adrenal hemorrhage is probably secondary.
- Neonatal hemorrhage due to delivery trauma, hypoxemia, and less fulminant episodes of septicemia may occur in the absence of Waterhouse–Friderichsen syndrome. In such cases, the adrenal hemorrhage is most often unilateral. Although many are asymptomatic, some patients may develop a large hematoma or may experience rupture of the gland with hemorrhage into the retroperitoneum. Surgery may be required to control bleeding or to treat secondary abscess formation. Resolution of adrenal hematomas may be associated with calcification and cyst formation.
- Adrenal hemorrhage in adults is often caused by anticoagulant therapy. Vascular manipulation and surgical trauma to the gland are other causative factors.

Pathology

Gross

- The adrenals are acutely congested and may be nearly effaced by hemorrhage, but are normal in size.

Histology

- The adrenal is massively hemorrhagic, with necrosis centered along the corticomedullary junction, which is most sensitive to hypoxemia.
- Fibrin thrombi in the sinusoids reflect the disseminated intravascular coagulation.

Treatment and prognosis

Although treatment with appropriate antibiotics may be aggressively instituted, the mortality rate from Waterhouse–Friderichsen syndrome is extremely high.

Table 13.4 Adrenal cysts
Parasitic cysts
Echinococcus granulosus
True epithelial cysts
Glandular (retention) cyst
Embryonal cyst
Endothelial cysts
Lymphangiomatous
Hemangiomatous
Pseudocysts (hemorrhagic cysts)

ADRENAL CYSTS[41–48]

Definition

These are rare lesions characterized by cystic alteration of the adrenal. The chief non-neoplastic cysts include retention and embryonal cysts and endothelial cysts, as well as the pseudocyst.

The classification of adrenal cysts is shown in Table 13.4.

Clinical

- Adrenal cysts are rare, with an autopsy incidence of 0.06%; most are incidental findings.
- Cysts occur over a wide age range, but are most common in the fifth and sixth decades and are very rare in children; they are more common in women than in men by a 3:1 ratio.
- Adrenal cysts are frequently asymptomatic; when symptoms occur, they are usually related to the mass effect of the lesion.
- Endothelial cysts and pseudocysts are the most common adrenal cysts, comprising over 85% of this group of lesions; epithelial-lined cysts of the adrenal include true glandular or retention cysts, and embryonal cysts, which are very rare. These lesions should be distinguished from adrenal cortical or medullary neoplasms with marked cystic degeneration.

Parasitic cysts

- Most parasitic cysts are associated with *Echinococcus granulosus* infection, though adrenal involvement is very rare in echinococcosis and is generally associated with widely disseminated disease.
- The cyst may be several centimeters in diameter and usually has a smooth fibrous wall with internal loculations.
- The cyst fluid contains sand-like grains that represent scolices of the parasite.

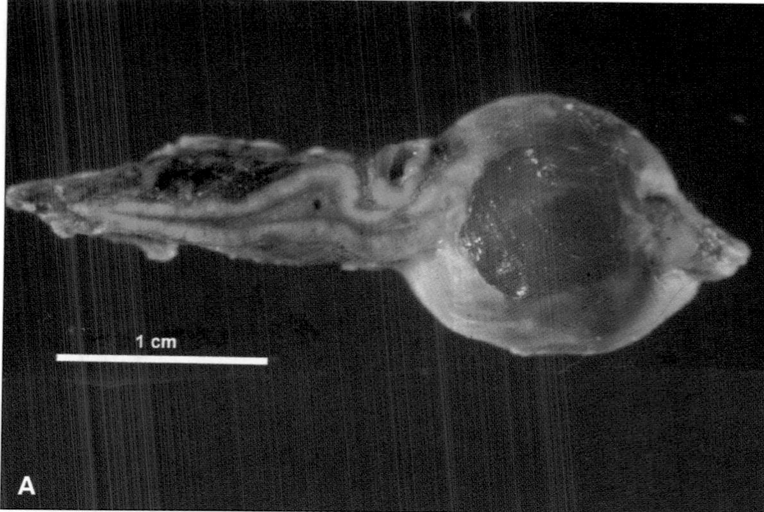

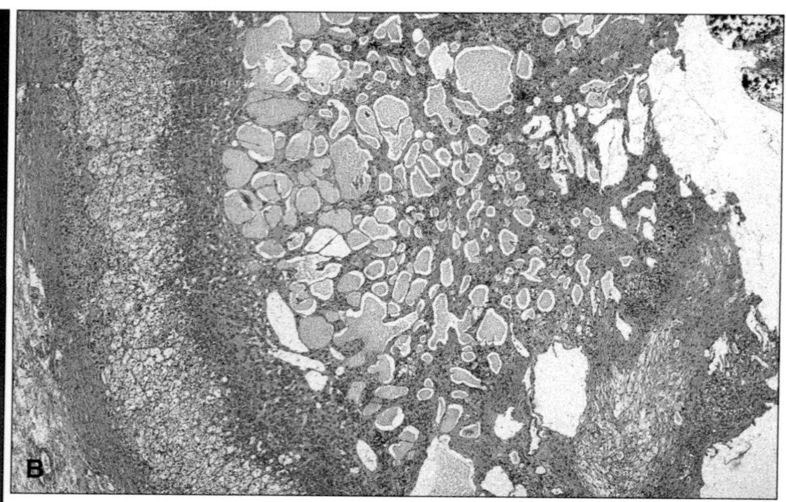

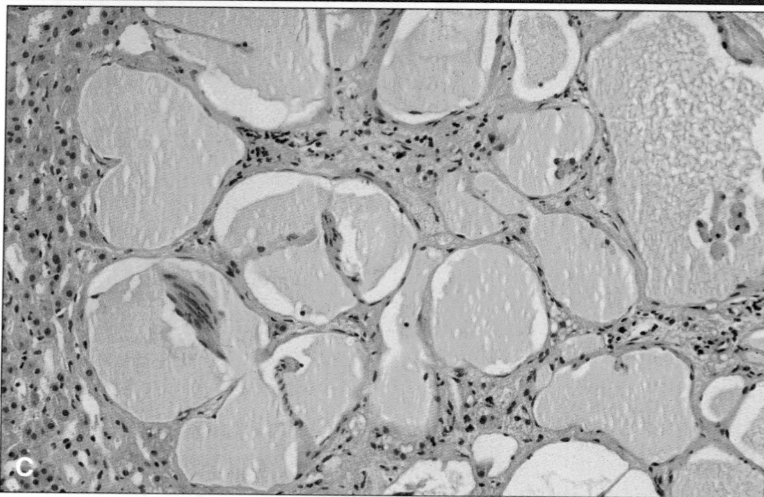

Fig. 13.11 Lymphangiomatous (or serous) cyst of the adrenal gland. (A) This lesion was incidentally identified by radiologic examination of the abdomen in a patient with non-adrenal abdominal disorder appearing as an intra-adrenal, translucent cyst. (B) Histologically, multiple, variably sized, fluid-filled cysts are seen within the adrenal gland. (C) The cysts are lined by a flattened layer of endothelium.

True epithelial cysts

- Usually small and incidental, these lesions are thought to be developmental accidents, possibly formed from rests of tissue of urogenital origin or from mesothelial inclusions.
- The cysts are lined by cuboidal or ciliated columnar epithelium and are filled with clear fluid.

Endothelial cysts

- These multiloculated cysts are lined by flat endothelium and are thought to be related to hemangiomas and lymphangiomas.
- Lymphangiomatous cysts are the more common of the two types, and are also known as 'serous' cysts. Though they are usually incidental, some cases attain a size adequate to become symptomatic surgical lesions.

(Fig. 13.11)

Pseudocysts

- In the past, pseudocysts were frequently incidental autopsy findings, but with radiographic advances and more widespread use of advanced diagnostic imaging techniques, the relative incidence in younger individuals and recognition of cysts as symptomatic lesions, usually causing abdominal pain, have increased.
- No etiology is discovered in many instances; possible etiologies proposed for pseudocysts include resolving adrenal hemorrhage for any of a variety of reasons or hemorrhage into a hemangiomatous or lymphangiomatous lesion. Adrenal hemorrhage occurs in a variety of situations, including trauma, sepsis, therapeutic anticoagulation, clotting disorders, steroid therapy or administration of ACTH, neoplasia, adrenal vein thrombosis, traumatic delivery, and pregnancy.
- Pseudocysts appear radiographically as a cyst with variable internal densities and peripheral calcification.
- Sizes range from 2 to 10 cm, except for a very rare example that attained a massive volume of 12 liters.
- The pseudocyst wall is well formed and fibrous and is filled with hemorrhagic material, organizing blood clot, and brown fluid. In some cases, smooth muscle has been seen in the wall.

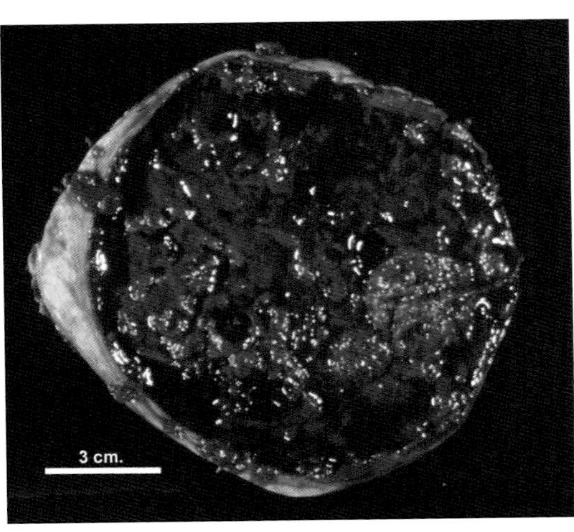

Fig. 13.12 Adrenal pseudocyst, also referred to as a hemorrhagic cyst. The cyst replaces most of the adrenal gland and is filled with organizing blood clot; residual adrenal gland is seen toward the left side of the illustration.

- Histologically, the cyst wall has no epithelial lining; the material in the cavity includes organizing clot, fibrous tissue, granulation tissue, and coagulated blood.
- There are descriptions of cysts with a partial endothelial lining, suggesting that some cysts may be the result of secondary hemorrhage in a vascular neoplasm or malformation; adrenal cortex may form a partial rim around the pseudocyst wall.
- Foci of adrenal cortical tissue have been described within the cavity of some lesions; the possibility of a hemorrhagic adrenal cortical adenoma must be considered in such cases.

(Fig. 13.12)

NONHYPERFUNCTIONAL ADRENAL CORTICAL NODULES[49–56]

Definition

This comprises multinodular adrenal cortical proliferation, almost always bilateral, without clinical, biochemical, or histologic evidence of hyperfunction.

Clinical

- Nonfunctional nodules are the most common cause of adrenal enlargement.
- They are a very common incidental finding at surgery or during radiographic procedures for other problems.
- These lesions have been classified in the past as 'nonfunctional adenomas'; however, the evidence supports a non-neoplastic origin.
- Nonhyperfunctional nodules are found over a wide age range, with incidence increasing with age; an increased incidence is seen in diabetes mellitus, hypertension, and in cardiovascular or peripheral vascular disease.
- Incidental nodules over 1.5 cm in diameter are found in 20% of hypertensive individuals at autopsy.
- The high incidence of incidental nodules with age, and the apparent close association with vascular disease, support the theory that these lesions are secondary to arteriopathy associated with hypertension and represent a regenerative hyperplastic response to localized ischemic injury.
- No clinical significance has been assigned to these lesions.
- Advances in radiologic imaging techniques have led to an apparent increase in nonhyperfunctioning nodules during life: CT and MRI demonstrate adrenal enlargement, usually bilateral, but sometimes quite asymmetric. A dominant nodule may have the appearance of a neoplasm, either primary or metastatic.

Pathology

Cytology

- Fine-needle aspiration (FNA) is an effective method for exclusion of metastatic disease in cases of adrenal enlargement due to nonfunctional nodules.
- The cytologic appearance is not distinguishable from normal cortex, or from a benign cortical neoplasm. Accurate localization is essential to assure sampling of the lesion.
- The cells are fragile, and the smears contain many naked nuclei in a background of foamy cytoplasmic material. The nuclei are round, with relatively dense chromatin.

Gross

- Nodules are usually multiple and bilateral; however, there may be significant disparity between glands regarding weight; in some cases, one nodule is large enough to overshadow the smaller ones around it, but additional small nodules can almost always be found upon close inspection.
- Size of individual nodules ranges from 1 mm to 3 cm, with most less than 1 cm.
- Larger nodules may contain foci of cystic degeneration or areas of calcification.

(Fig. 13.13)

Microscopic

- The cells have abundant, pale-staining, finely vacuolated cytoplasm, resembling the cells of the zona fasciculata; nodularity is quite obvious microscopically.
- The nodules are circumscribed, but not encapsulated.

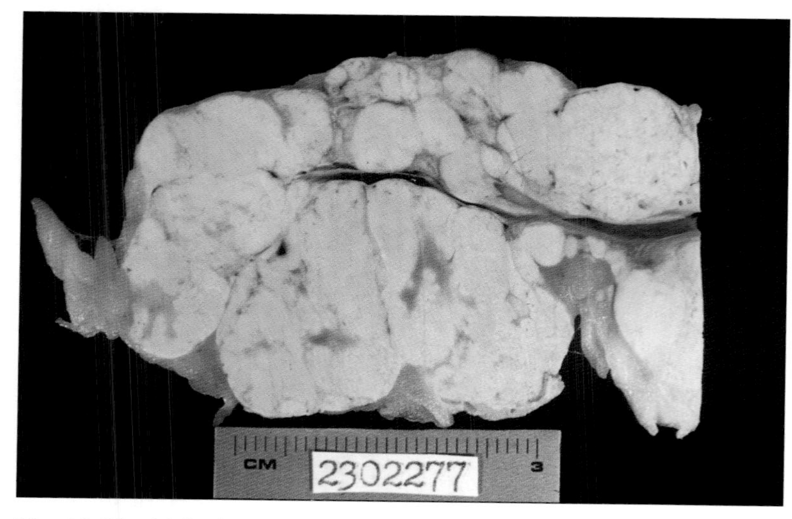

Fig. 13.13 Multiple, variably sized adrenal cortical nodules are seen in this gland. The nodules were incidental findings at autopsy, involved both glands, and were nonhyperfunctioning.

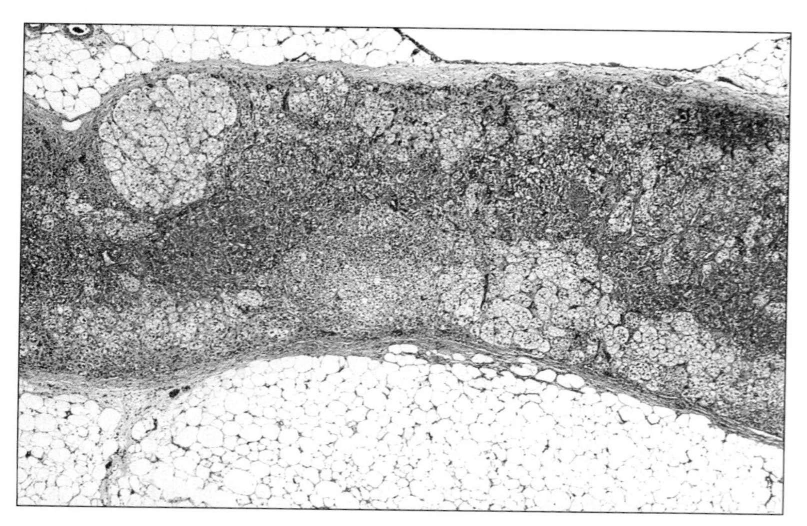

Fig. 13.14 Incidental, nonhyperfunctioning adrenal cortical nodules were identified in this gland. The small nodules are composed of lipid-rich cells resembling the zona fasciculata. These nodules, which are almost always multiple and bilateral, are seen with increased frequency in the elderly, and in patients with diabetes mellitus, vascular disease, and hypertension.

- Myelolipomatous foci may be present.
- Nuclear atypia and mitotic activity are not present.

(Figs 13.14 & 13.15)

Differential diagnosis

- Adrenal cortical adenoma.
- Nodular adrenal cortical hyperplasia with Cushing's disease.

Treatment and prognosis

No therapy is required; however, these lesions may be clinically mistaken for neoplasms and be resected.

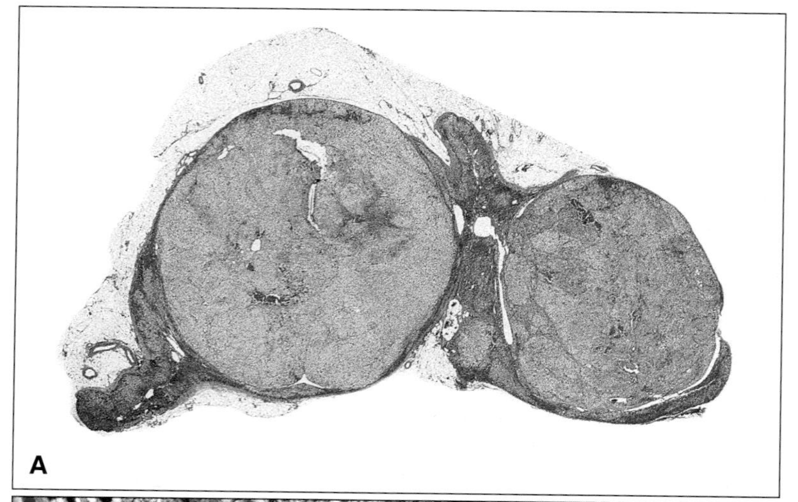

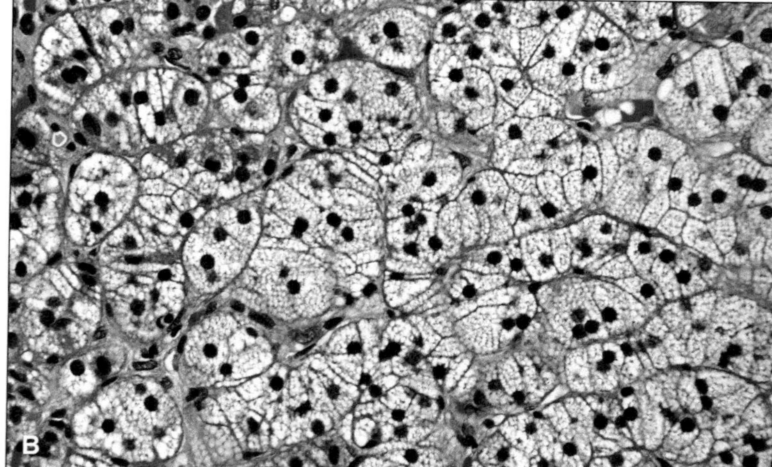

Fig. 13.15 (A) Large nonhyperfunctional cortical nodules. The etiology is thought to be a regenerative response to zonal ischemia in patients with arteriopathy due to hypertension. Note the areas of normal intervening cortical tissue between nodules. (B) At higher magnification, the nodules are composed of lipid-rich cells of the zona fasciculata type.

ADRENAL CORTICAL HYPERPLASIA WITH HYPERCORTISOLISM[22,53,55,57–71]

Definition

This comprises hypercortisolism with adrenal enlargement, usually bilateral, due to pituitary-based excess ACTH production, autonomous bilateral adrenal hyperplasia, or ectopic ACTH production (Table 13.5).

Clinical

- Eighty percent of cases of hypercortisolism are caused by overproduction of ACTH by the pituitary, usually due to an adenoma (Cushing's disease); 5–10%, by an adrenal cortical adenoma; 10–15%, by ectopic ACTH production by an extra-adrenal tumor; 4%, by adrenal cortical carcinoma; and a small number by

Table 13.5 Etiology of hypercortisolism – laboratory findings

	Pituitary-based	*Cortical neoplasm*	*Ectopic ACTH*	*Primary adrenal hyperplasia*
Plasma cortisol	High, no diurnal variation	High, no diurnal variation	High, no diurnal variation	High, no diurnal variation
Plasma ACTH	High	Low	High	Low
Response to ACTH with glucocorticoid production	Rise	None	Usually none	Variable, may rise
Dexamethasone suppression	Suppresses with high dose only	No suppression	No suppression	No suppression
Response to metyrapone	Rise in 12-deoxycortisol	No response	No response, usually	Variable, often rise in 12-deoxycortisol

autonomous adrenal cortical hyperplasia unrelated to ACTH.

- Cushing's disease in adults usually occurs in the third and fourth decades and is most often due to a pituitary adenoma.
- Pituitary-based hypercortisolism occurs more often in women than in men by a 3:1 ratio.
- Most patients with pituitary-dependent hypercortisolism have a pituitary adenoma that secretes ACTH; however, in a small number of patients no pituitary tumor can be identified; a pituitary hyperplasia or hypothalamic dysfunction is thought to be responsible for the small group without a demonstrable adenoma.
- Hypercortisolism is associated with a characteristic group of physical findings and related metabolic alterations known as Cushing's disease, which includes:
  truncal obesity;
  hirsutism;
  purple abdominal striae;
  osteoporosis;
  glucose intolerance;
  weakness and fatigue;
  amenorrhea;
  hypertension.
- Laboratory findings include:
  elevated plasma cortisol without diurnal fluctuation;
  increased glucocorticoid excretion, manifested by elevated urinary 17-ketosteroids, without diurnal fluctuation
  failure of low-dose dexamethasone to suppress cortisol levels.
- Further distinction among causes of hypercortisolism is achieved by the high-dose dexamethasone suppression test: cortisol levels are suppressed in pituitary-dependent Cushing's disease, while tumors producing ectopic ACTH and adrenal cortical hyperplasia rarely are suppressible, and adrenal cortical adenomas that produce cortisol are essentially never suppressible.

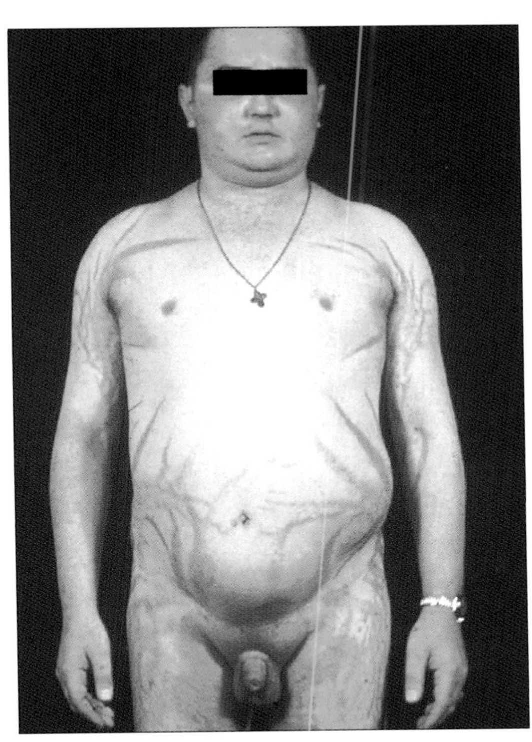

Fig. 13.16 Patient with longstanding hypercorticolism (Cushing's disease) showing the presence of large dark-purple striae on his trunk, truncal obesity, and 'moon facies'.

- Another distinguishing test is administration of metyrapone, which blocks the final step in cortisol production, stimulating ACTH secretion with an adrenal response of increase in 11-deoxycortisol: adrenal cortical hyperplasia is associated with a normal to exaggerated response, while adrenal cortical adenomas are not affected.
- Children under 8 years of age are much more likely to have an adrenal cortical adenoma.

(Figs 13.16–13.19)

Pathology

Difffuse hyperplasia, pituitary-dependent hypercortisolism

- Diffuse, symmetric hyperplasia due to an oversecretion of ACTH by the pituitary is the most common cause of hypercortisolism.
- Adrenal glands are usually no more than twice the normal weight.
- The cortex is diffusely, but usually mildly, thickened, with a yellow outer zone and a brownish inner zone. Scattered small nodules may be present.

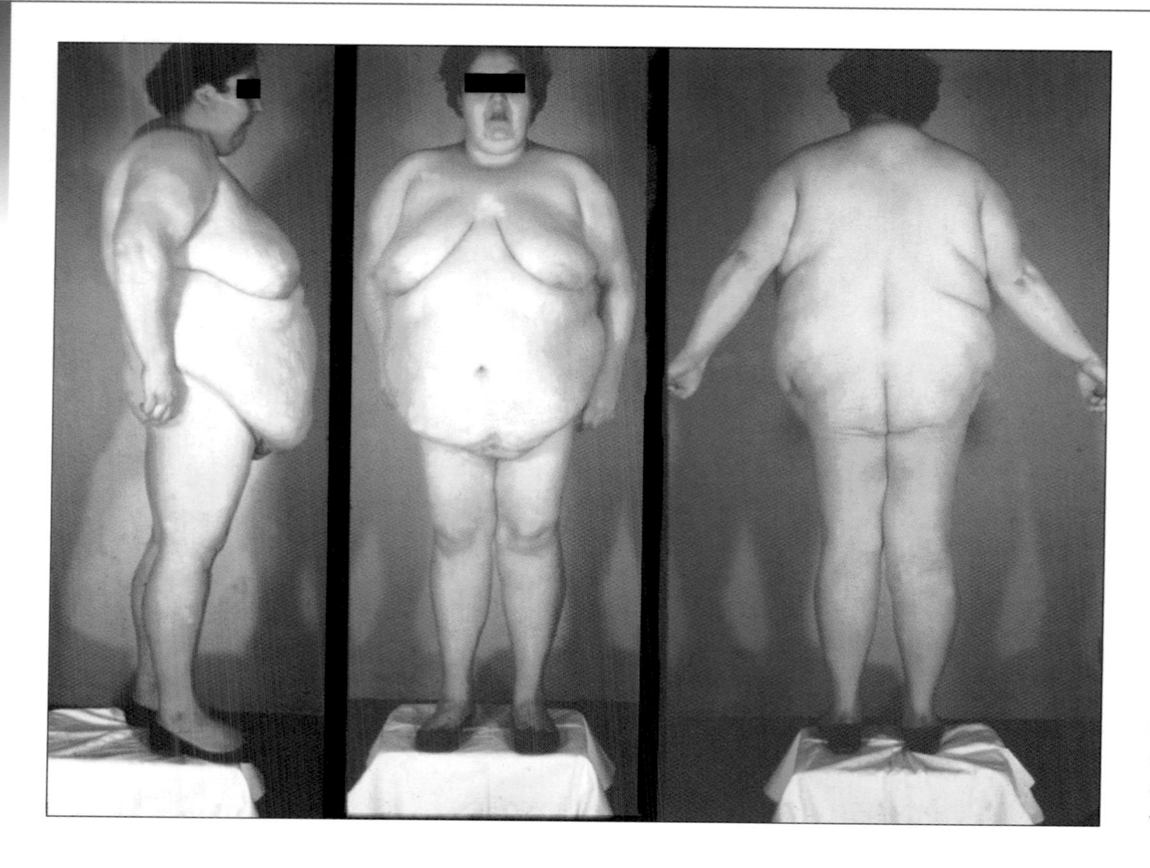

Fig. 13.17 Marked truncal obesity with a buffalo hump (accumulation of fat along the dorsum of the neck and shoulders) characterize the appearance of this patient with Cushing's syndrome.

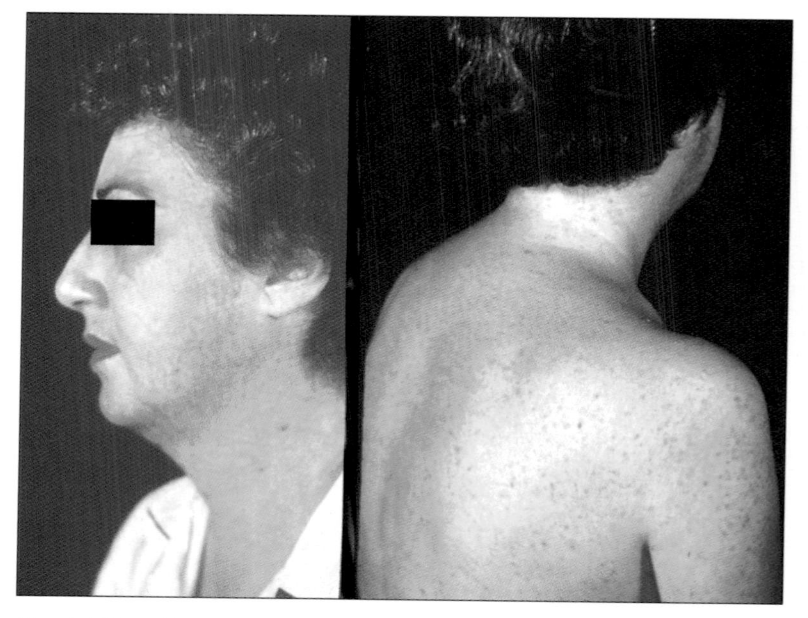

Fig. 13.18 Hirsutism in a patient with hypercortisolism due to an ACTH-producing pituitary adenoma (pituitary disease).

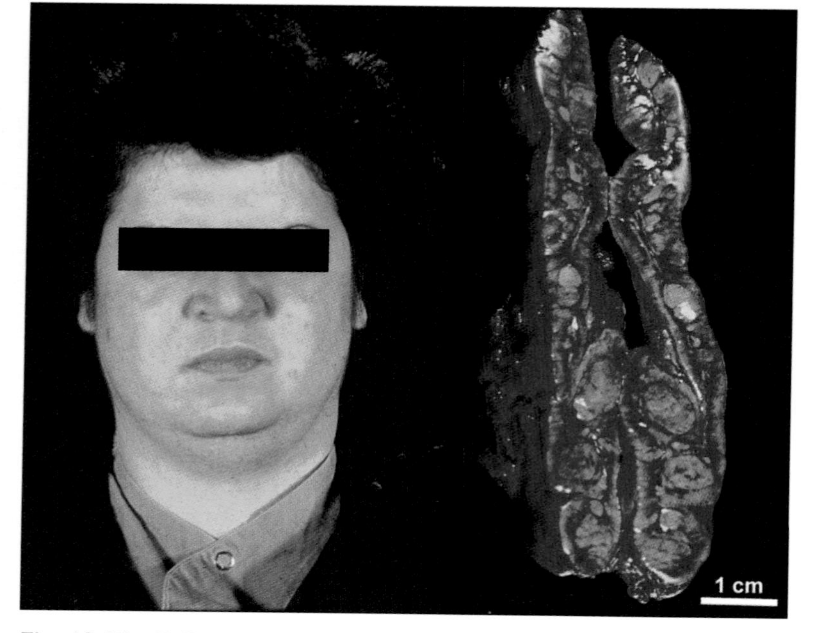

Fig. 13.19 Diffuse cortical hyperplasia in a patient with Cushing's disease. Left: Moon facies. Right: The cortex is diffusely widened. There are scattered small nodules, which may be seen in ACTH-based hypercortisolism. The nodules are distinctly different from the macronodular and microadenomatous patterns of nodular cortical hyperplasia that are usually seen in adrenal-dependent hypercortisolism, an uncommon cause of hypercortisolism.

- Larger nodules may be seen in patients with longstanding disease; they may achieve diameters of around 5 cm.
- The microscopic appearance reveals a widened inner zone of compact cells of the zona reticularis type (corresponding to the grossly brown zone), which comprises half of the volume of cortex. The outer zone is composed of lipid-rich cells; similar cells are seen in nodules that may be present. The relative thickening of the zona reticularis is important in recognizing subtle cases of diffuse hyperplasia.
- The changes in mild cases of diffuse hyperplasia closely resemble those seen in patients who have experienced chronic illness or prolonged

hospitalization. Demonstration of hypercortisolism with lack of diurnal rhythm is necessary for confirming cortical hyperplasia in such cases.

Diffuse hyperplasia due to ectopic ACTH syndrome

- Adrenal enlargement due to an ACTH-producing tumor, excluding pituitary adenoma, is characterized by cortical thickening that is greater than that seen in pituitary-based hypercortisolism, with gland weights commonly exceeding 12 g each. Adrenals usually do not exceed 30 g in this disorder.
- The cortex is diffusely brown, and usually 4 mm in thickness.
- The expanded cortex is composed of long fascicles of compact, lipid-poor cells. Nodules are not seen in most cases. The cortex lacks the distinct outer zone of clear cells seen in pituitary-based hypercortisolism.
- Metastases from the ACTH-producing tumor may be present in the glands. Nuclear pleomorphism is common in cortical cells adjacent to metastatic lesions.

Macronodular adrenal hyperplasia with hypercortisolism

- This small subset of patients, when distinguished from those with pituitary-based hypercortisolism with nodule formation by laboratory studies, is composed of those in whom the adrenal hyperplasia appears to be at least partially autonomous, similar to that seen in cortical neoplasms.
- Both micronodular ('microadenomatous') and macronodular forms occur: the micronodular pattern is more consistently associated with clear-cut autonomous behavior, and will be discussed separately.
- This group of patients is resistant to high-dose dexamethasone suppression, but usually responsive to ACTH and metyrapone. Plasma ACTH levels are variable, and are often somewhat elevated. The mechanism for this hyperplasia has not been defined, though there may be some relationship to the pituitary gland in its origin. Pituitary adenomas have not been described in this group.
- Adrenal glands usually weigh 30–50 g, but may approach 100 g.
- Multinodular adrenal hyperplasia is characterized grossly by nodularity that completely replaces the gland, unlike pituitary-based hyperplasia with nodules, in which there are areas of diffuse hyperplasia between scattered nodules. The nodules vary greatly in size, from a few millimeters to 3 cm. They are variegated, yellow–brown.
- The cells in multinodular hyperplasia are an admixture of groups of compact cells and lipid-rich cells. This admixture contrasts with simple diffuse hyperplasia associated with a pituitary adenoma, in which the nodules are composed of clear cells. In macronodular hyperplasia the cortex between distinct nodules is also hyperplastic, with subtle microscopic nodularity.

Microadenomatous adrenal hyperplasia with hypercortisolism

- Synonyms for this lesion include primary pigmented nodular adrenocortical disease, micronodular adrenal disease, and primary adrenocortical nodular disease.
- It is a very rare form of autonomous adrenal hyperplasia; both sporadic and familial cases are reported.
- Unlike macronodular cortical hyperplasia as described above, microadenomatous adrenal disease is clearly pituitary-independent. Plasma ACTH levels are extremely low; and the adrenals do not respond to administration of ACTH. Neither is there any response to metyrapone or dexamethasone.
- The adrenals are normal to slightly enlarged, and are dotted with 1–3-mm cortical nodules, which are usually darkly pigmented (brown to black). An occasional nodule may be larger than 3 mm; nodules as large as 1.8 cm have been described. Small nodules may protrude from the surface of the gland.
- The cortex between nodules appears atrophic, in contrast to that seen in macronodular hyperplasia.
- The cellular composition of the nodules is largely compact, lipid-poor cells, though scattered groups of lipid-rich cells are common. Slight nuclear pleomorphism may be seen. The pigment in the cytoplasm of the cells is thought to be lipofuscin, though neuromelanin has also been postulated to contribute to the color of these lesions.
- The etiology of this disorder is unknown; however, an autoimmune process with antibodies to ACTH receptors has been suggested.
- Bilateral adrenalectomy is the treatment of choice.

(Figs 13.20–13.22)

ADRENAL CORTICAL HYPERPLASIA WITH HYPERALDOSTERONISM[22,53,72–74]

Definition

This comprises a diffuse non-neoplastic proliferation of the zona glomerulosa of the adrenal cortex associated with excessive secretion of aldosterone.

Clinical

- In contrast to hypercortisolism, hyperaldosteronism is more often caused by an adrenal cortical adenoma than by hyperplasia of the adrenal cortex, with approximately 80% of patients with hyperaldosteronism harboring an adrenal cortical

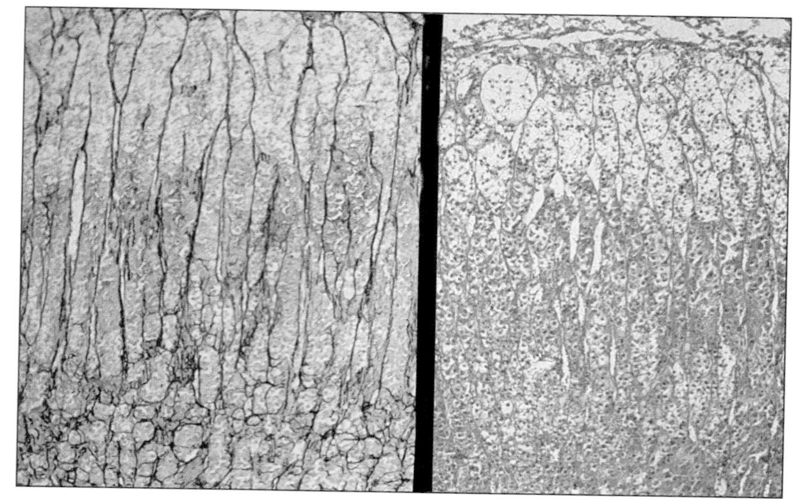

Fig. 13.20 Diffuse adrenal cortical hyperplasia associated with Cushing's disease. Compact cells make up more than half the thickness of the cortical ribbon, while an outer zone of lipid-rich cells is present. The expanded zone of compact (zona reticularis) cells is an important histologic feature of diffuse hyperplasia with hypercortisolism. The reticulin stain (left) shows the zona fasciculata, in which the normally lipid-rich cells have been converted into lipid-poor eosinophilic cells seen in the hematoxylin–eosin stain (right).

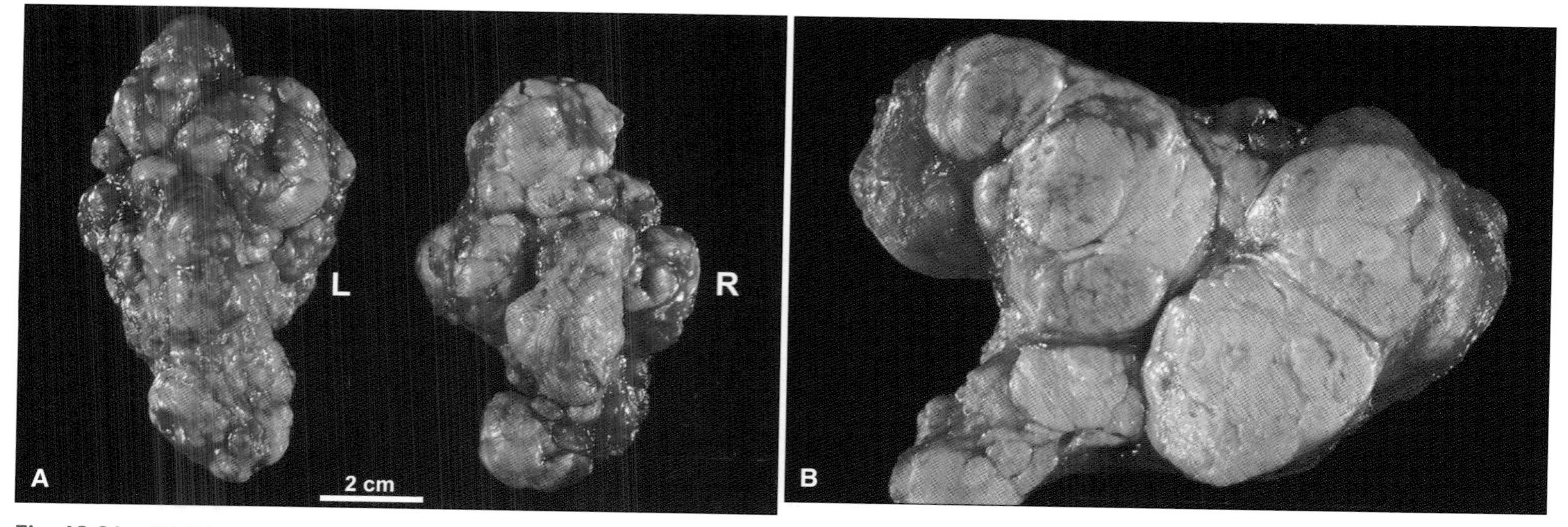

Fig. 13.21 (A) Bilateral macronodular hyperplasia in a patient with Cushing's syndrome (no pituitary adenoma was present). The large, variably sized nodules essentially replace the entire gland. No normal cortex is seen. This is an uncommon form of hypercortisolism. (B) A cross-section of one of the glands shows the presence of homogeneous orange–yellow nodules distorting the gland. No residual uninvolved gland is seen.

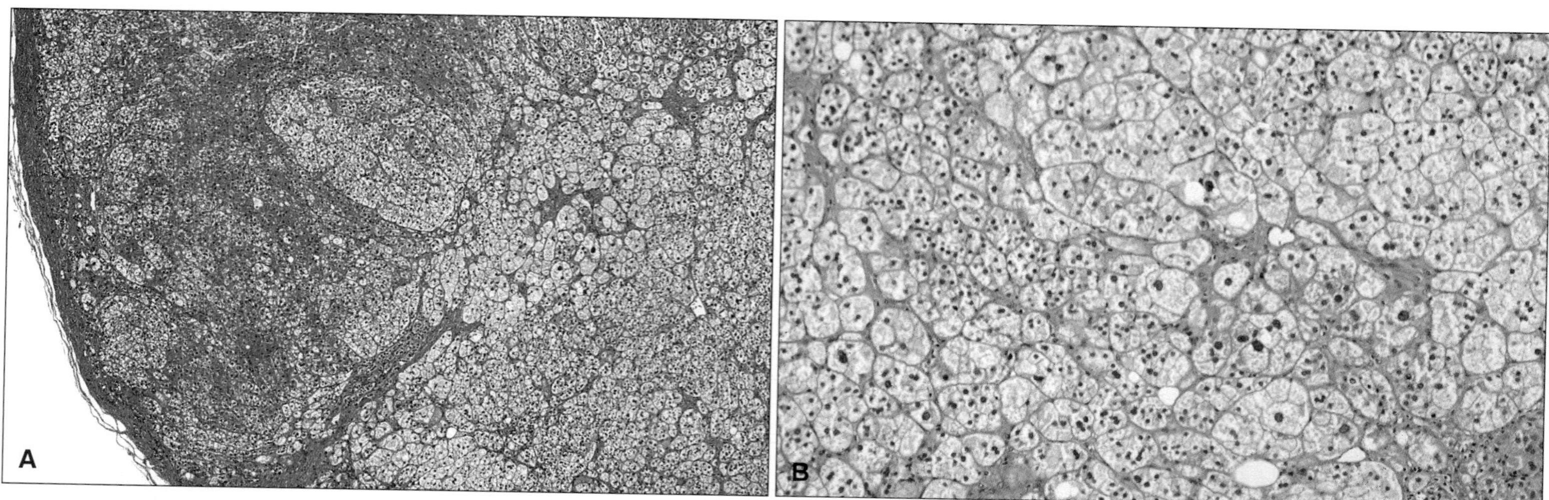

Fig. 13.22 (A) Bilateral macronodular cortical hyperplasia with Cushing's syndrome. Although the lipid-rich cells predominate, there are foci of eosinophilic compact cells within the nodules as well. (B) At higher magnification, the nodule is predominantly composed of lipid-rich cells.

adenoma; the remaining patients have bilateral hyperplasia of the zona glomerulosa.
- Age of presentation is usually in the fourth through sixth decades; the condition occurs more often in women than in men by a 3:1 ratio.
- The clinical presentation is hypertension with hypokalemia; plasma renin levels are low.

Pathology

Gross

- The adrenals are not enlarged, though nonfunctional cortical nodules may be present as a result of the hypertension.

Histology

- The histologic changes in diffuse hyperplasia with hyperaldosteronism are often very subtle; in the normal adrenal gland, the zona glomerulosa is extremely thin and discontinuous, and is often difficult to see.
- Hyperplasia of the zona glomerulosa is recognized by the presence of V-shaped proliferations of glomerulosa cells extending in a wedge-like fashion toward the center of the gland; the proliferation may be accompanied by an increase in delicate fibrous tissue within the zona glomerulosa. The zona glomerulosa may extend as a thin continuous band between the wedges of proliferating cells.
- Spironolactone bodies, small laminated spherical inclusions that are positive with periodic acid–Schiff (PAS)–diastase and Luxol fast blue, may be identified in patients who have recently been treated with spirololactone.
- Hyperplasia of the zona glomerulosa may accompany an aldosterone-producing cortical adenoma, which should be excluded before making a diagnosis of diffuse zona glomerulosa hyperplasia as the etiology for hyperaldosteronism.
- Small nonfunctional nodules composed of lipid-rich cells resembling the zona fasciculata frequently accompany both diffuse hyperplasia of the zona glomerulosa and aldosterone-producing adrenal cortical adenomas; these probably are secondary to the patient's hypertension.

(Fig. 13.23)

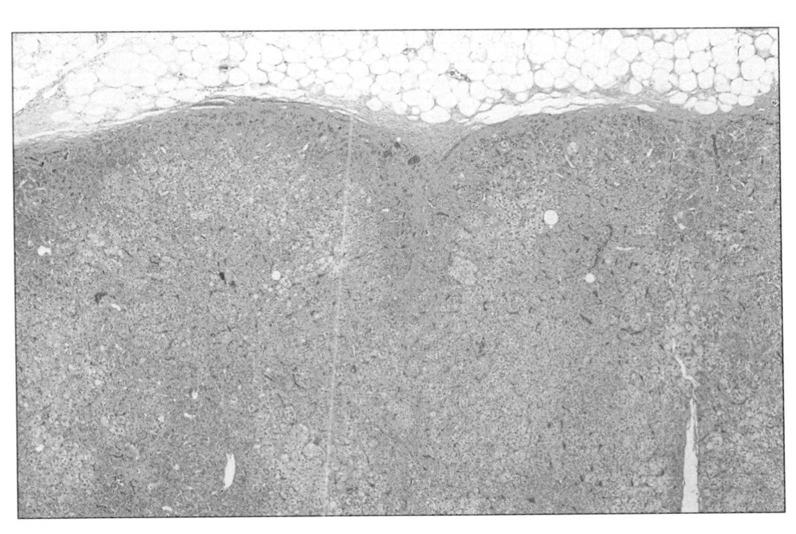

Fig. 13.23 Diffuse hyperplasia of the zona glomerulosa in a patient with hyperaldosteronism. The wedge-shaped proliferation angled toward the center of the gland is an essential feature of this disease. Continuity of the zona glomerulosa is also a helpful indicator of hyperplasia.

Differential diagnosis

- Aldosterone-producing adrenal cortical adenoma.

Treatment and prognosis

Response to bilateral adrenalectomy is somewhat unpredictable in patients with hyperaldosteronism. In many instances, there appear to be other factors influencing the aldosterone levels, independent of the adrenal. In such cases, hypertension is not cured by a rather radical surgical approach of resecting all of a patient's adrenal tissue. Patients in whom no cortical adenoma is found are generally treated conservatively with antihypertensives.

NEOPLASMS OF THE ADRENAL GLAND (Table 13.6)

Table 13.6 Classification of neoplasms of the adrenal gland
Neoplasms of the adrenal cortex
Adrenal cortical adenoma
Adrenal cortical carcinoma
Neoplasms of the adrenal medulla
Adrenal medullary hyperplasia
Pheochromocytoma
Neuroblastoma and ganglioneuroblastoma
Ganglioneuroma
Composite tumors of the adrenal medulla
Primary malignant melanoma
Miscellaneous neoplasms and tumor-like lesions
Myelolipoma
Adenomatoid tumor
Hemangioma
Nerve sheath tumors
Malignant lymphoma
Angiosarcoma
Metastatic or secondary neoplasms
Other rare neoplasms (smooth muscle tumors, gonadal stromal type tumors)

ADRENAL CORTICAL NEOPLASMS

ADRENAL CORTICAL ADENOMA[75–96]

Definition

Adrenal cortical adenoma comprises a benign neoplastic proliferation of adrenal cortical cells, almost always associated with endocrine hyperfunction discernible by clinical, biochemical, or histologic evidence.

Clinical

- Most adrenal cortical adenomas exhibit some evidence of hyperfunction, which is the feature that defines the separation of adenomas from the dominant nonhyperfunctioning adrenal cortical nodule. Although many adenomas are associated with clinical endocrine abnormalities, in others the secretory product may be so limited that it is detectable only by biochemical studies. Some adenomas may produce too little steroid hormone to produce biochemically diagnostic elevations; the only evidence of hyperfunction in such cases may be histologic evidence of atrophy in the adjacent cortex.
- Endocrine syndromes associated with adenomas include, in order of frequency: hyperaldosteronism (Conn's syndrome), hyperadrenocortisolism (Cushing's syndrome), virilization, and, very rarely, feminization.
- Most patients present either with pure hyperaldosteronism or Cushing's syndrome.
- The presence of virilization, feminization, or mixed syndromes increases the probability of malignancy in adrenal cortical neoplasms.
- Cortical adenomas are responsible for 80% of cases of hyperaldosteronism; the clinical findings include weakness, with hypertension and hypokalemia.
- The prevalence of Conn's syndrome (hyperaldosteronism associated with adrenal cortical adenoma) in the hypertensive population is approximately 0.5–8.0%. Most tumors are diagnosed in the fourth through sixth decades, with a predilection for females.
- Adrenal cortical adenomas are responsible for only 5–10% of cases of Cushing's syndrome, compared to 80% of cases associated with pituitary adenoma, and most of the remainder are related to ectopic ACTH secretion by other neoplasms.
- Hypercortisolism due to adrenal cortical adenoma is usually seen in young children. In children under 8 years of age, Cushing's syndrome is more often due to an adrenal cortical neoplasm; however, pituitary adenoma is more commonly the cause of hypercortisolism in children over the age 8 years.
- In adults, hypercortisolism is usually caused by pituitary adenomas in females (usually premenopausal) and by ectopic ACTH in men (increasing with age).
- Virilizing tumors are seen over a wide age range, including prepubertal children, and in adult females. They usually secrete dehydroepiandrosterone or dehyroepiandrosterone sulfate, and, less commonly, testosterone. The majority of virilizing adrenal cortical adenomas in adults are malignant, but they are often benign in children.
- Feminizing adrenal cortical neoplasms are usually seen in men between the ages of 25 and 45 years. The clinical findings include gynecomastia, decreased libido, feminized hair pattern, and testicular atrophy. The findings are due to increased estrogens. Most feminizing adrenal neoplasms are malignant.
- 'Mixed' endocrine syndromes usually include Cushing's syndrome with virilization or feminization, and are usually associated with malignant cortical neoplasms.
- Adrenal cortical adenoma with hyperaldosteronism is diagnosed biochemically by documenting low serum potassium levels (usually less than 4.0 mEq/l, though some individuals may be normokalemic), suppressed plasma renin level, and elevated plasma aldosterone level, though these studies are not entirely specific.
- Adrenal cortical adenoma with Cushing's syndrome must be distinguished biochemically from pituitary-dependent Cushing's disease. Both diseases are associated with elevated plasma cortisol and 17-hydroxycorticoid levels, which are not suppressed by low-dose dexamethasone. High-dose dexamethasone almost always suppresses pituitary-based hypercortisolism, but not that due to an adrenal cortical adenoma. Plasma ACTH is elevated in pituitary adenomas with hypercortisolism, but is usually undetectable in patients with adrenal cortical adenomas that produce Cushing's syndrome.
- Nonfunctional adrenal cortical adenomas are probably rare, while the nonfunctional and non-neoplastic adrenal cortical nodule described previously in this chapter is quite common. The distinction between these two entities rests upon subtle differences in the cortex adjacent to the nodule. The few true nonhyperfunctioning adenomas are most often incidental findings, though large examples may be associated with flank or abdominal pain.
- CT is very useful in localizing adrenal adenomas, particularly the larger lesions as typically seen in Cushing's syndrome. Adenomas associated with hyperaldosteronism, however, may be quite small and

difficult to identify. The frequent use of CT for evaluation of a variety of abdominal complaints has also increased the incidence of detection of adrenal masses during life; most incidentally discovered lesions are nonhyperfunctioning and represent cortical nodules rather than adenomas.

- MRI is also useful in localization, and has the added advantage of helping to categorize lesions by the signal intensity of the T2-weighted image: pheochromocytomas have a high intensity signal; metastases have an intermediate signal; nonhyperfunctioning cortical nodules or adenomas have a low intensity signal. Distinctions between hyperfunctioning and nonfunctioning adenomas cannot be made.
- Radionuclide scanning using cholesterol labeled with radioactive iodine is an indicator of steroid hormone secretion which demonstrates differential uptake between hyperfunctioning adenomas and the remaining cortex. The technique appears to be helpful in characterizing the nonhyperfunctional cortical nodules, which fail to exhibit differential uptake compared with the rest of the cortex.
- Radiographic images of adrenal cortical adenomas with extensive degenerative changes such as hemorrhage and cystic alterations may be misleading, suggesting the possibility of pheochromocytoma or adrenal cortical carcinoma.

Pathology

Cytology

- The typical smear contains predominantly naked nuclei scatted rather evenly in a background of foamy to slightly granular cytoplasm. Distinct borders are difficult to discern, but occasional intact cells with small, round nuclei with homogeneous chromatin, inconspicuous nucleoli, and vacuolated cytoplasm are seen. Focal enlarged and irregular nuclei may be present. Mitotic figures are not noted. Necrosis is not usually present. Some cases may be characterized by better preservation of the cortical cells, which are usually arranged in acinar groupings; the cytologic features are otherwise similar.
- The chief utility of FNA of adrenal masses is the exclusion of metastatic disease involving the adrenal. Distinction between benign and malignant adrenal cortical neoplasms may by very difficult based solely on cytologic criteria. The clinical and radiographic features, combined with such cytologic findings as necrosis and widespread marked nuclear atypia, may lend support to a malignant diagnosis.
- The close cytologic resemblance of most adenomas to normal cortex makes distinction between lesional and nonlesional samples difficult; reliance on careful radiologic localization for verification of the source of a sample is important.

Gross

- The gross appearance of adrenal cortical adenomas varies to some degree with the steroid hormone produced; however, overlap in size and appearance occurs between groups.
- Adenomas with hypercortisolism are unilateral and solitary, with an average size of 4.0 cm and a mottled yellow–brown color; they are usually encapsulated. The remaining cortex usually appears atrophic.
- Adenomas with hyperaldosteronism are unilateral and solitary, with an average size of 1.5 cm and a yellow color; they are frequently unencapsulated or incompletely encapsulated. The tumor may be accompanied by mild nodularity of the remaining cortex.
- Adenomas with virilization are unilateral and solitary, with an average size of 5 cm (some much larger) and a reddish-brown color; they are encapsulated.
- Adenomas associated with feminization are rare (most such neoplasms are malignant); they resemble tumors associated with virilization.
- Pigmented, or 'black', adenomas are rare adrenal cortical neoplasms that are distinguished from typical adenomas only by their diffusely brown to black gross appearance. The most common endocrine disorder associated with pigmented 'black' adenoma is Cushing's syndrome, but hyperaldosteronism has also been reported in a few patients. The pigment responsible for the gross appearance is visible as brown intracytoplasmic granular material by light microscopy. It is thought to represent primarily lipofuscin, though some may be neuromelanin.

(Figs 13.24 & 13.25)

Histology

Although there are some associations of cell type with secretory product in cortical neoplasms, tumors frequently exhibit a mixture of patterns that make specific classification of endocrine function based on histology difficult at best.

Adenoma with hypercortisolism

- More distinctly circumscribed than aldosteronomas, these adenomas are contained within a pseudocapsule of compressed cortex and connective tissue, or, if large, within the adrenal capsule.
- The tumor cells are most often quite large, with abundant finely vacuolated pale cytoplasm and

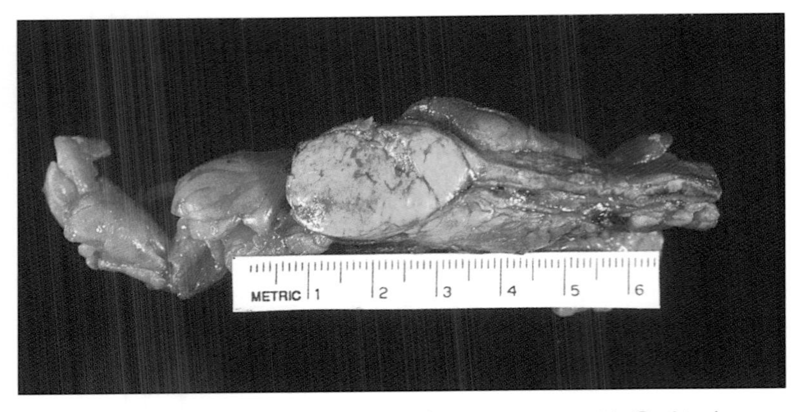

Fig. 13.24 Adrenal cortical adenoma from a patient with Cushing's disease. The adenoma is solitary, circumscribed, and yellow–orange, with associated thinning of the adjacent cortex.

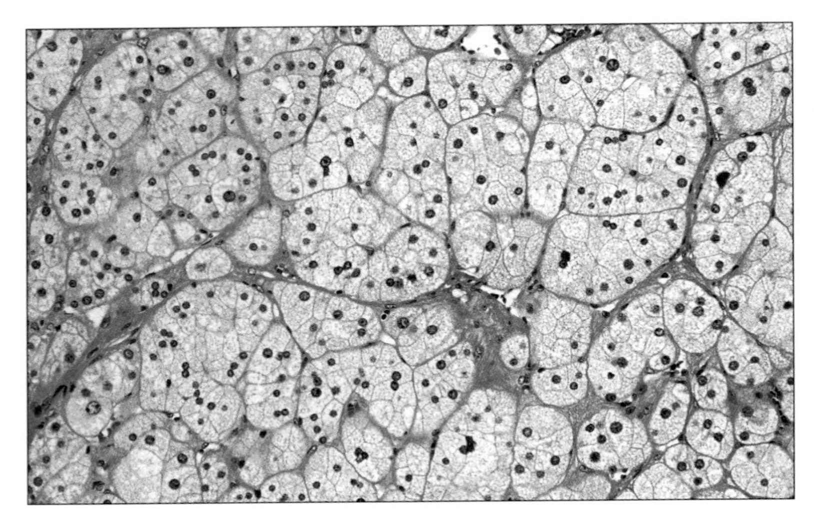

Fig. 13.26 Lipid-rich clear cells in a cortical adenoma with hypercortisolism. The cells resemble those of the normal zona fasciculata.

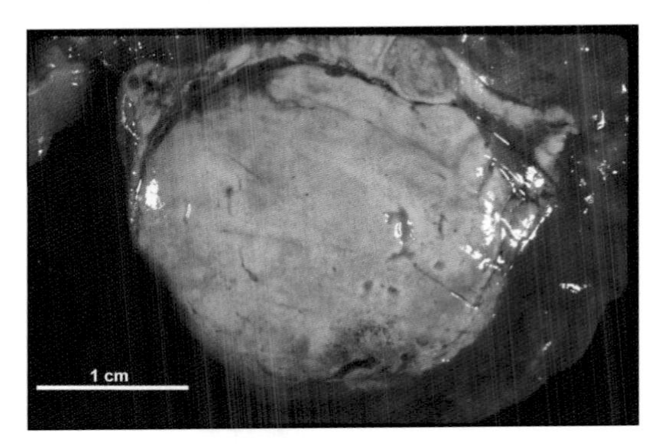

Fig. 13.25 Adrenal cortical adenoma with hyperaldosteronism ('aldosteronoma'). The tumor is circumscribed but lacks encapsulation, as is true for most aldosteronomas. The irregular thickening with vague nodularity of the adjacent cortex is a common finding, in contrast with the atrophic cortex seen with cortisol-producing adenomas.

vesicular nuclei (fasciculata-like), arranged in nests or cords. There are also smaller, more eosinophilic, lipid-poor cells resembling the zona reticularis. Lipofuscin may be prominent in some tumors.
- Enlarged atypical nuclei may be seen, but they are usually quite focal. Mitoses are rarely seen.
- The non-neoplastic adrenal cortex is usually atrophic, though there may be intervening nonfunctioning cortical nodules, which should be distinguished from nodular cortical hyperplasia. The cytologic features of the adenoma are usually different from the nonfunctional nodules in a given case.

(Fig. 13.26)

Adenoma with hyperaldosteronism

- The tumor is circumscribed, but a distinct fibrous capsule is usually lacking; the tumor cells usually appear different from the normal cortex by virtue of size and cytoplasmic staining features.
- The normal cortex may contain small cortical nodules that are probably secondary to the patient's hypertension. These nodules may confuse the issue of distinguishing between an adenoma and nodular cortical hyperplasia. It should be remembered, however, that hyperaldosteronism due to hyperplasia is a diffuse process involving the zona glomerulosa, rather than a multinodular process.
- There may be considerable variation in the cytologic features. Large, pale, vacuolated cells with abundant lipid and vesicular nuclei predominate; these cells resemble the cells of the zona fasciculata. In addition, a variety of cells, ranging from those with less cytoplasm but rich in lipid to small cells with a rim of eosinophilic cytoplasm and more condensed chromatin (similar to the zona glomerulosa and zona reticularis), may be seen.
- In addition to nonhyperfunctional cortical nodules, there may be hyperplasia of the zona glomerulosa in the adjacent or contralateral cortex. This expansion of the zona glomerulosa may be diffuse or regional.
- A unique feature of 'aldosteronomas' is the presence of '*spironolactone bodies*', which are eosinophilic laminated cytoplasmic inclusions surrounded by a clear space. They measure 2–12 μm in diameter. They are PAS-positive diastase-resistant, and are medium to dark blue with Luxol fast blue. The inclusions are found after treatment with spironolactone and may be seen for a few months after cessation of therapy. Spironolactone bodies contain phospholipids and may be derived from endoplasmic reticulum. The effect of spironolactone in controlling blood pressure lasts only 5–6 weeks; the number of spironolactone bodies diminishes as the efficacy of the medication wanes.

(Figs 13.27–13.31)

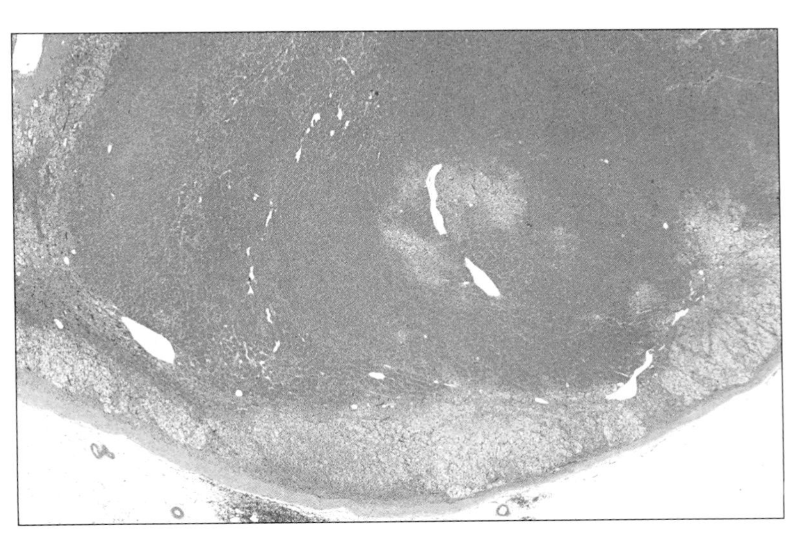

Fig. 13.27 Aldosterone-producing cortical adenoma is unencapsulated and 'merges' with the surrounding non-neoplastic cortex.

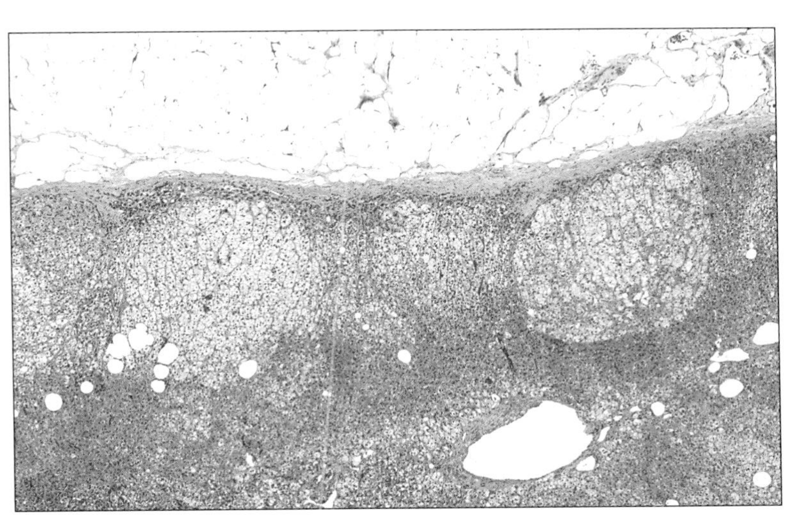

Fig. 13.30 The adrenal cortex adjacent to an aldosterone-producing cortical adenoma frequently contains nodules of clear cells that are cytologically distinct from those of the tumor; these nodules of clear cells are nonhyperfunctioning and are believed to be related to the patient's clinical hypertension.

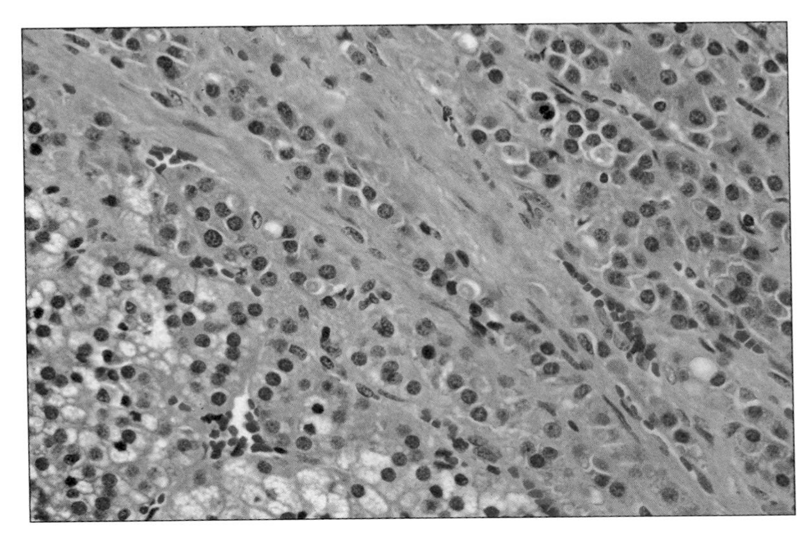

Fig. 13.28 Although compact or lipid-poor cells predominate in this aldosterone-producing adenoma, these neoplasms frequently have an admixture of clear and compact cells.

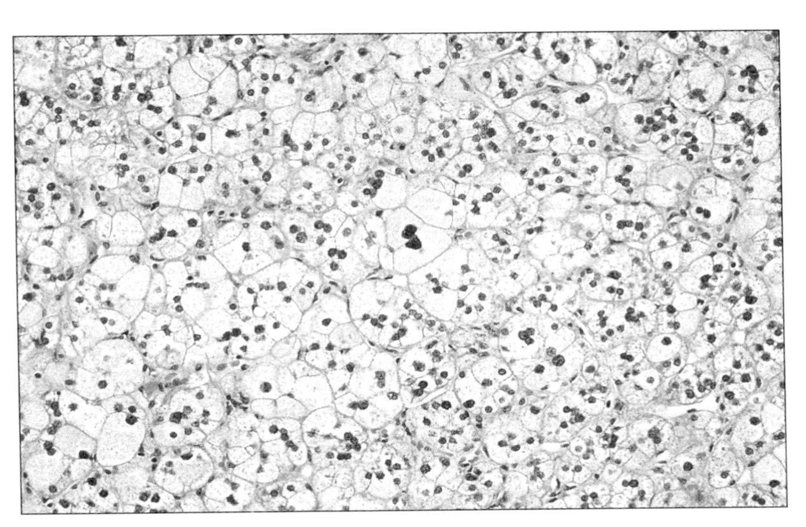

Fig. 13.31 Adrenal cortical adenomas may exhibit focal nuclear pleomorphism and hyperchromasia, as does this aldosterone-producing adenoma. These cells are not indicative of malignancy.

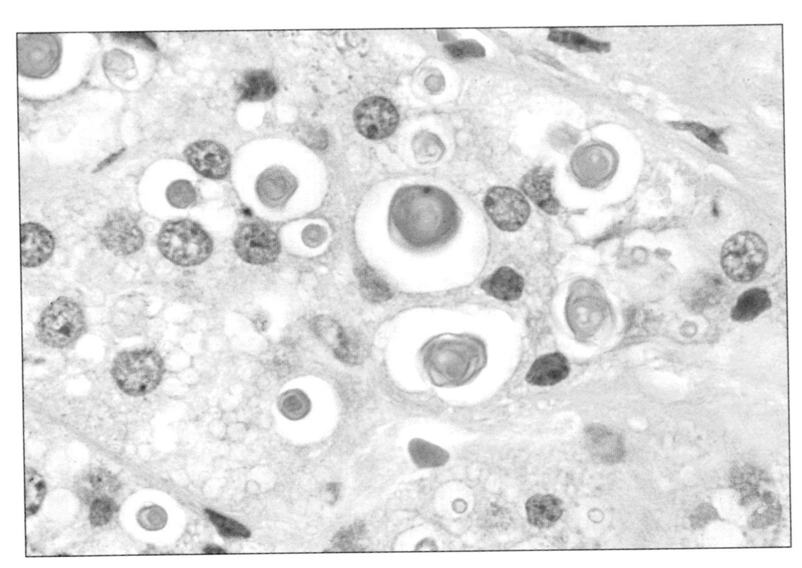

Fig. 13.29 Spironolactone bodies in an adrenal cortical adenoma associated with hyperaldosteronism. The patient had been treated with spironolactone for 3–4 weeks.

Adenomas with virilization

- The distinction between benign and malignant virilizing cortical neoplasms may be difficult. Half of these neoplasms occur in children; the criteria for malignanacy in childhood adrenal cortical neoplasms are not well defined, and the criteria utilized for adult tumors cannot be reliably applied. Many tumors with mitoses, marked nuclear atypia, and other features associated with malignancy in adults may be seen in childhood tumors that pursue a benign course.
- In adults, these tumors are more likely to behave aggressively, even if all of the histologic criteria of malignancy are not present.

- The usual histologic pattern is one in which small eosinophilic cells resembling the zona reticularis predominate; however, areas of lipid-rich cells may be seen as well.
- An unusual variant of virilizing adrenal cortical adenoma is associated with production of testosterone in some cases. The tumor cells are large and eosinophilic, and resemble ovarian theca-lutein cells.

Adenomas with feminization

- Feminizing adrenal cortical neoplasms are very rare. In adults, most of these tumors have the histologic features of malignancy and are classified as adrenal cortical carcinomas; however, there are reports of 'adenomas' with benign behavior in children.
- The histologic features are similar to those of virilizing tumors.

Degenerative and other changes associated with adrenal cortical adenomas

- Necrosis, although considered a criterion for malignancy, must be judged cautiously. Adenomas, particularly when large or following venographic studies, may undergo central necrosis. This finding is not indicative of malignancy. The necrosis observed in cortical carcinomas is usually patchy and is not localized to the center of the tumor. Other criteria of malignancy should be found to reinforce the significance of necrosis in a neoplasm.
- Central degenerative changes, when longstanding, may include resolving hemorrhage and necrosis with vascular proliferation and cystic alteration. These changes must be distinguished from a vascular neoplasm; the presence of residual viable cortical cells or ghost cells within the area of concern indicates an underlying adrenal cortical neoplasm.
- Hemorrhage in an adrenal cortical adenoma may be massive, greatly increasing the size and weight of adenomas, and sometimes masking the true neoplastic process involved.
- Myelolipomatous foci are common in cortical adenomas.

(Figs 13.32–13.35)

Differential diagnosis

- Adrenal cortical carcinoma.
- Adrenal cortical nodule (nonfunctional).
- Nodular adrenal cortical hyperplasia.
- Metastatic carcinoma, especially renal cell carcinoma.
- Pheochromocytoma with lipid degeneration.

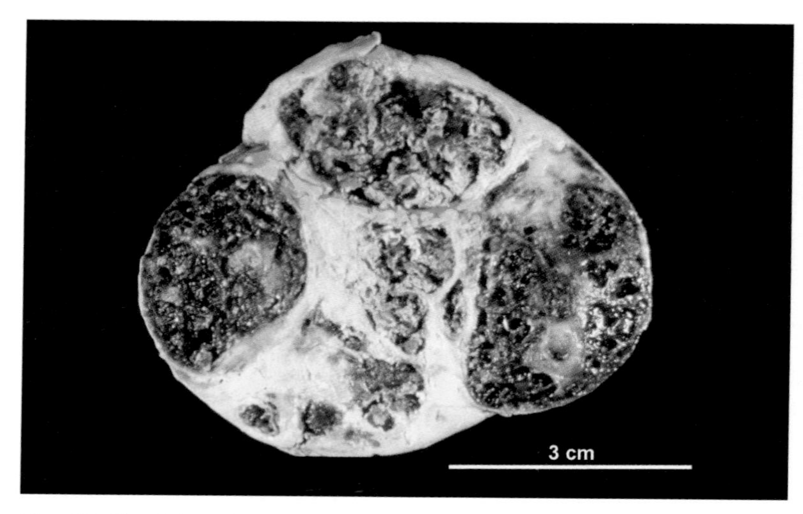

Fig. 13.32 Adrenal cortical adenoma with degenerative changes, including cystic change, hemorrhage, and fibrosis.

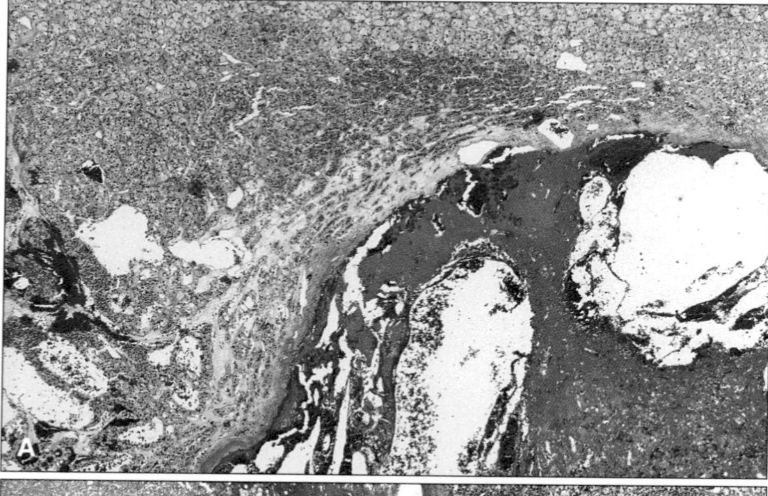

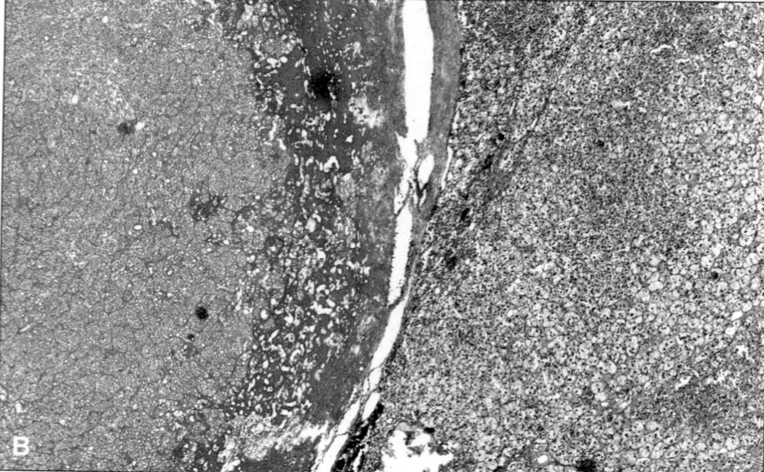

Fig. 13.33 Adrenal cortical adenoma with (A) cystic degeneration due to hemorrhage, and (B) necrosis. The latter is centrally located and lacks the patchy nature seen in association with adrenal cortical carcinomas.

Treatment and prognosis

- Surgical therapy for adrenal cortical adenoma associated with Cushing's syndrome is usually effective in reversing the clinical effects of hypercortisolism within 1 year of resection. There is a

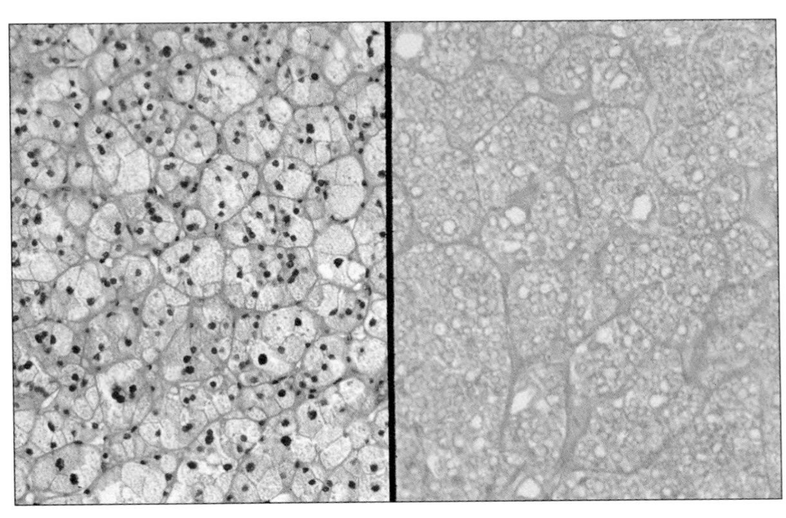

Fig. 13.34 Adrenal cortical adenoma with cystic degeneration and hemorrhage, infarction, and patchy tumor cell necrosis (left panel), in which the architecture of the tumor nests is retained, as highlighted by Masson trichrome stain (right panel). This type of necrosis differs from that seen in adrenal cortical carcinoma and should not be misinterpreted.

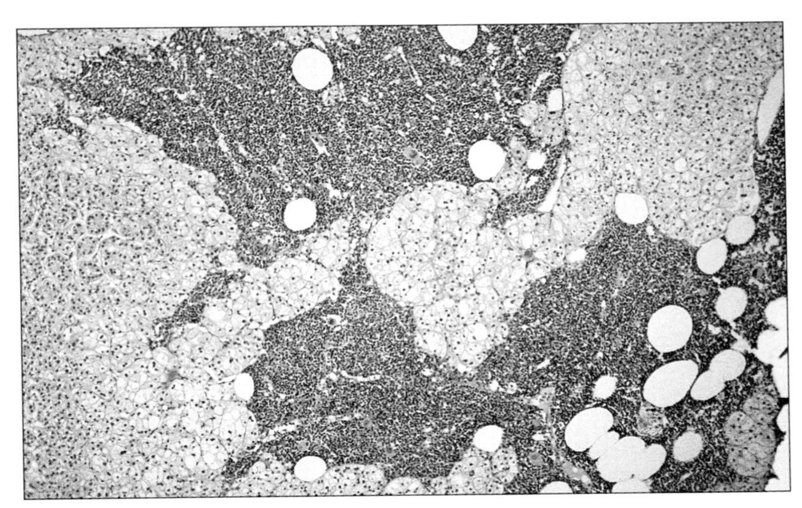

Fig. 13.35 Myelolipomatous foci are common in a wide variety of adrenal lesions, including adrenal cortical adenomas.

risk of adrenal cortical insufficiency due to longstanding suppression of the contralateral cortex by the tumor; supportive administration of mineralocorticoids and glucocorticoids, as well as ACTH, may be required for a year or longer.
- Hyperaldosteronism due to an adenoma usually responds quickly to resection of the involved gland; however, some patients may have persistent hypertension due to hyperplastic changes in the zona glomerulosa of the contralateral gland.
- Complete surgical resection (adrenalectomy) is the desired therapy for virilizing and feminizing cortical tumors; evaluation for evidence of metastases is essential due to the high incidence of malignancy, particularly in adults. Failure of the clinical syndrome to resolve is evidence of extra-adrenal spread.

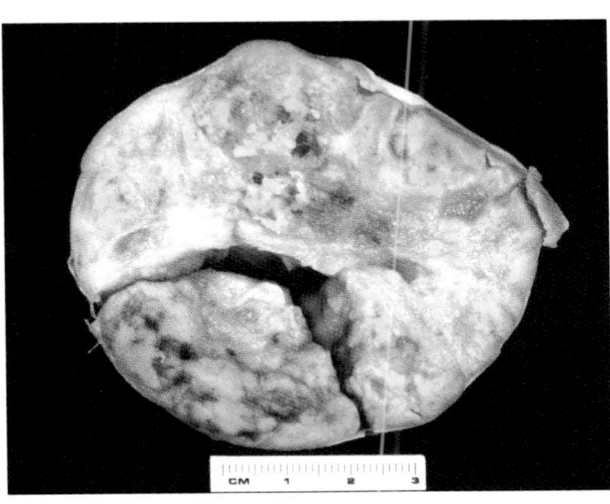

Fig. 13.36 Oncocytic adrenal cortical tumor with a tan to yellow color and foci of intratumoral fibrosis.

Oncocytic adrenal cortical neoplasms

Clinical
- Oncocytic adrenal cortical neoplasms are very uncommon, with only a few cases documented in the literature.
- Patient ages have been in the fifth through seventh decades, with no apparent gender predilection.
- Although most cases have been clinically nonfunctional, usually discovered incidentally, rarely these tumors may be associated with virilization.
- Initially these lesions were all thought to be benign; however, large oncocytic adrenal tumors (10 cm or greater) may exhibit locally aggressive behavior (invasion of the inferior vena cava, kidney, and liver) in the absence of definitive histologic features of malignancy.

Pathology

Gross
- Oncocytic adrenal cortical neoplasms are characterized grossly by a homogeneous tan to yellow-brown color.
- They range in size up to 10 cm and 865 g.

(Fig. 13.36)

Microscopic
- The histologic pattern is usually a diffuse proliferation of large polygonal cells with abundant granular eosinophilic cytoplasm, somewhat eccentrically placed and variably sized round vesicular nuclei, and one or more prominent nucleoli. Mitoses and necrosis are not usually seen.
- Electron microscopy has documented the presence of a vast number of mitochondria filling the cytoplasm.
- Of importance is the obligatory finding of three of Weiss' criteria for malignancy in all oncocytic adrenal tumors, including diffuse growth pattern, high nuclear grade, and predominance of eosinophilic cells; owing to the small number of cases, it is not clear whether a

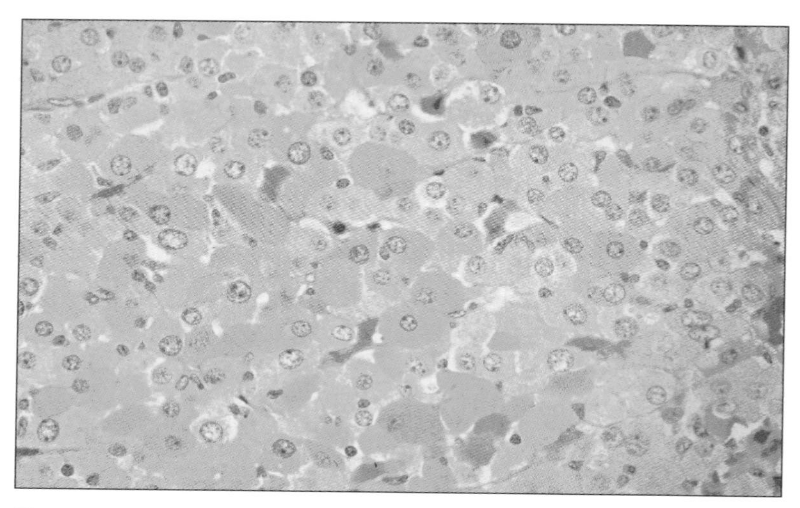

Fig. 13.37 Oncocytic adrenal cortical neoplasm characterized by the presence of cells with abundant brightly eosinophilic-appearing granular cytoplasm. The nuclei are relatively uniform with prominent nucleoli.

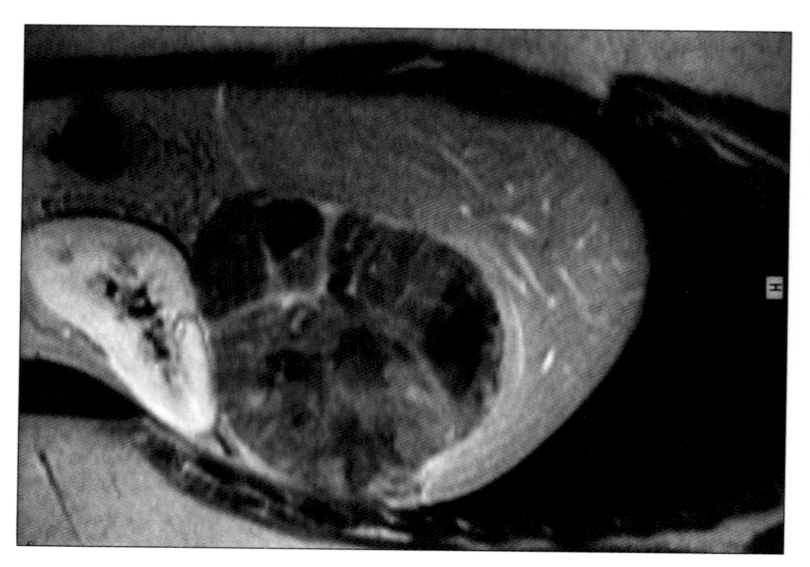

Fig. 13.38 Adrenocortical carcinoma appearing on magnetic resonance imaging as a large suprarenal mass with coarse fibrous septations and variable internal densities.

modification of these criteria would be predictive of behavior in these tumors.

(Fig. 13.37)

ADRENAL CORTICAL CARCINOMA[83,85,87,95,97–118]

Definition

This is a malignant neoplasm arising from the cells of the adrenal cortex, which may manifest pure or mixed endocrine syndromes (Cushing's syndrome, virilization, feminization), or which may be clinically nonfunctional.

Clinical

- Adrenal cortical carcinomas are rare, accounting for 0.02% of all cancers.
- A broad age distribution is seen, with cases concentrated in the first two decades and in the fifth through seventh decades.
- No definite gender or racial predilections are seen, though some series suggest a slight female predominance.
- Common presenting symptoms include a palpable abdominal mass, abdominal pain, weight loss, or evidence of endocrine hyperfunction.
- The overall incidence of endocrine manifestations in adrenal cortical carcinoma varies greatly in series of cases – from 24% to 96%. Cushing's syndrome is the most commonly encountered endocrine syndrome, usually as a mixed hypercortisolism/virilization syndrome. Pure virilizing or feminizing tumors are infrequently seen, and hyperaldosteronism as an isolated syndrome is exceedingly rare.
- Laboratory findings are dependent upon the endocrine function of the tumor. Cushing's syndrome is manifested by high levels of corticosteroids that are not suppressed by high-dose dexamethasone, and, unlike Cushing's syndrome seen in adenomas, carcinomas fail to increase cortisol levels in response to ACTH. The frequent mixture of Cushing's syndrome with virilization or hyperaldosteronism is also different from the pure Cushing's syndrome of adenomas. Marked elevation of urinary 17-ketosteroids due to the more frequent production of excess androgens is seen more often in carcinomas than in adenomas.
- In the past, many patients have had metastatic disease involving liver, lung, or bone at the time of presentation (24–50%), though the earlier discovery of these neoplasms with more advanced imaging in recent years may alter the epidemiology of cortical carcinoma.
- CT and MRI are the most widely utilized methods of localization. Cortical carcinomas are usually much larger than adenomas, and are more often partially necrotic or hemorrhagic.

(Fig. 13.38)

Pathology

Cytology

- The cytologic features are dependent upon the degree of differentiation, characterized by resemblance to normal cortical cells. More well-differentiated tumors may be difficult to distinguish from cortical adenomas, while more pleomorphic carcinomas may be difficult to distinguish from metastatic carcinomas.
- Smears are usually very cellular, and, unlike normal cortex and adenomas, the cytoplasm is usually intact.

There is loss of cohesiveness, with many single cells admixed with loose groups of cells.

- Though loss of cytoplasmic lipid vacuoles is common in carcinomas, some more 'well-differentiated' carcinomas may contain vacuolated cells, which are helpful in recognizing the neoplasm as being of cortical origin. The lipid-rich cells differ from those in adenomas in their nuclear features: the nuclei are enlarged and hyperchromatic and contain nucleoli. Mitoses, if present, are very suggestive of malignancy.
- Carcinomas in which the cells have little or no lipid are more difficult to distinguish from metastatic lesions. The cytoplasm is eosinophilic and granular, and varies greatly in amount; some tumor cells may have an abundance of cytoplasm, while others have a high nuclear:cytoplasmic (N:C) ratio. The nuclei tend to be quite atypical, with hyperchromasia and pleomorphism, which may become extremely bizarre. Nucleoli are usually prominent and large. Necrosis of tumor cells is helpful in supporting a malignant diagnosis.
- Immunohistochemistry and electron microscopy may be helpful in the differential diagnosis between adrenal cortical carcinoma and metastatic carcinoma, as discussed below.

(Fig. 13.39)

Gross

- Reported average weights of cortical carcinomas vary greatly, from 705 g to over 1210 g; however, the weight ranges are quite large – from less than 40 g to over 3000 g. The range of recorded weights overlaps significantly with the weight range of cortical adenomas. Although weight has in the past been used as a predictor of behavior in cortical neoplasms, it has become clear that weight is not, by itself, a reliable criterion for malignancy. This is particularly true with the increasing use of advanced radiologic imaging techniques, which are capable of detecting these neoplasms when they are much smaller, and sometimes incidental.
- Tumors as small as 38 g have metastasized, while others weighing as much as 1800 g have behaved in a benign fashion.
- Nonhyperfunctioning tumors tend to be larger at the time of diagnosis than those associated with clinical endocrine dysfunction.
- Cortical carcinomas may be grossly encapsulated or, especially if large, infiltrative; adjacent organs may be involved. Large tumors often completely efface the adrenal gland.
- The contour of the neoplasm is usually multinodular. The cut surface is yellow to brown, and is usually mottled by patches of hemorrhage and necrosis, which may be extensive. Degenerative changes lead to cystic areas.

(Figs 13.40 & 13.41)

Histology

- Although a variety of histologic patterns may be observed, including the typical nesting configuration of adrenal cortical adenomas, the presence of diffuse or solid and broad trabecular areas is common in carcinomas, and should alert one to the possibility of malignancy. Occasionally, pseudoglandular or myxoid patterns may seen.
- Broad bands of fibrous tissue often dissect the tumor into coarse irregular nodules.

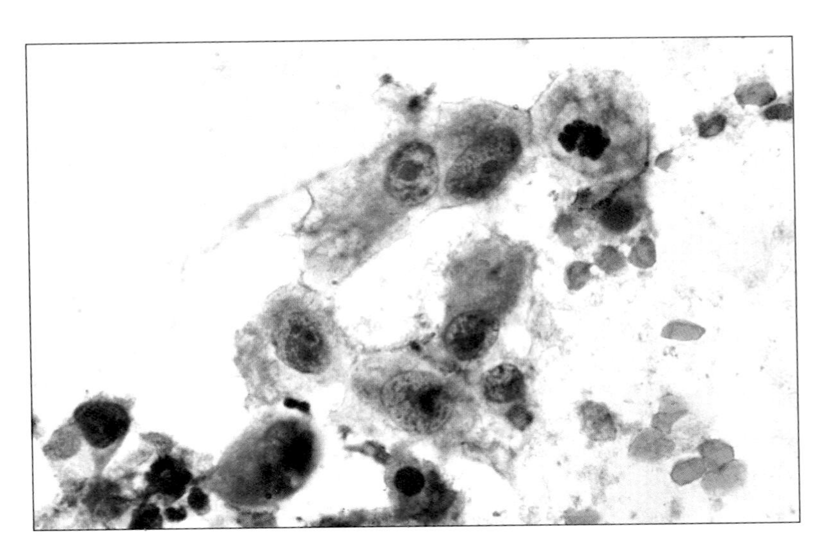

Fig. 13.39 Fine-needle aspiration biopsy of an adrenal cortical carcinoma, showing the presence of a highly pleomorphic cell population that is indistinguishable from a metastatic carcinoma.

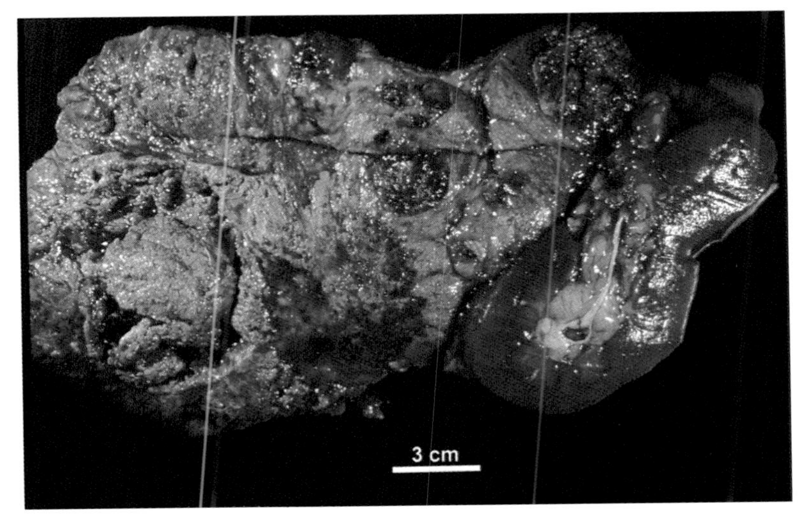

Fig. 13.40 Adrenal cortical carcinoma. This tumor has gross features commonly seen in adrenal cortical carcinoma, including hemorrhage, coarse nodularity, necrosis, and large size. The adjacent kidney is seen to the right and is separate from and uninvolved by the adrenal cortical carcinoma.

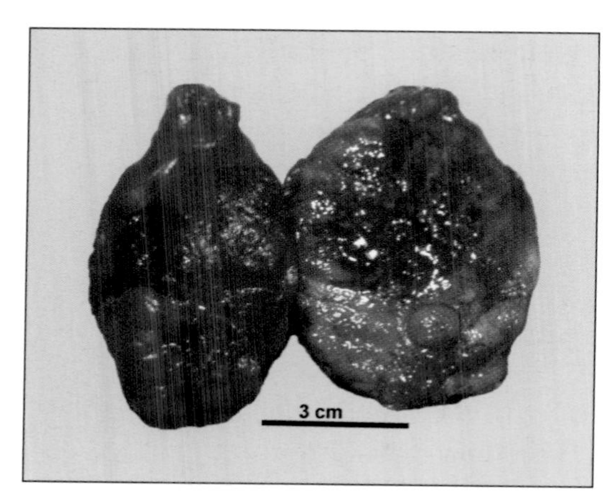

Fig. 13.41 Adrenal cortical carcinoma. Size is not necessarily a reliable criterion for malignancy. This relatively small, pigmented lesion histologically was an adrenal cortical carcinoma, aldosterone producing, with metastatic disease at the time of surgery.

- Necrosis may be absent in smaller tumors, but is a common finding overall; necrosis may be focal and involve only small clusters of tumor cells or it may be extensive, with confluent 'geographic' patches.
- Eosinophilic, lipid-poor tumor cells tend to predominate, though aggregates of cells with pale, vacuolated cytoplasm may be present as well. The amount of cytoplasm is quite variable. Pleomorphic cells with very atypical nuclei and abundant cytoplasm may be impressive, but these cells are not restricted to carcinomas. A more disturbing cell type is the rather monotonous cell with a high N:C ratio; these cells populate areas of intense cellularity and are usually fruitful areas for counting mitotic figures. The small cells have relatively large rounded hyperchromatic nuclei, with coarse chromatin and prominent nucleoli.
- Hyaline globules may be present in the cytoplasm of some carcinomas.
- The presence of readily identified mitotic figures is usually indicative of malignancy and is usually accompanied by other criteria for carcinoma. A rate of six or more mitoses per 50 high-power fields (HPF) has been suggested as an indicator of malignancy, though not all carcinomas will have such a high mitotic rate.
- Vascular invasion and extensive local capsular invasion are very suspicious for malignancy; involvement of true venous structures (in contrast to sinusoids) appears to be conclusive evidence of malignancy.

(Figs 13.42–13.49)

Criteria for malignancy in adrenal tumors

- The distinction between cortical adenoma and carcinoma is usually relatively simple; however, there are cases in which an unequivocal classification cannot be made. Several sets of criteria for malignancy have

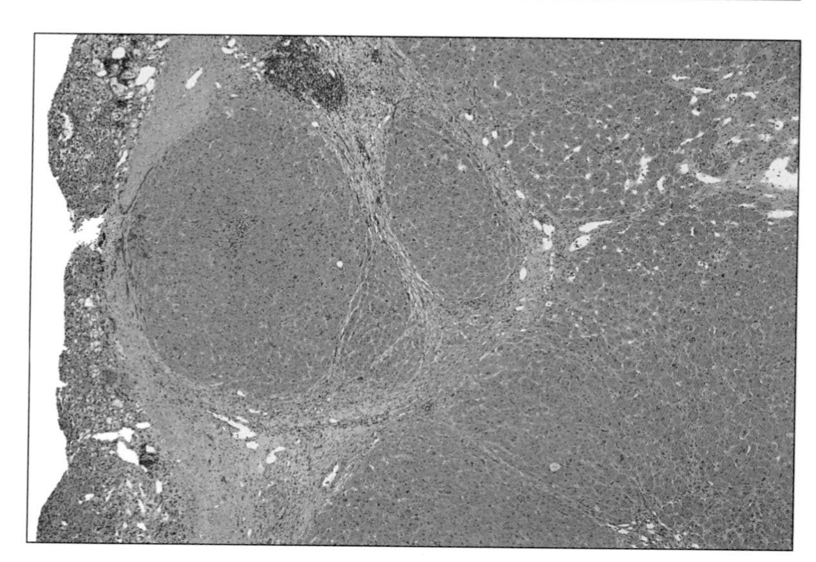

Fig. 13.42 Adrenal cortical carcinoma. Histologic features suggestive of malignancy in this field include dissection of the tumor into nodules by broad fibrous bands and tumor cell necrosis.

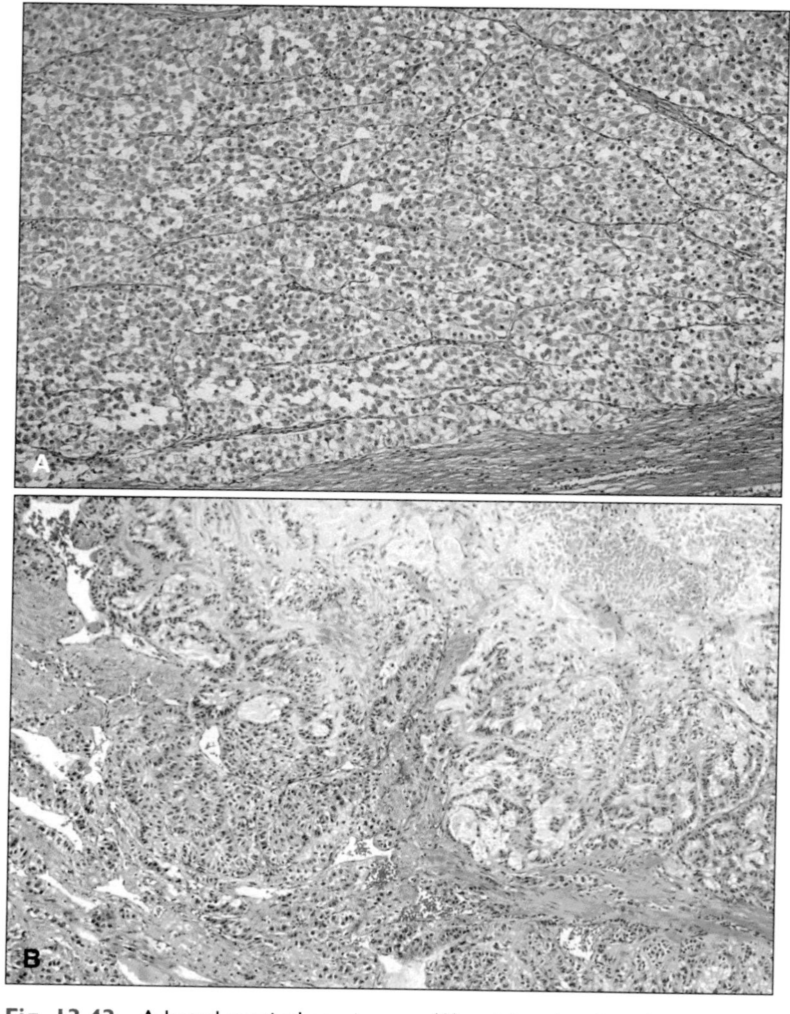

Fig. 13.43 Adrenal cortical carcinoma: (A) solid and trabecular growth patterns; (B) pseudoglandular pattern and myxoid degenerative changes.

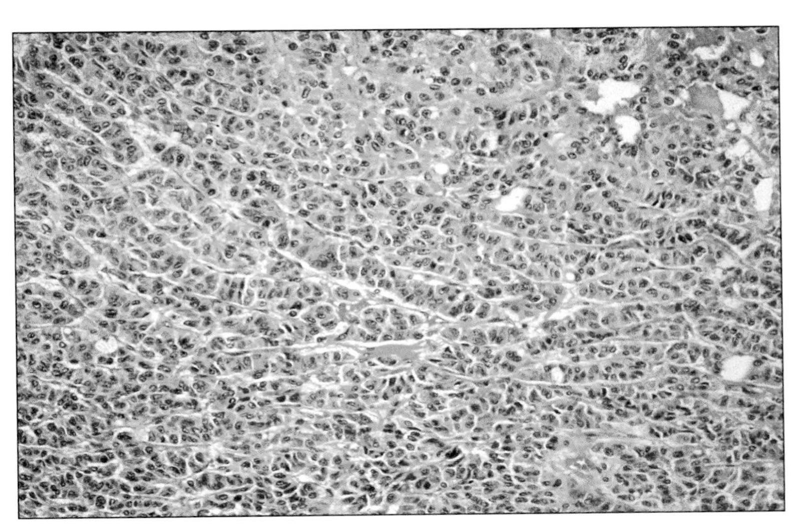

Fig. 13.44 Adrenal cortical carcinoma showing trabecular growth pattern. The cells are lipid-poor with an increased nuclear:cytoplasmic ratio.

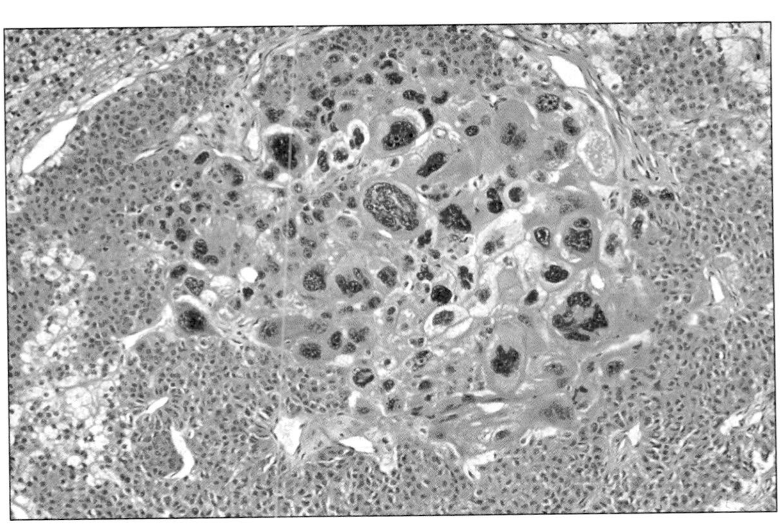

Fig. 13.46 Adrenal cortical carcinoma. Cellular neoplasm composed of compact, lipid-poor cells with an increased nuclear:cytoplasmic ratio, and markedly pleomorphic cells with prominent eosinophilic cytoplasm, high nuclear grade. Increased mitotic activity with atypical mitoses was present in this case (not shown). These findings are among the criteria for malignancy in adrenal cortical neoplasms.

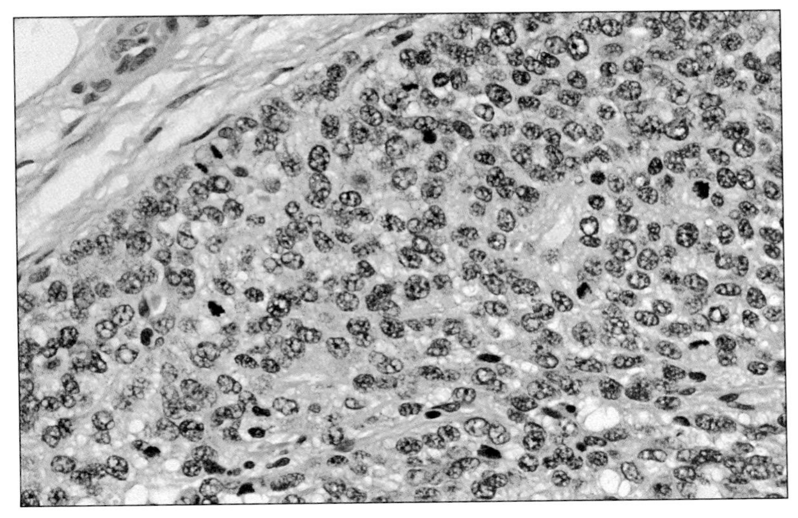

Fig. 13.45 Adrenal cortical carcinoma. This area of solid tumor shows small, lipid-poor cells with an increased nuclear:cytoplasmic ratio, and several mitotic figures.

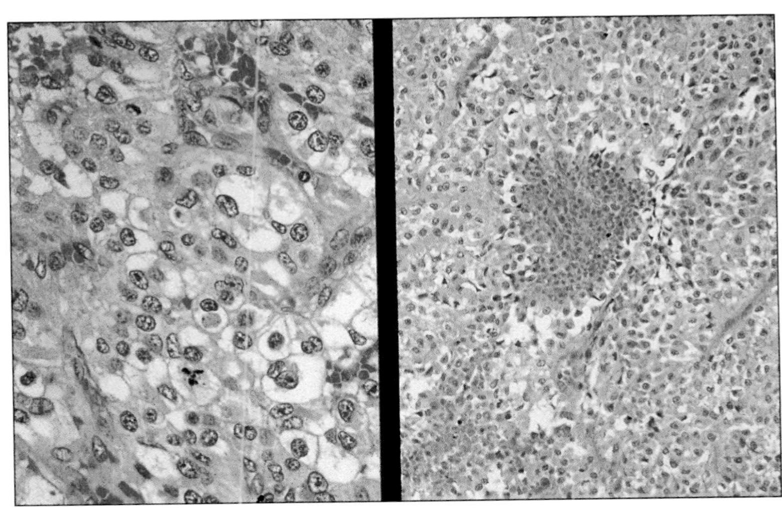

Fig. 13.47 Adrenal cortical carcinoma. Left: Increased mitotic figures including atypical mitoses are seen. Right: Solid cellular area showing small lipid-poor cells with an increased nuclear:cytoplasmic ratio and a confluent focus of tumor cell necrosis.

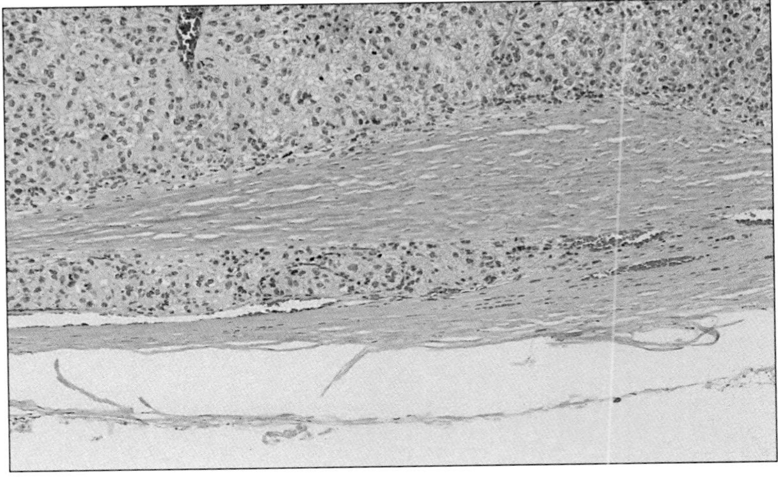

Fig. 13.48 Adrenal cortical carcinoma showing invasion of a capsular blood vessel, an important finding in the diagnosis of adrenal carcinomas.

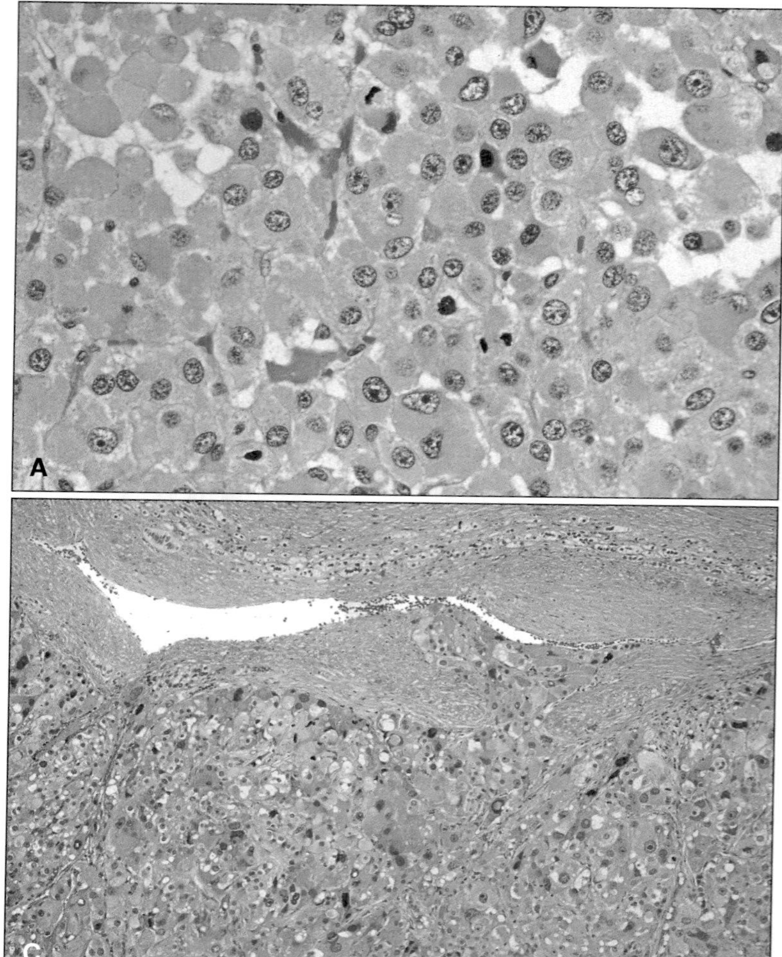

Fig. 13.49 A rare example of an oncocytic adrenal cortical carcinoma: (A) cells showing the presence of a prominent eosinophilic cytoplasm without an increase in the nuclear:cytoplasmic ratio but with scattered mitotic figures; (B) nuclear pleomorphism and intranuclear pseudoinclusions are seen; (C) invasion into a capsular blood vessel is diagnostic of malignancy in this case.

been compiled in conjunction with review of series of clinically benign and malignant adrenal cortical neoplasms. The criteria of Hough et al.[83] utilize both clinical and pathologic parameters, while Weiss[117] and van Slooten et al.[115] included only pathologic findings.

- *Immunohistochemistry* is not helpful in distinguishing between adrenal cortical adenoma and adrenal cortical carcinoma; however, it is useful in the differential diagnosis between cortical carcinoma and a variety of metastatic lesions. Cortical carcinomas may be positive for vimentin, Melan-A103, inhibin, synaptophysin, and neuron-specific enolase, but are usually negative for cytokeratin, epithelial membrane antigen, carcinoembryonic antigen (CEA), S-100 protein, HMB-45, chromogranin, and blood group isoantigens. It should be noted that use of some low molecular weight cytokeratins may yield scattered positive cells. The immunostaining pattern is helpful in distinguishing between adrenal cortical carcinoma and hepatocellular or renal cell carcinoma, which may be a histologic differential diagnostic problem.
- *Electron microscopy*: Few cytoplasmic lipid vacuoles are seen. Mitochondria are variable in shape, but usually elongated, and often have tubular cristae. Stacks of rough endoplasmic reticulum and myelin figures are usually present.
- *Flow cytometric DNA analysis*: Although aneuploidy tends to favor malignancy in cortical neoplasms, there is some overlap with adenomas, particularly larger ones.

(Tables 13.7–13.10)

Differential diagnosis

- Adrenal cortical adenoma.
- Metastatic carcinoma, especially hepatocellular or renal cell carcinoma.
- Pheochromocytoma.

Treatment and prognosis

- Adrenal cortical carcinomas are extremely aggressive, with over 60% of patients having metastatic disease at the time of diagnosis. Patients who develop metastatic disease rarely live beyond 1 year.
- The treatment includes resection of the primary lesion, followed by chemotherapy using mitotane.

Table 13.7 Criteria for malignancy in adrenal cortical neoplasms: Weiss

Histologic feature	*Definition*
High nuclear grade	Fuhrman's nuclear grade III or IV
Mitotically active*	>5 per 50 high-power fields
Atypical mitotic figures*	Abnormal spindles or chromosome distribution
Eosinophilic tumor cell cytoplasm	≥75% of tumor, rather than clear cells
Diffuse growth pattern	>1/3 of tumor area
Necrosis	Involving confluent nests of cells or larger areas
Venous invasion*	Vessel with smooth muscle in wall
Sinusoidal invasion	Vascular space without smooth muscle
Capsular invasion	Into or through capsule, with stromal reaction

*Found only in tumors with malignant clinical behavior.
Malignancy = 3 or more criteria.
After Weiss.[116]

Table 13.8 Nonhistologic criteria for malignancy in adrenal cortical neoplasms: Hough et al.

Tumor weight >100 g
Urinary 17-ketosteroids >100 mg/g creatinine/24 h
Nonresponsive to ACTH administration
Cushing's syndrome with virilization (mixed endocrine syndrome), virilism alone, or no clinical syndrome
Weight loss of >10 lb in 3 months

After Hough et al.[83]

Table 13.9 Histologic criteria for malignancy in adrenal cortical neoplasms: Hough et al.

Diffuse growth pattern predominates
Vascular invasion
Tumor cell necrosis (>2 HPF in diameter)
Broad fibrous bands (>1 HPF in diameter)
Capsular invasion
Mitotic rate >1/10 HPF
Moderate to marked cellular pleomorphism

HPF, high-power field.
After Hough et al.[83]

Table 13.10 Histologic criteria for malignancy in adrenal cortical neoplasms: van Slooten et al.

Extensive regressive changes, including necrosis, hemorrhage, fibrosis, or calcification
Loss of normal architecture
Moderate to marked nuclear atypia
Moderate to marked nuclear hyperchromasia
Abnormal nucleoli
Mitotic rate >2/10 HPF
Vascular or capsular invasion

HPF, high-power field.
After van Slooten et al.[115]

- Tumor stage is useful in predicting survival:
  stage I, tumor <5 cm and confined to adrenal;
  stage II, tumor >5 cm and confined to adrenal;
  stage III, tumor any size and confined to adrenal with regional lymph node involvement, or locally invasive without lymph node metastases;
  stage IV, tumor locally invasive with regional lymph node involvement, or tumor with involvement of adjacent organ, or any tumor with distant metastases.
- Approximately one-third of patients with stage I or II tumors survive 5 years.

Adrenal cortical neoplasms in children

- Adrenal cortical neoplasms in children cannot be categorized reliably utilizing the systems established for adult cortical neoplasms. Although childhood cortical tumors have been assigned a poor prognosis in the past, current detection methods, surgical technique, and endocrine replacement therapy appear to have altered the outcome significantly.
- Re-evaluation of criteria has shown that pediatric tumors may exhibit increased mitotic rate, atypical mitoses, necrosis, vascular and capsular invasion, fibrous bands, and marked nuclear pleomorphism, without aggressive clinical behavior.
- Tumor size may have prognostic significance, with a weight greater than 500 g usually associated with malignant behavior; however, as in adult tumors, there is overlap in the weights of benign and malignant tumors in different studies.

(Fig. 13.50)

NEOPLASMS OF THE ADRENAL MEDULLA

ADRENAL MEDULLARY HYPERPLASIA[119–124]

Definition

This comprises diffuse or nodular increases in medullary tissue and associated hypersecretion of catecholamines, most often as a precursor to pheochromocytoma in multiple endocrine neoplasia (MEN) syndromes.

Clinical

- Although most instances of adrenal medullary hyperplasia (AMH) are reported in patients with MEN, there are occasional patients who appear to have a

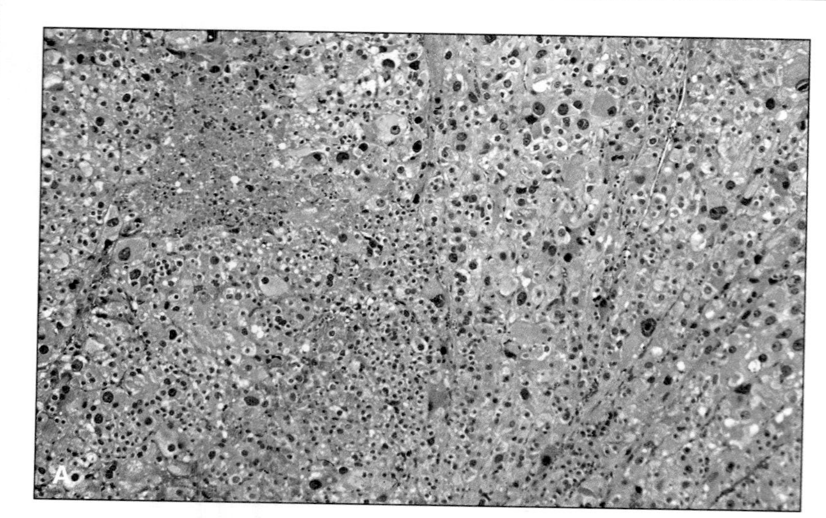

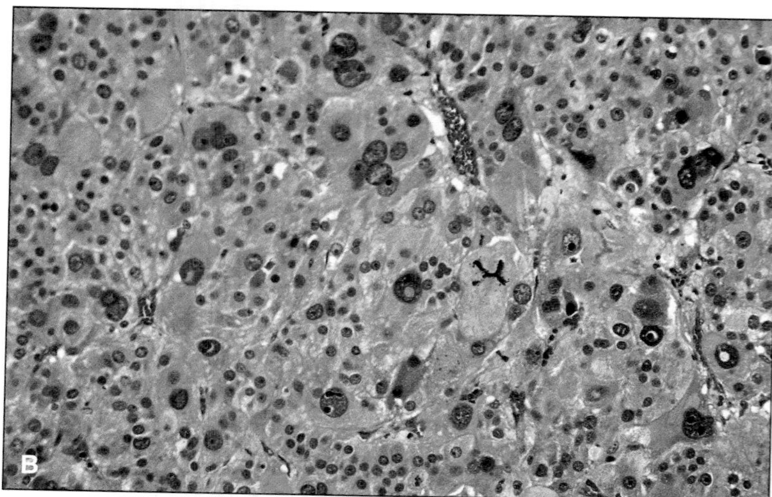

Fig. 13.50 This adrenal cortical neoplasm in a child shows histologic features that in adults are highly suspect for malignancy, including: (A) trabecular growth pattern, increased cellularity with small, lipid-poor cells, cells with prominent eosinophilic cytoplasm, nuclear pleomorphism, increased nuclear:cytoplasmic ratio, and focal tumor necrosis (upper left); (B) increased mitotic figures, including an atypical mitosis. However, these findings in pediatric adrenal cortical tumors are not necessarily indicative of malignancy.

sporadic form of hyperplasia, with similar clinical manifestations.

- *Sporadic* cases of AMH are characterized by:
  signs and symptoms of pheochromocytoma, including hypertension (paroxysmal or sustained), headaches, palpitations, and diaphoresis in the absence of a detectable tumor;
  no family history of MEN syndromes;
  elevated urinary levels of catecholamine or metanephrine.
- *Familial* AMH is usually associated with MEN 2 and is thought to be the precursor of pheochromocytomas in this setting. Unlike in patients with sporadic AMH, familial AMH may be detected before it is symptomatic, due to laboratory screening in families at risk. The earliest indication of AMH is elevation of the epinephrine-to-norepinephrine ratio in the urine. When symptoms become evident, they are generally those seen in pheochromocytoma.
- AMH has been reported in Beckwith–Wiedemann syndrome, which may be sporadic or familial.
- CT scans may show no abnormality or, in more advanced diffuse or nodular AMH, may demonstrate adrenal enlargement (bilateral in most cases).

Pathology

Gross

- Changes of AMH are usually bilateral, but may be asymmetric.
- Adrenal enlargement may not be evident grossly, requiring morphometric demonstration of an increase in medullary tissue. Normal medullary weights range from 0.37 to 0.48 g per gland.
- In more advanced cases of AMH, the medulla may be diffusely expanded or may be multinodular. The distinction of nodular AMH from multiple pheochromocytomas in MEN-associated medullary disease is somewhat arbitrary; nodules less than 1 cm are classified as hyperplastic, while those 1 cm or larger in diameter are considered pheochromocytomas.
- The hyperplastic medullary tissue may be gray to tan to dark red; the nodular areas tend to blend indistinctly with the surrounding medulla.

Histology

- The microscopic proliferation of medullary cells may be diffuse or variably nodular. The adjacent cortex may be compressed. As the hyperplasia advances, nodules become larger and more distinct.
- Various patterns may be seen, as in pheochromocytoma, including solid, trabecular, or the typical 'zellballen' nesting pattern.
- The cells may exhibit significant nuclear pleomorphism and hyperchromasia; the cytoplasm may be vacuolated or very granular. These changes are thought to reflect the hypersecretory activity of the hyperplastic medullary cells.
- Mitotic figures may be seen, though they are usually few in number.

Differential diagnosis

- Pheochromocytoma.

Treatment and prognosis

- Resection of one or both adrenal glands has resulted in resolution or improvement of symptoms in a large

proportion of patients with sporadic AMH; bilateral adrenalectomy has been used in many patients with MEN 2 with favorable results.
- AMH is considered a benign, pre-neoplastic disease by most; however, the clinical risks of hypersecretion of catecholamines and the potential for malignancy in pheochromocytoma are key concerns in clinical management decisions.

PHEOCHROMOCYTOMA[85,95,121,125–145]

Definition

Pheochromocytoma denotes a neoplastic proliferation of the neuroendocrine cells of the adrenal medulla and of their supporting, or 'sustentacular', cells. This term has specifically referred to paragangliomas of the adrenal medulla, but has also been used to designate all paragangliomas of the sympathoadrenal neuroendocrine system (the 'extra-adrenal' pheochromocytomas). Signs and symptoms are related to release of catecholamines, chiefly epinephrine and norepinephrine.

Synonyms

- Adrenal paraganglioma.
- Sympathoadrenal paraganglioma.
- Chromaffinoma.
- Chromaffin cell tumor.
- Chromophile tumor.
- Medullary adenoma.
- Adrenergic tumor.

Clinical

- Pheochromocytomas are uncommon, with an autopsy incidence of 0.005–0.1%. In the past, as many as 76% of pheochromocytomas were not diagnosed during life; these do not appear to have been nonfunctional or 'silent' tumors, however, since most of those patients died from sudden cardiac or cerebrovascular events, often related to a surgical procedure for an unrelated problem.
- Approximately 90% of cases are sporadic, while 10% are familial.
- Familial cases of pheochromocytoma may occur in the absence of other familial disease syndromes or may be seen in association with MEN 2A (most common), MEN 2B, von Recklinghausen's disease, and von Hippel–Lindau disease.
- Tumors occur over a very broad age range from infancy to old age, but the incidence peaks in the fifth decade; only approximately 10% of pheochromocytomas occur in children. Familial cases are usually diagnosed at an earlier age, usually within the first two decades.
- No definite gender predilection has been noted; however, some studies suggest a slight preponderance of females.
- Common presenting symptoms include headache (>90%), palpitations, diaphoresis, flushing of the skin, anxiety, nausea, and constipation. Dyspnea, chest pain, visual disturbances, abdominal pain, fatigue, and paresthesias are less frequent complaints. The triad of headache, palpitations, and sweating are particularly predictive of a diagnosis of pheochromocytoma.
- Hypertension, with or without tachycardia, is the key physical finding, with half of patients experiencing sustained hypertension with episodes of marked hypertension, while the remaining have paroxysmal hypertensive episodes. A few individuals with pheochromocytomas are normotensive.
- Approximately 10–15% of patients have a palpable abdominal mass.
- Laboratory biochemical evaluation is the cornerstone of diagnosis: 24-hour urine samples are assayed for elevations of epinephrine (E), norepinephrine (NE), and total catecholamines (CA), and for their metabolites, metanephrine (MN), normetanephrine (NMN), and vanillylmandelic acid (VMA). Plasma catecholamines (E and NE) may also be determined, and have a higher sensitivity for diagnosing pheochromocytoma than do urine assays. Urine MN and VMA levels are the most widely used assays and detect 80–90% of tumors.
- Clinical presentation reflects the pattern of catecholamine secretion: norepinephrine-secreting tumors produce sustained hypertension; tumors with significant epinephrine secretion in addition to norepinephrine produce episodic hypertension; pure epinephrine-secreting tumors may produce hypotension. Dopamine is the dominant product of a small number of pheochromocytomas; these patients are usually normotensive and may present a diagnostic dilemma.
- CT, I-MIBG (*m*-iodobenzylguanidine) scan, MRI, ultrasonography, and venous cannulation with sampling for catecholamine levels are all useful in localization of pheochromocytomas. CT is the most widely utilized imaging method for localization. The adrenal glands and sites of extra-adrenal paragangliomas are readily visualized. Pheochromocytomas are nonhomogeneous, well-circumscribed tumors. The lack of homogeneity is the result of areas of hemorrhage, necrosis, or cystic degeneration. MRI is similarly useful, with the added advantage of improved differential distinction among pheochromocytoma, metastases to the adrenal, and many adrenal cortical neoplasms.

- The ^{131}I-MIBG scan utilizes a radioactive material that is taken up by neuroendocrine tumors, including pheochromocytomas, neuroblastomas, parathyroid proliferative diseases, paragangliomas, and some carcinoids and medullary thyroid carcinomas. Almost all benign pheochromocytomas, but only half of malignant cases, are detectable with this procedure. I-MIBG is also useful in identifying metastatic disease in tumor with update of the radioisotope.
- Carney's triad is an unusual nonfamilial association of functioning paragangliomas (usually extra-adrenal), gastric epithelioid leiomyosarcoma, and pulmonary chondromas. Young females are usually affected. Adrenal pheochromocytomas have been seen in a few cases.

(Fig. 13.51)

Pathology

Cytology

- FNA of adrenal masses, as well as retroperitoneal extra-adrenal lesions, is a common preoperative diagnostic procedure that is helpful in distinguishing between metastatic and primary lesions. However, biochemical and clinical evidence of pheochromocytoma are usually adequate to make a preoperative diagnosis without resorting to FNA; indeed, aspiration of pheochromocytoma may result in life-threatening hemorrhage or in a hypertensive crisis. Most of the cytologic diagnoses of pheochromocytoma are made in patients with atypical clinical presentation or equivocal biochemical evidence.
- Smears are usually cellular, with loose clusters of polygonal to somewhat elongated cells with poorly defined cytoplasmic borders. Delicate wisp-like process may extend from some of the cells; the cytoplasm is finely granular.
- The nuclei are quite variable, with some marked anisonucleosis in some cases. Hyperchromasia is usually evident, with a coarse chromatin pattern. Nucleoli vary from cell to cell: inconspicuous to very prominent. Intranuclear cytoplasmic pseudoinclusions may be present, and are numerous in some cases. Naked nuclei are common.
- An unfortunate but helpful clue in the diagnosis may be noted during the procedure: hypertension, with palpitations, diaphoresis, or other manifestations.

(Fig. 13.52)

Gross

- Sporadic pheochromocytomas are usually single unilateral tumors, 3–5 cm in diameter. Multiple and bilateral tumors are common in a familial setting, particularly in MEN 2. The multiple neoplasms in MEN 2 may be accompanied by a diffuse increase in the medullary tissue due to AMH.
- Pheochromocytomas are circumscribed, with larger tumors possessing a definite capsule. Compressed adrenal cortex may be splayed over the capsule of large tumors.
- The cut surface is gray to pink–tan or red, with areas of hyperemia or recent hemorrhage. Areas of remote hemorrhage, fibrosis, cystic degeneration, and necrosis are more common in large tumors. The tumor may darken to a brown or mahogany color after exposure to air, due to oxidation of catecholamines.
- The *chromaffin reaction* is a gross method of demonstrating the presence of catecholamines. After immersion in a dichromate fixative, the tumor becomes

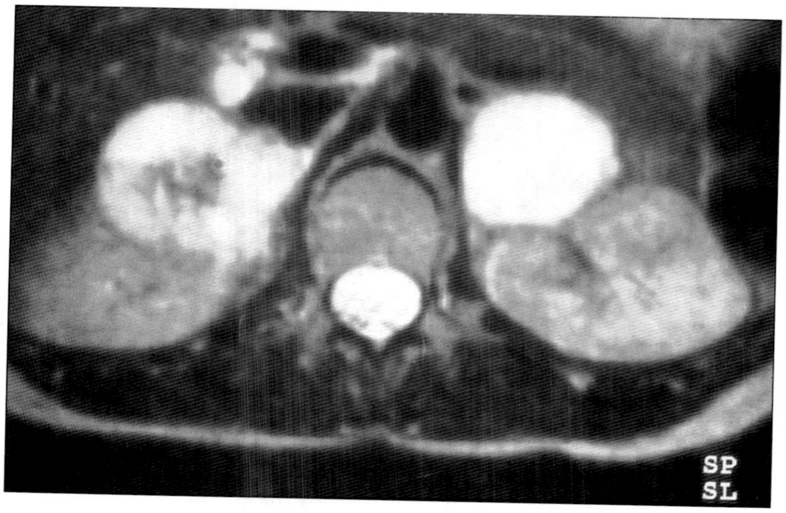

Fig. 13.51 Bilateral pheochromocytomas in a patient with multiple endocrine neoplasia, type 2A. The large tumors are bright on the T2-weighted image by magnetic resonance imaging.

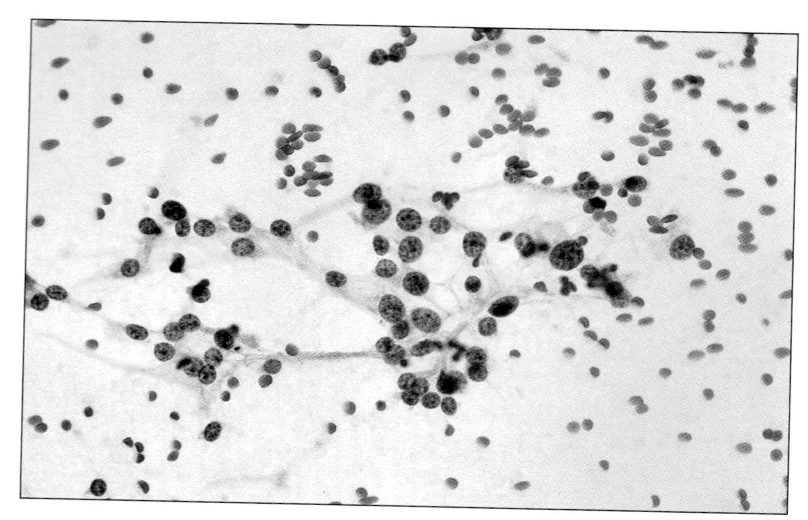

Fig. 13.52 Fine-needle aspiration biopsy of a pheochromocytoma. The tumor cells cluster in a loose acinar arrangement. Fibrillar cytoplasmic processes create a mesh-like background. The salt-and-pepper chromatin pattern reflects the neuroendocrine origin. Wisp-like processes of granular cytoplasm are present.

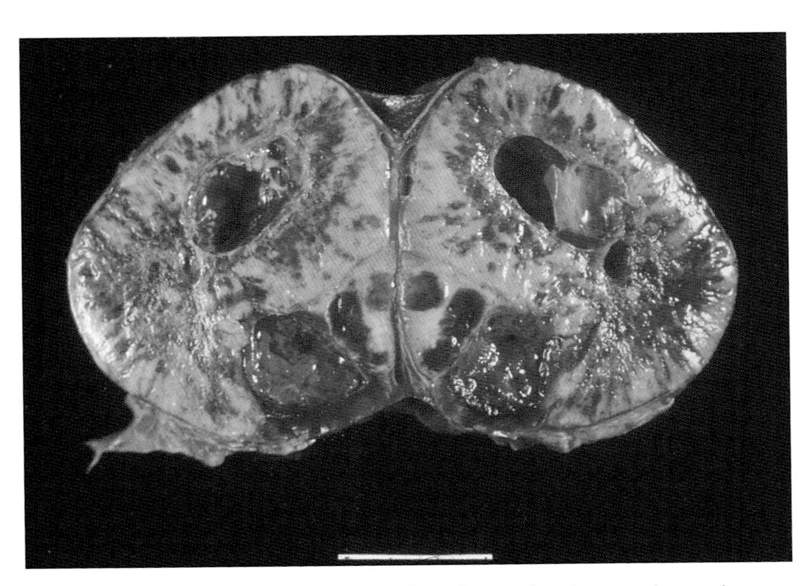

Fig. 13.53 Pheochromocytoma with variegated red–tan color and central area of cystic degeneration, a common finding in pheochromocytomas.

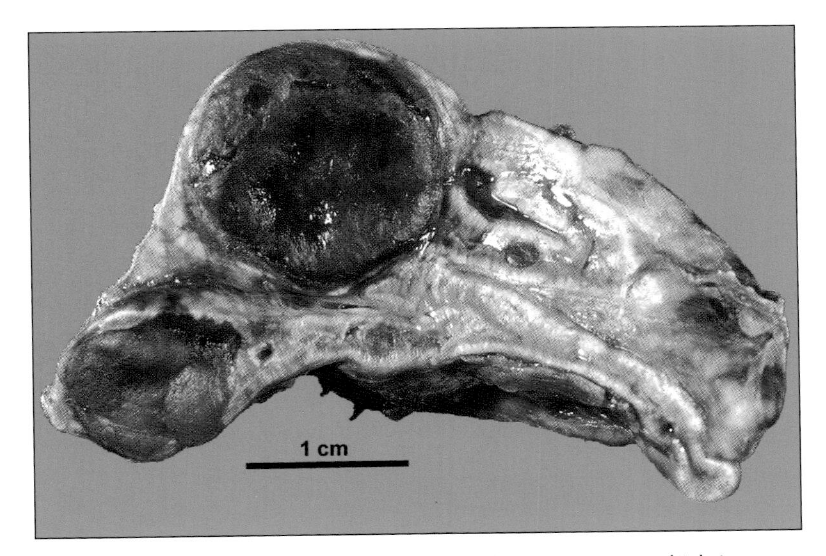

Fig. 13.54 Chromaffin reaction in a pheochromocytoma, which is a gross method of demonstrating the presence of catecholamines. After immersion in a dichromate fixative, the tumor becomes deep brown in color as a result of oxidation of epinephrine and norepinephrine. The pigments are visible microscopically, but are water-soluble and are thus largely removed in routine processing of tissue.

deep brown in color as a result of oxidation of epinephrine and norepinephrine. The pigments are visible microscopically, but are water-soluble and are thus largely removed in routine processing of tissue.

(Figs 13.53 & 13.54)

Histology

- Architectural patterns most frequently encountered are trabecular (most common), alveolar or nesting, and diffuse. Less often, pseudoacinar structures may be superimposed on an alveolar pattern. Focal spindling of cells is also reported; extensive spindling is thought by some to be more common in malignant pheochromocytomas, though not all studies support this impression.
- Vascularity is prominent, with capillaries in a delicate fibrovascular meshwork surrounding groups of tumor cells arranged in nest or cords. The vascularity in some cases is so prominent as to give the tumor an angiomatous appearance.
- Although most tumors are surrounded by at least a thin capsule of fibrovascular tissue, extension of tumor into the adrenal cortex may be seen; this does not imply invasion and malignancy.
- The cytologic features of pheochromocytomas vary greatly from case to case. Polygonal cells with finely granular eosinophilic to somewhat basophilic cytoplasm are most often seen; the N:C ratio is approximately 1:2. The nuclei are central to eccentric in position; they are ovoid, with stippled 'salt and pepper' chromatin and small nucleoli. From this typical cell, numerous variations emerge. Some tumors may contain small cells with a higher N:C ratio, while others have abundant granular cytoplasm that varies from pink to purple. Some tumor cells resemble ganglion cells, with prominent nucleoli and basophilic Nissl-like material. The cytoplasm may contain eosinophilic, PAS-positive globules, which appear to be related to a high level of secretory activity. Nuclear pleomorphism may be striking, with groups of cells with bizarre hyperchromatic nuclei many times the size of most surrounding pheochromocytes. Intranuclear cytoplasmic pseudoinclusions are common, and may be especially striking in pleomorphic nuclei.
- Degenerative changes are seen more often in large tumors: they include areas of sclerosis, hemosiderin accumulation, resolving hemorrhage, and cystic changes.
- Stromal amyloid has been reported in up to 70% of pheochromocytomas, and should be considered in the differential diagnosis of thyroid medullary carcinoma.
- *Histochemistry*: Argyrophilic granules can be demonstrated using a number of techniques, including the Grimelius, Pascual, and Churukian-Schenk stains.
- *Immunohistochemistry*: The most useful immunostains are for chromogranin, which stains the chief cells, and S-100, which stains the sustentacular cells found at the periphery of clusters of chief cells. Other markers that are positive in the chief cells include synaptophysin, neuron-specific enolase, and neurofilament proteins. Previous reports suggested that a decrease in the number of sustentacular cells, as demonstrated by S-100 staining, is associated with likelihood of malignant behavior in head and neck paragangliomas and in sympathoadrenal paragangliomas. However, some

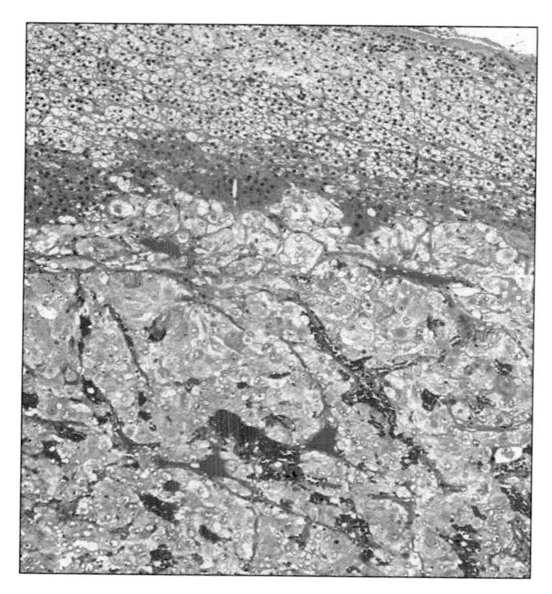

Fig. 13.55 Pheochromocytoma, surrounded by a rim of adrenal cortex (top). The capsule of a pheochromocytoma is often composed of the adrenal remnant and its capsule. The tumor shows a characteristic cell nest growth pattern.

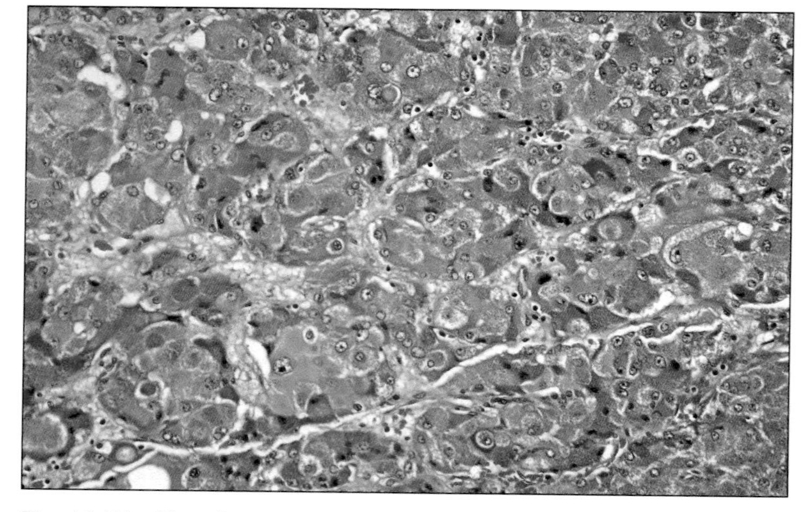

Fig. 13.56 Pheochromocytoma showing the classic cell nest ('zellballen') pattern: rounded nests of chief cells circumscribed by a fibrovascular network. The tumor cells are large and polygonal, with prominent cytoplasmic amphophilic granularity and mild nuclear pleomorphism.

recent reevaluations conclude that density of sustentacular cells is not a reliable predictor of behavior in either group of paragangliomas.

- *Flow cytometry/DNA measurement*: Although studies of normal medulla and AMH reveal a diploid or euploid DNA distribution, non-diploid and aneuploid DNA patterns were found in most benign and all malignant pheochromocytomas.
- *Electron microscopy*: The diagnostic feature is the presence of membrane-bound, dense-core neurosecretory granules. The granules range in size from 150 to 250 nm. In most pheochromocytomas, norepinephrine granules are most abundant; they differ from epinephrine granules by the presence of a large eccentric electron-lucent zone between the dense core and the granule membrane. In predominantly epinephrine-secreting tumors and in normal medullary cells, neurosecretory granules have only a uniform narrow halo surrounding the electron-dense core. Tumor cells may have poorly formed intercellular junctions, as well as variable basal lamina.
- Several studies have reported an association of brown adipose tissue in the periadrenal area, and elsewhere in the abdomen, with pheochromocytoma. Although explanations implicating activation of this fatty tissue by catecholamines have been proposed, a recent examination of periadrenal adipose tissue associated with pheochromocytoma and in control patients found no difference in incidence or amount of brown fat between the groups.

(Figs 13.55–13.59)

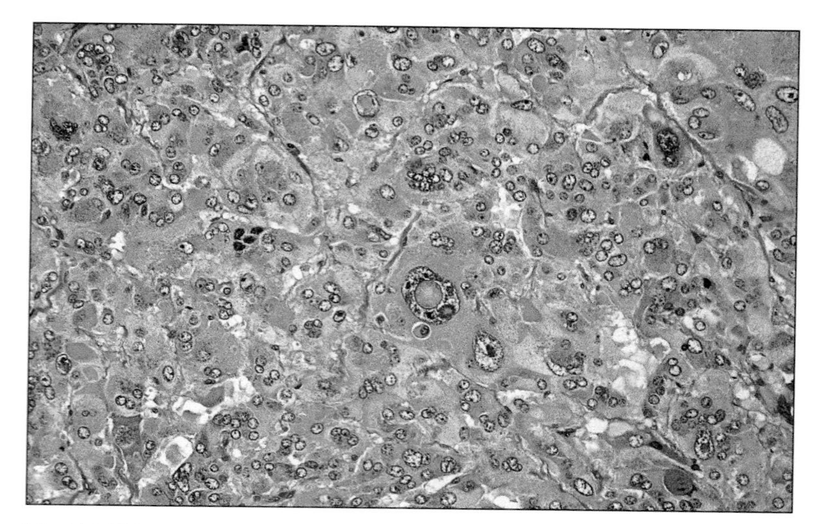

Fig. 13.57 Nuclear pleomorphism is more prominent in this pheochromocytoma with eosinophilic granular cytoplasm. Intranuclear cytoplasmic pseudoinclusions are common.

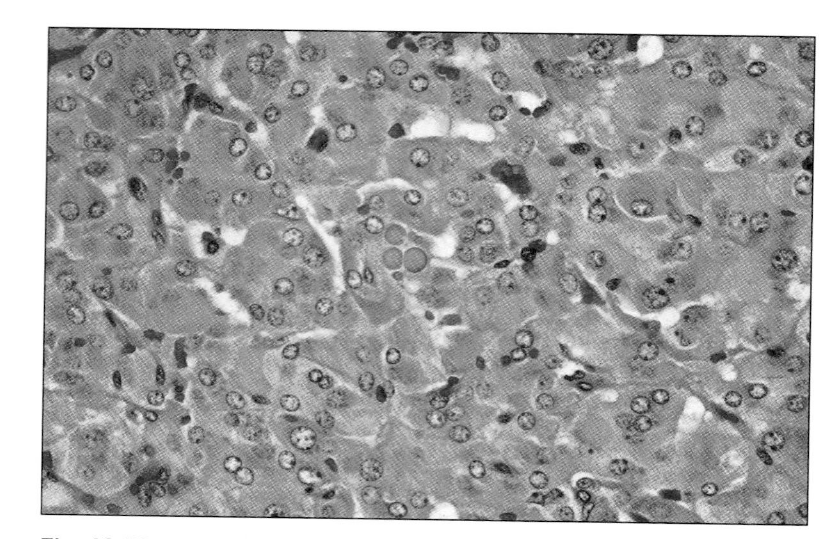

Fig. 13.58 Extracellular hyaline globules are present in this pheochromocytoma. The hyaline globules are PAS-positive, diastase-resistant. There is some evidence that their presence is a feature favoring a benign outcome. These globules are not specific and can be found in a variety of neoplasms.

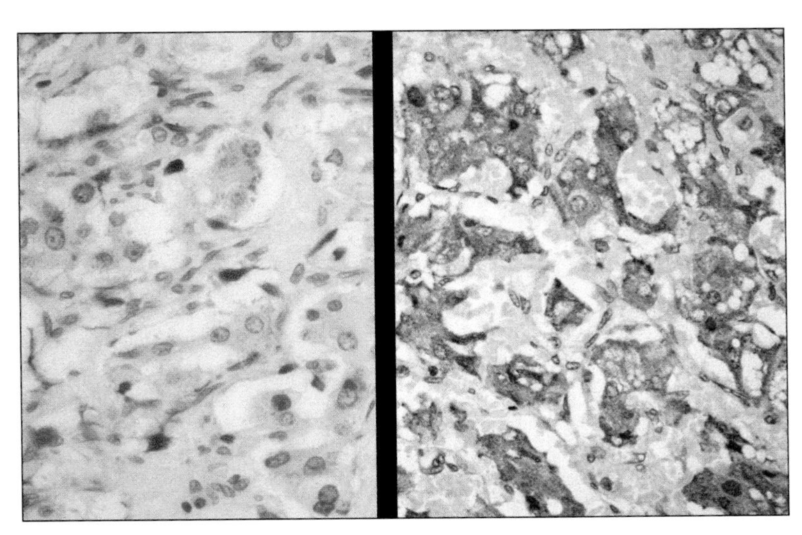

Fig. 13.59 Immunohistochemical pattern of pheochromocytoma. Left: Sustentacular cells are S-100-positive. Right: Chief cells are positive for chromogranin.

Malignancy in pheochromocytoma

- The reported incidence of malignancy in adrenal pheochromocytomas varies by series; however, the traditional 10% figure is near the average of most studies. Extra-adrenal pheochromocytomas have a significantly higher rate of malignancy, with reported rates ranging from 14% to 50%.
- The distinction between benign and malignant pheochromocytomas has long been problematic, with the only widely accepted and definitive proof of malignancy being metastasis to other organs. Sites of metastasis are usually liver, lymph nodes, bone, and lungs.
- Tumors with benign histologic features may metastasize, while tumors with bizarre pleomorphism may behave in a benign fashion. Metastatic deposits may likewise appear very atypical or may be histologically indistinguishable from benign paraganglioma. This unpredictability has frustrated pathologists and surgeons in spite of many attempts to define criteria for malignancy. The conclusions from several studies of pheochromocytoma have conflicted in many areas concerning malignant criteria. The following features have been associated with an increased incidence of malignant behavior, though there are some exceptions to each and no single criterion has proved entirely reliable:

  Tumor size: Malignant tumors averaged 383 g and 759 g versus 73 g and 156 g, respectively, for benign tumors in two large series. One malignant tumor, however, weighed only 35 g.

  Coarsely nodular or multinodular gross appearance: Benign tumors are more often unicentric and uniform, while gross nodularity is more common in malignant tumors. There is, however, overlap between benign and malignant categories.

  Confluent tumor necrosis: Necrosis involving contiguous groups of tumor cells is seen in one-third of malignant tumors.

  Mitotic rate: A mitotic rate of greater than 3/30 HPF favors malignancy; benign tumors usually have less than 1/30 HPF. Some malignant tumors, however, have very low mitotic rates. Atypical mitoses are uncommon, but very are a strong indicator of malignancy.

  Extensive local invasion and/or vascular invasion: Invasion is a helpful feature if extensive; however, tumors that do not behave aggressively may have some evidence of capsular invasion (or poor encapsulation) and may protrude into vessels in the area of the capsule.

  Large 'zellballen' with central degeneration: The nests seen in an alveolar pattern are usually small and compact; larger nests or nodules, when present, suggest malignancy.

  Lack of hyaline globules: The presence of numerous eosinophilic intracytoplasmic globules is very suggestive of benignity; however, globules are not readily apparent in all benign pheochromocytomas. Their absence, therefore, is not definitive evidence of malignancy.

  Dopamine secretion: Tumors that secrete predominantly or exclusively dopamine are more often malignant. This group of tumors is also difficult to diagnose due to lack of typical symptoms of pheochromocytoma.

  Small cells with a high N:C ratio: Malignant tumors have been noted in some studies to be composed predominantly of small cells; however, there is some overlap with benign tumors in this respect.

  Monotony of cytologic pattern: Nuclear pleomorphism is more often a feature of benign tumors; a monotonous cellular pattern is common in malignant pheochromocytomas.

  Spindle cell pattern: While some have reported an association of spindling of tumor cells with malignancy, others note a predominantly spindle cell pattern in rare clinically benign tumors. The presence of spindle cells should be evaluated in conjunction with other criteria of malignancy.

(Figs 13.60–13.65)

Differential diagnosis

- Adrenal cortical adenoma.
- Adrenal cortical carcinoma.
- Metastatic carcinoma, particularly renal cell carcinoma.
- Metastatic neuroendocrine neoplasms, including pancreatic islet cell tumors, thyroid medullary

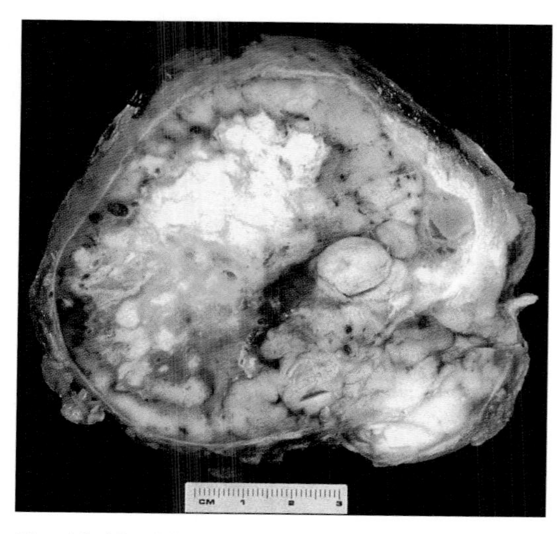

Fig. 13.60 This pheochromocytoma demonstrates the gross nodular pattern that is helpful in distinguishing between benign and malignant sympathoadrenal paragangliomas; histologic confirmation is needed.

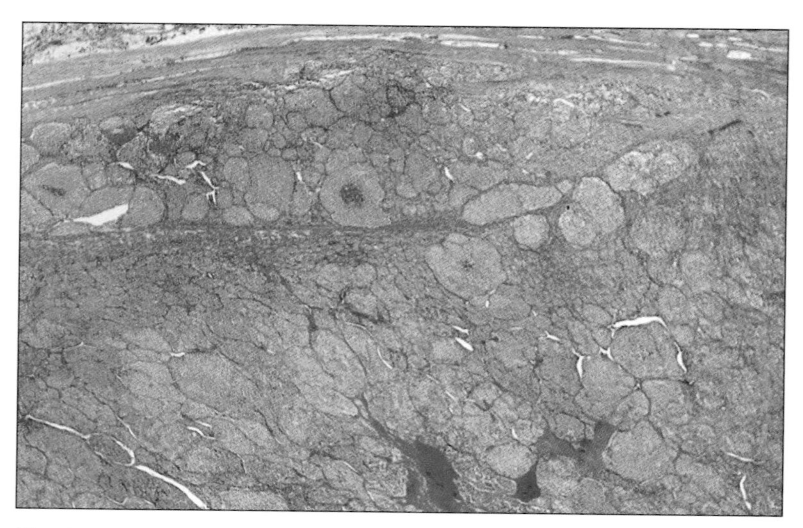

Fig. 13.61 Malignant pheochromocytoma with large, irregularly sized cell nests ('zellballen').

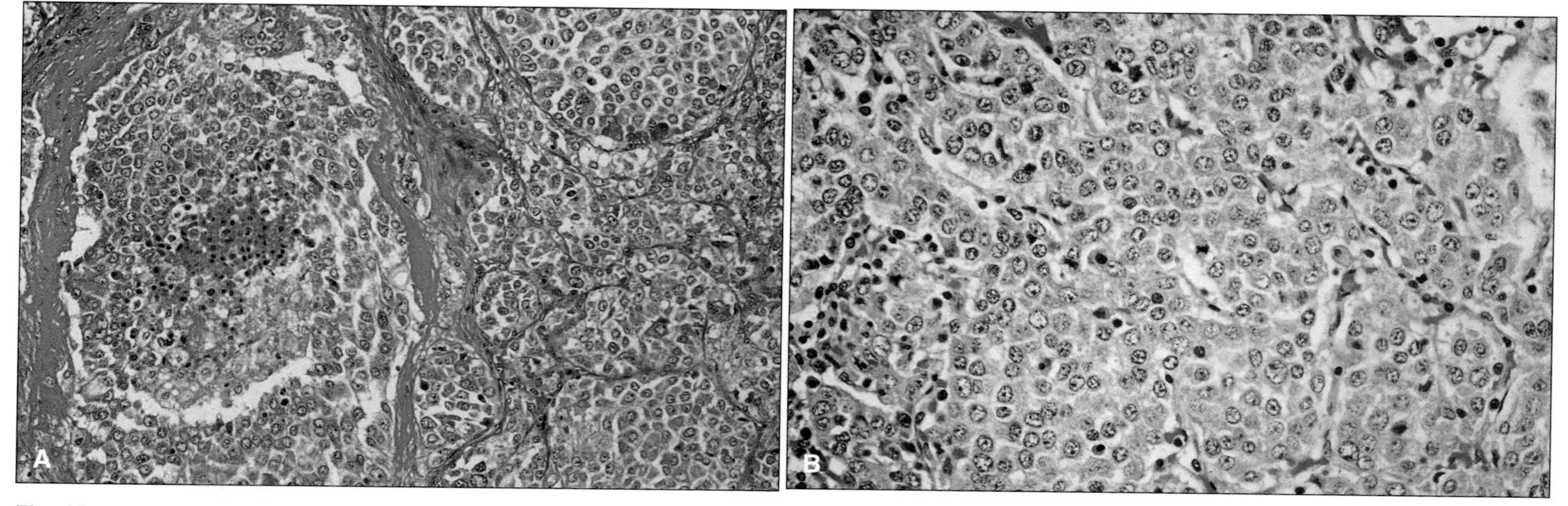

Fig. 13.62 Malignant pheochromocytoma: (A) large cell nests with central necrosis; (B) mitotic rate is very high in this lesion.

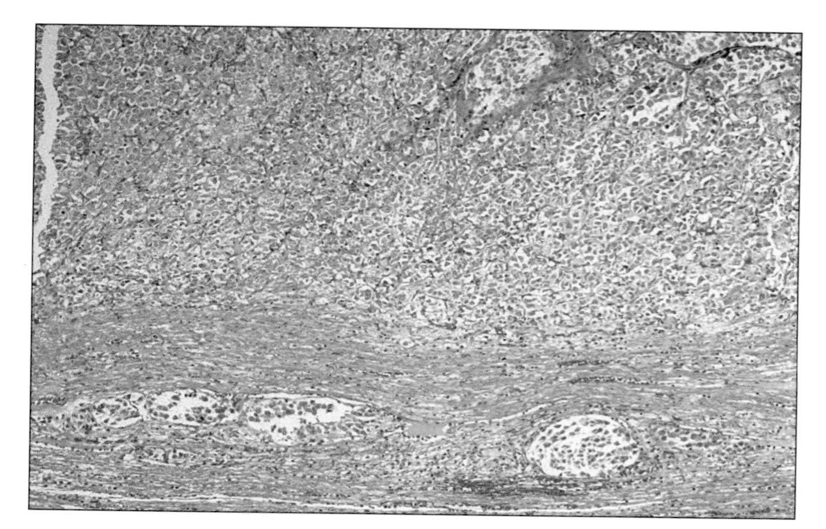

Fig. 13.63 Malignant pheochromocytoma with extensive regional vascular invasion. This patient developed regional lymph node metastases several months after resection of the adrenal tumor.

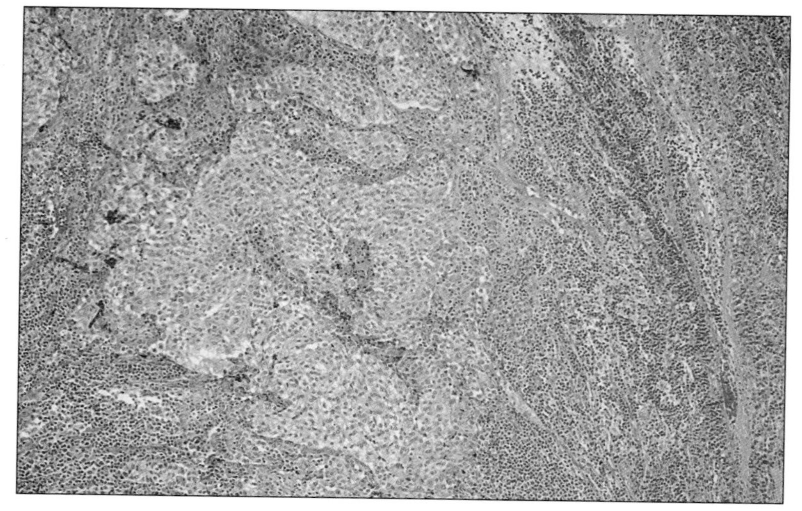

Fig. 13.64 Periaortic lymph node with metastatic malignant pheochromocytoma. Metastatic disease is the ultimate proof of malignancy in pheochromocytoma. Some pheochromocytomas with a benign histologic appearance metastasize, supporting the unpredictable reputation of these neoplasms.

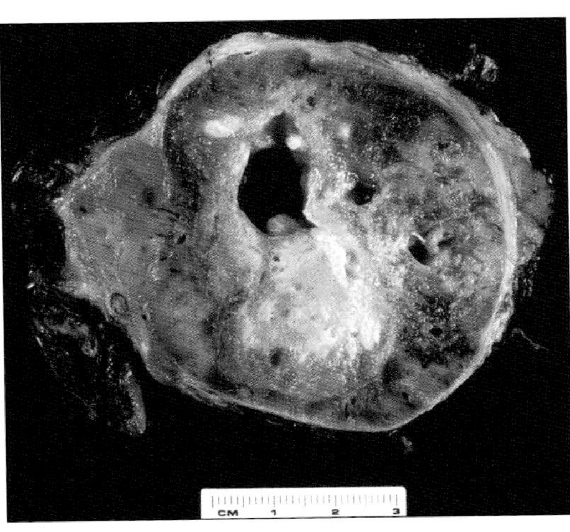

Fig. 13.65 Malignant pheochromocytoma metastatic to the lung.

carcinoma, and gastrointestinal and pulmonary carcinoid tumors.
- Alveolar soft part sarcoma.

Treatment and prognosis

- Preoperative management of hypertension is essential, and has contributed to a dramatic decrease in operative mortality.
- Surgical resection is the treatment of choice – adrenalectomy or, for extra-adrenal tumors, resection of the lesion. The possibility of multiple lesions or metastatic disease requires intraoperative evaluation of both adrenal glands, as well as the paracaval and para-aortic areas and regional lymph nodes.
- Because a diagnosis of malignancy may rely upon subsequent clinical behavior in the absence of definitive histologic evidence, close follow-up of patients with pheochromocytomas is needed.
- Treatment for malignant pheochromocytomas depends on extent of disease. Locally aggressive tumors with invasion of adjacent tissues or regional lymph node metastases may be adequately treated by radical surgery. If resection is incomplete or if distant metastases are present, radiation therapy and chemotherapy have been utilized; however, the limited number of cases makes results difficult to interpret.
- The 5-year survival rate of patients with malignant pheochromocytoma is reported as 43%, with approximately half of the patients dead after a rapidly progressive course, while the remainder may survive for many years with more indolent disease.
- Follow-up of serum and urinary catecholamines and their metabolites is an extremely useful method of monitoring patients for recurrent disease.
- Recurrent elevation of catecholamines in children or in patients with familial history of pheochromocytoma may indicate development of multifocal lesions rather than metastatic or recurrent disease.
- Other conditions that may manifest the clinical signs and symptoms of pheochromocytoma include coarctation of the abdominal aorta, adrenal myelolipoma, renal cysts, and acute mercury poisoning. 'Pseudopheochromocytoma' has been used to describe this clinical situation. Rare patients appear to have a hyperactive adrenergic system. Psychologic disorders must also be considered in the clinical differential of pheochromocytoma.

NEUROBLASTOMA AND GANGLIONEUROBLASTOMA[146–170]

Definition

Neuroblastoma and ganglioneuroblastoma are malignant neoplasms derived from the undifferentiated cells of the sympathetic nervous system. These lesions represent a spectrum from the primitive neuroblastoma to tumors in which differentiation into ganglion cells and schwannian stroma may be focal or nearly complete (ganglioneuroblastomas). The distinction between neuroblastoma and ganglioneuroblastoma has not been well defined. Clinically, the term 'neuroblastoma' is utilized in therapeutic protocols and staging to refer to the spectrum of pathologic entities that encompass neuroblastoma and ganglioneuroblastoma. A combination of histopathologic, molecular genetic, and clinical features separate the lesions into prognostic groups that sometimes overlap strict histologic nomenclature.

Clinical

- Neuroblastoma/ganglioneuroblastoma is the most common adrenal neoplasm in children, and represents the fourth most common malignant tumor in children. The incidence of neuroblastoma is 8.7 per million and the incidence of ganglioneuroblastoma is around 1.8 per million. The detection rate for neuroblastoma/ganglioneuroblastoma in infants is higher in Japan due to a mass screening program.
- There is no gender predilection, but the tumors are slightly less common in the black population.
- Familial cases are rare but do occur; also rare are the associations with von Recklinghausen's disease, Beckwith–Wiedemann syndrome, and Hirschsprung's disease.
- Approximately 85% of cases are diagnosed before 5 years of age; however, rare cases are reported in adults over a wide age range.
- Slightly over half of cases are intra-abdominal, with 36–38% arising in the adrenal; other sites include the

thorax (14–20%), neck (3.4–5%), pelvis (3.4–5%), and head (2%), but these tumors may occur in any location along the sympathetic chain or in the adrenal medulla.

- The most common presentation is an abdominal mass; however, paraspinal neuroblastomas, particularly those with a 'dumbell' configuration that extend through a vertebral foramen, may cause loss of neurologic function due to spinal cord impingement. Neuroblastomas and ganglioneuroblastomas may cause other 'location-dependent' symptoms related to their size. Children with metastatic disease at presentation may manifest more generalized symptoms and findings, such as fever, weight loss, irritability, bone pain, proptosis and periorbital ecchymosis due to orbital involvement, cutaneous metastatic nodules ('blueberry muffin baby'), anemia, or thrombocytopenia.
- A number of paraneoplastic phenomena may be seen, including hypertension out of proportion to measured catecholamine levels (in as many as 20% of patients), watery diarrhea syndrome due to vasoactive intestinal polypeptide, opsoclonus–myoclonus ('dancing eyes, dancing feet'), ectopic ACTH syndrome, Horner's syndrome, and heterochromia iridis. Opsoclonus–myoclonus is thought to be a paraneoplastic cerebellar dysfunction, probably autoimmune in origin. Found in approximately 5% of patients, it is associated with a favorable prognosis.
- Although there is much evidence to suggest that neuroblastoma and ganglioneuroblastoma are congenital tumors, rare cases have been reported in adults over a broad age range. The distribution of adult neuroblastoma/ganglioneuroblastoma is similar to that in children. Although adult tumors may pursue a longer course because of slower growth, they appear to be less responsive to chemotherapy than are childhood neuroblastoma/ganglioneuroblastoma. Bone marrow disease in adults is particularly resistant, resulting in difficulty in achieving clinical remissions of disease.
- Mass screening for neuroblastoma in children at age 6 months using a qualitative vanillylmandelic acid spot test has increased the incidence of this tumor in the more favorable age group (less than 1 year); however, the most recent consensus is that mass screening is not efficacious in reducing the population mortality due to neuroblastoma.
- Laboratory evaluation for suspected neuroblastoma includes quantitative urine levels of 3-methoxy-4-hydroxymandelic acid (VMA), a metabolite of norepinephrine, and 3-methoxy-4-hydroxyphenylacetic acid (HVA), a metabolite of dopamine. VMA is elevated in 75% of patients at the time of diagnosis and HVA is elevated in 80%.
- An elevated ratio of VMA to HVA is associated with a more aggressive course, as is the presence of vanillacetic acid (VLA).
- Clinical evaluation of patients with neuroblastoma routinely includes CT scan with contrast or MRI, chest X-ray, and radionuclide bone scan; bone marrow aspirate and biopsy are also essential due to the high incidence of bone marrow metastasis.
- CT and MRI are very useful in the preoperative evaluation of neuroblastoma.
- The tumors usually have well-defined margins that can be very effectively visualized by MRI, providing information on extent of disease (vascular structures and adjacent organs involved and laterality of the neoplasm). Neuroblastomas usually have a relatively uniform intensity, with low-density areas corresponding to necrosis. Calcifications may be seen by CT.
- By MRI, the tumors have a high signal intensity with T2-weighted images, and a low signal intensity with T1-weighted images.

Pathology

Cytology

- Neuroblastic areas of neuroblastoma/ganglio-neuroblastoma yield a monotonous population of small round nuclei with stipled chromatin. Individual cell borders are not distinct; the fibrillar cytoplasm of the cells forms a cobweb-like background.
- Ganglioneuromatous areas yield ganglion cells of variable maturity, some bi- or multi-nucleated. Ganglion cell differentiation is associated with an increase in cytoplasmic volume; elongated cytoplasmic processes may be seen. Fragments of eosinophilic stroma containing scattered spindle cells may be present; however, the cellularity of tumors with a predominance of mature ganglioneuromatous components is generally much lower than the cellular yield of those with abundant neuroblastic areas.

(Figs 13.66–13.68)

Gross

- Usually circumscribed, neuroblastomas and ganglioneuroblastomas may range in size from 5 to 10 cm, but may be larger.
- The appearance is quite variable – for example, a single circumscribed mass or a multinodular lesion may be seen.
- Encapsulation is variably present, and may simply reflect the adrenal investiture.

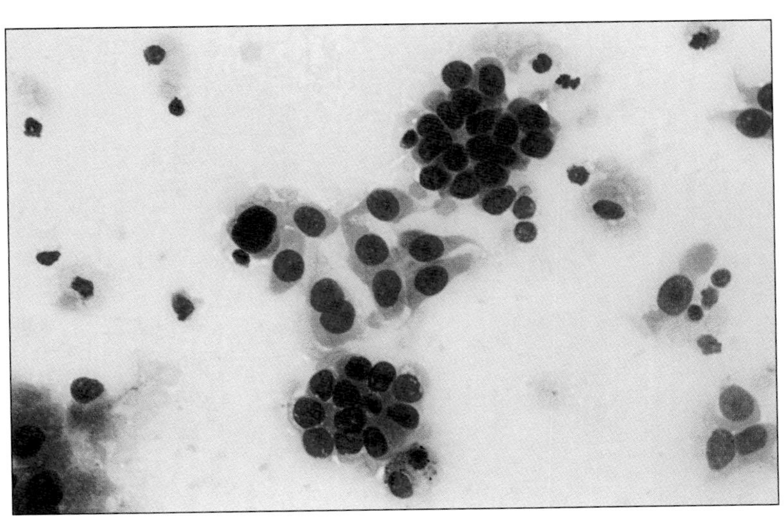

Fig. 13.66 Fine-needle aspiration biopsy of an adrenal neuroblastoma in a 1-year-old child. The small cells resemble those of many other small blue cell tumors of childhood, though the cytoplasmic processes in this example are helpful in suggesting the diagnosis (Diff-Quik).

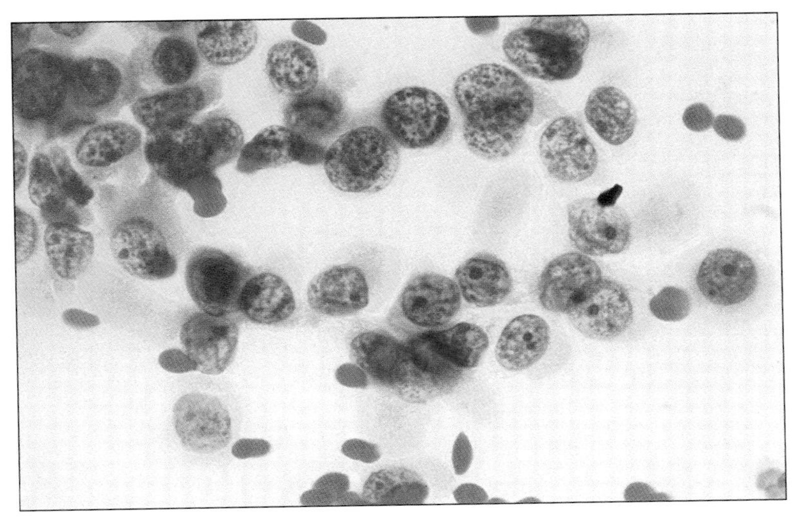

Fig. 13.67 Fine-needle aspiration biopsy of an adrenal neuroblastoma, demonstrating the 'salt-and-pepper' chromatin characteristic of many neuroendocrine tumors (Papanicolaou).

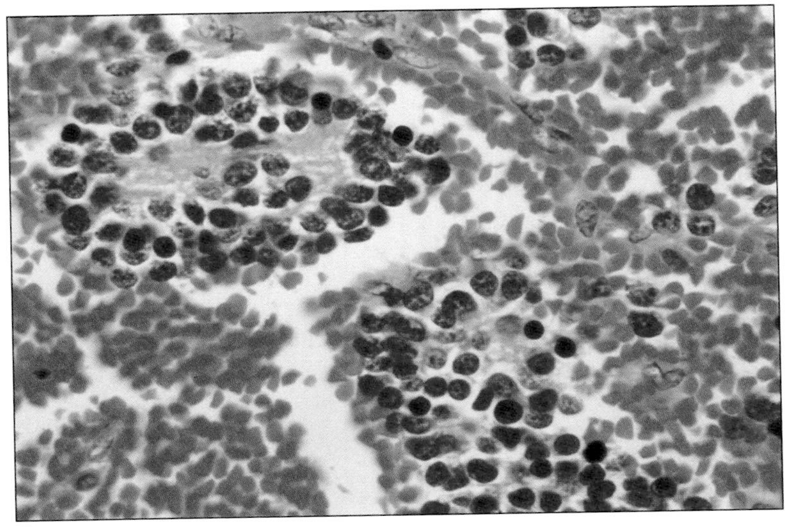

Fig. 13.68 Cell block of a fine-needle aspiration biopsy of an adrenal neuroblastoma. The tumor fragments are characteristic of neuroblastoma, showing the presence of Homer Wright rosettes.

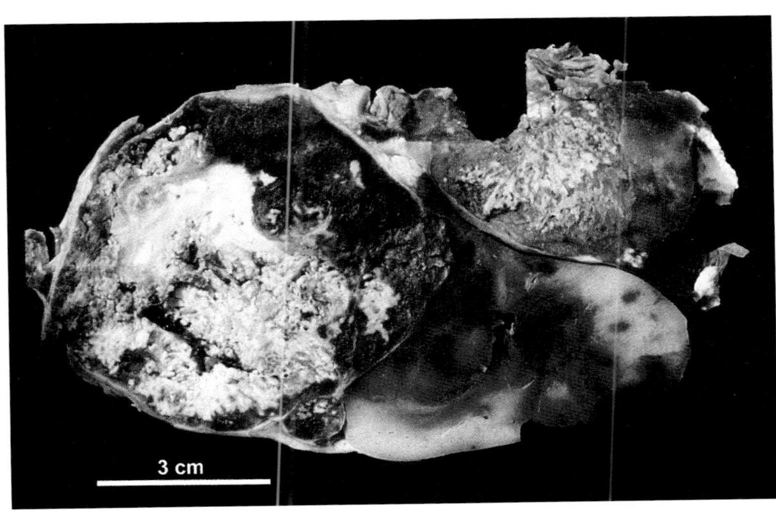

Fig. 13.69 A large adrenal neuroblastoma with the typical variegated appearance with areas of necrosis and hemorrhage. The chalky-appearing flecks represent foci of calcification.

- Since neuroblastoma/ganglioneuroblastoma represent a spectrum of tumors with variable proportions of primitive neuroblastic tissue and maturing stroma-rich ganglioneuromatous areas, the gross appearance may range from extremely soft gray tissue with extensive hemorrhage and necrosis, sometimes with chalky punctate calcifications, to more rubbery yellow–gray neoplasms which are similar to typical ganglioneuromas. An important gross feature is the presence of distinct nodule(s) of neuroblastoma in a tumor otherwise characteristic for ganglioneuroma; this 'nodular stroma-rich' pattern of ganglioneuroblastoma is associated with an unfavorable prognosis.

(Fig. 13.69)

Histology

- The microscopic appearance ranges from pure neuroblastomas to ganglioneuroblastomas in which primitive neuroblastic elements are mixed with maturing ganglion cells and schwannian stroma.
- *Neuroblastoma* is characterized by small, round nuclei with stippled (salt-and-pepper) chromatin, indistinct nucleoli, and cell borders that are not discernible. The cellular proliferation appears to be embedded in a mesh-like eosinophilic (neuro)fibrillary matrix. The nuclei may be randomly distributed in this neurofibrillary matrix or may be arranged in palisades or in rosettes around a center of fibrillary material, forming 'pseudorosettes' (or Homer Wright rosettes).
- *Maturation of ganglioneuroblastoma (differentiation into ganglion and Schwann cells)*: characterized by nuclear enlargement, an increase in eosinophilic cytoplasm with discernible cells borders, and, as maturation progresses, eccentric placement of the nucleus, vesicular chromatin pattern, prominent nucleoli, and

the appearance of granular basophilic Nissl substance in the cytoplasm. In most tumors, ganglionic maturation is associated with the appearance of a schwannian stroma with abundant fasciculated eosinophilic fibrillar material containing scattered spindle cells. The proportion of ganglioneuromatous tissue required to merit classification of a neuroblastic tumor as 'ganglioneuroblastoma' is not uniformly agreed upon; conventional terminology indicates that tumors with more than 5% ganglion cells should be considered ganglioneuroblastoma, while some authorities prefer to reserve the term for tumors in which the preponderant component is ganglioneuromatous tissue (tumors with minor components of ganglionic differentiation would be termed 'differentiating neuroblastoma'). Nomenclature is somewhat superseded by the Shimada age-linked histologic grading system discussed below.

- Neuroblastic and ganglioneuromatous areas may contain aggregates of small lymphocytes that may resemble neuroblasts. The distinction becomes important in ganglioneuromas and more differentiated ganglioneuroblastomas. Leukocyte common antigen immunohistochemistry is helpful in this regard.
- 'In situ neuroblastoma', a term coined to describe a small nodule of neuroblastic cells less than 1 cm in diameter in the adrenal with no other evidence of tumor, is found in 1 per 224 infants at autopsy. The incidence would appear to be greater than that for clinically evident neuroblastoma, suggesting that these lesions regress (involute or mature) spontaneously. All of these lesions have been located within the adrenal gland. The relationship of these lesions to the neuroblastic nodules observed in the normal developing adrenal gland is not clear; neither has their possible role as a precursor to overt neuroblastoma been defined.
- Some neuroblastomas exhibit such prominent cystic change that they may be confused with adrenal cysts or hematomas. These lesions generally fall within the favorable prognostic group using the Shimada age-linked histologic classification (see below).
- Spontaneous regression and maturation are common findings in neuroblastoma/ganglioneuroblastoma, and have been observed clinically and histologically.
- *Immunohistochemistry*: Although not reliable as specific markers of neural differentiation, neuron-specific enolase and synaptophysin are usually positive; Leu-7 and chromogranin are variably positive; broad-spectrum screening panels of 'cocktails' of antibodies against the range of subunits of neurofilament proteins are usually positive. Neuroblastomas are also cytokeratin-negative, and negative or minimally reactive for vimentin. Two antibodies that are reactive in neuroblastoma, though only in frozen sections or flow cytometric material, are HSAN 1.2 (very specific for neuroblastoma) and HLA epitope W6/32.
- *Electron microscopy*: Dense-core granules are most readily identified; neural tubules, neurofilaments, and neural processes may be seen, more abundantly in more differentiated tumors.
- *Molecular genetics*: N-*myc* oncogene amplification is associated with likelihood of disease progression. Amplification is rare in stages I and II, but is found in approximately half of cases of stages III and IV neuroblastoma. Amplification of N-*myc* is not usually seen in stage IV-S neuroblastoma or in patients with opsoclonus–myoclonus, two settings associated with a very favorable prognosis. Proto-oncogenes *ras*, *ret*, and c-*src* have been linked with neuroblastoma, too; however, the prognostic implications are not as strong as with N-*myc*. The N-*myc* oncogene in neuroblastoma is translocated from its normal position on chromosome 2 to 1p.
- *Flow cytometric DNA analysis*: Aneuploidy and a low percentage of cells in the S, G2, and M phases of the cell cycle are associated with a favorable prognosis and correlate with favorable histologic patterns and stages.

Histologic grading

Several histologic grading systems have been developed for neuroblastoma/ganglioneuroblastoma. The currently most widely used system was developed by Shimada and includes the following.

Stroma-rich tumors

With abundant schwannian stroma, these tumors encompass the spectrum of ganglioneuroblastomas. Three subgroups include:

- *Well differentiated*: lacks gross nodules of neuroblastic cells; largely ganglioneuromatous, with only occasional scattered groups of primitive neuroblasts that do not form microscopic nodules that disrupt the stroma; favorable histology – 100% survival.
- *Intermixed*: lacks gross nodules of neuroblastic cells; however, there are microscopic aggregates of primitive neuroblasts displacing the stroma; favorable histology – 92% survival.
- *Nodular*: grossly visible nodules distinguish between the primitive neuroblastic and mature ganglioneuromatous components of the neoplasm; unfavorable histology – 18% survival.

Stroma-poor tumors

Grade based on age at diagnosis, correlated with mitosis–karyorrhexis index (MKI), and quantity of differentiating elements (undifferentiated: <5% of neuroblasts with ganglionic maturation).

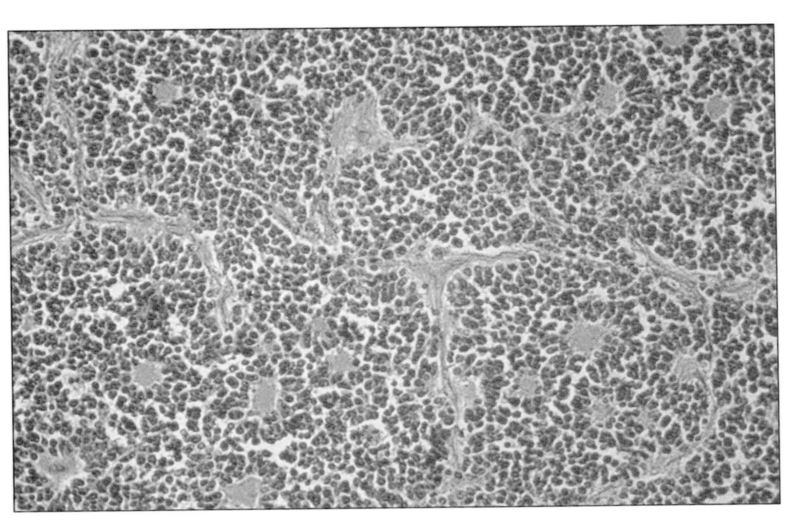

Fig. 13.70 The classic pattern of neuroblastoma, with well-developed Homer Wright rosettes in a background of small cells with a very high nuclear:cytoplasmic ratio.

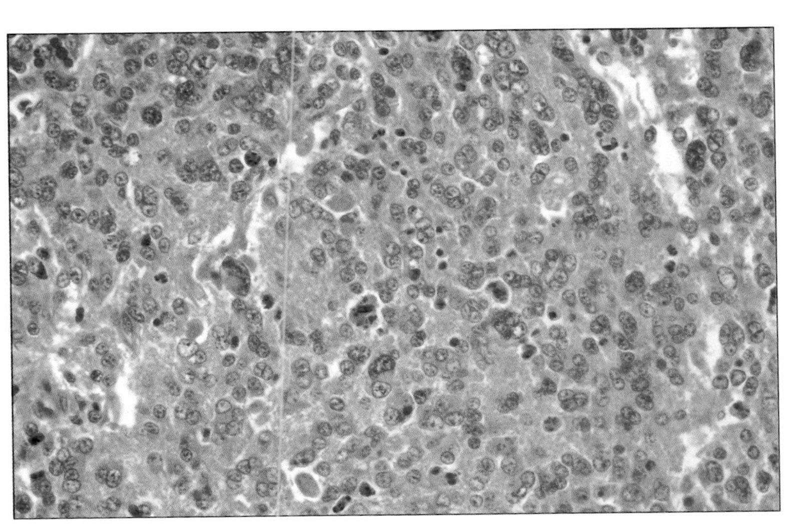

Fig. 13.72 Neuroblastoma with areas of more prominent stroma and neuronal differentiation. Other areas of this neoplasm had higher cellularity with little fibrillar stroma.

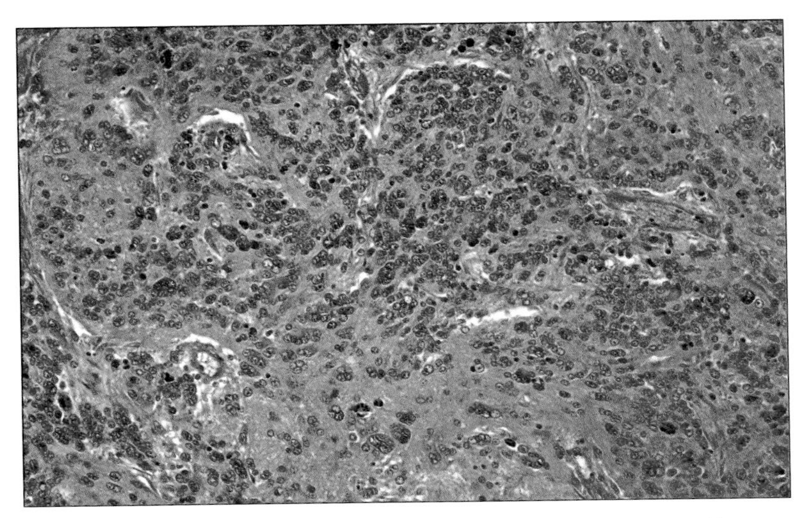

Fig. 13.71 The Homer Wright rosette of neuroblastoma formed by a cluster of tumor cells arranged around a central core of neurofibrillary material.

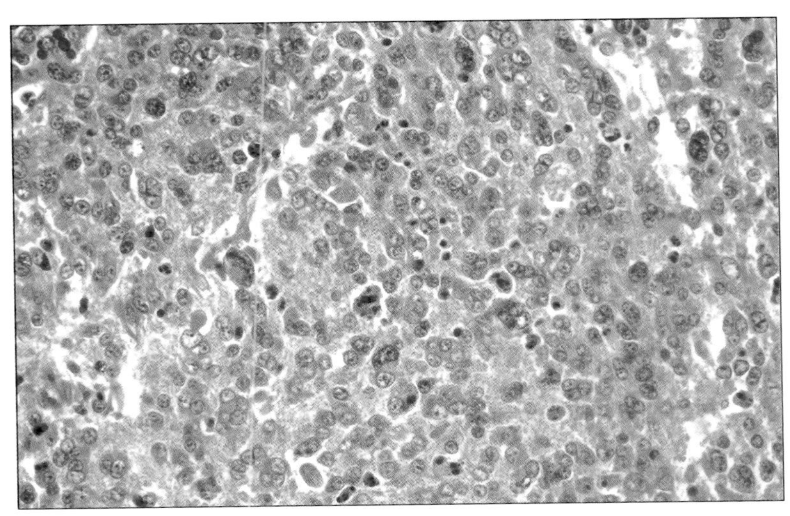

Fig. 13.73 Neuronal differentiation in neuroblastoma is characterized by nuclear enlargement with a more vesicular chromatin pattern and a more prominent nucleolus. The eosinophilic cytoplasm becomes more obvious and cell borders are visible. Karyorrhexis is present.

- *Favorable prognosis groups* (84% survival):
  <1.5 years old with MKI <200;
  1.5–4 years old, differentiating tumor, with MKI <100.
- *Unfavorable prognosis groups* (4.5% survival):
  <1.5 years old with MKI >200;
  1.5–4 years old, differentiating tumor, with MKI >100;
  >1.5 years old with undifferentiated tumor;
  >5 years old.

(Figs 13.70–13.78)

Differential diagnosis

- Pheochromocytoma.
- Neuroblastoma (Wilms' tumor).
- Lymphoma/leukemia.
- Rhabdomyosarcoma.

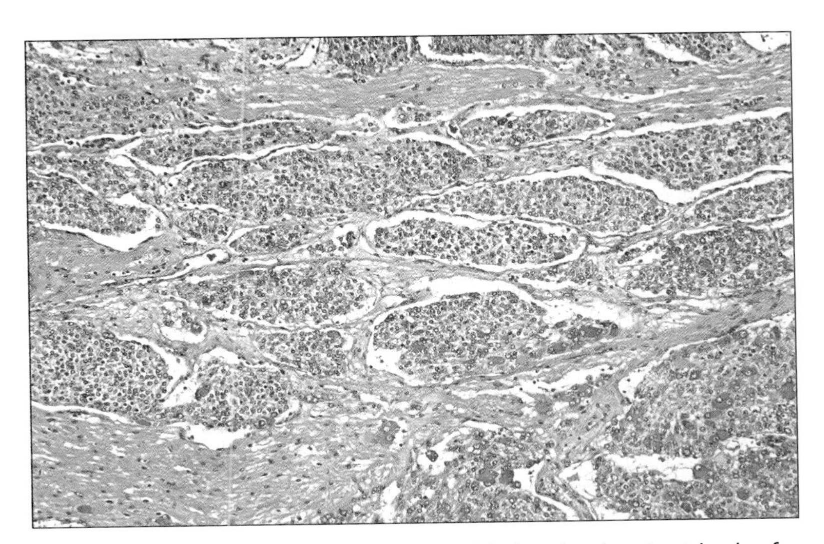

Fig.13.74 Ganglioneuroblastoma in an adult female, showing islands of neuroblasts scattered among differentiated ganglioneuromatous areas.

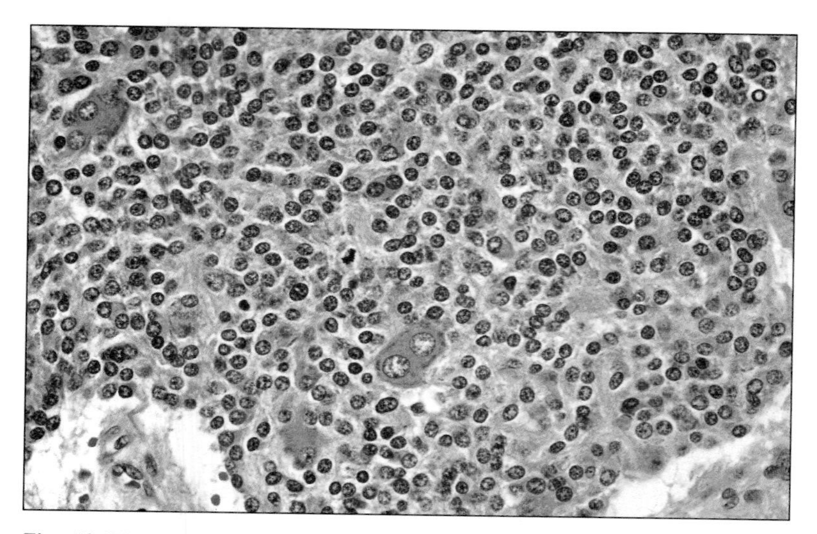

Fig. 13.75 Neuroblastic areas in the ganglioneuroblastoma, showing cells with distinct neuronal differentiation.

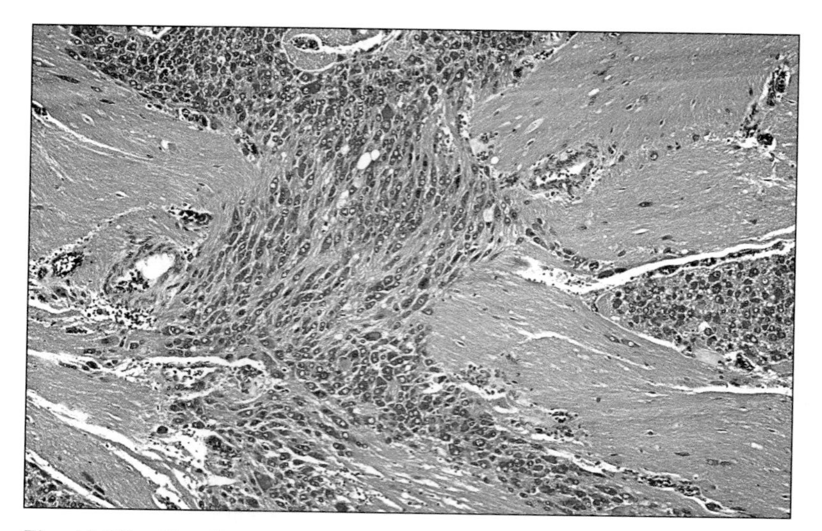

Fig. 13.76 Ganglioneuromatous areas with bands of schwannian stroma admixed with ganglion cells in various stages of maturation.

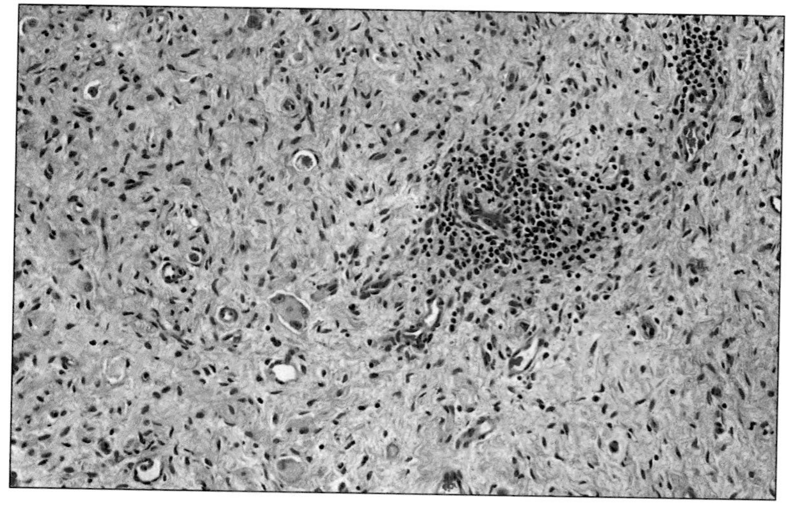

Fig. 13.77 A paraspinous ganglioneuroblastoma in a 1-year-old child, predominantly composed of a ganglioneuromatous pattern comprised of aggregates of small lymphocytes, which should not be confused with neuroblasts.

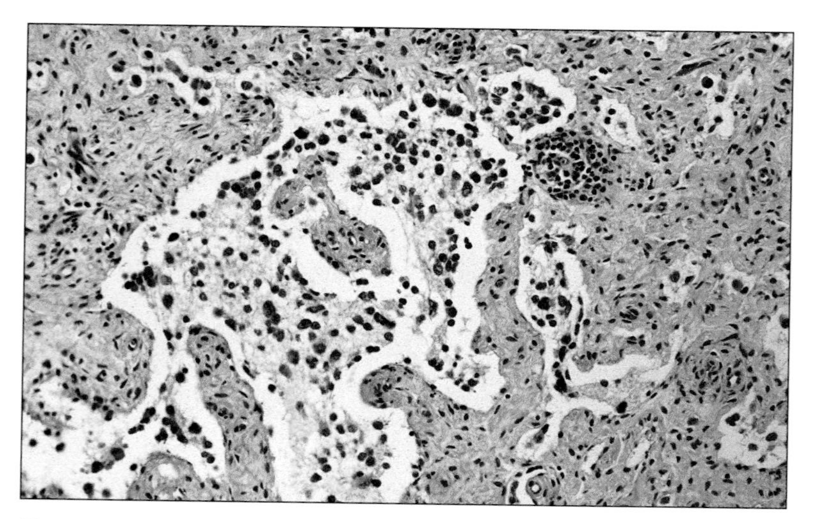

Fig. 13.78 Ganglioneuroblastoma containing rare microscopic islands of neuroblastic cells with fibrillar stroma.

- Ewing's sarcoma (ES; see below).
- Primitive neuroectodermal tumor (PNET; see below).

PNET and ES are two small cell malignant neoplasms with evidence of neuroectodermal differentiation that may be difficult to distinguish from classic neuroblastoma histologically. Particularly PNET, which by definition contains at least occasional Homer Wright rosettes, may pose difficulties in the differential diagnosis. Immunohistochemistry may be quite helpful. Although PNET, like neuroblastoma, expresses neuron-specific enolase, neurofilament proteins, and S-100, PNET also expresses vimentin, HNK-1, HBA-71, and sometimes cytokeratin, unlike neuroblastoma. ES is also positive for HBA-71 and vimentin, but does not express neurofilaments or S-100; it is variably positive for neuron-specific enolase. Most cases of PNET and ES are associated with the genetic translocation t(11; 22)(q24; q12), which has not been found in neuroblastoma.

Treatment and prognosis

- Several systems for staging have been utilized. The Evans Staging System and a recent modification, the International Staging System (Table 13.11), are frequently utilized in the United States.
- Surgery alone may be adequate therapy for stages I and IIa; the addition of chemotherapy and/or radiation is required in higher-stage disease.
- Approximately 65% of patients have disseminated disease at the time of diagnosis; 60% of those are classified as stage IV; 5% are considered stage IV-S, which has a very favorable prognosis in spite of dissemination (Table 13.12).
- Stage IV-S patients are usually infants, with a median age of 3 months. Although most have an adrenal primary, some have no identifiable primary tumor. If an adrenal primary tumor is present, it must be no

Table 13.11 International staging system for neuroblastoma and ganglioneuroblastoma

Stage I	Localized tumor confined to the area of origin; complete gross excision, with or without microsopic residual disease; identifiable ipsilateral and contralateral lymph nodes negative microscopically
Stage IIa	Unilateral tumor with incomplete gross excision; identifiable ipsilateral and contralateral lymph nodes negative microscopically
Stage IIb	Unilateral tumor with complete or incomplete gross excision; with positive ipsilateral regional lymph nodes; identifiable contralateral lymph nodes negative microscopically
Stage III	Tumor infiltrating across the midline with or without regional lymph node involvement; or, unilateral tumor with contralateral regional lymph node involvement; or, midline tumor with bilateral regional lymph node involvement
Stage IV	Dissemination of tumor to distant lymph nodes, bone, bone marrow, liver, and/or other organs (exclusive of cases defined as stage IV-S)
Stage IV-S	Localized primary tumor as defined for stages I or II with dissemination limited to the liver, skin, and/or bone marrow

After Brodeur et al.[148]

Table 13.12 Neuroblastoma and ganglioneuroblastoma: clinical and laboratory prognostic factors

	Favorable	*Unfavorable*
Age at diagnosis	<1 year	>1 year
Stage	I, II, IV-S	III, IV
Location	Thoracic	
Symptoms/signs	Opsoclonus–myoclonus	
Serum ferritin		>142 ng/ml
Serum neuron-specific enolase		>100 ng/ml
Urinary catecholamines	Elevated VMA/ HVA	Low VMA/HVA; + VLA
N-*myc* amplification	1 diploid copy	>3 copies
Quantitative DNA analysis	Hyperdiploid or aneuploid	Diploid (linked to N-*myc* amplification)

VMA, vanillylmandelic acid; HVA, homovanillic acid; VLA, vanillacetic acid.

higher than stage II. These patients commonly have massive hepatomegaly secondary to metastases. Bone marrow involvement (true bone metastases place the patient in stage IV), cutaneous metastatic nodules, and regional lymph node metastases are frequently present as well. The cutaneous nodules are often blue–purple, earning the clinical appellation 'blueberry muffin baby'. Infants less than 1 year of age with stage IV-S neuroblastoma/ganglioneuroblastoma are typically long-term survivors. Because of the frequency of spontaneous regression in children under 1 year old, surgical resection is often the sole initial treatment modality; chemotherapy and radiation may be withheld if there is no evidence of disease progression. The prognosis is poor in children over 1 year of age.

- The most effective drugs in the treatment of neuroblastoma/ganglioneuroblastoma are cyclophosphamide, cisplatin, doxorubicin, teniposide, vincristine, Peptichemio, and melphalan.
- High-dose chemotherapy with or without radiation, followed by allogeneic or autologous bone marrow transplantation, and immunotherapy are areas of research interest in stage IV neuroblastoma/ganglioneuroblastoma.
- Long-term survival is affected by several clinical, histologic, and genetic factors; however, overall long-term survival by stage of disease is a useful parameter: stage I, >90%; stage II, 70–80%; stage III, 25%. Survival of stage IV patients is exquisitely age-sensitive: >60% if <1 year old at diagnosis; 20% if between 1 and 2 years old at diagnosis; and 10% if greater than 2 years old at diagnosis. Survival of stage IV-S patients is >80% (most of these patients are less than 1 year old).

GANGLIONEUROMA[158,171–177]

Definition

Ganglioneuroma is a benign neoplasm composed of mature sympathetic ganglion cells and neurites (with variable myelination), with Schwann cells and collagen. These lesions represent the mature end of the histologic spectrum from neuroblastoma to ganglioneuroblastoma to ganglioneuroma.

Clinical

- Ganglioneuromas are uncommon neoplasms, occurring in an older age group than neuroblastomas or ganglioneuroblastomas.
- Most are diagnosed in patients in the first three decades of life, though they occur over a broad age range; adrenal ganglioneuromas are more common in the third through fifth decades.
- They tend to predilect to females.
- Ganglioneuromas are associated with the sympathetic nervous system, occurring along the length of the sympathetic chains, often paravertebral, and in association with related structures. They are found in the posterior mediastinum > retroperitoneum> adrenal gland (30%) > pelvic cavity > neck > parapharyngeal area. Unusual reported locations include the gastrointestinal tract, kidney, skin, uterus, ovary, orbit, and upper respiratory tract mucosa.
- Adrenal ganglioneuromas are usually smaller than those found in the mediastinum or retroperitoneum, and are usually asymptomatic; occasional patients express complaints of vague abdominal or flank pain. The larger masses of the mediastinum or retroperitoneum more often present with symptoms related to compression of adjacent structures. Rarely, hypertension, watery diarrhea syndrome (with elevated vasoactive intestinal peptide), virilization, or

myasthenia gravis has been reported. Occasional patients have elevation of urinary catecholamines.
- Rare examples of virilizing ganglioneuromas have been reported. The presence of Leydig cells with crystalloids of Reinke may rarely occur, suggesting that cells of the adrenal gland may transform into gonadal stromal cells. More commonly, virilization is associated with adrenal cortical neoplasms.
- Ganglioneuromas are often incidentally discovered during routine radiographic studies; calcifications present in 41% of tumors may be seen on plain X-ray films.

Pathology

Cytology

- Limited material may be obtained due to the preponderance of stroma with collagen and Schwann cells.
- Ganglion cells of variable size, and somewhat dysmorphic, are usually present in a few scattered groups. They may be bi- or multi-nucleated.
- Surrounding the ganglion cells is an eosinophilic fibrillar matrix containing spindled nuclei with somewhat corrugated nuclear contour. Collagen bundles are scattered through the matrix.
- FNA of these lesions is somewhat tenuous, since small immature neuroblastic areas may be missed in sampling.

Gross

- Usually circumscribed, ganglioneuromas often appear to be encapsulated, particularly the extra-adrenal examples; however, they usually are surrounded by a fibrous pseudocapsule rather than a true capsule.
- The average size for all ganglioneuromas is 8 cm; however, adrenal tumors tend to be smaller than mediastinal and retroperitoneal tumors, which may become very large.
- The light gray to tan cut surface is rubbery to gelatinous; it may be homogeneous, fasciculated, or whorled.
- Degenerative alterations, often with cyst formation, hemorrhage, or myxoid change, may occur, particularly in larger tumors.
- Close attention to the gross features is extremely important. Note should be made of grossly distinctive areas or nodules of different color or texture, particularly if they appear darker or purplish, or if they are hemorrhagic. Such areas should be sampled to exclude neuroblastic foci, as stroma-rich ganglioneuroblastomas may be grossly quite similar to ganglioneuroma.

(Fig. 13.79)

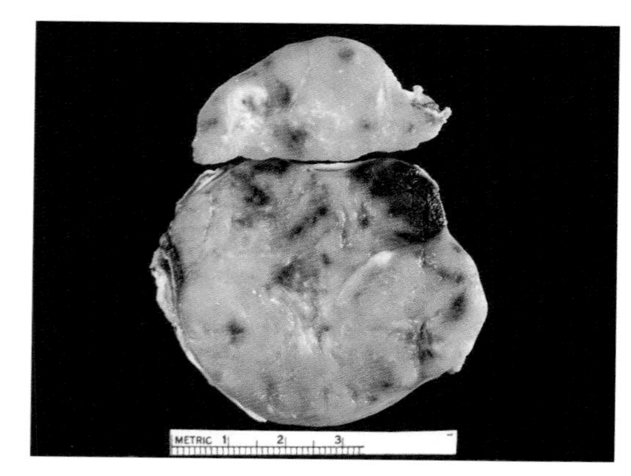

Fig. 13.79 Ganglioneuroma with typical gray and fairly homogeneous cut surface. The texture was rubbery, which contrasts to the soft texture of a neuroblastoma, the latter reminiscent of fetal brain tissue.

Histology

- Ganglion cells are present in variable numbers. They are round to polygonal, with eccentrically placed vesicular nuclei and a single prominent nucleolus. Bi- and multi-nucleated forms are often seen, and are helpful in distinguishing between entrapped non-neoplastic ganglion cells in a peripheral nerve sheath tumor and the neoplastic ganglion cells of ganglioneuroma. Nissl substance is often seen in larger ganglion cells; and brown, finely granular 'neuromelanin' may be observed.
- Neuritic processes are readily demonstrated using a silver stain. Myelin may or may not be present.
- The more voluminous component of ganglioneuroma consists of proliferating Schwann cells with spindled nuclei, and a variable quantity of collagen fibers. The Schwann cells and collagen often form interlacing bundles. Ganglion cells are usually distributed in small groups within the schwannian stroma. Individual ganglion cells may be surrounded by a rim of satellite cells.
- Mature adipose tissue may be incorporated into the schwannian stroma at the advancing edge of the tumor. Blunt fingers of tumor may protrude into surrounding tissue from the periphery of a ganglioneuroma.
- *Immunohistochemistry*: Aggregates of mature lymphocytes are commonly found within ganglioneuromas. These must be distinguished from immature neuroblastic cells of a ganglioneuroblastoma. Leukocyte common antigen may be helpful in problem cases. As expected, the ganglion cells express neural markers such as neurofilament proteins, synaptophysin, S-100, and neuron-specific enolase. The schwannian component is also S-100-positive.
- *Electron microscopy*: The bulky stromal component is represented by numerous nerve bundles, which are

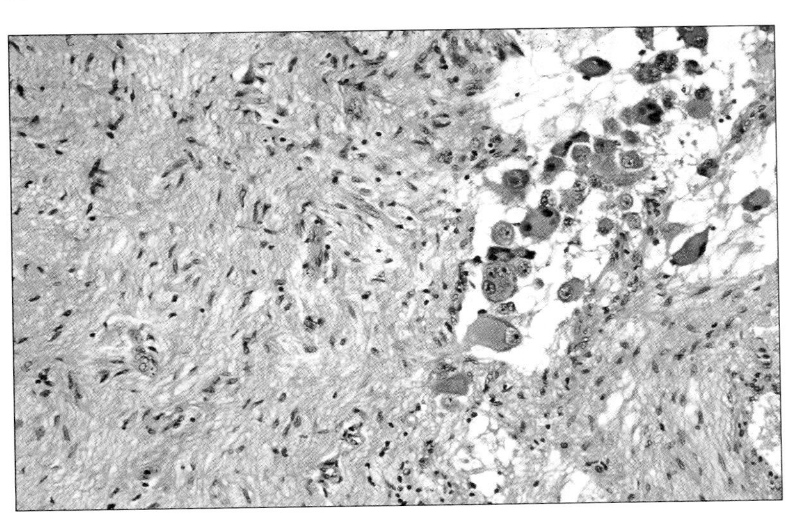

Fig. 13.80 Ganglioneuroma is characterized by well-developed abundant schwannian stroma and patches of ganglion cells, which are often slightly dysmorphic.

largely unmyelinated, and mature Schwann cells, which are completely surrounded by basal lamina. Each Schwann cell is associated with multiple axons. The collagen bundles are not long-spacing collagen.

(Fig. 13.80)

Differential diagnosis

- Ganglioneuroblastoma.
- Neurilemmoma.
- Neurofibroma.

Treatment and prognosis

- Surgical excision is the treatment of choice.
- Ganglioneuromas are benign and slow-growing tumors, though they may become quite large.
- Rare cases of malignant transformation of ganglioneuroma into a neurofibrosarcoma (malignant schwannoma) or malignant peripheral nerve sheath tumor have been reported. In some cases there has been a previous history of radiation or chemotherapy, but others appear to represent spontaneous malignant transformation. Histologic features seen in malignant nerve sheath tumors include increased cellularity, mitotic activity, and tumor necrosis.
- Ganglioneuromas appear to occur either de novo, or as the result of maturation of neuroblastoma or ganglioneuroblastoma. Patients who have been treated for confirmed neuroblastoma may be found to have residual mass lesions, either in the site of the primary or in metastatic sites. In many instances, excision of such lesions has revealed pure mature ganglioneuroma; in other cases, consecutive biopsies have demonstrated a progressive pattern of maturation from neuroblastic neoplasms to ganglioneuroma. A similar maturation sequence may occur spontaneously, without chemotherapy or radiation. Although some support the theory that apparently de novo ganglioneuromas are actually the endpoint of maturation of an unrecognized congenital or childhood neuroblastoma/ganglioneuroblastoma, the differences in anatomic distribution and delay in presentation lend credence to the possibility of two mechanisms of origin for ganglioneuroblastoma.

COMPOSITE TUMOR OF THE ADRENAL MEDULLA[178–185]

Definition

This is a neoplasm in which there are components of pheochromocytoma and neuroblastoma, ganglioneuroblastoma, or ganglioneuroma. The occurrence of 'composite' tumors with both neuronal and neuroendocrine differentiation is logical in light of the neural crest origin of both cell lines.

Clinical

- These neoplasms represent approximately 3% of sympathoadrenal paragangliomas.
- Most occur in the adrenal gland; however, an extra-adrenal location is reported.
- Age and gender distribution are similar to those for pheochromocytoma.
- Rarely, these tumors may be associated with von Recklinghausen's disease or with MEN 2A (Sipple's syndrome).
- Symptoms associated with catecholamine hypersecretion as seen in typical pheochromocytomas are common: hypertension, palpitations, diaphoresis, headaches, etc. A few patients have presented with watery diarrhea syndrome due to secretion of excess vasoactive intestinal peptide (VIP). Symptoms related to the mass effect of the neoplasm may predominate.
- Laboratory evaluation reveals results similar to those in patients with pure pheochromocytoma, except in the instances of VIP excess.

Pathology

Cytology

- Limited sampling may fail to illustrate the biphasic nature of this neoplasm. Since pheochromocytoma is usually the dominant component in needle aspiration of composite tumors, fine-needle aspirates are more likely to yield pheochromocytes.

- The areas of pheochromocytoma are characterized by loose aggregates of polygonal cells with variably granular cytoplasm and poorly defined cell borders. Wispy projections of cytoplasm may be seen. The chromatin is clumped and rather coarse. Anisonucleosis and rare bizarre nuclei may be present; some cells have prominent nucleoli.
- The ganglioneuroma/ganglioneuroblastoma yields elongated spindled nuclei in an eosinophilic and somewhat fibrillar background. Scattered ganglion cells with abundant cytoplasm, vesicular nuclei, and a single prominent nucleolus are present. If an immature neuroblastic component is sampled, groups of small cells with a very high N:C ratio are seen; the chromatin is somewhat stippled but evenly distributed; a fine fibrillar background may be noted. It is important to distinguish between small round lymphocytes, which are often present in ganglioneuromas, and neuroblastic cells.

Gross

- Diameters of up to 15 cm have been reported.
- Usually circumscribed, the gross appearance is dependent upon the relative proportions of pheochromocytoma and neuroblastoma/ganglio-neuroblastoma/ganglioneuroma. The color ranges from gray–white to tan to purple, often with areas of hemorrhage.
- The texture is usually firm to rubbery, but larger areas of immature neuroblastic tumor may be soft, and sometimes necrotic.
- A thin rim of yellow adrenal cortex may be seen at the periphery of the tumor.

Histology

- Composite tumors show areas with any of the variety of patterns typically seen in pheochromocytomas. The pheochromocytoma is usually the predominant component. Occasionally, pheochromocytomas exhibit focal neuronal differentiation.
- Admixed with the areas of pheochromocytoma are histologically distinct areas that may have features of neuroblastoma, ganglioneuroblastoma, or ganglioneuroma, as previously described.
- Transitional areas in which the features of pheochromocytes and ganglionic cells seem to blend may be difficult to categorize.
- *Immunohistochemistry*: Chromogranin staining is strong and diffuse in pheochromocytes; it is absent or weak in the perikarya of ganglion cells, but concentrated in the distal neuronal processes. S-100 is present in a sustentacular cell distribution in the pheochromocytoma component, but is much more abundant in ganglioneuromatous areas with schwannian differentiation. S-100 distribution may also be helpful in differentiating between areas of pheochromocytoma and neuroblastoma: neuroblastoma lacks the sustentacular cell pattern of S-100 staining.

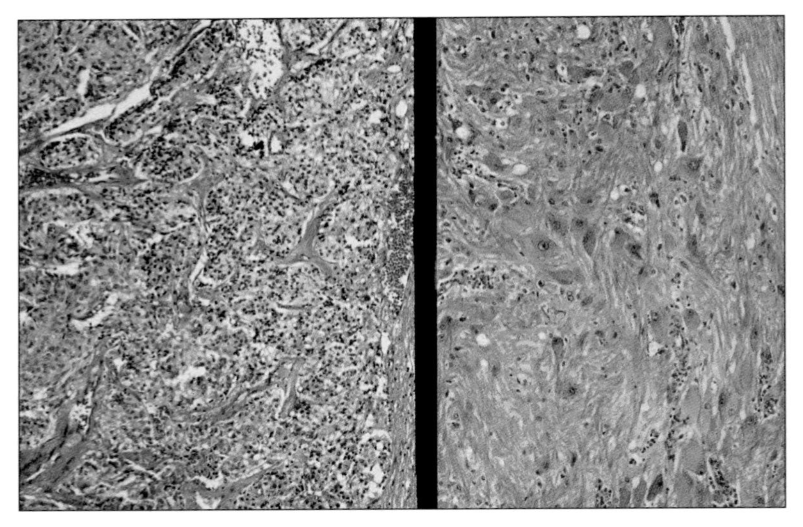

Fig. 13.81 Compound tumor of the adrenal medulla, with pheochromocytoma (left) and ganglioneuroblastoma (right).

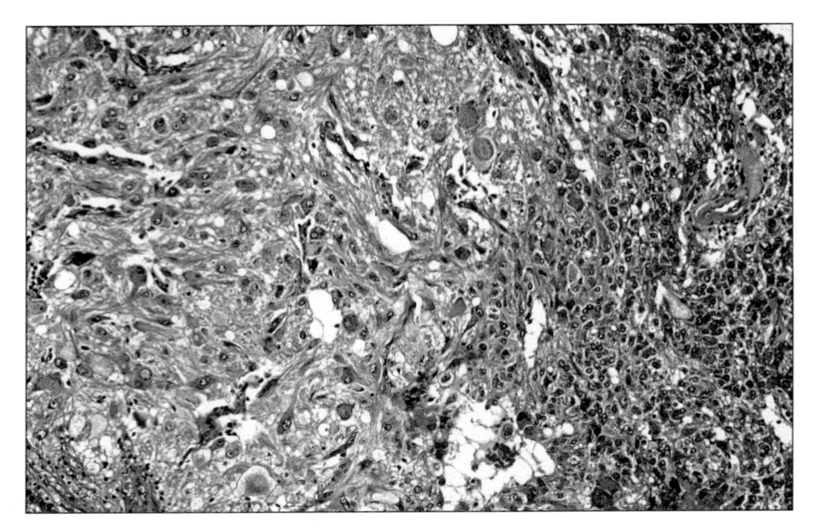

Fig. 13.82 Compound tumor of the adrenal medulla, with areas of pheochromocytoma (left) merging with ganglioneuromatous areas (right).

(Figs 13.81 & 13.82)

Differential diagnosis

- Pheochromocytoma.
- Ganglioneuroblastoma/ganglioneuroma.

Treatment and prognosis

- The clinical course of composite tumors has not been well delineated due to the tumor's rarity. Most have occurred in adults; therefore it is not clear whether the

histologic grading and stage have the same implications as in childhood neuroblastoma/ ganglioneuroblastoma.
- Aggressive behavior with metastasis and poor clinical outcome has been reported in approximately half of the reported cases with a neuroblastic component, including one in which both a malignant pheochromocytomatous and a neuroblastic component metastasized.
- Complete surgical removal is desirable; radiation and chemotherapy have been used with inconclusive results.

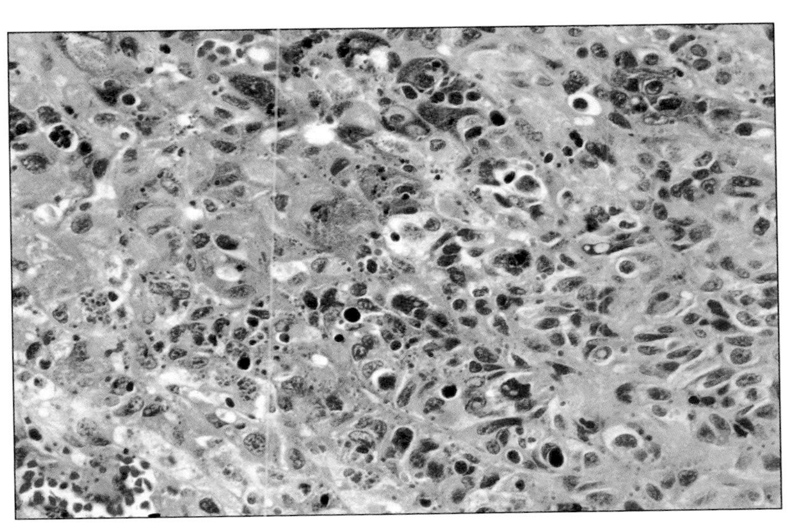

Fig. 13.83 Primary malignant melanoma of the adrenal gland. Pleomorphic epithelioid cell proliferation with prominent nucleoli and nuclear molding are seen. The presence of melanin in this example is very helpful in suggesting the correct diagnosis.

PRIMARY MALIGNANT MELANOMA[186–189]

Definition

This is a malignant neoplasm composed of cells with light microscopic, immunohistochemical, or ultrastructural evidence of melanocytic differentiation. The diagnostic criteria for primary adrenal melanoma require in addition: unilateral adrenal involvement, no current or prior history of suspicious pigmented lesions of the skin, eye, or mucosal surfaces, and absence of extra-adrenal primary melanoma after a thorough search. The origin of primary adrenal melanomas is not clear; however, the common neural crest origin of the adrenal chromaffin cells that populate the medulla and of melanocytes lends credence to the concept of melanoma arising in the adrenal medulla.

Clinical

- The few reported cases have occurred in adults, with no gender predilection.
- Common presenting symptoms include abdominal or flank pain, weight loss, malaise, or a palpable abdominal mass.
- Patients should be studied carefully to exclude other more common sites of primary melanoma, such as the skin, mucous membranes, and eye.
- By CT, ultrasonography, or arteriography, the lesions are hypovascular, and may contain large necrotic or cystic areas.

Pathology

Gross

- The tumor is usually large, measuring up to 17 cm in greatest dimension.
- The cut surface is usually brown to black, and may be partially cystic, hemorrhagic, and necrotic.

Histology

- The tumor cells may vary in size from small and monotonous to large, bizarre cells.
- The presence of a nesting or a biphasic pattern with epithelioid cells alternating with spindle cells may provide helpful clues to the diagnosis.
- Brown to black pigment is usually present, but varies in quantity; a Fontana–Masson stain may help highlight pigment.
- *Immunohistochemistry*: S-100 protein, HMB-45, typosinase, and Melan-A are positive.
- *Electron microscopy*: Premelanosomes in various stages of development are seen.

(Figs 13.83 & 13.84)

Differential diagnosis

- Pigmented adrenal cortical nodules.
- Bilateral pigmented micronodular hyperplasia.
- Pigmented ganglioneuroblastoma.
- Black adenomas of the adrenal cortex.
- Pigmented pheochromocytomas.

Treatment and prognosis

- Resection of tumors localized to the adrenal may be helpful in controlling symptoms.
- The prognosis is very poor, with death due to disseminated disease occurring within a year of diagnosis.

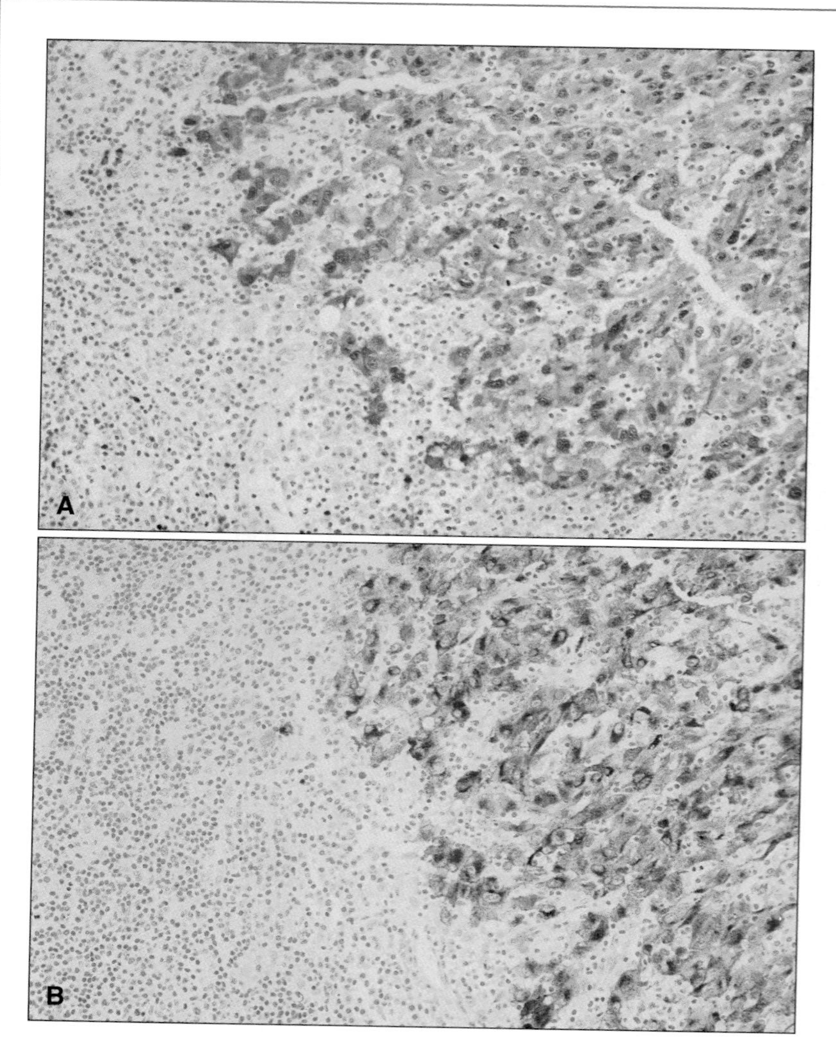

Fig. 13.84 Amelanotic primary malignant melanoma of the adrenal gland. Diagnostic confirmation is achieved by immunohistochemical staining, including diffuse (A) S-100 protein and (B) HMB-45 staining. Other melanocytic cell stains such as Melan-A (A103) and tyrosinase were positive, too.

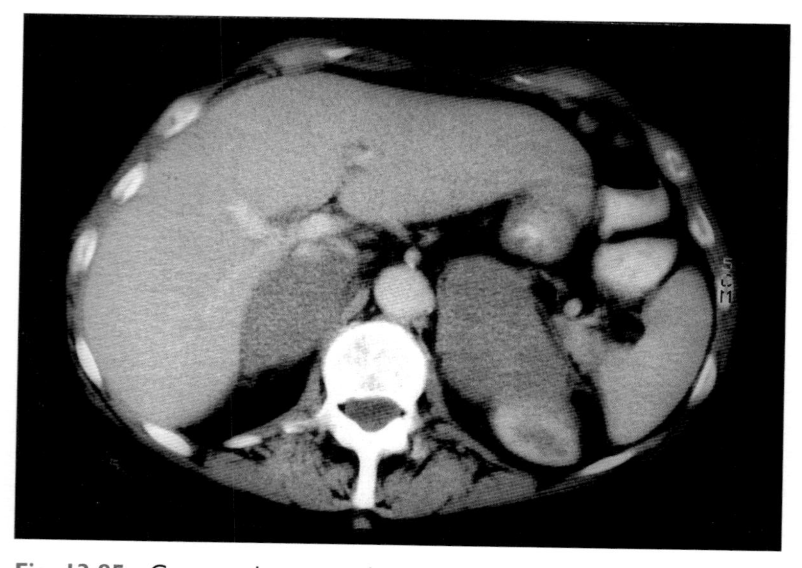

Fig. 13.85 Computed tomographic scan demonstrating bulky suprarenal masses with homogeneous density, representing primary adrenal lymphoma. Bilaterality is a peculiar common attribute of adrenal gland lymphomas.

MISCELLANEOUS NEOPLASMS OF THE ADRENAL GLAND

MALIGNANT LYMPHOMA[190–196]

Definition

This comprises a malignant neoplastic proliferation of any of a variety of lymphoid cell lines. Primary lymphomas of the adrenal are very rare; some of the reported cases must be viewed critically, as it is difficult to exclude secondary involvement of the adrenal by the much more common lymphoma arising in retroperitoneal lymph nodes. The report of pure bilateral adrenal involvement without regional lymph node involvement supports the concept of a true primary adrenal malignant lymphoma.

Clinical

- Primary non-Hodgkin lymphomas of the adrenal gland are reported almost exclusively in adults, in the fifth through ninth decades, with a mean age of 60 years and a 3:1 male-to-female ratio of occurrence.
- Presenting symptoms include abdominal pain, fever, anemia, weight loss, and manifestations of adrenal insufficiency.
- Involvement is bilateral in approximately 50% of cases.
- CT and ultrasonography are useful in localization for percutaneous needle biopsy or FNA, but do not readily exclude adrenal cortical neoplasms or metastases to the adrenal gland.

(Fig. 13.85)

Pathology

Cytology

- FNA provides a useful diagnostic alternative to laparotomy, since resection is not the treatment of choice.
- The presence of a monotonous large cell lymphoid population is the most common finding, and is readily diagnosed as malignant lymphoma.
- Small cell and mixed small and large cell lymphomas may be more difficult to classify based solely on the cytomorphology. Cell suspensions for flow cytometric immunophenotyping or immunohistochemical phenotyping may provide definitive classification if adequate material is obtained.

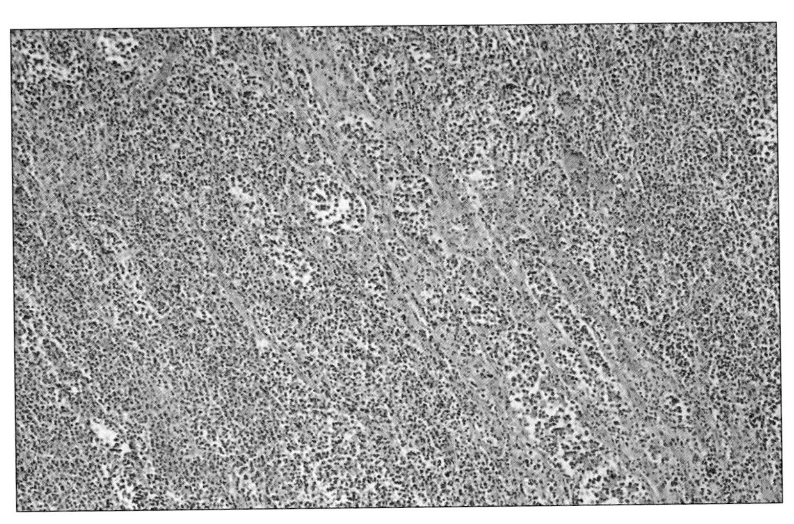

Fig. 13.86 Primary adrenal lymphoma showing diffuse effacement of the adrenal parenchyma.

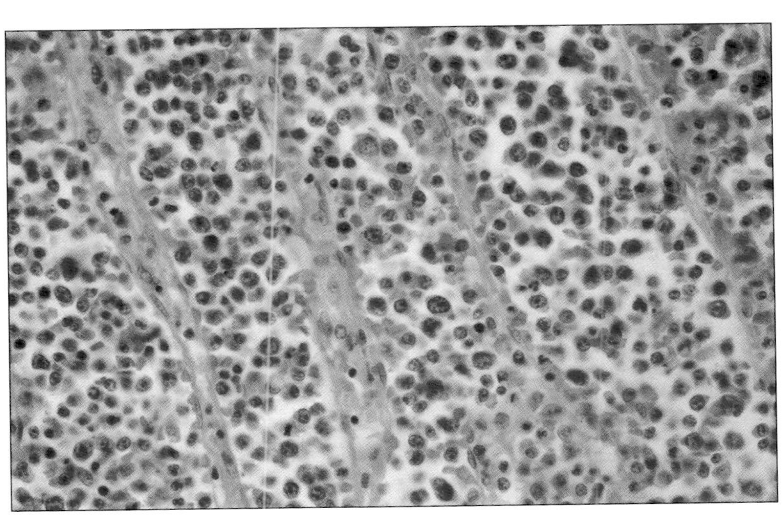

Fig. 13.87 Primary adrenal lymphoma, large cell B-cell type, the most common pattern of primary lymphomas in this location. Immunomarkers were confirmatory of a B-cell type.

Gross

- Adrenal lymphomas are frequently bilateral and range in size from 2 to 17 cm.
- The cut surface is white–gray and fleshy, and may be partially necrotic.
- Extension out of the adrenal gland into surrounding soft tissue in many cases makes difficult the exclusion of a retroperitoneal lymphoma secondarily involving the adrenal.

Histology

- The histologic pattern is dependent on the type of malignant lymphoma present. All cases of primary adrenal lymphoma have been non-Hodgkin lymphoma. Large cell lymphoma is the most common pattern reported in this location.
- The malignant lymphoid cells infiltrate and replace the adrenal medullary and cortical tissue, resulting in adrenal insufficiency in advanced bilateral cases.
- *Immunohistochemistry*: Most adrenal lymphomas are of the B-cell phenotype, and are positive for leukocyte common antigen and B-cell markers (e.g. L26); rarely, T-cell lymphomas may occur, which are positive for T-cell markers (e.g. UCHL-1, CD3).

(Figs 13.86 & 13.87)

Differential diagnosis

- Poorly differentiated adrenal cortical carcinoma.
- Metastatic poorly differentiated carcinoma.
- Malignant melanoma (either primary adrenal or metastatic).
- Malignant pheochromocytoma.

Treatment and prognosis

- Chemotherapeutic regimens and radiation therapy are selected based on the histologic classification of the lymphoma.
- Surgical resection does not improve survival.
- The prognosis of primary adrenal lymphoma is very poor, with death usually within several months of diagnosis despite aggressive therapy.

MYELOLIPOMA[197–200]

Definition

Myelolipoma is a benign tumor-like lesion composed of both mature adipose tissue and hematopoietic elements.

Clinical

- Myelolipoma is most often discovered in the fifth to seventh decades of life.
- There is no gender predilection.
- Its incidence in adults between the ages of 36 and 65 years is 1 in 7600.
- It is most often found in the adrenal, but is also reported in the mediastinum, perirenal/periadrenal region, presacral area, liver, and gastrointestinal tract.
- Most commonly, it is an incidental finding in an asymptomatic patient; however, patients may complain of abdominal or flank pain, or rarely may present with massive retroperitoneal hemorrhage. Other findings include hematuria, hypertension, and hormonal dysfunction.
- Endocrine dysfunction reported in association with myelolipomas includes Cushing's syndrome, Conn's syndrome, Addison's disease, virilization, diabetes

mellitus, and congenital adrenal hyperplasia. Because secondary myelolipomatous foci are common (and may be quite extensive) in many adrenal neoplasms and hyperplastic lesions, an underlying causative lesion other than myelolipoma must be excluded. It is likely that many reports of syndromes such as Cushing's and Conn's syndrome and virilization linked to myelolipomas actually represent myelolipomatous changes overshadowing an underlying cortical adenoma or hyperplastic process.
- The improved resolution and frequency of use of imaging techniques such as CT and MRI have increased the detection rate of myelolipomas, often as incidental findings.
- The radiographic appearance does not distinguish between metastatic lesions and adrenal myelolipomas.
- CT-directed FNA cytology can be very useful in distinguishing between metastases and myelolipoma of the adrenal.
- Although the etiology and nature of myelolipoma is not well defined, they do not appear to represent true neoplasms.
- Theories regarding the presence of myelolipomatous masses in the adrenal, either alone or associated with adrenal cortical proliferations, suggest the following possibilities: metaplastic changes in adrenal stromal cells, metaplastic changes in adrenal cortical cells, bone marrow emboli lodging in the adrenal gland, and embryonic rests of bone marrow in the adrenal gland. Metaplastic change in stromal cells is the favored origin of myelolipomatous proliferations in the adrenal.

Pathology

Cytology
- An admixture of mature adipocytes and hematopoietic cells, including myeloid and erythroid precursors and megakaryocytes, is characteristic of myelolipoma.
- The chief cytologic differential diagnosis in CT-directed FNA of myelolipoma is inadvertent sampling of normal bone marrow from vertebral body or rib.

Gross
- Sizes range from small incidental findings in autopsy or surgical specimens to masses measuring up to 34 cm in diameter.
- Circumscribed, but not usually encapsulated, the border of the myelolipoma often blends with a thin rim of compressed adrenal tissue.
- The cut surface is yellow and fatty, with variably sized patches of mottled red to purple tissue.
- Areas of hemorrhage and infarction are more common in larger examples.

(Figs 13.88 & 13.89)

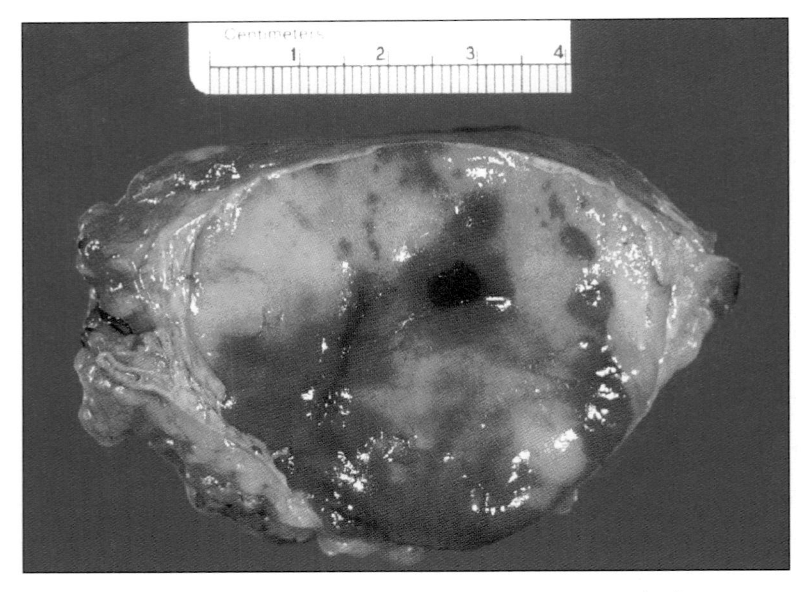

Fig. 13.88 Adrenal myelolipoma appearing as a circumscribed mass surrounded by a thin rim of golden-appearing residual (normal) adrenal cortical tissue. The yellow cut surface resembles adipose tissue; the reddish areas represent foci of hematopoietic elements.

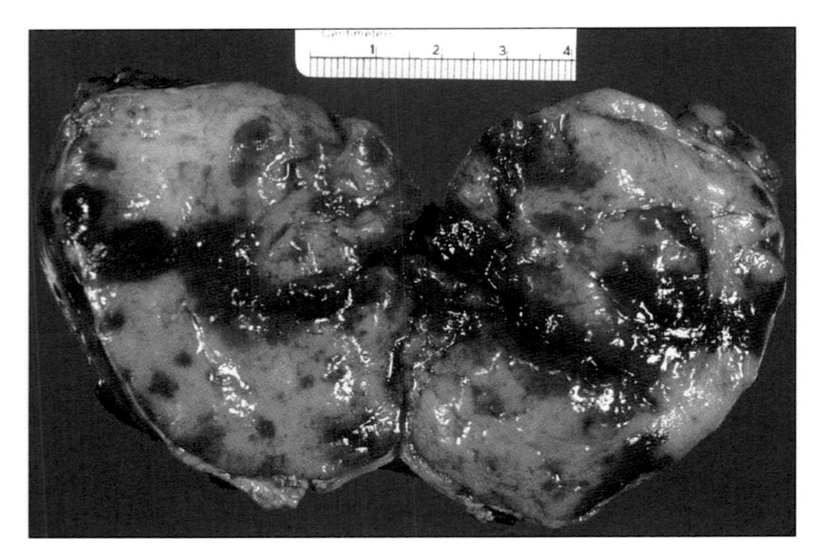

Fig. 13.89 Another example of an adrenal myelolipoma, in which residual (normal) adrenal tissue is not evident. The cut surface of this tumor shows an admixture of yellow-appearnig adipose tissue and reddish areas representing foci of hematopoietic elements.

Histology
- Mature adipocytes are admixed with aggregates of hematopoietic cells representing myeloid, erythroid, and megakaryocytic elements.
- The relative proportions of adipose and hematopoietic tissue vary; the marrow elements may be inconspicuous in some cases.
- Metaplastic bone or areas of fibrosis or hyalinization may be present.

(Fig. 13.90)

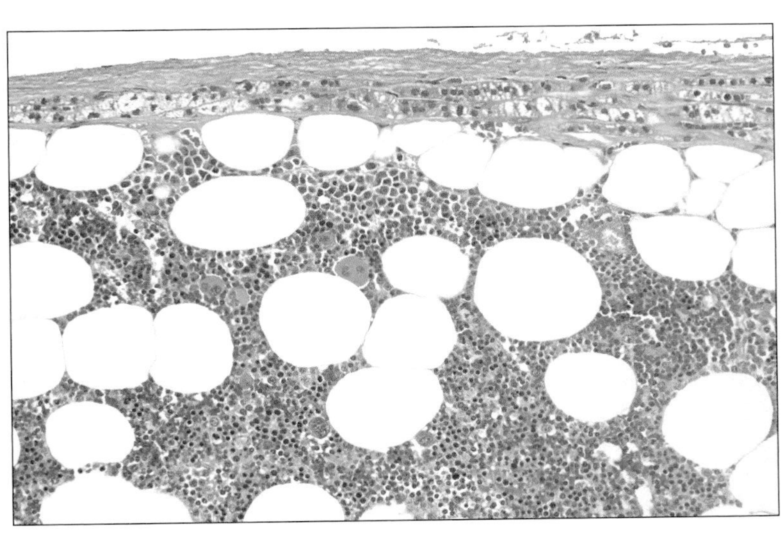

Fig. 13.90 Adrenal myelolipoma composed of an admixture of adipose cells and hematopoietic elements, including myeloid, erythroid, and megakaryocytic components. Note the thinned adrenal cortical parenchyma (top) surrounding the myelolipoma.

Table 13.13 Myelolipomatous lesions of the adrenal gland
As an isolated entity:
Myelolipoma
Secondarily associated with other lesions:
Adrenal cortical hyperplasia
Adrenal cortical nodule
Adrenal cortical adenoma

Differential diagnosis

- Myelolipomatous foci in adrenal cortical neoplasm or hyperplasia (Table 13.13).
- Extramedullary hematopoiesis.

Treatment and prognosis

- Surgical excision is the treatment of choice for symptomatic or large incidental lesions. Observation is acceptable for small, clinically silent lesions.
- Myelolipomas are benign and do not recur after complete excision.
- Large myelolipomas are at risk for rupture and massive retroperitoneal hemorrhage.

ADENOMATOID TUMOR[201–203]

Definition

Adenomatoid tumor is a rare benign neoplasm of probable mesothelial origin characterized by vacuolated epithelioid cells that form gland-like structures.

Clinical

- Only a few examples of adenomatoid tumor of the adrenal gland have been reported. They are characteristically found in the genital tract, particularly involving the epididymis, uterus, or fallopian tube.
- Most adenomatoid tumors are small and incidental.

Pathology

Gross

- Most adenomatoid tumors measure only a few centimeters in diameter.
- Poorly circumscribed, the tumor may have an infiltrative border.
- The cut surface is white to gray; the lesion may appear solid or may contain punctate to slightly larger cystic spaces.
- Foci of calcification may be present.

Histology

- The border may appear infiltrative, with microscopic projections into the surrounding adrenal or periadrenal soft tissue.
- The tumor is composed of nest and cords of epithelioid cells with uniform round nuclei and frequent intracytoplasmic vacuoles. The vacuoles may be quite large and lend a signet ring appearance to the cells. Tubular or gland-like spaces are seen in many areas; the epithelioid cells may be flattened in these tubule-like areas.
- The stroma varies in quantity and consists of fibroblastic cells and collagen. Some areas may be hyalinized. Foci of calcification may be present in the stroma.
- *Histochemical stains*: Mucicarmine and PAS (with and without diastase) are negative.
- *Immunohistochemistry*: The tumor cells have the staining characteristics of mesothelial cells – positive for cytokeratin, epithelial membrane antigen, and vimentin. Neuroendocrine markers are negative.
- *Electron microscopy*: Tumor cells with well-formed desmosomes, elongated thin microvilli typical of mesothelial cells, and tonofilaments are seen.

(Figs 13.91 & 13.92)

Differential diagnosis

- Lymphangioma.
- Metastatic adenocarcinoma, especially signet ring cell type.

Treatment and prognosis

Adenomatoid tumors are benign, and do not recur after surgical excision.

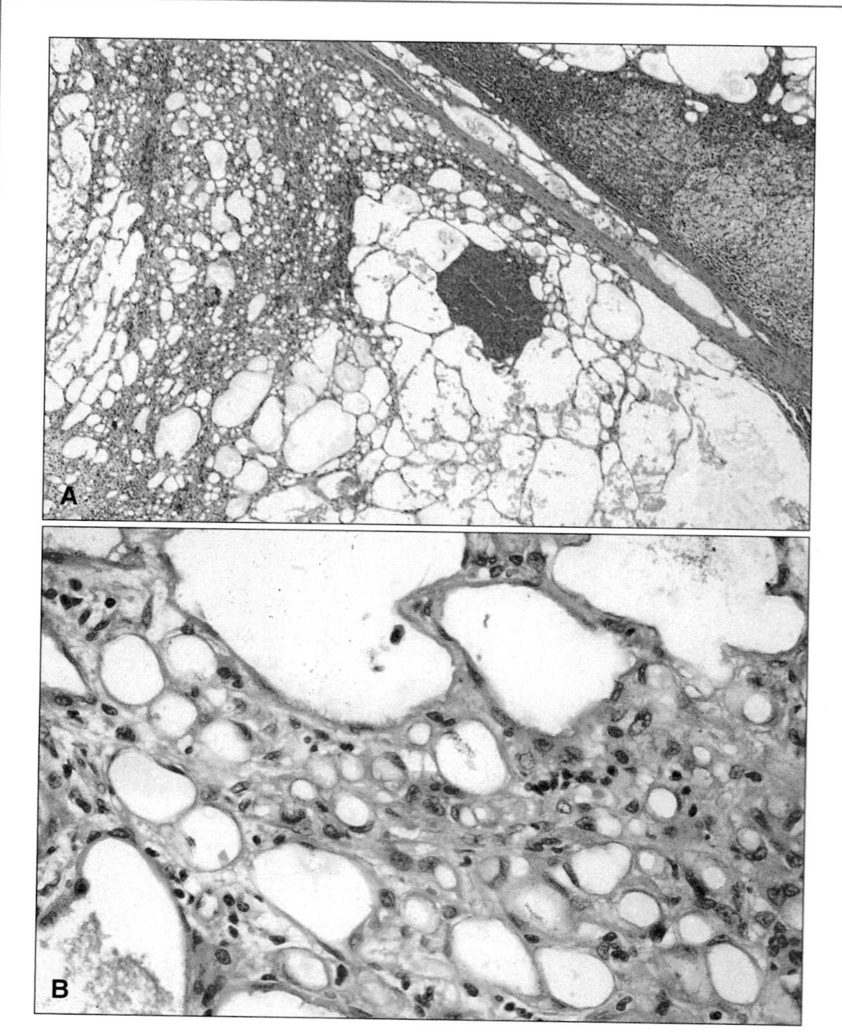

Fig. 13.91 (A) Adenomatoid tumor within the adrenal gland, composed of variably sized gland-like structures. Adrenal cortical tissue is seen in the upper right. (B) Higher magnification shows the gland-like structures lined by flattened epithelioid cells. Cords and nests of these cells are also seen; in these areas, large intracytoplasmic vacuoles may be seen, giving some of the cells a signet ring appearance.

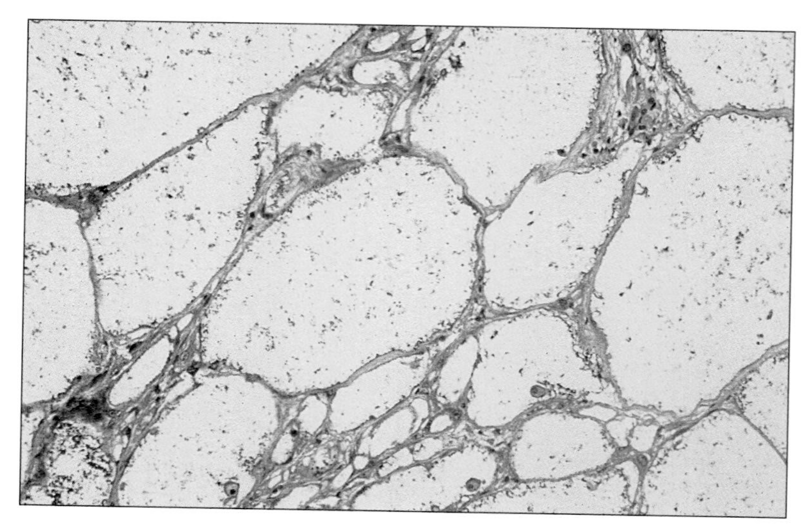

Fig. 13.92 The neoplastic cells of the adenomatoid tumor have staining characteristics of mesothelial cells, as seen by the presence of cytokeratin immunoreactivity.

HEMANGIOMA[189,204–206]

Definition

Hemangioma is a very rare benign neoplastic proliferation of blood vessels; the predominant pattern is cavernous, though capillary-type hemangiomas occur as well.

Clinical

- Adrenal hemangioma is most commonly an incidental autopsy finding; even surgical cases are usually asymptomatic and incidental.
- It is found over a broad age range, from 25 to 79 years.
- It is more common in females.
- The few symptomatic cases are related to large tumor size and local mass effect.
- Radiography is a common means of incidental discovery of adrenal hemangiomas. CT reveals a hypodense lesion with contrast enhancement. Ultrasonographic images have variable echogenicity related to the size of the proliferating vessels and the extent of thrombosis. The lesions may be identified on plain radiographs if calcification is present.

Pathology

Gross

- Sizes range from 2 cm (most incidental tumors) to 22 cm for symptomatic lesions.
- Most are solitary and unilateral, but bilateral examples do occur.
- Tumors are encapsulated; smaller examples may be surrounded, at least partially, by a rim of residual adrenal gland.
- The cut surface is hemorrhagic, with variably sized blood-filled spaces. The color is red–purple, with yellow areas if necrosis is present. Calcification, phleboliths, and areas of fibrosis are common, especially in larger tumors.

Histology

- Proliferating, well-formed vascular spaces of variable size are arranged in an orderly fashion, sometimes forming distinct lobules. The supportive stroma is predominantly fibrous, but may appear more cellular in capillary-type hemangiomas. Large dilated vascular spaces are more common – the cavernous pattern of hemangioma.
- The endothelial cells may be plump, but they are uniform and lack nuclear pleomorphism and hyperchromasia. They form a complete, even lining within the vascular spaces.

Differential diagnosis

- Adrenal cortical adenomas with marked degenerative changes and secondary vascular proliferation are often mistaken for hemangiomas, or occasionally for angiosarcoma. Central hemorrhage or infarction in cortical adenomas resolves with loss of cortical cells, which are replaced by areas of variably dense fibrosis and vascular proliferation that may be quite pronounced. The vessels in such cases are usually variable in size, often resembling the components of a cavernous hemangioma; they are usually associated with hemosiderin deposits, fibrosis, and sometimes with cholesterol granulomas. Close observation of the remaining adrenal cortical tissue may reveal an abnormally thickened rim of cortical cells surrounding the vascular proliferation; often islands of preserved cortical cells or 'ghosts' of necrotic cortical cells are found deep within the fibrovascular process, indicating the underlying cortical neoplasm, which represents the primary lesion. Degenerative change with neovascularization in cortical adenomas is much more common than adrenal hemangiomas.
- Lymphangiomas (see Fig. 13.11) also occur rarely in the adrenal gland. Like hemangiomas, lymphangiomas are frequently incidental findings, though some may become quite large and replace much of the cortex. They are distinguished from hemangiomas by the presence of serous fluid within the vascular spaces and frequently by associated lymphoid tissue. Treatment and behavior are similar to hemangiomas.
- Angiosarcoma.
- Pheochromocytoma with vascular ectasia.

Treatment and prognosis

Hemangiomas are benign; if treatment is required for alleviation of symptoms, surgical resection is preferred.

ANGIOSARCOMA[81,207-210]

Definition

Angiosarcoma is a rare malignant vasoformative neoplasm in which the neoplastic cellular component exhibits endothelial cell differentiation, usually with epithelioid features when encountered in the adrenal.

Clinical

- Most commonly encountered in the sixth and seventh decades, angiosarcomas are seen over an age range from 45 to 85 years.
- There is no gender predilection.

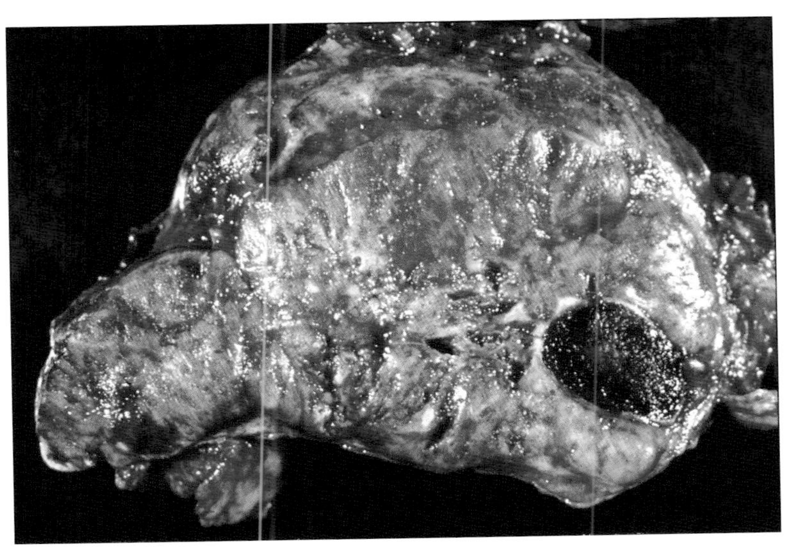

Fig. 13.93 Primary adrenal angiosarcoma. The cut surface shows a yellow to red appearance with areas of necrosis and hemorrhage. The cut surface does not immediately suggest the vascular nature of the neoplasm.

- Presenting symptoms include a palpable abdominal mass, flank or abdominal pain, weight loss, fever, and weakness, over a period of weeks to several months. The tumors may be asymptomatic and incidentally discovered.
- Rarely, paraneoplastic endocrine abnormalities are reported.
- CT or ultrasonography demonstrates retroperitoneal or suprarenal, partially cystic to solid neoplasms with contrast enhancement.

Pathology

Gross

- Size ranges from 6 to 10 cm.
- The tumors may be circumscribed to grossly infiltrative.
- The cut surface is gray to yellow to red, variably cystic to solid, with hemorrhage and necrosis.

(Fig. 13.93)

Histology

- An infiltrative border is usually evident in spite of gross circumscription. The residual adrenal cortex, as well as periadrenal soft tissue, is often invaded by tumor.
- Hemorrhage is usually extensive, as is necrosis.
- The tumor cells are arranged in solid sheets or nests, which merge with vasoformative areas. The vascular spaces are lined by cells identical to those in the more solid areas; they form an endothelial lining which varies from single cells to tufts of tumor cells projecting into the vascular lumina.

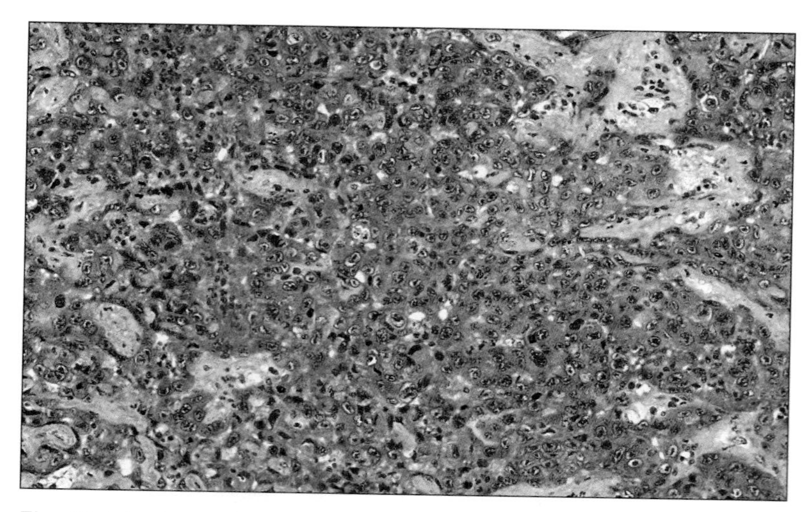

Fig. 13.94 Adrenal epithelioid angiosarcoma. The solid growth and epithelioid cytomorphology raise concern for a diagnosis of an epithelial malignancy (e.g. adrenal cortical carcinoma or metastatic carcinoma) rather than a vascular neoplasm. The sheets of cells have eosinophilic cytoplasm with hyperchromatic nuclei and prominent nucleoli; numerous mitoses are seen.

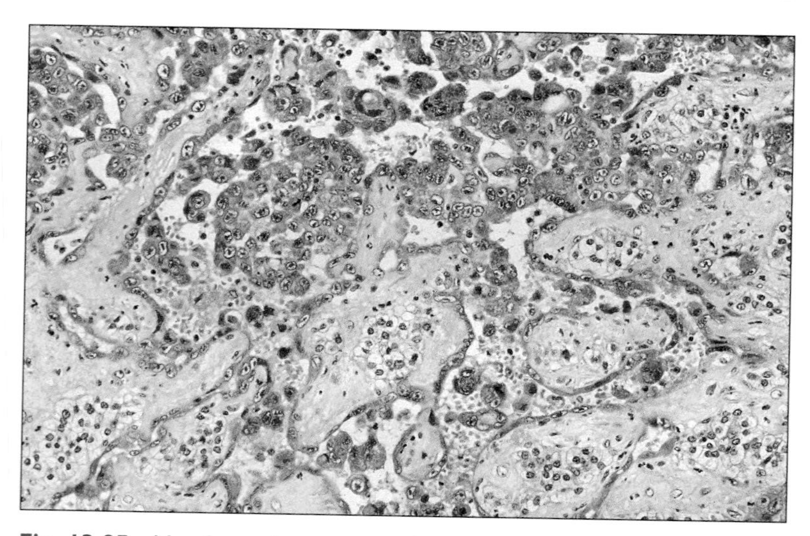

Fig. 13.95 Vasoformative areas in adrenal epithelioid angiosarcoma are more diagnostic. The endothelial cells are large and very atypical, with crowded papillary tufts projecting into the vascular lumen.

- The tumor cells are often epithelioid in appearance, characterized by the presence of polygonal cells with abundant eosinophilic cytoplasm, round to oval vesicular nuclei with hyperchromasia, and prominent central nucleoli. Nuclear pleomorphism and mitotic activity are common findings. Some cells contain intracytoplasmic lumina in which red blood cells may be seen.
- A background stroma is composed of fibrous tissue with areas of acute and chronic inflammation.
- *Histochemistry*: Mucicarmine and PAS with and without diastase are negative.
- *Immunohistochemistry*: Neoplastic cells are positive for factor VIII-related antigen, CD34 (QBEND), CD31, vimentin, cytokeratin (most cases), B72.3, and *Ulex europaeus* lectin (only one-third of cases); no staining is seen with smooth muscle actin, S-100 protein, chromogranin, desmin, or epithelial membrane antigen.
- *Electron microscopy*: The epithelioid tumor cells are found in sheets, or may line vascular lumina. Occasional cells contain intracytoplasmic lumina, in which red blood cells may be seen. Basal lamina surrounds the tumor cells, and pinocytotic vesicles may be identified. Weibel–Palade bodies, if found, are characteristic of endothelial differentiation; they appear as intracytoplasmic rod-shaped bodies with an internal parallel array of microtubules.

(Figs 13.94–13.97)

Differential diagnosis

- Adrenal cortical carcinoma.
- Metastatic adenocarcinoma.

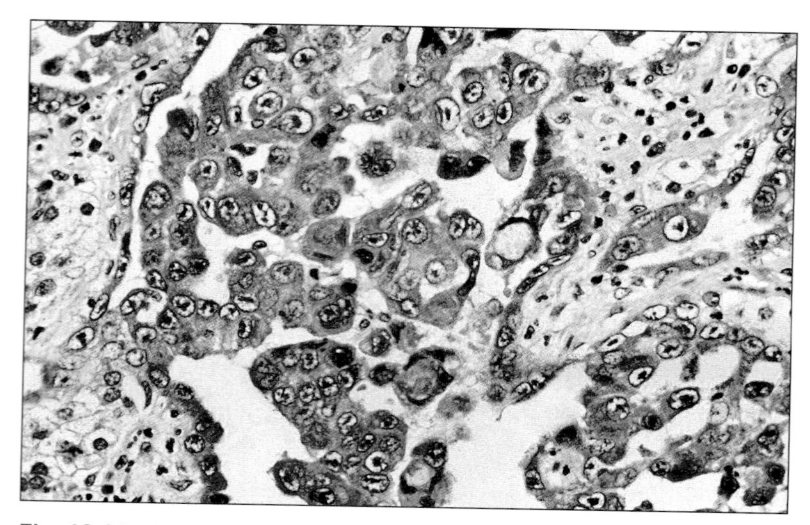

Fig. 13.96 In addition to epithelioid tumor cells with eosinophilic cytoplasm and marked nuclear atypia, some cells show characteristic intracytoplasmic lumina.

- Pheochromocytoma.
- Primary or metastatic melanoma.

Note: The epithelioid appearance of the tumor cells in adrenal angiosarcoma, combined with the positive immunohistochemistry for cytokeratin, may cause confusion with the much more common epithelial malignancies of the adrenal, including adrenal cortical carcinoma and metastatic carcinoma. Immunohistochemical markers of endothelial cell differentiation, factor VIII-associated antigen, CD31, CD34, and *Ulex europaeus* lectin are helpful discriminators in this differential diagnosis.

Treatment and prognosis

- Surgical resection is the preferred therapy.
- Approximately one-third of patients develop metastatic disease, usually involving the lungs, and die within 2

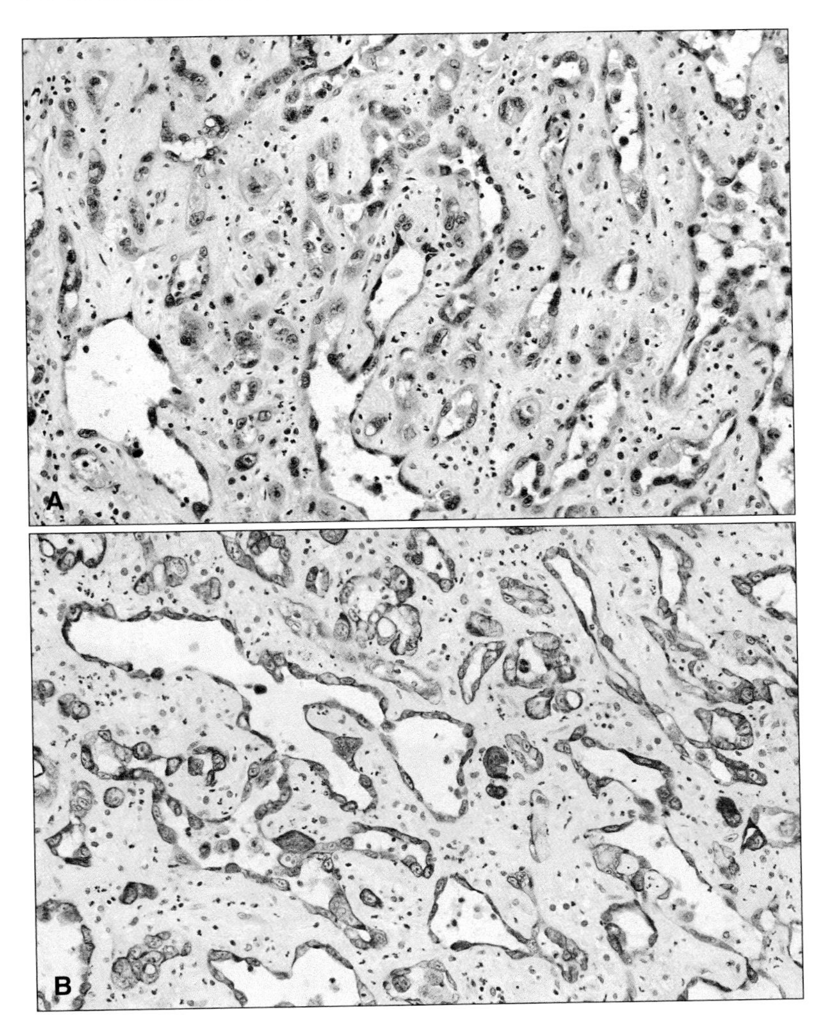

Fig. 13.97 Immunohistochemical staining in adrenal epithelioid angiosarcoma includes the presence of (A) factor VIII-associated antigen, and (B) strong cytokeratin reactivity. The latter, in face of solid growth and epithelioid cell morphology, may be confused with adrenal cortical carcinoma or metastatic carcinoma. The tumor cells are also positive for a variety of endothelial-related stains, including CD34 and *Ulex europaeus* lectin.

years; however, long-term survival is reported in an equal number of patients.

NERVE SHEATH TUMORS[177,189,211,212]

Definition

Nerve sheath tumors comprise a spectrum of benign and malignant neoplasms, all uncommon in the adrenal gland, characterized by a proliferation of schwannian cells with or without a neuritic component. Included in this group are neurilemmoma, neurofibroma, and malignant peripheral nerve sheath tumors (MPNSTs).

Clinical

- Although all nerve sheath tumors are rare in the adrenal gland, cases are reported over a wide age range.
- No gender predilection is evident.
- Nerve sheath tumors, benign and malignant, may be seen in association with von Recklinghausen's disease.
- Most MPNSTs have been associated with ganglioneuromas, either in patients with a history of irradiation for neuroblastoma/ganglioneuroblastoma or as a de novo occurrence.
- Both incidental and symptomatic cases are reported. Symptomatology is usually related to mass effect of the lesion, and includes abdominal or flank pain.
- Incidental proliferations of neural tissue in the adrenal gland may be found at autopsy or seen in adrenal glands resected for another disease process. These lesions consist of a single nodule or multiple small nodules, which may be circumscribed or, occasionally, have an infiltrative border. The spindle cells have wavy nuclei and variable cellularity; they may resemble a neurofibroma, neurilemmoma, or even a traumatic neuroma. Most are centered in the medulla. Though the natural history of these lesions is a mystery, they may represent incipient neurofibromas or neurilemmomas.

Pathology

Neurofibroma

- Grossly, the tumor is unencapsulated, with a white to gray–yellow rubbery cut surface, and variable cystic or myxoid changes.
- The histologic pattern is one of a mixture of neurites, fibroblasts, and collagen fibers.
- Scattered spindle cells are positive for S-100 protein.

Neurilemmoma, or schwannoma

- Grossly, the tumor is encapsulated, with a white to pink–yellow rubbery cut surface, and variable cystic changes and focal calcification.
- The spindle cell proliferation may be compact, orderly and cellular in areas (Antoni A area), with foci of nuclear palisading; other areas are less cellular and orderly, and have a myxoid background (Antoni B area). The cellular component is predominantly Schwann cells, with few, if any, neurites. Occasional mitotic figures may be seen. Scattered pleomorphic nuclei may be seen, especially in degenerated or 'ancient' neurilemmomas.
- '*Cellular schwannomas*' represent a more cellular variant in which the Antoni A areas predominate; mitotic activity (usually less than 4/10 HPF) is common; the cellularity and mitoses may cause confusion with malignant nerve sheath tumors, fibrosarcoma, or leiomyosarcoma.
- S-100 protein is strongly and diffusely positive in neurilemmomas; this feature is particularly helpful in

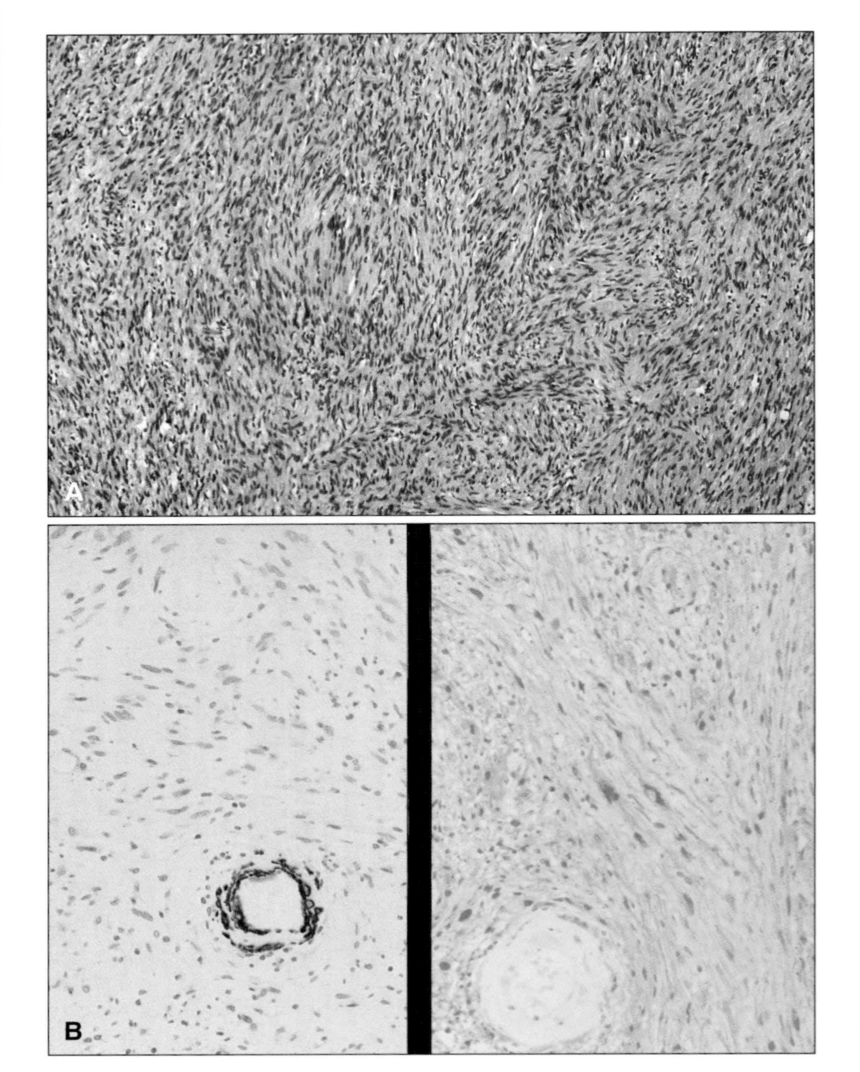

Fig. 13.98 (A) Intra-adrenal gland cellular benign spindle cell neoplasm showing wavy-appearing nuclei suggesting neural differentiation. (B) Immunohistochemical staining shows the neoplastic cells to be nonreactive with smooth muscle actin (left) but diffusely positive for S-100 protein (right). The light microscopic findings in conjunction with the immunohistochemical results confirm the diagnosis of an adrenal gland neurilemmoma.

excluding malignant nerve sheath tumors (in which S-100 protein staining is weaker and usually focal) and other soft tissue sarcomas.

(Fig. 13.98)

Malignant peripheral nerve sheath tumor

- This is sometimes seen arising as a fusiform mass from a peripheral nerve.
- The cut surface is usually fleshy white–tan and may be somewhat hemorrhagic or necrotic.
- The very cellular spindle cell proliferation is characterized by wavy nuclei and indistinct cell borders: fascicular, whorled, or loose myxoid patterns may be seen. Nuclear palisading, as seen in neurilemmomas, is uncommon and focal. Pleomorphism and mitotic activity are commonly seen, and are helpful in excluding neurofibroma. Neurilemmoma, also in the differential diagnosis, may exhibit atypical nuclei and mitoses; the distinction between MPNST may be made on the basis of lack of the Antoni A/Antoni B patterns and on the S-100 protein staining pattern in MPNST.
- S-100 protein stains only scattered cells or groups of cells, and is present in 50–90% of cases.

Differential diagnosis

- Ganglioneuroma.
- Ganglioneuroblastoma.
- Smooth muscle neoplasms.
- Secondary adrenal involvement by a variety of primary soft tissue sarcomas of the retroperitoneum.
- Malignant melanoma, primary or metastatic, of adrenal.

Treatment and prognosis

- Benign nerve sheath tumors may be treated, if symptomatic, by surgical excision, which is curative.
- MPNSTs frequently recur locally and metastasize in spite of aggressive surgical therapy.

METASTATIC NEOPLASMS[189,213–218]

Definition

These comprise secondary deposits from a malignant neoplasm primary to another site, exclusive of contiguous infiltration of the adrenal by a neoplasm in an adjacent organ or soft tissue. The adrenal is the fourth most common targeted organ of metastatic disease, after lung, liver, and bone.

Clinical

- Adrenal metastases are present in 9–27% of patients with cancer; involvement is bilateral in 41%.
- Lung and breast carcinomas are the most common tumors to metastasize to the adrenal.
- Most metastatic lesions are clinically silent with regard to adrenal function; however, rare instances of Addison's disease as a result of metastases from a variety of primary malignancies, including carcinomas of the lung and breast, renal cell carcinoma, carcinomas of the gastrointestinal tract, seminoma, pancreatic carcinoma, transitional cell carcinoma, and melanoma, have been reported. Adrenal cortical carcinoma may also metastasize to the contralateral gland and cause adrenal insufficiency.
- Destruction of 90% of the cortex must occur before overt adrenal insufficiency occurs; however, the

symptoms of Addison's disease may be subtle and may be overlooked in the chronically ill cancer patient. Laboratory testing for hypoadrenalism is helpful in patients with bilateral metastatic lesions.
- Manifestations of adrenal insufficiency include weakness, wasting, intolerance of physical stress, and hyperpigmentation of the skin and mucous membranes.
- Metastatic disease, even relatively small lesions, is readily detected by CT; however, unilateral metastatic lesions cannot easily be distinguished from primary adrenal neoplasms.
- CT-directed FNA is an effective method for preoperative exclusion of metastatic disease in the event of a unilateral adrenal lesion, and may be helpful in identifying the source of metastases when the primary site is undetermined.

Pathology

Gross

- Lesions may be unilateral or bilateral; though frequently multiple, they may be solitary.
- Gross lesions are usually readily identified, and, if large, are often partially necrotic. Some lesions are subtle, replacing the medulla and causing enlargement of the gland without a distinct nodule.

(Fig. 13.99)

Histology

- Although most metastatic lesions are readily recognized as secondary lesions, some neoplasms may be difficult to distinguish from primary adrenal neoplasms such as adrenal cortical carcinoma or pheochromocytoma. The differential diagnosis between some poorly differentiated metastatic carcinomas and adrenal cortical carcinoma can be especially problematic. In contrast to primary adrenal gland neoplasms, metastases to the adrenal gland may have an associated neutrophilic infiltrate. This finding may be helpful in identifying or at least considering the possibility of metastatic disease to the adrenal gland.
- Metastatic neuroendocrine malignancies may mimic pheochromocytoma (particularly malignant ones).
- *Immunohistochemistry*: Adrenal cortical carcinomas are usually positive for vimentin, but negative or only weakly positive for cytokeratin and negative for epithelial membrane antigen. These stains may be helpful in the differential with metastatic carcinoma if the carcinoma is strongly positive for cytokeratin and/or epithelial membrane antigen.

(Figs 13.100 & 13.101)

Treatment and prognosis

- The outlook for patients with adrenal metastases is dismal.
- Treatment is dependent on the primary source and tumor type.

OTHER RARE NEOPLASMS[219–221]

- *Smooth muscle tumors*: Leiomyomas and leiomyosarcomas of the adrenal are extremely rare, and are thought to arise from vascular smooth muscle.

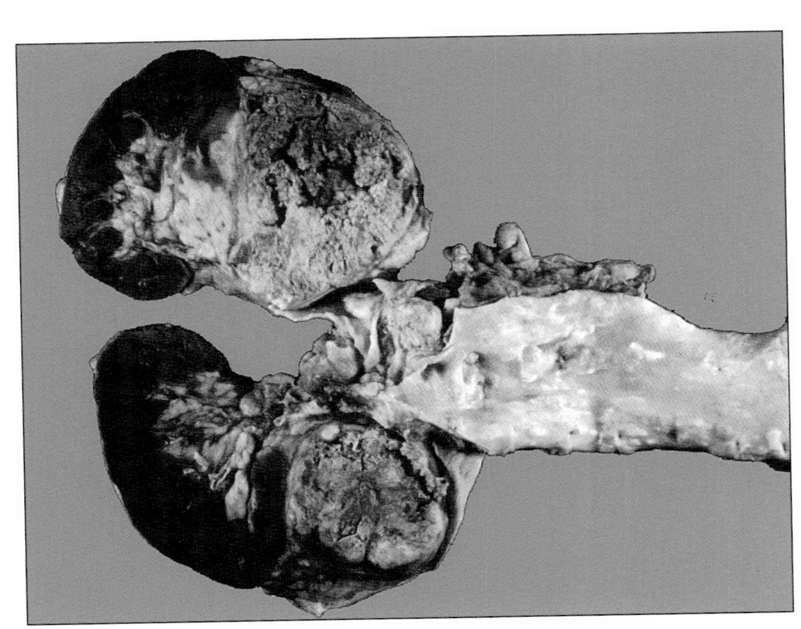

Fig. 13.99 Bilateral adrenal gland metastases from a primary pulmonary adenocarcinoma.

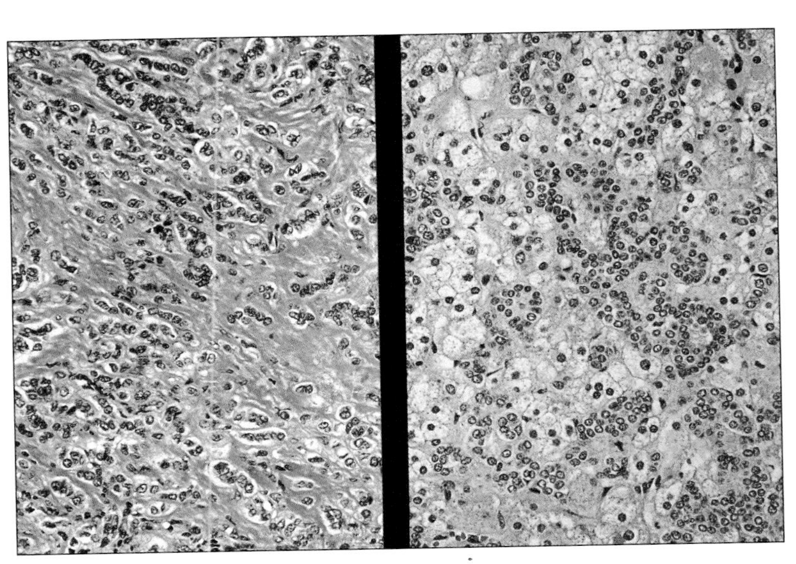

Fig. 13.100 Metastatic lobular breast carcinoma that was metastatic to both adrenal glands. Left: Linear (single file) arrangement of tumor cells with sclerotic collagenous stroma is seen. Right: The tumor was diffusely infiltrative into the adrenal glands, growing in cords and clusters; residual adrenal cortical cells can be seen.

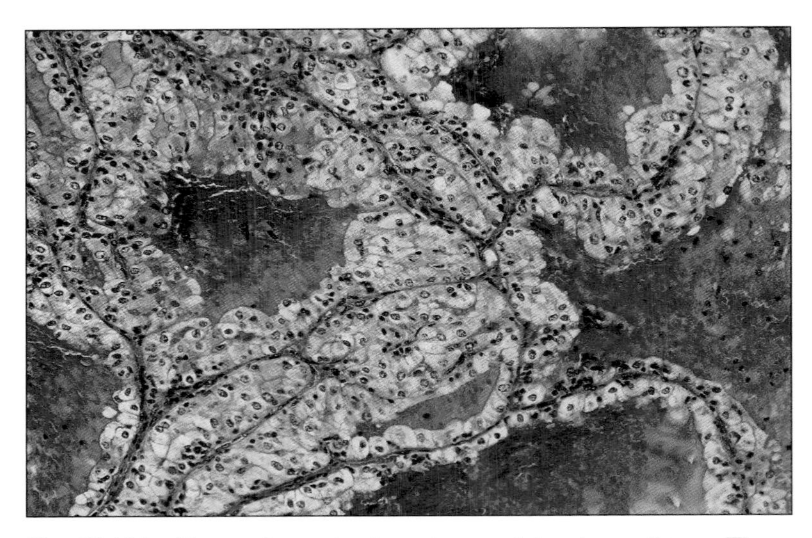

Fig. 13.101 Metastatic renal cell carcinoma of the clear cell type. The pooling of blood within the glandular spaces is typical of renal cell carcinoma.

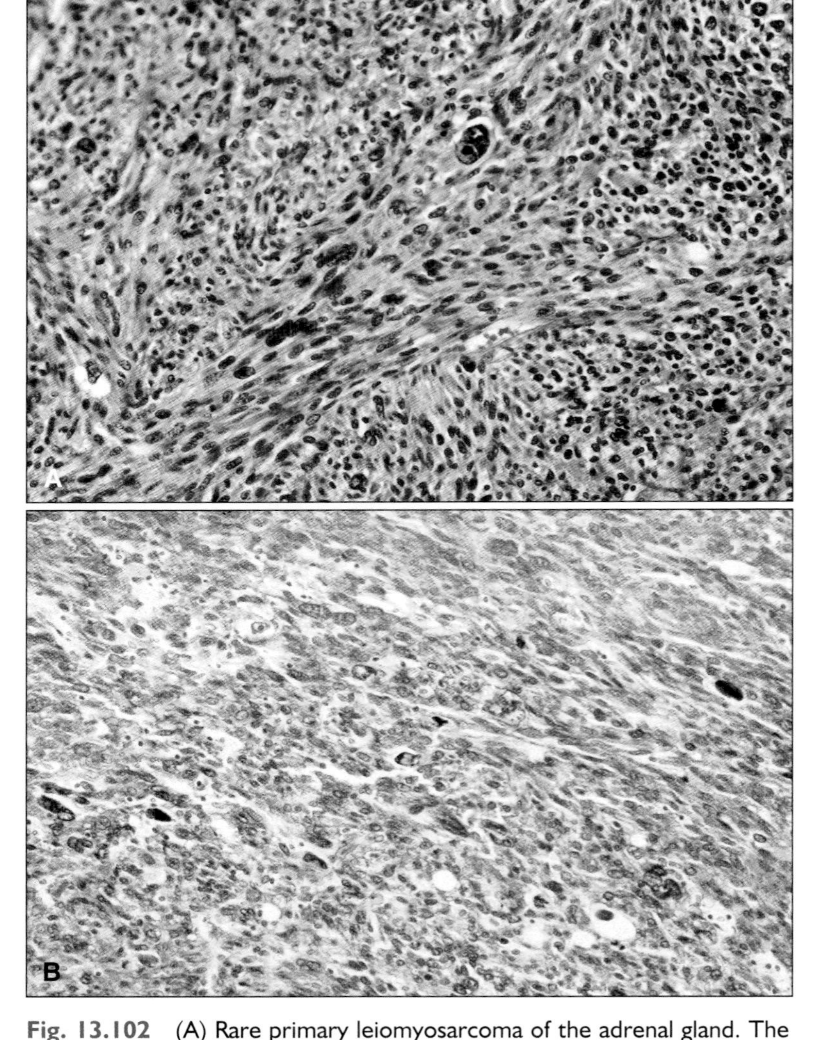

Fig. 13.102 (A) Rare primary leiomyosarcoma of the adrenal gland. The tumor shows fascicular growth and is comprised of a hypercellular spindle cell proliferation with pleomorphic, hyperchromatic nuclei. (B) The neoplastic cells are diffusely immunoreactive for smooth muscle actin.

- *Gonadal stromal-type tmors*: Tumefactive spindle cell lesions resembling ovarian thecal metaplasia, granulosa-theca cell tumor, and Leydig cell tumor with crystalloids of Reinke have been described, but are exceedingly rare.

(Fig. 13.102)

REFERENCES

1. Busuttil A. Ectopic adrenal within the gallbladder wall. J Pathol 1974;113:231–233.
2. Dolan MF, Janovski N. Adreno-hepatic union. Arch Pathol 1968;86: 22–24.
3. Falls JL. Accessory adrenal cortex in the broad ligament. Incidence and functional significance. Cancer 1955;8:143–150.
4. Graham LS. Celiac accessory adrenal glands. Cancer 1953;114:149–152.
5. Lack EE, Kozakewich HPW. Embryology, developmental anatomy, and selected aspects of non-neoplastic pathology. In: Lack EE, ed. Pathology of the adrenal glands. Vol. 14. New York: Churchill Livingstone; 1990:1–74.
6. Schechter DC. Aberrant adrenal tissue. Ann Surg 1968;167:421–426.
7. Symonds DA, Driscoll SG. An adrenal cortical rest within the fetal ovary. Am J Clin Pathol 1973;60:562–564.
8. Wiener MF, Dallgard SA. Intracranial adrenal gland. Arch Pathol 1959;67:228–233.
9. Lack EE. Congenital adrenal heterotopia, hyperplasia and Beckwith–Weidmann syndrome. In: Rosai J, Sobin LH, eds. Tumors of the adrenal gland and extra-adrenal paraganglia. Fascicle 19, third series. Washington, DC: Armed Forces Institute of Pathology; 1997:33–48.
10. Hay ID, Smail PJ, Forsyth CC. Familial cytomegalic adrenocortical hypoplasia: an X-linked syndrome of pubertal failure. Arch Dis Child 1981;56:715–721.
11. Kruse K, Sippell WG, Schnakenburg KV. Hypogonadism in congenital adrenal hypoplasia: evidence for a hypothalamic origin. J Clin Endocrinol Metab 1984;58:12–17.
12. Silla IN, Voorhess ML, MacGillivray MH, et al. Prolonged survival without therapy in congenital adrenal hypoplasia. Am J Dis Child 1983;137:1186–1188.
13. Wise JE, Matalon R, Morgan AM, McCabe ERB. Phenotypic features of patients with congenital adrenal hypoplasia and glycerol kinase deficiency. Am J Dis Child 1987;141:744–747.
14. Borit A, Kosek J. Cytomegaly of the adrenal cortex. Arch Pathol 1969;88:58–64.
15. Oppenheimer EH. Adrenal cytomegaly: studies by light and electron microscopy. Arch Pathol 1970;90:57–64.
16. Pettinati MJ, Haines JL, Higgins RR, et al. Wiedemann–Beckwith syndrome: presentation of clinical and cytogenetic data on 22 new cases and review of the literature. Hum Genet 1986;74:143–148.
17. Sotelo-Avila C, Gooch WM. Neoplasms associated with the Beckwith–Wiedemann syndrome. Perspect Pediatr Pathol 1976;3:255–262.
18. Wiedemann HR. Tumors and hemihypertrophy associated with Wiedemann–Beckwith syndrome. Eur J Pediatr 1983;141:129.
19. Brook CGC, Zachmann M, Prader A, Murset G. Experience with long-term therapy in congenital adrenal hyperplasia. J Pediatr 1974;85:12–19.
20. Mininberg DT, Levine LS, New MI. Current concepts in congenital adrenal hyperplasia. Pathol Annu 1982;2:179–195.
21. New MI, Levine LS. Congenital adrenal hyperplasia. Adv Hum Genet 1973;4:251–326.
22. Page DL, DeLellis RA, Hough AJ. Hyperplasia. In: Page DL, DeLellis RA, Hough AJ, eds. Tumors of the adrenal. Fascicle 23, second series. Washington, DC: Armed Forces Institute of Pathology; 1986:56–80.
23. Rutgers JL, Young RH, Scully RE. The testicular "tumor" of the adrenogenital syndrome. A report of six cases and review of the literature on testicular masses in patients with adrenocortical disorders. Am J Surg Pathol 1988;12:503–513.
24. Van Seters AP, Van Aalderen W, Moolenaar AJ, et al. Adrenocortical tumour in untreated congenital adrenal hyperplasia associated with inadequate ACTH suppressibility. Clin Endocrinol 1981;14:325–334.
25. White PC, New MI, Dupont B. Congenital adrenal hyperplasia. N Engl J Med 1987;316:1519–1524, 1580–1586.

26. Dunlop D. Eighty-six cases of Addison's disease. Br Med J 1963;5362:887–896.
27. Griffel B. Focal adrenalitis. Its frequency and correlation with similar lesions in the thyroid and kidney. Virchows Arch A Pathol Anat Histol 1974;364:191–188.
28. Lack EE. Lymphoid "hypophysitis" with end organ insufficiency. Arch Pathol 1975;99:215–219.
29. Nerup J. Addison's disease – clinical studies. A report of 108 cases. Acta Endocrinol 1974;76:127–141.
30. Neufeld M, Maclaren NK, Blizzard RM. Two types of autoimmune Addison's disease associated with different polyglandular autoimmune (PGA) syndromes. Medicine 1981;60:355–362.
31. Vita JA, Silverberg SJ, Goland RS, et al. Clinical clues to the cause of Addison's disease. Am J Med 1985;78:461–466.
32. Goodwin RA Jr, Shapiro JL, Thurman GH, et al. Disseminated histoplasmosis: clinical and pathologic correlations. Medicine 1980;59:1–33.
33. Greene LW, Cole W, Greene JB, et al. Adrenal insufficiency as a complication of the acquired immunodeficiency syndrome. Ann Intern Med 1984;101:497–499.
34. Guttman PH. Addison's disease. A statistical analysis of five hundred and sixty-six cases and a study of the pathology. Arch Pathol 1930;10:742–785, 896–935.
35. Klatt EC, Shibata D. Cytomegalovirus infection in the acquired immunodeficiency syndrome. Clinical and autopsy findings. Arch Pathol Lab Med 1988;112:540–544.
36. Singer DB. Pathology of neonatal herpes simplex virus infection. In: Rosenberg S, Bernstein J, eds. Perspectives in pediatric pathology. Vol. 6. New York: Masson Publishing; 1981:243–262.
37. Heller EL, Camarata SJ. Addison's disease from amyloidosis of the adrenal glands. Arch Pathol 1950;49:601–604.
38. Khuri FJ, Alton DJ, Hardy BE, et al. Adrenal hemorrhage in neonates: report of 5 cases and review of the literature. J Urol 1980;124:684–687.
39. Kuhajda F, Hutchins GM. Adrenal cortico-medullary junction necrosis: a morphologic marker for hypotension. Am Heart J 1979;98:294–297.
40. Mostoufizadeh M, Lack EE, Gang DL, et al. Postmortem manifestations of echovirus 11 sepsis in five newborn infants. Hum Pathol 1983;14:818–823.
41. Cerny JC, Warshawsky A, Hall J, et al. The preoperative diagnosis of adrenal cysts. J Urol 1970;104:787–790.
42. Cheema P, Cartagena R, Stanbitz W. Adrenal cysts: diagnosis and treatment. J Urol 1981;126:393–399.
43. Foster DG. Adrenal cysts: review of the literature and report of a case. Arch Surg 1966;92:131–143.
44. Gaffey MJ, Mills SE, Fechner RE, et al. Vascular adrenal cysts: a clinicopathologic and immunohistochemical study of endothelial and hemorrhagic (pseudocystic) variants. Am J Surg Pathol 1989;13:740–747.
45. Incze JS, Lui PS, Merriam JC, et al. Morphology and pathogenesis of adrenal cysts. Am J Pathol 1979;95:423–432.
46. Medieros LJ, Lewandrowshi KB, Vickery AL. Adrenal pseudocyst: a clinical and pathologic study of eight cases. Hum Pathol 1989;20:660–665.
47. Medeiros LJ, Weiss LM, Vickery AL. Epithelial-lined (true) cyst of the adrenal gland: a case report. Hum Pathol 1989;20:491–492.
48. Page DL, DeLellis RA, Hough AJ. Cysts. In: Page DL, DeLellis RA, Hough AJ, eds. Tumors of the adrenal. Fascicle 23, second series. Washington, DC: Armed Forces Institute of Pathology; 1986:175–178.
49. Cohen RB. Observations on cortical nodules in human adrenal glands. Cancer 1966;19:552–556.
50. Copeland PM. The incidentally discovered adrenal mass. Ann Surg 1984;199:116–122.
51. Dobbie JW. Adrenocortical nodular hyperplasia: the aging adrenal. J Pathol 1969;99:1–18.
52. Geelhoed GW, Druy EM. Management of the adrenal "incidentaloma". Surgery 1982;92:866–874.
53. Lack EE, Travis WD, Oertel JE. Adrenal cortical nodules, hyperplasia, and hyperfunction. In: Lack EE, ed. Pathology of the adrenal glands. Vol. 14. New York: Churchill Livingstone; 1990:75–113.
54. Neville AM. The nodular adrenal. Invest Cell Pathol 1978;1:99–111.
55. Neville AM, O'Hare MJ. Aspects of structure, function, and pathology. In: James VHT, ed. The adrenal gland. NewYork: Raven Press; 1979:1–65.
56. Page DL, DeLellis RA, Hough AJ. The multinodular adrenal. In: Page DL, DeLellis RA, Hough AJ, eds. Tumors of the adrenal. Fascicle 23, second series. Washington, DC: Armed Forces Institute of Pathology; 1986:73–78.
57. Arce B, Licea M, Hung S, Padron R. Familial Cushing's syndrome. Acta Endocrinol 1978;87:139–147.
58. Burke CW. Disorders of cortisol production: diagnostic and therapeutic progress. Recent Adv Endocr Metab 1978;1:61–90.
59. Choi Y, Werk EE Jr, Sholiton LJ. Cushing's syndrome with dual pituitary-adrenal control. Arch Intern Med 1970;125:1045–1049.
60. Cohen RB, Chapman WB, Castleman B. Hyperadrenocorticism (Cushing's disease); a study of surgically resected adrenal glands. Am J Pathol 1959;35:537–561.
61. Hidai H, Fujii H, Otsuka K, Abe K, Shimizu N. Cushing's syndrome due to huge adrenocortical multinodular hyperplasia. Endocrinol Jpn 1975;22:555–560.
62. Jex RK, van Herden JA, Carpenter PC, Grant CS. Ectopic ACTH syndrome. Am J Surg 1985;149:276–282.
63. Neville AM, Symington T. Bilateral adrenocortical hyperplasia in children with Cushing's syndrome. J Pathol 1972;107:65–106.
64. Orth DN. The old and the new in Cushing's syndrome. N Engl J Med 1984;310:649–651.
65. Plotz CM, Knowlton AI, Ragan C. The natural history of Cushing's syndrome. Am J Med 1952;13:597–614.
66. Prinz RA, Brooks MH, Lawrence AM, Paloyan E. The continued importance of adrenalectomy in the treatment of Cushing's disease. Arch Surg 1979;114:481–484.
67. Ruder HJ, Loriaux DL, Lipsett MB. Severe osteopenia in young adults associated with Cushing's syndrome due to micronodular adrenal disease. J Clin Endocrinol Metab 1974;39:1138–1147.
68. Schweizer-Cagianut M, Froesch ER, Hedinger C. Familial Cushing's syndrome with primary adrenocortical microadenomatosis (primary adrenocortical nodular dysplasia). Acta Endocrinol 1980;94:529–535.
69. Shenoy BV, Carpenter PB, Carney JA. Bilateral primary pigmented nodular adrenocortical disease. Am J Surg Pathol 1984;8:335–344.
70. Singer W, Kovacs K, Ryan N, Horvath E. Ectopic ACTH syndrome: clinicopathological correlations. J Clin Pathol 1978;31:591–598.
71. Smals AGH, Pieters GFFM, van Haelst UJG, Kloppenborg PWC. Macronodular adrenocortical hyperplasia in long-standing Cushing's disease. J Clin Endocrinol Metab 1984;58:25–31.
72. Ferris JB, Brown JJ, Fraser R, et al. Hypertension with aldosterone excess and low plasma-renin: preoperative distinction between patients with and without adrenocortical tumor. Lancet 1970;2:995–1000.
73. Grant CS, Carpenter P, van Heerden JA, et al. Primary aldosteronism. Clinical management. Arch Surg 1984;119:585–590.
74. Weinberger MH, Grim CE, Hollifield JW, et al. Primary aldosteronism. Diagnosis, localization, and treatment. Ann Intern Med 1979;90:386–395.
75. Bhettay E, Bonnici F. Pure oestrogen-secreting feminizing adrenocortical adenoma. Arch Dis Child 1977;52:241–243.
76. Caplan RH, Virata RL. Functional black adenoma of the adrenal cortex. Am J Clin Pathol 1974;62:97–103.
77. Conn JW, Hinerman DL. Spironolactone-induced inhibition of aldosterone biosynthesis in primary aldosteronism: morphological and functional studies. Metabolism 1977;26:1293–1307.
78. Erlandson RA, Reuter VE. Oncocytic adrenal cortical adenoma. Ultrastruct Pathol 1991;15:539–547.
79. Favre L, Jacot-des-Combes E, Morel P, et al. Primary aldosteronism with bilateral adrenal adenomas. Virchows Arch A Pathol Anat Histol 1980;388:229–236.
80. Garret R, Ames RP. Black-pigmented adenoma of the adrenal gland. Arch Pathol 1973;95:349–353.
81. Granger JK, Houn H-Y, Collins C. Massive hemorrhagic functional adrenal adenoma histologically mimicking angiosarcoma. Report of a case with immunohistochemical study. Am J Surg Pathol 1991;15:699–704.
82. Hamwi GJ, Gwinup G, Mostow JH, Besch PK. Activation of testicular adrenal rest tissue by prolonged excessive ACTH production. J Clin Endocrinol Metab 1963;23:861–869.
83. Hough AJ, Hollifield JW, Page DL, Hartmann WH. Prognostic factors in adrenal cortical tumors. A mathematical analysis of clinical and morphologic data. Am J Clin Pathol 1979;72:390–399.
84. Kable WT, Yussman MA. Testosterone-secreting adrenal adenoma. Fertil Steril 1979;32:610–611.
85. Katz RL. Kidney, adrenal and retroperitoneum. In: Bibbo M, ed. Comprehensive cytopathology. Philadelphia: WB Saunders; 1991:771–805.
86. Kovacs K, Horvath E, Feldman PS. Pigmented adenoma of adrenal cortex associated with Cushing's syndrome. Urology 1979;7:641–645.
87. Lack EE, Travis WD, Oertel JE. Adrenal cortical neoplasms. In: Lack EE, ed. Pathology of the adrenal glands. Vol. 14. New York: Churchill Livingstone; 1990:115–171.
88. Macadam RF. Black adenoma of the human adrenal cortex. Cancer 1971;27:116–119.
89. Orth DN, Liddle GW. Results of treatment in 108 patients with Cushing's syndrome. N Engl J Med 1971;285:243–247.

90. Page DL, DeLellis RA, Hough AJ. Adrenal cortical adenoma. In: Page DL, DeLellis RA, Hough AJ, eds. Tumors of the adrenal. Fascicle 23, second series. Washington, DC: Armed Forces Institute of Pathology; 1986: 81–114.
91. Reidbord H, Fisher ER. Aldosteronoma and nonfunctioning adrenal cortical adenoma. Arch Pathol 1969;88:155–161.
92. Ross NS, Aron DC. Hormonal evaluation of the patient with an incidentally discovered adrenal mass. N Engl J Med 1990;323:1401–1405.
93. Sasano H, Suzuki T, Sano T, et al. Adrenocortical oncocytoma. A true nonfunctioning adrenocortical tumor. Am J Surg Pathol 1991;15:949–956.
94. Sasano N, Ojima M, Masuda T. Endocrinologic pathology of functioning adrenocortical tumors. Pathol Annu 1980;15:105–142.
95. Wadih GE, Nance KV, Silverman JF. Fine-needle aspiration cytology of the adrenal gland. Fifty biopsies in 48 patients. Arch Pathol Lab Med 1991;116:841–846.
96. Young WF, Hogan MJ, Klee GG, et al. Primary aldosteronism: diagnosis and treatment. Mayo Clin Proc 1990;65:96–110.
97. Alsabeh R, Mazoujian G, Coates J, Medeiros LJ, Weiss LM. Adrenal cortical tumors clinically mimicking pheochromocytoma. Am J Clin Pathol 1995;104:382–390.
98. Bugg MF, Ribeiro RC, Roberson PK, et al. Correlation of pathologic features with clinical outcome in pediatric adrenocortical neoplasia. Am J Clin Pathol 1994;101:625–629.
99. Busam KJ, Iversen K, Coplan KA, et al. Immunoreactivity for A103, an antibody to melan-A (Mart-1), in adrenocortical and other steroid tumors. Am J Surg Pathol 1998;22:57–63.
100. Cibas ES, Medeiros LJ, Weinberg DS, et al. Cellular DNA profiles of benign and malignant adrenocortical tumors. Am J Surg Pathol 1990;14:948–955.
101. Cagle PT, Hough AJ, Pysher TJ, et al. Comparison of adrenal cortical tumors in children and adults. Cancer 1986;57:2235–2237.
102. El-Naggar AK, Evans DB, Mackay B. Oncocytic adrenal cortical carcinoma. Ultrastruct Pathol 1991;15:549–556.
103. Evans HL, Vassilopoulou-Sellin R. Adrenal cortical neoplasms. A study of 56 cases. Am J Clin Pathol 1996;105:76–86.
104. Fuhrman SA, Lasky LC, Limas C. Prognostic significance of morphologic parameters in renal cell carcinoma. Am J Surg Pathol 1982;6:655–663.
105. Gandour MJ, Grizzle WE. A small adrenocortical carcinoma with aggressive behavior. An evaluation of criteria for malignancy. Arch Pathol Lab Med 1986;110:1076–1079.
106. King DR, Lack EE. Adrenal cortical carcinoma. A clinical and pathologic study of 49 cases. Cancer 1979;44:239–244.
107. Komminoth P, Roth J, Schröder S, et al. Overlapping expression of immunohistochemical markers and synaptophysin mRNA in pheochromocytomas and adrenocortical carcinomas. Implications for the differential diagnosis of adrenal gland tumors. Lab Invest 1995;72:424–431.
108. Lack EE, Mulvihill JJ, Travis WD, Kozakewich HPW. Adrenal cortical neoplasms in the pediatric and adolescent age group. Clinicopathologic study of 30 cases with emphasis on epidemiological and prognostic features. Pathol Annu 1992;27:1–53.
109. Li M, Wenig BM. Oncocytic adrenal cortical carcinoma. Am J Surg Pathol 2001;24:1552–1557.
110. Luton J-P, Cerdas S, Billaud L, et al. Clinical features of adrenocortical carcinoma, prognostic factors, and the effect of mitotane therapy. N Engl J Med 1990;322:1195–1201.
111. Medeiros LJ, Weiss LM. New developments in the pathologic diagnosis of adrenal cortical neoplasms. A review. Am J Clin Pathol 1992;97:73–83.
112. Miettinen M. Neuroendocrine differentiation in adrenocortical carcinoma. New immunohistochemical findings supported by electron microscopy. Lab Invest 1992;66:169–174.
113. Nader S, Hickey RC, Sellin RV, Samaan NA. Adrenal cortical carcinoma. A study of 77 cases. Cancer 1983;552:707–711.
114. Ribeiro RC, Neto RS, Schell MJ, et al. Adrenocortical carcinoma in children: a study of 40 cases. J Clin Oncol 1990;8:67–74.
115. van Slooten H, Schaberg A, Smeenk D, Moolenaar A. Morphologic characteristics of benign and malignant adrenocortical tumors. Cancer 1985;55:766–773.
116. Weiss LM Comparative histologic study of 43 metastasizing and nonmetastasizing adrenocortical tumors. Am J Surg Pathol 1984;8:163–169.
117. Weiss LM, Medeiros LJ, Vickery AL. Pathologic features of prognostic significance in adrenal cortical carcinoma. Am J Surg Pathol 1989;13:202–206.
118. Wick MR, Cherwitz DL, McGlennen RC, Dehner LP. Adrenocortical carcinoma. An immunohistochemical comparison with renal cell carcinoma. Am J Pathol 1986;122:343–352.
119. Carney JA, Sizemore GW, Tyce GM. Bilateral adrenal medullary hyperplasia in multiple endocrine neoplasia, type II: the precursor of bilateral pheochromocytoma. Mayo Clin Proc 1975;50:3–10.
120. DeLellis RA, Wolf HJ, Gagel RT, et al. Adrenal medullary hyperplasia: a morphometric analysis of patients with familial medullary thyroid carcinoma. Am J Pathol 1976;83:177–190.
121. Lack EE. Adrenal medullary hyperplasia and pheochromocytoma. In: Pathology of adrenal and extra-adrenal paraganglia. Major problems in pathology. Vol. 29. Philadelphia: WB Saunders, 1994:220–272.
122. Montalbano FP, Barnovsky ID, Ball H. Hyperplasia of the adrenal medulla: a clinical entity. JAMA 1962;182:264–267.
123. Rudy FR, Bates RD, Cimorelli AJ, et al. Adrenal medullary hyperplasia: a clinicopathologic study of four cases. Hum Pathol 1980;11:650–657.
124. Visser JW, Axt R. Bilateral adrenal medullary hyperplasia: a clinicopathologic entity. J Clin Pathol 1975;28:298–304.
125. Bravo EL. Pheochromocytoma: new concepts and future trends. Kidney Int 1991;40:544–556.
126. Bravo EL, Gifford RW Jr. Pheochromocytoma: diagnosis, localization, and management. N Engl J Med 1984;311:1298–1303.
127. Feldman JM, Blalock JA, Zern RT, et al. Deficiency of dopamine-beta-hydroxylase: a new mechanism for normotensive pheochromocytomas. Am J Clin Pathol 1979;72:175–185.
128. Greene JP, Guay AT. New perspectives in pheochromocytomas. Urol Clin North Am 1989;16:487–503.
129. Linnoila RI, Keiser HR, Steinberg SM, Lack EE. Histopathology of benign versus malignant sympathoadrenal paragangliomas: clinicopathologic study of 120 cases including unusual histologic features. Hum Pathol 1990;21:1168–1180.
130. Medeiros LJ, Katsas GG, Balogh K. Brown fat and adrenal pheochromocytoma: association or coincidence? Hum Pathol 1985;16:970–972.
131. Medeiros LJ, Wolf BC, Balogh K, Federman M. Adrenal pheochromocytoma: a clinicopathologic review of 60 cases. Hum Pathol 1985;16:580–589.
132. Melicow MM. One hundred cases of pheochromocytoma (107 tumors) at the Columbia-Presbyterian Medical Center, 1926–1976: a clinicopathologic analysis. Cancer 1977;40:1987–2004.
133. Modlin IM, Farndon JR, Shepherd A, et al. Phaeochromocytomas in 72 patients: clinical and diagnostic features, treatment, and long term results. Br J Surg 1979;66:456–465.
134. Padberg B-C, Garbe E, Achilles E, et al. Adrenomedullary hyperplasia and phaeochromocytoma. DNA cytomorphometric findings in 47 cases. Virchows Arch A Pathol Anat Histopathol 1990;416:443–446.
135. Proye MAC, Fossati P, Fontaine P, et al. Dopamine-secreting pheochromocytoma: an unrecognized entity? Classification of pheochromocytomas according to their type of secretion. Surgery 1986;100:1154–1161.
136. Ramsay JA, Asa SL, van Nostrand AWP, et al. Lipid degeneration in pheochromocytomas mimicking adrenal cortical tumors. Am J Surg Pathol 1987;11:480–486.
137. Samaan NA, Hickey RC, Shutts PE. Diagnosis, localization, and management of pheochromocytoma: pitfalls and follow-up in 41 patients. Cancer 1988;62:2451–2460.
138. Sheps SG, Jiang N-S, Klee GG, van Heerden JA. Recent developments in the diagnosis and treatment of pheochromocytomas. Mayo Clin Proc 1990;65:88–95.
139. Steinhoff MM, Wells SA Jr, Deschryver-Kecskemeti K. Stromal amyloid in pheochromocytomas. Hum Pathol 1992;23:33–36.
140. Stenstrom G, Svardsudd K. Pheochromocytoma in Sweden 1958–1981: an analysis of the National Cancer Registry data. Acta Med Scand 1986;220:225–232.
141. Sutton MGS, Sheps SG, Lie JT. Prevalence of clinically unsuspected pheochromocytoma. Review of a 50-year autopsy series. Mayo Clin Proc 1981;56:354–360.
142. Swenson SJ, Brown ML, Sheps SG, et al. Use of ^{131}I-MIGB scintigraphy in the evaluation of suspected pheochromocytoma. Mayo Clin Proc 1985;60:299–304.
143. Van Heerden JA, Sheps SG, Hamberger B, et al. Pheochromocytoma: current status and changing trends. Surgery 1982;91:367–373.
144. Webb TA, Sheps SG, Carney JA. Differences between sporadic pheochromocytoma and pheochromocytoma in multiple endocrine neoplasia, type 2. Am J Surg Pathol 1980;4:121–126.
145. Welbourn RB. Early surgical history of phaeochromocytoma. Br J Surg 1987;74:594–596.

146. Brodeur GM. Molecular pathology of human neuroblastomas. Semin Diagn Pathol 1994;11:118–125.
147. Brodeur GM, Nakagawara A. Molecular basis of clinical heterogeneity in neuroblastoma. Am J Surg Pathol 1992;14:111–116.
148. Brodeur GM, Seeger RC, Barrett A, et al. International criteria for diagnosis, staging, and response to treatment in patients with neuroblastoma. J Clin Oncol 1988;6:1874–1881.
149. Carlsen NLT. Neuroblastoma: epidemiology and pattern of regression. Problems in interpreting results of mass screening. Am J Pediatr Hematol Oncol 1992;14:103–110.
150. Davis S, Rogers MAM, Pendergrass TW. The incidence and epidemiologic characteristics of neuroblastoma in the United States. Am J Epidemiol 1987;126:1063–1074.
151. Dehner LP. Primitive neuroectodermal tumor and Ewing's sarcoma. Am J Surg Pathol 1993;17:1–13.
152. Evans AE, D'Angio GJ, Randolph J. A proposed staging for children with neuroblastoma. Cancer 1980;27:374–378.
153. Gansler T, Chatten J, Varello M, et al. Flow cytometric DNA analysis of neuroblastoma. Correlation with histology and clinical outcome. Cancer 1986;58:2453–2458.
154. Joshi VV, Chatten J, Sather HN, Shimada H. Evaluation of the Shimada classification in advanced neuroblastoma with a special reference to the mitosis-karyorrhexis index: a report from the Children's Cancer Study Group. Mod Pathol 1991;4:139–148.
155. Joshi VV, Silverman JF. Pathology of neuroblastic tumors. Semin Diagn Pathol 1994;11:107–117.
156. Kaye JA, Warhol MJ, Kretschmar C, Landsberg L, Frei E III. Neuroblastoma in adults. Three case reports and a review of the literature. Cancer 1986;58:1149–1157.
157. Kretschmar CS. Childhood neuroblastoma: clinical and prognostic features. In: Lack EE, ed. Pathology of the adrenal glands. Vol. 14. New York: Churchill Livingstone; 1990:257–275.
158. Lack EE. Neuroblastoma, ganglioneuroblastoma, and related tumors. In: LiVolsi VA, ed. Pathology of adrenal and extra-adrenal paraganglia. Major problems in pathology. Vol. 29. Philadelphia: WB Saunders; 1994:315–370.
159. Look T, Hayes A, Shuster JJ, et al. Clinical relevance of tumor cell ploidy and N-*myc* gene amplification in childhood neuroblastoma: a Pediatric Oncology Group study. J Clin Oncol 1991;9:581–591.
160. McGahey BE, Moriarty AT, Nelson WA, Hull MT. Fine-needle aspiration biopsy of small round blue cell tumors of childhood. Cancer 1992;69:1067–1073.
161. Murphy SB, Cohn SL, Craft AW, et al. Do children benefit from mass screening for neuroblastoma? Consensus statement from the American Cancer Society workshop on neuroblastoma screening. Lancet 1991;337:344–345.
162. Oppedal BR, Storm-Mathisen I, Lie S, Brandtzaeg P. Prognostic factors in neuroblastoma. Clinical, histopathologic, and immunohistochemical features and DNA ploidy in relation to prognosis. Cancer 1988;62: 772–780.
163. Philip T. Overview of current treatment of neuroblastoma. Am J Pediatr Hematol Oncol 1992;14:97–102.
164. Rosen EM, Cassady JR, Frantz CN, et al. Neuroblastoma: the joint Center for Radiation Therapy/Dana-Farber Cancer Institute/Children's Hospital experience. J Clin Oncol 1984;2:719–732.
165. Shimada H, Chatten J, Newton WA, et al. Histopathologic prognostic factors in neuroblastic tumors: definition of subtypes of ganglioneuroblastoma and an age-linked classification of neuroblastomas. J Natl Cancer Inst 1984;73:405–416.
166. Shochat SJ, Corbelletta NL, Repman MA, Schengrund C-L. A biochemical analysis of thoracic neuroblastomas: a Pediatric Oncology Group Study. J Pediatr Surg 1987;22:660–667.
167. Silverman JF, Dabbs DJ, Ganick DJ, et al. Fine needle aspiration cytology of neuroblastoma, including peripheral neuroectodermal tumor, with immunocytochemical and ultrastructural confirmation. Acta Cytol 1988;32:367–376.
168. Triche TJ. Differential diagnosis of neuroblastoma and related tumors. In: Lack EE, ed. Pathology of the adrenal glands. Vol. 14. New York: Churchill Livingstone; 1990:323–350.
169. Tsuda T, Obara M, Hirano H, et al. Analysis of N-*myc* amplification in relation to disease stage and histologic types in human neuroblastoma. Cancer 1987;60:820–826.
170. Tsuda H, Shimosato Y, Upton MP, et al. Retrospective study on amplification of N-*myc* and c-*myc* genes in pediatric solid tumors and its association with prognosis and tumor differentiation. Lab Invest 1988;59:321–327.
171. Aguirre P, Scully RE. Testosterone-secreting adrenal ganglioneuroma containing Leydig cells. Am J Surg Pathol 1983;7:699–703.
172. Carpenter WB, Kernohan JW. Retroperitoneal ganglioneuromas and neurofibromas: a clinicopathological study. Cancer 1963;16:788–797.
173. Fletcher CDM, Fernando IN, Braimbridge MV, et al. Malignant nerve sheath tumor arising in a ganglioneuroma. Histopathology 1988;12:445–454.
174. Ghali VS, Gold JE, Vincent RA, Cosgrove JM. Malignant peripheral nerve sheath tumor arising spontaneously from retroperitoneal ganglioneuroma: a case report, review of the literature, and immunohistochemical study. Hum Pathol 1992;23:72–75.
175. Hayes FA, Green AA, Rao BN. Clinical manifestations of ganglioneuroma. Cancer 1989;63:1211–1214.
176. Keller SM, Papazoglou S, McKeever P, et al. Late occurrence of malignancy in a ganglioneuroma 19 years following radiation therapy to a neuroblastoma. J Surg Oncol 1984;25:227–231.
177. Ricci A Jr, Parham DM, Woodruff JM, et al. Malignant peripheral nerve sheath tumors arising from ganglioneuromas. Am J Surg Pathol 1984;8:19–29.
178. Fernando PB, Cooray GH, Thanabalasundram RS. Adrenal pheochromocytoma with neuroblastomatous elements: report of a case with autopsy. Arch Pathol 1951;52:182–188.
179. Franquemont DW, Mills SE, Lack EE. Immunohistochemical detection of neuroblastomatous foci in composite adrenal pheochromocytoma–neuroblastoma. Am J Clin Pathol 1994;102:163–170.
180. Layfield LJ, Glasgow BJ, Du Puis MH, Bhuta S. Aspiration cytology and immunohistochemistry of a pheochromocytoma–ganglioneuroma of the adrenal gland. Acta Cytol 1987;31:33–39.
181. Lewis D, Geschickter CF. Tumors of the sympathetic nervous system. Arch Surg 1934;28:16–58.
182. Nakagawara A, Ikeda K, Tsuneyoshi M, et al. Malignant pheochromocytoma with ganglioneuroblastomatous elements in a patient with von Recklinghausen's disease. Cancer 1985;55:2794–2798.
183. Tischler AS, Dayal Y, Balogh K, et al. The distribution of immunoreactive chromogranins, S-100, and vasoactive intestinal peptide in compound tumors of the adrenal medulla. Hum Pathol 1987;18:909–917.
184. Trump DL, Livingston JN, Baylin SB. Watery diarrhea syndrome in an adult with ganglioneuroma–pheochromocytoma: identification of vasoactive intestinal peptide, calcitonin, and catecholamines in assessment of their biologic activity. Cancer 1977;40:1526–1532.
185. Wahl HR, Robinson D. Neuroblastoma of the mediastinum with pheochromoblastomatous elements. Arch Pathol 1943;35:571–578.
186. Carstens PHB, Kuhns JG, Ghazi C. Primary malignant melanomas of the lung and adrenal. Hum Pathol 1984;15:910–914.
187. Das Gupta T, Brasfield RD, Paglia MA. Primary melanomas in unusual sites. Surg Gynecol Obstet 1969;128:841–844.
188. Sasidharan K, Babu AS, Pandey AP, et al. Primary melanoma of the adrenal gland: a case report. J Urol 1977;117:663–665.
189. Travis WD, Oertel JE, Lack EE. Miscellaneous tumors and tumefactive lesions of the adrenal gland. In: Lack EE, ed. Pathology of the adrenal glands. Vol. 14. New York: Churchill Livingstone; 1990:351–378.
190. Bauduer F, Delmer A, Le Tourneau, et al. Primary adrenal lymphoma. Acta Hematol 1992;88:213–215.
191. Harris GJ, Tio FO, von Hoff DD. Primary adrenal lymphoma. Cancer 1989;63:799–803.
192. Hayes JA, Christensen OE. Primary adrenal lymphoma. J Pathol Bacteriol 1961;82:193–219.
193. Ohsawa M, Tomita Y, Hashimoto M, et al. Malignant lymphoma of the adrenal gland: its possible correlation with Epstein–Barr virus. Mod Pathol 1996;9:534–543.
194. Schnitzer B, Smid D, Lloyd RV. Primary T-cell lymphoma of the adrenal glands with adrenal insufficiency. Hum Pathol 1986;17:634–636.
195. Shea TC, Spark R, Kane B, Lange RF. Non-Hodgkin's lymphoma limited to the adrenal gland with adrenal insufficiency. Am J Med 1985;78:711–714.
196. Sparagana M. Addison's disease due to reticulum-cell sarcoma apparently confined to the adrenals. J Am Geriatr Soc 1970;18:550–554.
197. Bennett BD, McKenna TJ, Hough AJ, et al. Adrenal myelolipoma associated with Cushing's disease. Am J Clin Pathol 1980;73:443–447.
198. Gee WF, Chikos PM, Greaves JP, et al. Adrenal myelolipoma. Urology 1975;5:562–566.
199. Olsson CA, Krane RJ, Klugo RC, Selikowitz SM. Adrenal myelolipoma. Surgery 1973;73:665–670.
200. Page DL, DeLellis RA, Hough AJ. Myelolipoma and related lesions. In: Page DL, DeLellis RA, Hough AJ, eds. Tumors of the adrenal gland.

Fascicle 23, second series. Washington, DC: Armed Forces Institute of Pathology; 1986:162–182.

201. Craig JR, Hart WR. Extragenital adenomatoid tumor: evidence for the mesothelial theory of origin. Cancer 1979;43:1678–1681.
202. Simpson PR. Adenomatoid tumor of the adrenal gland. Arch Pathol Lab Med 1990;114:725–727.
203. Travis WD, Lack EE, Azumi N, et al. Adenomatoid tumor of the adrenal gland with ultrastructural and immunohistochemical demonstration of a mesothelial origin. Arch Pathol Lab Med 1990;114:722–724.
204. Orringer RD, Lynch JA, McDermott WV. Cavernous hemangioma of the adrenal gland. J Surg Oncol 1983;22:106–108.
205. Rothberg M, Bastidas J, Mattey, Bernas E. Adrenal hemangiomas: angiographic appearance of a rare tumor. Radiology 1978;126: 341–344.
206. Vargas AD. Adrenal hemangioma. Urology 1980;16:389–390.
207. Bosco PJ, Silverman ML, Zinman LM. Primary angiosarcoma of adrenal gland presenting as a paraneoplastic syndrome: case report. J Urol 1991;146:1101–1103.
208. Kareti LR, Katlein S, Siew S, Blauvelt A. Angiosarcoma of the adrenal gland. Arch Pathol Lab Med 1988;112:1163–1165.
209. Livaditou A, Alexiou G, Floros D, et al. Epithelioid angiosarcoma of the adrenal gland associated with chronic arsenical intoxication? Pathol Res Pract 1991;187:284–289.
210. Wenig BM, Abbondanzo SL, Heffess CS. Epithelioid angiosarcoma of the adrenal glands. A clinicopathologic study of nine cases with a discussion of the implications of "epithelial-specific" markers. Am J Surg Pathol 1994;18:62–73.
211. Bedard YC, Horvath E, Kovacs K. Adrenal schwannoma with apparent uptake of immunoglobulin. Ultrastruct Pathol 1986;10:505–509.
212. Oliver WR, Reddick RL, Gillespie GY, Siegel GP. Juxtaadenal schwannoma: verification of the diagnosis by immunohistochemistry and ultrastructural studies. J Surg Oncol 1985;30:259–261.
213. Campbell CM, Middleton RG, Rigby OF. Adrenal metastasis in renal cell carcinoma. Urology 1983;21:403–405.
214. Cedermark BJ, Blumenson LE, Pickren JW, Elias EG. The significance of metastases to the adrenal gland from carcinoma of the stomach and esophagus. Surg Gynecol Obstet 1977;145:41–48.
215. Cedermark BJ, Blumenson LE, Pickren JW, et al. The significance of metastasis to the adrenal glands in adenocarcinoma of the colon and rectum. Surg Gynecol Obstet 1977;144:537–546.
216. Foucar E, Dehner LP. Renal cell carcinoma occurring with contralateral adrenal metastasis. Arch Surg 1979;114:959–963.
217. Seidenwurm DJ, Elmer EB, Kaplan LM, et al. Metastases to the adrenal glands and the development of Addison's disease. Cancer 1984;54:552–557.
218. Vieweg WVR, Reitz RE, Weinstein RL. Addison's disease secondary to metastatic carcinoma: an example of adrenocortical and adrenomedullary insufficiency. Cancer 1973;31:1240–1243.
219. Choi SH, Liu K. Leiomyosarcoma of the adrenal gland and its angiographic features: a case report. J Surg Oncol 1981;16:145–148.
220. Lack EE, Graham CW, Azumi N, et al. Primary leiomyosarcoma of the adrenal gland. Case report with immunohistochemical and ultrastructural study. Am J Surg Pathol 1991;15:899–905.
221. Pollock WJ, McConnell CF, Hilton C, Lavine RL. Virilizing Leydig cell adenoma of adrenal gland. Am J Surg Pathol 1986;10:816–822.

HEMATOPOIETIC NEOPLASMS

Scott Ely and April Chiu

INTRODUCTION

The histologic and immunophenotypic features of hematologic neoplasms in the genitorurinary tract (GU) are identical to those in other sites. Because most represent secondary involvement, clinical history is of great help in diagnosis. As in other sites, hematologic neoplasms in the GU are mostly B-cell non-Hodgkin lymphomas (B-NHLs); the majority are diffuse large B-cell lymphoma (DLBCL) or extranodal marginal zone lymphoma (EMZL, also referred to as mucosa-associated lymphoid tissue [MALT] lymphoma).[1]

HEMATOLOGIC NEOPLASMS BY SITE

KIDNEY AND URETER

Renal involvement by NHL is found in up to 50% of autopsied secondary cases.[2,3] Primary renal lymphoma (PRL), on the other hand, is extraordinarily rare, representing 0.7% of all extranodal lymphomas in North America.[4,5] Up to 43% of PRL patients have bilateral involvement. Almost all PRLs are B-NHLs. DLBCL is by far the most common type (64–75%). Rare cases of 'plasmacytoma' have been reported but are typically associated with bony lesions and, therefore, usually are best classified as extramedullary involvement by multiple myeloma.

Secondary involvement of a ureter by NHL has been reported in 16% of carefully autopsied NHL patients.[2,3] Primary lymphoma of the ureter has been reported, but is very rare.

URINARY BLADDER

Secondary bladder involvement has been documented in 10–25% of autopsied patients with NHL. Primary bladder lymphoma (PBL) represents only 15% of bladder lymphomas.[6-8] In contrast to primary NHL in other sites, which has a slight male predominance, PBLs are more common in women, with a male-to-female ratio (M:F) of 1:6.5. EMZL is by far the most common type.[6] Given the well-documented occurrence of EMZL arising in the background of infection in the stomach and skin, the female predilection likely reflects the higher incidence of urinary tract infections in women. DLBCL is also seen, sometimes arising from preexisting EMZL.[7]

Unlike primary bladder lymphoma, secondary bladder involvement by lymphomas is slightly more common in male patients (M:F = 1.5:1), again, most likely reflecting the slight male sex predilection for most NHLs.[8]

URETHRA

The urethra is the least common site of GU lymphoma. Most patients are described in isolated case reports. Like bladder lymphomas, primary urethral lymphomas are more common in female than in male patients (M:F = 1:2–3), again likely reflecting the female predilection for infections at this site.[9]

PROSTATE

Lymphoma involving the prostate is rare and usually secondary spread from other sites. Even so, <1% of patients with NHL have prostatic involvement.[10] The most common histologic subtypes, in decreasing order of frequency, are DLBCL, chronic lymphocytic leukemia/small lymphocytic lymphoma (CLL/SLL), and follicular lymphoma (FL) in both primary and secondary forms.[11]

TESTIS

Testicular lymphoma is usually secondary.[12,13] However, the testis is more commonly involved by lymphomas than are other GU sites. Testicular lymphoma accounts for 5% of testicular neoplasms and represents the most common primary and secondary testicular tumor in patients over 60 years of age.[13-15] Other extranodal locations commonly involved by primary testicular lymphomas, either at presentation or recurrence, include the contralateral testicle, central nervous system, and skin. The most common histologic type is DLBCL in adults and Burkitt lymphoma (BL) in children.[12,15–17]

Acute leukemia, especially precursor B- or T-cell acute lymphoblastic leukemia/lymphoma (ALL/LBL), commonly involves the testis; the incidence ranges between 40% and 65% in autopsy studies.[18,19] A testicular biopsy may detect leukemic infiltrates in 5–10% of ALL patients and is predictive of subsequent systemic relapse.[20–22] Bilateral involvement is common.

ADRENAL GLAND

Systemic NHL involves the adrenal in 25% of patients.[23,24] Massive bilateral adrenal involvement may result in Addison's disease. Primary adrenal lymphoma is extremely rare.[25] The majority of the reported cases are bilateral, among which 50% manifest signs of adrenal insufficiency, even with small tumors. The most common type is DLBCL.

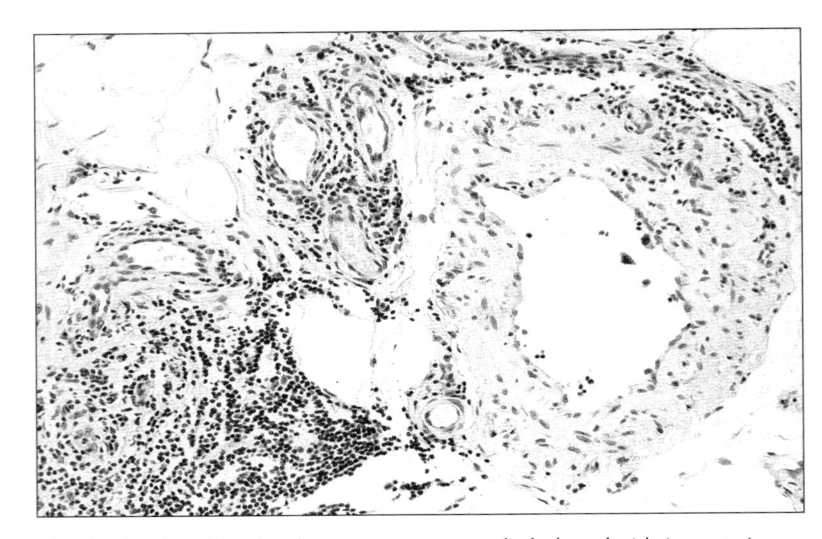

Fig. 14.1 Outside the disease setting, very little lymphoid tissue exists in the genitourinary tract. Normal lymphoid tissue is limited to sparse infiltrates composed of small lymphocytes in the subcapsular area of the prostate and the vascular pole of the testis.[26] The normal testicular lymphoid tissue, shown here, consists primarily of T cells. Lymphoid follicles are not seen. (Hematoxylin–eosin, 100×.)

NORMAL LYMPHOID TISSUE IN THE GENITOURINARY TRACT

(Figs 14.1 & 14.2)

HEMATOPOIETIC NEOPLASMS ENCOUNTERED IN THE GENITOURINARY TRACT

B-NHLs are the most commonly encountered hematopoietic neoplasms in the GU. Diagnostic criteria for hematopoietic neoplasms of all types are delineated in the World Health Organization (WHO) classification.[27] The diagnostic modalities available for GU biopsies are typically limited to histology and immunohistochemistry (IHC).[28]

The diagnostic algorithm for hematopoietic cancers in the GU does not differ from that in lymph nodes or other extranodal sites. A key concept is that biologic behavior – and therefore the treatment – is dictated by the intrinsic biology of the neoplasm, not by the site of presentation. As such, distinction between 'leukemia' and 'lymphoma' is of little consequence. Stage for stage, the chemotherapeutic treatment for DLBCL of the bladder is no different from that for nodal DLBCL. Likewise, CLL and SLL are now known to be the same disease, the only difference being the site of initial detection. Thus, even when CLL presents in the prostate, the diagnostic terminology and general therapeutic approach are essentially unaltered.

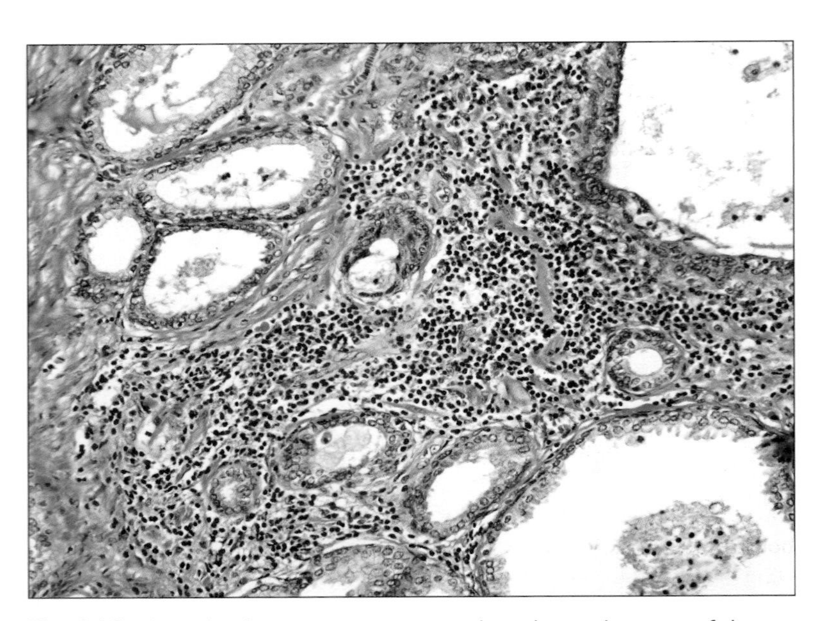

Fig. 14.2 Lymphoid tissue is common in the subcapsular zone of the prostate. Some degree of chronic inflammatory infiltration is virtually a universal feature of the aging prostate.

With the exception of follicular lymphoma (FL), which is characteristically nodular, and rare cases of mantle cell lymphoma (MCL), all commonly encountered NHLs are diffuse. Although great emphasis has been placed on the nodular versus diffuse distinction in the past, this feature is now considered to have limited diagnostic utility. Furthermore, the pattern of infiltration cannot always be assessed in small biopsies. The diagnosis ultimately depends on cytologic features and the immunophenotype. (Figs 14.3 & 14.4)

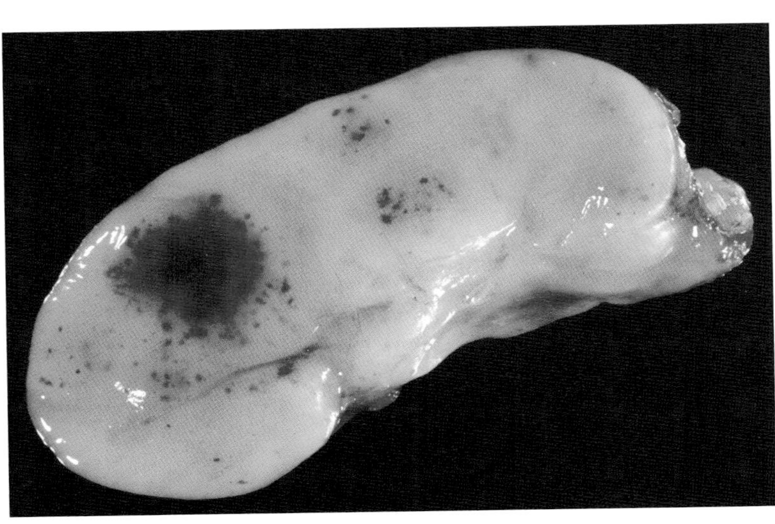

Fig. 14.3 With rare exceptions (e.g. nodular sclerosing Hodgkin lymphoma, which is white and fibrotic), all lymphomas have the same 'fish flesh' gross appearance.

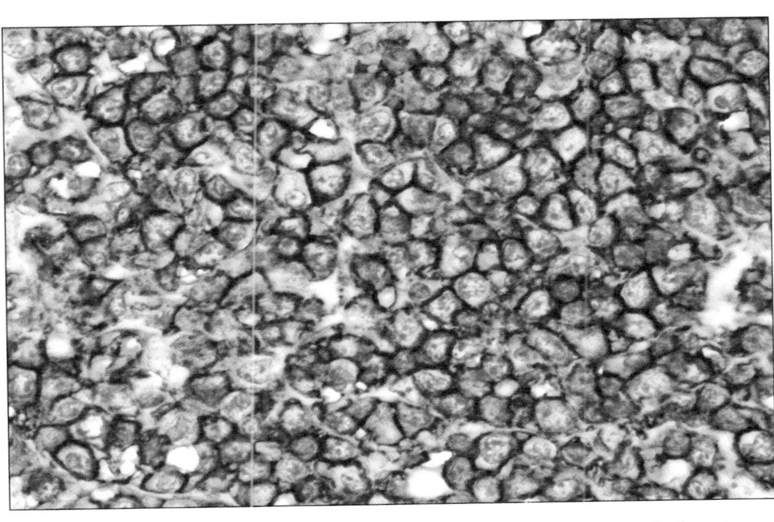

Fig. 14.5 This immunohistochemical stain (same specimen of chronic lymphocytic leukemia as in Fig. 14.15) for CD20, a pan-B-cell antigen, shows strong membranous expression. (CD20 immunohistochemistry, 400×.)

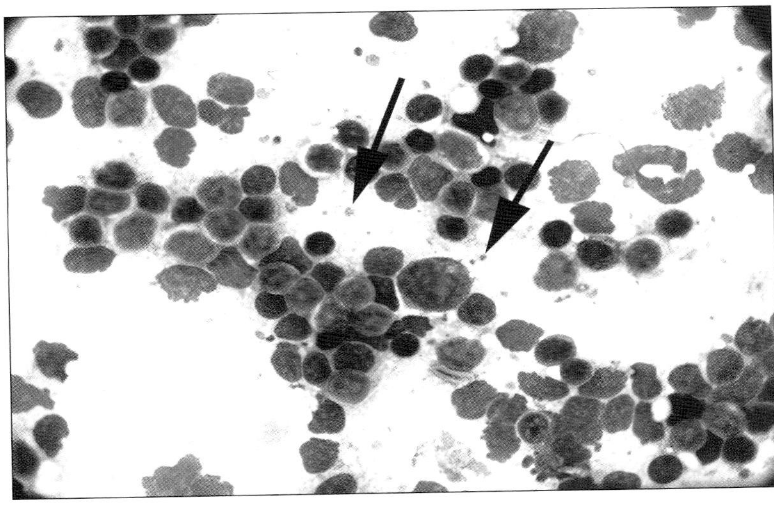

Fig. 14.4 Smeared touch preparation, bladder biopsy (Diff-Quick, 1000×). When a 'fish flesh' appearance is noted in a gross specimen, a smear preparation, performed by sliding the specimen across the glass, shows dyshesive cells with lymphoid morphology and lymphoglandular bodies in the background (arrows); these findings are consistent with a lymphoid lesion rather than a carcinoma.

LOW-GRADE B-CELL LYMPHOMAS

DIAGNOSTIC ALGORITHM FOR LOW-GRADE B-CELL LYMPHOMAS

A low-grade lymphoma is suspected based on the presence of a monotonous infiltrate composed of small mature-appearing lymphocytes with clumped chromatin. The B-cell origin can be confirmed with IHC by expression of a pan-B-cell antigen, such as CD20 or PAX5, by the neoplastic cells.

In small biopsies, monotypic immunoglobulin light chain expression can sometimes be used to establish clonality, and thus B-cell neoplasia. Most low-grade B-NHLs express surface immunoglobulin, which can be difficult to detect in paraffin-embedded biopsies because of background immunoglobulin staining. Cytoplasmic immunoglobulin (cIg) is usually a more satisfactory target for paraffin IHC, but only B-cell lymphomas with plasmacytoid differentiation express cIg. The normal ratio of $\kappa : \lambda$ cIg light chain-bearing cells is ~3 : 1 in benign infiltrates. A significant alteration of the ratio suggests a B-cell lymphoma. (Fig. 14.6)

Another marker that can be quite useful is membranous CD43. This antigen is not expressed in any benign B cells. So, in a biopsy that might otherwise be too small to provide a conclusive diagnosis, clear and unequivocal co-expression of CD43 along with a pan-B-cell antigen is diagnostic of a lymphoma. CD43 also can be of use in lymphoma classification: CD43 is positive in 100% of BLs, >90% of CLLs and MCLs, 30% of EMZLs, and only rarely in FL.[29] (Figs 14.5 & 14.6)

To assign a diagnostic category, the critical next step is assessment of CD5 expression. Membranous CD5 is expressed by CLL and MCL. Although neoplastic marginal zone cells are CD5–, all EMZLs contain scattered CD5+ T cells in the background).

CLL and MCL can then be distinguished on the basis of membranous CD23 (CLL+, MCL–) and nuclear cyclin D1/bcl-1 (CLL–, MCL+) protein expression by IHC.

If the low-grade lymphoma cells lack expression of CD5, nuclear bcl-6 and membranous CD10 expression can be used to distinguish FL (bcl-6+ in all cases; CD10+ in two-thirds of cases), from EMZL (bcl-6– and CD10– in all cases). Although BL cells are also CD10+ and bcl-6+, they are easily distinguished from FL on the basis of morphology and CD43 expression (see below). Exceptions to these rules are rare.

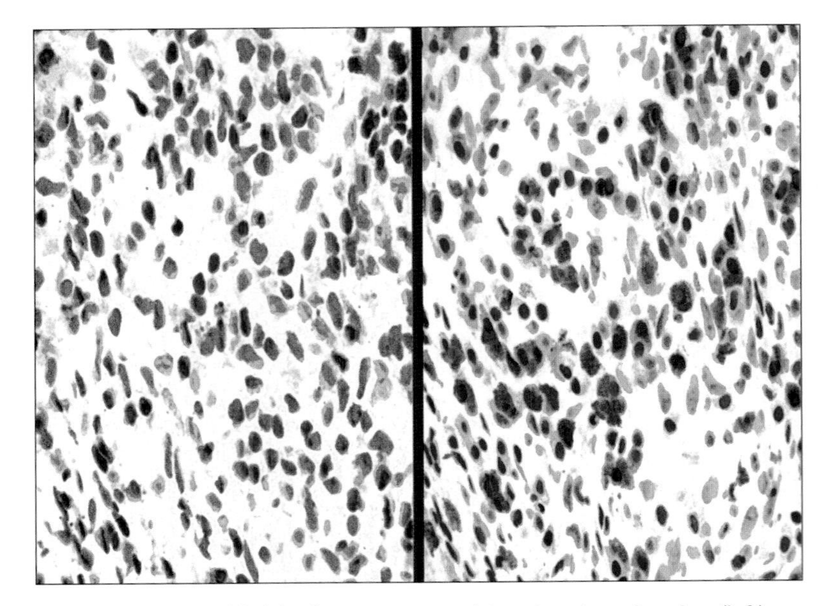

Fig. 14.6 In this bladder biopsy, immunohistochemistry for cIgκ (left) shows only rare positive cells. Stain for cIgλ (right) shows many plasmacytoid cells with strong cytoplasmic immunoglobulin (cIg) λ expression (red). The κ : λ ratio is greatly skewed in favor of cIgλ+ cells, a finding that denotes a clonal population and thus is diagnostic of a B-cell neoplasm. (cIgκ [left], cIgλ [right] immunohistochemistry, 400×.)

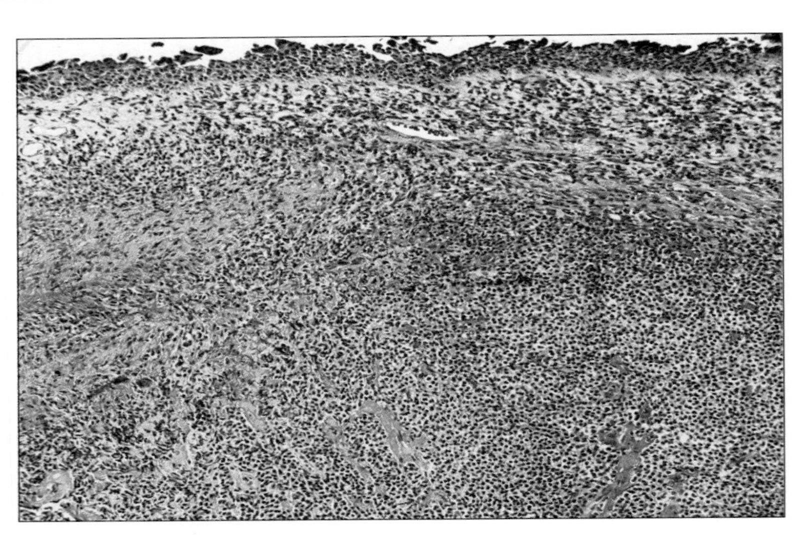

Fig. 14.7 In the bladder, extranodal marginal zone lymphoma is often most conspicuous in the lamina propria, underlying eroded or ulcerated transitional epithelium. Lymphoepithelial lesions (LELs) are best detected with pan-B-cell immunohistochemistry and careful assessment of whether the B cells lie within the epithelium (typical of LEL) or deep to the basement membrane (typical of benign). Between the epithelium and the deeper area of most dense infiltration, a zone of plasmacytoid differentiation often is found. (Hematoxylin–eosin, 200×.)

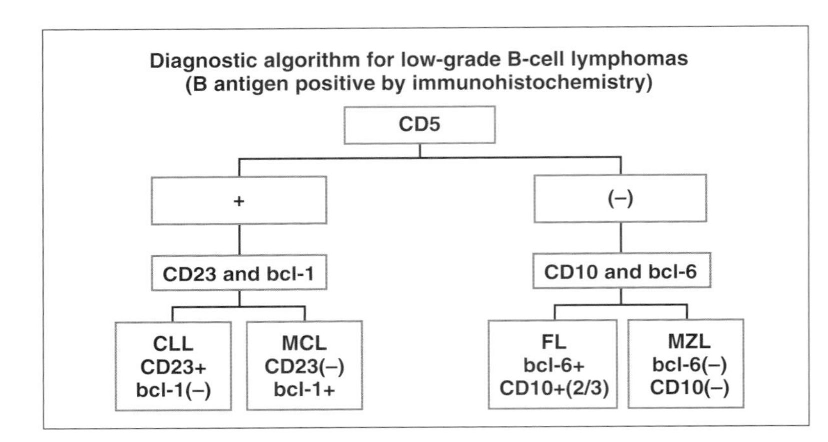

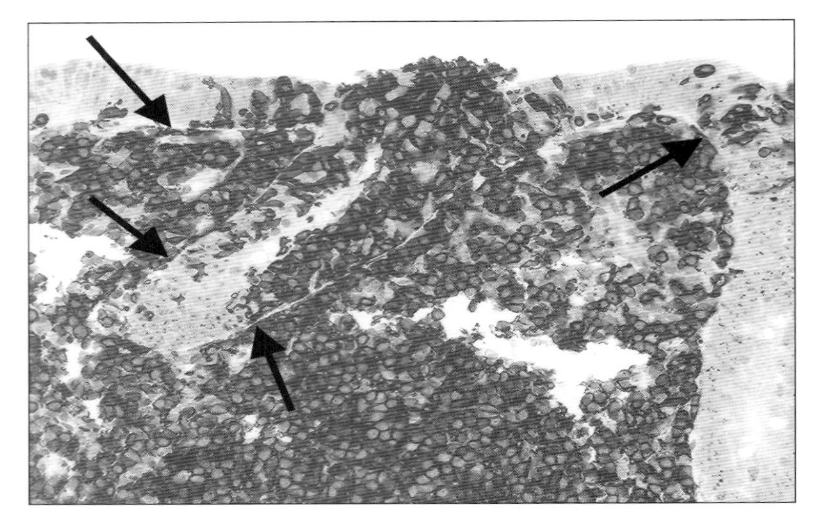

Fig. 14.8 Extranodal marginal zone lymphoma. There is a copious B-cell (CD20+) infiltrate deep to the epithelium; however, the B cells also form intraepithelial aggregates (lymphoepithelial lesions [LELs]); LELs are most easily detected by making a careful assessment of where the B cells are in relation to the basement membrane (arrows). (CD20 immunohistochemistry, 400×.)

EXTRANODAL MARGINAL ZONE LYMPHOMA/LYMPHOPLASMACYTIC LYMPHOMA

EMZL (also referred to as MALT lymphoma) can occur in any epithelial site. In the GU, it is most common in the bladder. Although the lymphoepithelial lesions characteristic of EMZL in the stomach are well known, epithelial invasion is not as significant outside the stomach.

EMZL is composed of monocytoid B cells, 'centrocyte-like' cells, or a mixture of the two. The EMZL cells are positive for pan-B-cell antigens, negative for CD5, CD10, CD23, and bcl-6, and are CD43+ in 30% of cases.[29]

Most cases formerly described as 'lymphoplasmacytoid' or 'lymphoplasmacytic' lymphoma (LPL),[27] are now considered to be EMZLs with plasmacytoid differentiation. The LPL designation is generally not appropriate for GU lesions. (Figs 14.7–14.14)

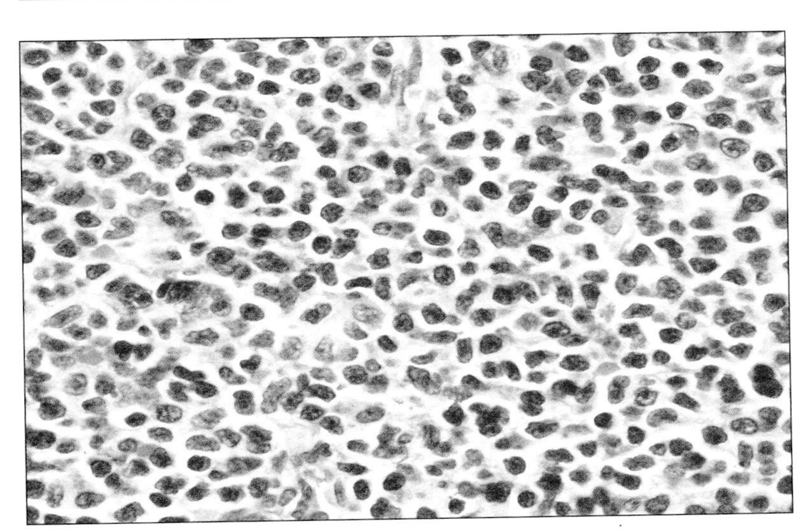

Fig. 14.9 'Centrocyte-like' extranodal marginal zone lymphoma (EMZL) cells are small with little cytoplasm and irregular, 'cleaved' nuclear contours. These cells are thought to be derived from bcl-6– post-germinal center memory B cells. By contrast, true (benign) centrocytes are bcl-6+ germinal center cells ('cleaved cells'). 'Centrocyte-like' EMZL cells are cytologically similar to benign centrocytes, except that their nuclear contours are not as irregular. (Hematoxylin–eosin, 400×.)

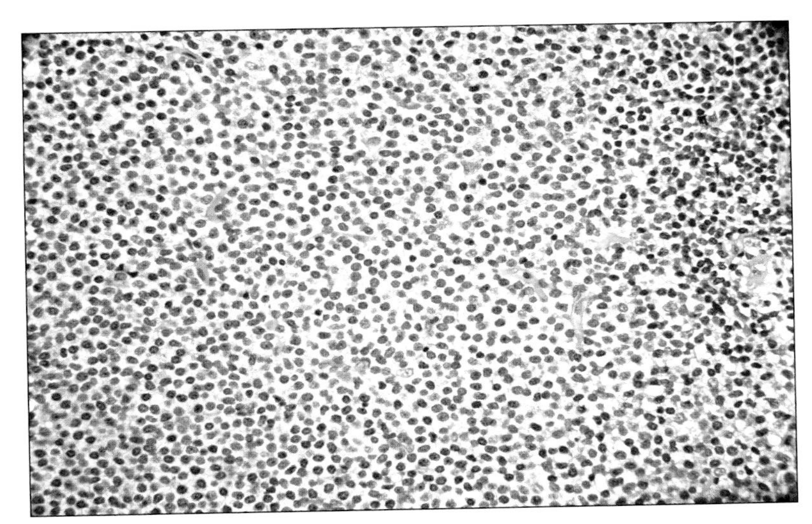

Fig. 14.10 In this bladder biopsy, a monotonous infiltrate of small monocytoid B lymphocytes is present, another appearance typical of extranodal marginal zone lymphoma. (Hematoxylin–eosin, 200×.)

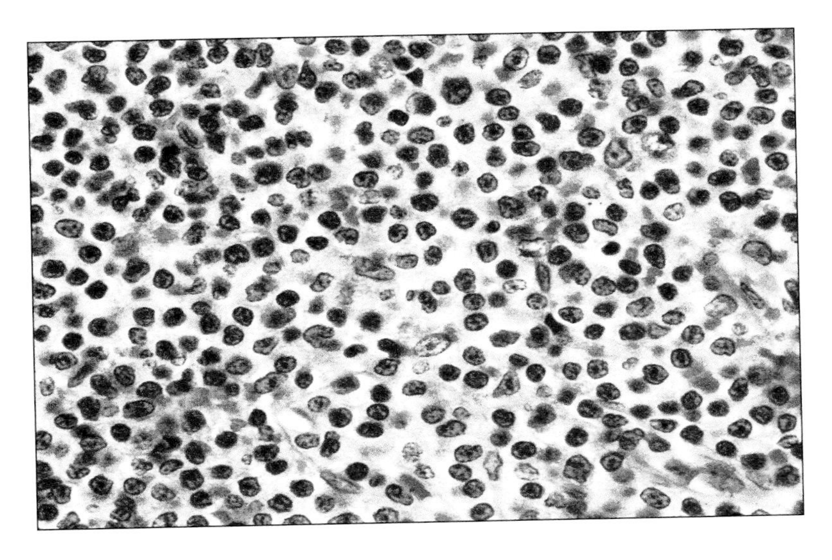

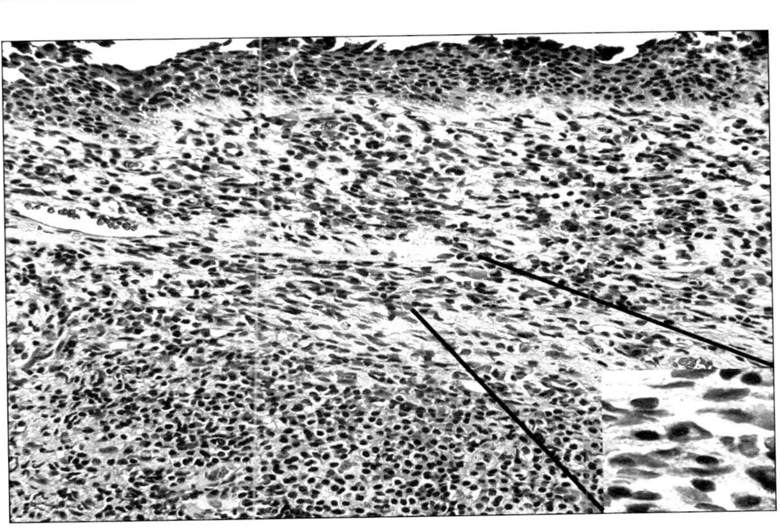

Fig. 14.12 In extranodal marginal zone lymphoma, there is often an area of plasmacytoid differentiation between the epithelium (top) and the deeper, more dense area of infiltration. The plasmacytoid component shows cytoplasmic immunoglobulin light chain restriction (see Fig. 14.6), a finding that both proves clonality and is pathognomonic of plasmacytoid differentiation in a low-grade B-cell non-Hodgkin lymphoma. (Hematoxylin–eosin, 400×, inset 1000×.)

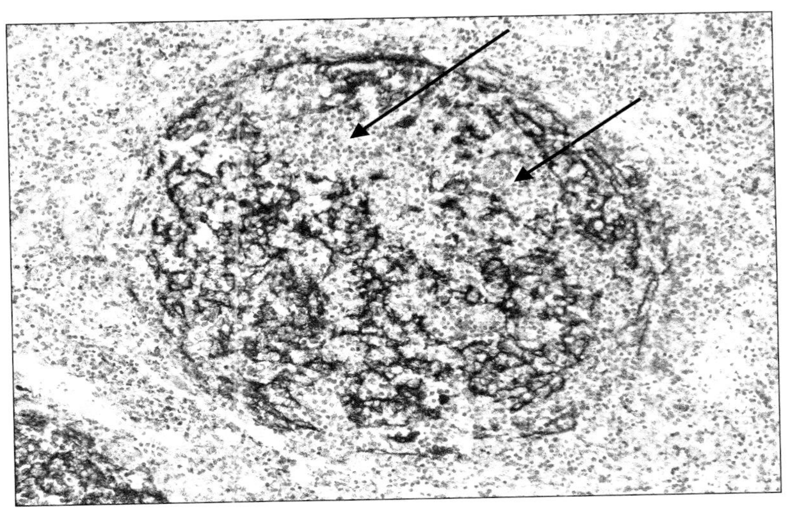

Fig. 14.13 Extranodal marginal zone lymphoma (EMZL) cells may surround and invade benign background follicles. This behavior can impart a pseudofollicular appearance at low power. Immunohistochemistry (IHC) for CD21, which highlights follicular dendritic cells (FDCs) of benign germinal centers, can distinguish follicular invasion from true nodular growth. In this bladder biopsy with EMZL, the FDC meshwork is typically dense and uniform, but areas where it is absent (arrows) represent follicular invasion by lymphoma cells. (CD21 IHC, 100×.)

Fig. 14.11 Monocytoid B cells with the characteristic abundant pale-staining cytoplasm, reminiscent of myeloid-derived monocytes. Due to the greater amount of cytoplasm, the nuclei are farther apart than in a typical small lymphocyte infiltrate. (Hematoxylin–eosin, 400×.)

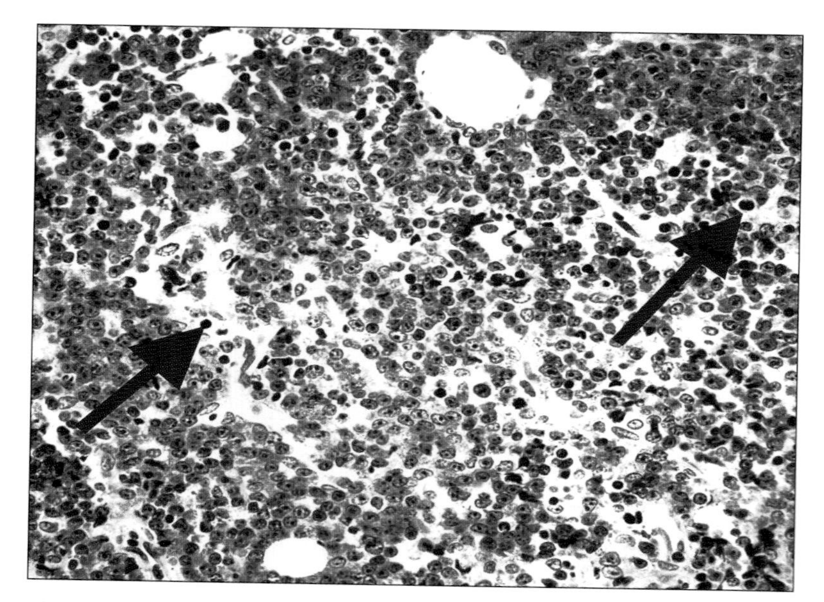

Fig. 14.14 Extranodal marginal zone lymphoma (EMZL) is low grade by definition, and the World Health Organization classification specifically discourages grading.[1,27] If a lymphoma consists of sheets of large, transformed cells outside germinal centers, the correct diagnosis is diffuse large B-cell lymphoma (DLBCL), regardless of the presence of some EMZL-like features. This bladder biopsy with DLBCL shows large transformed cells with little cytoplasm, vesicular nuclei, mitotic figures (arrows) and prominent nucleoli; contrast this appearance with that of EMZL. (Hematoxylin–eosin, 100×.)

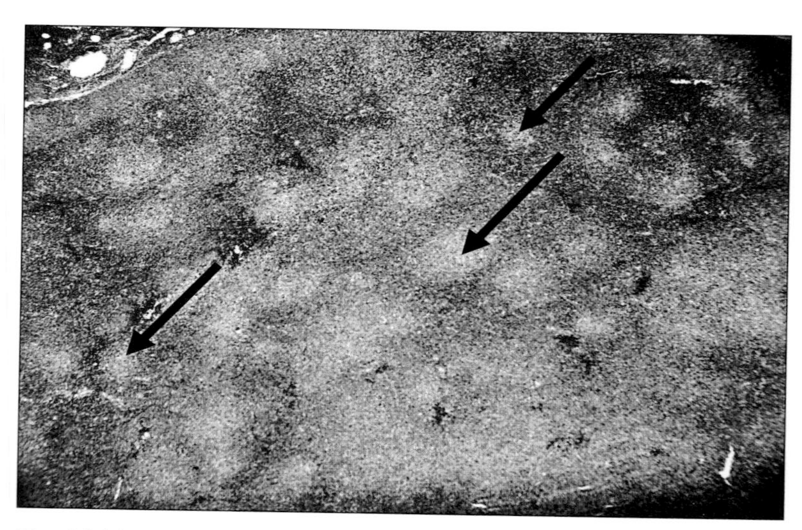

Fig. 14.16 A prostatectomy specimen in a patient with chronic lymphocytic leukemia shows massive involvement. The infiltrate is diffuse, but, at low power, numerous proliferation centers are evident (arrows). Proliferation centers can be distinguished from germinal centers by their vague borders and their component cells, which are variable in size but have generally round nuclei, unlike germinal center cells. (Hematoxylin–eosin, 40×.)

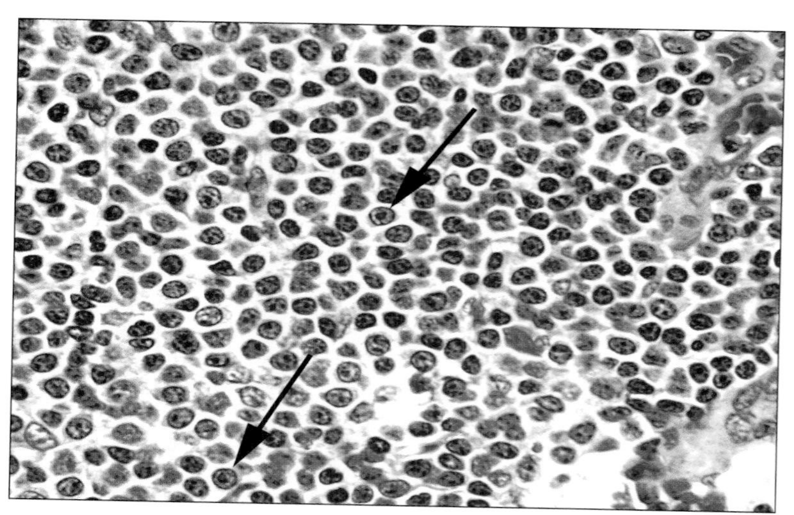

Fig. 14.15 A case of chronic lymphocytic leukemia involving the prostate. Unlike the mixed infiltrate seen in reactive lymphoid proliferations, the cells are monotonous and small with little cytoplasm, round nuclei, lightly clumped chromatin, and inconspicuous nucleoli. Prolymphocytes (arrows) are scattered throughout. (Hematoxylin–eosin, 400×.)

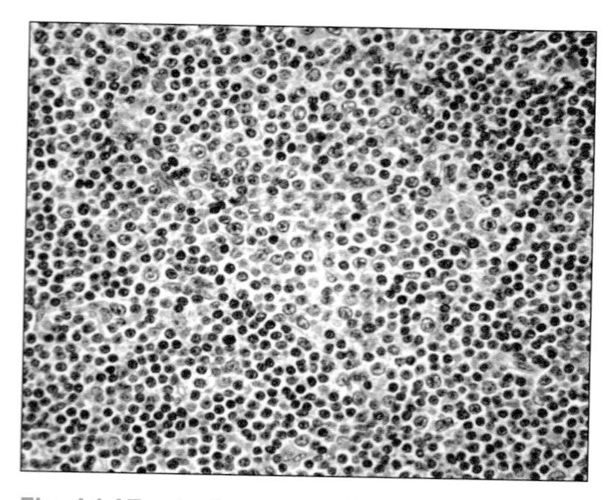

Fig. 14.17 At the center of the image is a proliferation center, paler than the surrounding small chronic lymphocytic leukemia cells. Prolymphocytes (intermediate-sized cells with prominent, large nucleoli) and large transformed lymphocytes are clustered together in proliferation centers. The nuclei of prolymphocytes are rounder than those of germinal center cells. (Hematoxylin–eosin, 400×.)

CHRONIC LYMPHOCYTIC LEUKEMIA/ SMALL LYMPHOCYTIC LYMPHOMA[27,28]

CLL is composed of diffuse sheets of small lymphocytes with little cytoplasm, and round nuclei with clumped chromatin and indistinct nucleoli. The immunophenotype of CLL is distinctive (pan-B antigen+, CD5+, CD23+, cyclin D1–). When a large cell lymphoma is encountered with a similar immunophenotype, it might be a Richter's transformation (i.e. large cell transformation of CLL). (Figs 14.15–14.17)

MANTLE CELL LYMPHOMA

MCL is clinically an intermediate-grade lymphoma. However, due to its histologic resemblance to low-grade NHLs, it is best considered along with them in the differential diagnosis – even though encountered far less frequently (MCL composes only 3–10% of NHLs).[30] MCL is generally diffuse, although the 'mantle zone pattern' and 'nodular pattern' have been described. The immunophenotype is pan-B+, CD5+, CD43+, CD23–, cyclin D1/BCL+.

MCL may rarely transform to a 'blastoid' variant, histologically resembling ALL, or even more rarely to a large cell variant. However, the immunophenotype is nearly identical to that of untransformed MCLs, except that nuclear p53 is expressed. (Figs 14.18 & 14.19)

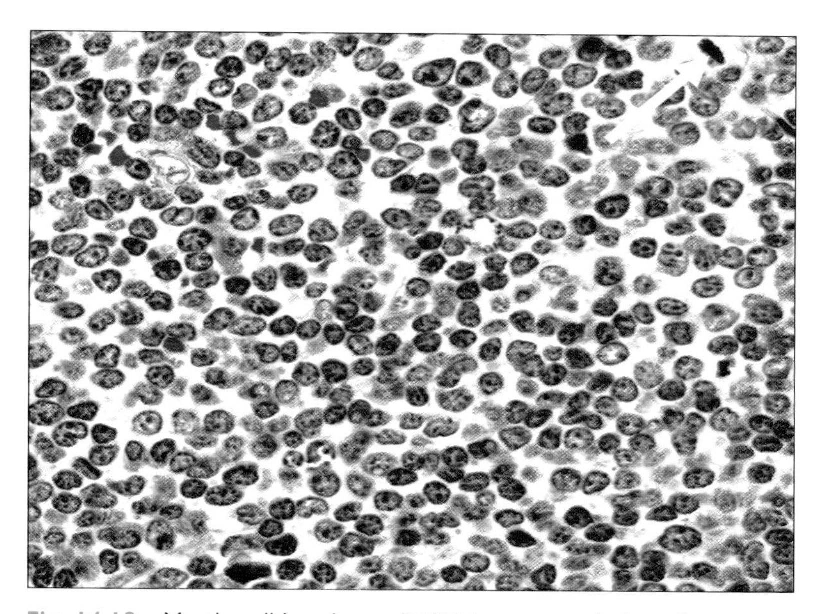

Fig. 14.18 Mantle cell lymphoma (MCL) is composed of small to intermediate-size cells. If difficulty is encountered in deciding on cell size in a monotonous population of lymphocytes, it is best described as 'intermediate'. In such lesions, MCL should be considered. MCL cells have little cytoplasm and mildly irregular nuclear contours (i.e. generally less round than chronic lymphocytic leukemia cells but not as cleaved as follicular lymphoma cells). The chromatin is lightly clumped and nucleoli are indistinct. (Hematoxylin–eosin, 1000×.)

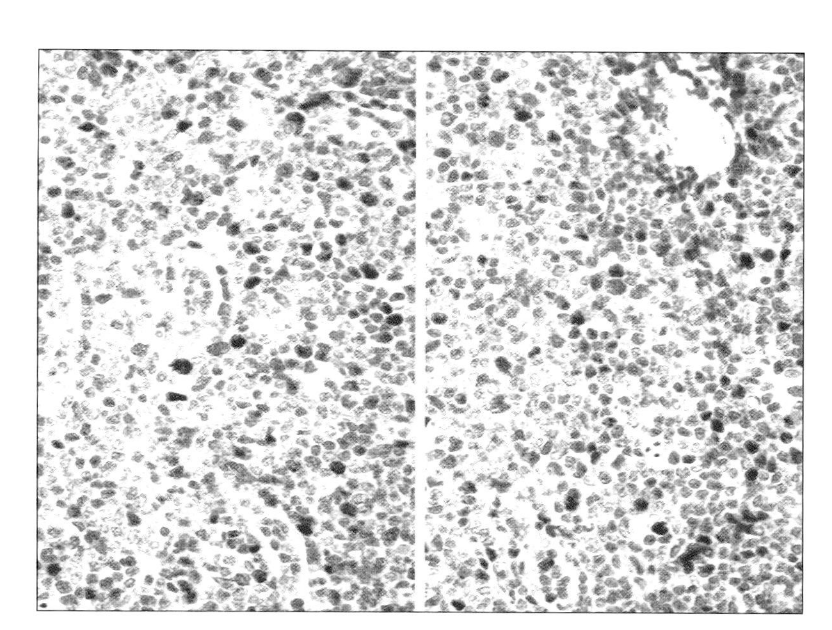

Fig. 14.19 Mantle cell lymphoma (MCL) involving the prostate shows coordinate expression of cyclin D1 (left) and PAX5 (right). Among B-cell-derived neoplasms, only MCL, hairy cell leukemia, and a minority (20%) of plasma cell neoplasms express cyclin D1. Like chronic lymphocytic leukemia cells, MCL cells co-express CD5 and CD43 along with pan-B-cell antigens. However, they are negative for CD23. (Cyclin D1 [left], PAX5 [right] immunohistochemistry, 400×.)

FOLLICULAR LYMPHOMA

FL cells express pan-B-cell antigens and are negative for CD5; they show nuclear expression of the bcl-6 protein and two-thirds of cases show membranous expression of CD10. CD23 expression is variable. CD43 expression is seen only in rare cases of grade 3 FL.[29] (Figs 14.20 & 14.21)

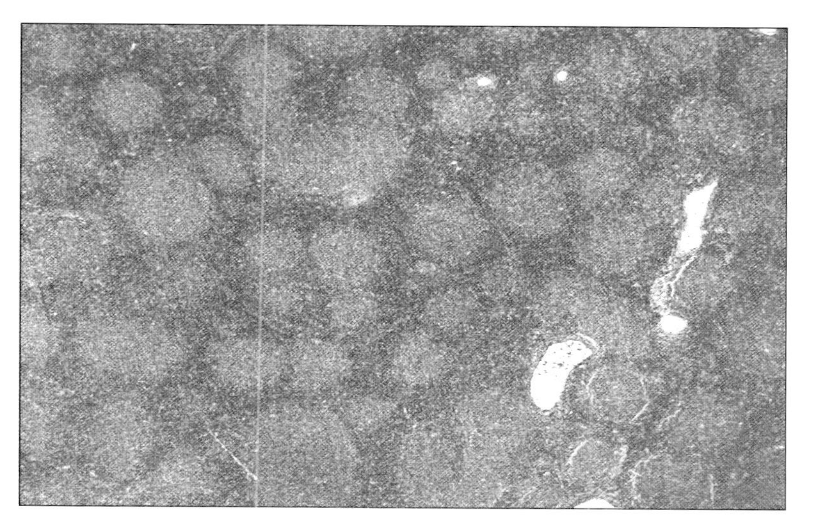

Fig. 14.20 Follicular lymphoma (FL) always shows some degree of nodular architecture. In most cases, the majority of the infiltrate is nodular. Unlike the proliferation centers seen in chronic lymphocytic leukemia, the FL nodules are typically well circumscribed. If a lesion contains diffuse areas composed mainly of large cells, it should be diagnosed as diffuse large B-cell lymphoma, not FL. (Hematoxylin–eosin, 40×.)

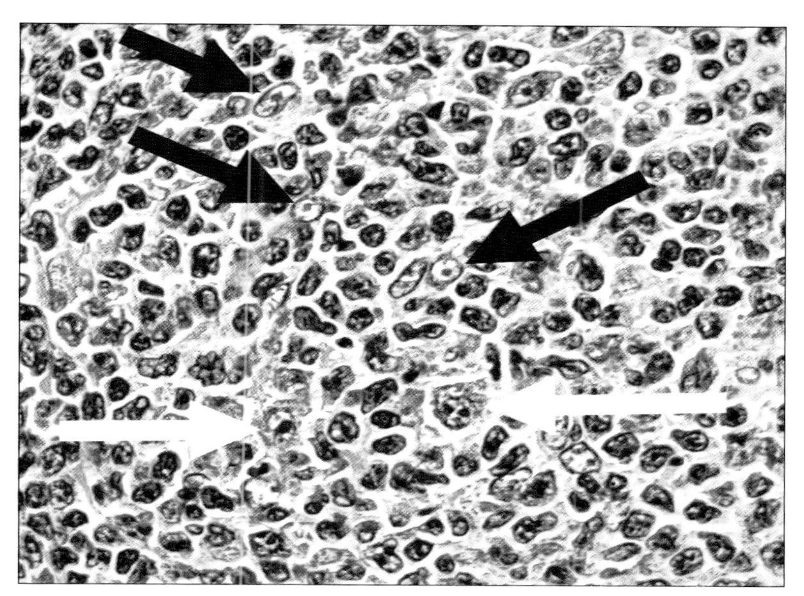

Fig. 14.21 Follicular lymphoma (FL) is composed of a mixture of small cleaved centrocytes and large transformed centroblasts (white arrows). FL is graded by the number of centroblasts per high-power field,[27] and can be estimated as grade 1 (predominantly small cleaved cells), grade 2 (mixed small and large cells), and grade 3 (predominantly large cells). For grading, do not count follicular dendritic cells (black arrows), which have round or ovoid, not irregularly shaped, nuclei and a single punctate red nucleolus. (Hematoxylin–eosin, 1000×.)

HIGH-GRADE B-CELL LYMPHOMAS

DIAGNOSTIC ALGORITHM FOR HIGH-GRADE LYMPHOMAS

A lymphoma is considered to be high grade if, when left untreated, patients typically succumb to the disease in weeks or months. The high-grade B-NHLs include DLBCL, BL, Burkitt-like lymphoma (B-LL), and precursor B-cell ALL. Aside from B-LL, these entities are usually easily distinguished by histology alone. If a precise diagnosis is difficult due to poor fixation or a small limited tissue, a simple immunophenotypic algorithm can be employed.

Starting with a lesion that has high-grade histologic features and shows unequivocal expression of a pan-B-cell antigen (e.g. CD20 or PAX5), terminal deoxynucleotidyl transferase (TdT) is almost always positive in ALL/LBL and is never positive in any other neoplasms, with the rare exception of acute myelogenous leukemia (AML) (<5% of cases).

If the lesion is TdT-negative and composed of medium-sized cells with lightly clumped chromatin (see below), it is BL. If the cells are larger or have vesicular nuclei and prominent nucleoli, it is DLBCL.

If the morphologic features are intermediate between BL and DLBCL, B-LL should be considered. Ki-67 expression is helpful. If the percentage of Ki-67+ cells is >90%, it is best categorized as B-LL. If Ki-67 is expressed by <60% of cells, DLBCL is the best diagnosis.

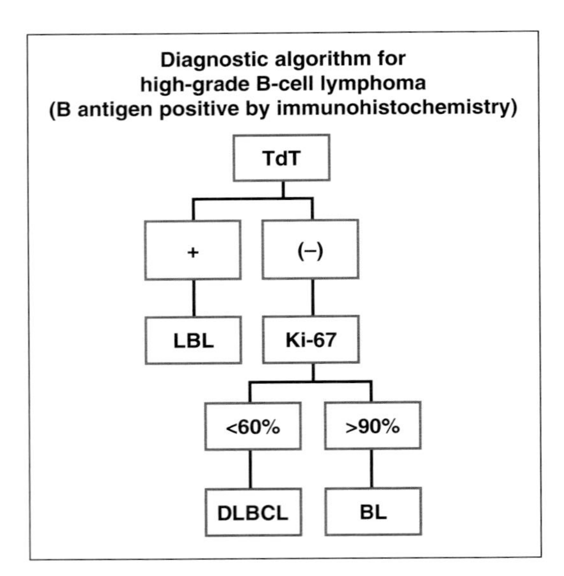

DIFFUSE LARGE B-CELL LYMPHOMA AND BURKITT-LIKE LYMPHOMA

The most commonly encountered high-grade B-cell lymphoma in the GU (as in all other extranodal sites) is DLBCL. On the basis of hematoxylin–eosin (H&E) morphology, it is easily distinguished from the low-grade lymphomas but bears cytologic resemblance to some poorly differentiated carcinomas, especially in a small biopsy where architectural features cannot be appreciated. The diagnosis can be established on the basis of B-cell antigen expression (CD20 or PAX5). Immunohistochemistry for leukocyte common antigen (LCA; CD45) is not recommended, because it is not lineage-specific (e.g. does not distinguish a B-NHL from an extramedullary myeloid tumor) and because it is weak or negative in a significant number of B-NHLs. (Figs 14.22–14.24)

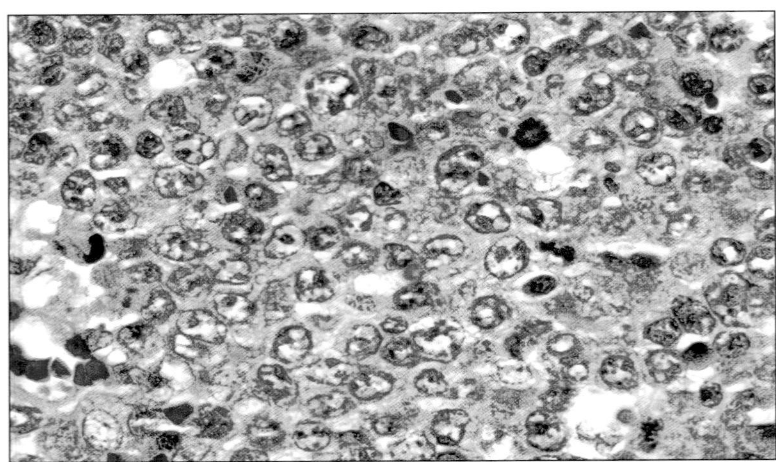

Fig. 14.22 Diffuse large B-cell lymphoma in the kidney is composed of large cells with a moderate amount of pale cytoplasm. Nuclei are ovoid with evenly dispersed (vesicular) chromatin and prominent nucleoli, often resting on the nuclear rim. It is distinguished from the low-grade lymphomas by the chromatin (evenly dispersed instead of clumped) and by nuclear size (usually greater than twice the size of that of a normal lymphocyte). (Hematoxylin–eosin, 1000×.)

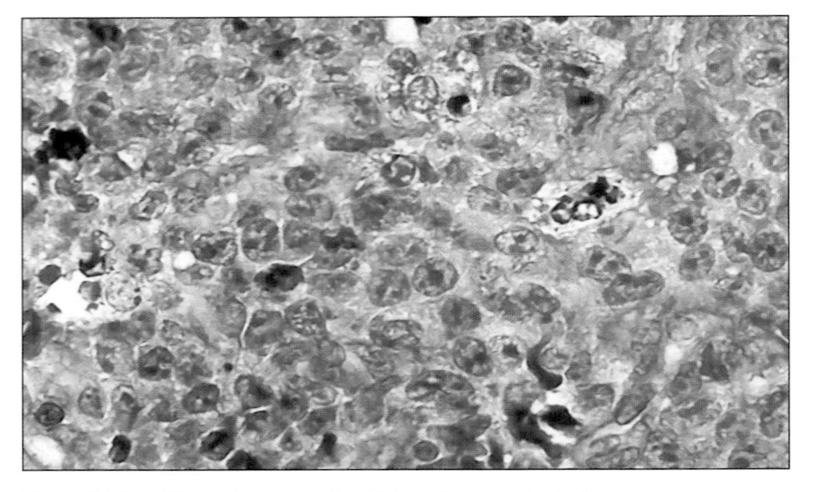

Fig. 14.23 This infiltrate in the kidney has cytologic features intermediate between those of diffuse large B-cell lymphoma (DLBCL) and Burkitt lymphoma (BL). In such cases, the designation Burkitt-like lymphoma (B-LL) should be considered. The cells are intermediate to large in size, with cytologic membranes less distinct than typically encountered in BL. The nuclei are round, like BL, but have prominent nucleoli, like DLBCL. (Hematoxylin–eosin, 400×.)

BURKITT LYMPHOMA

BL is rare in the GU. When present, it is indistinguishable from BL in other sites. BL cells express pan-B-cell antigens and are CD5–, CD10+, CD43+, and bcl-6+. (Figs 14.25–14.27)

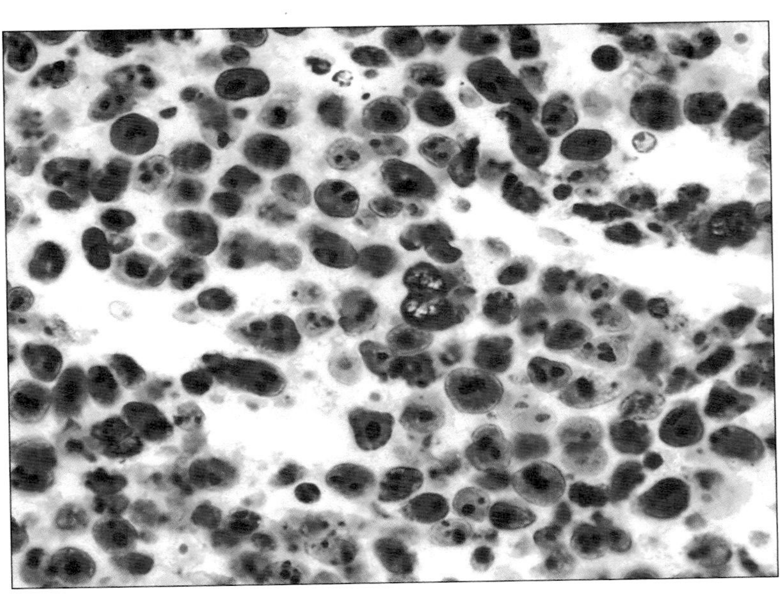

Fig. 14.24 Studies have shown that Burkitt-like lymphomas (B-LLs) with <60% Ki-67+ cells typically behave like diffuse large B-cell lymphoma (DLBCL).[31] The biologic behavior is more akin to Burkitt lymphoma (BL) when >90% of the cells express the Ki-67 proliferation antigen. The distinction is important because treatment for B-LL is the same as for BL and differs from that for DLBCL. In this case, the Ki-67+ cells are >99%, portending behavior like that of BL rather than DLBCL, even though the histologic features are not classic. (Ki-67 immunohistochemisty (red), 400×.)

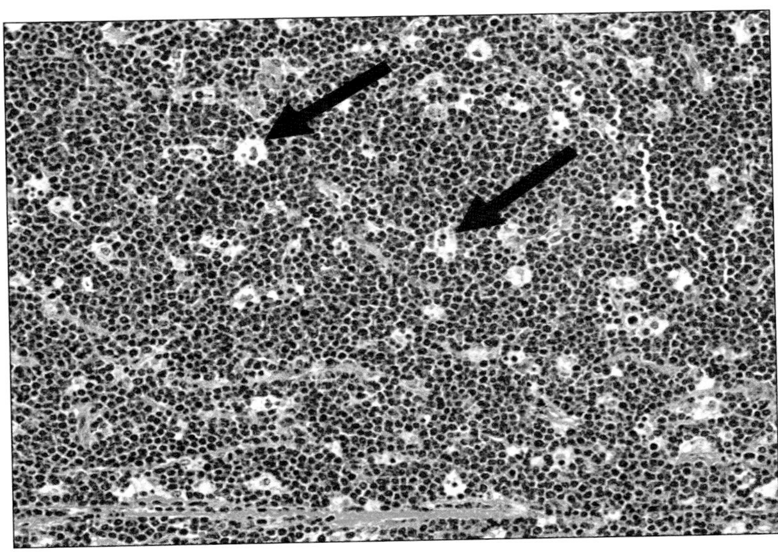

Fig. 14.25 In this case of Burkitt lymphoma in the kidney, tingible-body macrophages (arrows) are scattered throughout the infiltrate, giving the characteristic 'starry sky' appearance. (Hematoxylin–eosin, 200×.)

PRECURSOR B-CELL ACUTE LYMPHOBLASTIC LEUKEMIA/LYMPHOBLASTIC LYMPHOMA

Precursor B-cell ALL may involve a variety of extranodal sites. In a GU lesion, TdT expression is pathognomonic of a precursor ALL. However, because TdT is expressed by both pre-B and pre-T ALLs, lineage-specific lymphoid antigens should also be assessed. Pre-B ALLs typically show strong expression of PAX5, while CD20 is negative or weak.

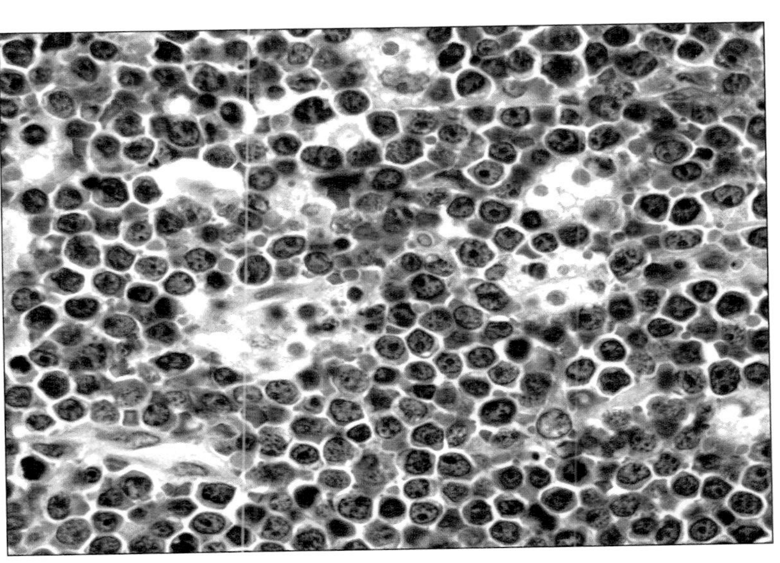

Fig. 14.26 Burkitt lymphoma cells are typically intermediate in size (larger than small lymphocytes, smaller than transformed lymphocytes), with finely clumped chromatin and small or inconspicuous nucleoli. Distinct cytoplasmic membranes impart a 'tile and grout' appearance. Nuclei are round with small or indistinct nucleoli. Tingible-body macrophages are present. (Hematoxylin–eosin, 1000×.)

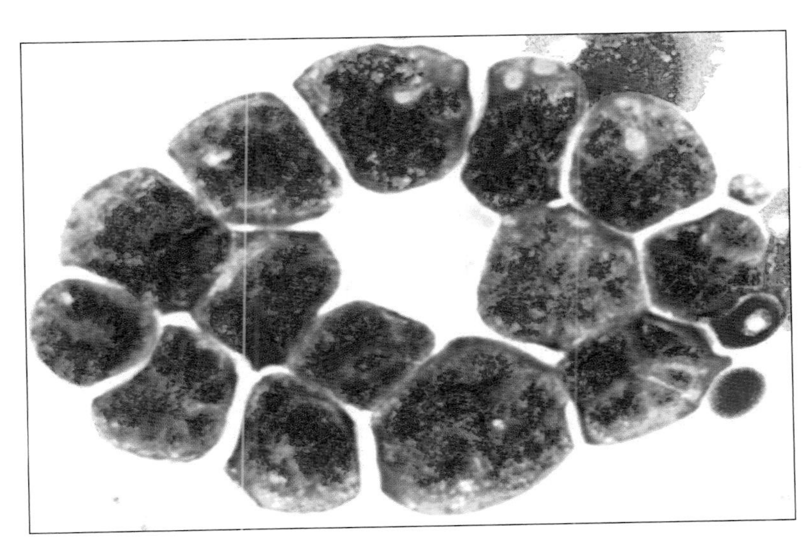

Fig. 14.27 In smear preparations, Burkitt lymphoma (BL) cells have a dark-blue, vacuolated appearance. Although this appearance is typical of BL, it can also be seen in diffuse large B-cell lymphoma or Burkitt-like lymphoma. (Diff-Quick, 1000×.)

Pre-T ALLs typically express CD7 and cytoplasmic CD3. CD99 is positive in both neuroendocrine lesions and ALL. (Figs 14.28 & 14.29)

RARELY ENCOUNTERED HEMATOPOIETIC CANCERS

HODGKIN LYMPHOMA

Both types of Hodgkin lymphoma, classic Hodgkin lymphoma and nodular lymphocyte-predominant Hodgkin lymphoma, are exceedingly rare in the GU.

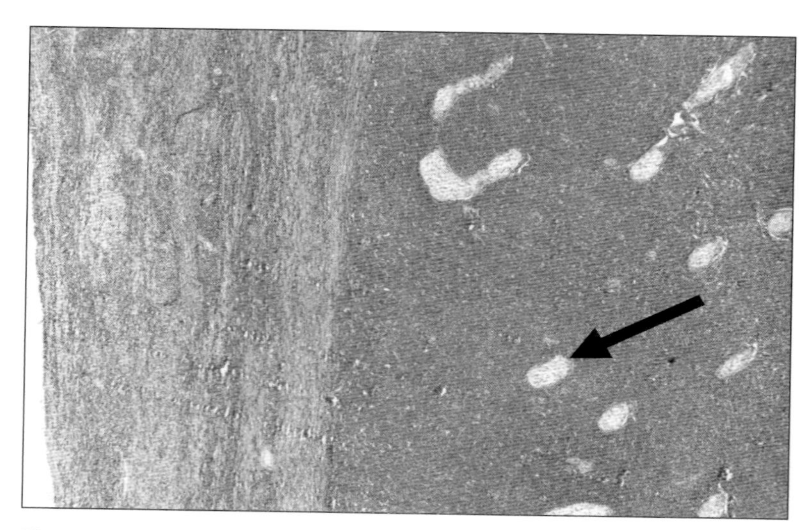

Fig. 14.28 The testis is infiltrated by a monotonous population of small blue cells, separating the seminiferous tubules (arrow) and diffusely involving the capsule (left side of image). Precursor B-cell acute lymphoblastic leukemia/lymphoma has the morphologic appearance of a small blue cell tumor. As such, it can easily be confused with a low-grade lymphoma or with a neuroendocrine small cell cancer. (Hematoxylin–eosin, 40×.)

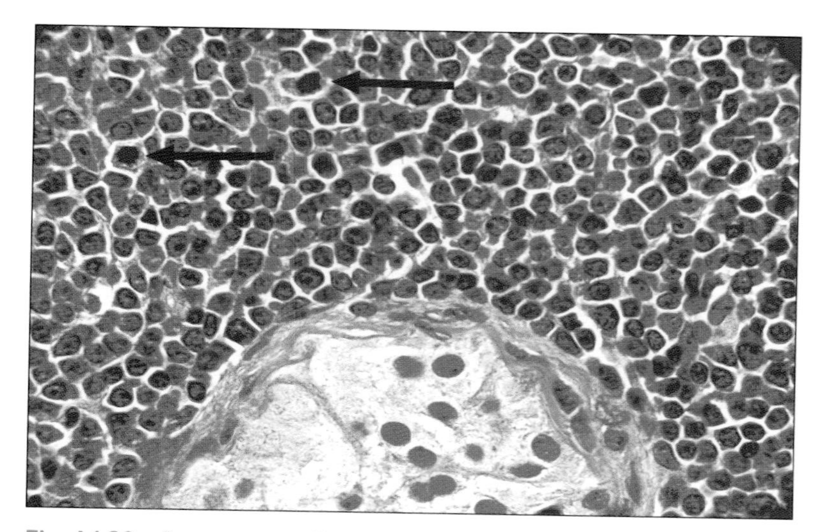

Fig. 14.29 For precursor B-cell acute lymphoblastic leukemia/ lymphoma, the key to diagnosis is the chromatin pattern, which is characteristically speckled, rather than clumped as in mature lymphocytes. The neoplastic cells surround a seminiferous tubule. They are small with mildly irregular nuclear contours and the characteristic speckled chromatin pattern. Mitotic figures are abundant (arrows). (Hematoxylin–eosin, 1000×.)

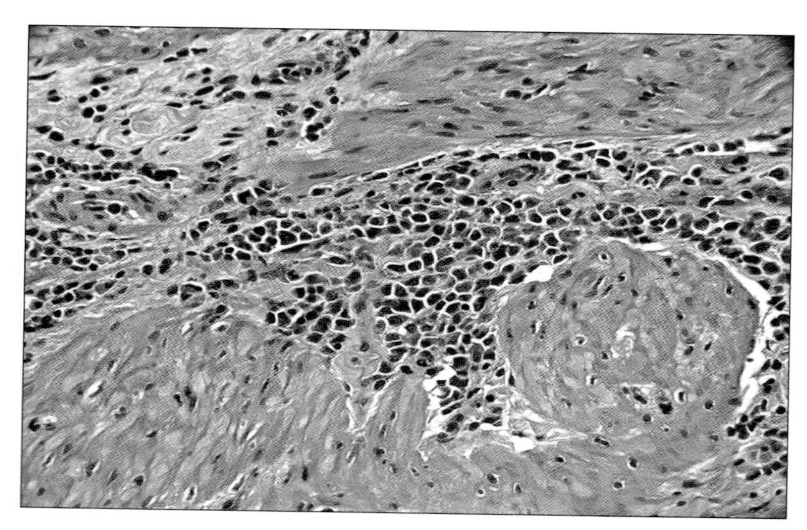

Fig. 14.30 In this bladder biopsy from a patient with acute myelogenous leukemia, malignant cells invade bladder smooth muscle. (Hematoxylin–eosin, 400×.)

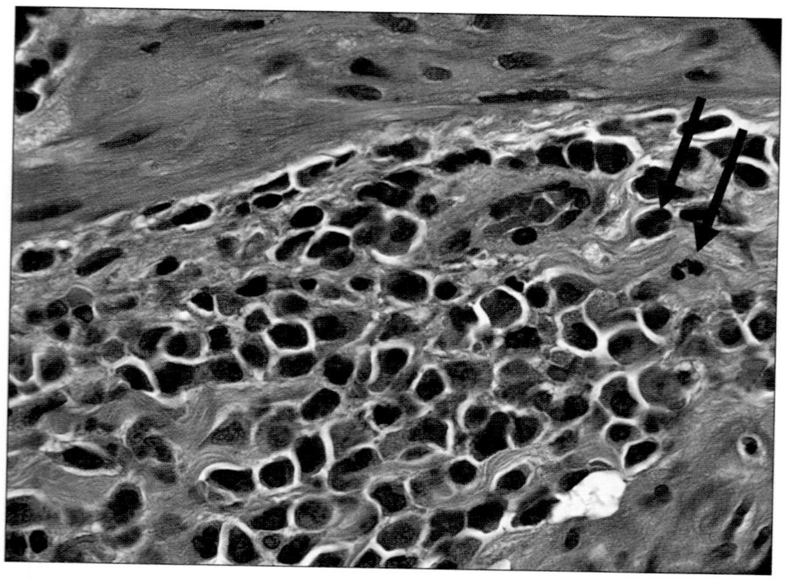

Fig. 14.31 **Extramedullary myeloid tumor.** The neoplastic cells are large with abundant pink cytoplasm and have rounded nuclei with evenly dispersed chromatin (blastic appearance) and variably prominent nucleoli. Mature myeloid cells (neutrophils) are easily found within the infiltrate (arrows). The immunophenotype is characteristic (CD20–, CD3–, CD7+/–, CD43+, CD117+/–, myeloperoxidase +/–, lysozyme +/–). (Hematoxylin–eosin, 1000×.)

T-CELL NON-HODGKIN LYMPHOMA

T-cell NHLs also are exceedingly rare in the GU. The key to the diagnosis lies in IHC, showing expression of a pan-T-cell antigen (CD2, CD3, CD5, and/or CD7). For a complete discussion, please see the referenced texts.[30,31]

NATURAL KILLER CELL LYMPHOMA

These lesions also are extremely rare in the GU. Diagnosis depends on showing a natural killer (NK) immunophenotype by IHC (CD2+, CD3–, CD5–, CD7+/–, CD43+/–, CD16+, CD56+, CD57+/–).

EXTRAMEDULLARY MYELOID TUMOR (CHLOROMA; MYELOID SARCOMA; GRANULOCYTIC SARCOMA)

Myeloid sarcomas are rare in the GU, and usually occur in a background of known AML. The morphology is variable, but similar to that of DLBCL – except that the cytoplasm is often more eosinophilic, and the nuclei have dispersed chromatin but are less often vesicular. (Figs 14.30 & 14.31)

REFERENCES

1. Ely S. The distinction between high grade MALT and diffuse large B cell lymphoma. Gut 2002;51:893.
2. Martinez-Maldonado M, Ramirez D, Arellano GA. Renal involvement in malignant lymphomas. A survey of 49 cases. J Urol 1966;95:485–488.
3. Xiao JC, Walz-Mattmuller R, Ruck P, et al. Renal involvement in myeloproliferative and lymphoproliferative disorders. A study of autopsy cases. Gen Diagn Pathol 1997;142:147–153.
4. Freeman C, Berg JW, Cutler SJ. Occurrence and prognosis of extranodal lymphomas. Cancer 1972;29:252–260.
5. Kandel LB, McCullough DL, Harrison LH, et al. Primary renal lymphoma. Does it exist? Cancer 1987;60:386–391.
6. Al-Maghrabi J, Kamel-Reid S, Jewett M, et al. Primary low-grade B-cell lymphoma of mucosa-associated lymphoid tissue type arising in the urinary bladder: report of 4 cases with molecular genetic analysis. Arch Pathol Lab Med 2001;125:332–336.
7. Bates AW, Norton AJ, Baithun SI. Malignant lymphoma of the urinary bladder: a clinicopathological study of 11 cases. J Clin Pathol 2000;53:458–461.
8. Kempton CL, Kurtin PJ, Inwards DJ, et al. Malignant lymphoma of the bladder: evidence from 36 cases that low-grade lymphoma of the MALT-type is the most common primary bladder lymphoma. Am J Surg Pathol 1997;21:1324–1333.
9. Masuda A, Tsujii T, Kojima M, et al. Primary mucosa-associated lymphoid tissue (MALT) lymphoma arising from the male urethra. A case report and review of the literature. Pathol Res Pract 2002;198:571–575.
10. Patel DR, Gomez GA, Henderson ES, et al. Primary prostatic involvement in non-Hodgkin lymphoma. Urology 1988;32:96–98.
11. Bostwick DG, Iczkowski KA, Amin MB, et al. Malignant lymphoma involving the prostate: report of 62 cases. Cancer 1998;83:732–738.
12. Paladugu RR, Bearman RM, Rappaport H. Malignant lymphoma with primary manifestation in the gonad: a clinicopathologic study of 38 patients. Cancer 1980;45:561–571.
13. Sussman EB, Hajdu SI, Lieberman PH, et al. Malignant lymphoma of the testis: a clinicopathologic study of 37 cases. J Urol 1977;118:1004–1007.
14. Doll DC, Weiss R. Malignant lymphoma of the testis. Am J Med 1986;81:515–524.
15. Ferry JA, Harris NL, Young RH, et al. Malignant lymphoma of the testis, epididymis, and spermatic cord. A clinicopathologic study of 69 cases with immunophenotypic analysis. Am J Surg Pathol 1994;18:376–390.
16. Fonseca R, Habermann TM, Colgan J, et al. Testicular lymphoma is associated with a high incidence of extranodal recurrence. Cancer 2000;88:154–161.
17. Turner RR, Colby TV, MacKintosh FR. Testicular lymphomas: a clinicopathologic study of 35 cases. Cancer 1981;48:2095–2102.
18. Givler RL. Testicular involvement in leukemia and lymphoma. Cancer 1969;23:1290–1295.
19. Kuhajda FP, Haupt HM, Moore GW, et al. Gonadal morphology in patients receiving chemotherapy for leukemia. Evidence for reproductive potential and against a testicular tumor sanctuary. Am J Med 1982;72: 759–767.
20. Askin FB, Land VJ, Sullivan MP, et al. Occult testicular leukemia: testicular biopsy at three years continuous complete remission of childhood leukemia: a Southwest Oncology Group Study. Cancer 1981;47:470–475.
21. Nesbit M Jr, Robison LL, Ortega JA, et al. Testicular relapse in childhood acute lymphoblastic leukemia: association with pretreatment patient characteristics and treatment. A report for Children's Cancer Study Group. Cancer 1980;45:2009–2016.
22. Tiedemann J, Chessells JM, Sandland RM. Isolated testicular relapse in boys with acute lymphoblastic leukaemia: treatment and outcome. Br Med J (Clin Res Ed) 1982;285:1614–1616.
23. Bostwick DG. Urologic surgical pathology. St. Louis: Mosby Year Book; 1997.
24. Lack EE. Tumors of the adrenal gland and extra-adrenal paraganglia. Washington, DC: Armed Forces Institute of Pathology; 1997.
25. Wang J, Sun NC, Renslo R, et al. Clinically silent primary adrenal lymphoma: a case report and review of the literature. Am J Hematol 1998;58:130–136.
26. Isaacson PG, Norton AJ. Extranodal lymphomas. New York: Churchill Livingstone; 1994.
27. Jaffee ES, Harris NL, Stein H, et al. Tumours of hematopoietic and lymphoid tissues. Lyon, France: IARC Press; 2001.
28. Knowles DM. Neoplastic hematopathology. New York: Lippincott Williams & Wilkins; 2001.
29. Lai R, Weiss LM, Chang KL, et al. Frequency of CD43 expression in non-Hodgkin lymphoma. A survey of 742 cases and further characterization of rare CD43+ follicular lymphomas. Am J Clin Pathol 1999;111:488–494.
30. The Non-Hodgkin's Lymphoma Classification Project. A clinical evaluation of the International Lymphoma Study Group classification of non-Hodgkin's lymphoma. Blood 1997;89:3909–3918.
31. Braziel RM, Arber DA, Slovak ML, et al. The Burkitt-like lymphomas. A Southwest Oncology Group study delineating phenotypic, genotypic, and clinical features. Blood 2001;97:3713–3720.

Index